Prefix
MTW

01031

D1325307

Every Decker book

is
a C

BcD
Book Club

decker.com

BC DECKER INC

The Library, Ed & Trg Centre   KTW
Tunbridge Wells Hospital
Tonbridge Rd, PEMBURY
Kent TN2 4QJ
01892 635884 and 635489

The di   t.
Affixe

**Books are to be returned on or before
the last date below.**

"**Book**

* check CD-rom on return *

The di   n fully
search   e;
neither   he
items i

27. NOV. 2003

13. APR. 2004

1 2 SEP 2005

BC De
publica
method

7 MAY 2009

DISCARDED

ckage
ents

LIBREX —

er

Glasscock-Shambaugh
SURGERY
of the
EAR
Fifth Edition

Michael E. Glasscock III, MD, FACS
Department of Otolaryngology
Vanderbilt University
Nashville, Tennessee

Aina Julianna Gulya, MD
Department of Surgery
The George Washington University
Washington, District of Columbia

£125.00

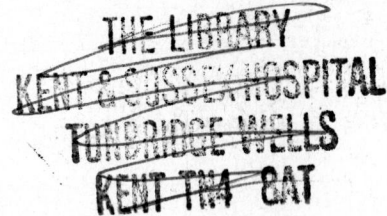

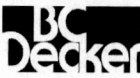

THE LIBRARY
KENT & SUSSEX HOSPITAL
TUNBRIDGE WELLS
KENT TN4 8AT

BC Decker Inc

P.O. Box 620, L.C.D. 1
Hamilton, Ontario L8N 3K7
Tel: 905-522-7017; 800-568-7281
Fax: 905-522-7839; 888-311-4987
E-mail: info@bcdecker.com
www.bcdecker.com

© 2003 BC Decker Inc

All rights reserved. No part of this publication may be reproduced, stored in a retrieval system, or transmitted, in any form or by an means, electronic, mechanical, photocopying, recording, or otherwise, without prior written permission from the publisher.

Previously published by WB Saunders Company 1990 under ISBN 0–7216–2063–9.

02 03 04 05/GSA/9 8 7 6 5 4 3 2 1

ISBN 1–55009–151–4

Printed in Spain

Sales and Distribution

United States
BC Decker Inc
P.O. Box 785
Lewiston, NY 14092-0785
Tel: 905-522-7017; 800-568-7281
Fax: 905-522-7839; 888-311-4987
E-mail: info@bcdecker.com
www.bcdecker.com

Canada
BC Decker Inc
20 Hughson Street South
P.O. Box 620, LCD 1
Hamilton, Ontario L8N 3K7
Tel: 905-522-7017; 800-568-7281
Fax: 905-522-7839; 888-311-4987
E-mail: info@bcdecker.com
www.bcdecker.com

Foreign Rights
John Scott & Company
International Publishers' Agency
P.O. Box 878
Kimberton, PA 19442
Tel: 610-827-1640
Fax: 610-827-1671
E-mail: jsco@voicenet.com

Japan
Igaku-Shoin Ltd.
Foreign Publications Department
3-24-17 Hongo
Bunkyo-ku, Tokyo, Japan 113-8719
Tel: 3 3817 5680
Fax: 3 3815 6776
E-mail: fd@igaku-shoin.co.jp

U.K., Europe, Scandinavia, Middle East
Elsevier Science
Customer Service Department
Foots Cray High Street
Sidcup, Kent
DA14 5HP, UK
Tel: 44 (0) 208 308 5760
Fax: 44 (0) 181 308 5702
E-mail: cservice@harcourt.com

Singapore, Malaysia,Thailand, Philippines, Indonesia, Vietnam, Pacific Rim, Korea
Elsevier Science Asia
583 Orchard Road
#09/01, Forum
Singapore 238884
Tel: 65-737-3593
Fax: 65-753-2145

Australia, New Zealand
Elsevier Science Australia
Customer Service Department
STM Division
Locked Bag 16
St. Peters, New South Wales, 2044
Australia
Tel: 61 02 9517-8999
Fax: 61 02 9517-2249
E-mail: stmp@harcourt.com.au
www.harcourt.com.au

Mexico and Central America
ETM SA de CV
Calle de Tula 59
Colonia Condesa
06140 Mexico DF, Mexico
Tel: 52-5-5553-6657
Fax: 52-5-5211-8468
E-mail: editoresdetextosmex@prodigy.net.mx

Argentina
CLM (Cuspide Libros Medicos)
Av. Córdoba 2067 - (1120)
Buenos Aires, Argentina
Tel: (5411) 4961-0042/(5411) 4964-0848
Fax: (5411) 4963-7988
E-mail: clm@cuspide.com

Brazil
Tecmedd
Av. Maurílio Biagi, 2850
City Ribeirão Preto - SP - CEP: 14021-000
Tel: 0800 992236
Fax: (16) 3993-9000
E-mail: tecmedd@tecmedd.com.br

WV 200
A031051

Notice: The authors and publisher have made every effort to ensure that the patient care recommended herein, including choice of drugs and drug dosages, is in accord with the accepted standard and practice at the time of publication. However, since research and regulation constantly change clinical standards, the reader is urged to check the product information sheet included in the package of each drug, which includes recommended doses, warnings, and contraindications. This is particularly important with new or infrequently used drugs. Any treatment regimen, particularly one involving medication, involves inherent risk that must be weighed on a case-by-case basis against the benefits anticipated. The reader is cautioned that the purpose of this book is to inform and enlighten; the information contained herein is not intended as, and should not be employed as, a substitute for individual diagnosis and treatment.

Dedication

This book is dedicated to the three most influential otologists of the twentieth century, Julius Lempert, John J. Shea Jr, and William F. House. These pioneers fought the status quo of the medical establishment to advance the diagnosis and surgical treatment of otologic disease.

Lempert was a Jewish immigrant who came to the United States in the early part of the Twentieth Century to settle in New York City. He should be considered the father of modern otology because of his many contributions to this specialty.

Lempert established his surgical techniques based on the work of Gunnar Holmgren and Maurice Sourdille to develop the one-stage fenestration procedure for otosclerosis. While other New York otologists were advising hearing aids for their patients, Lempert was opening the lateral semicircular canal and improving hearing. In some cases, hearing was brought to a 20- or 25-dB level.

He routinely used magnification (loupes) in otologic surgery and was the first to employ a dental drill to open the mastoid in place of a gouge and mallet. His techniques reduced the incidence of facial nerve injuries in radical and modified radical procedures. Lempert's approach to the petrous apex via the carotid artery established the basis for modern skull base surgery.

Lempert was willing to share his knowledge and surgical techniques with other surgeons, and that may well be his greatest contribution to the specialty of otology. He established the first temporal bone laboratory for teaching the one-stage fenestration procedure and ran a 6-week course in his private hospital. Lempert single-handedly trained the entire first echelon of otologists, such as Howard House, George Shambaugh Jr, and Gordon Hoople, who went on to follow their mentor's example by training a second generation of young otologists.

Lempert overcame a poor medical education (third-rate medical school and no formal residency in otolaryngology), rampant anti-Semitism, and the wrath of the academic medical community to become a respected and renowned otologist who treated patients from all over the world.

In the mid- to late 1950s, John Shea Jr took the bold step of removing the stapes of an individual with otosclerosis and replaced it with a polyethylene prosthesis, thereby performing the first successful stapedectomy. He should also be credited with the first stapedotomy because early on he placed a wire through the intact stapes and obtained a hearing improvement.

Working with Harry Treace of the old Richards Company, he developed a whole new line of surgical instruments for middle ear surgery. He did a great deal to popularize the operating microscope in his teaching activities. Shea, along with Harold Tabb, performed the first transcanal, under-surface tympanoplasty using connective tissue (vein). This contribution opened the way for fascia grafts and essentially did away with using skin in an overlay technique for tympanoplasty.

A charismatic and daring young surgeon, Shea traveled the world teaching his techniques, and the world came to his clinic for treatment — all of this when he was still in his thirties. He had his picture on the cover of *Life* magazine and was the most famous ear surgeon in the United States. Doctors from far and wide came to study with him, and at medical meetings, he had a whole entourage following him and hanging on to his every word. This notoriety and the excellent results of the stapedectomy procedure stimulated an entire generation of otolaryngologists to enter the subspecialty of otology.

Like Lempert, Shea had to dispel the naysayers who told him that he would destroy hearing by removing the stapes and subject his patients to meningitis and possible death.

The last 40 years of the Twentieth Century belong to William F. House. The list of his accomplishments and contributions to otology is legendary. He is considered the father of neurotology and is credited with introducing the operating microscope to the field of neurosurgery.

Working with an electrical engineer, Jack Urban, House developed the first practical teaching system for the microscope, starting with a viewing tube (side arm) so that a student could follow every move the operating surgeon made. Soon followed a 16-mm movie camera and a black and white television that preceded the color system.

An innovator, House was constantly developing new surgical procedures to deal with specific medical problems. He championed the intact canal wall mastoidectomy for chronic ear disease and cholesteatoma. In an attempt to control the symptoms of Meniere's disease, he perfected the endolymphatic shunt procedure and introduced the middle fossa vestibular nerve section.

In the early 1960s, working with the neurosurgeon William Hitselberger, House changed forever the course of acoustic neuroma surgery. Before his groundbreaking techniques were adopted, the mortality rate ran 15 to 17%, facial nerves were sacrificed 90 to 100% of the time, and hearing was almost always destroyed. Today most large series report mortality rates of 1% or less, preservation of facial nerve function in 90%, and hearing preservation of 35 to 40% in small tumors. Some institutions report hearing conservation in as much as 75% of their cases.

In the early 1970s, House, again working with Jack Urban, developed the first cochlear implant. I remember going to a meeting in San Francisco during this period, which was attended by most of the department heads of university otolaryngology programs along with the directors of their research laboratories. The consensus from this group held that it was impossible to stimulate the auditory nerve electrically and produce intelligible sound in an individual with a profound sensorineural hearing loss. They were wrong.

Throughout his incredible career, William F. House courageously fought the medical establishment every step of the way. He was told repeatedly that what he wanted to do was impossible, and he was accused on more than one occasion of experimenting on humans simply because he believed in clinical research.

Otologists today owe a great debt to these three pioneers because they overcame tremendous odds to advance the specialty. It shocks me when I talk to young otologic surgeons and realize how little they understand of the history of their chosen field of practice.

Michael E. Glasscock III, MD, FACS
Nashville, Tennessee
August 2002

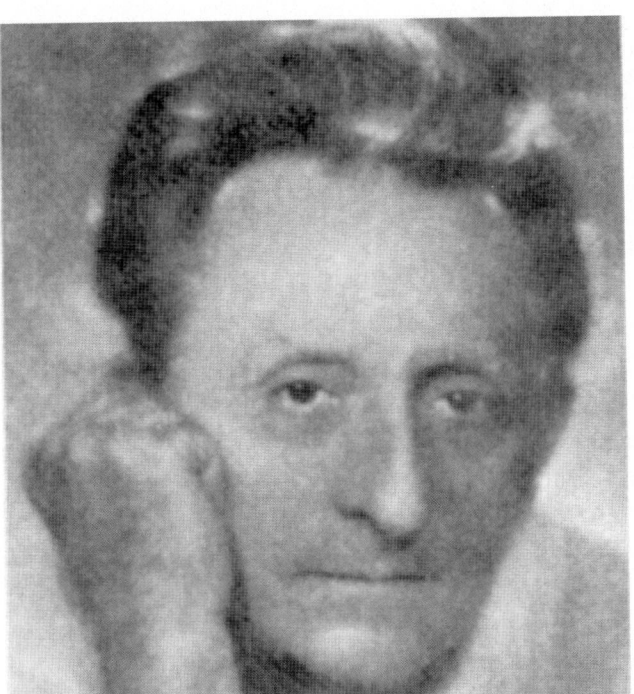

Julius Lempert (1890–1968).
Foremost advocate of the endaural approach to the temporal bone. His one-stage fenestration operation led to the renaissance of reconstructive surgery for conductive hearing loss.

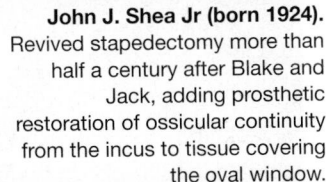

John J. Shea Jr (born 1924).
Revived stapedectomy more than half a century after Blake and Jack, adding prosthetic restoration of ossicular continuity from the incus to tissue covering the oval window.

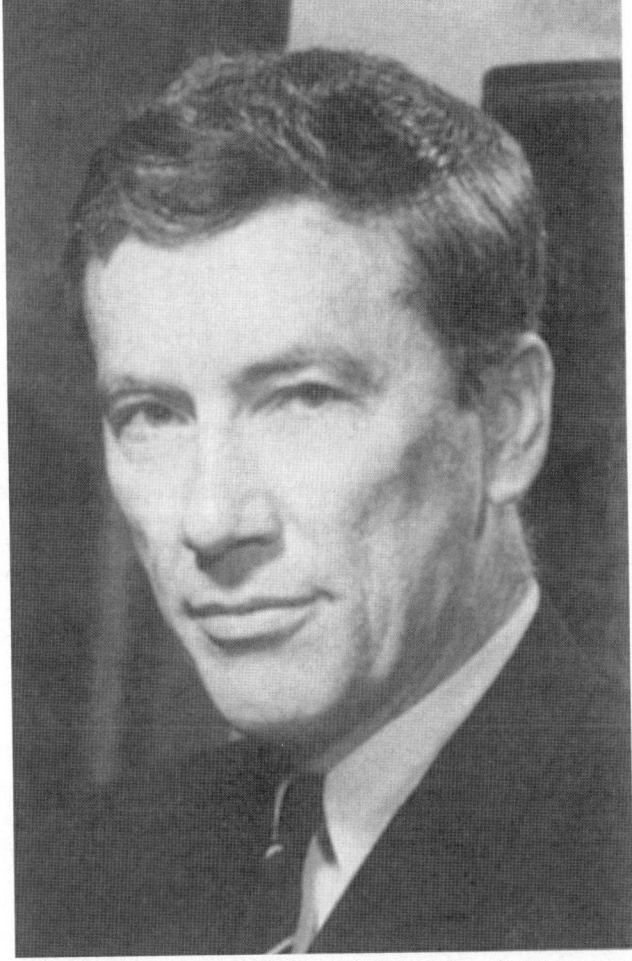

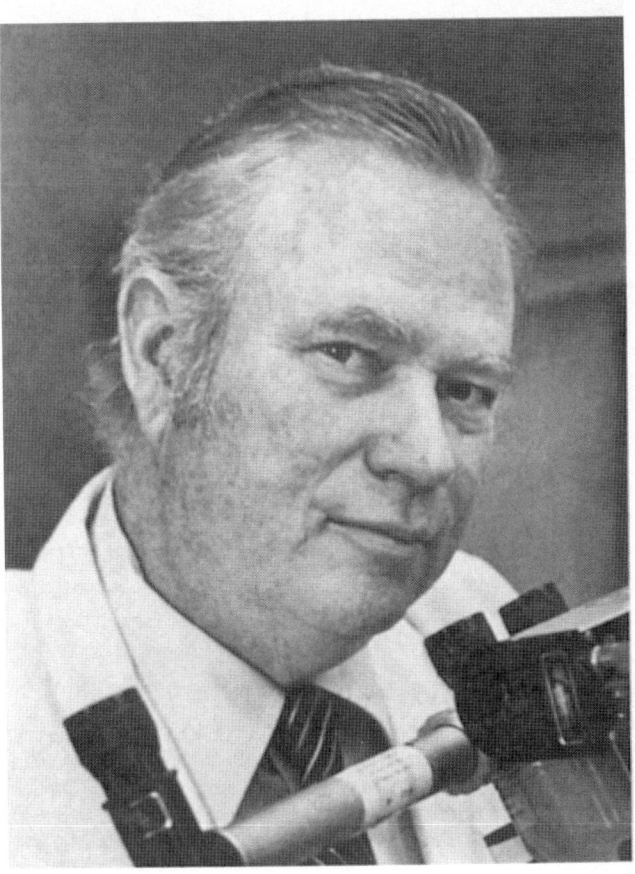

William F. House, MD (born 1923).
The "father of neurotology." He pioneered the early diagnosis and translabyrinthine removal of vestibular schwannomas and the development of the cochlear implant.

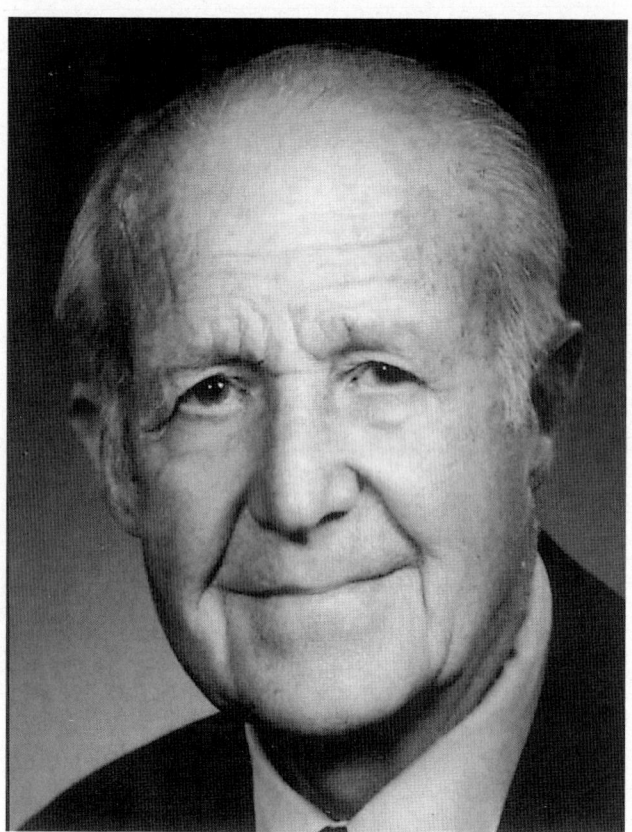

George E. Shambaugh Jr, MD (1903–1999).
Author of the first and second editions of
Surgery of the Ear and senior coauthor of the
third edition.

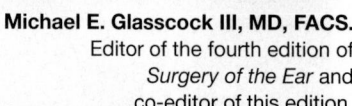

Michael E. Glasscock III, MD, FACS.
Editor of the fourth edition of
Surgery of the Ear and
co-editor of this edition.

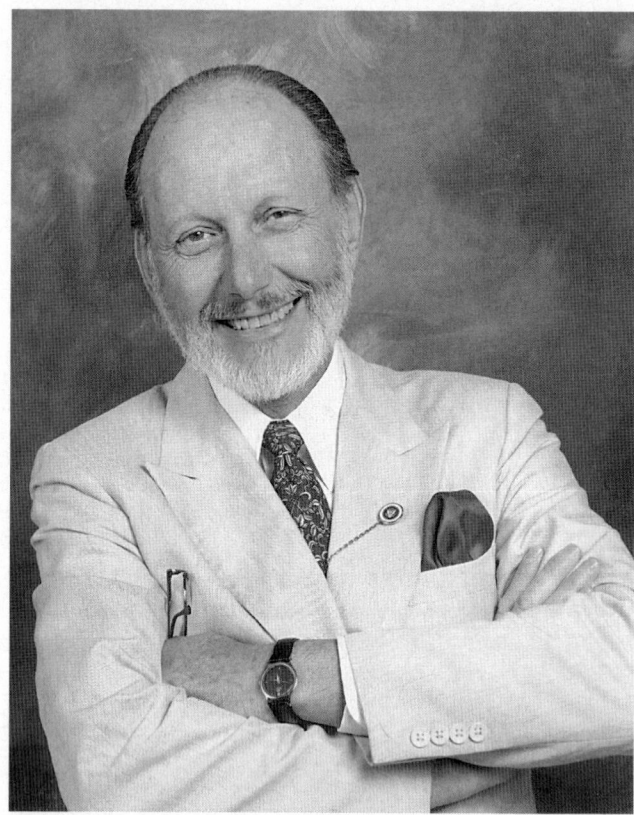

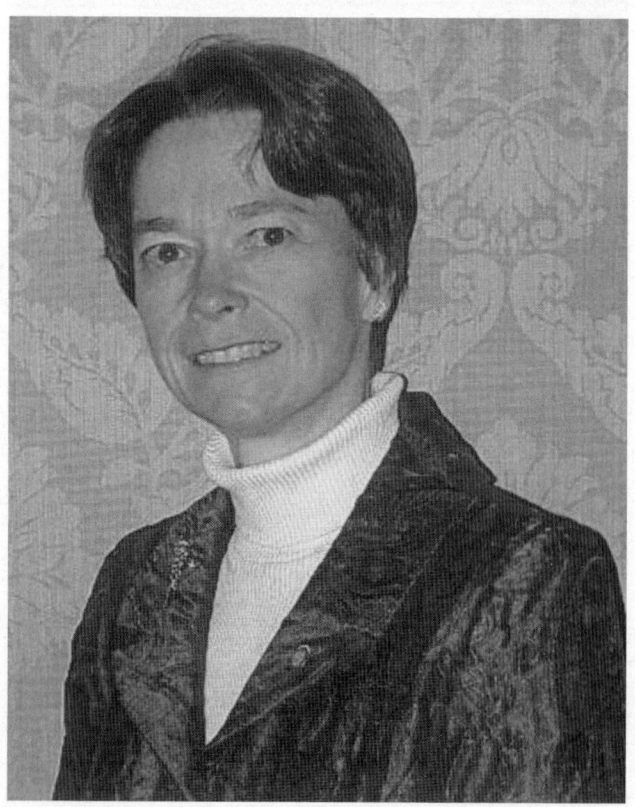

Aina Julianna Gulya, MD.
Co-editor of this edition of
Surgery of the Ear. Photo
by Jennifer Flesher, American
Academy of Otolaryngology
Head and Neck Surgery.

Contents

VI   Surgery of the Inner Ear

VII   Surgery of the IAC/CPA/Petrous Apex

VIII Surgery of the Skull Base

Appendix

Index

Editor's Note

Through four editions, spanning nearly 50 years, *Glasscock & Shambaugh's Surgery of the Ear* has been recognized not only as *the* primer for the neophyte otologist but also as a trusted reference for the experienced surgeon. The practical, easy-to-read content of the book belied the wealth and complexity of information conveyed by the text.

It was therefore with some trepidation that I accepted Michael Glasscock's challenge to update this classic. A sustaining motivation throughout this endeavor has been the desire to honor the mentors who have so profoundly influenced my career, Harold F. Schuknecht, MD, and Michael E. Glasscock III, MD, as well as to recognize the support and encouragement of my husband, William R. Wilson, MD, and my parents, Aladar and Sylvia Gulya.

Working with Michael Glasscock and Brian C. Decker, I sought to revamp the content of the book to reflect the modern surgical practice of otology/neurotology. Accordingly, those familiar with *Surgery of the Ear* will detect changes in the table of contents, both in organization and in subject matter. For example, the "Auditory Physiology (Mechanics of Hearing)" chapter has been moved to the lead section, "Scientific Foundations"; the "Cochlear Implantation" chapter has been greatly expanded; and new chapters have been added, for example, "Surgery for Middle Ear Implants." In contrast, a few chapters, such as "The Simple Mastoid Operation," remain much as in previous editions, requiring only the updating of a few details.

Hopefully, this fifth edition of *Surgery of the Ear* will serve otologic surgeons as well as its predecessor did.

Aina Julianna Gulya, MD
Washington, District of Columbia
August 2002

Acknowledgment

Many thanks to Andy Rideout for all his help with the illustrations and to Jamie White for all her hard work and dedication.

Preface

Sometime in 1957, George E. Shambaugh Jr took 6 months out of his busy otologic practice to write what was to become a classic text on surgery of the ear. There have now been four editions of *Surgery of the Ear:* 1959, 1967, 1980, and 1990. I was fortunate to have been asked to assist in the 1980 edition and was responsible for the 1990 effort.

The hallmark of this text has always been its simplicity and straightforwardness. It has always been an easy read. My goal is to keep it that way.

I bought my 1959 edition in 1963 when I was a resident in otolaryngology at the University of Tennessee. It formed the basis of my knowledge of temporal bone anatomy, and I kept it open while I drilled my first cadaver specimens. I routinely referred to the text when I ran into a difficult diagnostic problem and continued to use later editions when I went into practice.

Much has changed in our specialty since 1959. We still perform radical and modified radical mastoidectomies and tympanoplasties as they are described in the first *Surgery of the Ear*, but gone are the fenestration and stapes mobilization procedures. These have been replaced by a variety of new surgical procedures, such as stapedotomies, middle fossa approaches, translabyrinthine removal of acoustic tumors, intact canal wall mastoidectomies, skull base tumor removal, endolymphatic shunt operations, vestibular nerve sections, cochlear implants, and totally implanted hearing aids.

Any text on otology must be revised on a regular basis for it is impossible to keep current otherwise. As it has worked out, a new edition of *Surgery of the Ear* has been published about every 10 years. Given the rapid expansion of knowledge in this day of data processing, that interval is probably too long. I am not really sure what the proper time period is, but my guess would be somewhere between 6 and 8 years. For truly current literature, the student should depend on the many fine journals in this field.

In the first edition, Dr. Shambaugh made a point of stating that physicians should remain students for the remainder of their professional careers. I can remember going to meetings and seeing Dr. Shambaugh sitting on the front row taking notes furiously. This was when he was in his late eighties. He practiced what he taught, and that should be an example for all of us.

I am deeply indebted to Julie Gulya for overseeing the development of this fifth edition. Without her help, this edition of *Surgery of the Ear* would never have come to fruition. Numerous chapters in this book were written by my ex-fellows. I am grateful to all of them. I wish to thank the other authors, as well, for their fine contributions. My input has been minimal because it is my feeling that a surgeon no longer in active practice cannot truly be considered on the cutting edge of the specialty.

It is my sincere desire that subsequent editions of *Surgery of the Ear* will be forthcoming in the future. As I write this Preface to the fifth edition, the field of otology appears to be in good hands. I continue to be impressed by the moral and ethical quality of our modern young otologists. I will leave the reader with this one thought: *All of us benefit from the knowledge passed on by the pioneers in our chosen field.*

Michael E. Glasscock III, MD, FACS
Nashville, Tennessee
August 2002

Contributors

Ben J. Balough, MD
Naval Medical Center
San Diego, California

Dennis I. Bojrab, MD
Department of Otolaryngology-Head
　and Neck Surgery
Wayne State University
Detroit, Michigan

Derald E. Brackmann, MD
School of Medicine
University of Southern California
Los Angeles, California

Roberto A. Cueva, MD, FACS
Department of Otolaryngology-Head
　and Neck Surgery
University of California
San Diego, California

Chris De Souza, MD, FACS
Tata Memorial Hospital
Bandra, Mumbai, India

John R. E. Dickins, MD
Arkansas Otolaryngology Center
Little Rock, Arkansas

Carlos Esquivel, MD
Department of Otolaryngology
Northwestern University Medical School
Chicago, Illinois

John C. Flickinger, MD
Department of Radiation Oncology
University of Pittsburgh School of Medicine
Pittsburgh, Pennsylvania

Lendra M. Friesen, MA
Department of Speech and Hearing Sciences
University of Washington
Seattle, Washington

Bruce J. Gantz, MD
Department of Otolaryngology
University of Iowa
Iowa City, Iowa

M. Miles Goldsmith, MD, FACS
University of North Carolina
Chapel Hill, North Carolina

Sharon S. Graham, MS
Arkansas Otolaryngology Center
Little Rock, Arkansas

Neil D. Gross, MD
Department of Otolaryngology-Head
　and Neck Surgery
Oregon Health and Science University
Portland, Oregon

Aina Julianna Gulya, MD
Department of Surgery
The George Washington University
Washington, District of Columbia

Mark L. Gustafson, MD
Department of Otolaryngology
Tanner Medical Center of Carrollton
Carrollton, Georgia

David S. Haynes, MD
Department of Otolaryngology
Vanderbilt University
Nashville, Tennessee

Gayle H. Hicks, PhD, FASM
South California Permanente Medical Group
San Diego, California

William E. Hitselberger, MD
House Ear Institute
Los Angeles, California

Dick Hoisted, MD
Department of Otolaryngology
Northwestern University Medical School
Chicago, Illinois

Gordon B. Hughes, MD
Department of Otolaryngology
Cleveland Clinic Foundation
Cleveland, Ohio

Timothy E. Hullar, MD, FACS
Department of Otolaryngology-Head
    and Neck Surgery
Johns Hopkins University School of Medicine
Baltimore, Maryland

C. Gary Jackson, MD, FACS
Temple University
Philadelphia, Pennsylvania

Robert A. Jahrsdoerfer, MD
Department of Otolaryngology-Head
    and Neck Surgery
University of Virginia
Charlottesville, Virginia

Glenn D. Johnson, MD, FACS
Department of Surgery
Dartmouth Medical School
Hanover, New Hampshire

B. Maya Kato, MD
Department of Otolaryngology-Head
    and Neck Surgery
The Permanente Medical Group
Union City, California

David F. Kroon, MD
Department of Otolaryngology-Head
    and Neck Surgery
Eastern Virginia Medical School
Norfolk, Virginia

John F. Kveton, MD
Department of Surgery
Yale University
New Haven, Connecticut

Anil K. Lalwani, MD
Department of Otolaryngology-Head
    and Neck Surgery
University of California San Francisco
San Francisco, California

John M. Lasak, MD
Department of Surgery
Wichita Ear Clinic
University of Kansas School of Medicine
Wichita, Kansas

Joung Lee, MD
Department of Neurosurgery
Cleveland Clinic Foundation
Cleveland, Ohio

S. George Lesinski, MD
Midwest Ear Foundation
Cincinnati, Ohio

Samuel C. Levine, MD, FACS
Department of Otolaryngology
University of Minnesota
Minneapolis, Minnesota

Spiros Manolidis, MD
Department of Otolaryngology-Head
    and Neck Surgery
Baylor College of Medicine
Houston, Texas

Michael J. McKenna, MD
Department of Otology and Laryngology
Harvard Medical School
Boston, Massachusetts

Sean O. McMenomey, MD
Departments of Otolaryngology-Head
    and Neck Surgery and Neurosurgery
Oregon Health and Science University
Portland, Oregon

Saumil N. Merchant, MD
Department of Otology and Laryngology
Harvard Medical School
Boston, Massachusetts

Anand N. Mhatre, PhD
Department of Otolaryngology-Head
    and Neck Surgery
University of California San Francisco
San Francisco, California

Lloyd B. Minor, MD, FACS
Department of Otolaryngology-Head
    and Neck Surgery
Johns Hopkins University School of Medicine
Baltimore, Maryland

Aage R. Møller, PhD
School of Human Development
University of Texas at Dallas
Dallas, Texas

Steven R. Otto, MA
Department of Auditory Implants and Perception
House Ear Institute
Los Angeles, California

Myles L. Pensak, MD, FACS
Department of Otolaryngology
University of Cincinnati Medical Center
Cincinnati, Ohio

Dennis S. Poe, MD, FACS
Department of Otology and Laryngology
Harvard Medical School
Boston, Massachusetts

Peter S. Roland, MD
Department of Otolaryngology
University of Texas
Southwestern Medical Center
Dallas, Texas

John J. Rosowski, PhD
Department of Otology and Laryngology
Harvard Medical School
Boston, Massachusetts

Paul M. Ruggieri, MD
Department of Radiology
Cleveland Clinic Foundation
Cleveland, Ohio

Ravi N. Samy, MD
Department of Otolaryngology
University of Texas
Southwestern Medical Center at Dallas
Dallas, Texas

David A. Schessel, PhD, MD
Departments of Otolaryngology and Neurosurgery
The George Washington University
Washington, District of Columbia

Laligam N. Sekhar, MD, FACS
Mid-Atlantic Brain and Spine Institutes
Annandale, Virginia

Robert V. Shannon, PhD
Department of Auditory Implants and Perception
House Ear Institute
Los Angeles, California

John J. Shea Jr, MD
Department of Otolaryngology
    and Maxillofacial Surgery
University of Tennessee Center
    for the Health Sciences
Memphis, Tennessee

Paul F. Shea, MD
Department of Otology/Neurotology
Shea Ear Clinic
Memphis, Tennessee

Aristides Sismanis, MD
Department of Otolaryngology-Head
    and Neck Surgery
Virginia Commonwealth University Health System
Richmond, Virginia

William H. Slattery III, MD
Department of Otolaryngology
University of Southern California
Los Angeles, California

Brad A. Stach, PhD
Department of Speech and Hearing
Washington University
St. Louis, Missouri

Barry Strasnick, MD, FACS
Department of Otolaryngology-Head
    and Neck Surgery
Eastern Virginia Medical School
Norfolk, Virginia

Elizabeth H. Toh, MD
Department of Otolaryngology
University of Pittsburgh School of Medicine
Pittsburgh, Pennsylvania

Galdino E. Valvassori, MD
Departments of Radiology and Otolaryngology
University of Illinois
Chicago, Illinois

D. Bradley Welling, MD
Department of Otolaryngology
The Ohio State University
Columbus, Ohio

Richard Wiet, MD
Department of Otolaryngology
Northwestern University Medical School
Chicago, Illinois

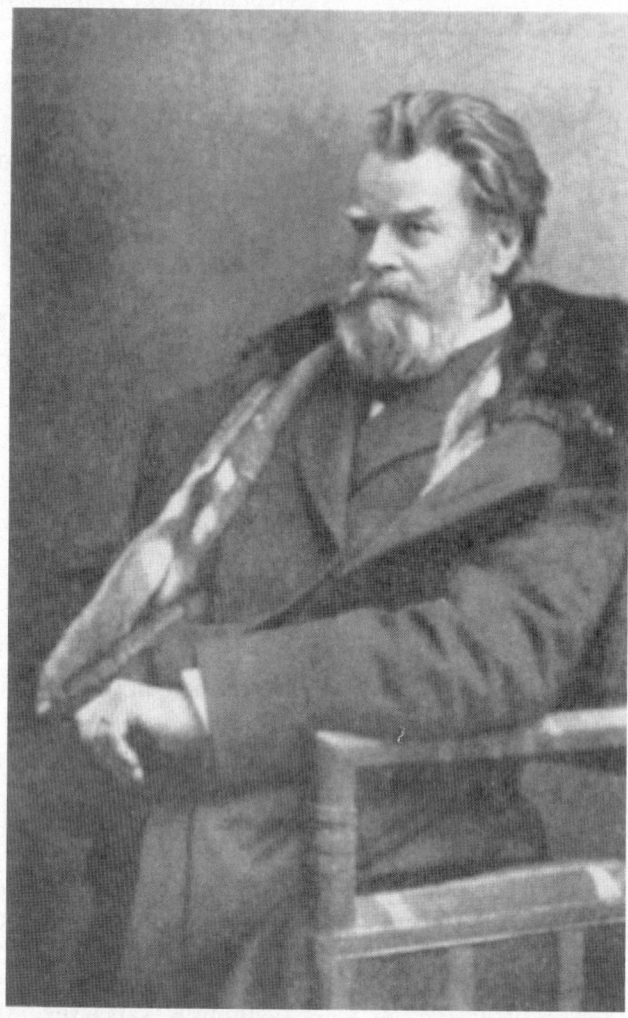

Friedrich Bezold (1842–1908). Clarified the differentiation by tuning fork tests of conductive and sensorineural hearing losses and the clinical diagnosis of otosclerosis. His clear and concise *Textbook of Otology* served as a model for Shambaugh as he wrote his *Surgery of the Ear.*

I

Scientific Foundations

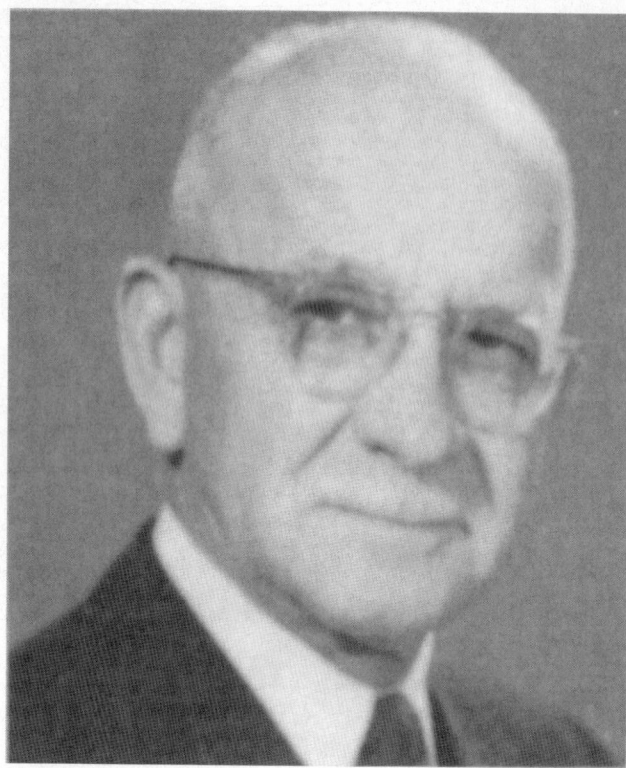

Theodore H. Bast (1890–1959). First described the utriculoen-dolymphatic valve and with Barry Anson studied the developmental anatomy of the temporal bone.

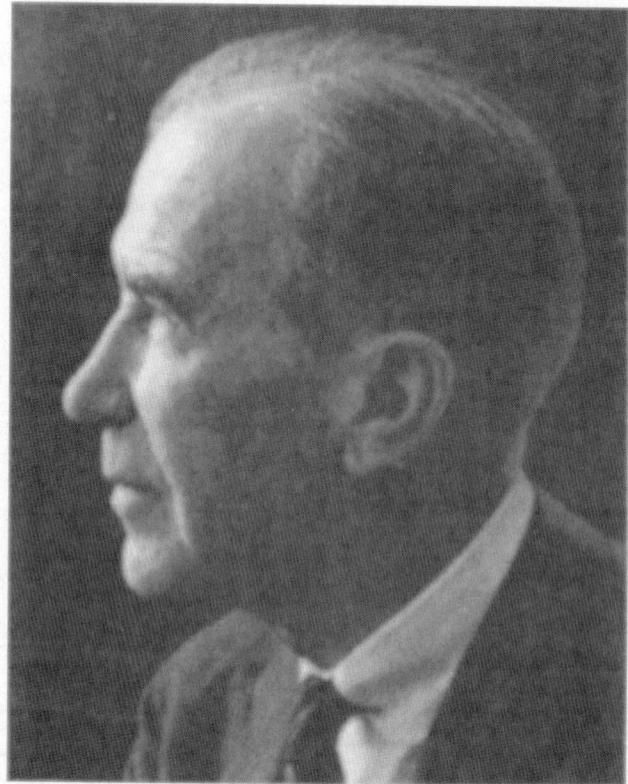

Barry J. Anson (1894–1974). Student and investigator par excellence of the gross and microscopic anatomy of the temporal bone.

1

Developmental Anatomy of the Temporal Bone and Skull Base

AINA JULIANNA GULYA, MD

The complexity of nature's machinations is exemplified in the development of the ear, both in phylogenetic and ontogenetic terms. The labyrinth represents a parsimonious salvage and modification of the lateral line system of fish, whereas the ossicles originally participated in the masticatory apparatus of ancestral vertebrates.

As intriguing as the phylogeny of the ear is in an abstract sense, knowledge of its embryologic development is of crucial, concrete importance to the modern-day neurotologic surgeon. Management of major malformations of the ear, such as the manifestations of aural dysmorphogenesis, obviously demands such knowledge if a rational approach to the alleviation of associated hearing handicaps is to prevail. The surgeon who is able to anticipate more subtle irregularities of development, such as persistent stapedial arteries and high jugular bulbs, can confidently negotiate such potential hazards rather than fall prey to them.

This chapter presents a focused discussion of the development of the ear, emphasizing those features of particular surgical importance. The discussion begins with the most lateral structures of the temporal bone and progresses medially, just as a surgeon encounters these structures. The fetal ages are based on conversion of crown-rump measurements to postconceptual ages and thus may show some variations from figures based on alternative dating methods.

The reader interested in reviewing the pioneer works of Bast, Anson, Donaldson, Streeter, and Padget is referred to their referenced works. Comprehensive overviews of both phylogeny and anatomy are extant in such works as those by Gulya and Schuknecht,[1] Anson and Donaldson,[2] Pearson,[3] and Bast and Anson.[4]

DEVELOPMENT OF THE EXTERNAL EAR AND TEMPORAL BONE

External Ear

The development of the pinna commences at 4 weeks as tissue condensations of the mandibular and hyoid arches appear at the distal portion of the first branchial groove. Within 2 weeks, six ridges, known as the hillocks of His, arise from the tissue condensations (Figure 1–1). The significance of these hillocks varies, according to the investigator, from coincidental to integral to the development of the pinna. Accompanying these divergent views are studies that, on the one hand, suggest that

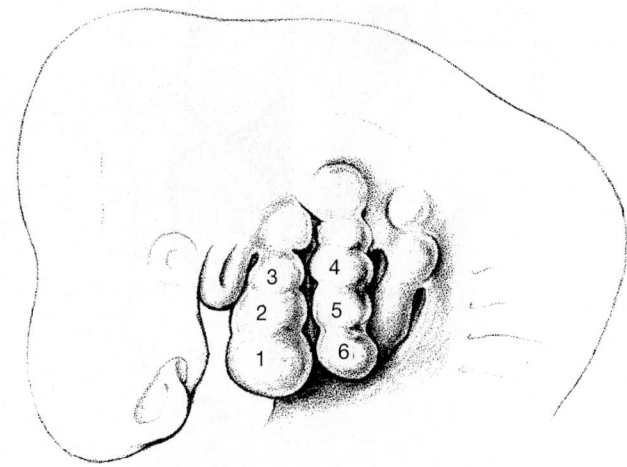

Figure 1–1 The six hillocks of His at approximately 6 weeks. After Levine.[6] Reproduced with permission from Gulya AJ, Schuknecht HF. Anatomy of the temporal bone with surgical implications. 2nd ed. Pearl River (NY): Parthenon Publishing Group; 1995.

3

the entire pinna except the tragus and anterior external auditory canal (of mandibular arch origin) arises from the hyoid (second branchial) arch.[5] Other studies demonstrate a balanced participation of both the first and second branchial arches in the development of the pinna.[3,6]

The hillocks fuse into an anterior fold of mandibular arch origin and a posterior fold of hyoid arch origin, oriented about the first branchial groove. The folds unite at the upper end of this groove (Figure 1–2).

Adult configuration (Figure 1–3) is achieved by the fifth month, independent of developmental progress in the middle and inner ears. The darwinian tubercle, corresponding to the tip of the pinna in lower mammals, makes its appearance at roughly 6 months.

Temporal Bone, External Auditory Canal, Tympanic Ring, and Tympanic Membrane

The adult temporal bone is an amalgam of the squamous, petrous, mastoid, tympanic, and styloid bones. The close association of the external auditory canal, tympanic ring, and tympanic membrane justifies the inclusion of their developmental process in conjunction with that of the temporal bone as a whole. The development of the bony labyrinth and petrosa, however, because of its

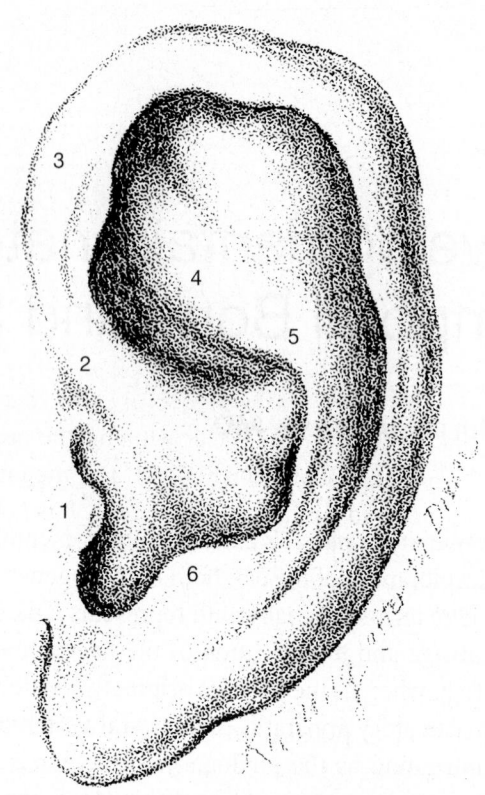

Figure 1–3   The adult auricle with the derivatives of the six hillocks numbered. After Levine.[6] Reproduced with permission from Gulya AJ, Schuknecht HF. Anatomy of the temporal bone with surgical implications. 2nd ed. Pearl River (NY): Parthenon Publishing Group; 1995.

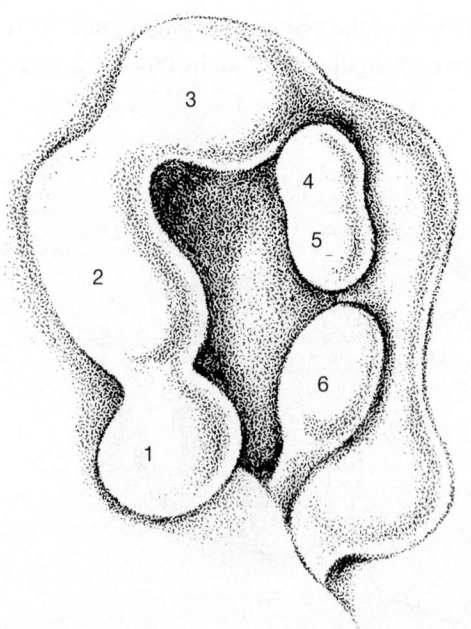

Figure 1–2   At approximately 7 weeks, the six hillocks are fusing to form two folds, which will later fuse superiorly. After Levine.[6] Reproduced with permission from Gulya AJ, Schuknecht HF. Anatomy of the temporal bone with surgical implications. 2nd ed. Pearl River (NY): Parthenon Publishing Group; 1995.

intricacy, warrants separate discussion. The following account of the development of the external auditory canal, tympanic ring, tympanic membrane, and temporal bone is derived from the works of Anson and associates[7] as well as Pearson.[3]

The dorsal part of the first branchial groove, which gives rise to the external auditory canal, progressively deepens during the second month. The ectoderm of the groove briefly abuts on the endoderm of the tubotympanic recess (first pharyngeal pouch), but during the sixth week, a mesodermal ingrowth breaks this contact. Beginning at 8 weeks, the inferior portion of the first branchial groove deepens again, forming the primary external auditory canal, which corresponds to the fibrocartilaginous canal of the adult. At the same time, development of the squama begins, marked by the appearance of a membranous bone ossification center. In the next week of development, a cord of epithelial cells at the depths of the primary external auditory canal grows medially into the mesenchyme to terminate in a solid (meatal) plate (Figure 1–4). The mesenchyme adjacent to the meatal plate gives rise to the lamina propria (fibrous layer) of the tympanic membrane and at 9 weeks is surrounded by the four membranous bone ossification centers of the tympanic ring. In addition to supporting the tympanic membrane, it has been theorized that the tympanic ring also functions to inhibit inward epithelial migration. Failure of this function may lead to cholesteatoma formation (ie, congenital cholesteatoma) at the junction of the first and second branchial arches.[8]

By the tenth week, the tympanic ring elements fuse except superiorly, where a defect remains, the notch of Rivinus. These elements then expand, accompanied by growth of the solid epithelial cord of cells. It is not until after the fifth month that the cord splits open, initially at its medial terminus, forming the bony external auditory canal by the seventh month. The cells remaining at the periphery form the epithelial lining of the bony external auditory canal, whereas those remaining medially form the superficial layer of the tympanic membrane. The medial layer of the tympanic membrane derives from the epithelial lining of the first pharyngeal pouch. These developmental changes in the external auditory canal occur at a time when the outer, middle, and inner ears are already well developed.

Meanwhile, beginning at 4 months, the squama projects posterior to the tympanic ring, forming what will become the lateral (squamous) portion of the mastoid, roof of the external auditory canal, and lateral wall of the antrum. The medial (petrous) portion of the mastoid develops as air cells invade the periosteal layer of the bony labyrinth. The external petrosquamous fissure marks the junction of the petrosa with the squama and generally disappears by the second year of life.

The hypotympanum develops between 22 and 32 weeks as a tripartite bony amalgam[9] composed of the tympanic bone (membranous bone), the canalicular otic capsule (enchondral bone), and a petrosal ledge (periosteal bone). This variegated structure is thought to predispose this area to anomalous development, such as that which leaves bare the jugular bulb in the middle ear.

After the eighth month, the tympanic ring begins to fuse with the otic capsule, a process that is not completed until birth. Postnatally, lateral extensions of the tympanic ring and the squama (Figure 1–5) extend the external auditory canal and carry the tympanic membrane from the horizontal angulation of the neonate to the acute angulation of the adult (see Figure 1–5). The styloid process does not make its appearance until after birth, arising in an ossification center at the upper aspect of Reichert's cartilage.

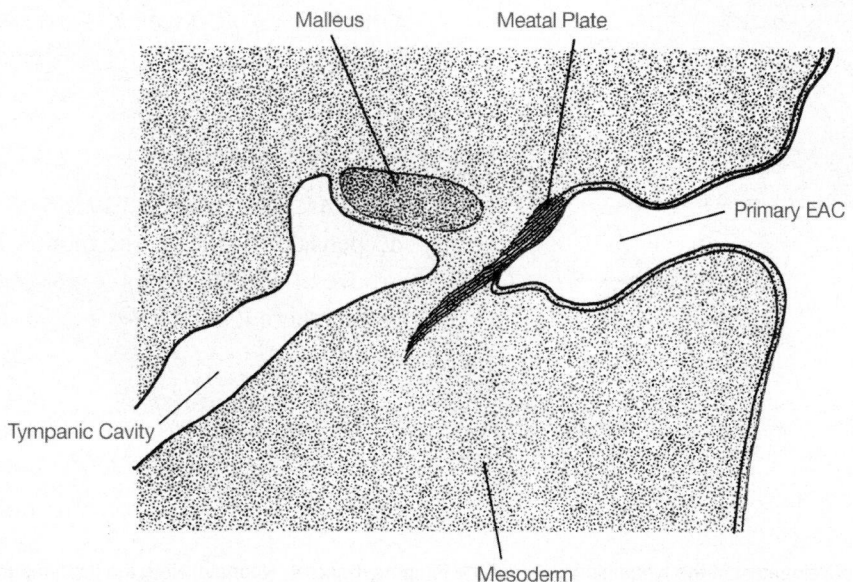

Malleus   Meatal Plate

Primary EAC

Tympanic Cavity

Mesoderm

Figure 1–4 The primary external auditory canal (EAC) is formed at 9 weeks with deepening of the first branchial groove. The meatal plate develops as epithelial cells grow medially toward the tympanic cavity. After Anson and Donaldson.[2] Reproduced with permission from Gulya AJ, Schuknecht HF. Anatomy of the temporal bone with surgical implications. 2nd ed. Pearl River (NY): Parthenon Publishing Group; 1995.

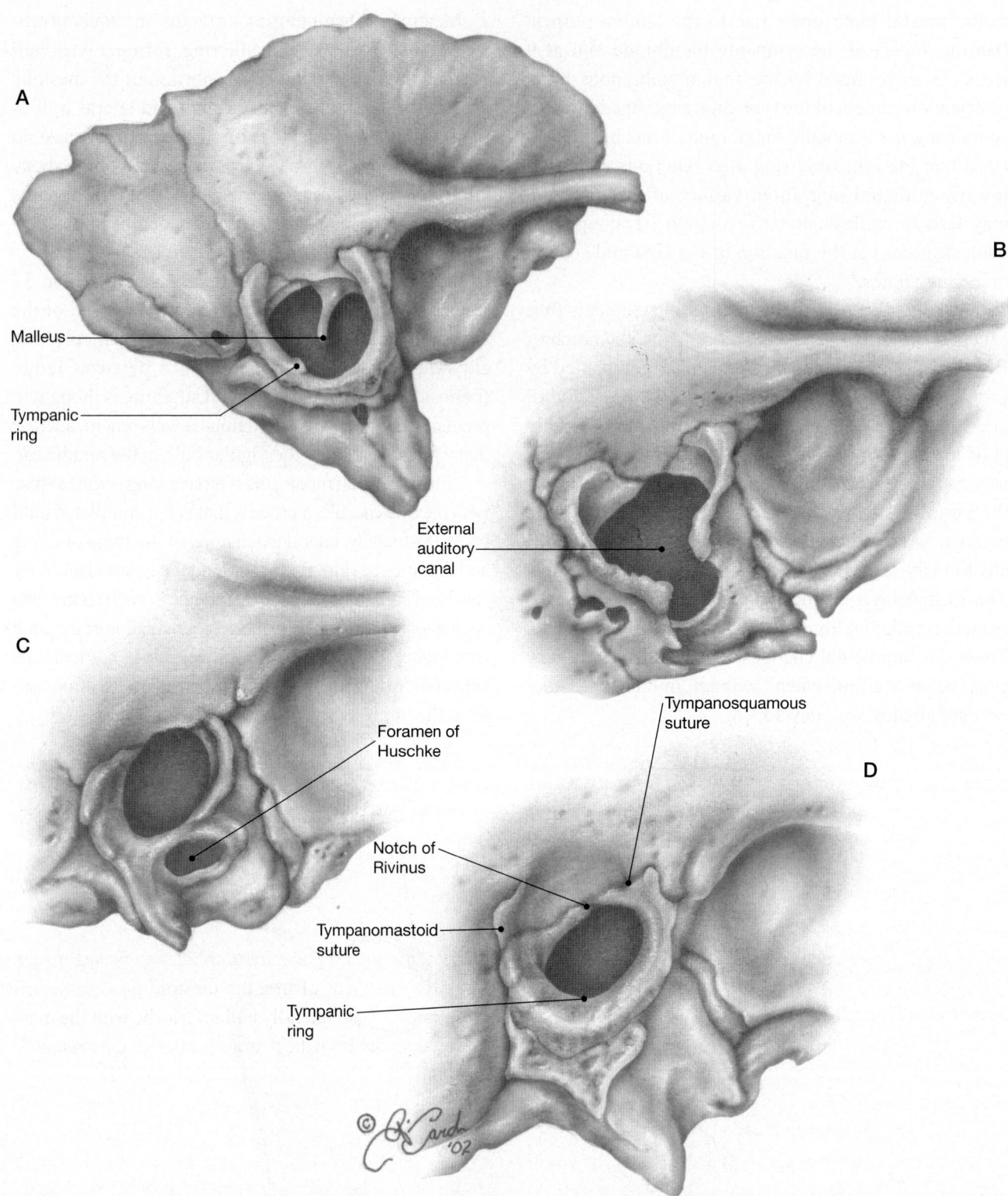

A

Malleus

Tympanic
ring

B

External
auditory
canal

C

Foramen of
Huschke

Tympanosquamous
suture

D

Notch of
Rivinus

Tympanomastoid
suture

Tympanic
ring

Figure 1–5 Postnatal development of the tympanic portion of the temporal bone. *A*, Neonate. Note the flat tympanic ring and the exposed stylomastoid foramen. *B*, Infant, 11 months. The notch of Rivinus and the foramen of Huschke are becoming evident. *C*, Infant, 1 year. *D*, Adolescent. After Anson BJ, Donaldson JA. Surgical anatomy of the temporal bone and ear. Philadelphia: WB Saunders; 1981.

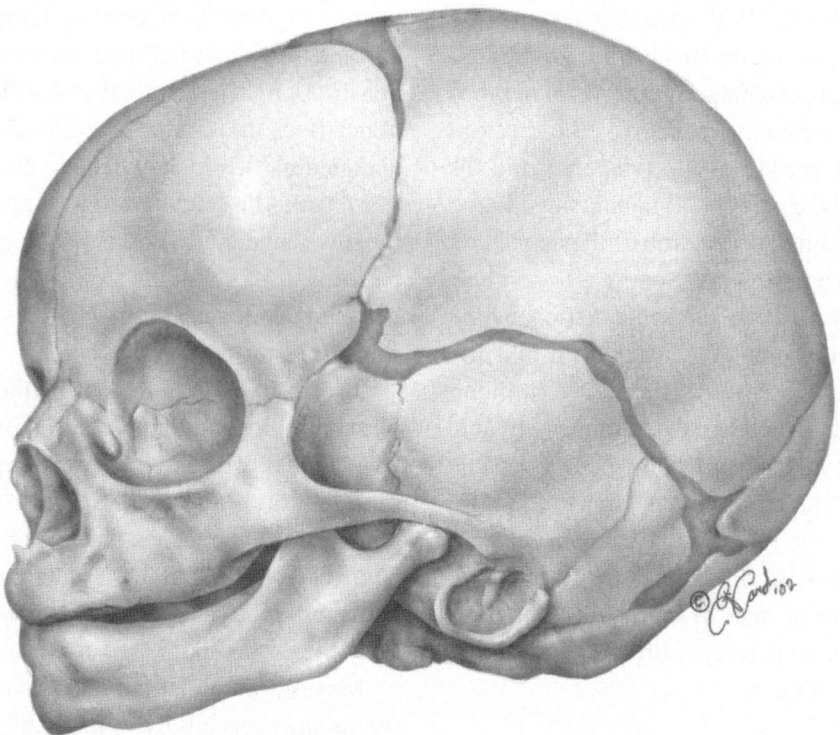

Figure 1–6   The temporal bone of the infant, absent a mastoid process and laterally extending external auditory canal, is located more inferiorly on the skull than that of the adult.

Microtia, anotia, and aberrant positioning of the pinna derive from abnormal development of the first and second branchial arches. Developmental failure of the first branchial groove results in stenosis or atresia of the external auditory canal, based on either a lack of canalization of the meatal plate or a deficiency in epithelial ingrowth. The presence or absence of accompanying defects in the middle and inner ears depends on the time period at which development was disrupted.

Postnatal Development of the Temporal Bone

Although inner and middle ear structures have completed development long before birth, the mastoid and tympanic bones, in particular, manifest postnatal growth and development. Knowledge of these developmental changes is imperative for the otologic surgeon contemplating operative intervention in the very young pediatric patient or cochlear implantation in the profoundly deaf infant or child.

In the neonate, the squama is disproportionately large in comparison with that of the adult (Figure 1–6). The mastoid process is essentially nonexistent, and the tympanic bone is a relatively flat ring, rather than a cylinder. The relative position of the entire temporal bone in the neonate (see Figure 1–6) is inferolateral in comparison with the temporal bone in the adult and its more lateral orientation.

The facial nerve, in the absence of a mastoid process, exits the stylomastoid foramen to emerge on the lateral aspect of the skull and thus is especially vulnerable to injury if a standard postauricular incision is performed. After the first year of life, the mastoid process begins development both laterally and inferiorly, with the mastoid tip deriving from the petrous portion of the mastoid.[10] Similarly, the tympanic ring extends laterally, completing the formation of the bony external auditory canal, the sheath of the styloid process, and the nonarticular part of the glenoid fossa (see Figure 1–5). In the 1-year-old infant, opposing spurs of growing bone at the ventral aspect of the bony external auditory canal fuse, dividing the original external auditory canal into the adult external auditory canal and an inferior channel, known as the foramen of Huschke. The adult external auditory canal is cranial to, and larger than, the foramen of Huschke (see Figure 1–5). This secondary foramen closes in late childhood.[7] With these changes in the mastoid and tympanic bones, the lateral aspect of the temporal bone is vertically oriented, and the facial nerve is buried beneath the protective barrier of the mastoid process. The lateral growth of the tympanic ring, as mentioned previously, carries the tympanic membrane from the nearly horizontal orientation of the neonate to the adult angulation by age 4 or 5 years.

With a view toward cochlear implantation in the infant or young child, one study suggested that the dimensions that show significant growth, continuing into the teenage years, include the depth of the tympanic cavity (as measured by the distance between the tympanic membrane and the stapes footplate) and the length, width, and depth of the mastoid.[11] Cochlear wires, if reaching to the lateral skull, should be placed with approximately 2.5 cm of slack to accommodate anticipated growth. The facial recess, on the other hand, should be adult size at birth.[12]

DEVELOPMENT OF THE TYMPANOMASTOID COMPARTMENT AND EUSTACHIAN TUBE

The tympanomastoid compartment represents the phylogenetic salvage and functional adaptation of the aquatic gill apparatus, which transiently appears in the ontogeny of the human. As life forms evolved from a water environment to a terrestrial environment, a mechanism for matching the sound impedance of water with that of air became essential to auditory function. The middle ear and its contained ossicular chain serve this purpose. The first vestige of such an impedance-matching mechanism emerged as the spiracular diverticulum of the eusthenopteron (a crossopterygian fish).[13]

In the developing human, the tympanomastoid compartment appears at the 3-week stage as an outpouching of the first pharyngeal pouch known as the tubotympanic recess. The endodermal tissue of the dorsal end of this pouch eventually becomes the eustachian tube and tympanic cavity (Hammar, as cited in Proctor[14]). Expansion of the pouch begins at the inferior aspect of the definitive tympanic cavity and progresses by invasion of the adjacent mesenchyme, a loose, gelatinous derivative of mesoderm. By 7 weeks, concomitant growth of the second branchial arch constricts the midportion of the tubotympanic recess; according to Hammar (as

cited in Proctor[14]), the primary tympanic cavity lies lateral and the primordial eustachian tube lies medial to this constriction. The terminal end of the first pharyngeal pouch buds into four sacci (anticus, posticus, superior, and medius[14]), which expand to progressively pneumatize the middle ear and the epitympanum. Expansion of the sacci envelops the ossicular chain and lines the tympanomastoid compartment, whereas the interface between two sacci gives rise to mesentery-like mucosal folds, transmitting blood vessels.

The further development of the eustachian tube is marked by its lengthening and narrowing, with mesodermal chondrification establishing the fibrocartilaginous eustachian tube. By the twenty-first week, pneumatization reaches the antrum. Although the tympanic cavity is essentially complete by 30 weeks, some configurational changes occur with finalization of the bony hypotympanum (see above).

Mastoid pneumatization is evident as early as 33 weeks and proceeds by well-established tracts.[15] Heredity, environment, nutrition, bacterial infection, and adequate ventilation provided by the eustachian tube are all thought to play a role in the interindividual variability of temporal bone pneumatization.[1]

By birth, the antrum approximates that of the adult. However, mesenchymal resolution may continue as late as 1 year postnatally,[16] or even later in some rare cases. Remnants of embryonic connective tissue in the adult are manifest as connective tissue strands draped over the oval and round windows.[10] Similarly, the mastoid continues to grow for up to 19 years after birth.[11]

Epitympanic fixation of the head of the malleus is a clinically encountered condition rooted in the incomplete pneumatization of the epitympanum.[17] Such bony fixation of the malleus is a normal occurrence in certain mammals.[18]

Alternative theories for the development of the middle ear have been proposed. Fraser (cited in Proctor[14]) suggested that the first, second, and third branchial arches, as well as the second branchial groove, give rise to the primitive tympanic cavity. Other workers suggested that the first pharyngeal pouch forms only the eustachian tube, whereas the remainder of the tympanomastoid compartment develops by the cavitation of mesenchyme.[19] In this scheme, mesenchymal derivatives, rather than the respiratory mucosa of the first pharyngeal pouch, form the lining of the middle ear.

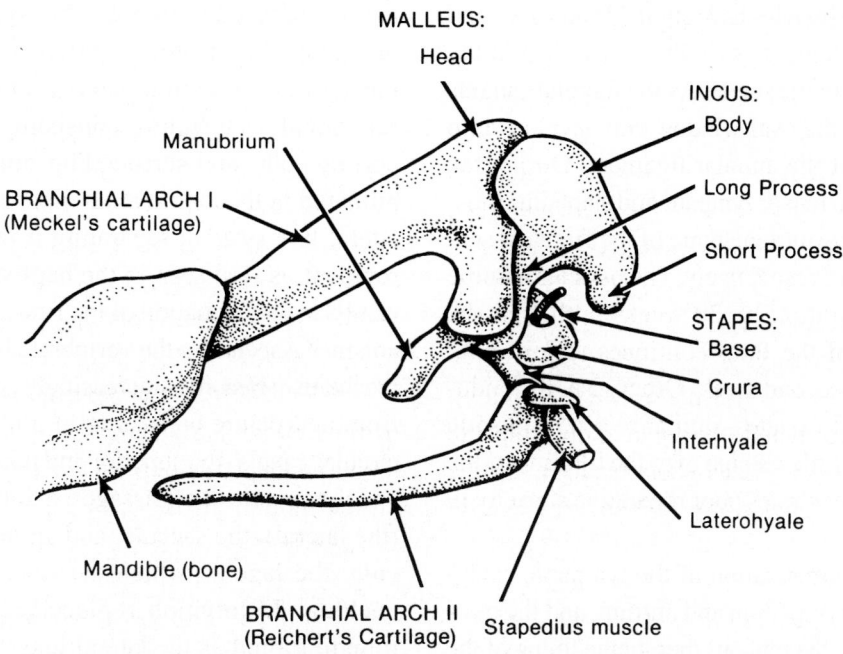

Figure 1–7   The branchial arch origin of the ossicles at 8 to 9 weeks as seen in a left lateral view. The interhyale marks the site of development of attachment of the stapedius tendon, which is its derivative. The laterohyale, eventually migrating to lie posterior to the stapes, temporarily acts as part of the facial nerve canal. After Hanson and colleagues.[21] Reproduced with permission from Gulya AJ, Schuknecht HF. Anatomy of the temporal bone with surgical implications. 2nd ed. Pearl River (NY): Parthenon Publishing Group; 1995.

DEVELOPMENT OF THE OSSICULAR CHAIN

The ossicular chain, a functional component of the middle ear impedance-matching mechanism, for the most part traces its phylogenetic roots to the branchial arch (gill slit) apparatus. In early vertebrates, the mesenchyme of branchial arches I (Meckel's cartilage, mandibular arch) and II (Reichert's cartilage, hyoid arch) was destined to become part of the masticatory apparatus. Evolutionary modifications that reduced the stresses on the jaw rendered certain of its components, namely, the articular and the quadrate, superfluous.[20] The malleus and the incus, respectively, are derived from these jaw components, whereas the origin of the stapes has been traced back to the columella auris of reptiles.

The first evidence of ossicular development in the human embryo occurs at approximately 4 weeks as an interbranchial bridge appears, connecting the upper end of that portion of the first branchial arch referred to as the mandibular visceral bar and the central region of the hyoid (second branchial arch) visceral bar. It is this condensed mesenchymal bridge, consisting of both first and second branchial arch elements, that through cartilaginous differentiation gives rise to the primordial malleus and incus.[21] All of the stapes blastema derives from the hyoid bar except for the medial surface of the footplate and its annular ligament, which are of otic capsular (lamina stapedialis) origin (Gradenigo, 1889, cited in Gulya and Schuknecht[1]) (Figure 1–7).

Over the following 11 weeks, the future ossicular chain continues growth and development as a cartilaginous model (see Figure 1–7); such formation of bone from a cartilage model is termed enchondral bone development (see "Development of the Otic Capsule"). The anterior process of the malleus is unique in that it develops as membranous bone without a cartilaginous model. Development of the stapes blastema involves progressive encirclement of the stapedial artery. The obturator foramen represents the completed ring left empty after the stapedial artery involutes (see "Development of the Arteries"). Growth of the lamina stapedialis, an otic capsule structure, involves retrogressive changes in the cartilaginous rim of the oval window.

By 15 weeks, the ossicles have attained adult size, and ossification soon begins, first in the incus, then in the malleus, and finally in the stapes. As the footplate attains adult size, tissue at the oval window rim develops into the fibrous tissue of the annular ligament. During the same time frame, the tensor tympani and stapedius muscles develop from the mesenchyme of the first and second branchial arches, respectively. The ossicles assume their adult configuration by 20 weeks, although the megalithic stapes of the fetus continues to lose bulk well into the thirty-second week. Otherwise, the endochondral bone of the ossicles, similar to that of the otic capsule, undergoes little change over the lifetime of the individual and demonstrates poor reparative capacity in response to trauma.

Meanwhile, pneumatization of the tympanic cavity extends into the epitympanum and antrum, and the ossicles are enveloped in the mucous membrane lining of the tubotympanic recess.

DEVELOPMENT OF THE OTIC LABYRINTH

The precursor of the mammalian otic labyrinth is the cranial portion of the lateral line system of fish,[22] a water-motion detection system. This system of fluid-filled pits (ampullae) features epidermal placode derivation; innervation by cranial nerves VII, IX, and X; and a functional architecture consisting of hair cells, supporting cells, and surrounding fluid (sea water), recapitulated in the mammalian inner ear. Enclosure of the lateral line system, separating it from the ocean environment, is first seen in the hagfish (*Myxinoidea*) and results in the formation of the first true vestibular mechanism.[22] Ascending the vertebrate ladder, the vestibular mechanism becomes increasingly complex as it changes from a structure consisting of a utricle and two semicircular canals (the superior and posterior) by adding the endolymphatic duct passages; a third semicircular canal (the lateral), the saccule; and an outgrowth of the saccule, the lagena, which eventually gives rise to the cochlea. Endolymph replaced seawater as the surrounding fluid as the lateral line system evolved from use in aquatic to terrestrial organisms.

The development of the otic labyrinth in the human embryo faithfully follows much the same sequence as did the development of the mechanism in our vertebrate ancestors; hence, the phylogenetically older semicircular canals and utricle (pars superior) precede the

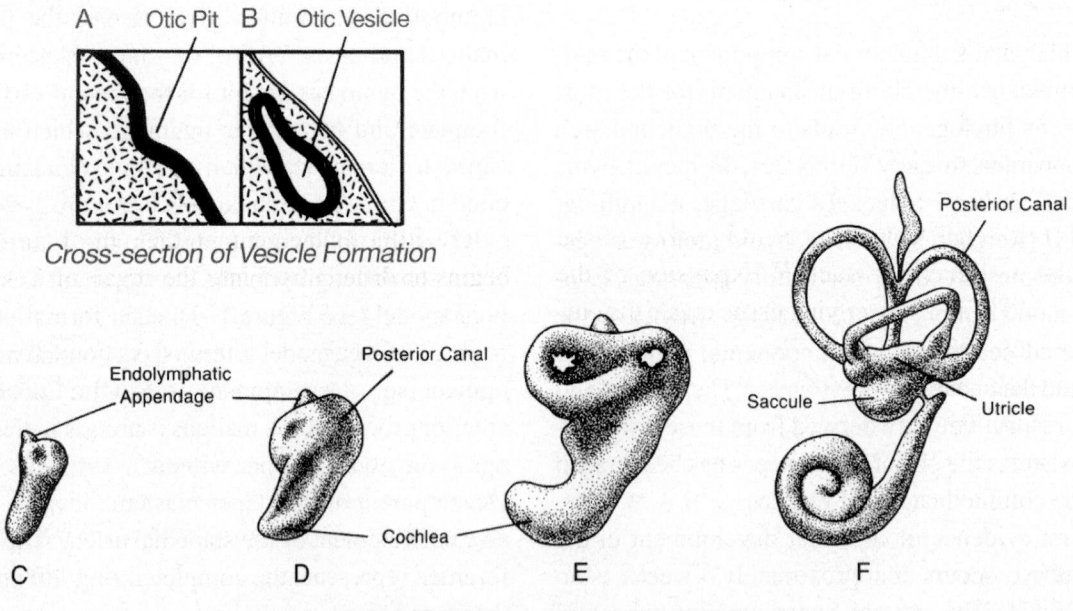

Figure 1–8   The evolution of the endolymphatic (otic) labyrinth. *A* = 22 days, *B* = 4 weeks, *C* = 4½ weeks, *D* = 5½ weeks, *E* = 6 weeks, and *F* = 8+ weeks. After Streeter.[23] Reproduced with permission from Gulya AJ, Schuknecht HF. Anatomy of the temporal bone with surgical implications. 2nd ed. Pearl River (NY): Parthenon Publishing Group; 1995.

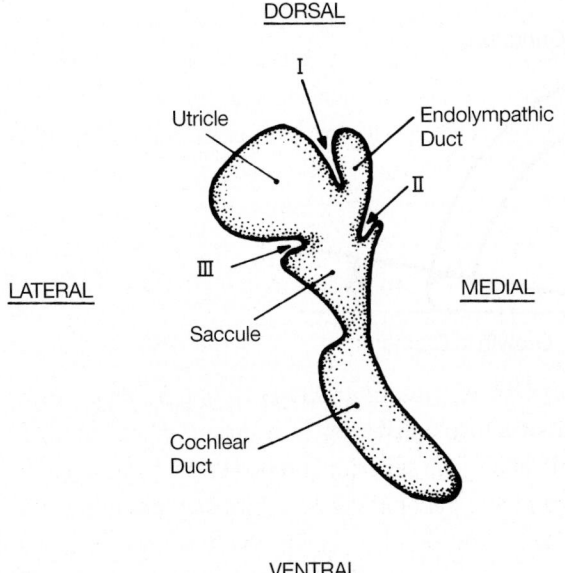

DORSAL

Utricle

Endolympathic
Duct

I

II

LATERAL

III

MEDIAL

Saccule

Cochlear
Duct

VENTRAL

Figure 1–9   The otic labyrinth at the 6- to 8-week stage. Folds I, II, and III begin to indent the otocyst. After Bast and Anson.[4] Reproduced with permission from Gulya AJ, Schuknecht HF. Anatomy of the temporal bone with surgical implications. 2nd ed. Pearl River (NY): Parthenon Publishing Group; 1995.

development of the saccule and the cochlear duct (pars inferior). The phylogenetic seniority of the pars superior is thought to underlie its relative resistance to developmental malformations when contrasted with the newer pars superior.

The otic placode, a plaquelike thickening of surface ectoderm dorsal to the first branchial groove, appears at the end of the third week. Invagination into the underlying mesenchyme occurs within days, forming the auditory pit (Figure 1–8). The endolymphatic appendage appears at this stage, considerably in advance of the semicircular and cochlear ducts.[23] Expansion of the auditory pit and fusion of overlying tissue create the otocyst (otic vesicle), separated from the surface. The mesenchymal tissue that surrounds and differentiates in conjunction with the otocyst is the future otic capsule (bony labyrinth). By the fourth week, two flanges (the future semicircular ducts) arise from the otocyst. Development then involves elongation of the otocyst and the appearance of three deepening folds (I, II, and III), which demarcate the utricle with its three semicircular ducts, the endolymphatic duct and sac, and the saccule with its cochlear duct (Figure 1–9). The utriculoendolymphatic valve (of Bast) is a derivative of fold III,

functionally separating the utricle and the dilated proximal aspect, or sinus, of the endolymphatic duct.[24]

In the 6-week embryo, the lumina of the semicircular ducts have formed, and the macula communis (the primordial macula at the medial wall of the otocyst) has divided into superior and inferior segments. The macula of the utricle and the ampullary crests of the superior and lateral semicircular ducts are derivatives of the superior segment, whereas the macula of the saccule and the ampullary crest of the posterior semicircular duct are derived from the inferior segment. At the same time, the cochlear duct has extended from the saccule, completing one turn during the course of the week.

As the semicircular ducts increase in both the radius of the arc of curvature and in luminal diameter (Figure 1–10), progressive deepening of the three folds (Figure 1–11) delineates the ductal connections of the utricle, saccule, and endolymphatic sac as well as of the cochlea and saccule. Meanwhile, the cochlear duct continues its spiraling growth, rapidly completing its 2½ turns by the eighth week (see Figure 1–8). A number of cochlear anomalies are recognized and are believed to reflect the stage at which normal development is disrupted.[25]

Between 8 and 16 weeks, the otic labyrinth approaches its adult configuration (Figure 1–12). The epithelium of the cristae ampullaries of the semicircular ducts differentiates to a sensory neuroepithelium with hair cells and gelatinous cupula as the semicircular ducts continue expansion. Similarly, the maculae of the otolithic organs (utricle and saccule) differentiate as hair cells and otolithic membranes appear. The proximal endolymphatic sac begins to develop a rugose epithelium. The primitive circular cochlear duct assumes a more triangular outline as the neuroepithelium of the basal turn begins to differentiate into the organ of Corti (Figure 1–13).

At 20 weeks, the superior semicircular duct has reached adult size. In a phylogenetically determined sequence, the posterior and lateral ducts complete growth, and the cristae ampullares are completely differentiated. The endolymphatic duct, up to this stage, has followed a straight course, paralleling the crus commune to reach the endolymphatic sac; now the duct begins to develop a bend as it is dragged inferiorly and laterally along with the endolymphatic sac by the continuing growth of the sigmoid sinus and posterior fossa. The first part of the endolymphatic duct, then, is an anatomically constant

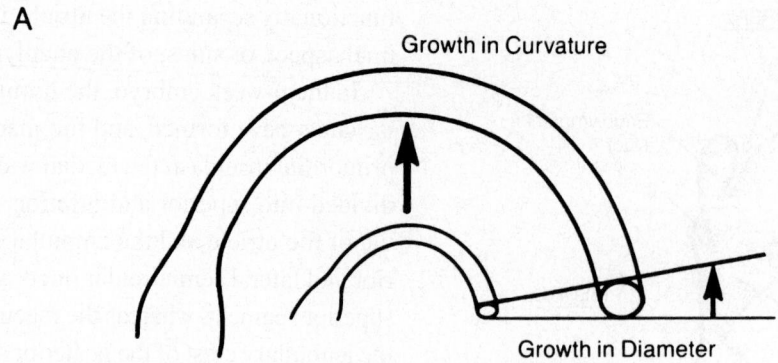

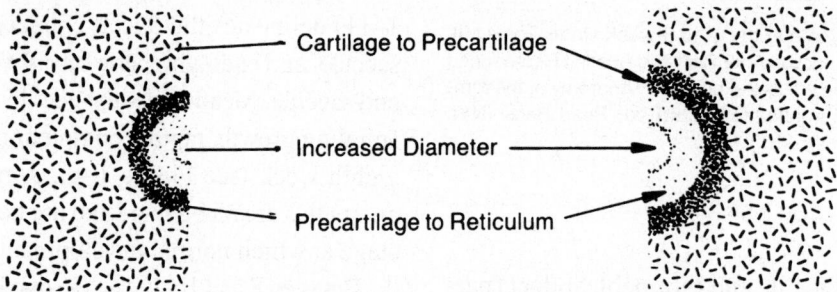

Figure 1–10 Growth of the semicircular ducts involves retrogressive changes in the surrounding cartilage and precartilage. After Pearson.[3] Reproduced with permission from Gulya AJ, Schuknecht HF. Anatomy of the temporal bone with surgical implications. 2nd ed. Pearl River (NY): Parthenon Publishing Group; 1995.

structure in close relationship to the crus commune; the distal duct and sac, however, vary in position according to the degree of sigmoid sinus migration and posterior fossa development.[1] The sac continues to grow, with its size at term attaining quadruple that seen at midterm and with its lining further differentiating. The lining epithelium of the saccular, utricular, and endolymphatic ducts ranges from simple squamous to cuboidal. As demonstrated by Lundquist,[26] the proximal endolymphatic sac (Figure 1–14), located within the vestibular aqueduct, and the distal third, completely enveloped in dura adjacent to the lateral venous sinus, similarly possess a simple cuboidal lining. In contrast, the intermediate one-third, or rugose portion, which lies partly within the vestibular aqueduct and partly within folds of dura mater, has a highly differentiated epithelium. The tall, cylindrical cells of the epithelium possess microvilli and pinocytotic vesicles, are ruffled into papillae and crypts, and overlie a rich, subepithelial capillary network.

All of these features suggest resorptive and phagocytic functions, with the latter function providing for local immune defense.[27]

The organ of Corti is differentiated to such a degree by 20 weeks that the fetus can "hear" and respond to fluid-borne sounds.[28] The organ of Corti approximates the adult structure by 25 weeks.[3]

DEVELOPMENT OF THE PERILYMPHATIC (PERIOTIC) LABYRINTH

The perilymphatic (periotic) labyrinth comprises the fluid-tissue space interposed between the membranous otic (or endolymphatic) labyrinth and its bony covering—the otic capsule. The perilymphatic cistern (of the vestibule), scala tympani, scala vestibuli, perilymphatic space of the semicircular canals, fissula ante fenestram, fossula post fenestram, and periotic duct are all considered part of the perilymphatic labyrinth.

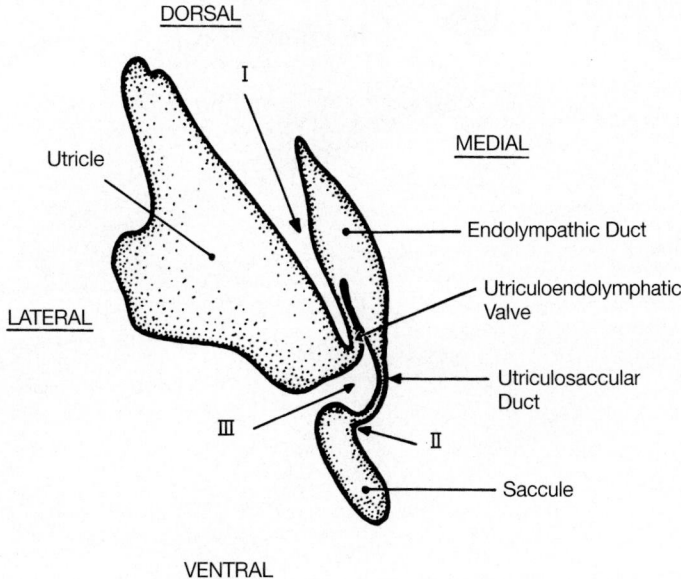

Figure 1–11   The otic labyrinth at 9 weeks. Deepening of folds I, II, and III (compare with Figure 1–9) more clearly distinguishes the utricle, saccule, and endolymphatic duct. After Bast and Anson.[4] Reproduced with permission from Gulya AJ, Schuknecht HF. Anatomy of the temporal bone with surgical implications. 2nd ed. Pearl River (NY): Parthenon Publishing Group; 1995.

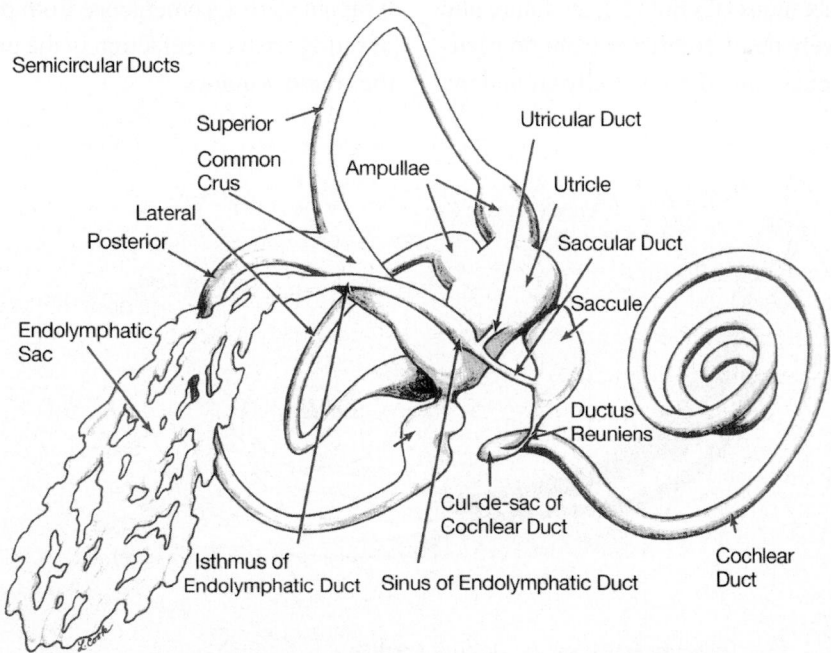

Figure 1–12   The adult membranous labyrinth, medial aspect. The endolymphatic duct initially parallels the common crus and posterior semicircular duct but then diverges to the posterior cranial fossa location of the endolymphatic sac. After Anson and Donaldson.[2] Reproduced with permission from Gulya AJ, Schuknecht HF. Anatomy of the temporal bone with surgical implications. 2nd ed. Pearl River (NY): Parthenon Publishing Group; 1995.

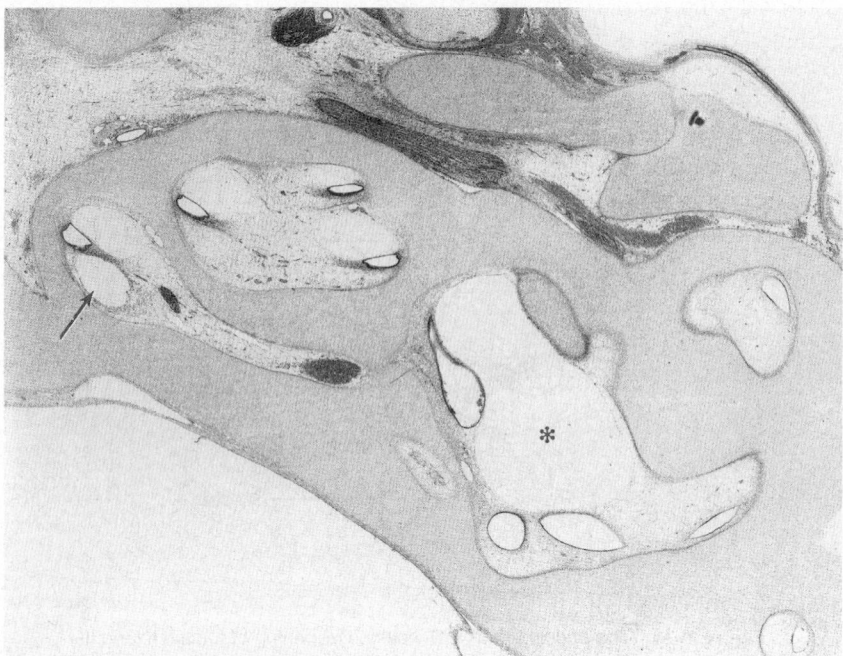

Figure 1–13   In this 12-week fetus, the vestibule (*) is advanced in development and the scala tympani (*arrow*) is evident in the basal turn of the cochlea. The cochlear duct of the basal turn assumes a more triangular configuration, whereas the apical turn still retains its circular outline. Reproduced with permission from Gulya AJ, Schuknecht HF. Anatomy of the temporal bone with surgical implications. 2nd ed. Pearl River (NY): Parthenon Publishing Group; 1995.

It is not until the eighth week that the first sign of perilymphatic space formation is seen. Mesodermal tissue surrounding the membranous labyrinth (ie, the future otic capsule) retrogressively dedifferentiates from precartilage into a loose, vascular reticulum, initially around the ampullae of the semicircular ducts and in the region of the perilymphatic cistern of the vestibule. The scala tympani starts its emergence from precartilage as an area of retrogressive rarefaction in the precartilage just under the round window.

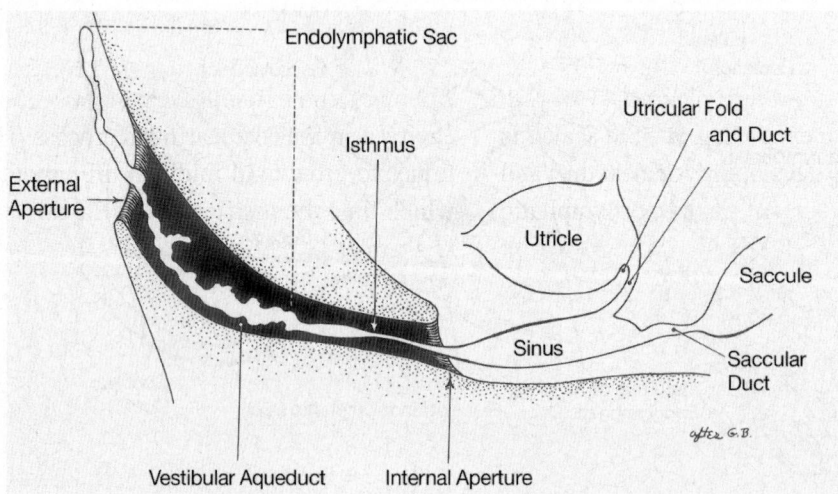

Figure 1–14   The osseous relationships of the endolymphatic duct and sac. After Anson and Donaldson.[2] Reproduced with permission from Schuknecht HF. Pathology of the ear. Boston: Harvard University Press; 1974.

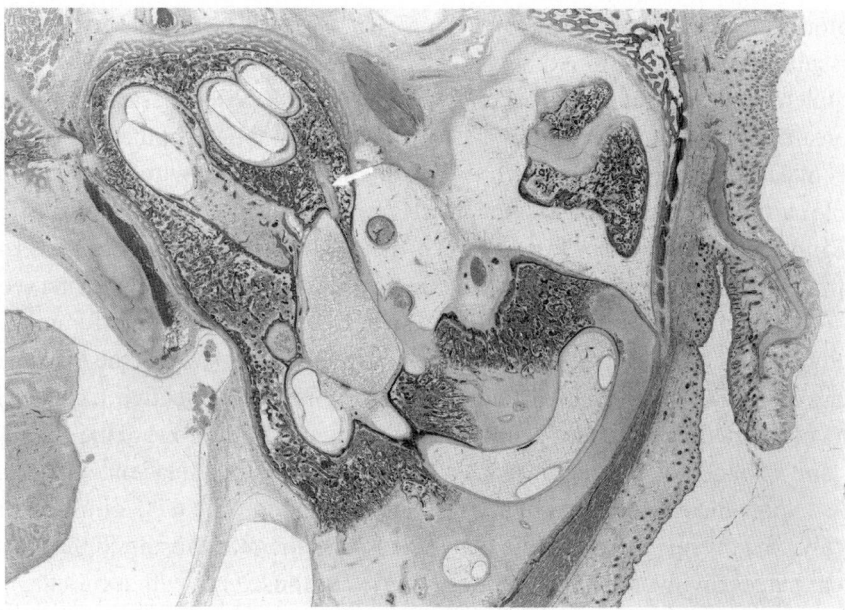

Figure 1–15 This photomicrograph, from a 16-week specimen, shows the fissula ante fenestram (*arrow*). Reproduced with permission from Gulya AJ, Schuknecht HF. Anatomy of the temporal bone with surgical implications. 2nd ed. Pearl River (NY): Parthenon Publishing Group; 1995.

Rapidly changing over the next several weeks, the reticulum of the primordial perilymphatic labyrinth becomes highly vacuolated, its spaces traversed by supporting fibers for the walls of the saccule and the utricle and for the vascular and neural supplies of the inner ear.[3] The perilymphatic cistern of the vestibule, adjacent to the oval window, is the first recognizable space of the perilymphatic labyrinth, appearing late in the twelfth week (see Figure 1–13). The scala tympani appears soon afterward, with the scala vestibuli appearing somewhat later as a diverticulum of the perilymphatic cistern near the oval window. The expansion of both scalae is closely linked to that of the developing cochlear duct and cochlea. The canalicular portion of the perilymphatic labyrinth is relatively delayed in development. Only at 16 weeks does vacuolization begin; however, development is usually completed by 20 weeks.

Fissula Ante Fenestram

The fissula ante fenestram and the fossula post fenestram, although part of the perilymphatic labyrinth, undergo a different developmental sequence and hence merit separate discussion (Figure 1–15).

Apparently, the fissula ante fenestram is unique to humans, although Anson and Bast[10] detected a rudimentary, incomplete fissula in the rhesus monkey. The fissula is first apparent in the 9-week embryo as a strip of precartilage in the lateral wall of the cartilaginous otic capsule immediately anterior to the oval window (ante is Latin for "in front of," fenestram is Latin for "window"). In the course of the next 3 weeks, this extension of periotic tissue stretches as a connective tissue ribbon from the vestibule to the middle ear. Vertically, the ribbon extends from the scala vestibuli to the tympanic cavity, near the cochleariform process. The fissula continues to grow until midfetal life (about 21 weeks), at which time the ossification of the otic capsule is nearing completion.

Although the fissula is a constant tract in humans, it shows interindividual variation both in capacity and in form and undergoes alteration of its lining cartilage over the life of the individual. The cartilage border that separates the connective tissue of the fissula from the bone of the otic capsule is gradually replaced by intrachondral bone (see "Development of the Otic Capsule"). Because of the metamorphosis of the lining cartilage, fissulae in general and large fissulae in particular are thought to be areas of histologic instability.[29]

Several investigators have focused on the histologic instability of the fissula in an attempt to explain the etiopathology of otosclerosis in general and its peculiar affinity for the region anterior to the oval window.[4,30–35] Anson and Bast and colleagues etiologically related the histologically unstable cartilage in the fissular region to the development of otosclerosis.[29,36,37] These workers frequently noted pathologic tissue occupying the fissular region, especially if the fissula was large. Such pathologic tissue consisted of either newly formed cartilage or its derivative, a mass of newly formed gnarled bone.[37] Anson and coworkers contended that the newly formed bone may remodel and expand to become an active focus of otosclerosis.[37] Spontaneous cessation of activity before stapes involvement results in histologic otosclerosis only, whereas stapes involvement precipitates clinical otosclerosis. Independent concurrence[30–32,34] is countered by the findings that small otosclerotic foci can be found anterior to the oval window, "separate and distinct from" the fissula.[33] An autoimmune reaction to type II collagen present in the cartilage of the fissula has been proposed as the underlying cause of otosclerosis.[38] More recent research findings regarding the etiology of otosclerosis can be found in Chapter 27.

Fossula Post Fenestram

The fossula post fenestram, an evagination of periotic tissue from the vestibule into the otic capsule (see Figure 1–15) posterior to the oval window, undergoes a developmental sequence similar to that of the fissula ante fenestram. The fossula (fossula is Latin for "little ditch," post is Latin for "behind") is first seen in the fetus of 10½ weeks as an area of dedifferentiating precartilage. As early as 4½ weeks later, the fossula can be distinguished as a zone of connective tissue, which soon becomes surrounded by the bone of the otic capsule. Differing from the fissula, the fossula is an inconstantly occurring structure found in only 67% of all ears studied and extends through the otic capsule to the tympanic cavity in only 25% of those ears with a fossula.[4]

Although the fossula is an area of histologic instability for reasons similar to those for the fissula, cartilaginous and bony changes affect only 5% of all fossulae.[4]

Cochlear Aqueduct

The primordial (bony) cochlear aqueduct first appears at 7 weeks as a rarefaction of precartilage at the medial

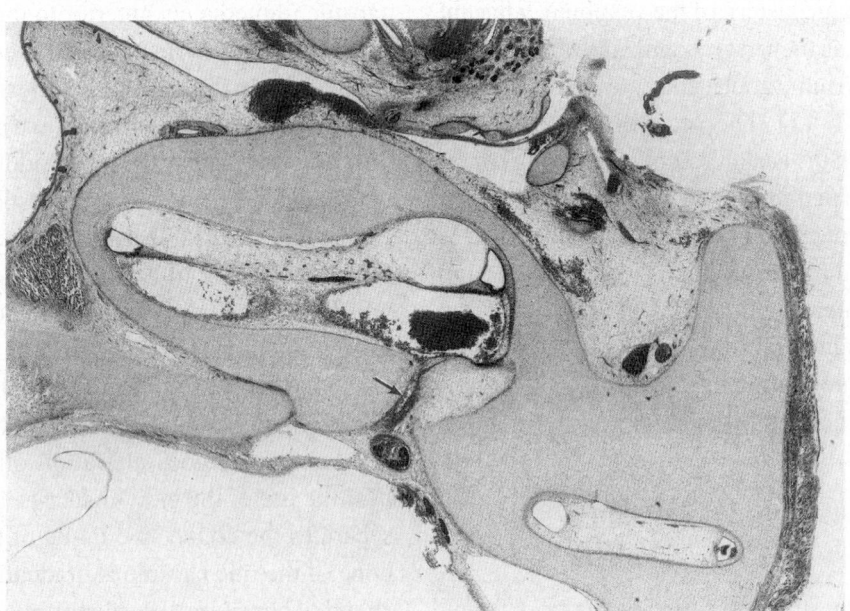

Figure 1–16 As seen in a 12-week fetus, the cochlear aqueduct (*arrow*) reaches from the posterior cranial fossa to the scala tympani of the basal turn. Reproduced with permission from Gulya AJ, Schuknecht HF. Anatomy of the temporal bone with surgical implications. 2nd ed. Pearl River (NY): Parthenon Publishing Group; 1995.

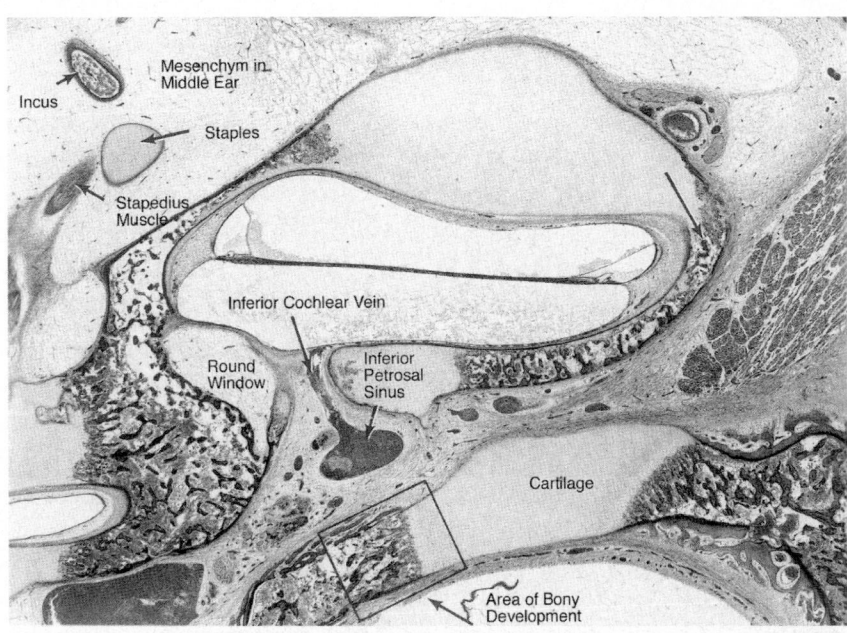

Figure 1–17 The inferior cochlear vein occupies the primitive cochlear aqueduct, as seen in a fetus of approximately 17 weeks. The boxed area is enlarged in Figure 1–22. Reproduced with permission from Gulya AJ, Schuknecht HF. Anatomy of the temporal bone with surgical implications. 2nd ed. Pearl River (NY): Parthenon Publishing Group; 1995.

wall of the cochlear basal turn. The cochlear aqueduct extends from the area of the developing round window to the posterior cranial fossa. The reticulum of the primordial aqueduct links the loose mesenchyme of the round window niche with the connective tissue of the posterior cranial fossa dura, ninth cranial nerve, and inferior petrosal sinus (Figure 1–16).

By the ninth week, the inferior cochlear vein emerges from the syncytium of the cochlear aqueduct. Meanwhile, a cartilaginous bar, as it extends from the round window

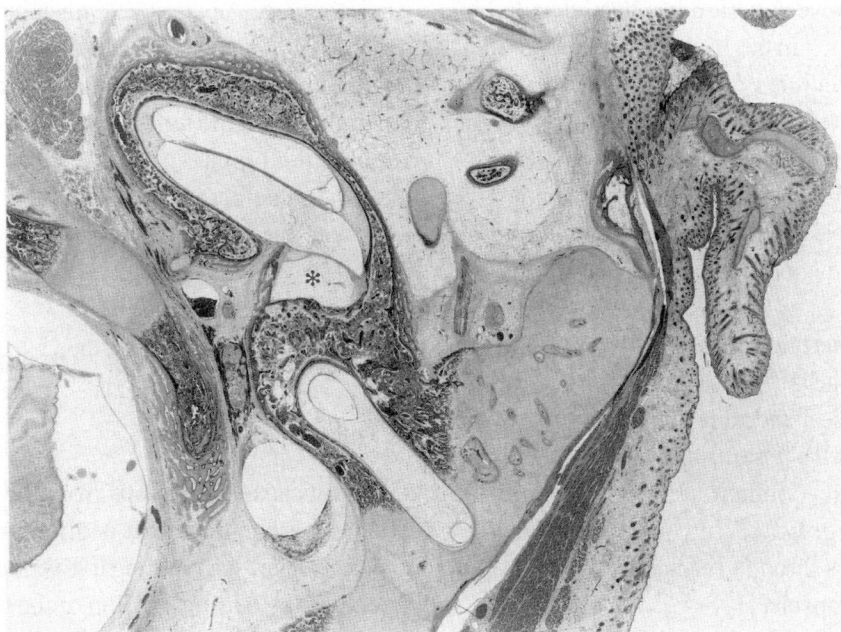

Figure 1–18 Although younger than the fetus shown in Figure 1–17, this fetus shows more advanced ossification of the rim of the round window niche (*) in particular, breaking the communication of the round window niche with the posterior cranial fossa (fetus, 16 weeks). Reproduced with permission from Gulya AJ, Schuknecht HF. Anatomy of the temporal bone with surgical implications. 2nd ed. Pearl River (NY): Parthenon Publishing Group; 1995.

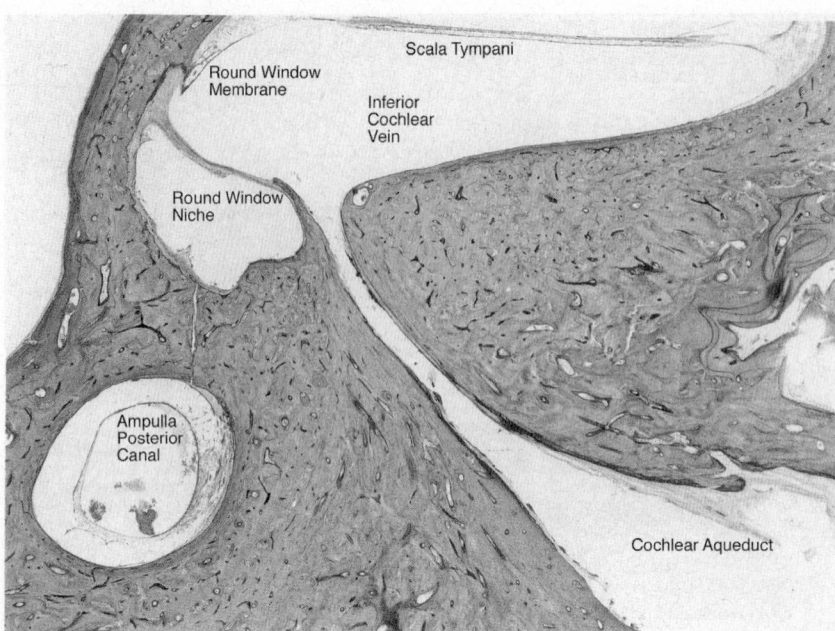

Figure 1–19 The widely patent cochlear aqueduct is thought to underlie the "perilymph oozer" seen in stapes surgery (man, age 67 years). A microfissure is visible between the posterior semicircular canal ampulla and the round window niche. Reproduced with permission from Schuknecht HF, Seifi AE. Experimental observations on the fluid physiology of the inner ear. Ann Otol Rhinol Laryngol 1963;72:687.

niche and ampulla of the posterior canal toward the opening of the cochlear aqueduct, gives rise to the floor and medial rim of the round window.

The development of the periotic duct and surroundings in the 16- to 40-week period has been detailed by Spector and associates.[39] In the 16- to 18-week stage (Figure 1–17), three structures are seen in the primitive cochlear aqueduct: the inferior cochlear vein (vein at the cochlear aqueduct), the tympanomeningeal hiatus (Hyrtl's fissure), and the periotic duct. There is still connective tissue continuity between the posterior cranial fossa and the tissue of the round window niche, especially through Hyrtl's fissure.

Ossification of the otic capsule, progressing to the round window by the 18- to 26-week stage (Figure 1–18), fuses the cochlear and canalicular segments of the otic capsule, caps Hyrtl's fissure, and relegates the round window niche to the tympanic cavity. The inferior cochlear vein is segregated into its own canal (of Cotugno) at 20 weeks through further growth and ossification of the otic capsule.

Completion of the cochlear aqueduct occurs between 32 and 40 weeks and entails elongation of the cochlear aqueduct with its contained periodic duct, widening of the cranial apertures of the cochlear aqueduct and peri-

otic duct, and ingrowth of arachnoid tissue, which forms a lining membrane and meshwork. A widely patent cochlear aqueduct (Figure 1–19) is thought to underlie the "perilymph oozer"[1] occasionally encountered in stapes surgery. A persistent tympanomeningeal hiatus represents incomplete ossification. The hiatus extends from the depths of the round window niche to the posterior cranial fossa at the junction of the inferior petrosal sinus and jugular bulb (Figure 1–20).[1] The hiatus is a potential route that cerebrospinal fluid and brain tissue may follow to the middle ear.[39–42]

DEVELOPMENT OF THE OTIC CAPSULE

The otic capsule develops from the precartilage (compacted mesenchyme that is differentiating into embryonic cartilage) surrounding it. Eventually, the otic capsule becomes the petrous portion of the temporal bone.[4] The initial step in development of the otic capsule, as described by Bast and Anson,[4] occurs at the end of the fourth week as the cell density of the mesenchyme enveloping the otic capsule increases. By the eighth week, the mes-

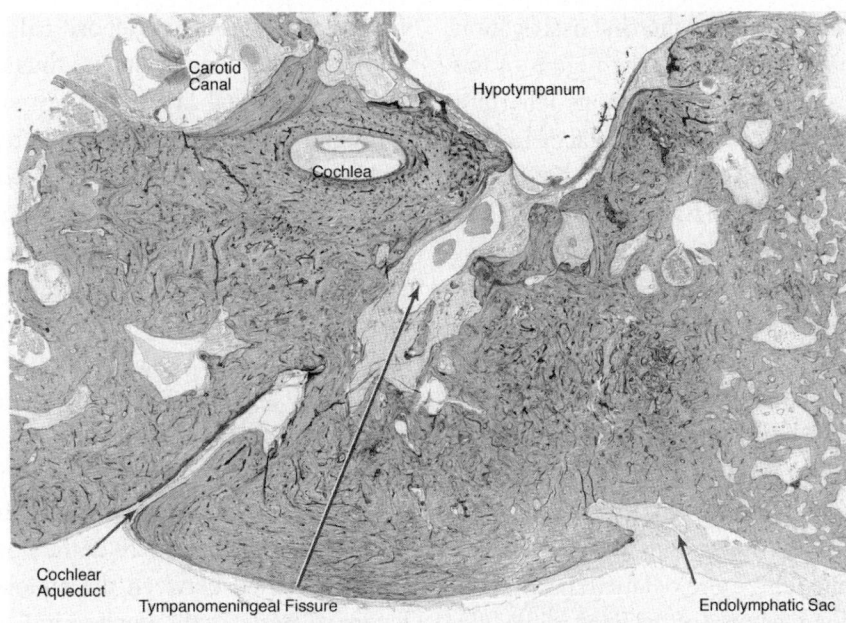

Figure 1–20   The tympanomeningeal fissure (hiatus), occasionally persisting in the adult, is paralleled by the cochlear aqueduct (man, age 44 years). Reproduced with permission from Gulya AJ, Schuknecht HF. Anatomy of the temporal bone with surgical implications. 2nd ed. Pearl River (NY): Parthenon Publishing Group; 1995.

enchymal condensation has formed a cartilaginous model of the otic capsule. At this stage, although the membranous labyrinth, which the cartilaginous otic capsule surrounds, has attained adult configuration, it does not attain adult size until nearly midterm. Retro-gressive dedifferentiation of otic capsular cartilage to a loose reticulum accommodates the expansion of the membranous labyrinth. Redifferentiation to cartilage occurs at the inner, trailing edge of the semicircular ducts (see Figure 1–10).

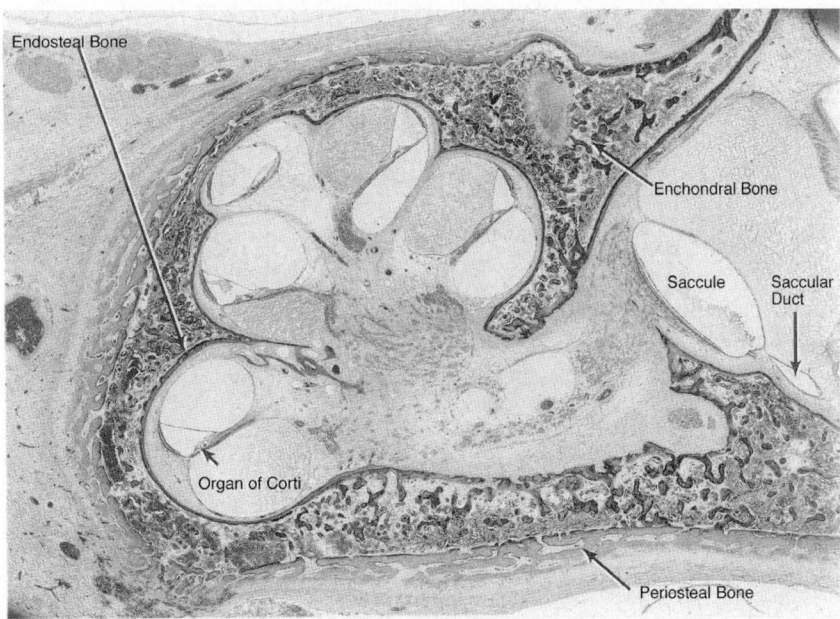

Figure 1–21   With ossification of the otic capsule, three layers of bone are created (fetus, 16 weeks). Reproduced with permission from Gulya AJ, Schuknecht HF. Anatomy of the temporal bone with surgical implications. 2nd ed. Pearl River (NY): Parthenon Publishing Group; 1995.

According to Bast and Anson,[4] the first ossification center of the otic capsule appears at the region of the cochlea only as the contained membranous labyrinth reaches adult size, usually by 16 weeks. A total of 14 centers eventually appear and fuse to complete the ossification of the otic capsule despite its small size. The last ossification center appears at 20 to 21 weeks in the posterolateral region of the posterior semicircular canal. The only areas that remain cartilaginous are those at the region of the fissula ante fenestram and an area that overlies part of the posterior and lateral semicircular ducts, where ossification does not begin until 2 weeks later.[4]

A detailed discussion of the ossification sequence of the otic capsule is beyond the scope of this chapter, and the interested reader is referred to Bast and Anson[4] and Gulya and Schuknecht[1] for a more detailed discussion. However, several unique features of the bone of the otic capsule are of clinical significance and are outlined below.

Three layers of bone emerge from the ossification of the cartilaginous otic capsule (Figure 1–21). The perichondrial membrane lining the external and the internal (facing the membranous labyrinth) surfaces of the otic capsule becomes a periosteal membrane as newly dif-

ferentiated osteoblasts deposit calcium. The periosteal and endosteal bone layers are thus formed.

The endosteal layer does not significantly change throughout adult life, although in response to infection or trauma (including perhaps electrical stimulation), it may proliferate to such a degree as to obliterate the lumen of the labyrinth.[1] Alternatively, it has been proposed that undifferentiated mesenchymal cells, located around capillaries, are the true source of such obliterative, bony growths.[43] The periosteal layer, in contrast, does change, by lamellar addition of bone and by pneumatization, until early adult life.[10] This layer has the capability of good osteogenic repair in response to trauma and infection and remodels throughout life, similar to periosteal bone elsewhere in the body.

Sandwiched between the endosteal and periosteal layers of bone is the enchondral layer, consisting of both intrachondral (intrachondrial) and endochondral bone. Intrachondral bone (globuli interossei) comprises persistent islands of calcified hyaline cartilage, the lacunae of which are occupied by osteocytes and on which endochondral bone is deposited. Initial steps in the formation of intrachondral bone (Figure 1–22) are hypertrophy of cartilage cells in their lacunae, calcification of

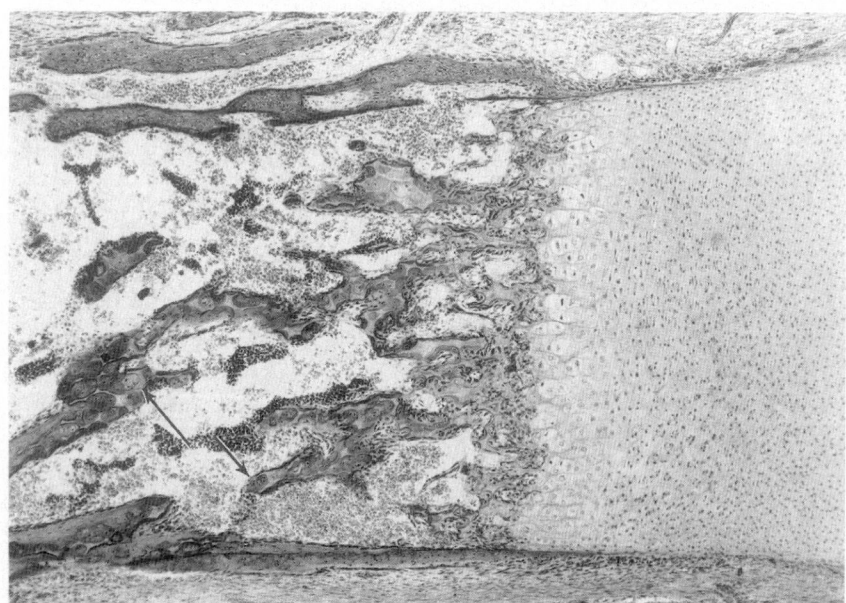

Figure 1–22 This detailed view of the boxed area of Figure 1–17 illustrates the steps of enchondral bone formation. Going from right to left, cartilage cells multiply, enlarge, and are ossified. Globuli interossei (*arrows*) represent persisting islands of cartilage (fetus, age 17 weeks). Reproduced with permission from Gulya AJ, Schuknecht HF. Anatomy of the temporal bone with surgical implications. 2nd ed. Pearl River (NY): Parthenon Publishing Group; 1995.

the cartilaginous matrix, and vascular bud invasion. Much of the calcified cartilage is removed, but scattered islands remain. Osteocytes repopulate the formerly cartilaginous lacunae and begin bone deposition.

Osteoblasts lining the surface of the calcified cartilage islands deposit layers of endochondral bone. This bone deposition nearly obliterates the vascular spaces and establishes the layer of very dense, poorly vascular bone characteristic of the petrous (rocklike) pyramid known as the enchondral layer.

The enchondral layer, similar to the endosteal layer, once formed in midfetal life undergoes little change save for conversion to increasingly dense bone.[10] Enchondral bone, also similar to endosteal bone, exhibits a minimal reparative response to insults, such as trauma and infection, at best healing by fibrous union. Because of the poor reparative capacity of the endosteal and enchondral layers, the ravages of stress and trauma leave indelible marks on the architecture of the bony labyrinth. Major trauma, sufficient to fracture the temporal bone, results in large fissures that may traverse the entire temporal bone.

So-called microfissures are commonly encountered disruptions in the endosteal and enchondral layers of the bony labyrinth.[1] A microfissure found in all ears after the age of 6 years is located between the round window niche and the ampulla of the posterior canal (see Figure 1–19).[44] Additionally, microfissures can be found about the oval window region in 25% of ears examined, usually extending vertically above and below the oval window without involving the footplate, more commonly after the age of 40 years.[45] Typically, these microfissures are obstructed by fibrous tissue in association with an acellular matrix resembling osteoid. Why these microfissures occur remains unclear. It has been hypothesized that the microfissures represent stress fractures resulting from structural changes of the labyrinth[45] or from the transferred stresses of mastication.[46] Alternatively, the microfissures bridging the round window niche and the posterior canal ampulla may be related to an embryologic communication.[44] Although, by term, cartilage replaces the mesenchyme of this transient channel, this area may remain structurally weak and readily fractured.

The microfissures of the bony labyrinth have been thought to play a role in the contamination of the inner ear by inflammatory processes or ototoxic substances applied to the middle ear. Similarly, these microfissures have been theorized to give rise to spontaneous perilymph fistulae.

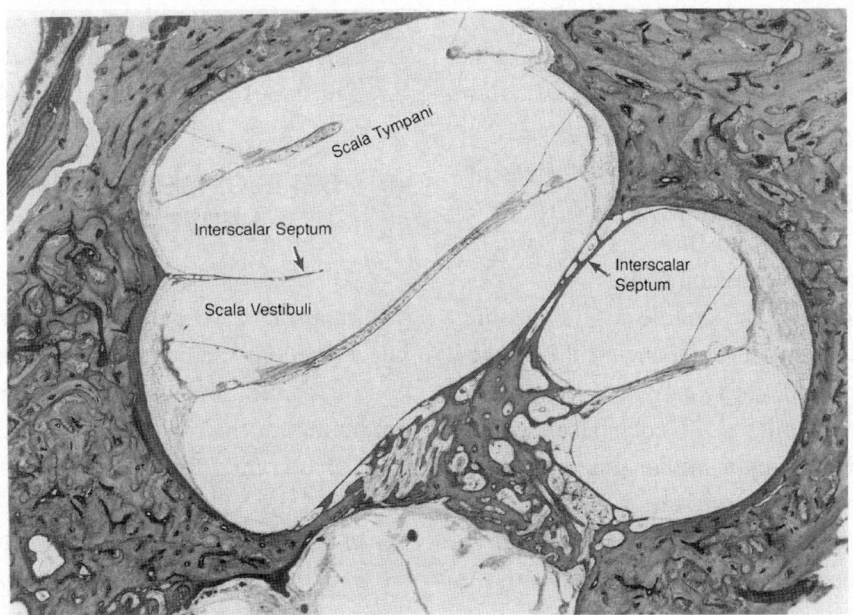

Figure 1–23 Partial absence of the interscalar septum, as shown in this micrograph, is known as scala communis (woman, age 63 years). Reproduced with permission from Gulya AJ, Schuknecht HF. Anatomy of the temporal bone with surgical implications. 2nd ed. Pearl River (NY): Parthenon Publishing Group; 1995.

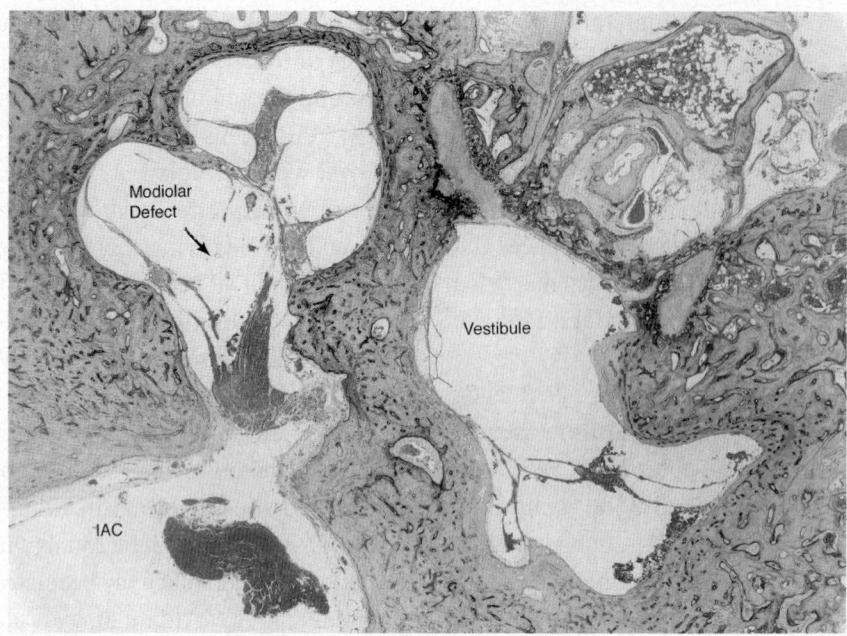

Figure 1–24   The modiolar defect in the cochlea of this 2½-year-old child with a congenital conductive hearing loss results in a wide communication of the subarachnoid space of the internal auditory canal (IAC) with the scala vestibuli of the basal turn. Stapedectomy in such cases results in a "perilymph gusher." Reproduced with permission from Shi S-R. Temporal bone findings in a case of otopalatodigital syndrome. Arch Otolaryngol 1985;111:120. Copyright 1985, American Medical Association.

Attaching such clinical implications to microfissures remains a matter of conjecture. In an examination of 34 temporal bones, El Shazly and Linthicum were unable to find any relationship between the presence or absence of microfissures to sudden sensorineural hearing loss.[47]

Distinct from and independent of the formation of the otic capsule from a cartilaginous model is the formation of the cochlear modiolus as membranous bone. The deposition of bone within the modiolus, housing the cochlear nerve, first occurs at 20 to 21 weeks in the region between the basal and second turns.[4] By 25 weeks, modiolar ossification is nearly complete.

Osseous extensions of the cochlear otic capsule, known as interscalar septa, serve to anchor the modiolus. The first septa appear in the twenty-second week and within 5 weeks have stabilized the cochlear modiolus from base to apex. Following a similar time frame, the osseous spiral lamina begins ossification in the twenty-third week and completes this process by the twenty-fifth.

Aberrations in the finer developmental steps of the cochlea may appear as structural anomalies that occasionally attain surgical importance. Partial absence of the interscalar septum (scala communis) is a relatively common developmental anomaly that does not interfere

with normal cochlear function (Figure 1–23). Absence of the modiolus results in a wide communication between the subarachnoid space of the internal auditory canal and the scala vestibuli of the basal turn. This anomaly may represent the anatomic correlate of the "perilymph gusher," the voluminous outflow occasionally encountered in stapes surgery (Figure 1–24).

DEVELOPMENT OF THE ACOUSTIC NERVE AND GANGLION

The acoustic nerve, ganglion, and Schwann sheath cells begin development in the fourth week as cells of otic placode derivation begin to stream ventrally between the epithelium of the otocyst and its basement membrane. After penetrating the basement membrane, these cells reach the area at which the acoustic ganglion forms,[3,48] ventral and slightly medial to the otocyst.[49]

Over the remainder of the fourth and fifth weeks, the acoustic ganglion divides into superior and inferior segments.[23] The superior segment gives rise to the fibers that innervate the crista of the superior and lateral semicircular ducts as well as the utricular macula. Slightly later, the inferior segment divides into upper and lower portions. The upper portion supplies fibers to the saccular macula and to the crista of the posterior semicircular duct, whereas the lower portion innervates the organ of Corti.

By the end of 8 weeks, the acoustic nerve approaches full maturity. The ganglia of the vestibular division are spread along the nerve trunks, and its terminal branches, derived from the bipolar ganglion cells, develop as fairly long, discretely individual nerve fibers. The cochlear ganglion, in contrast, ends up at the distal terminus of the nerve trunk, and its terminal branches are short, anastomosing fibers.[23] Similarly, central connections (to the brainstem) are established, initially by the vestibular nerve and then later by the cochlear nerve fibers.[49] As soon as central connections (to the brainstem) are estab-

lished, migration of glial cells from the brain tube begins to envelop the proximal portion of the acoustic nerve fibers, but it is only later in development that Schwann cells begin to migrate centrally. Thus, the central glial sheath extends for a considerable distance laterally along the acoustic nerve before Schwann cells migrate medially. Moreover, the distance covered by glial cells is greater on the vestibular nerve than on the cochlear nerve because of the earlier initiation of migration, the former when compared with the latter.[49] The junction of the Schwann cell and glial sheaths occurs variably about the region of the fundus of the internal auditory canal.

It is thought that the sensory neuroepithelium develops in those areas of the membranous labyrinth at which neural contact is established.[3] Such contact may not be

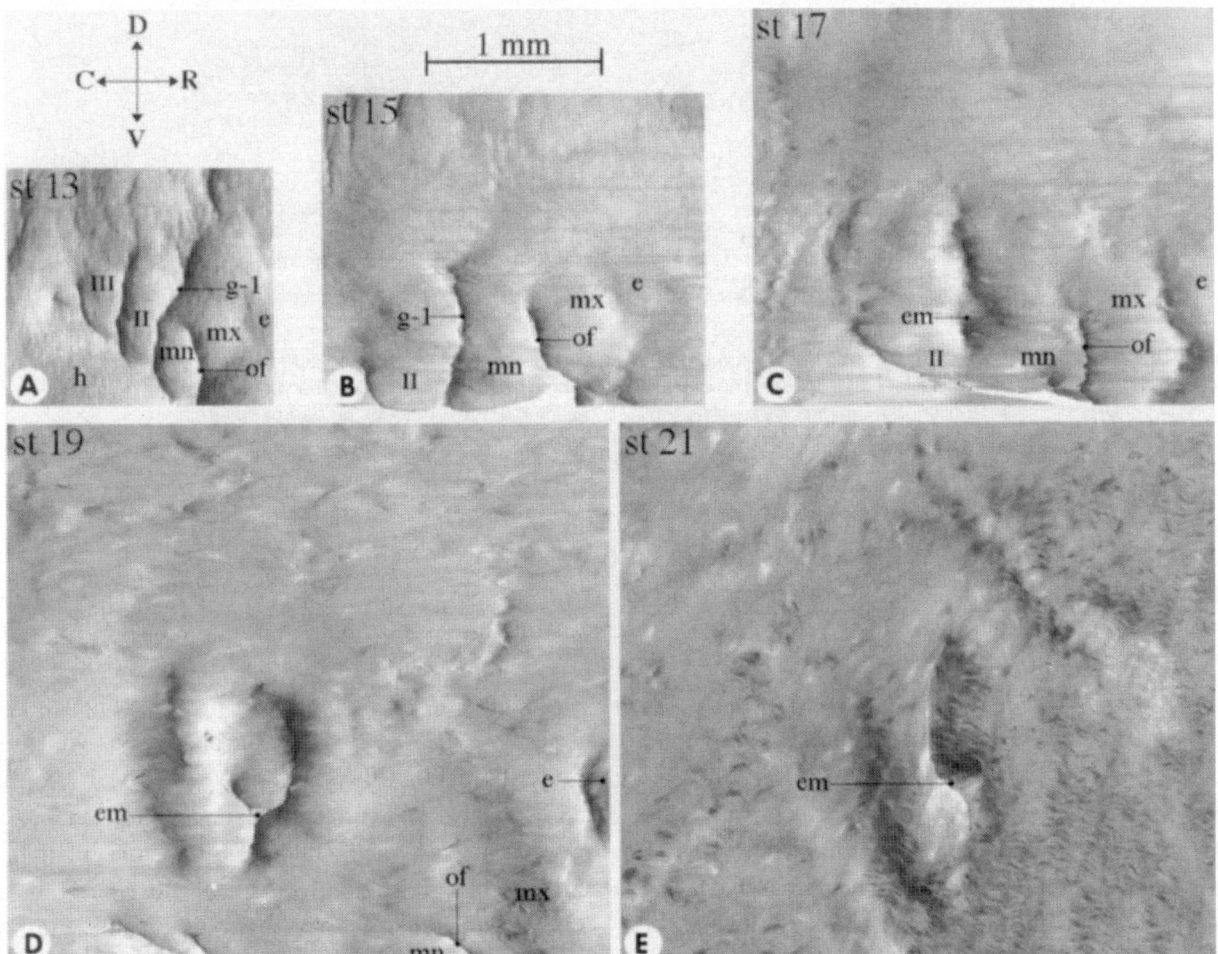

Figure 1–25 Computer reconstructions of the ectoderm of the right external ear region at approximate ages 28 days (*A*), 33 days (*B*), 41 days (*C*), 48 days (*D*), and 52 days (*E*). Dorsal is superior, ventral is inferior, rostral is to the right, and caudal is to the left. This view, companion to Figure 1–26, reveals the structures anatomically related to the lateral aspect of the developing facial nerve. II = second arch; III = third arch; e = eye; em = external auditory meatus; g-1 = first groove; h = heart; mn = mandibular part of first arch; mx = maxillary part of first arch; of = oral fissure. Reproduced with permission from Gasser RF, Shigihara S, Shimada K. Three-dimensional development of the facial nerve path through the ear region in human embryos. Ann Otol Rhinol Laryngol 1994;103:395–403.

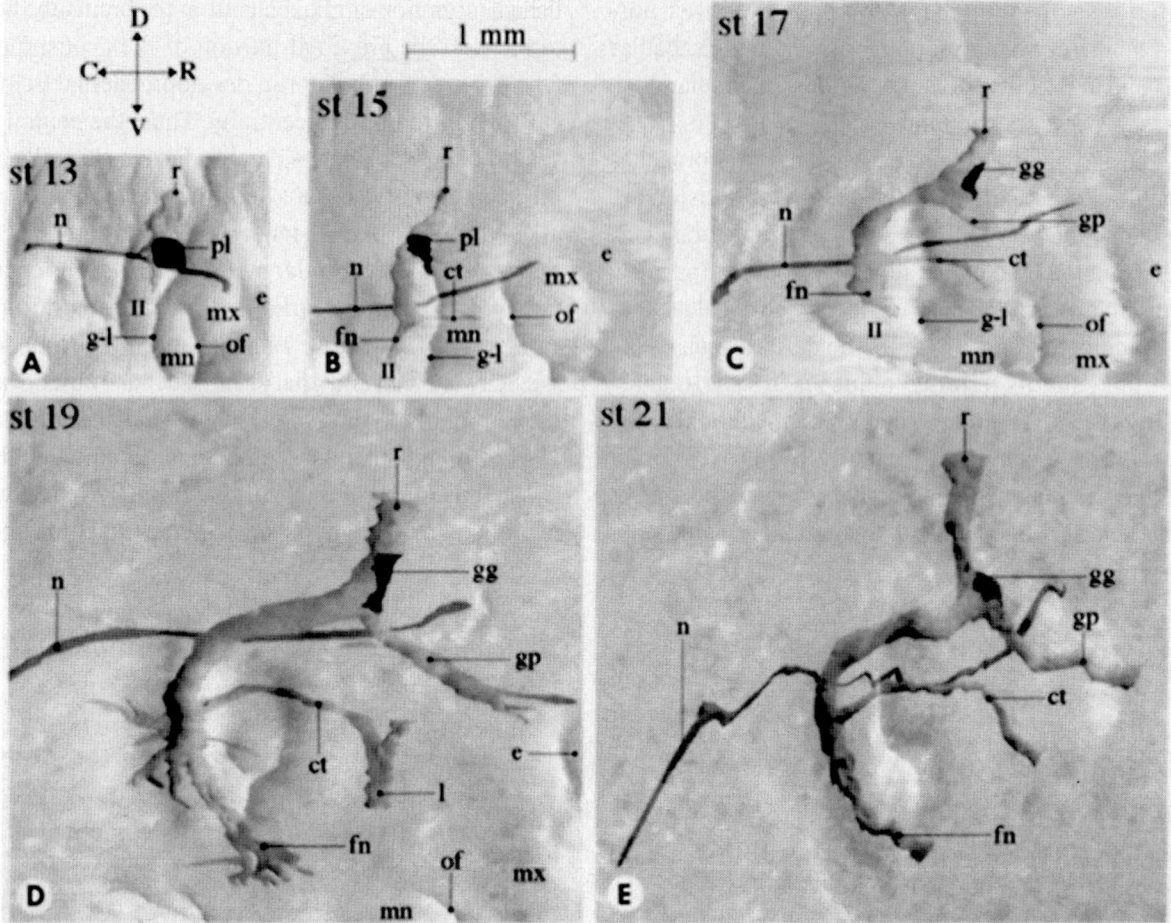

Figure 1–26   Same specimens as Figure 1–25 but with computer reconstruction making the surface ectoderm relatively transparent, allowing visualization of the developing facial nerve. II = second arch; III = third arch; ct = chorda tympani nerve; e = eye; fn = facial nerve; g-1 = first groove; gg = geniculate ganglion; gp = greater petrosal nerve; l = lingual nerve; mn = mandibular part of first arch; mx = maxillary part of first arch; of = oral fissure; pl = placode; n = notocord; r = facial nerve root. Reproduced with permission from Gasser RF, Shigihara S, Shimada K. Three-dimensional development of the facial nerve path through the ear region in human embryos. Ann Otol Rhinol Laryngol 1994;103:395–403.

required for neuroepithelial differentiation but may play a role in maintaining such specialization.[50,51]

DEVELOPMENT OF THE FACIAL NERVE AND GENICULATE GANGLION

At about 4 weeks, the facial nerve and its geniculate ganglion begin to develop from primordial tissue, arising from the rhombencephalon, which impinges on the deep aspect of the second branchial arch epibranchial placode,[52] a thickened area of surface ectoderm just caudal to the first branchial groove (Figures 1–25, A and B, and 1–26, A and B).

The later stages of facial nerve and geniculate ganglion development have been described by Gasser and

colleagues.[52–54] Neuroblast differentiation in the region at which the primordial facial nerve tissue is in contiguity with the epibranchial placode results in a distinguishable geniculate ganglion by 6 weeks (Figures 1–25, C, and 1–26, C). Meanwhile, the chorda tympani nerve, the first branch of the facial nerve to appear, is clearly evident. At approximately the same time, the facial motor nucleus appears in the future metencephalon; its intramedullary fibers are displaced by the abducens nucleus as the metencephalon grows, creating the internal genu of the facial nerve.

The chorda tympani nerve, at 6 weeks approximating the size of the facial nerve, dives into the mandibular arch to terminate in the same region as the lingual nerve ends and the submandibular ganglion develops.

The chorda tympani and lingual nerves clearly unite just proximal to the ganglion by the seventh week (Figures 1–25, D, and 1–26, D). Also at approximately 6 weeks, the greater petrosal nerve, the second branch of the facial nerve to form, develops from the ventral aspect of the geniculate ganglion. The nervus intermedius (nerve of Wrisberg, the sensory fibers of the facial nerve) develops independently from the geniculate ganglion and extends to the brainstem bordered by the motor root of the facial nerve and the eighth cranial nerve. The main trunk of the facial nerve establishes its definitive intratemporal relationships within the cartilaginous otic capsule.

In sequence, the posterior auricular nerve and the fibers to the posterior belly of the digastric muscle appear. Branches of the posterior auricular nerve communicate with nerves of the second and third cervical ganglia, resulting in the formation of the transverse cervical and lesser occipital nerves.

At 7 weeks, a ventral offshoot from the geniculate ganglion reaches the glossopharyngeal ganglion. In the next week, the tympanic plexus and the lesser petrosal nerve form along this offshoot. At approximately the same time, the branch to the stapedius muscle has developed. The facial nerve grows and develops peripheral (muscular) branches, which appear in close conjunction with and just deep to the primitive facial muscle masses. These peripheral branches establish communications with the branches of the trigeminal nerve. Similarly, anastomotic linkages with other peripheral facial nerve fibers appear. With the growth of the facial nerve, the chorda tympani nerve diminishes in relative size (Figures 1–25, E, and 1–26, E).

Between the twelfth and thirteenth weeks, two twigs from the dorsomedial surface of the facial nerve (between the stapedius and the chorda tympani nerves) fuse and extend to the superior ganglia of the vagus and glossopharyngeal nerves. The nerve fiber emerging from this intermingling is Arnold's nerve (the auricular branch of the vagus), which traverses the primitive tympanomastoid fissure to innervate the subcutaneous tissue of the posterior aspect of the external auditory canal.

By 17 weeks, the definitive communications of the facial nerve, including those with the second and third cervical nerves, the three divisions of the trigeminal nerve, and the vagus and the glossopharyngeal nerves, are established.

The facial canal, originally a sulcus in the cartilaginous otic capsule, becomes a bony canal as it ossifies. Spector and Ge detailed the ossification of the tympanic segment of the fallopian canal, a process that involves two ossification centers: an anterior one developing at the apical cochlear ossification center at the end of 20 weeks gestation and a posterior one arising at the pyramidal eminence at 25 weeks gestation.[55] Each ossification center emits two bony projections that (ideally) encircle the facial nerve in its entirety. Each ossification center also extends from its point of origin, the anterior one posteriorly and the posterior one inferiorly, to envelop progressively more of the length of the facial nerve. By term, about 80% of the tympanic segment of the fallopian canal is present and is completely developed by roughly 3 months after birth. According to Spector and Ge, most of the surgically encountered dehiscences of the tympanic segment of the fallopian canal can be related to varying degrees of failure of fusion of the two ossification centers and to failure of fusion of their bony projections.[55] Additionally, they report that the pattern of ossification of the tympanic segment is symmetric in 80% of the paired bones studied.

The mastoid process and tympanic ring grow postnatally, medially displacing and thus protecting the facial nerve.

DEVELOPMENT OF THE ARTERIES

The fetal circulatory system first appears in the third week of development as mesenchymal vascular islands coalesce.[56] The primordial vascular supply to the brain derives from presegmental branches of the paired ("dorsal") aortae. A total of six aortic arches arise successively from the dilated region of the truncus arteriosus known as the aortic sac and course ventrally through their corresponding branchial arches into the ipsilateral dorsal aorta.[56] The primitive internal carotid artery is a branch of the first aortic arch. During this branchial phase of arterial development, there is a correspondence between each branchial arch and its aortic arch. However, not all of the aortic arch arteries exist at the same time. The first and second arch arteries disappear before the more caudal arch arteries develop. The following details of cranial arterial development are based on the comprehensive study of Padget.[57]

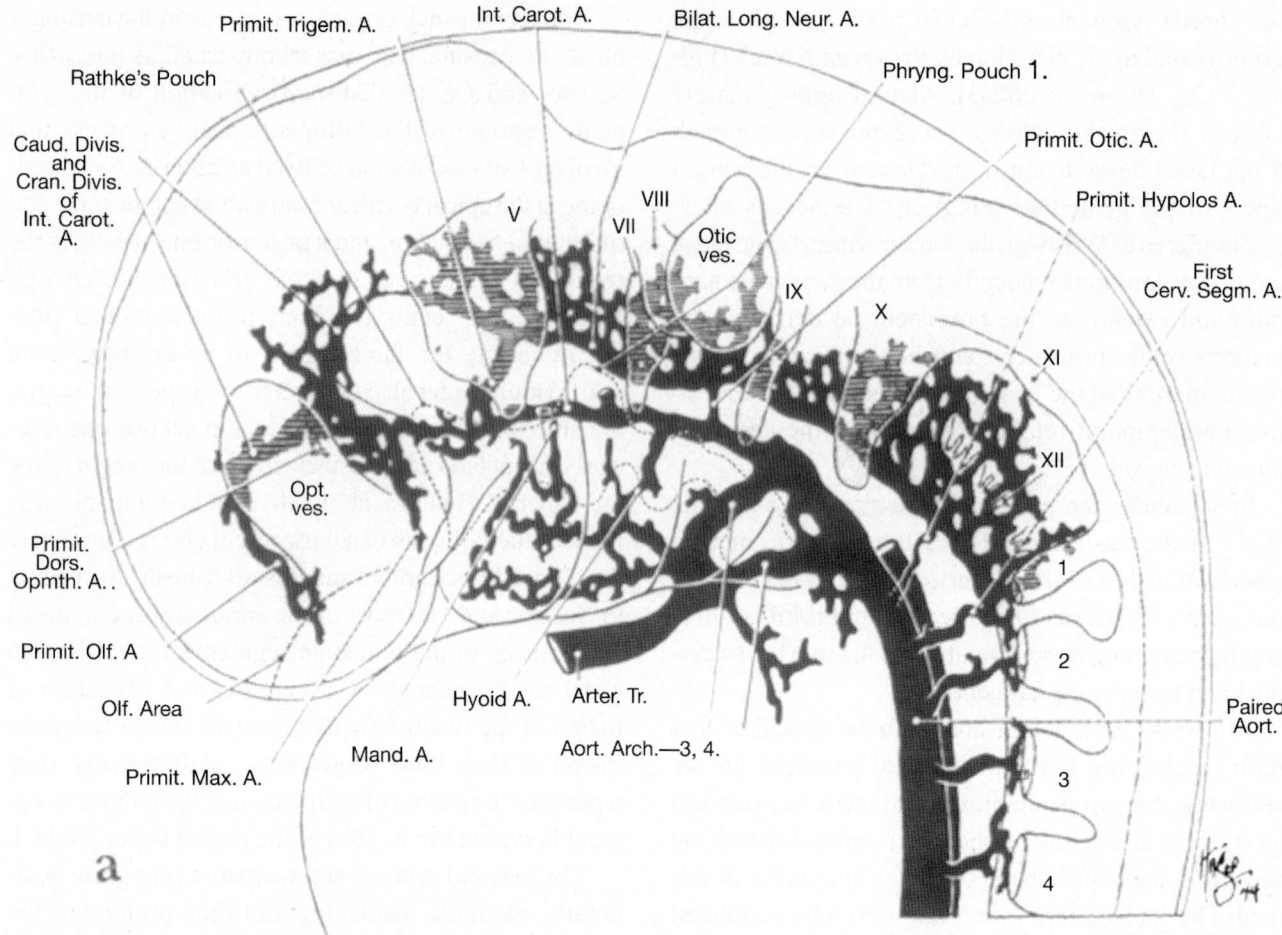

Figure 1–27   Graphic reconstruction of the cranial arteries in a 4-week embryo. The mandibular and hyoid arteries are remnants of the first two aortic arches; the internal carotid artery originates from the third arch, and the bilateral neural arteries are starting to emerge. Reproduced with permission from Padget DH. The development of the cranial arteries in the human embryo. Contrib Embryol 1948;32:205.

In the fourth week, as the first and second aortic arches begin to involute, they leave behind dorsal fragments, the mandibular and hyoid arteries, respectively, and the portion of the paired dorsal aortae extending anteriorly from the third arch artery becomes the adult internal carotid artery (Figure 1–27). In the hindbrain region, the bilateral longitudinal neural arteries emerge, supplied at the level of the otocyst and acoustic nerve by the primitive otic artery, a remnant of a presegmental branch of the paired aortae (see Figure 1–27).

In the 4- to 5-week stage, the ventral pharyngeal artery, which parallels the internal carotid artery, arises in the area formerly occupied by the ventral aspects of the first and second arch arteries. This artery supplies the bulk of the first two pharyngeal bars and subsequently is involved in the formation of the stapedial and external carotid arteries. At the same time, the bilateral longitudinal neural arteries fuse to form the basilar artery.

At 6 weeks, as the transition from branchial phase to postbranchial phase takes place, the stapedial artery appears as a small offshoot of the hyoid artery and passes through the stapes blastema to enter the mandibular bar; here the stapedial artery anastomoses with the distal remnant of the shrinking ventral pharyngeal artery. The maxillomandibular division of the stapedial artery is the result of this anastomosis, and it divides into maxillary and mandibular branches. The proximal remnant of the ventral pharyngeal artery evolves into the root of the external carotid artery, whereas the common carotid artery develops from the ventral union of the third and fourth arch arteries.

The development of the labyrinthine and anterior inferior cerebellar arteries during the fourth through sixth weeks passes through a ring configuration, with the abducens nerve in the center. Whether the labyrinthine artery arises from the anterior inferior cerebellar artery

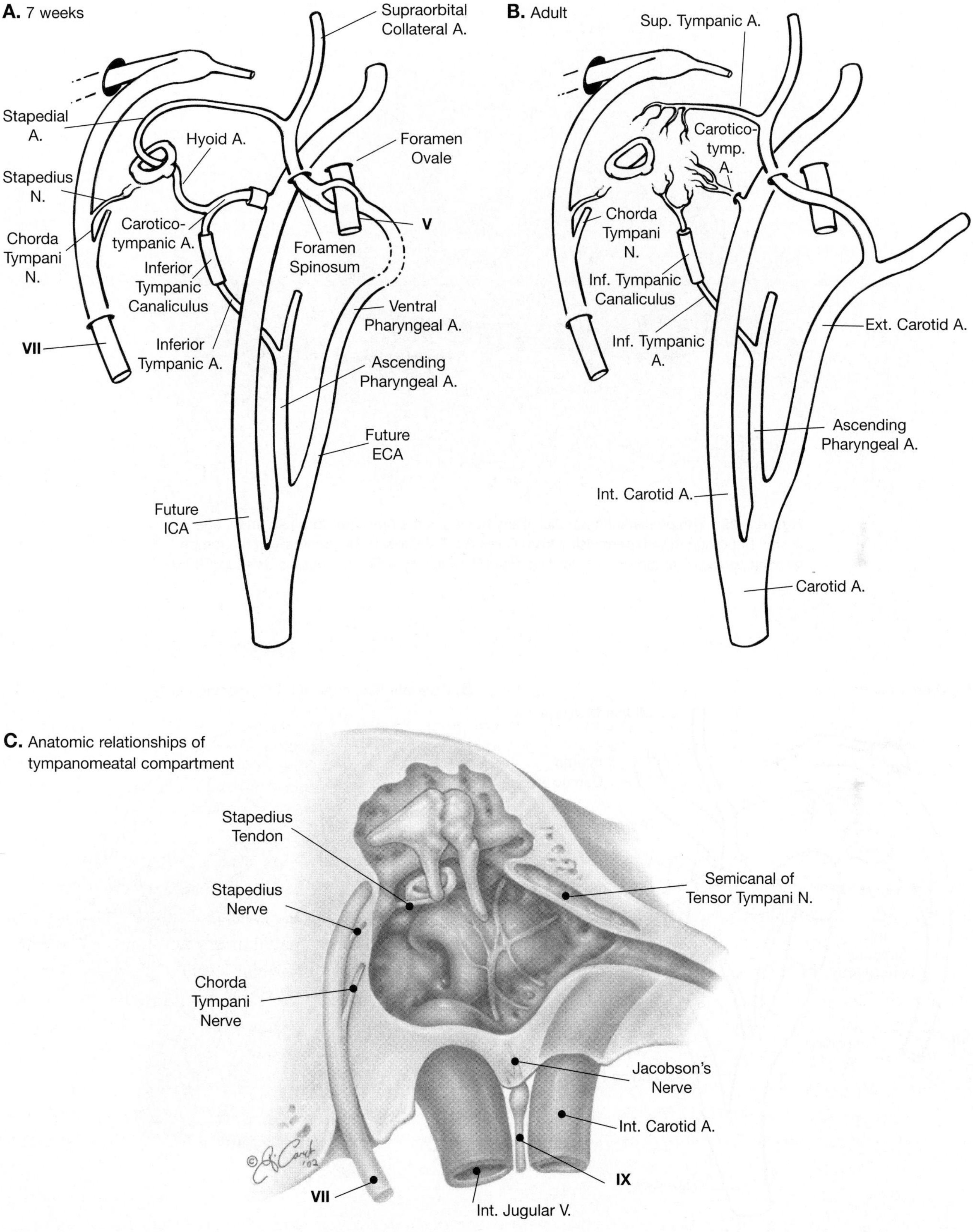

A. 7 weeks

Supraorbital
Collateral A.

Stapedial
A.

Hyoid A.

Foramen
Ovale

Stapedius
N.

Carotico-
tympanic A.

V

Chorda
Tympani
N.

Foramen
Spinosum

Inferior
Tympanic
Canaliculus

VII

Inferior
Tympanic A.

Ventral
Pharyngeal A.

Ascending
Pharyngeal A.

Future
ECA

Future
ICA

B. Adult

Sup. Tympanic A.

Carotico-
tymp.
A.

Chorda
Tympani
N.

Inf. Tympanic
Canaliculus

Inf. Tympanic
A.

Ext. Carotid A.

Ascending
Pharyngeal A.

Int. Carotid A.

Carotid A.

C. Anatomic relationships of
tympanomeatal compartment

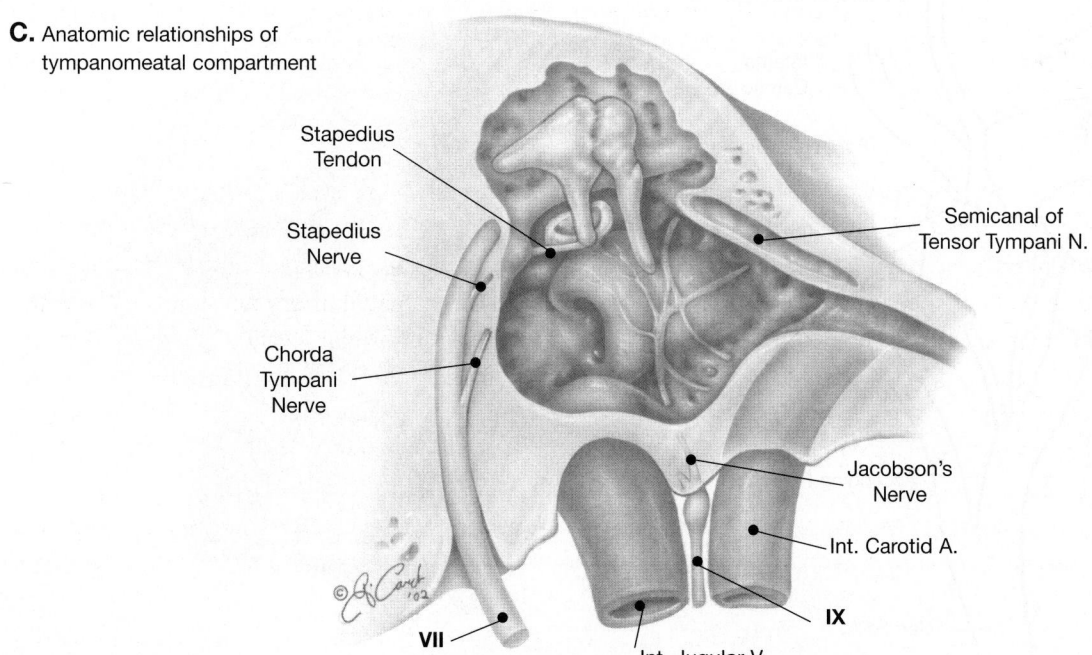

Stapedius
Tendon

Stapedius
Nerve

Chorda
Tympani
Nerve

Semicanal of
Tensor Tympani N.

Jacobson's
Nerve

Int. Carotid A.

IX

VII

Int. Jugular V.

Figure 1–28 Development of the cranial arteries. *A*, Approximately 7 weeks. *B*, Adult configuration. *C*, The internal carotid artery, internal jugular vein, and their interrelationships with the tympanomastoid compartment. After Moret and colleagues. Abnormal vessels in the middle ear. J Neuroradiol 1982;9:227.

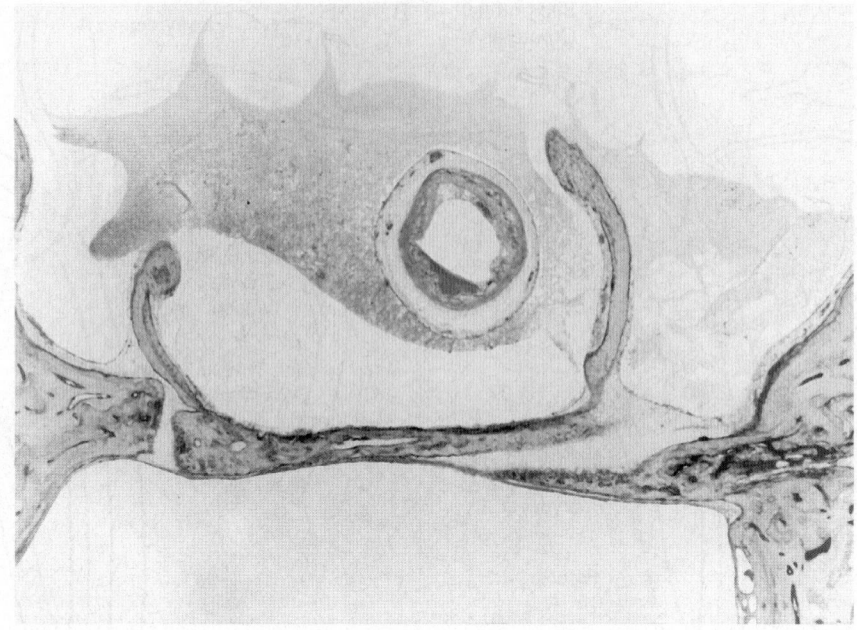

Figure 1–29 The persistent stapedial artery traverses the obturator foramen (man, age 84 years). Reproduced with permission from Gulya AJ, Schuknecht HF. Anatomy of the temporal bone with surgical implications. 2nd ed. Pearl River (NY): Parthenon Publishing Group; 1995.

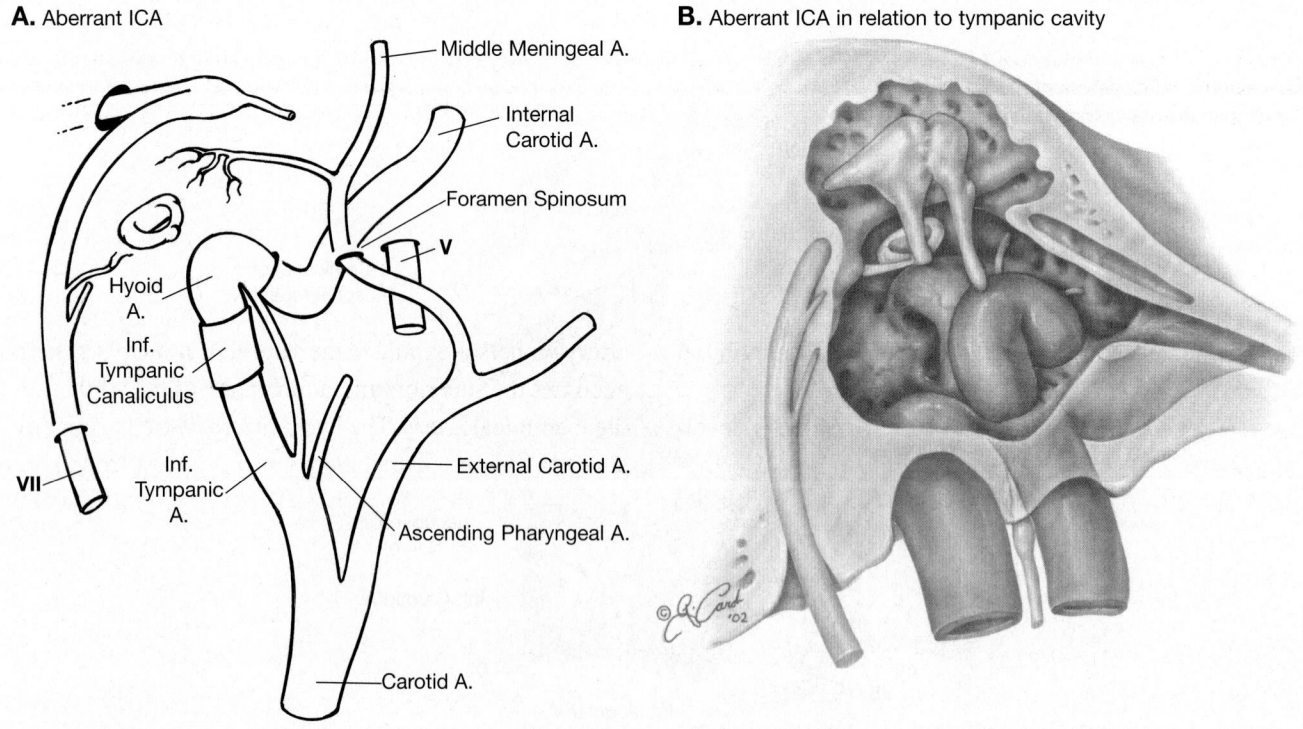

Figure 1–30 *A*, The aberrant internal carotid artery, feeding into the horizontal portion of the intrapetrous internal carotid artery, is seen in association with the inferior tympanic artery and a persisting hyoid artery. *B*, The aberrant internal carotid artery is seen protruding into the tympanic cavity. After Moret and colleagues. Abnormal vessels in the middle ear. J Neuroradiol 1982;9:227.

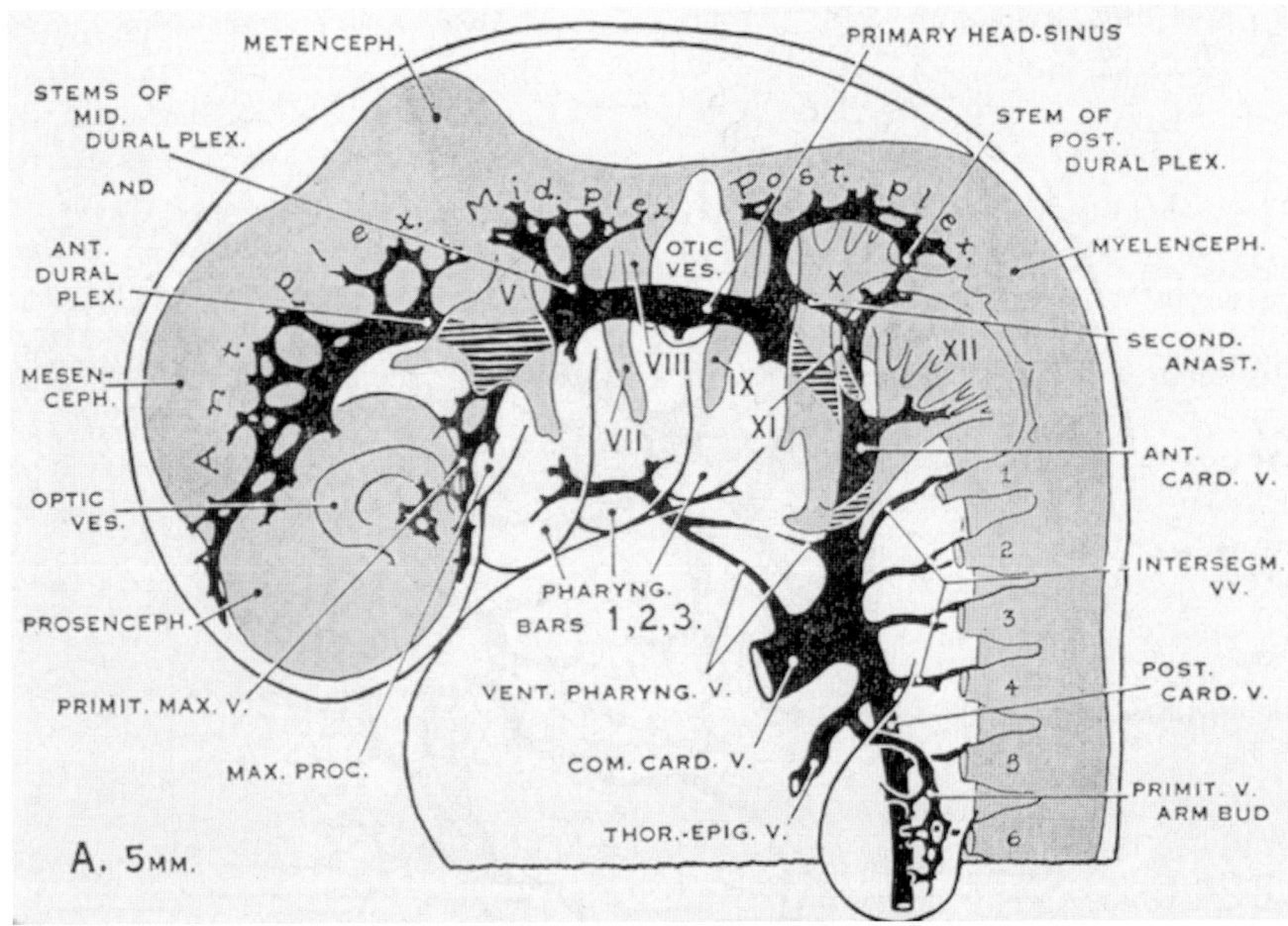

Figure 1–31 The cranial venous system at approximately 4 weeks. Venous blood of the brain drains to the primary head sinus through three stems. The primary head sinus is in continuity with the anterior cardinal vein. Reproduced with permission from Padget DH. Development of the cranial venous system in man, from the viewpoint of comparative anatomy. Contrib Embryol 1957;36:79.

or from the basilar artery is determined by the point at which the vascular ring atrophies.

The stapedial artery reaches the height of its development at 7 weeks (Figure 1–28, A) and has two divisions, the maxillomandibular and the supraorbital; the latter division supplies the primitive orbit. Branches of the external carotid artery that can be identified now are the thyroid, lingual, occipital, and external maxillary arteries. Over the next week, the two major divisions of the stapedial artery are annexed by the internal maxillary artery of the external carotid artery and the ophthalmic artery, respectively. The trunk of the maxillomandibular division becomes the stem of the middle meningeal artery (Figure 1–28, B). As the stapedial

artery withers proximal to the stapes, its more distal stem becomes the superior tympanic branch of the adult middle meningeal artery. The hyoid artery, which originally gave rise to the stapedial artery, dwindles to a mere twig and is partially retained as a caroticotympanic branch of the adult internal carotid artery (Figure 1–28, C). Remnants of the stapedial artery also are thought to play a role in the development of the caroticotympanic arteries, anterior tympanic artery, and superior petrosal artery (Tandler, as cited in Gulya and Schuknecht[1] and Altmann[58]).

The subarcuate artery, traversing the subarcuate fossa, develops as a branch of either the labyrinthine or anterior inferior cerebellar artery by the end of the eighth

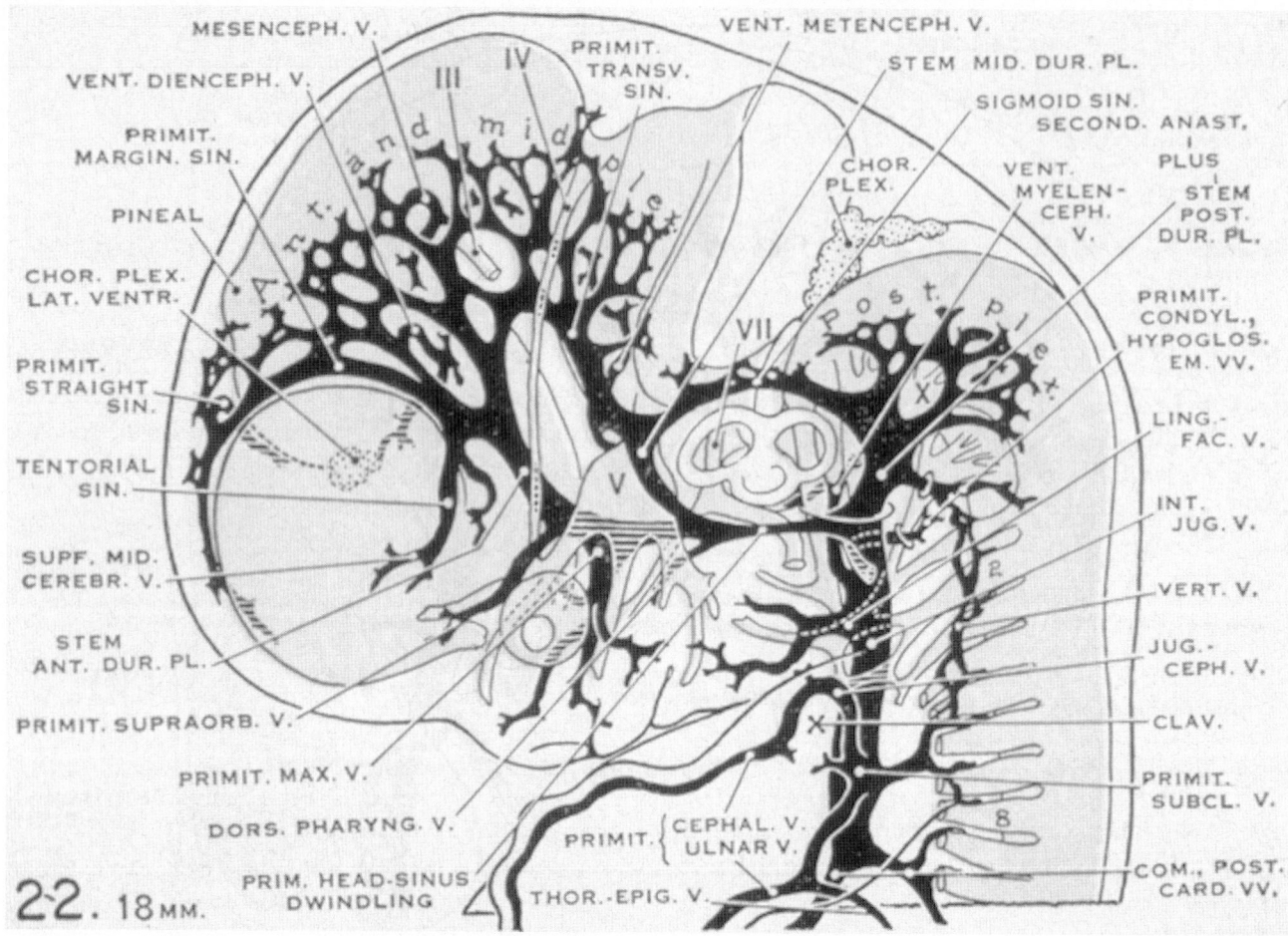

Figure 1–32 The venous system at approximately 8 weeks shows the development of the sigmoid sinus from the anastomotic linkage of the middle and posterior dural plexuses. Reproduced with permission from Padget DH. Development of the cranial venous system in man, from the viewpoint of comparative anatomy. Contrib Embryol 1957;36:79–140.

week and supplies part of the otic capsule and mastoid. The adult pattern of origin of all of the cranial arteries is visible by the ninth week.

The stapedial artery, usually a transient structure, may abnormally persist into adulthood, interfering with stapes operations especially (Figure 1–29). After passing through the stapes, the stapedial artery branches; bifurcation of the stapedial artery proximal to the stapes, with both branches penetrating the stapes blastema, may give rise to a three-legged stapes.[59] The stapedial artery, either directly or indirectly through a branch, may fix the developing internal carotid artery so as to pull it into the middle ear (Figure 1–30, A and B) more posteriorly and laterally than it ordinarily would run.[59] Such aberrant internal carotid arteries occasionally are encountered clinically as pulsatile middle ear masses.

DEVELOPMENT OF THE VEINS

The following account of the development of the venous circulation of the human is largely based on the exhaustive reviews of Padget.[60,61] In general, the venous system lags behind the arterial system in approaching adult configuration; in fact, adult configuration of the cranial venous system is not usually present at birth.[61]

In the developing human of 3 to 4 weeks, most of the neural tube is covered by a primitive capillary plexus, which drains dorsolaterally into a more superficial plexus. Through anterior, middle, and posterior venous stems, the superficial plexus drains into the primary head sinus (also known as the lateral capital vein), a channel that is medial to cranial nerves V and X and lateral to cranial nerves VII, VIII, and IX and the otocyst. The primary head sinus is the first true drainage channel of the craniocervical region and is present by 4 weeks (Figure 1–31). The primary head sinus is continuous with the anterior cardinal vein (the primitive internal jugular vein), which lies medial to cranial nerves X, XI, and XII. The anterior cardinal vein joins the posterior cardinal vein to form the common cardinal vein (duct of Cuvier), draining into the sinus venosus of the embryonic heart.

In the fifth and sixth weeks of development, the primary head sinus encircles and then completes its migration to lie lateral to the vagus nerve. The medial aspect of the ring around the vagus nerve forms the ventral myelencephalic vein. As the primary head sinus moves laterally, the posterior stem moves caudally, becoming continuous with the primitive internal jugular vein and thus constituting the caudal end of the definitive sigmoid sinus. The anterior cardinal (internal jugular) vein also moves to lie lateral to cranial nerves X, XI, and XII.

The jugular foramen, demarcating the internal jugular vein inferiorly and the sigmoid sinus superiorly, is completed by the seventh week. At the same time, a plexiform channel develops, parallel and dorsal to the primary head sinus. This channel links the anterior, middle, and posterior stems and lies dorsal to the trigeminal nerve and the otocyst. Also during the seventh week, the primary head sinus begins to involute, being replaced by the dorsal channel, and the direction of flow reverses in the middle stem as it becomes the pro-otic sinus (Figure 1–32). The definitive sigmoid sinus is composed of the channel connecting the middle and posterior stems and the ventral remainder of the posterior stem. The transverse sinus develops from the anastomotic channel between the anterior and middle stems.

In embryos of approximately 8 weeks, the primary head sinus has essentially disappeared except for three remnants. The cranial remnant medial to the trigeminal nerve (part of the pro-otic sinus) becomes the lateral wing of the cavernous sinus. A caudal remnant contributes to the formation of the veins accompanying the superficial petrosal and stylomastoid arteries and draining the middle ear region, whereas yet another remnant of the primary head sinus accompanies the facial nerve extracranially, ventral to the otic capsule. Also at this stage, for the first time, the tendency of the venous drainage to pass more to the right than to the left is apparent and is accompanied by greater developmental maturity of the venous system of the right side when compared with that of the left side.

In the ninth and tenth weeks, the ventral myelencephalic vein receives the hypoglossal emissary and inferior cochlear veins. The inferior petrosal sinus is thus established.

By 12 weeks, cerebral expansion pushes the transverse sinus into its adult position. A medial tributary of the pro-otic sinus, the ventral metencephalic vein, becomes recognizable as the superior petrosal sinus.

After birth, anastomoses develop that add cavernous and inferior petrosal sinus drainage routes to the drainage of the cerebral and cerebellar veins into the junction of the transverse and sigmoid sinuses.[61]

REFERENCES

1. Gulya AJ, Schuknecht HF. Anatomy of the temporal bone with surgical implications. 2nd ed. Pearl River (NY): Parthenon Publishing Group, Inc.; 1995.

2. Anson BJ, Donaldson JA. Surgical anatomy of the temporal bone. 3rd ed. Philadelphia: WB Saunders; 1981.

3. Pearson AA. Developmental anatomy of the ear. In: English GM, editor. Otolaryngology. Philadelphia: Harper & Row Publishers; 1984. p. 1–68.

4. Bast TH, Anson BJ. The temporal bone and the ear. Springfield (IL): Charles C. Thomas; 1949.

5. Wood-Jones F, Wen I-C. The development of the external ear. J Anat 1934;68:525–33.

6. Levine H. Cutaneous carcinoma of the head and neck: management of massive and previously uncontrolled lesions. Laryngoscope 1983;93:87–105.

7. Anson BJ, Bast TH, Richany SF. The fetal and early postnatal development of the tympanic ring and related structures in man. Ann Otol Rhinol Laryngol 1955;64:802–23.

8. Aimi K. Role of the tympanic ring in the pathogenesis of congenital cholesteatoma. Laryngoscope 1983;93:1140–6.

9. Spector GJ, Ge X-X. Development of the hypotympanum in the human fetus and neonate. Ann Otol Rhinol Laryngol 1981; 90 Suppl 88:2–20.

10. Anson BJ, Bast TH. Developmental anatomy of the ear. In: Shambaugh GE Jr, Glasscock ME III, editors. Surgery of the ear. 3rd ed. Philadelphia: WB Saunders; 1980. p. 5–29.

11. Eby TL, Nadol JB Jr. Postnatal growth of the human temporal bone: implications for cochlear implants in children. Ann Otol Rhinol Laryngol 1986;95:356–64.

12. Eby TL. Development of the facial recess: implications for cochlear implantation. Laryngoscope 1996;106 Suppl 80:1–7.

13. van Bergeijk WA. Evolution of the sense of hearing in vertebrates. Am Zoologist 1966;6:371–7.

14. Proctor B. Embryology and anatomy of the eustachian tube. Arch Otolaryngol 1967;86:503–14.

15. Allam AF. Pneumatization of the temporal bone. Ann Otol Rhinol Laryngol 1969;78:49–64.

16. Takahara T, Sando I, Hashida Y, et al. Mesenchyme remaining in human temporal bones. Otolaryngol Head Neck Surg 1986;95:349–57.

17. Davies DG. Malleus fixation. J Laryngol Otol 1968;82:331–51.

18. Pye A, Hinchcliffe R. Comparative anatomy of the ear. In: Hinchcliffe R, Harrison D, editors. Scientific foundations of otolaryngology. London: William Heinemann Medical Books; 1976.

19. Marovitz WF, Porubsky ES. The embryological development of the middle ear: a new concept. Ann Otol Rhinol Laryngol 1971;80:384–9.

20. Van de Water TR, Maderson PFA, Jaskoll TF. The morphogenesis of the middle and external ear. Birth Defects 1980;16:147–80.

21. Hanson JR, Anson BJ, Strickland EM. Branchial sources of the auditory ossicles in man. Part II: Observations of embryonic stages from 7 mm to 28 mm (CR length). Arch Otolaryngol 1962;76:200–15.

22. Guggenheim L. Phylogenesis of the ear. Culver City (CA): Murray and Gee; 1948.

23. Streeter GL. On the development of the membranous labyrinth and the acoustic and facial nerves in the human embryo. Am J Anat 1906;6:139–65.

24. Schuknecht HF, Belal AA. The utriculoendolymphatic valve: its functional significance. J Laryngol Otol 1975;89:985–96.

25. Jackler RK, Luxford WM. Congenital malformations of the inner ear. Laryngoscope 1987;97 Suppl 40:2–14.

26. Lundquist P-G. The endolymphatic duct and sac in the guinea pig: an electron microscopic and experimental investigation. Acta Otolaryngol Suppl (Stockh) 1965;201:1–108.

27. Rask-Andersen H, Bredberg G, Stahle J. Structure and function of the endolymphatic duct. In: Vosteen K-H, Schuknecht HF, Pfaltz C, et al, editors. Meniere's disease. New York: Thieme-Stratton; 1981.

28. Smith RJH. Medical diagnosis and treatment of hearing loss in children. In: Cummings CW, Fredrickson JM, Harker LA, et al, editors. Otolaryngology—head and neck surgery. St. Louis: CV Mosby; 1986.

29. Anson BJ, Cauldwell EW, Bast TH. The fissula ante fenestram of the human otic capsule. I. Developmental and normal adult structure. Ann Otol Rhinol Laryngol 1947;56:957–85.

30. Schoetz W. Gibt es eine kongenitale ortliche Disposition zur Bildung otosklerotischer Knochenherde? Arch Ohren-Nasen-u Kehlkopfh 1914;95:239–48.

31. Manasse P. Neue Untersuchungen zur Otosklerosenfrage. Ztchr Ohren 1922;82:76–95.

32. Guggengeim LK. Otosclerosis. St. Louis: Author; 1935.

33. Guild SR. Histologic otosclerosis. Ann Otol Rhinol Laryngol 1944;53:246–66.

34. Cawthorne T. Otosclerosis. J Laryngol Otol 1955;69:437–56.

35. Schuknecht HF, Barber W. Histologic variants in otosclerosis. Laryngoscope 1985;95:1307–17.

36. Bast TH. Development of the otic capsule. V. Residual cartilages and defective ossification and their relation to otosclerotic foci. Arch Otolaryngol 1940;32:771–82.

37. Anson BJ, Cauldwell EW, Bast TH. The fissula ante fenestram of the human otic capsule. II. Aberrant form and contents. Ann Otol Rhinol Laryngol 1948;57:103–28.

38. Yoo TJ. Etiopathogenesis of otosclerosis: a hypothesis. Ann Otol Rhinol Laryngol 1984;93:28–33.

39. Spector GJ, Lee D, Carr C, et al. Later stages of development of the periotic duct and its adjacent area in the human fetus. Laryngoscope 1980;90 Suppl 20:1–31.

40. Gacek RR, Leipzig B. Congenital cerebrospinal otorrhea. Ann Otol Rhinol Laryngol 1979;88:358–65.

41. Neely JG, Neblett CR, Rose JE. Diagnosis and treatment of spontaneous cerebrospinal fluid otorrhea. Laryngoscope 1982;92:609–12.

42. Gulya AJ, Glasscock ME III, Pensak ML. Neural choristoma of the middle ear. Otolaryngol Head Neck Surg 1987;97:52–6.

43. Schuknecht HF. Pathology of the ear. Cambridge (MA): Harvard University Press; 1974.

44. Okano Y, Myers EN, Dickson DB. Microfissure between the round window niche and posterior canal ampulla. Ann Otol Rhinol Laryngol 1977;86:49–57.

45. Harada T, Sando I, Myers EN. Microfissure in the oval window area. Ann Otol Rhinol Laryngol 1981;90:174–80.

46. Proops DW, Hawke WM, Berger G. Microfractures of the otic capsule: the possible role of masticatory stress. J Laryngol Otol 1986;100:749–58.

47. El Shazly MAR, Linthicum FH Jr. Microfissures of the temporal bone: do they have any clinical significance? Am J Otol 1991;12:169–71.

48. Batten EH. The origin of the acoustic ganglion in sheep. J Embryol Exp Morph 1958;6:597–615.

49. Skinner HA. The origin of acoustic nerve tumors. Br J Surg 1928–1929;16:440–63.

50. Van De Water TR, Ruben RJ. Organogenesis of the ear. In: Hinchcliffe R, Harrison D, editors. Scientific foundations of otolaryngology. London: William Heinemann Medical Books; 1976.

51. Hilding DA. Electron microscopy of the developing hearing organ. Laryngoscope 1969;79:1691–704.

52. Gasser RF, Shigihara S, Shimada K. Three-dimensional development of the facial nerve path through the ear region in human embryos. Ann Otol Rhinol Laryngol 1994;103:395–403.

53. Gasser RF. The development of the facial nerve in man. Ann Otol Rhinol Laryngol 1967;6:37–56.

54. Gasser RF, May M. Embryonic development of the facial nerve. In: May M, editor. The facial nerve. New York: Thieme; 1986. p. 3–19.

55. Spector JG, Ge X. Ossification patterns of the tympanic facial canal in the human fetus and neonate. Laryngoscope 1993;103: 1052–65.

56. Pansky B. Review of medical embryology. New York: Macmillan; 1982.

57. Padget DH. The development of the cranial arteries in the human embryo. Contrib Embryol 1948;32:205–61.

58. Altmann F. Anomalies of the internal carotid artery and its branches. Their embryological and comparative anatomical significance. Report of a new case of persistent stapedial artery in man. Laryngoscope 1947;57:313–39.

59. Steffen TN. Vascular anomalies of the middle ear. Laryngoscope 1968;78:171–97.

60. Padget DH. Development of the cranial venous system in man, from the viewpoint of comparative anatomy. Contrib Embryol 1957;36:79–140.

61. Padget DH. The cranial venous system in man in reference to development, adult configuration, and relation to the arteries. Am J Anat 1956;98:307–55.

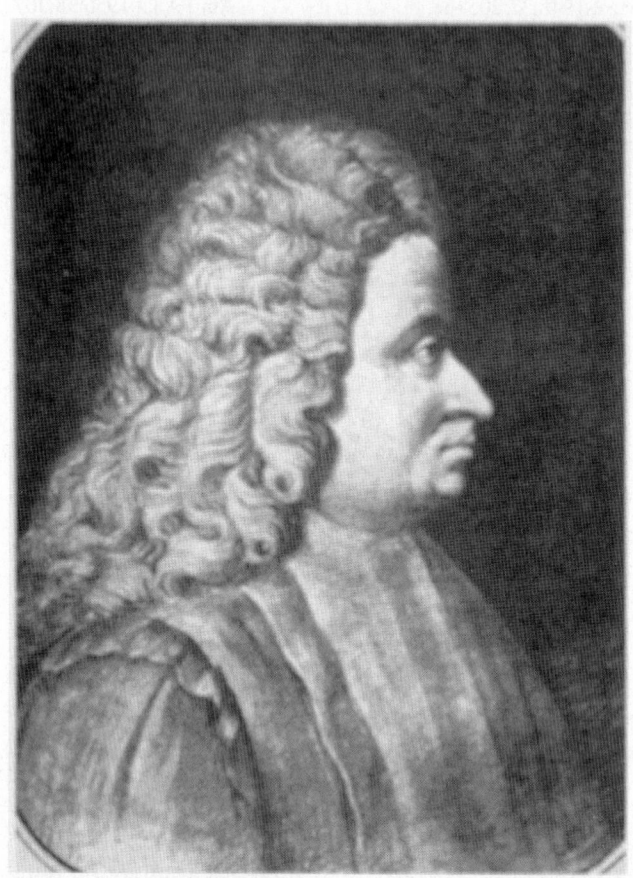

Antonio Maria Valsalva (1666–1723). Described autoinflation of the eustachian tube and middle ear by the patient and in 1707 first observed fluid within the labyrinth.

2

Anatomy of the Ear and Temporal Bone

AINA JULIANNA GULYA, MD

The temporal bone is a fascinating, intricate, and complex structure, and developing a three-dimensional appreciation of the anatomic interrelationships of its components is an intellectually demanding task. To the otologic/neurotologic surgeon, such a three-dimensional grasp is critical to understanding the pathophysiology of, and skillfully diagnosing and managing, otologic disorders. This chapter presents a brief overview of those features of the anatomy of the temporal bone and its environs critical to the otologist; the interested reader is referred to *Anatomy of the Temporal Bone with Surgical Implications*[1] for detail beyond the scope of this chapter. In addition, since there is (as yet) no substitute for supplementing the acquisition of anatomic facts by careful dissection of a wide variety of temporal bone specimens, the reader is strongly encouraged to review the Appendix, "Surgical Anatomy of the Temporal Bone through Dissection," and to practice the described dissections.

PINNA AND EXTERNAL AUDITORY CANAL

Pinna

The pinna acts to focus and aid in the localization of sound. Its shape, showing considerable interindividual variability, reflects its multicomponent embryologic origin. Nonetheless, there are constant features.

The contour of the pinna is determined by the configuration of its elastic cartilage frame. The lateral surface of the pinna is dominated by concavities, in particular the concha (Figure 2–1). The skin of the lateral and medial surfaces of the pinna possesses hair and both seba-

ceous and sudoriferous glands; however, the attachment of the skin differs, being tightly bound down to the perichondrium on the lateral aspect and only loosely attached on the medial.

The pinna is securely attached to the tympanic bone by the continuity of its cartilage with that of the cartilaginous external auditory canal (EAC). Otherwise, the pinna loosely attaches to the skull by its skin, connective tissue, ligaments, and three extrinsic and six intrinsic muscles. A branch of the facial nerve, the posterior auricular nerve, innervates the intrinsic muscles, in general poorly developed in the human.

External Auditory Canal

The lateral one-third of the EAC comprises a continuation of the cartilage of the pinna and is deficient superiorly at the incisura terminalis (see Figure 2–1); the extracartilaginous endaural incision for access to the underlying temporal bone capitalizes on this gap. The two or three variably present perforations in the anterior aspect of the cartilaginous canal are the fissures of Santorini. The remaining medial two-thirds of the approximately 2.5-cm length of the canal are bony. The isthmus, the narrowest portion of the EAC, lies just medial to the junction of the bony and cartilaginous canals.

The skin of the cartilaginous canal has a substantial subcutaneous layer, replete with hair follicles, sebaceous glands, and cerumen glands. The skin of the osseous canal, in contrast, is very thin and its subcutaneous layer is bereft of the usual adnexal structures. Accordingly, the absence of hair serves to distinguish the bony and cartilaginous canals.

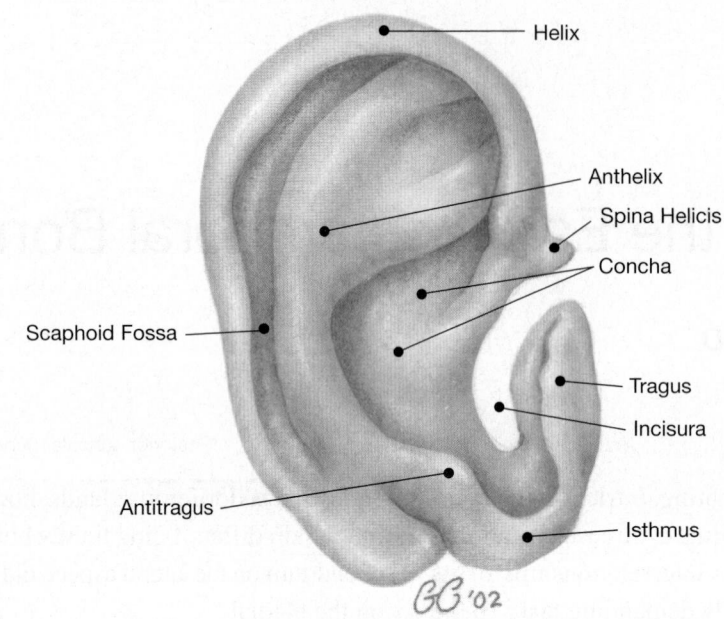

Figure 2–1   Auricular cartilage.

Innervation

The auriculotemporal branch of the trigeminal nerve, greater auricular nerve (a branch of C3), lesser occipital nerve (of C2 and C3 derivation), auricular branch of the vagus nerve (Arnold's nerve), and twigs from the facial nerve all contribute to the sensory innervation of the pinna and EAC (Figures 2–2 and 2–3).

Effective local anesthesia can be obtained by 1 to 2% lidocaine infiltration of the postauricular region accompanied by infiltration of the cartilaginous canal in a four-quadrant (ie, at the 2, 4, 8, and 10 o'clock positions) fashion. Infiltration of the bony canal must be done gently to avoid troublesome bleb formation; if done properly, the anchoring of the skin of the bony EAC "outlines" the tympanomastoid and tympanosquamous sutures, which are the landmarks for the "vascular strip" incisions (see below). Inflammation, as with infection of the middle ear or external ear, reduces the efficacy of local anesthesia.

Vascular Supply

Two branches of the external carotid artery, the posterior auricular artery and the superficial temporal artery, are the sources of arterial blood supply to the pinna and EAC (see Figure 2–2). The posterior auricular artery, as it courses superiorly on the mastoid portion of the temporal bone, supplies the skin of the pinna and the skin and bone of the mastoid; its stylomastoid branch enters the fallopian canal to supply the inferior segment of the facial nerve. Anteriorly, a few twigs of the superficial temporal artery provide additional supply to the pinna and EAC. The veins accompanying the arteries drain into the internal jugular vein by either the facial or external jugular veins.

TEMPORAL BONE, SKULL BASE, AND RELATED STRUCTURES

Temporal Bone and Skull Base

The temporal bone is a composite structure consisting of the tympanic bone, mastoid process, squama (also known as the squamous portion of the temporal bone, and petrosa (also known as the petrous portion of the temporal bone). Although the styloid process is closely related to the temporal bone, it is not considered a portion of it.

The tympanic, squamous, and mastoid portions of the temporal bone are evident on a lateral view (Figure 2–4). The tympanic bone forms the anterior, inferior, and

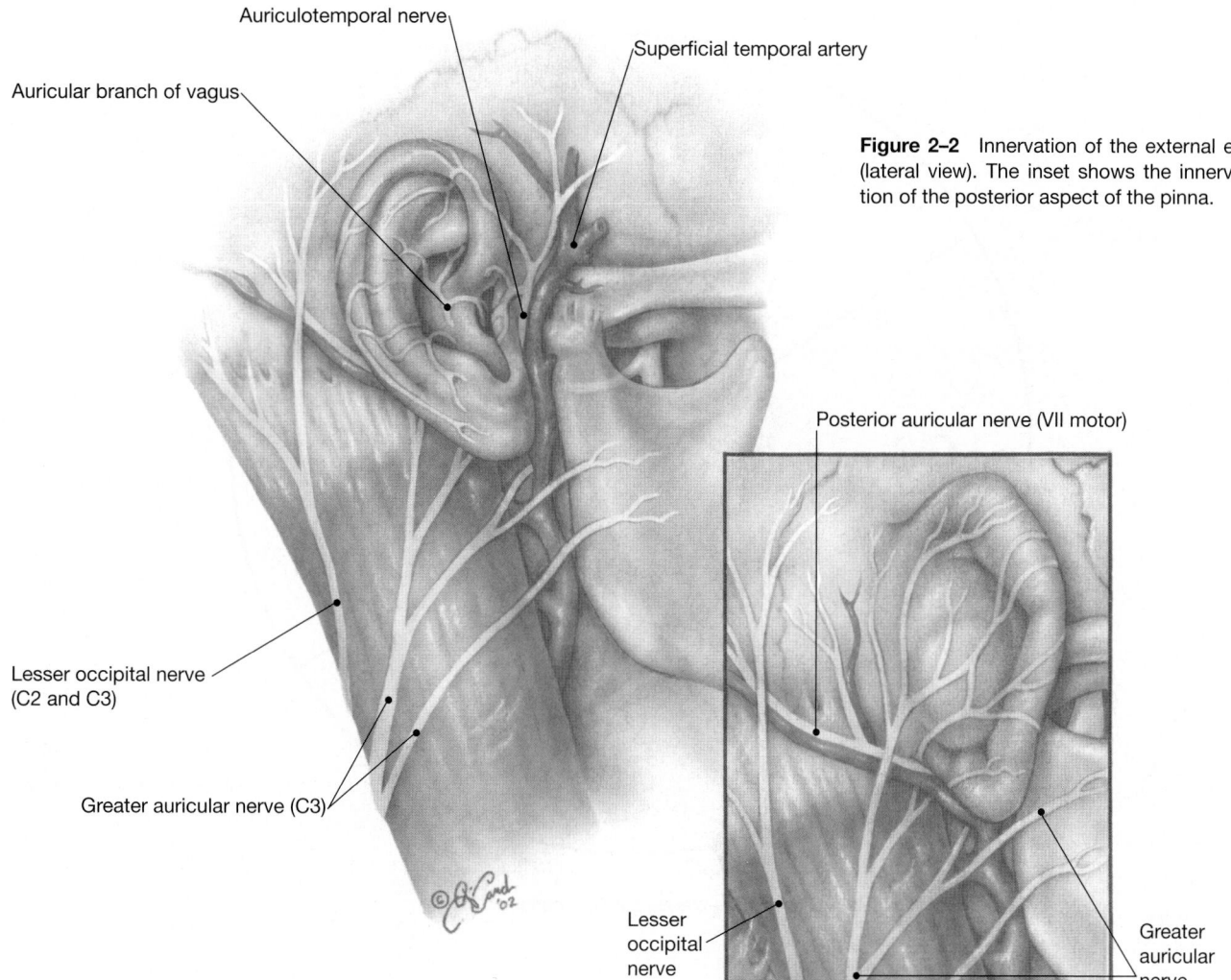

Auriculotemporal nerve

Superficial temporal artery

Auricular branch of vagus

Figure 2–2 Innervation of the external ear (lateral view). The inset shows the innervation of the posterior aspect of the pinna.

Posterior auricular nerve (VII motor)

Lesser occipital nerve (C2 and C3)

Greater auricular nerve (C3)

Lesser occipital nerve

Greater auricular nerve

parts of the posterior wall of the EAC. It interfaces with the squama at the tympanosquamous suture, the mastoid at the tympanomastoid suture, and the petrosa at the petrotympanic fissure and constitutes the posterior wall of the glenoid fossa for the temporomandibular joint (TMJ). The tympanomastoid suture is traversed by Arnold's nerve, whereas the chorda tympani nerve, anterior process of the malleus, and anterior tympanic artery traverse the petrotympanic fissure. Henle's spine is a projection of variable prominence at the posterosuperior aspect of the EAC. Inferiorly, the vaginal process, a projection of tympanic bone, forms the sheath of the styloid bone. Laterally, the tympanic bone borders the cartilaginous EAC, whereas medially it bears a circular groove, the annular sulcus. The annular sulcus houses the annulus of the tympanic membrane except superiorly, where it is deficient; at this point, known as the notch of Rivinus, the tympanic membrane attaches directly to the squama.

The tympanosquamous and tympanomastoid sutures are landmarks for the "vascular strip" incisions used in tympanomastoid surgery. The elevation of EAC skin and periosteum at these two sutures often requires sharp dissection to divide the contained periosteum, particularly at the tympanosquamous suture. Elevation of the tympanic membrane, as for a transcanal exploratory tympanotomy, typically commences just above the notch of Rivinus; the surgeon is thus able to identify and elevate the annulus in continuity with the tympanic membrane. The apparent size of the EAC may be diminished by excessive prominence of the bone at the tympanosquamous suture; access to the EAC in such cases can be improved by removal of the offending spur. Henle's spine marks the anterior limit of dissection in a canal wall up mastoidectomy. On occasion, posterior bulging of the anterior canal wall may obscure full visualization of the tympanic membrane. Anterior canalplasty can improve surgical visualization but if overzealous may

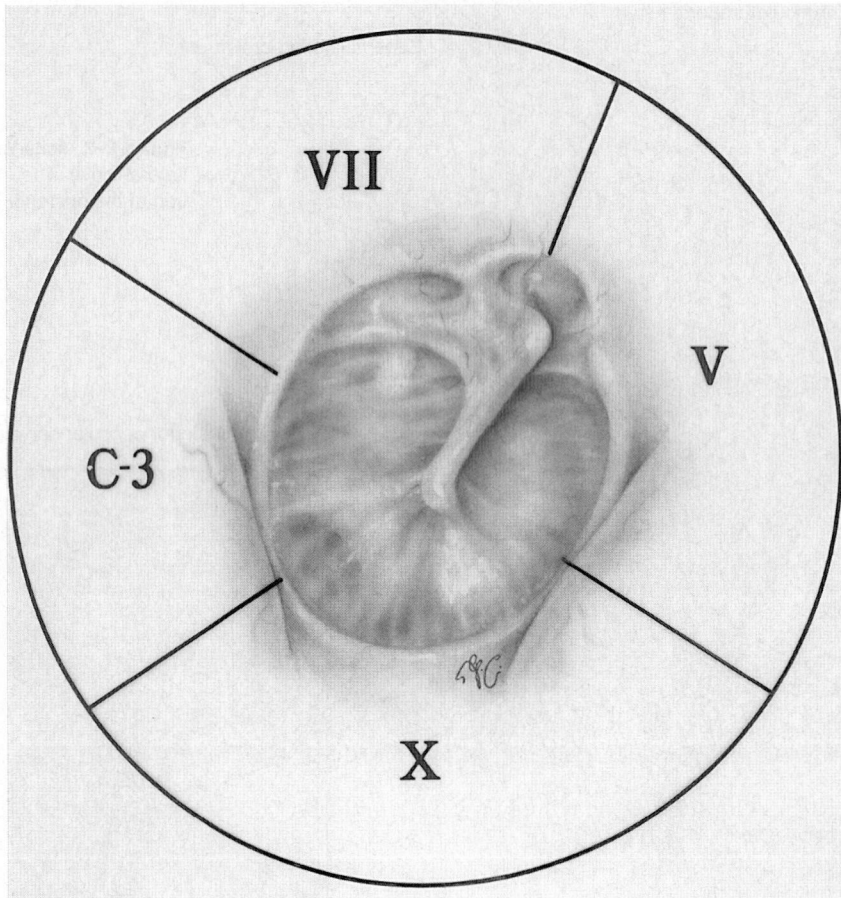

Figure 2–3   The innervation of the external auditory canal.

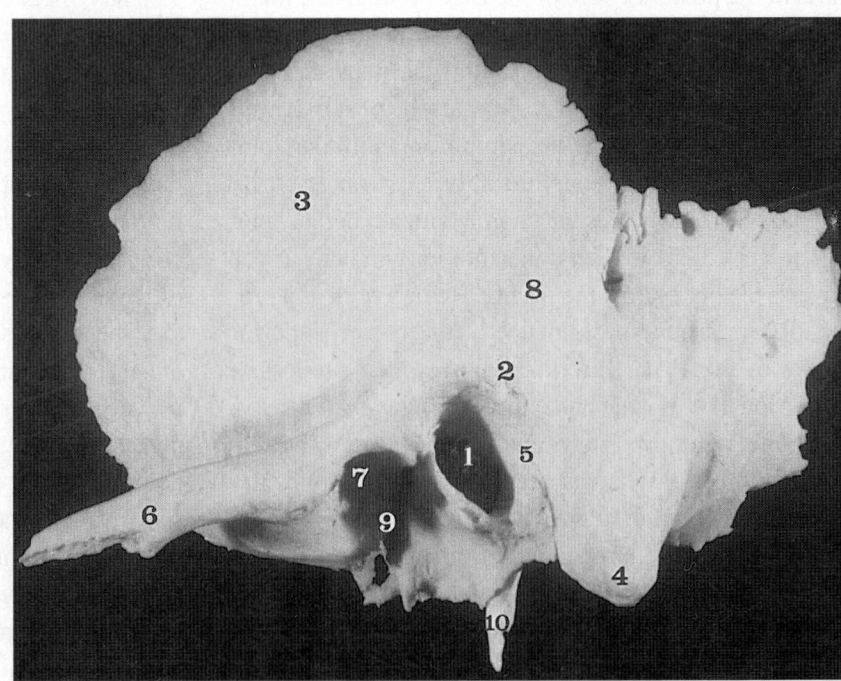

Figure 2–4   Left adult temporal bone, lateral aspect. 1 = external auditory canal; 2 = fossa mastoidea; 3 = squama; 4 = mastoid tip; 5 = tympanomastoid suture; 6 = zygoma; 7 = glenoid fossa; 8 = temporal line; 9 = petrotympanic fissure; 10 = styloid process. Reproduced with permission from Hughes GB, Pensak ML, editors. Clinical otology. 2nd ed. New York: Thieme Medical Publishers; 1997.

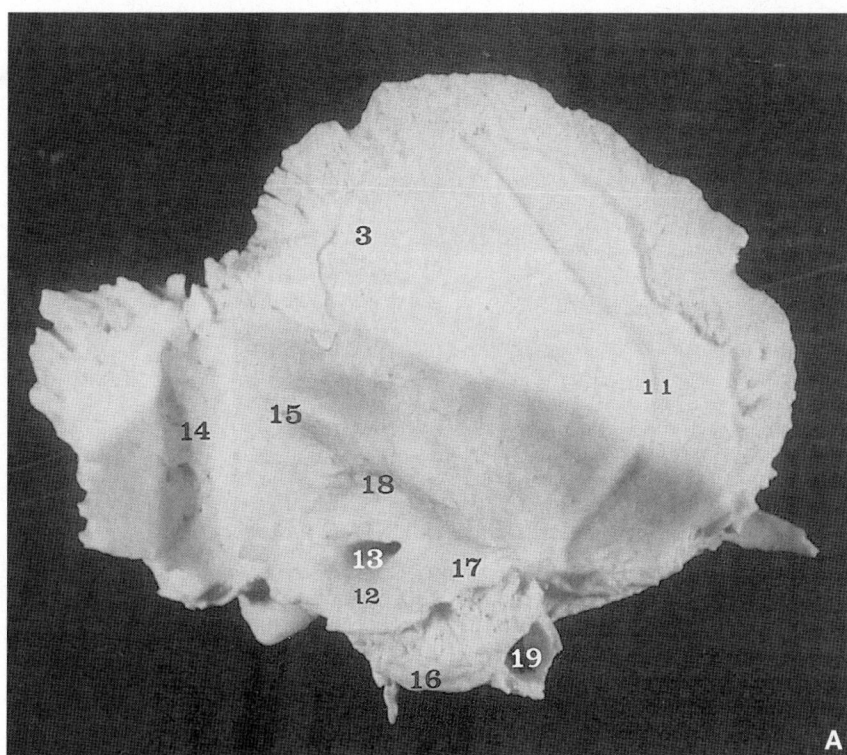

Figure 2–5 *A*, Left adult temporal bone, medial aspect. 3 = squama; 11 = middle meningeal arterial sulcus; 12 = petrous bone; 13 = internal auditory canal; 14 = sigmoid sulcus; 15 = superior petrosal sulcus; 16 = inferior petrosal sulcus; 17 = petrous apex; 18 = arcuate eminence; 19 = internal carotid artery foramen. Reproduced with permission from Hughes GB, Pensak ML, editors. Clinical otology. 2nd ed. New York: Thieme Medical Publishers; 1997. *B*, Drawing indicating approximate anatomic relationships of the internal carotid artery, superior petrosal sinus, facial nerve, bony labyrinth, and ossicular chain (right temporal bone). Inset shows the anatomic interrelationships at the fundus of the internal auditory canal.

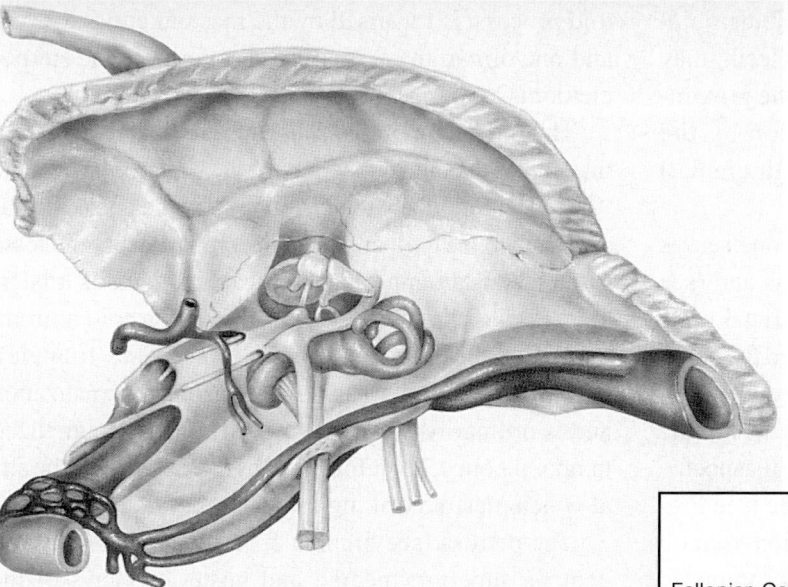

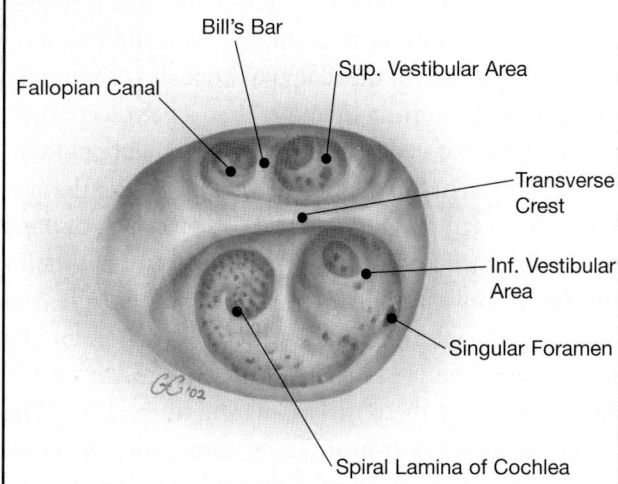

B

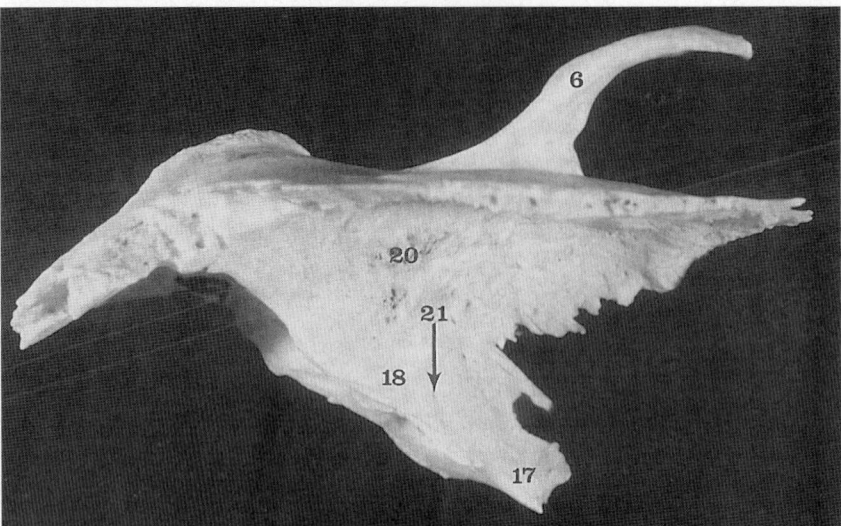

Figure 2–6   Left adult temporal bone, superior aspect. 6 = zygoma; 17 = petrous apex; 18 = arcuate eminence; 20 = tegmen; 21 = facial hiatus. Reproduced with permission from Hughes GB, Pensak ML, editors. Clinical otology. 2nd ed. New York: Thieme Medical Publishers; 1997.

result in prolapse of the TMJ into the EAC with, for example, opening the mouth. Temporomandibular joint dysfunction, as well as disease of the molar teeth, may manifest in referred otalgia, owing both to the proximity of the EAC and the shared innervation by the mandibular division of the trigeminal (fifth cranial) nerve.

The squamous portion of the temporal bone serves as the lateral wall of the middle cranial fossa and (see Figures 2–4 and 2–5) interfaces with the parietal bone superiorly and with the zygomatic process and the sphenoid anteriorly. Its medial surface is grooved by a sulcus for the middle meningeal artery, whereas the middle temporal artery runs in a groove on its lateral aspect.

The mastoid portion of the temporal bone (see Figure 2–4) is the inferiorly extending projection seen on the lateral surface of the temporal bone. It is composed of a squamous portion (laterally) and a petrous portion (medially) separated by Körner's (petrosquamous) septum. The fossa mastoidea (Macewen's triangle) is defined by the linea temporalis (temporal line), a ridge of bone extending posteriorly from the zygomatic process (marking the lower margin of the temporalis muscle and approximating the inferior descent of the middle cranial fossa dura), the posterosuperior margin of the EAC, and a tangent to the posterior margin of the EAC. The fossa mastoidea, a cribrose (cribriform) area, is identified by its numerous, perforating small blood vessels.

The mastoid foramen, located posteriorly on the mastoid process, is traversed by the mastoid emissary vein and one or two mastoid arteries. Inferiorly, the sternocleidomastoid muscle attaches to the mastoid tip.

The linea temporalis is an avascular plane, a feature that makes it an ideal location for the superior limb of the "T" musculoperiosteal incision used in the postauricular approach to the tympanomastoid compartment. The fossa mastoidea is an important surgical landmark as it laterally overlies the mastoid antrum. The mastoid antrum, medial to the fossa mastoidea (Macewen's triangle), develops in the earliest stages of mastoid pneumatization and is ordinarily present in even the least pneumatized temporal bones. Therefore, the fossa mastoidea is the site at which mastoid drilling ordinarily commences.

The petrosa (see Figures 2–5, 2–6, and 2–7) is evident on superior, medial, and posterior views of the temporal bone; the term "petrous" (Greek for "rocklike") stems from the extreme density of its bone, which guards the sensory organs of the inner ear. Important landmarks seen on a superior view (see Figure 2–6) are the arcuate eminence (roughly corresponding to the superior semicircular canal), meatal plane (indicative of the internal auditory canal), foramen spinosum for the middle meningeal artery, and facial hiatus (marking the departure of the greater petrosal nerve from the anterior aspect of the geniculate ganglion). The lesser petrosal nerve, accompanied by the superior tympanic artery,

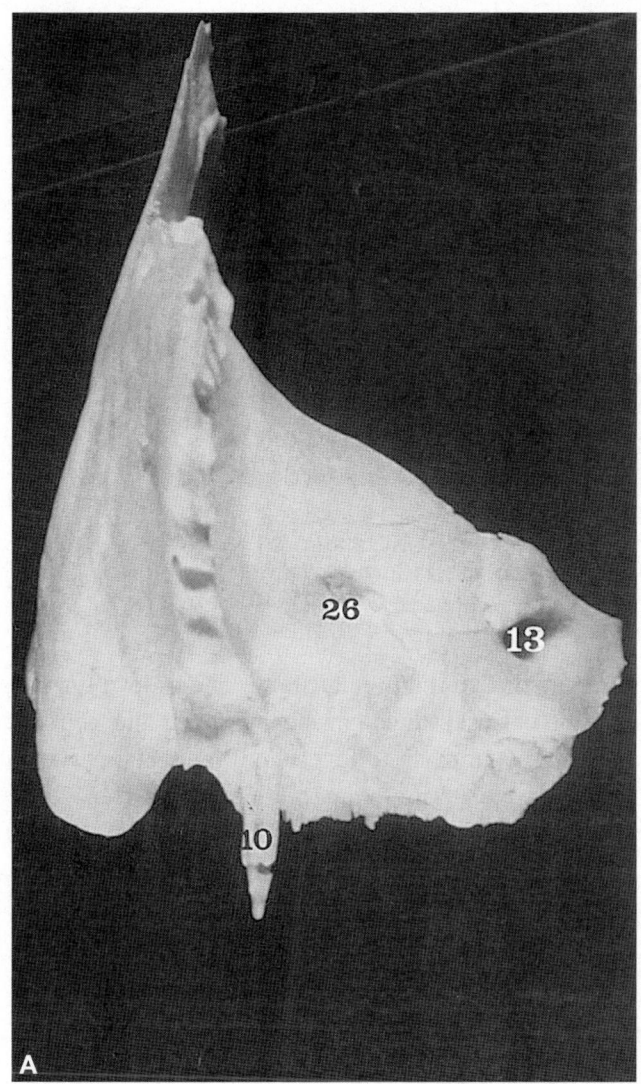

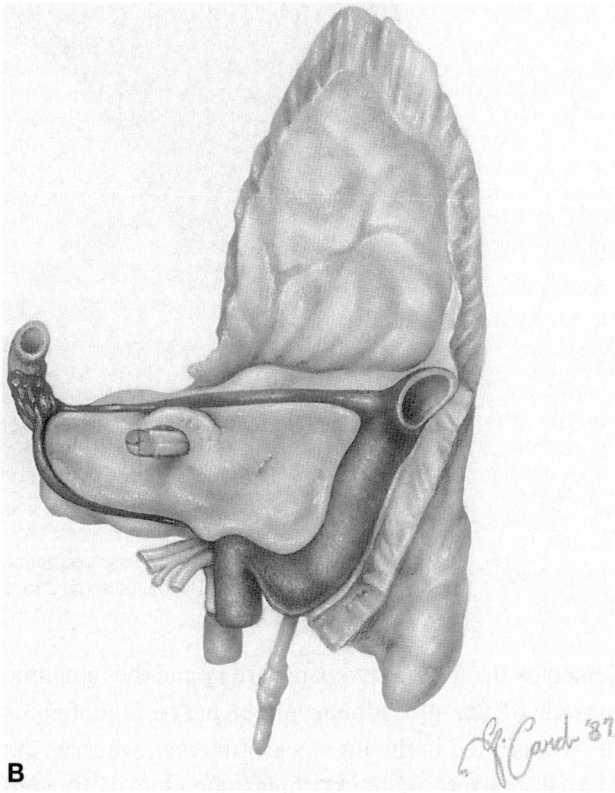

Figure 2–7 *A,* Left adult temporal bone, posterior aspect. 10 = styloid process; 13 = internal auditory canal; 26 = endolymphatic fossette. Reproduced with permission from Hughes GB, Pensak ML, editors. Clinical otology. 2nd ed. New York: Thieme Medical Publishers; 1997. *B,* Artist's depiction of the posterior aspect of the right temporal bone, with neurovascular structures.

occupies the superior tympanic canaliculus, lying lateral to and paralleling the path of the greater petrosal nerve to the petrous apex. The petrous apex points anteromedially and is marked by the transition of the intrapetrous to the intracranial internal carotid artery, orifice of the bony eustachian tube, and, anterolaterally, ganglion of the trigeminal nerve in Meckel's cave.

The medial view of the temporal bone (see Figure 2–5) features the porus of the internal auditory canal (IAC). The foramen seen at the petrous apex is the internal carotid foramen, by which the internal carotid artery exits the temporal bone. The sigmoid portion of the lateral venous sinus runs in the deep sulcus seen posteriorly, whereas the superior petrosal sinus runs in the sulcus located at the junction of the posterior and middle fossa faces of the temporal bone.

The vertically oriented posterior face of the petrosa dominates the posterior view of the temporal bone (see Figure 2–7) as it delimits the anterolateral aspect of the posterior cranial fossa and lies between the superior and inferior petrosal sinuses. The porus of the IAC, operculum, endolymphatic fossette cradling the endolymphatic sac, and subarcuate fossa are the key anatomic features on this surface.

The inferior surface of the temporal bone (Figure 2–8) figures prominently in skull base anatomy as it interfaces with the sphenoid and occipital bones. It provides attachment for the deep muscles of the neck and is perforated by a multitude of foramina. The jugular fossa, housing the jugular bulb, is separated from the internal carotid artery by the jugulocarotid crest. The aperture of the inferior tympanic canaliculus, tra-

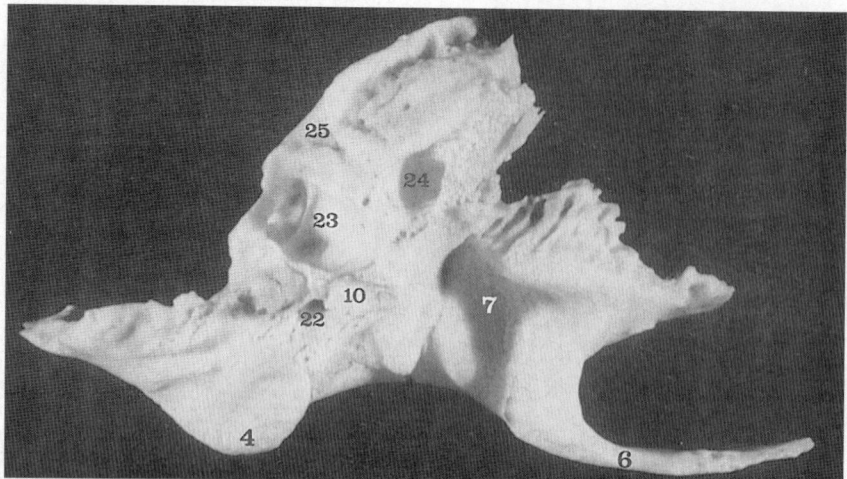

Figure 2–8 Left adult temporal bone, inferior aspect. 4 = mastoid process; 6 = zygoma; 7 = glenoid fossa; 10 = styloid process; 22 = stylomastoid foramen; 23 = jugular fossa; 25 = external opening of the cochlear aqueduct. Reproduced with permission from Hughes GB, Pensak ML, editors. Clinical otology. 2nd ed. New York: Thieme Medical Publishers; 1997.

versed by the inferior tympanic artery and the tympanic branch of the glossopharyngeal nerve (Jacobson's nerve), is sited in the jugulocarotid crest, whereas the cranial aperture of the cochlear aqueduct is located anteromedial to the jugular fossa. The groove for the inferior petrosal sinus can be seen near the petrous apex. The stylomastoid foramen of the facial nerve is located just posterior to the styloid process. The occip-

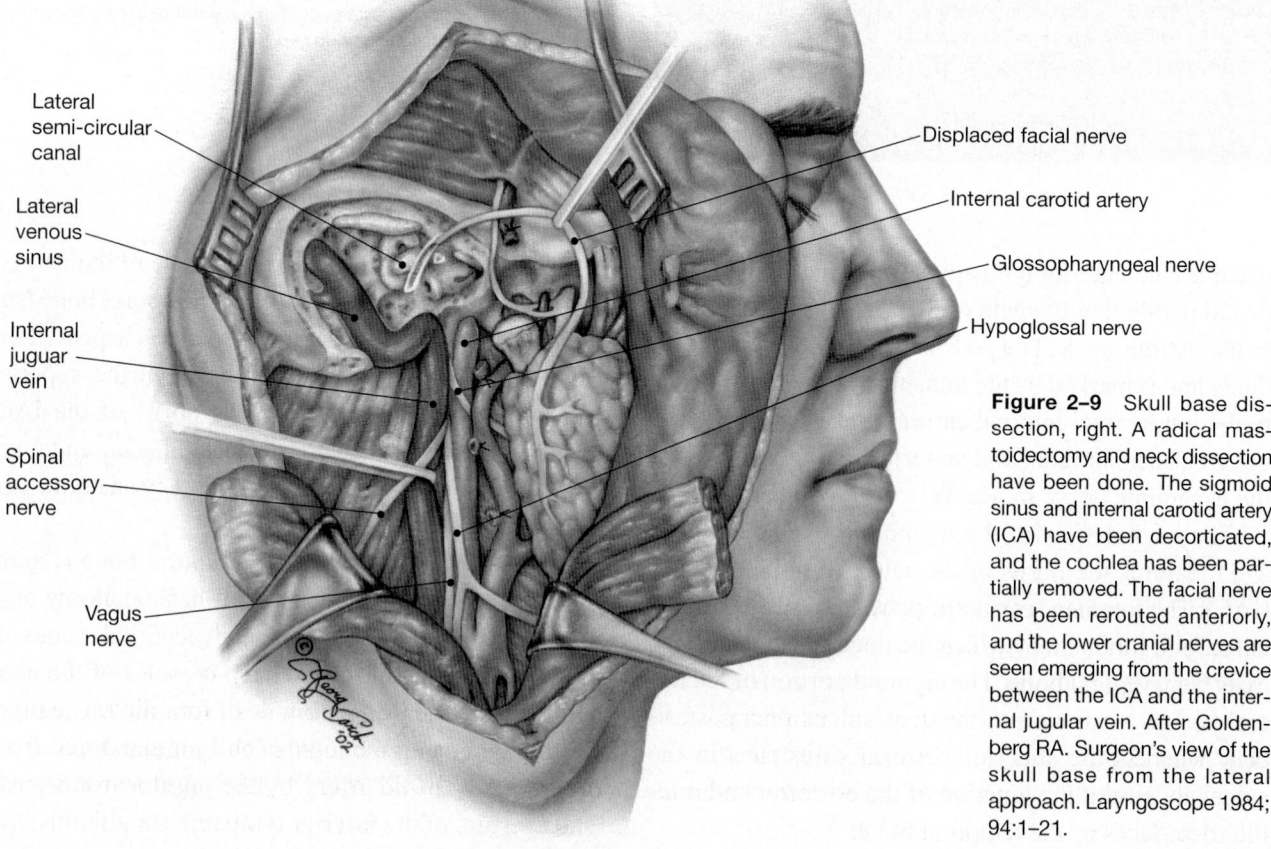

Lateral semi-circular canal

Lateral venous sinus

Internal juguar vein

Spinal accessory nerve

Vagus nerve

Displaced facial nerve

Internal carotid artery

Glossopharyngeal nerve

Hypoglossal nerve

Figure 2–9 Skull base dissection, right. A radical mastoidectomy and neck dissection have been done. The sigmoid sinus and internal carotid artery (ICA) have been decorticated, and the cochlea has been partially removed. The facial nerve has been rerouted anteriorly, and the lower cranial nerves are seen emerging from the crevice between the ICA and the internal jugular vein. After Goldenberg RA. Surgeon's view of the skull base from the lateral approach. Laryngoscope 1984; 94:1–21.

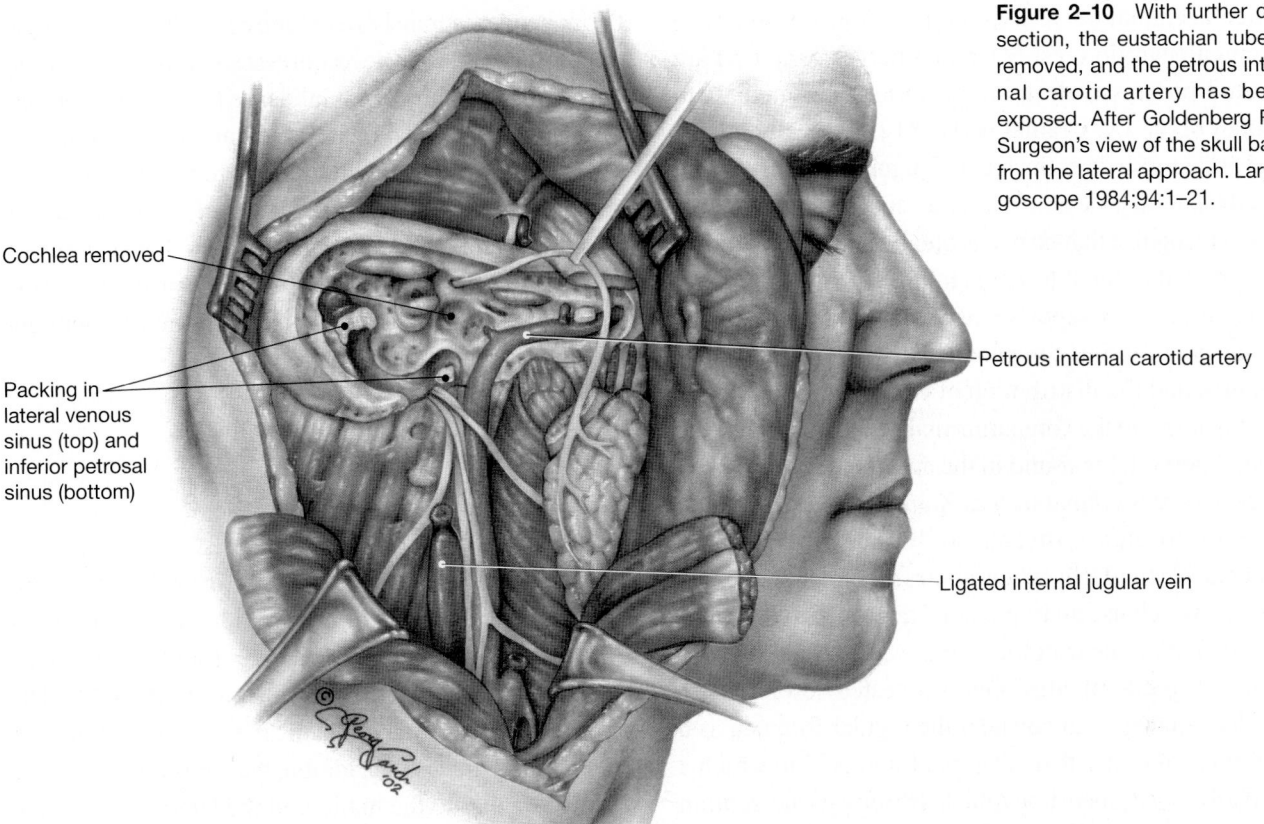

Cochlea removed

Packing in
lateral venous
sinus (top) and
inferior petrosal
sinus (bottom)

Petrous internal carotid artery

Ligated internal jugular vein

Figure 2–10 With further dissection, the eustachian tube is removed, and the petrous internal carotid artery has been exposed. After Goldenberg RA. Surgeon's view of the skull base from the lateral approach. Laryngoscope 1984;94:1–21.

Figure 2–11 Left skull base dissection. Removal of the internal jugular vein and the jugular bulb exposes the exit of the lower cranial nerves from the posterior fossa. Asterisk = jugular fossa; 1 = internal carotid artery; 2 = glossopharyngeal nerve; 3 = vagus nerve; 4 = hypoglossal nerve; 5 = spinal accessory nerve. Photo courtesy of John Kveton, MD; reproduced with permission from Kveton JF. Anatomy of the jugular foramen: the neurotologic perspective. Op Tech ORL-HNS 1996;7:95–8.

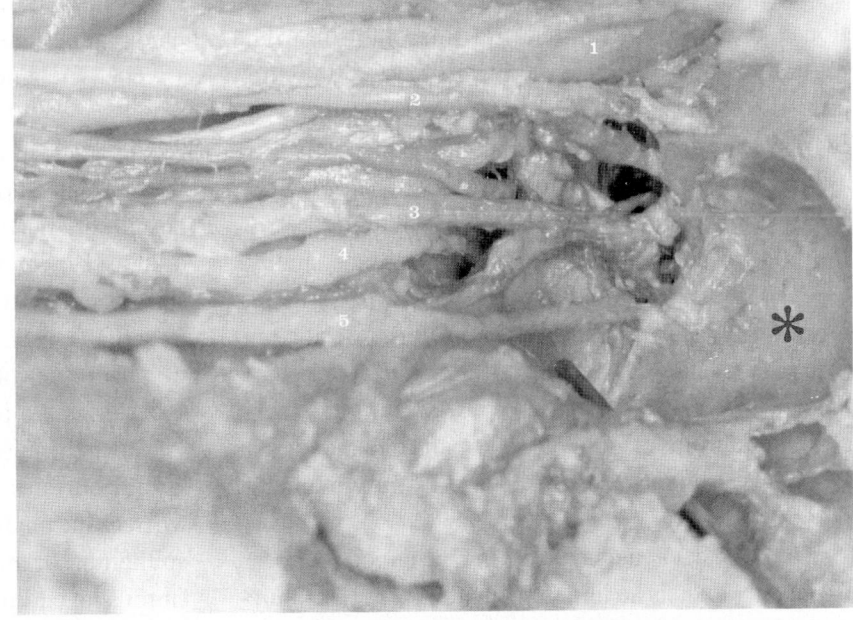

ital artery and the digastric muscle occupy the temporal groove and the mastoid incisure, respectively, at the medial aspect of the tip.

The jugular foramen is of particular importance in skull base surgery as it is traversed by the glossopharyngeal (ninth), vagus (tenth), and spinal accessory (eleventh) cranial nerves as they exit the skull (Figures 2–9, 2–10, and 2–11). In the course of posterolateral skull base exposure, decortication and fibrous tissue dissection reveal the internal jugular vein, its bulb, and the internal carotid artery. Posterior retraction of the internal jugular vein and resection of the jugular bulb allow visualization of the lower cranial nerves exiting the skull (see Figure 2–11), the most anterior and lateral of which is cranial nerve IX, as it passes just posterior to the jugulocarotid crest.[2,3] Cranial nerves X and XI are located progressively more posterior (and medial) to cranial nerve IX. Cranial nerve XI is generally identified as it crosses over the internal jugular vein in the neck and the lateral process of the atlas; however, it is important to recognize that nearly as often cranial nerve XI can pass medial to the internal jugular vein.[4]

Contradictory reports exist in the literature regarding the bony/fibrous compartmentalization of the jugular foramen and the distribution of contained neurovascular structures; in the compartmentalized jugular foramen, cranial nerve IX is found in the anteromedial compartment, whereas cranial nerves X and XI and the jugular bulb are located posterolaterally. The contradiction appears particularly when contrasting neurosurgical studies, which use an intracranial approach to the jugular foramen, to neurotologic studies, in which a lateral approach predominates. One suggested resolution to the discrepancy is to consider the jugular foramen as a "short canal rather than a simple foramen"[4] in which a medially positioned bony/thick fibrous tissue septum thins as one approaches the lateral aspect of the foramen.

The hypoglossal canal, located in the anterior portion of the occipital condyle and anteroinferior to the jugular foramen, carries cranial nerve XII, which courses medial to cranial nerve X and inferior to the jugular foramen.[3]

The inferior petrosal sinus is in close anatomic relation to cranial nerves IX through XI as it drains, in two-thirds of cases via multiple openings, into the anterior aspect of the jugular bulb (see Figure 2–10). Most commonly, the inferior petrosal sinus runs inferior and medial to cranial nerve IX and superior and lateral to cranial nerves X and XI.[4] The condylar emissary vein, draining the suboccipital plexus, opens into the jugular bulb inferiorly and posteriorly, in proximity to cranial nerves X and XI.[4]

The cochlear aqueduct, carrying the periotic (or perilymphatic) duct, is an important landmark for the neuro-otologist. As the cochlear aqueduct runs from the medial aspect of the scala tympani of the basal cochlear turn to terminate anteromedial to the jugular bulb, it parallels, and lies inferior to, the IAC. From the transmastoid perspective, the aqueduct is encountered when drilling medial to the jugular bulb; opening the aqueduct results in the flow of cerebrospinal fluid into the mastoid, a useful maneuver in translabyrinthine cerebellopontine angle tumor surgery as it decompresses cerebrospinal fluid pressure. In addition, cranial nerve IX, the inferior petrosal sinus, and, in some cases, cranial nerves X and XI can be found immediately inferior to the lateral terminus of the cochlear aqueduct.[5] Therefore, the cochlear aqueduct can be used as a guide to the lower limits of IAC dissection in, for example, the translabyrinthine approach as it allows full exposure of the IAC without risking the lower cranial nerves.

Related Structures

Tympanic Membrane

The tympanic membrane (see Figure 2–3) emulates an irregular cone, the apex of which is formed by the umbo (at the tip of the manubrium). The adult tympanic membrane is about 9 mm in diameter and subtends an acute angle with respect to the inferior wall of the EAC. The fibrous annulus of the tympanic membrane anchors it in the tympanic sulcus. In addition, the tympanic membrane firmly attaches to the malleus at the lateral process and at the umbo; between these two points, only a flimsy mucosal fold, the plica mallearis, connects the tympanic membrane to the malleus.

The tympanic membrane is separated into a superior pars flaccida (Shrapnell's membrane) and a pars inferior by the anterior and posterior tympanic stria, which run from the lateral process of the malleus to the anterior and posterior tympanic spines, respectively. Shrapnell's membrane serves as the lateral wall of Prussak's space (the superior recess of the tympanic membrane); the head and neck of the malleus, the lateral malleal ligament, and anterior and posterior malleal folds form the medial, anterosuperior, and inferior limits of Prussak's space.

The tympanic membrane is a trilaminar structure. The lateral surface is formed by squamous epithelium, whereas the medial layer is a continuation of the mucosal epithelium of the middle ear. Between these layers is a fibrous layer, known as the pars propria. The pars propria at the umbo splits to envelop the distal tip of the manubrium.

Ossicles

The ossicular chain (Figure 2–12), made up of the malleus, incus, and stapes, serves to conduct sound from the tympanic membrane to the cochlea.

The malleus, the most lateral of the ossicles, has a head (caput), manubrium (handle), neck, and anterior and lateral processes. The lateral process has a cartilaginous "cap" that imperceptibly merges with the pars propria of the tympanic membrane. The anterior ligament of the malleus, extending from the anterior process, passes through the petrotympanic fissure and, with the posterior incudal ligament, creates the axis of ossicular rotation.

The incus, the largest of the three ossicles, is immediately medial to the malleus. The incus has a body and three processes: a long, a short, and a lenticular. The body of the incus articulates with the head of the malleus in the epitympanum. The short process of the incus is anchored in the incudal fossa by the posterior incudal ligament. The long process extends inferiorly, roughly paralleling and lying posterior to the manubrium. The lenticular process, at the terminus of the long process, articulates with the stapes.

The stapes is the smallest and most medial of the ossicles. Its head articulates with the lenticular process of the incus, whereas its footplate sits in the oval window, surrounded by the stapediovestibular ligament. The arch of the stapes, composed of an anterior and a posterior crus, links the head and the footplate.

In the course of tympanic membrane elevation, as for instance in tympanoplasty, since the cartilaginous "cap" of the lateral process of the malleus blends into the pars propria of the drum, it is more expedient to sharply dissect it from the malleus rather than tediously attempting to dissect the drum from the "cap." The long process of the incus, perhaps owing to its tenuous blood supply, is particularly prone to osteitic resorption in the face of chronic otitis media. Although the ossicles are held in position by their ligaments and tendons, the force of injudicious surgical manipulation can easily overcome these restraints, resulting in subluxation or complete luxation. When dissecting disease from the stapes, one should parallel the plane of the stapedius tendon, in a posterior to an anterior direction, so that the tendon resists displacement of the stapes.

Middle Ear Muscles

The tensor tympani muscle, innervated by the trigeminal nerve, originates from the walls of its semicanal,

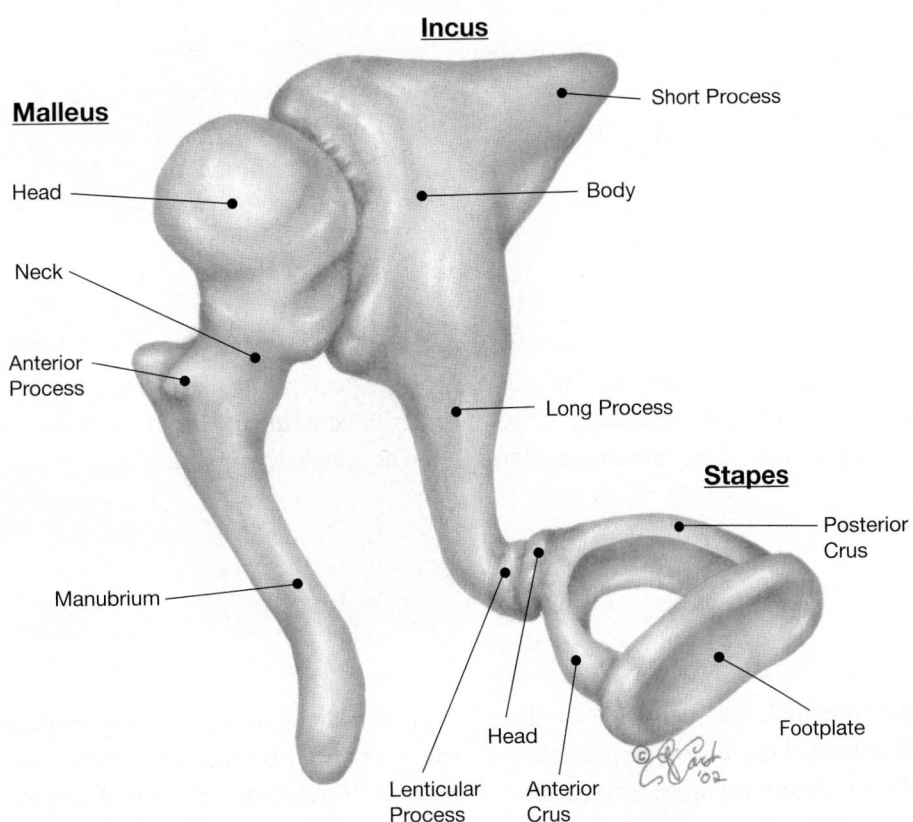

Figure 2–12   The ossicular chain, medial aspect.

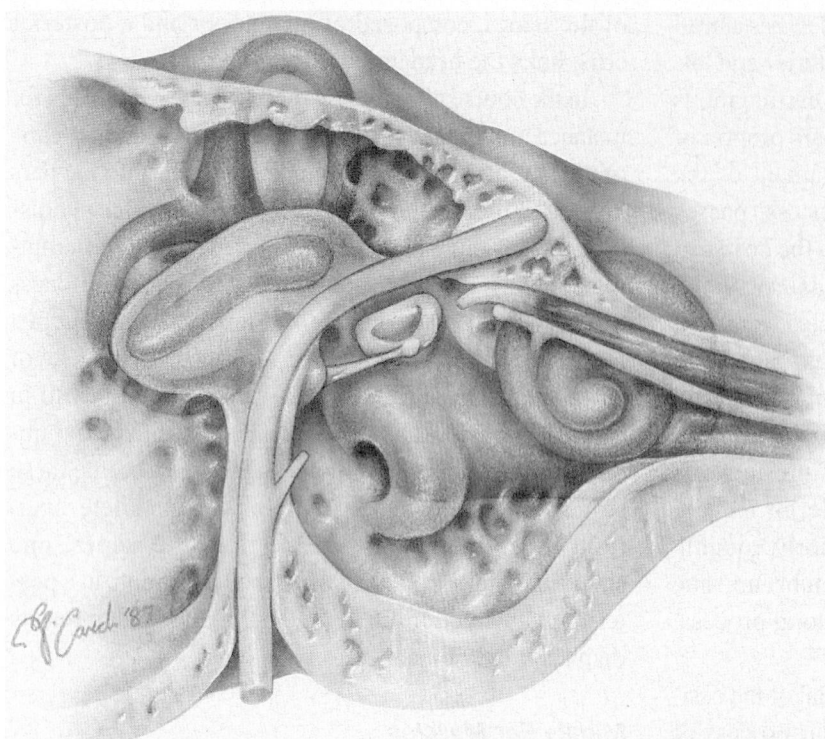

Figure 2–13   The facial nerve is seen in its vertical and tympanic segments. Anterosuperiorly, the facial nerve passes superior to the tensor tympani tendon, which is seen sectioned just after it exits the cochleariform process.

Figure 2–14   Radical mastoid dissection view of a right temporal bone. The three semicircular canals have been opened. The anatomic interrelationships between the internal carotid artery (1), eustachian tube (2), promontory (3), and geniculate ganglion (4) are seen. Reproduced with permission from Gulya AJ, Schuknecht HF. Anatomy of the temporal bone with surgical implications. 2nd ed. Pearl River (NY): Parthenon Press; 1995.

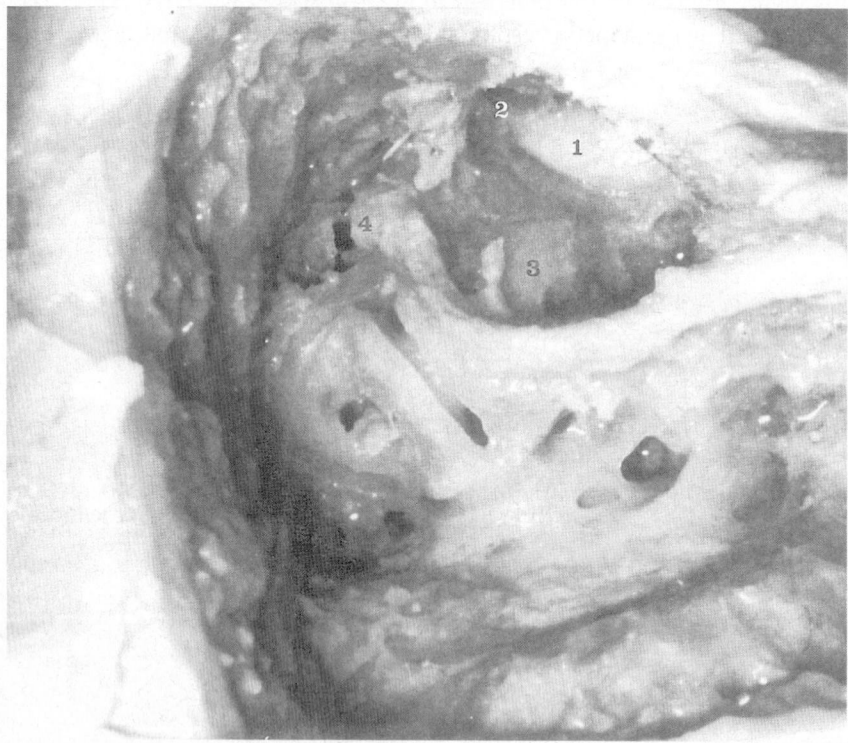

greater wing of the sphenoid, and cartilage of the eustachian tube. The tendon of the tensor tympani muscle sweeps around the cochleariform process and across the tympanic cavity to attach to the medial aspect of the neck and manubrium of the malleus.

The medial pull of the tensor tympani muscle is ordinarily opposed by the intact tympanic membrane. In the case of a chronic, substantial perforation of the tympanic membrane, the unopposed action of the tensor tympani muscle can medialize the manubrium, effectively

Figure 2–15 The sinus tympani is bordered superiorly by the ponticulus and inferiorly by the subiculum. Reproduced with permission from Schuknecht HF. Pathology of the ear. Cambridge (MA): Harvard University Press; 1974.

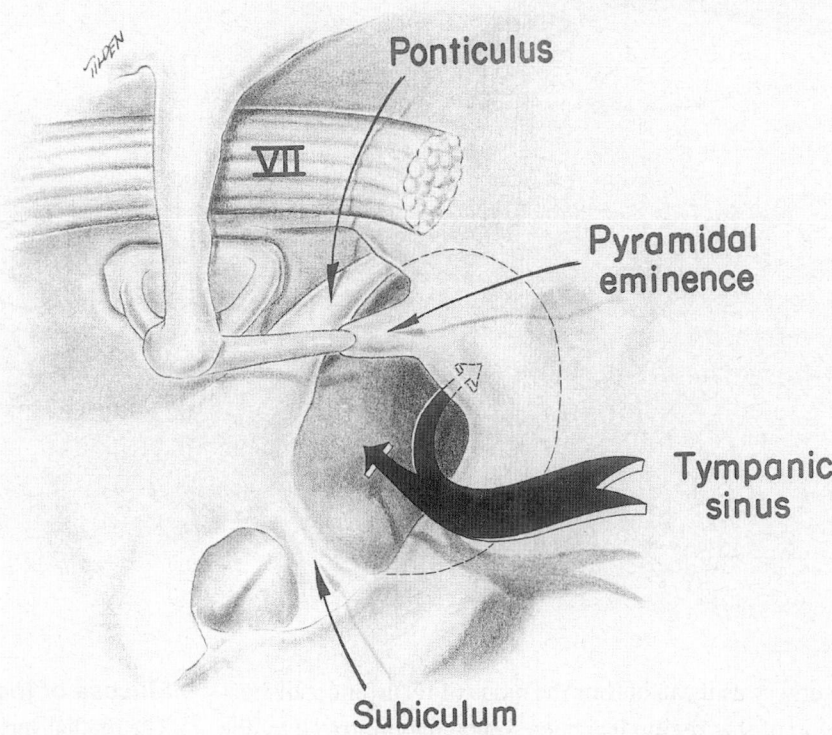

contracting the depth of the tympanic cavity. Forcible lateralization of the malleus, or even sectioning of the tensor tympani tendon, may be required to allow the surgeon to perform tympanic membrane grafting or ossiculoplasty. The cochleariform process is a landmark to the anterior aspect of the tympanic segment of the facial nerve as the nerve runs immediately superior to this process (Figure 2–13).

The stapedius muscle runs in a vertical sulcus in the posterior wall of the tympanic cavity adjacent to the facial nerve, from which it receives its innervation. Its tendon traverses the pyramidal eminence to attach to the posterior crus, and occasionally the head, of the stapes.

Middle Ear Spaces

The tympanic cavity is a sagittally oriented slit that lies immediately medial to the tympanic membrane. Its roof, or tegmen, also serves as part of the floor of the middle cranial fossa, whereas its irregularly contoured floor features the jugular bulb and, posteriorly, the root of the styloid process. The tympanic cavity is in continuity with the eustachian tube anteriorly and with the mastoid air cells via the aditus and antrum. It is traversed by the ossicular chain and is lined with a mucosal epithelium. Planes extended from the tympanic annulus subdivide the tympanic cavity into a mesotympanum, hypotym-

panum, protympanum, and posterior tympanic cavity. The epitympanum lies above the plane of the anterior and posterior tympanic spines.

Anteriorly, the mesotympanum is dominated by the bulge of the semicanal of the tensor tympani muscle; the tympanic orifice of the eustachian tube is immediately inferior to this bulge (Figure 2–14). Posteriorly, the key anatomic features are the pyramidal eminence and, lateral to it, the chordal eminence. The chordal eminence houses the iter chordae posterius by which the chorda tympani nerve enters the tympanic cavity.

The medial wall (the surgical "floor" of the middle ear) features three depressions: the sinus tympani, oval window niche, and round window niche (Figure 2–15). The sinus tympani is defined by the ponticulus superiorly, the subiculum inferiorly, the mastoid segment of the facial nerve laterally, and the posterior semicircular canal medially; there is substantial variability in the posterior extension (surgical "depth") of the sinus tympani, ranging from "shallow" to "deep." The oval window niche, occupied by the stapes footplate, is located anterosuperior to the ponticulus. The round window niche can be found posteroinferior to the promontory, the bulge created by the basal turn of the cochlea.

The sinus tympani evades direct surgical visualization, which is particularly worrisome in cholesteatoma

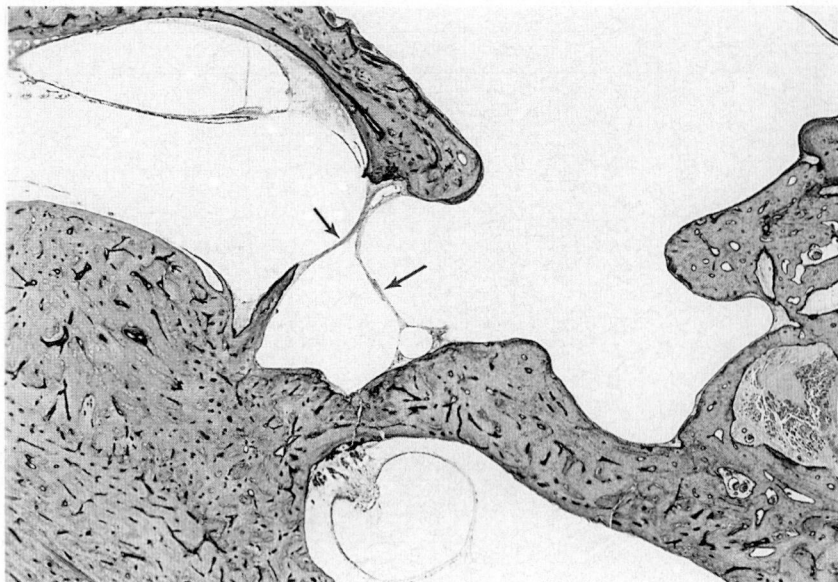

Figure 2–16 The true round window membrane (*left arrow*) is covered by a veil of mucosa (*right arrow*). There is a microfissure extending from the medial aspect of the round window niche to the ampulla of the posterior semicircular canal. Right temporal bone; reproduced with permission from Gulya AJ, Schuknecht HF. Anatomy of the temporal bone with surgical implications. 2nd ed. Pearl River (NY): Parthenon Press; 1995.

surgery as it can harbor the nidus of recurrence. Inspection of this region has been somewhat improved by the advent of endoscopes appropriate for otologic surgery. The oval window niche may be the site of a perilymphatic fistula. Similarly, the round window niche may be implicated in perilymph leakage. In assessing the round window, it is important to realize that in the vast majority of cases, the true round window membrane is obscured by some kind of mucosal veil (Figure 2–16); most often, the veil is perforated, giving the false impression of seeing a defect in the round window membrane.[6]

Eustachian Tube

The eustachian tube extends approximately 35 mm from the anterior aspect of the tympanic cavity to the posterior aspect of the nasopharynx and serves to ventilate, clear, and protect the middle ear (see Figures 2–9 and 2–14). The lining mucosa of the tube has an abundance of mucociliary cells, important to its clearance function. The anteromedial two-thirds of the eustachian tube are fibrocartilaginous, whereas the remainder is bony. The tympanic orifice is in the anterior wall of the middle ear, a few millimeters above the floor. In its normal resting position, the tube is closed; opening of the tube is accomplished by the tensor veli palatini muscle, innervated by the trigeminal nerve. A body of fat, the lateral fat pad of Ostmann, abuts the lateral aspect of the fibrocartilaginous tube and aids in maintaining the resting closure of the tube.

Mucosa of the Tympanomastoid Compartment

The medial surface of the tympanic membrane, tympanic cavity, and mastoid air cells are all lined with a mucosal epithelium, reflecting their common heritage from the tubotympanic recess. The predominant cell type varies with location in the tympanomastoid compartment. Ciliated cells intermingle with secretory cells on the promontory, in the hypotympanum, and in the epitympanum[7]; the mucociliary tracts thus formed act in concert with the mucociliary clearance system of the eustachian tube.

Pneumatization

The extent of pneumatization of the temporal bone varies according to heredity, environment, nutrition, infection, and eustachian tube function. There are five recognized regions of pneumatization: the middle ear, mastoid, perilabyrinthine, petrous apex, and accessory (Figure 2–17). The middle ear region, as described above, is divided into epitympanic, hypotympanic, mesotympanic, protympanic, and posterior tympanic areas. The mastoid region is subdivided into the mastoid antrum, central mastoid, and peripheral mastoid. The bony labyrinth divides the perilabyrinthine region into supralabyrinthine and infralabyrinthine areas. The apical area and the peritubal area comprise the petrous apex region. The accessory region encompasses the zygomatic, squamous, occipital, and styloid areas. There are five recognized air cell tracts. The posterosuperior tract runs at the juncture of the posterior and middle fossa

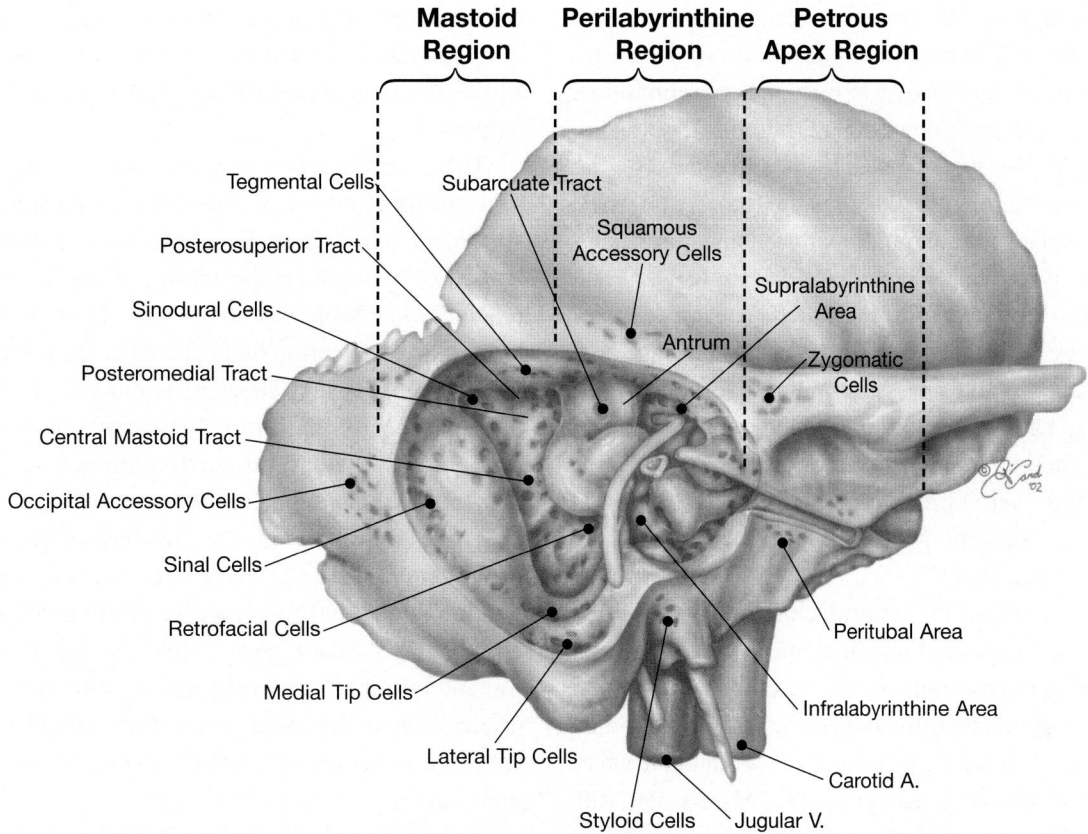

Figure 2–17 Pneumatization of the temporal bone, with regions, areas, and tracts indicated. After Nadol JB Jr, Schuknecht HF, editors. Surgery of the ear and temporal bone. New York: Raven Press; 1993.

aspects of the temporal bone. The posteromedial cell tract parallels and runs inferior to the posterosuperior tract. The subarcuate tract passes through the arch of the superior semicircular canal. The perilabyrinthine tracts run superior and inferior to the bony labyrinth, whereas the peritubal tract surrounds the eustachian tube.

The anterior petrous apex is pneumatized in only 10 to 15% of specimens studied.[8] Most often, it is diploic; in a small percentage of cases, it is sclerotic.

Troublesome cerebrospinal fluid leakage, persisting after translabyrinthine vestibular schwannoma resection despite apparently adequate tympanomastoid obliteration, has been linked to the presence of peritubal cells that open directly into the eustachian tube anterior to its tympanic orifice.[9]

Inner Ear

The bony labyrinth (see Figure 2–17) houses the sensory organs and soft tissue structures of the inner ear and consists of the cochlea, three semicircular canals, and vestibule. Its bone has three layers: an inner, or endosteal, layer; an outer, or periosteal, layer; and a middle layer consisting of enchondral and intrachondral bone. Intrachondral bone (globuli interossei) is characterized by cartilage islands, the lacunae of which have a thin bony layer owing to their invasion by osteoblasts.

The cochlea spirals 2½ turns about its central axis, the modiolus, and has a height of 5 mm. The base of the cochlea abuts the fundus of the IAC and is perforated (cribrose), allowing for the passage of cochlear nerve fibers. The apex lies medial to the tensor tympani muscle. The osseous spiral lamina winds about the modiolus and, along with the basilar membrane, separates the scala media (the cochlear duct) from the scala tympani. Adjacent turns of the cochlea are separated by an interscalar septum.

The three semicircular canals (see Figure 2–14) are the lateral (horizontal), superior (anterior vertical), and posterior (posterior vertical). The three canals are orthogonally related to one another and arc over a span of 240 degrees. Each canal has an ampullated limb, measuring 2 mm in diameter, and a nonampullated limb, which is

1 mm in diameter. The ampulla is cribrose for passage of nerve fibers. The nonampullated limbs of the posterior and superior canals fuse to form the crus commune. The ampullated and nonampullated limbs all open into the vestibule. The angle formed by the three semicircular canals is the solid angle, whereas the triangle bounded by the bony labyrinth, sigmoid sinus, and superior petrosal sinus is known as Trautmann's triangle.

Thinning, or frank dehiscence, of the bone of the superior semicircular canal is recognized as underlying some cases of sound- and/or pressure-induced vertigo.[10] Such dehiscence has been found in 0.5% of temporal bones studied, whereas thinning was encountered in 1.4%; both findings were "frequently" bilateral.[11] A failure in postnatal development of the bony labyrinth has been theorized to be the cause.[11]

The vestibule is the central chamber of the bony labyrinth and measures 4 mm in diameter. Its medial wall is marked by depressions for the saccule (the spherical recess), utricle (the elliptical recess), and cochlear duct (the cochlear recess). Cribrose areas accommodate nerve fiber access to their sensory organs. "Mike's dot" (the macula cribrosa superior) marks the passageway for superior vestibular nerve fibers to the cristae ampullares

of the lateral and superior semicircular canals. As it corresponds to the extreme lateral aspect of the IAC, Mike's dot is an important landmark in translabyrinthine surgery.

There are three fissures of the bony labyrinth. The fissula ante fenestram is an evagination of the perilymphatic space that is invariably found extending anterosuperior to the oval window; in the adult, fibrous tissue and cartilage fill the fissula. The fossula post fenestram is a perilymphatic evagination that extends posterior to the oval window; it is a less constant feature of the temporal bone. Hyrtl's fissure (or the tympanomeningeal hiatus) is a remnant of embryologic development and is rarely present (see Chapter 1 for additional details).

There are two commonly encountered microfissures of the temporal bone. One extends between the round window niche and the ampulla of the posterior semicircular canal (see Figure 2–16). The other runs superior and inferior to the oval window. Both microfissures, or breaks in the endosteal and endochondral layers of the temporal bone, are filled with fibrous tissue and acellular matrix.

A persistent Hyrtl's fissure has been implicated as a route for cerebrospinal fluid leakage into the middle

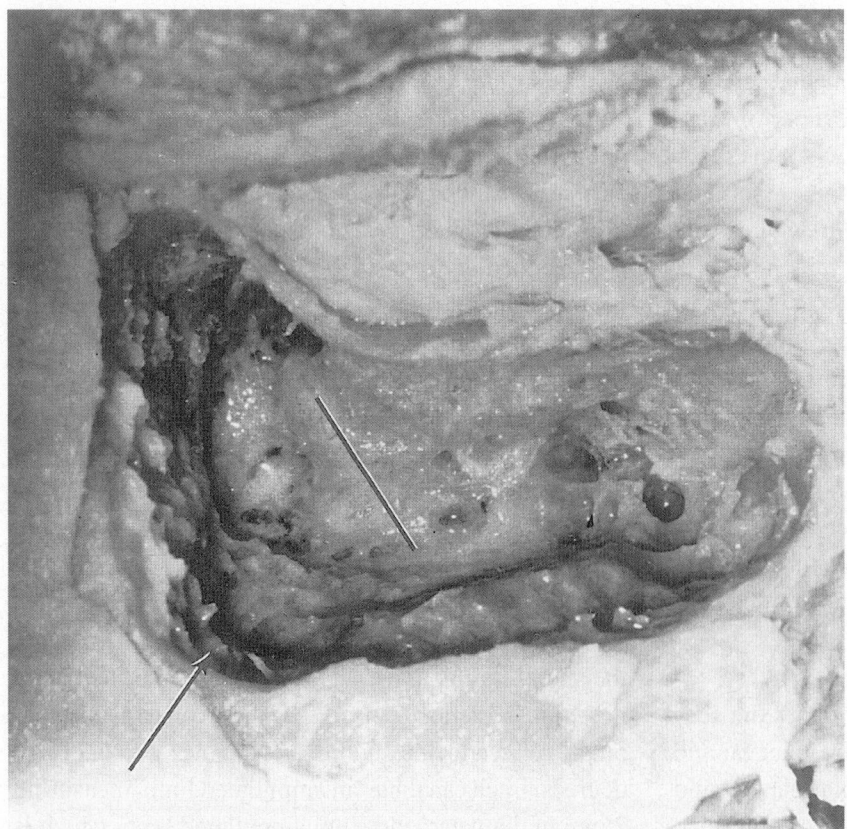

Figure 2–18 Complete mastoidectomy view of a right temporal bone. The lateral and posterior semicircular canals form Donaldson's line (*line*). The angle of Citelli is indicated (*arrow*). Reproduced with permission from Gulya AJ, Schuknecht HF. 2nd ed. Pearl River (NY): Parthenon Press; 1995.

ear.[12] Although the oval and round window microfissures have been hypothesized to be the site of perilymph leakage, evidence refutes this theory.[13]

The membranous (endolymphatic) labyrinth housed within the bony labyrinth consists of the cochlear duct (scala media), the three semicircular ducts and their cristae ampullares, the otolithic organs (the utricle and the saccule), and the endolymphatic duct and sac. Generally interposed between the bony and membranous labyrinths are the connective tissue, blood vessels, and fluid of the perilymphatic space, including the scala tympani, scala vestibuli, perilymphatic cistern of the vestibule, perilymphatic duct, and perilymph spaces surrounding the semicircular ducts.

The endolymphatic duct originates in the medial wall of the vestibule. It first parallels the crus commune and then the posterior semicircular canal as it heads to the endolymphatic sac, anterior and medial to the sigmoid sinus. The endolymphatic sac lies approximately 10 mm inferior and lateral to the porus of the IAC; the sac has an intraosseous portion, which is covered by the operculum, and a more distal intradural portion (see Figure 1–14).

Donaldson's line, a surgical landmark in endolymphatic sac surgery, is derived by extending the plane of the lateral semicircular so that it bisects the posterior semicircular canal and contacts the posterior fossa dura (Figure 2–18); the endolymphatic sac lies inferior to this line. The precise position of the sac shows considerable variability.

Internal Auditory Canal

The IAC is the bony channel that shelters the superior and inferior vestibular, cochlear, facial, and intermediate nerves, as well as the labyrinthine artery and vein, as they course from the posterior cranial fossa to the labyrinth. On average, the canal measures 3.4 mm in diameter and 8 mm in length; these dimensions display

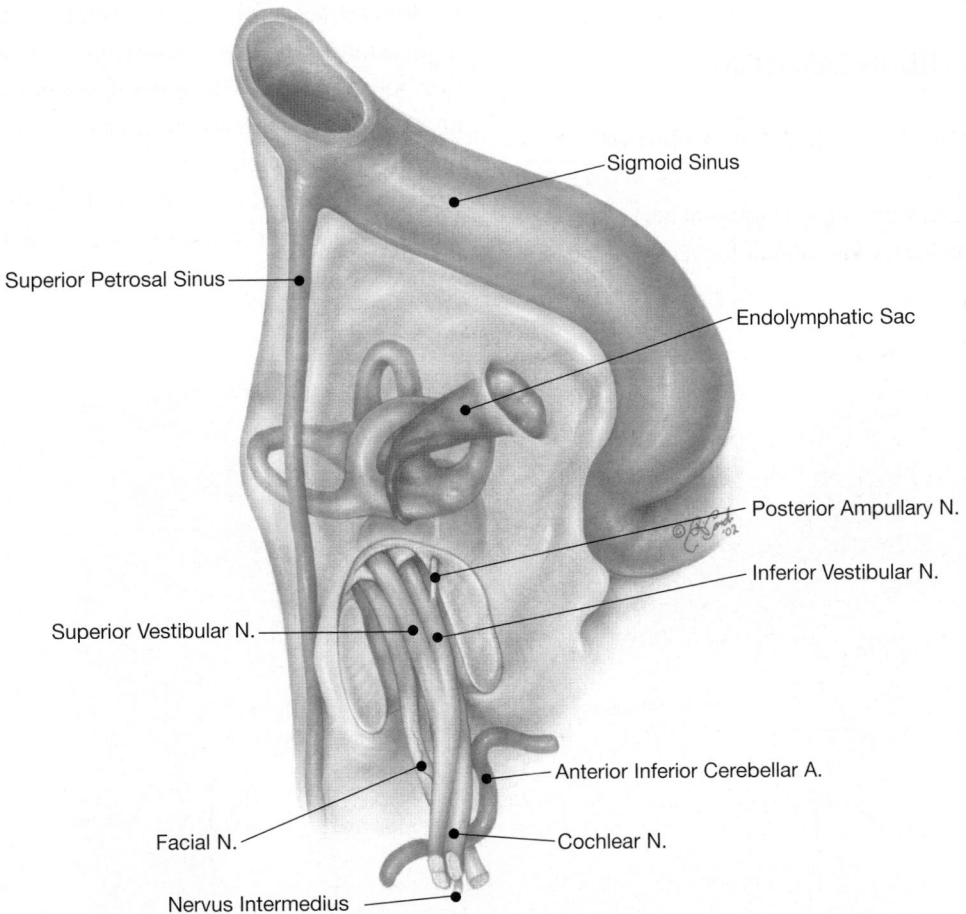

Sigmoid Sinus

Superior Petrosal Sinus

Endolymphatic Sac

Posterior Ampullary N.

Inferior Vestibular N.

Superior Vestibular N.

Anterior Inferior Cerebellar A.

Facial N.

Cochlear N.

Nervus Intermedius

Figure 2–19 The rotation of the facial, cochlear, and vestibular nerves as they traverse the internal auditory canal. After Nadol JB Jr, Schuknecht HF, editors. Surgery of the ear and temporal bone. New York: Raven Press; 1993.

considerable interindividual variability. The porus is the posterior cranial fossa opening of the canal, whereas the canal abuts the bony labyrinth at its fundus. At the fundus, the vestibular, facial, and cochlear nerves are in a constant anatomic relationship that is determined by the horizontal (falciform) crest and the vertical crest ("Bill's bar") (see Figure 2–5, B). Progressing medially from the fundus, the nerves rotate, with fusion of the cochlear and vestibular nerves (Figure 2–19), so that the facial nerve assumes a location anterior to the cochleovestibular nerve bundle, whereas the cochlear nerve moves to lie inferior to the vestibular nerve.

Bill's bar is a useful landmark in translabyrinthine surgery of the cerebellopontine angle as it separates the superior vestibular nerve from the anteriorly located facial nerve. Although the medial anatomic relationships of the cochlear, vestibular, and facial nerves are useful in vestibular nerve section surgery, these relationships can undergo considerable distortion in the face of a cerebellopontine angle tumor.

NEUROANATOMY

Trigeminal and Abducens Nerves

The gasserian ganglion of the trigeminal nerve occupies Meckel's cave on the middle cranial fossa face of the tem-

poral bone, anterolateral to the petrous apex. The abducens (sixth cranial) nerve runs in Dorello's canal beneath the posterior petroclinoid (Gruber's) ligament. Petrous apicitis, with its attendant dural and venous inflammation, can manifest with purulent otorrhea, retro-orbital pain, and abducens palsy.

Facial Nerve

The facial nerve (the seventh cranial nerve) innervates structures derived from Reichert's cartilage. Three nuclei give rise to the fibers of the facial nerve: its motor nucleus in the caudal pons, the superior salivatory nucleus that is dorsal to the motor nucleus, and the nucleus of the solitary tract in the medulla oblongata. The superior aspect of the motor nucleus, innervating the frontalis and orbicularis oculi muscles, receives both crossed and uncrossed input from the motor cortex, whereas the inferior portion receives only ipsilateral input.

Five fiber types make up the trunk of the facial nerve. Its special visceral efferent fibers supply the facial expression, stapedius, stylohyoid, and digastric (posterior belly) muscles. Its general visceral efferent fibers go to the lacrimal, nasal cavity seromucinous, submaxillary, and sublingual glands. The taste (sensory) fibers of the facial nerve derive from the anterior two-thirds of the tongue, tonsillar fossae, and posterior palate, whereas its somatic sensory fibers emanate from the EAC

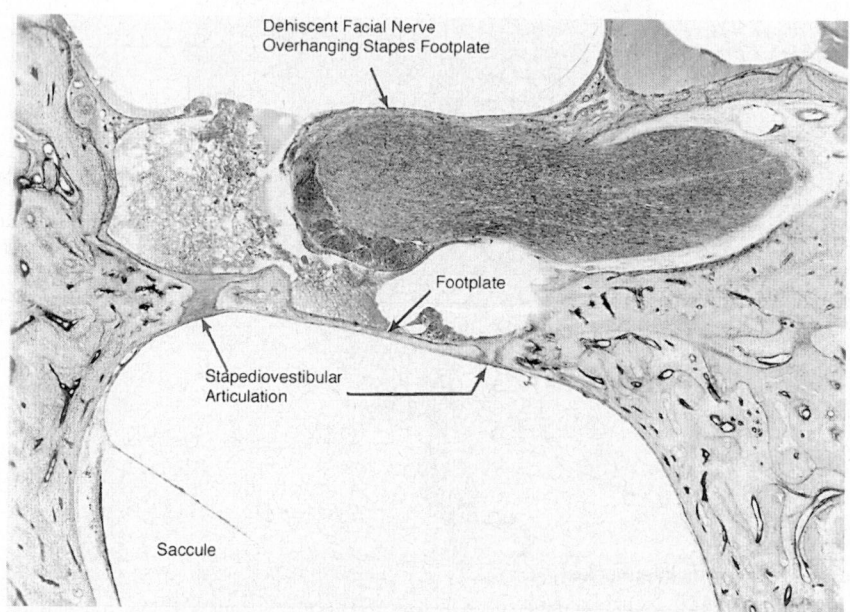

Figure 2–20   The facial nerve is dehiscent at the oval window. Reproduced with permission from Gulya AJ, Schuknecht HF. Anatomy of the temporal bone with surgical implications. 2nd ed. Pearl River (NY): Parthenon Press; 1995.

and concha. Visceral afferent fibers arise from the mucosa of the nose, pharynx, and palate.

The course of the facial nerve is divided into five segments. Its intracranial segment stretches 24 mm from the pons to the porus of the IAC. The intracanalicular segment traverses the IAC; at the fundus, it occupies the anterosuperior quadrant, where it is joined by the nervus intermedius. The shortest segment is the labyrinthine segment, running 4 mm from the beginning of the fallopian canal to the geniculate ganglion. The tympanic segment is roughly 13 mm long and courses in the medial wall of the tympanic cavity, superior to the cochleariform process and oval window. The mastoid segment spans the 20-mm distance from the second genu (at the lateral semicircular canal) to the stylomastoid foramen.

The facial nerve may follow an anomalous course. One such alternate path takes the tympanic segment of the facial nerve anterior and inferior to the oval window.[14] In another variant, the mastoid segment of the facial nerve bulges more posteriorly and laterally than usual as it runs inferior to the prominence of the lateral semicircular canal.[15] Rarely, the vertical segment of the facial nerve may be bipartite or even tripartite.

The fallopian canal has numerous gaps, or dehiscences, which render the facial nerve liable to injury. The tympanic segment over the oval window is the most likely site to be dehiscent; in one series, this site comprised 66% of dehiscences.[16] In approximately 75% of cases, the dehiscence at the oval window is bilateral.[17] On occasion, the facial nerve can protrude through the gap (Figure 2–20) to present as a middle ear mass.[18]

The subarachnoid space of the facial nerve usually extends no further than the junction of its labyrinthine and tympanic segments.[19] Occasionally, it extends into the geniculate ganglion and, rarely, onto the lateral aspect of the tympanic segment. Gacek theorized that the subarachnoid space extending onto the tympanic segment may spontaneously fistulize into the middle ear, resulting in cerebrospinal fluid otorrhea.[19] Alternatively, he suggested that it may gradually enlarge, presenting as a mass lesion with erosion or enlargement of the fallopian canal.

There are three intratemporal branches of the facial nerve: the greater petrosal nerve, nerve to the stapedius muscle, and chorda tympani nerve. The greater petrosal nerve arises from the anterior aspect of the geniculate gan-

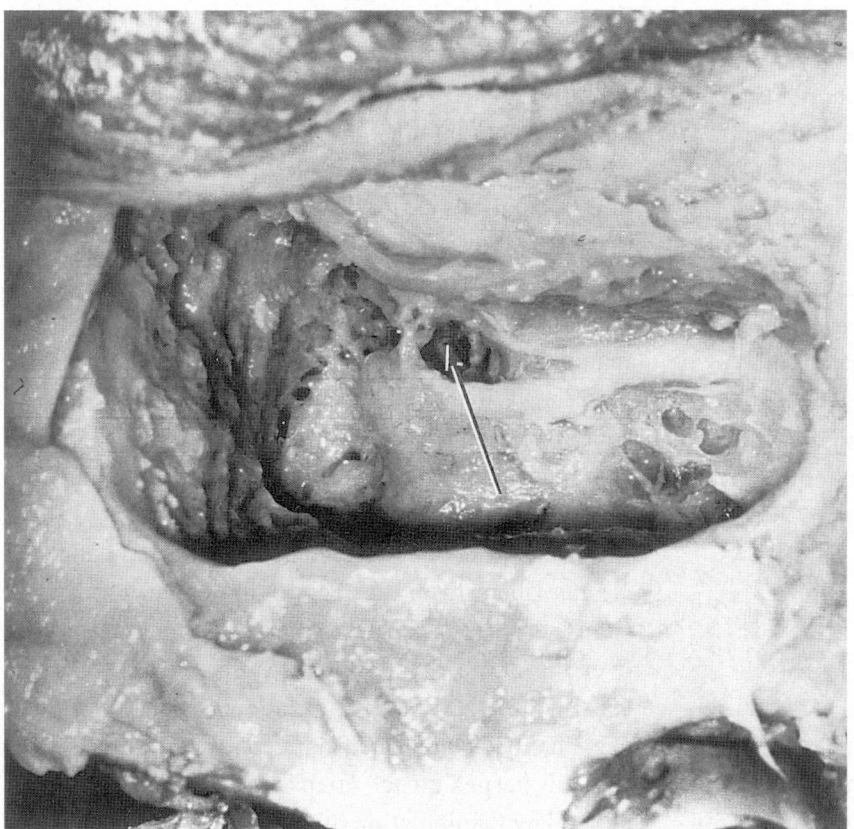

Figure 2–21 The facial recess (*arrow*) lies between the facial and chorda tympani nerves. The incudostapedial joint is visible just to the right of the arrowhead. Reproduced with permission from Gulya AJ, Schuknecht HF. Anatomy of the temporal bone with surgical implications. 2nd ed. Pearl River (NY): Parthenon Press; 1995.

glion (see Figure 2–14) and emerges onto the floor of the middle cranial fossa via the facial hiatus; in some cases, the geniculate ganglion and the greater petrosal nerve may lie exposed in the floor of the middle cranial fossa, lacking their usual bony covering. The nerve to the stapedius muscle arises from the mastoid segment of the facial nerve near the pyramidal eminence. The chorda tympani nerve, the sensory bundle making up some 10% of the cross-sectional area of the facial nerve, usually separates from the main trunk of the facial nerve approximately 4 mm proximal to the stylomastoid foramen (Figure 2–21); rarely, the chorda tympani and facial nerves separate extratemporally, and the chorda tympani re-enters the temporal bone via its own canal. Alternatively, the chorda may not separate from the facial nerve until it reaches the level of the lateral semicircular canal. After vertically ascending the temporal bone in a canal that lies lateral and anterior to the facial nerve, the chorda enters the tympanic cavity at the iter chordae posterius. It crosses lateral to the long process of the incus and medial to the malleus to exit the tympanic cavity via the iter chordae anterius (canal of Huguier) and the petrotympanic (glaserian) fissure. Rarely, the chorda may pass lateral to the malleus and the tympanic membrane.

The facial recess (see Figure 2–21) is a triangular area inferior to the incudal fossa, lateral to the facial nerve (vertical segment), and medial to the chorda tympani nerve; it is used in intact canal wall mastoidectomy to gain access to the middle ear.

The nervus intermedius (nerve of Wrisberg) carries the taste, secretory, and sensory fibers of the facial nerve. In the IAC, the nervus intermedius runs as a separate nerve between the facial and superior vestibular nerves. In the temporal bone, the nervus intermedius is within the facial nerve, occupying its dorsal aspect in the tympanic segment and its posterolateral aspect in the mastoid segment. The chorda tympani nerve represents the separation of the sensory fibers at the inferior mastoid segment.

Cochlear Nerve

The cochlear nerve arises from the spiral ganglion neurons. At the fundus of the IAC, the cochlear nerve is in the anteroinferior compartment. It rotates as it heads toward the porus and enters the brainstem a few mil-limeters caudal to the root entry zone of the trigeminal nerve.

Vestibular Nerves

The superior and inferior vestibular nerves occupy the posterior half of the IAC. The structures innervated by the superior vestibular nerve are the superior and lateral semicircular canals, utricular macula, and superior portion of the saccular macula. The inferior vestibular nerve innervates the inferior saccular macula and, by its posterior ampullary branch, the posterior semicircular canal. The posterior ampullary nerve separates from the main trunk of the inferior vestibular nerve a few millimeters from the porus of the IAC and traverses the singular canal to the posterior canal ampulla.

Sensory Nerves of the Tympanomastoid Compartment

Jacobson's nerve (the tympanic branch of cranial nerve IX) arises from the inferior (petrosal) ganglion of cranial nerve IX, which is located in the petrosal fossula of the jugulocarotid crest. It enters the tympanic cavity, accompanied by the inferior tympanic artery, through the inferior tympanic canaliculus. Subsequently, the nerve climbs the promontory and medial wall of the tympanic cavity to meet with the caroticotympanic nerves originating from the pericarotid plexus. The union of the preganglionic parasympathetic fibers of Jacobson's nerve and the postganglionic sympathetic caroticotympanic nerves at the tympanic plexus results in the formation of the lesser petrosal nerve. The lesser petrosal nerve heads to the floor of the middle cranial fossa adjacent to, or even within, the semicanal of the tensor tympani muscle. Jacobson's nerve mediates otalgia referred from the pharynx.

Arnold's nerve, the auricular branch of cranial nerve X, has fibers from the facial, glossopharyngeal, and vagus nerves. It originates in the jugular foramen, passes over the dome of the jugular bulb (via the mastoid canaliculus), and enters the fallopian canal. Arnold's nerve has been implicated in herpetic involvement of the EAC in herpes zoster oticus[20] and the cough reflex elicited by manipulation of the skin of the EAC.

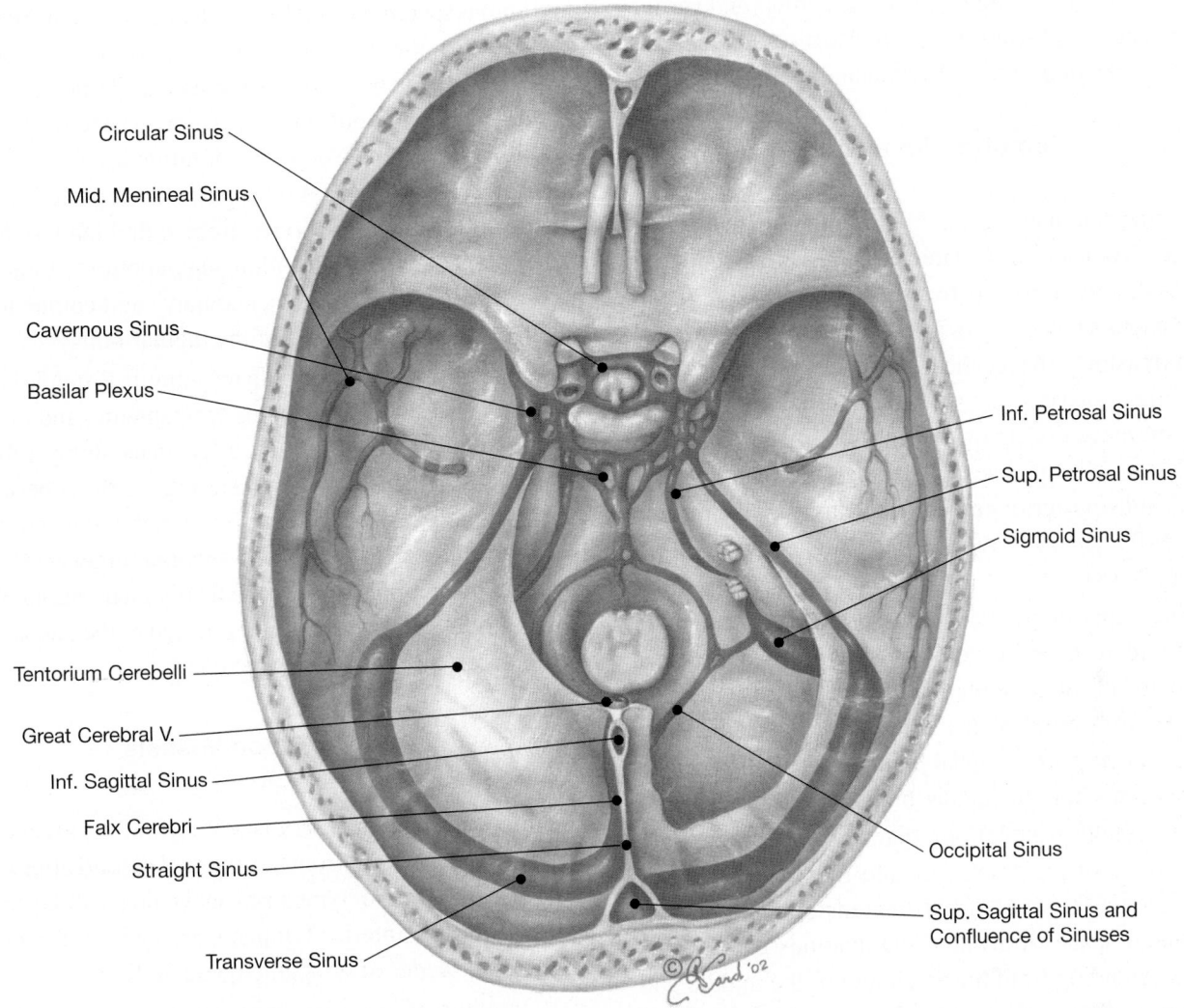

Circular Sinus

Mid. Menineal Sinus

Cavernous Sinus

Basilar Plexus

Inf. Petrosal Sinus

Sup. Petrosal Sinus

Sigmoid Sinus

Tentorium Cerebelli

Great Cerebral V.

Inf. Sagittal Sinus

Falx Cerebri

Straight Sinus

Occipital Sinus

Sup. Sagittal Sinus and Confluence of Sinuses

Transverse Sinus

Figure 2–22 The cranium has been opened and its contents removed to reveal the sinuses and related structures.

VASCULAR ANATOMY

Temporal Bone Arteries

The internal carotid artery enters the temporal bone through the external carotid foramen, located just anteromedial to the styloid process. As it ascends in its intrapetrous segment, it passes first anterior to the tympanic cavity and cochlea and then bends (its "knee") to run medial to the eustachian tube and inferomedial to the semicanal of the tensor tympani muscle (see Figures 2–9 and 2–10). The artery climbs to exit the temporal bone at the internal carotid foramen. Accompanying the artery throughout its intrapetrous course are a venous

and a neural (sympathetic) plexus. The bony shell protecting the artery is thin (often less than 0.5 mm thick) and can be dehiscent in 6% of cases.[21] In the course of surgery for chronic otitis media or cholesteatoma, the potential for injuring the internal carotid artery mandates gentle dissection in the medial wall of the eustachian tube.

Aberrant development of the carotid artery (see Chapter 1) can result in an artery that follows an anomalous course lateral and posterior to the vestibular line (a vertical line through the lateral aspect of the vestibule in the coronal plane).

The anterior inferior cerebellar artery (AICA) often extends a loop into the IAC. Its role of such a loop in the generation of symptoms such as tinnitus and vertigo is debatable.[22] Disruption of AICA causes hemorrhage in and infarction of the labyrinth and brainstem.

Temporal Bone Veins

The three dominant sinuses of the temporal bone are the sigmoid (portion of the lateral venous sinus), superior petrosal, and inferior petrosal (Figure 2–22). The lateral venous sinus occupies an S-shaped sulcus in the posterior mastoid—hence the term sigmoid—as it extends from the transverse sinus to the internal jugular vein. This drainage system on the right is larger than that on the left in 75% of cases.[23] The angle between the sigmoid sinus/posterior cranial fossa dura and the middle cranial fossa dura is known as the angle of Citelli (see Figure 2–18).

The superior petrosal sinus drains the cavernous sinus into the lateral venous sinus as it runs in the superior petrosal sulcus at the junction of the posterior and middle fossa dural plates. The inferior petrosal sinus courses in the petro-occipital suture line. It drains the cavernous sinus into the jugular bulb.

Arachnoid granulations (pacchionian bodies) are projections of pia-arachnoid into the venous sinuses and venous lacunae and are extensions of the subarachnoid space. Arachnoid granulations can also be found extending from the arachnoid of the middle and posterior cranial fossae into the adjacent mastoid air cells. Gacek has linked arachnoid granulations to adult-onset spontaneous cerebrospinal fluid otorrhea.[24,25]

The jugular bulb is interposed between the sigmoid sinus and internal jugular vein; in contrast to the thick wall of the sigmoid sinus, which quite readily contracts with bipolar cautery, the thin wall of the bulb does not and is prone to rupture with manipulation. The venous hemorrhage of a torn or incised sigmoid sinus can be controlled with pressure applied via a large square of gelatin sponge (Gelfoam®) surmounted by a neurosurgical cottonoid; several minutes after the bleeding has stopped, the cottonoid can be removed safely, and, leaving the Gelfoam in place, surgery can be resumed.

The jugular bulb displays considerable variability in its position relative to the facial nerve and in its penetration into the tympanic cavity. A high-riding jugular bulb (one extending to or above the level of the inferior tympanic annulus) has been reported in 3.5 to 5% of temporal bone specimens studied[26,27] and may occur more frequently on the right side.[27] Its bony covering is very thin— only 0.1 to 0.3 mm. An alternate definition of the high-riding jugular bulb encompasses one encroaching to within 2 mm or less on the inferior aspect of the IAC.[28] Using this definition, one study reported that two-thirds of temporal bones from individuals older than 6 years housed a high-riding jugular bulb.[28] A jugular diverticulum is a "venous anomaly" and comprises an "irregular outpouching" of the jugular bulb.[29]

The high-riding jugular bulb may mimic a middle ear vascular mass, such as a glomus tympanicum, and may be the source of hemorrhage in tympanostomy tube insertion. Jugular bulbs reaching as high as the superior aspect of the IAC have been encountered in the course of posterior fossa vestibular schwannoma surgery,[23] rendering exposure of the IAC technically challenging. A jugular diverticulum has been implicated as the etiology of Meniere's disease–like symptoms.[29]

Middle Ear Blood Vessels

The inferior tympanic artery is a branch of the ascending pharyngeal artery (from the external carotid artery). It traverses the inferior tympanic canaliculus with Jacobson's nerve. The inferior tympanic artery is an important arterial feeder of tympanic paragangliomas.

A number of branches from the external carotid artery contribute to the anastomotic network of the tympanic cavity, including the anterior tympanic artery, deep auricular artery, mastoid artery, stylomastoid artery, superficial petrosal artery, and tubal artery.

Labyrinthine Vessels

The majority of the blood supply to the membranous labyrinth stems from the labyrinthine artery, a branch of the AICA. The subarcuate artery arises either as a branch of the labyrinthine artery, or of the AICA, or as multiple branches of both; it passes within the arch of the superior semicircular canal.

Facial Nerve Vessels

The facial nerve has both an intrinsic and an extrinsic vascular system. The extrinsic system consists of the

AICA, supplying the intracranial segment of cranial nerve VII; the labyrinthine artery, supplying the intracanalicular segment; the superficial petrosal artery, which supplies the geniculate ganglion and the superior portion of the mastoid segment of the facial nerve; and the stylomastoid artery, which supplies the inferior mastoid segment of the nerve.

The intrinsic network, running within the nerve, is generally thought to be most poorly developed at its labyrinthine segment, in contrast to the tympanic and mastoid segments.[30]

REFERENCES

1. Gulya AJ, Schuknecht HF. Anatomy of the temporal bone with surgical implications. 2nd ed. Pearl River (NY): Parthenon Publishing Group, Inc.; 1995.

2. Kveton JF, Cooper MH. Microsurgical anatomy of the jugular foramen region. Am J Otol 1988;9:109–12.

3. Kveton JF. Anatomy of the jugular foramen: the neurotologic perspective. Op Tech ORL-HNS 1996;7:95–8.

4. Saleh E, Naguib M, Aristegui M, et al. Lower skull base: anatomic study with surgical implications. Ann Otol Rhinol Laryngol 1995;104:57–61.

5. Aslan A, Falcioni M, Balyan FR, et al. The cochlear aqueduct: an important landmark in lateral skull base surgery. Otolaryngol Head Neck Surg 1998;118:532–6.

6. Nomura Y. Otological significance of the round window. Adv Otorhinolaryngol 1984;33:1–162.

7. Lim DJ. Functional morphology of the lining membrane of the middle ear and eustachian tube. An overview. Ann Otol Rhinol Laryngol 1974;83 Suppl 11:5–22.

8. Lindsay JR. Suppuration in the petrous pyramid. Ann Otol Rhinol Laryngol 1938;47:3–36.

9. Saim L, McKenna MJ, Nadol JB Jr. Tubal and tympanic openings of the peritubal cells: implications for cerebrospinal fluid otorrhea. Am J Otol 1996;17:335–9.

10. Minor LB, Solomon D, Zinreich JS, Zee DS. Sound- and/or pressure-induced vertigo due to bone dehiscence of the superior semicircular canal. Arch Otolaryngol Head Neck Surg 1998;124:249–58.

11. Carey JP, Minor LB, Nager GT. Dehiscence or thinning of bone overlying the superior semicircular canal in a temporal bone survey. Arch Otolaryngol Head Neck Surg 2000;126:137–47.

12. Gacek RR, Leipzig B. Congenital cerebrospinal fluid otorrhea. Ann Otol Rhinol Laryngol 1979;88:358–65.

13. El Shazly MAR, Linthicum FH Jr. Microfissures of the temporal bone: do they have any clinical significance? Am J Otol 1991;12:169–71.

14. Hough JVD. Malformations and anatomical variations seen in the middle ear during the operation for mobilization of the stapes. Laryngoscope 1958;68:1337–79.

15. Procter B, Nager GT. The facial canal: normal anatomy, variations and anomalies. Ann Otol Rhinol Laryngol 1982;91 Suppl 97:33–61.

16. Baxter A. Dehiscence of the fallopian canal: an anatomical study. J Laryngol Otol 1971;85:587–94.

17. Moreano EH, Paparella MM, Zelterman D, Goycoolea MV. Prevalence of facial canal dehiscence and of persistent stapedial artery in the human middle ear: a report of 1000 temporal bones. Laryngoscope 1994;104:309–20.

18. Johnsson L-G, Kingsley TC. Herniation of the facial nerve in the middle ear. Arch Otolaryngol 1970;91:598–602.

19. Gacek RR. Anatomy and significance of the subarachnoid space in the fallopian canal. Am J Otol 1998;19:358–64.

20. Eshraghi AA, Buchman C, Telischi FF. Facial nerve branch to the external auditory canal. American Neurotology Society 2001 Annual Meeting abstracts. http://itsa.ucsf.edu/~ajo/ANS/ANSspr21ab.html (accessed Mar 31, 2001).

21. Moreano EH, Paparella MM, Zelterman D. Goycoolea MV. Prevalence of carotid canal dehiscence in the human middle ear: a report of 1000 temporal bones. Laryngoscope 1994;104:612–8.

22. Makins AE, Nikolopoulus TP, Ludman C, O'Donoghue GM. Is there a correlation between vascular loops and unilateral auditory symptoms? Laryngoscope 1998;108:1739–42.

23. Kennedy DW, El-Sirsy HH, Nager GT. The jugular bulb in otologic surgery: anatomic, clinical, and surgical considerations. Otolaryngol Head Neck Surg 1986;94:6–15.

24. Gacek RR. Arachnoid granulation cerebrospinal fluid otorrhea. Ann Otol Rhinol Laryngol 1990;99:854–62.

25. Gacek RR. Evaluation and management of temporal bone arachnoid granulations. Arch Otolaryngol Head Neck Surg 1992;118:327–32.

26. Overton SB, Ritter FN. A high placed jugular bulb in the middle ear: a clinical and temporal bone study. Laryngoscope 1973;83:1986–91.

27. Subotic R. The high position of the jugular bulb. Acta Otolaryngol (Stockh) 1979;87:340–4.

28. Rausch SD, Xu W-Z, Nadol JB Jr. High jugular bulb: implications for posterior fossa neurotologic and cranial base surgery. Ann Otol Rhinol Laryngol 1993;102:100–7.

29. Jahrsdoerfer RA, Cain WS, Cantrell RW. Endolymphatic duct obstruction from a jugular bulb diverticulum. Ann Otol Rhinol Laryngol 1981;90:619–23.

30. Balkany T, Fradis M, Jafek BW, Rucker NC. Intrinsic vasculature of the labyrinthine segment of the facial nerve—implications for site of lesion in Bell's palsy. Otolaryngol Head Neck Surg 1991;104:20–3.

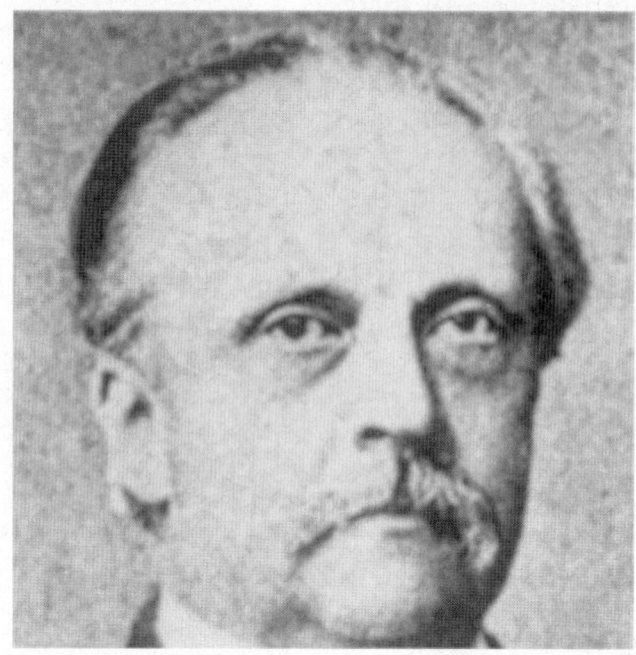

Hermann von Helmholtz (1821–1894). Foremost physiologist of the 19th century, who developed the theory of the mechanics of the middle ear transformer.

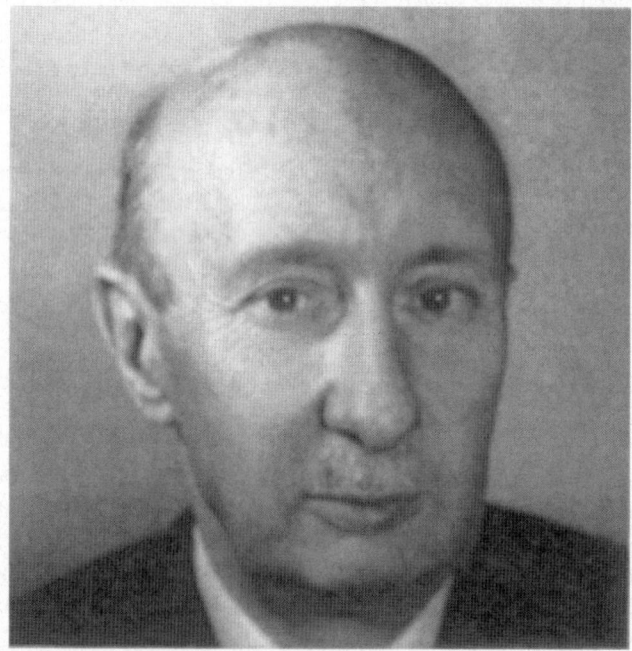

Georg von Békésy (1899–1972). Awarded the Nobel Prize in 1961 for his fundamental studies of the physiology of the middle and inner ears.

3

Auditory Physiology

SAUMIL N. MERCHANT, MD
JOHN J. ROSOWSKI, PhD

Two of the primary tasks of the otologic surgeon include *diagnosis*, the understanding of how pathologic variations in external and middle ear structure lead to hearing loss, and *surgical treatment* of external and middle ears ravaged by disease, such that the reconstructed ear has near-normal mechanical and acoustic function. The authors believe that a basic knowledge of physiology of the normal ear and pathophysiology of the diseased ear is necessary for proper diagnosis and surgical treatment of otologic disorders. This chapter provides a review of some fundamental principles of acoustics that are relevant to sound transmission in normal, diseased, and reconstructed middle ears. The review concentrates on middle ear mechanics and does not cover the physiologic maintenance of middle ear gases or static air pressures. The chapter is meant as a guide rather than an exhaustive treatise and has been written with clinicians as its primary audience.

HISTORICAL ASPECTS

The history of otology, audiology, and acoustics has been documented by several authors.[1–5] The early events may be summarized as follows[6]:

Early Greek physicians (fifth century BC) knew of the tympanic membrane and middle ear space. The Greeks considered the middle ear space to be the seat of hearing. Galen (131 to 201 AD) described the auditory nerve but suggested that it originated in the middle ear. The Renaissance produced several great anatomists who described the ear in detail. Vesalius, in 1543, described the malleus and incus. In 1546, Ingrassia described the stapes and the oval and round windows. In 1561, Fallopius named the cochlea, the labyrinth, and the canal for the facial nerve. Eustachius described the auditory tube, which bears his name, in 1564.

These anatomic discoveries formed the basis for tracing the pathway of sound through the ear by Coiter in 1566 and the later, more elaborate description of Duverney in 1683. Neither Coiter nor Duverney appreciated the impedance-matching function of the middle ear because both thought the inner ear was filled with air. That the labyrinth contained fluid was established by Meckel, who, in 1777, demonstrated that frozen temporal bones were always filled with ice. The microscopic structures of the inner ear were first described by Corti in 1851, followed by Retzius's description of hair cells and their innervation by auditory nerve fibers in 1892.

Helmholtz, in 1868,[7] initiated the period of modern auditory physiology by defining the principles of impedance matching and how the middle ear served this function. Stating the problem of matching the transmission of sound in low-impedance air to the high impedance of the fluid-filled cochlea, Helmholtz conceived of three means by which this pressure transformation takes place: a lever action that resulted from the shape of the drumhead itself, a lever effect of the ossicular chain, and a hydraulic action of the large tympanic membrane acting on the small stapes footplate.

In the twentieth century, many investigators expanded, corrected, or quantified these basic concepts. Notable contributors to our knowledge of middle ear mechanics include Nobel laureate Georg von Békésy, Ernst Glenn Wever, Merle Lawrence, Juergen Tonndorf, Shyam Khanna, William Peake, Aage Møller, and Josef

Zwislocki. Clinical observations and surgical advances that have stimulated physiologic investigations have included the question of altered sound conduction as a result of middle ear diseases and the restoration of hearing in pathologic middle ears through tympanoplasty and stapedectomy procedures.

SOUND AND ITS MEASUREMENT

Sound results when particles of a medium are set into vibration. For example, the vibrating tines of a struck tuning fork produce backward and forward motions of the air particles that surround the tines (Figure 3–1). The particles set in motion by the vibrating tines then push on adjacent air particles, where the push is proportional to the sound pressure, setting the next layer of particles into back and forth motion. The physical disturbance of sound pressure and particle motion, not the particles themselves, propagates through the medium as succeeding layers of air particles are set into vibration. The *frequency* of the resulting sound is the number of cycles per second of the back and forth motion of the air particles. The unit of frequency is Hertz (with 1 Hz = 1 cycle per second). The amplitude of the propagating physical disturbance can be quantified either in terms of the sound pressure acting on the particles or the amplitude of the particle motion. In practice, it is easier to measure pressure variations than to measure the motion of the particles; hence, sound pressure is the primary measure of sound.

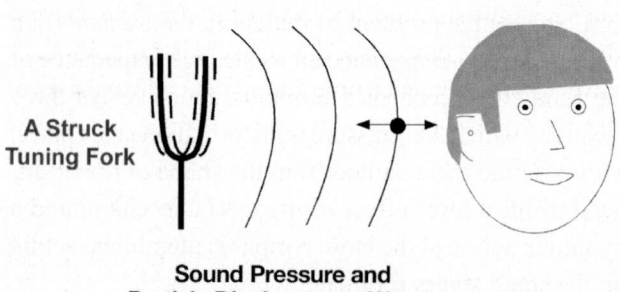

**Sound Pressure and
Particle Displacement Waves**

Figure 3–1 The vibrating tines of a struck tuning fork set nearby air particles into motion with a frequency equal to the natural frequency of the fork. The air particles that are set in motion push on adjacent particles and so forth, resulting in a propagating physical disturbance that is perceived as sound. The *black dot with the arrow* is a hypothetical air particle set into back and forth motion by the waves (*curved lines*) propagating from the struck fork.

Sound pressure refers to the magnitude of the temporal variations in pressure produced around ambient static pressure (Figure 3–2). A pressure is a force per area. The international unit of pressure is the pascal, where 1 Pa = one newton of force per square meter of area. The quietest sounds heard by a human ear are of very low pressure; the change in pressure associated with sound at the threshold of hearing for a 1,000-Hz tone is about 20 μPa (or two-tenths of a billionth atmospheres). There are many ways to quantify sound pressure, the most common being in terms of the root mean square (rms) or the root of the mean squared deviation in pressure. For a sinusoidal pure tone like that in Figure 3–2, A, the sound pressure can be quantified in terms of the peak, peak-to-peak, or rms measures of amplitude. In the case of sinusoids, there is a fixed relationship between the three different measures, and for the tone shown in Figure 3–2, A, these different measures yield values of 1, 2, or 0.71 Pa, respectively. The intensity or power within a complex sound waveform, as illustrated in Figure 3–2, B, is not readily quantified by peak measures but is well described by the rms value of the sound pressure. In fact, the rms sound pressure of this complex sound is 0.71 Pa, a value identical to that of the tonal sound pressure shown in Figure 3–2, A. In general, then, sound pressure measurements are usually quantified in terms of the rms pressure.

The human auditory system is sensitive to a wide range of sound pressures. Conversational speech is typically 100 to 500 times threshold, music often contains sound pressures that are 10,000 times threshold, and jet engines, guns, and fireworks can produce pressures that are more than 1 million times threshold. Because of the ear's sensitivity to pressures that vary by more than a million times, and because the human ear can discriminate fractional changes in pressure, it is common to use a logarithmic scale to grade sound pressures.[8] The decibel (one-tenth of a Bell) is a logarithmic measure of relative energy where 10 dB (1 Bell) represent an increase over a given reference energy level of 1 order of magnitude (ie, 1 common log unit or a factor of 10). The reference level for sound pressure level (SPL) is 2×10^{-5} rms Pa, and since energy is proportional to pressure squared,

Sound level in dB SPL=

$$10\log_{10}\left[\frac{X}{0.00002\,rmsPa}\right]^{2}=20\log_{10}\left[\frac{X}{0.00002\,rmsPa}\right]$$

A

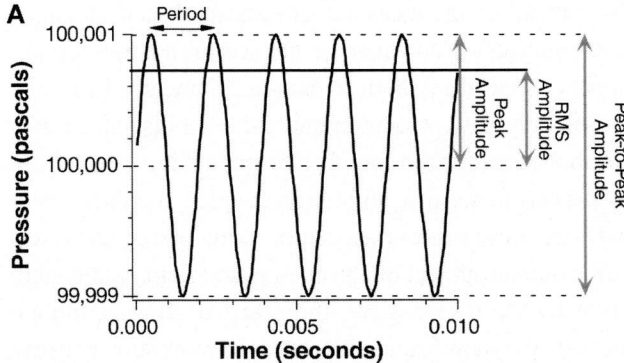

B

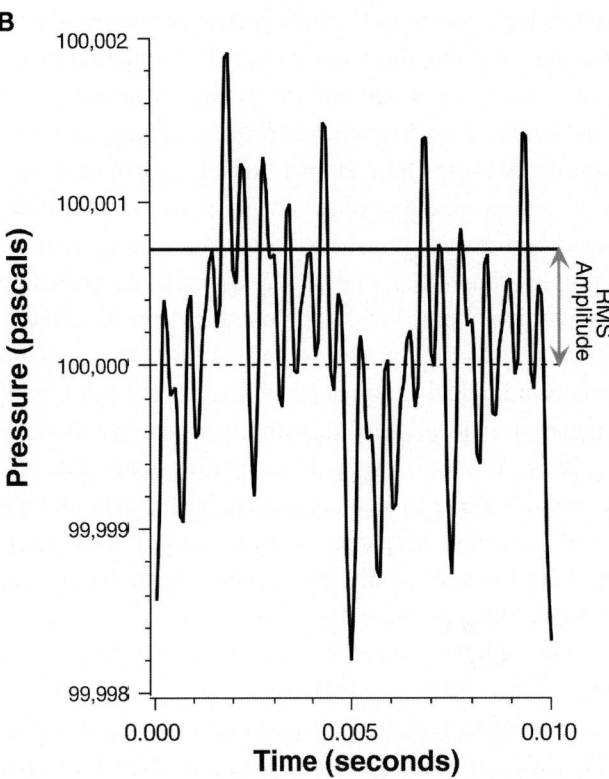

Figure 3–2 Two patterns of temporal variations in air pressure produced by sounds. The schematic in *A* depicts that produced by a 512-Hz pure tone, whereas *B* depicts that produced by a complex sound. The absolute value of pressure is scaled in both plots; therefore, the sound-induced variations occur around a static value of 100,000 Pa = 1 atmosphere. The sound pressure corresponds to amplitude of variations around the static value. In both *A* and *B*, although the static atmospheric pressure is 100,000 Pa, the amplitude of the sound pressure is on the order of 1 Pa. *A*, The pressure variations are those of a 512-Hz pure tone. The pressure varies sinusoidally with a period of $1/512 = 0.00195$ s. The amplitude of pressure variations around the static value can be quantified in terms of the peak-to-peak value of 2 Pa, the peak value of 1 Pa, or the root mean square (rms) value of 0.71 Pa. (The rms value is the square root of the mean of the squared pressure deviations from static values averaged over some time. In the case of a sinusoid, a convenient averaging time is an integral number of periods of the sine wave. With sinusoidal sound pressures, the rms value equals the peak amplitude/$\sqrt{2}$.) *B*, The pressure variations are those of a complex sound with many irregular risings and fallings of the sound pressure. With this kind of sound, peak amplitude and peak-to-peak amplitude are poor indicators of the average sound level. However, rms is an excellent measure as long as one specifies an averaging time. In the case depicted, the rms sound pressure was computed over the 0.01-second time window. Note that the sound pressure in *B* has the same rms value as the sound pressure in *A*.

where *X* is the sound pressure in rms Pa and 0.00002 rms Pa = 2×10^{-5} rms Pa is the reference pressure. Different dB sound pressure scales use different reference pressures. For example, the dB hearing level (dB HL) scale of the clinical audiogram uses the average sound pressure threshold of the normal population at a given frequency as the reference pressure. The sound pressure level of both sounds shown in Figure 3–2 is 91 dB SPL, where $91 = 20 \log_{10} (0.71/0.00002)$. The loudness of a sound is a monotonic function of the sound pressure; for mid-level sounds, a 20-dB increase in sound pressure produces about a factor of six increase in loudness.[9] The sound pressures of various commonly experienced sounds are noted in terms of rms Pa and dB SPL in Table 3–1.

Sound is a variation in pressure with time. A pure tone, as in Figure 3–2, A, is a sound in which the relationship between sound pressure and time can be described by a sine function; for example,

$$p(t) = A \cos(2\pi ft + \phi)$$

where we use the cosine function that is the common standard in engineering applications, *p(t)* describes the variation in sound pressure with time, *A* describes the peak amplitude or magnitude of the pressure, *f* is the *frequency* of the sinusoid, and ϕ is the *phase*. The phase ϕ determines the time when the pressure is maximum relative to some reference time zero. The relative phases of the sound pressure in the ear canal and the mechanical and neural responses within the ear are useful in deter-

Table 3–1 SOUND PRESSURES OF COMMON SOUNDS		
Approximate Sound Level		
rms Pa	**dB SPL**	**Sound Source**
0.0001–0.0002	14–20	Just audible whisper
0.002–0.02	40–60	Conversational speech
0.02–0.6	60–90	Noisy room
0.6–20	90–120	Loud music
> 20	> 120	Gunfire

mining the physical and biologic processes associated with hearing.[10,11] Also, the relative timing information in the phase is critical when waveforms are combined; two waves of the same frequency added together can sum constructively if they have similar phases, sum to near zero if the waves are out of phase and of identical amplitude, or can be somewhere in between for intermediate phases. Complex sounds (eg, Figure 3–2, B) can be described by the addition of pure tones of different frequencies and different phases. A complex sound can be broken down into its individual components (individual sinusoids with magnitude and phase information) by using a Fourier analysis. Although the ear is insensitive to the absolute phase of a single tone, a complex acoustic signal with a fixed number of frequency components of fixed magnitude can sound quite different depending on the relative phases of the components.

Although the human ear can hear sound frequencies ranging from 20 to 20,000 Hz, the ear is differentially sensitive to sounds of different frequencies, and measurements of the hearing threshold vary depending on how the sound stimulus is specified. Sound pressure thresholds (the lowest sound pressures that are audible) measured in normal young adults with pure tones of different frequencies under two different measurement conditions are shown in Figure 3–3. The lower curve depicts thresholds determined with subjects in an open space or free field,[12] where the sound pressure measurement was made at the location of the subject's head when the subject was not present. The upper curve is the American National Standards Institute[13] (ANSI) standard measurement of thresholds made under earphones, where the sound pressures are those generated by the earphones in a calibration coupler. The differences between these two curves can be explained by the effect of the human subject on the open sound field, sound gathering by the external ear, the effect of closing the ear canal by earphones, and differences in calibration between the two circumstances.[14] Both curves clearly show that normal young adult humans are most sensitive to sound frequencies of 500 to 8,000 Hz. The best frequency differs depending on the measurement circumstance, being 1,500 Hz under earphones and 4,000 Hz in the free field. At higher and lower frequencies, more sound pressure is required to be audible, and the thresholds increase steeply below 500 Hz and above 8,000 Hz.

Clinicians are most interested in how an individual's hearing threshold differs from normal; in practice, normal is defined by the ANSI standard earphone measurements shown in Figure 3–3. A powerful graphical tool for comparing two different functions is to plot their difference. The *clinical audiogram* (Figure 3–4, discussed more in Chapter 8) uses this difference technique by plotting an individual's threshold relative to the ANSI standard normal hearing level (HL). For example, a person whose hearing threshold at 1,000 Hz is 10 dB greater than the ANSI standard is assigned an HL of 10 dB at that

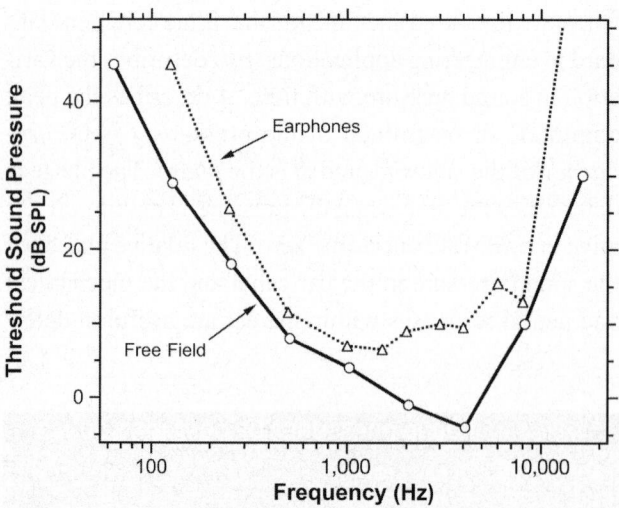

Figure 3–3 Sensitivity of the ear to sounds of different frequencies. The figure depicts measurements of auditory threshold made under earphones (ANSI standards, 1969[13]) and those made in the free field (Sivian and White, 1933[12]). The mean normal threshold at 1,000 Hz under both measurement conditions is about 0 dB SPL.

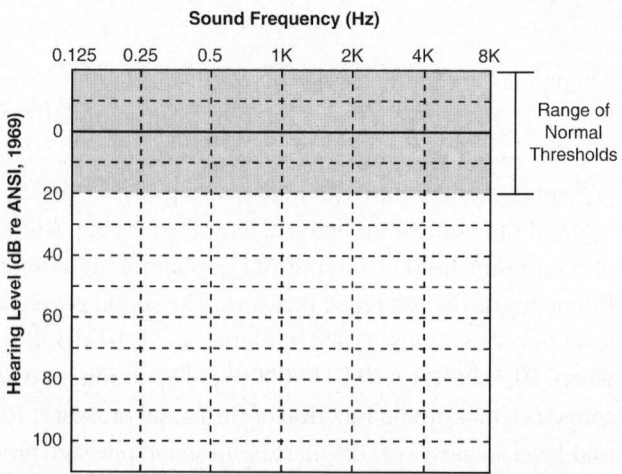

Figure 3–4 Clinical audiogram, in which an individual's hearing threshold relative to the ANSI standard normal hearing level is plotted versus frequency. The ordinate scale is inverted so that higher thresholds are plotted lower on the graph.

frequency. In clinical audiograms, threshold SPL relative to the standard HL is quantified in dB relative to normal at frequencies of octave or half-octave intervals. It is important to remember that the normal curve is based on mean hearing thresholds in normal subjects and that there is normal variation ($\pm$ 20 dB) around the mean.

The *speed or propagation velocity* of sound through a medium determines the sound *wavelength* for a given frequency, which is the distance it takes a propagating sound wave to repeat itself. Specifically, the wavelength λ equals the propagation velocity divided by sound frequency. The wavelength describes how a tone varies in space, and the relative size of the wavelength and an object's dimensions determines how sound interacts with the object. If the wavelength of a sound is at least five times larger than the largest dimension of an object, the object will have little effect on the sound; that is, as the sound propagates around the object, the sound pressure at the front and back sides of the object will be very similar to the sound pressure measured when the object is not present. On the other hand, if the wavelength is similar to or smaller than the dimensions of an object, variations in sound pressure will be introduced by the object. In general, as short-wavelength sound interacts with the object, the sound pressure along the front surface of the object will increase because of reflection of sound, and sound pressure along the back surface will be decreased because the object shields that location from the sound. A common analogy is between light and sound, where in the small-wavelength case, the object casts a sound shadow.

The size of body and ear structures relative to sound wavelength plays a significant role in determining the interaction of the ear with sounds of different frequencies.[14] A 20-Hz sound wave (wavelength of 17 meters) is affected very little by the head or body. A 200-Hz sound (wavelength of 1.7 meters) can be effectively scattered by the head and torso so that there is a small gain in sound pressure at the ear. A 2,000-Hz tone (wavelength of 17 cm) is diffracted by the head so that there is a doubling of sound pressure on the side of the head directed toward the sound source and a shadow on the opposite side of the head. A 4,000-Hz tone (8.5-cm wavelength) is scattered by the pinna such that there is an increase in sound pressure for sound sources pointing directly at the meatus and decreases in sound pressure for other directions. Another kind of wavelength interaction occurs in the external ear canal; resonances occur within the ear at frequencies where the length of the ear canal and depth of the concha are odd multiples of $\lambda/4$.[14] Table 3–2 lists some of the critical frequencies above which sound wavelengths allow interactions with various parts of the body and ear. In general, the interaction of the structures of the external ear and sound is restricted to sound frequencies of 2,000 Hz and above.

SOUND TRANSMISSION IN THE NORMAL EAR

Problem of Transferring Airborne Sound Power to the Fluids of the Inner Ear: Air-Fluid Impedance Mismatch

Acoustic signals are transmitted from the air of the external environment to the fluid-filled inner ear. The transmission of sound power at an air–fluid interface depends on the relative impedances of air and fluid. In the case of the inner ear, only about 0.1% of the power density of an incident sound wave is transmitted to the fluid, and this is equivalent to a 30-dB loss. The external and middle ears act to better match the sound-conducting properties of air and cochlear fluid by increasing the sound pressures that reach the inner ear at certain frequencies, as described below. The discussion that fol-

Frequency (Hz)	Wavelength	Anatomic Structure	Structural Dimensions
340	1 m	Torso	0.5 m
2,000	17 cm	Head	10 cm
4,000	8.5 cm	Pinna	4 cm
		Ear canal length	2.5 cm
20,000	1.7 cm	Diameter of ear canal and tympanic membrane	0.8 cm

Table 3–2 WAVELENGTHS OF SOUND AND BODY STRUCTURES WITH WHICH WAVE INTERACTIONS ARE IMPORTANT

lows is meant to be an overview, and readers seeking more detailed descriptions are referred to other sources.[15–17]

External Ear

The external ear, along with the head and body, has a significant influence on the sounds that reach the middle ear. This acoustic function of the external ear, sometimes called the *external ear gain*, can be described by a frequency- and directionally dependent alteration in the sound pressure at the tympanic membrane when compared to the sound pressure in the free field. As illustrated in Figure 3–5, when a sound source is positioned facing the ear, the external ear produces a gain of as much as 20 dB at 2,500 Hz, with less gain at lower and higher frequencies. As also illustrated in Figure 3–5, this gain results from the combination of sound scattering and diffraction around the head and torso, as well as the acoustic influence of the pinna, concha, ear canal, and middle ear load impedance. The figure illustrates the frequency dependence of these different contributions and shows how the gains add (in dB terms) to define the total external ear gain. Not shown in Figure 3–5 is how this external ear gain is directionally dependent for frequencies above 1,000 Hz. In fact, for sounds coming from the opposite side of the head, the sound pressure at the tympanic membrane can be less than the sound pressure in the stimulus (ie, the external ear gain in dB is negative).

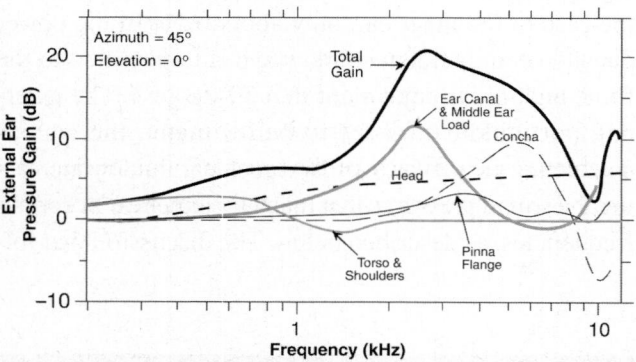

Figure 3–5 Schematic representation of the external ear gain. The total gain and the gain of individual components in dB are plotted versus frequency. The plots describe the gains for a sound source that is positioned on the same horizontal plane as the interaural axis (elevation of 0 degrees) and that is 45 degrees off the midline toward the ear that is measured (azimuth of 45 degrees). The gains of the different components are all multiplied (added in dB) together to achieve the total gain (after Shaw, 1974[14]).

Middle Ear

The middle ear couples sound signals from the ear canal to the cochlea primarily through the action of the tympanic membrane and the ossicular chain. Figure 3–6 is a schematic depicting the important structures in the

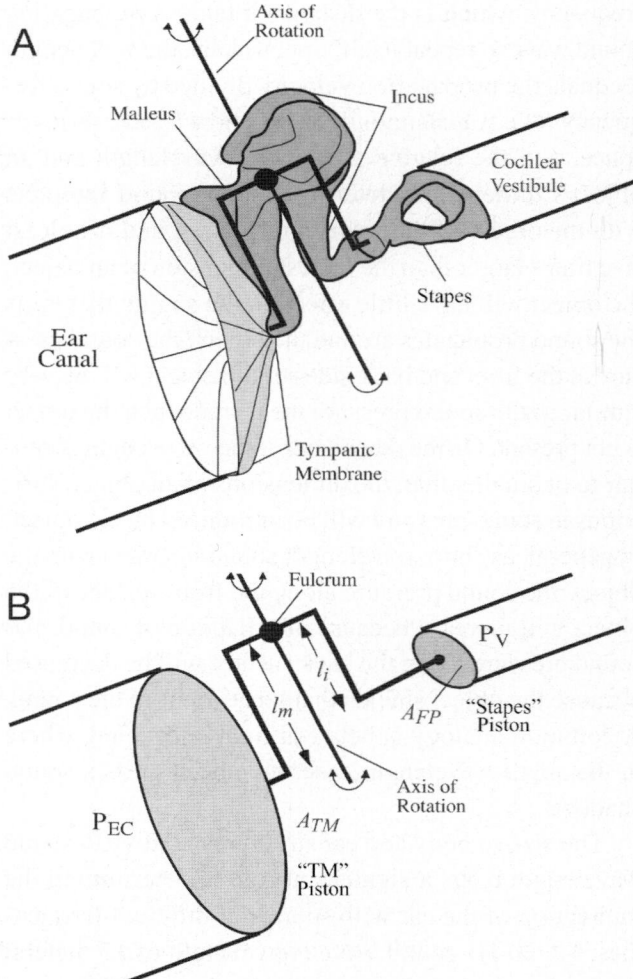

Figure 3–6 Schematics of the tympano-ossicular system (*A*) and a mechanical analog (*B*) depicting important structures in the transformation of sound power from the middle ear to the inner ear. The key transformer within the middle ear is the ratio of the tympanic membrane area (A_{TM}) to the area of the stapes footplate (A_{FP}). Another transformer is the ossicular lever: this is the lever action caused by differing lengths of the manubrium (l_m) and long process of incus (l_i) around the axis of rotation of the ossicles. This axis of rotation is an imaginary line joining the anterior malleal ligament to the incudal ligament that anchors the short process of the incus. The total middle ear sound pressure gain, which is the result of the area ratio and the ossicular lever, can be quantified and measured using the ratio of sound pressure in the vestibule (**P_V**) to the sound pressure in the ear canal (**P_{EC}**). As described in the text, the theoretical (ideal) middle ear gain is 28 dB, whereas the actual (measured) middle ear gain is only about 20 dB.

transformation of sound power from the external ear to the inner ear. (Power is a product of pressure and volume velocity. Volume velocity refers to how much particle volume flows through a given area and is equal to the product of the average linear velocity across a surface and surface area. An acoustic transformer increases either pressure or volume velocity while decreasing the other, thereby equalizing the sound power at the input and output.) The middle ear acts as a transformer to increase sound pressure at the footplate relative to that at the tympanic membrane at the expense of a decrease in stapes volume velocity relative to the tympanic membrane volume velocity. The major transformer mechanism within the middle ear is the ratio of the tympanic membrane area to the stapes footplate area (*the area ratio*). The tympanic membrane gathers force over its entire surface and then couples the gathered force to the smaller footplate of the stapes. Since pressure is force per area, and the human tympanic has an area that is 20 times larger than the footplate,[2] if the transformer action of the area ratio is "ideal," the sound pressure applied to the inner ear by the stapes footplate should be 20 times or 26 dB larger than the sound pressure at the tympanic membrane. Another transformer within the middle ear is the ossicular lever: the lever action that results from the different lengths of the rotating malleus and incus arms around the axis of rotation of the ossicles. The axis of rotation is an imaginary line joining the anterior malleal ligament to the incudal ligament that anchors the short process of the incus. The malleus and incus lever arms in humans are nearly the same length. Hence, the ratio of these lengths, which is 1.3,[18] predicts only a small, 2-dB increase in sound pressure applied by the stapes to the inner ear. Thus, if these transformers acted ideally, then the *theoretical middle ear sound pressure gain* is about 28 dB (26-dB area ratio + 2-dB ossicular lever).

Measurements of the *actual middle ear sound pressure gain* of the human middle ear performed in normal temporal bones under physiologic conditions[19] are illustrated in Figure 3–7. The data demonstrate that the pressure gain is frequency dependent, with a maximum gain of only about 20 dB near 1,000 Hz, with lower gains at other frequencies. Similar findings have also been reported by other investigators.[20,21] Thus, the measured middle ear gain is less than the 28-dB gain predicted by the ideal anatomic transformer model of Figure 3–6. The difference between the measured and theoretical

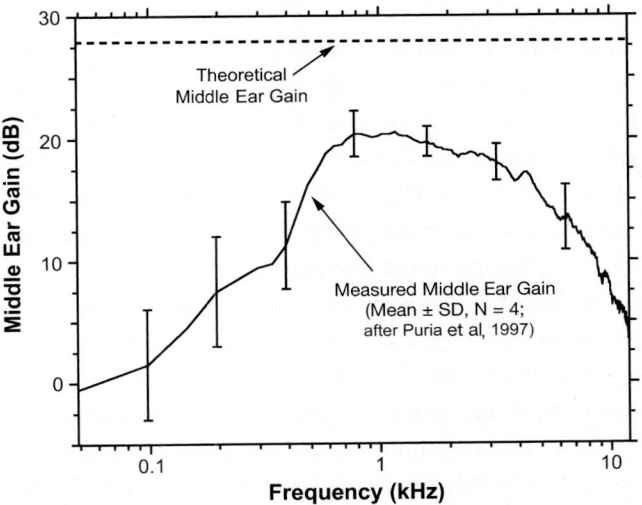

Figure 3–7 Middle ear sound pressure gain. The *dashed line* at the top shows the theoretical (ideal) transformer ratio produced by the tympanic membrane to footplate area ratio and the ossicular lever. The theoretical middle ear gain, which is approximately 28 dB, is independent of frequency. The curve represents the mean ± standard deviation (SD) of measurements of middle ear gain made in four normal temporal bones (after Puria and colleagues, 1997[19]). The measurements consist of the increase in magnitude of the sound pressure in the cochlear vestibule over the sound pressure at the tympanic membrane. It is evident that the actual middle ear gain is frequency dependent and is only about 20 dB at best (around 1,000 Hz).

gains is the result of several nonideal conditions within the middle ear: (1) The anatomic transformer model assumes that the entire tympanic membrane moves as a rigid body. However, measurements of tympanic membrane motion[22,23] show that portions of the membrane move differently than others. At low frequencies, the entire tympanic membrane moves with the same phase, but the magnitude varies. At frequencies above 1,000 Hz, the patterns of vibration become more complicated with the tympanic membrane, breaking up into smaller vibrating portions that vibrate with different phases. This decreases the efficacy of the tympanic membrane as a coupler of sound pressure. (2) The simple transformer model does not account for the forces and pressures needed to stretch the tympanic membrane and ossicular ligaments and accelerate the mass of the middle ear components. Part of the force generated by a sound pressure in the ear canal is used to move the tympanic membrane and ossicles themselves, and this force is lost before it reaches the cochlea. (3) Other acoustic structures of the ear such as the middle ear air spaces load the motion of the tympanic membrane and ossicles and use up some of the pressure increase produced by the middle ear transformer. (4) The anatomic transformer model implies that the ossicular system acts as a rigid body. In reality, there is slippage in the ossicular system, particularly at frequencies above 1,000 to 2,000 Hz, which reduces the motion of the stapes relative to that of the manubrium. This slippage has been associated with translational movement in the rotational axis of the ossicles[24] or flexion in the ossicular joints.[10]

As will be discussed later, the effective stimulus to the inner ear is a difference in sound pressure between the oval and round windows. The middle ear maximizes this window pressure difference via two mechanisms.[25,26] First, as described above, the tympano-ossicular system preferentially increases the sound pressure at the oval window of the inner ear. At the same time, the intact tympanic membrane reduces the sound pressure in the tympanic cavity by 10 to 20 dB compared with the sound pressure in the ear canal,[27,28] thereby protecting or shielding the round window from the sound in the ear canal. A third function of the middle ear related to the protective function is that the presence of middle ear air outside the round window permits the window to move freely when the inner ear is stimulated by motion of the footplate. These concepts of middle ear sound pressure gain, round window protection, and round window mobility have important practical implications for tympanoplasty.

Inner Ear

The cochlea is a coiled tube made of three fluid-filled chambers. The fluid is essentially incompressible, so that any movement of the stapes footplate within the oval window must be accompanied by fluid motion elsewhere. Over the auditory frequency range, the small fluid-filled cochlear and vestibular aqueducts and other connections between the cochlea and cerebrospinal fluid space are effectively closed,[29] and it is the compliant membrane covering the round window that permits large motions of the footplate. When the stapes footplate moves in, the round window moves out. (The footplate and round window have approximately the same volume velocities but move with opposite phase.) It is this coupling of the round and oval windows by the incompressible cochlear fluids that leads to the importance of the *difference* in sound pressure at the two cochlear windows in stimulating the inner ear.[30,31]

The cochlear partition within the inner ear includes the basilar membrane, the organ of Corti, scala media, and Reissner's membrane. The mechanical properties of the cochlear partition are heavily influenced by the mechanics of the basilar membrane; the latter is narrow, stiff, and thick at the base and wider, compliant, and thin at the apex. Because the fluid is essentially incompressible, inward motion of the stapes causes a nearly instantaneous transfer of the motion through the cochlear fluids, resulting in outward motion of the round window. Associated with this displacement of the fluid is a nearly instantaneous pressure distribution across the cochlear partition. The reaction of the cochlear partition with its graded mechanical properties to this pressure distribution results in a *traveling wave* of cochlear partition displacement.[32] The maximum displacement of this wave is tonotopically organized in a manner consistent with place-dependent differences in partition mechanics. High-frequency sounds produce displacement maxima near the stiff and thick base, whereas low-frequency sounds produce displacement maxima near the compliant and thin apex.

Because the wave appears to travel from the base toward the apex and also appears to stop just past the location of maximum displacement, there is an asymmetry in the motion of the cochlear partition. All sounds produce some motion of the basal portions of the cochlear partition, whereas only low-frequency sounds produce significant partition motion in the apex. This asymmetry has implications in our perception of complex sounds (where low-frequency sounds can interfere with our perception of high-frequency sounds but not vice versa[33]) and has also been suggested to play a role in the sensitivity of the high-frequency base to noise trauma and in presbycusis.[34] Motion of the cochlear partition stimulates hair cells of the organ of Corti, where larger stimuli result from larger motions.

Phase Difference between the Cochlear Windows

As stated earlier, the cochlea responds to the *difference* in sound pressure between the cochlear windows,[30,31] where the sound pressure at the oval window is a sum of the pressure produced by the tympano-ossicular system and the acoustic pressure within the middle ear air space. It is important to understand how this difference (the essential stimulus to the inner ear) depends on the relative magnitude and phase of the individual sound pressures at the two windows. When there is a significant difference in magnitude between the oval and round window sound pressures (as in the normal ear and after successful tympanoplasty when the tympano-ossicular system amplifies the pressure acting at the oval window), *differences in phase have little effect* in determining the window pressure difference.[35,36] The lack of importance of phase when the magnitudes differ is illustrated in Figure 3–8, which shows a hypothetical situation in which the magnitude of the oval window sound pressure is 10 times (20 dB) greater than the round window sound pressure. The range of possible window pressure difference is shown by two curves: one with an amplitude of 9 representing the difference when the two window pressures are in phase (0-degree phase difference) and the other curve with an amplitude of 11 representing the difference when the window pressures are completely out of phase (180-degree phase difference). Even with

this maximum effect of varying the phase difference, the two curves shown in Figure 3–8 are similar in magnitude, within 2 dB of each other. With larger magnitude differences such as factors of 100 to 1,000 (40 to 60 dB) that occur in the normal ear and in ears that have undergone successful tympanoplasty, variations in phase have a negligible effect.

However, phase differences can become important under conditions when the magnitudes of the sound pressures at the oval and round windows are similar (eg, with an interrupted ossicular chain). When the individual window pressures are of similar magnitude and similar phase, they tend to cancel each other and produce only a small net window pressure difference. On the other hand, if the individual window pressures are of similar magnitude but opposite phase, then they will add to each other, resulting in a window pressure difference that is similar in magnitude to the applied pressures.

Multiple Pathways for Sound Stimulation of the Inner Ear

The contribution of the middle ear to the window pressure difference that stimulates the inner ear can be split into several stimulus pathways. A previous section described how the tympano-ossicular system transforms sound pressure in the ear canal to sound pressure at the oval window. This pathway has been termed *ossicular coupling*.[37] There is another mechanism, called *acoustic coupling*,[37] through which the middle ear can stimulate the inner ear (Figure 3–9). Motion of the tympanic membrane in response to ear canal sound creates sound pressure in the middle ear cavity. Because the cochlear windows are separated by a few millimeters, the acoustic sound pressures at the oval and round windows, respectively, are similar but *not* identical. Small differences between the magnitudes and phases of the sound pressures outside the two windows result in a small but measurable difference in sound pressure between the two windows. In the normal ear, the magnitude of this acoustically coupled window pressure difference is small, on the order of 60 dB less than ossicular coupling.[36] Hence, ossicular coupling dominates normal middle ear function, and one can ignore acoustic coupling. However, as will be seen later, acoustic coupling can play an important role when ossicular coupling is compromised, as in some diseased and reconstructed ears.

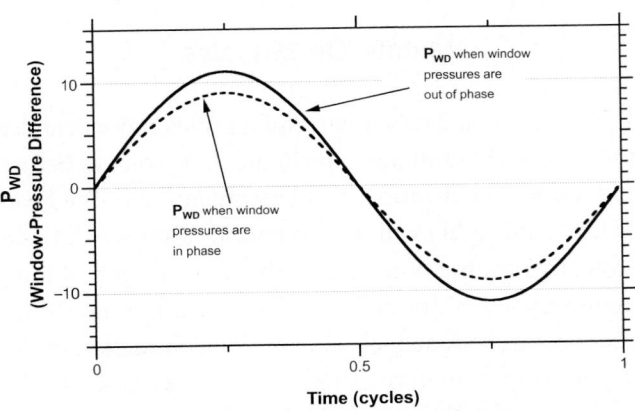

Figure 3–8 Schematic showing that if there is a significant difference in magnitude between window pressures, then differences in phase are of little importance in determining the difference between the two sound pressures. In this specific case, the oval window sound pressure is 10 times (20 dB) greater than the round window sound pressure. One cycle of the wave form of the window pressure difference (P_{WD}) is plotted for two circumstances. The *dashed line* shows P_{WD} when the oval window and round window pressures are in phase, and the result is a P_{WD} wave of peak amplitude 9 = 10−1. The *solid line* shows P_{WD} when the individual window pressures are completely out of phase, and the result is a P_{WD} wave of amplitude 11 = 10−(−1). Note that the two P_{WD} pressures differ by less than 2 dB ($20\log_{10}11/9$ = 1.7 dB), even though this phase variation produces the largest possible magnitude difference. Thus, in the normal ear and after successful tympanoplasty when the sound pressure at the oval window is large because of significant ossicular conduction of sound, differences in phase of sound pressures at the oval and round windows have little effect in determining the hearing outcome.

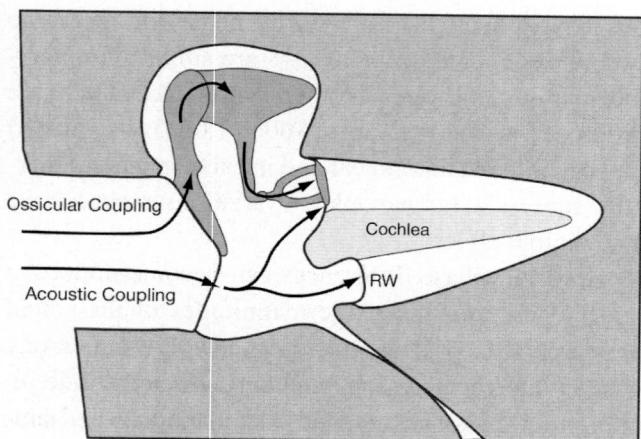

Figure 3–9 Schematic showing the pathways of ossicular coupling and acoustic coupling. Ossicular coupling is produced by the coupled motion of the tympanic membrane, ossicles, and stapes footplate. Acoustic coupling results from middle ear sound pressure that is produced by ear canal sound pressure and motion of the tympanic membrane. Because the cochlear windows are spatially separated, the sound pressures within the middle ear cavity that act at the oval and round windows (RW), respectively, are *not* identical. The small differences between the magnitudes and phases of the two window pressures result in a small but measurable *difference* in sound pressure between the two windows. This difference is called acoustic coupling. In the normal ear, acoustic coupling is quite small, and its magnitude is approximately 60 dB less than ossicular coupling.[36,37]

Environmental sound can also reach the inner ear by producing vibrations of the whole body and head, so-called *whole-body sound conduction.*[38] This is a more general process than audiologic *bone conduction,* where a vibrator acts only on the mastoid portion of the skull. Sound-induced vibrations of the whole body and head can stimulate the inner ear by (1) generating external ear or middle ear sound pressures via compressions of the ear canal and middle ear walls, (2) producing relative motions between the ossicles and inner ear, and (3) direct compression of the inner ear. Little is known about the contribution of whole-body sound conduction to normal auditory function. However, measurements of hearing loss caused by pathology such as congenital aural atresia suggest that the whole-body route can provide a stimulus to the inner ear that is about 60 dB smaller than that provided by normal ossicular coupling.[38]

Audiologic Bone Conduction

Sound energy transmitted to the skull by a bone vibrator (eg, a tuning fork or the electromagnetic vibrator of an audiometer) sets the basilar membrane in motion and is perceived as sound. Clinical bone conduction testing is used as a means to determine the functionality of the cochlea. The mechanisms by which a bone vibrator can stimulate the inner ear have been described by Tonndorf[39] and are similar to those described earlier for whole-body sound transmission. It is important to realize that all of the hypothesized bone conduction mechanisms involve relative motion between the ossicles and inner ear and that bone conduction hearing is influenced by pathologies in the external and middle ears. The so-called "occlusion effect" (easily demonstrated by occlusion of the external ear canal while talking, which results in increased loudness of sound heard in the occluded ear) occurs because vibrations of the ear canal wall produce significant sound pressures in the closed ear canal. Furthermore, a classic pattern in bone conduction audiometry known as the Carhart notch (see Chapter 8) is used to help identify cases of stapes footplate fixation.[40] The mechanical processes that underlie the Carhart notch phenomenon are not well understood. Therefore, the idea that vibrating the skull directly stimulates the cochlea in a manner that is independent of the middle ear is not strictly true.

Middle Ear Muscles

The stapedius and tensor tympani muscles contract under a variety of circumstances, including loud sounds, before and during vocalization, tactile stimulation of the head or face, and fight or flight behavioral responses.[41] Such protective contractions reduce the transmission of low-frequency sound through the middle ear but have little effect on high-frequency sound.[2,42,43] Contraction of the stapedius muscle in response to sound is known as the *acoustic reflex.* The reflex is thought to help in speech discrimination (the reflex reduces masking by low-frequency sound of high-frequency stimuli[44,45]) and in protecting the inner ear from acoustic trauma of loud continuous sound.[46] Contractions of the tensor tympani have also been associated with opening of the eustachian tube, where the inward motion of the tympanic membrane that results from the contraction produces an overpressure in the middle ear that helps open the tube.[47]

Middle Ear Joints

The incudomalleal and incudostapedial joints add flexibility to the ossicular system, which allows the middle ear to withstand large variations in the static pressure difference across the tympanic membrane without producing damage to the ear. Middle ear static pressure variations that occur regularly in day-to-day activities (eg, those produced by sneezing and swallowing) generate millimeter-sized motions of the tympanic membrane; such large motions are not transmitted to the stapes because of the flexibility of the incudomalleal and incudostapedial joints.[48,49]

The ossicular joints also permit independent control of tympanic membrane and stapes motion by the middle ear muscles. Large contractions of the stapedius muscle that cause 0.1-mm changes in the position of the stapes head have been shown to have little effect on the position of the other ossicles because of sliding in the incudostapedial joint.[50] Similarly, the tensor tympani can pull the malleus inward by a millimeter or more but has little effect on the stapes because of the incudomalleal joint. There are some data from studies of ossicular motion in animals and human temporal bones to suggest that a consequence of the joint-induced flexibility is a decrease in the high-frequency response of the middle ear.[10,51]

Investigation of Middle Ear Mechanics

Broadly speaking, investigations of middle ear mechanics have employed one or more of four approaches: behavioral and other assessments of hearing in normal and diseased ears, physiologic studies of the middle ears of animals, quantitative physics-based models, and acoustic measurements in cadaveric temporal bones.

The use of animal models to study the middle ear was pioneered by Wever and Lawrence in a series of studies of the effects of middle ear modifications on cochlear potentials in cats.[2] Other landmark studies include investigations of middle ear impedance and ossicular motion,[10,52–55] investigations of the effect of middle ear muscles,[56] and investigations of simulated pathologies on middle ear transmission.[57–59] Animal studies continue to provide new insights into middle ear function, including recent evidence that the ossicles are not completely rigid,[60] evidence of wave motion in the tympanic membrane itself,[61] and new evidence of contractile elements within the support of the tympanic membrane.[62]

A "model" of the middle ear is essentially a set of mathematical equations that relate the physical structure

of the ear to its acoustic function. The degree and complexity of the association of model elements with anatomic structures vary widely within models, ranging from simple "black box" models of the ear,[63] through models for which simple elements are associated with specific structures of the ear,[64] to complex three-dimensional finite-element models that include detailed depictions of middle ear shape and approximations of the mechanical properties of the structural elements.[65] A wide variety of middle ear models have been described, dealing with sound transmission in normal as well as in pathologic ears. A discussion of such models is outside the scope of this review, and the reader is referred to other sources.[17,63–65]

Cadaveric temporal bones (the "temporal bone preparation") are also useful in studying middle ear mechanics. It has been shown that the mechanical properties of the middle ear in carefully prepared temporal bones are indistinguishable from those measured in living human ears.[66,67] The temporal bones must be in a fresh state and kept moist, and static pressure must not be allowed to build up within the middle ear. Besides its utility in studying normal middle ear function, the temporal bone preparation allows one to make repeated measurements of acoustic and mechanical function after precise modifications that simulate specific pathologies or tympanoplasties. Measurements in such preparations have provided valuable insight into the mechanics of sound transmission in a variety of diseased and reconstructed ears.

ACOUSTICS AND MECHANICS OF DISEASED MIDDLE EARS

The concepts discussed in the previous section help us to understand sound transmission in various pathologic middle ear conditions. In this review, we have chosen the "air–bone gap" as determined by standard clinical audiometry to describe the loss of middle ear sound transmission in various pathologic conditions. Our choice of the air–bone gap measure is a matter of ease and convenience since the gap can be easily calculated from a clinical audiogram and allows one to compare ears with disparate levels of sensorineural function. However, one must remember that the air–bone gap is not always an accurate measure of middle ear sound transmission loss because bone conduction thresholds can be influenced by middle ear pathologies, as mentioned previously.

Ossicular Interruption with an Intact Tympanic Membrane

When there is ossicular interruption in the presence of an intact drum, ossicular coupling is lost, and sound input to the cochlea via the middle ear would occur as a result of acoustic coupling.[37] Since acoustic coupling is about 60 dB smaller than ossicular coupling, one would predict that complete ossicular interruption would result in a 60-dB conductive hearing loss. This prediction is consistent with clinical observations as shown in Figure 3–10, where there is good agreement between the predicted and actual air–bone gap as measured in eight surgically confirmed cases of ossicular interruption with an intact tympanic membrane. Note that the consistency of the clinical results with the model of acoustic coupling suggests that stimuli reaching the inner ear through whole-body or bone conduction mechanisms in this particular condition are small enough to be ignored.

Loss of the Tympanic Membrane, Malleus, and Incus

In cases in which the tympanic membrane, malleus, and incus are lost, the conductive hearing loss is on the order of 40 to 50 dB; that is, this condition results in hearing sensitivities that are 10 to 20 dB superior to cases with an intact tympanic membrane and complete ossicular interruption. The 40- to 50-dB loss can be explained by a loss of ossicular coupling together with an enhancement of acoustic coupling by about 10 to 20 dB, as compared to the normal ear.[37] The enhancement of acoustic coupling results from loss of the shielding effect of the tympanic membrane, which in the normal ear attenuates middle ear sound pressure by 10 to 20 dB relative to ear canal sound pressure. The air–bone gap predicted by loss of ossicular coupling and enhanced acoustic coupling is similar to that measured in patients as shown in Figure 3–11. The increase in acoustic coupling caused by loss of tympanic membrane shielding also explains why the hearing of a patient with an interrupted ossicular chain and an intact drum is improved by 10 to 20 dB when a perforation is created in the tympanic membrane.

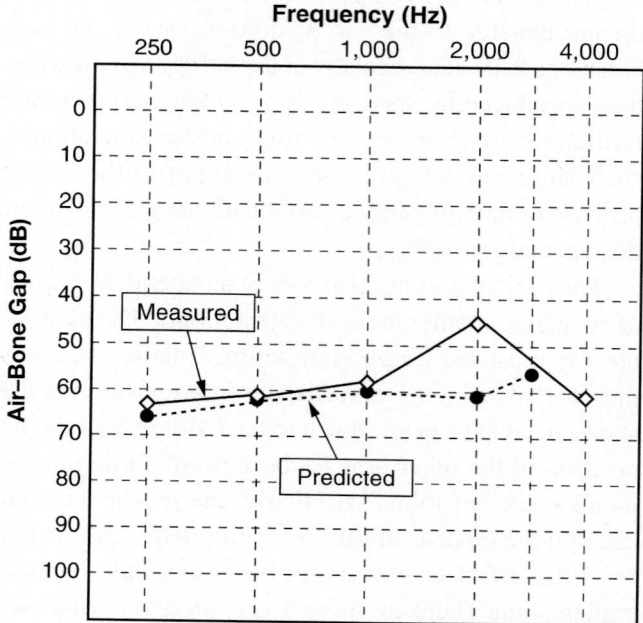

Interrupted Ossicular Chain

Figure 3–10 Comparison of air–bone gaps measured in eight cases with surgically confirmed complete ossicular chain interruption with an intact tympanic membrane to air–bone gaps predicted on the basis of hearing resulting from acoustic coupling. In this pathologic state, there is no ossicular coupling. Since acoustic coupling is about 60 dB smaller than ossicular coupling, the prediction is a 60-dB conductive hearing loss, which is consistent with the measured air–bone gaps. The standard deviation for each of the measured points is about ± 10 dB. After Peake and colleagues.[37]

Ossicular Fixation

Partial or complete fixation of the stapes footplate (eg, otosclerosis, tympanosclerosis, etc.) results in conductive hearing losses that range from 5 to 60 dB depending on the degree of fixation.[68] The losses are greater for the lower frequencies (Figure 3–12). Fixation of the footplate reduces ossicular coupling by hindering stapes motion, resulting in a conductive hearing loss. The amount of hearing loss depends on the degree of decreased stapes motion. The primary effect of the otosclerotic lesion is an increase in the stiffness of the annular ligament that supports the stapes, where the normal ligament stiffness is a major constraint on the ossicular coupling route in the normal ear. Increases in ligament stiffness should first affect the low-frequency response of the ear, which is consistent with the observation that in early otosclerosis, the hearing loss is mainly in the low frequencies.[68]

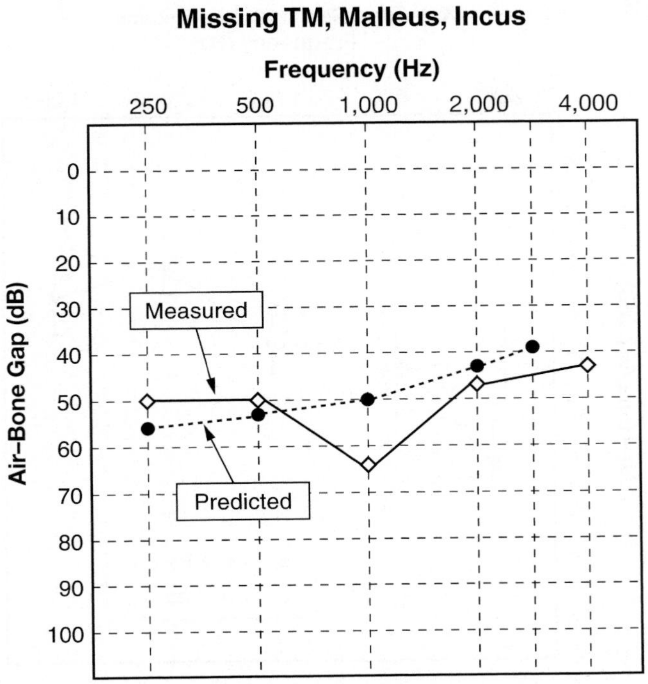

Missing TM, Malleus, Incus

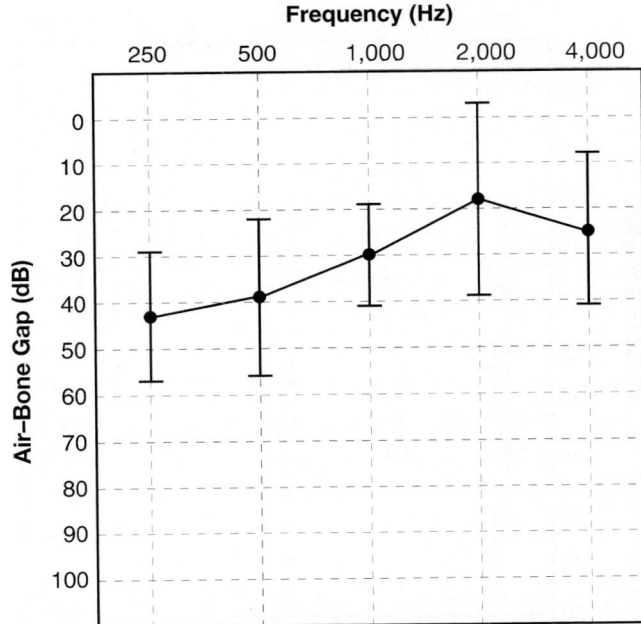

Figure 3–11 Comparison of air–bone gaps measured in five cases with missing tympanic membrane (TM), malleus, and incus to air–bone gaps predicted on the basis of acoustic coupling. With loss of the tympanic membrane, there is enhancement of acoustic coupling by about 10 to 20 dB compared to the normal ear. The predicted and measured gaps are similar. After Peake and colleagues.[37]

Stapes Fixation due to Otosclerosis

Figure 3–12 Air–bone gaps measured in 75 cases of surgically confirmed stapes fixation of varying degrees caused by otosclerosis. The mean ±1 standard deviation (SD) of the air–bone gap at each frequency is shown. The conductive hearing loss is greater for the lower frequencies.

In contrast to stapes fixation, the conductive hearing loss associated with so-called "malleus fixation" is only 15 to 25 dB.[69,70] Malleus fixation is generally the result of a bony spur that extends from the epitympanic wall to the malleus head.[69] The point of fixation lies near the axis of rotation of the malleus where displacements of the malleus should be small. Furthermore, since the spur is rather small compared to the malleus head, it is likely that complete fixation of the malleus does not occur and some motion is still transmitted across the incudomalleal joint. Hence, we suggest that malleus fixation leads to only a mild reduction in ossicular coupling, consistent with the 15- to 25-dB conductive hearing losses observed clinically.[69,70]

Tympanic Membrane Perforation

Perforations of the tympanic membrane cause a conductive hearing loss that can range from negligible to 50 dB (Figure 3–13). The primary mechanism of conductive loss caused by a perforation is a reduction in ossicular coupling caused by a loss in the sound pressure difference across the tympanic membrane.[57,71–74] The sound pressure difference across the tympanic membrane provides the primary drive to the motion of the drum and ossicles. Perforation-induced physical changes such as reduction in tympanic membrane area or changes in coupling of tympanic membrane motion to the malleus do not appear to contribute significantly to the hearing loss caused by a perforation.[72–74]

Perforations cause a loss that depends on frequency, perforation size, and middle ear air space volume.[72–74] Perforation-induced losses are greatest at the lowest frequencies and generally decrease as frequency increases. Perforation size is an important determinant of the loss; larger perforations result in larger hearing losses (see Figure 3–13, A). The volume of the middle ear air space (combined tympanic cavity and mastoid air volume) is also an important parameter that determines the amount of hearing loss caused by a perforation; small middle ear air space volumes result in larger air–bone gaps. Other things being equal, for a given sound pressure in the ear canal and a given perforation, the resulting sound pres-

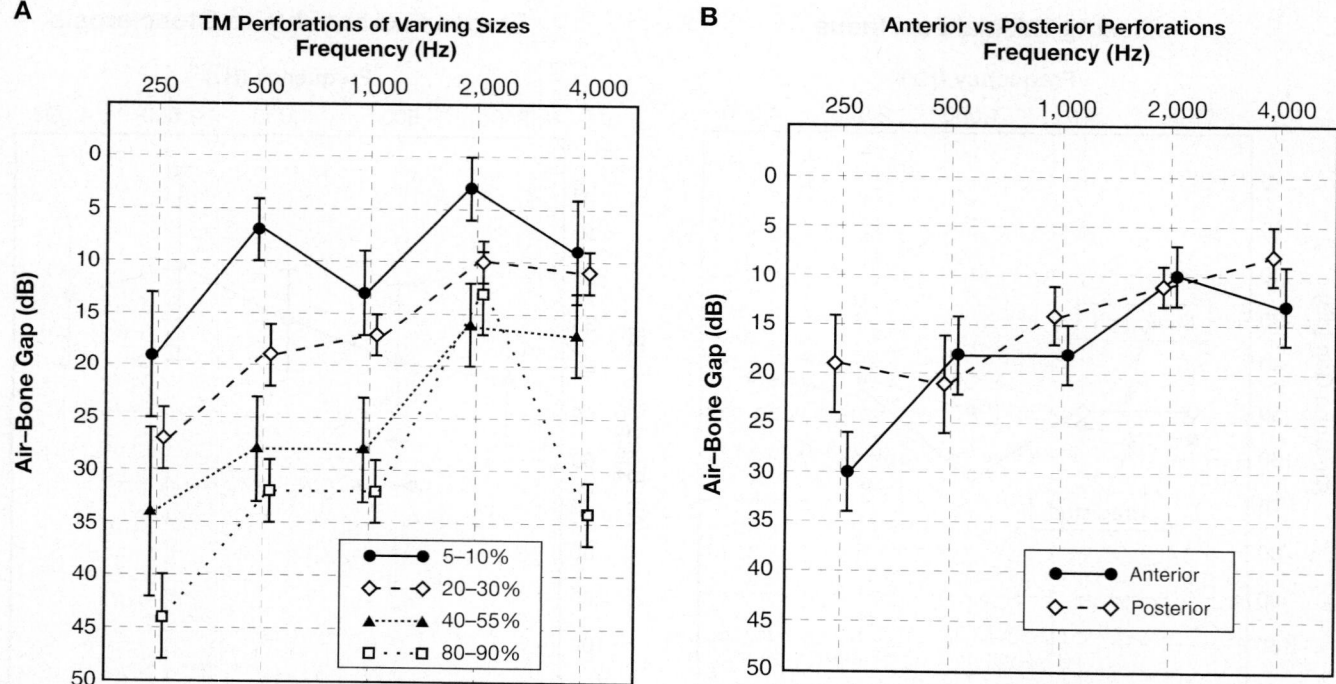

Figure 3–13   Air–bone gaps measured in 42 ears with tympanic membrane (TM) perforations. In each case, the conductive hearing loss was caused solely by the perforation because the ossicular chain was found to be intact and mobile at subsequent tympanoplasty surgery done to repair the perforation and there was closure of the air–bone gap after the surgery. *A,* Air–bone gaps (mean ± 1 standard error of mean [SEM]) are shown for perforations of varying sizes. Perforation size was estimated as a percentage of the area of the tympanic membrane. There were four groups of perforations, based on their size: 5 to 10% (5 ears), 20 to 30% (22 ears), 45 to 55% (6 ears), and 80 to 90% (9 ears). Air–bone gaps are greater at the lower frequencies, and the gaps increase as the perforations get larger. The largest perforation-induced air–bone gaps are about 40 to 50 dB. *B,* Air–bone gaps (mean ± 1 SEM) are shown for anterior versus posterior perforations of the same size. The ears of perforation size equal to 20 to 30% of tympanic membrane area from the dataset shown in (*A*) were subdivided into anterior (11 ears) and posterior (8 ears) groups, based on the location of the perforation with respect to the manubrium. There are no statistically significant differences between the two means at any frequency. (In 3 ears with 20 to 30% perforations, the perforation was directly inferior to the umbo, and they were excluded from the anterior versus posterior analysis.)

sure within the middle ear cavity will vary inversely with middle ear volume. Hence, the transtympanic membrane sound pressure difference will be smaller (and the conductive loss correspondingly greater) with smaller middle ear volumes. Identical perforations in two different ears can have conductive losses that differ by up to 20 to 30 dB if the middle ear air space volumes differ substantially (within normal ears, middle ear air space volume can range from 2 cm³ to 20 cm³).[75]

The dependence of perforation-induced hearing loss on the transtympanic membrane sound pressure difference also suggests that there should be *no* systematic differences in the air–bone gaps caused by perforations of identical size at different locations. The notion that the location of a perforation should not influence the resulting hearing loss is supported by the following evidence to date.

1. *Theoretical calculations.* While it has been demonstrated that perforations of the tympanic membrane lead to increases in the sound pressure outside the cochlear windows, since the wavelengths of sound are generally larger than the middle ear dimensions, the acoustically coupled window pressure difference should not depend on perforation location.

2. *Experimental data.* Measurements in a temporal bone preparation have shown that the location of a perforation affects neither the resulting loss in sound transmission nor the magnitude or phase of the sound pressures acting at the oval and round windows.[72–74]

3. *Clinical data.* Figure 3–13, B, compares air–bone gaps between same-sized perforations situated in anterior versus posterior locations, and there is no significant difference between the two groups.

We speculate that the common clinical perception that perforations of similar size but different locations produce different hearing losses may result from interear differences in the volume of the middle ear and mastoid air space.[72–74]

Finally, measurements in temporal bones[72–74] demonstrate that tympanic membrane perforations lead to an increase in acoustic coupling by 10 to 20 dB caused by loss of the shielding effect of the intact tympanic membrane. The increase in acoustic coupling allows one to predict that the maximum conductive loss following a perforation will be about 40 to 50 dB, which is consistent with clinical observations (see Figure 3–13, A).

Middle Ear Effusion

Fluid in the middle ear, a primary feature of otitis media with effusion (OME), is associated with a conductive hearing loss of up to 30 to 35 dB,[76] though the degree and frequency dependence of individual losses vary (Figure 3–14). The conductive loss occurs because of a reduction in ossicular coupling caused by several mechanisms.[77] At frequencies greater than 1,000 Hz, the loss is caused primarily by mass loading of the tympanic membrane by fluid, with decreases in sound transmission of up to 20 to 30 dB. The effect increases as more of the tympanic membrane surface area is covered with fluid. At frequencies below 1,000 Hz, the hearing loss is caused by an increase in impedance of the middle ear air space resulting from reduced middle ear air volume and possibly from negative middle ear static pressure, which is often associated with OME. Increasing the viscosity of the middle ear fluid does not appear to have a significant effect on the overall hearing loss.

Tympanic Membrane Atelectasis

Atelectasis of the tympanic membrane occurring without a tympanic membrane perforation (and in the presence of intact and mobile ossicles) can result in conductive hearing losses that vary in severity from negligible to 50 dB.[35] The conductive loss can be explained on the basis of a reduction in ossicular coupling caused by the tympanic membrane abnormality. As long as the area outside the round window remains aerated and is shielded from the sound pressure in the ear canal by the tympanic membrane, the conductive hear-

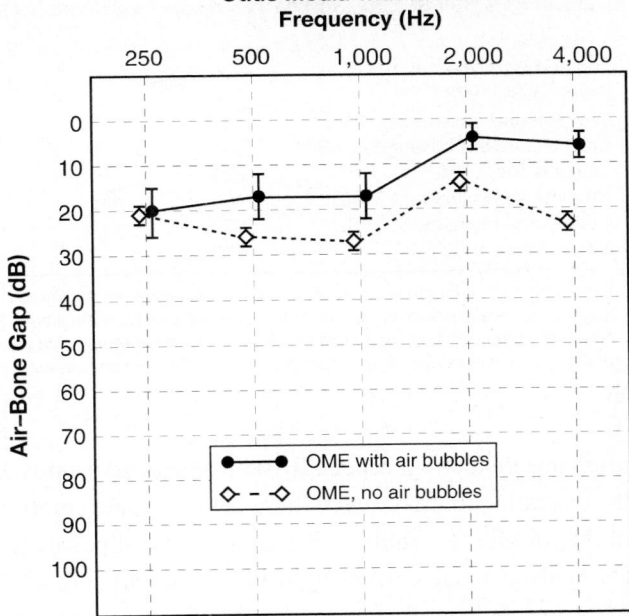

Figure 3–14 Air–bone gaps (mean ± 1 standard error of mean [SEM]) measured in 29 adult ears with otitis media with effusion (OME). In each case, the air–bone gap disappeared when the OME resolved, either spontaneously or after myringotomy. Two groups of ears are displayed, based on absence (n = 24) or presence (n = 5) of visible air bubbles behind the tympanic membrane at otoscopy at the time the air–bone gaps were measured. Ears with air in the tympanic cavity show a smaller conductive loss than ears with no visible air bubbles. The differences between the two groups are statistically significant at the 5% level for 1,000, 2,000, and 4,000 Hz.

ing loss caused by the atelectasis should not exceed the amount of middle ear sound pressure gain in normal ears, that is, air–bone gaps of up to 25 dB. If the atelectasis results in invagination of the tympanic membrane into the round window niche, the protective effect of the tympanic membrane and middle ear air space on round window motion is lost, and larger (40 to 50 dB) air–bone gaps should result. This prediction is consistent with the amount of acoustic coupling in cases in which there is loss of the tympanic membrane, malleus, and incus.

ACOUSTICS AND MECHANICS OF RECONSTRUCTED MIDDLE EARS

Although tympanomastoid surgery for chronic otitis media is quite successful in controlling infection with reported success rates in excess of 80 to 90%, it is well recognized that post-tympanoplasty hearing results are

Table 3–3 HEARING RESULTS AFTER OSSICULAR RECONSTRUCTION CASES (%) WITH POSTOPERATIVE AIR–BONE GAPS ≤ 20 dB

Study	No. of Cases	Minor Columellas, Including PORPs	Major Columellas, Including TORPs
Lee and Schuknecht, 1971[78]	936	40	—
Pennington, 1973[79]	216	70	—
Jackson and colleagues, 1983[80]	417	64	43
Brackmann and colleagues, 1984[81]	1,042	73	55
Lau and Tos, 1986[82]	229	54	40
Ragheb and colleagues, 1987[83]	455	52	37
Colletti and colleagues, 1987[84]	832	48–80*	28–70*
Goldenberg, 1992[85]	262	57	58

Minor columella refers to an ossicular strut or prosthesis from the stapes head to the tympanic membrane/manubrium.
Major columella refers to an ossicular strut or prosthesis from the stapes footplate to the tympanic membrane/manubrium.
*Results varied with time interval after surgery: results got worse with increasing length of follow-up.
PORP = partial ossicular replacement prosthesis; TORP = total ossicular replacement prosthesis.

often unsatisfactory, especially with advanced lesions of the ossicular chain or when there is inadequate aeration of the middle ear. Table 3–3 is a summary of postsurgical hearing results from eight large clinical series[78–85] spanning the past three decades that demonstrates that the results are often less than satisfactory. When the ossicular chain has to be reconstructed, long-term closure of the air–bone gap to ≤ 20 dB occurs in only 40 to 70% of cases when the stapes is intact and only in 30 to 60% of cases when the stapes superstructure is missing.

One factor responsible for the modest nature of posttympanoplasty hearing results is a lack of quantitative understanding of structure-function relationships in the mechanical response of reconstructed ears. The need for improved understanding of middle ear mechanics is clearly shown by the clinical occurrence of many instances in which the structural differences between a good and poor hearing result are not apparent or where seemingly minor variations in structure are associated with large differences in function. For example, Liston and colleagues, with the use of intraoperative monitoring by auditory evoked responses during ossiculoplasty, found that changes in prosthesis position of 0.5 to 1.0 mm had effects on hearing as large as 20 dB.[86] It is also a common clinical observation that postsurgical ears, which seem identical in structure, can exhibit markedly different degrees of conductive hearing loss. Better quantitative understanding of the factors that determine the hearing response (eg, graft stiffness and tension and the mechanical properties of the prosthesis) should permit us to understand what the important structural differences are that might account for these seemingly unexplainable results.

Other major factors contributing to unsatisfactory postsurgical hearing results are incomplete knowledge of the biology of chronic middle ear disease (including pathology of middle ear aeration and eustachian tube function) and a lack of control over the histopathologic and tissue responses of the middle ear to surgery. These factors are outside the scope of this chapter.

Reconstruction of the Sound Conduction Mechanisms

The goal of tympanoplasty is to restore sound pressure transformation at the oval window by coupling an intact tympanic membrane with a mobile stapes footplate via an intact or reconstructed ossicular chain and to provide sound protection for the round window membrane by means of a closed, air-containing, mucosa-lined middle ear. As previously mentioned, the mean sound pressure gain provided by the normal ear is only about 20 dB. Consequently, a mechanically mobile but suboptimal tympanoplasty, combined with adequate stapes mobility, adequate middle ear aeration, and round window sound protection, can result in no middle ear gain but still produce a relatively good hearing result. For example, a tympanoplasty that gives a middle ear gain of 5 dB but leaves the middle ear aerated and allows round window motion will result in an air–bone gap of only 15 dB. (Of course, an immobile, rigid tympanoplasty graft will result in very little stapes motion and much larger hearing losses.) As previously discussed, the magnitude of the ossicularly coupled sound pressure at the oval window is significantly greater than the acoustically coupled sound pressure at the round window in the normal ear, and we suspect a similar pressure gain after successful tympanoplasty. Under these circumstances, differences in phase of sound pressures at the oval and round windows have little effect in determining the hearing outcome. Therefore, the goal of a tympanoplasty should be to increase the magnitude of sound pressure at the oval window relative to the round window, without regard to phase.

The following subsections attempt to describe the structural parameters that are thought to be important to hearing results after middle ear surgery.

Aeration of the Middle Ear

Aeration of the middle ear (including the round window) is *critical* to the success of any tympanoplasty procedure. Aeration allows the tympanic membrane, ossicles, and round window to move. Clinical experience has shown that nonaerated ears often demonstrate 40- to 60-dB air–bone gaps.[36] The large gap in nonaerated ears occurs because ossicular coupling is greatly reduced and stapes motion is reduced because the round window membrane (which is coupled to the stapes by incompressible cochlear fluids) cannot move freely.

How much air is necessary behind the tympanic membrane (ie, within the middle ear and mastoid)? Model analyses of the effects of varying the volume of the middle ear and mastoid predict an increasing low-frequency hearing loss as air volume is reduced (Figure 3–15).[87] The normal, average volume of the middle ear and mastoid is 6 cc; a combined middle ear and mastoid volume of 0.4 cc is predicted to result in a 10-dB conductive hearing loss. Volumes smaller than 0.4 cc should lead to progressively larger gaps, whereas increases in volume above about 1.0 cc should provide little additional acoustic benefit. Experimental studies using a human temporal bone preparation in which the middle ear and mastoid volume was reduced progressively show results consistent with the model prediction.[27,88]

Another parameter of the middle ear air space that can influence middle ear mechanics is the static air pressure within the space. Experiments in human perception dating back to the 19th century,[89] numerous animal studies,[2,53] and measurements of ossicular motion in human temporal bones[90] have demonstrated that middle ear static pressure can have different effects on sound transmission at different frequencies. Generally, transtympanic membrane static pressure differences produce decreases in sound transmission through the middle ear for frequencies less than 1,000 Hz and have less effect at higher frequencies. Also, the effects of such static pressure differences are asymmetric, with larger decreases observed when the middle ear pressure is negative relative to that in the ear canal. The mechanisms by which pressure changes reduce middle ear sound transmission are not well defined, and possible sites of pressure sensitivity include the tympanic membrane, annular ligament, incudomalleal joint, and suspensory ligaments of the ossicles. Some of these structures are drastically altered as a result of tympanoplasty, and the acoustic effects of negative and positive middle ear static pressure in reconstructed ears have not been characterized.

Tympanoplasty Techniques without Ossicular Linkage: Types IV and V

A type IV tympanoplasty[91] is a surgical option in cases in which the tympanic membrane and ossicles are missing, the stapes footplate is mobile, and there is a canal wall down mastoid cavity. Incoming sound from the

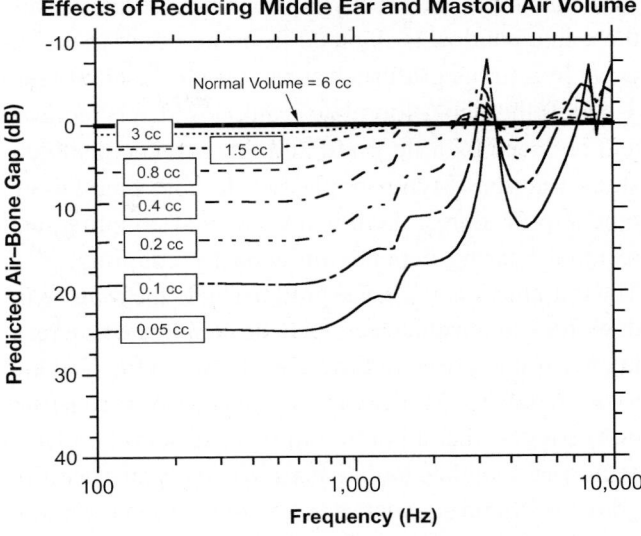

Figure 3–15   Model predictions of the effects of reducing the volume of the middle ear and mastoid. The normal baseline volume is taken to be 6 cc. Note that reduction of the volume to 0.4 cc is predicted to result in an air–bone gap < 10 dB. Volumes smaller than 0.4 cc are predicted to lead to progressively larger gaps. After Rosowski and Merchant.[87]

ear canal impinges directly on the stapes footplate while the round window is shielded from the sound in the ear canal by a tissue graft such as temporalis fascia (Figure 3–16). If the stapes footplate is ankylosed, it is removed and replaced by a fat graft, and this arrangement constitutes a type V tympanoplasty.[92] In both type IV and type V procedures, there is no ossicular coupling, and residual hearing depends on acoustic coupling.[37,93–95] The introduction of a tissue graft to shield the round window from sound enhances acoustic coupling by increasing the sound pressure difference between the oval and round windows. Model analyses of type IV reconstructions suggest that an optimum reconstruction (defined by normal footplate mobility, a sufficiently stiff acoustic graft shield, and adequate aeration of the round window) results in *maximum* acoustic coupling with a predicted residual conductive hearing loss of only 20 to 25 dB.[93,94] This optimum result is consistent with the best type IV hearing results (Figure 3–17). These analyses also predict that decreased footplate mobility, inadequate acoustic shielding, or inadequate round window aeration can lead to hearing losses as large as 60 dB.

Since the literature demonstrates that less than 50% of ears after type IV surgery have air–bone gaps less than 30 dB,[94] it is clear that many type IV reconstructions are nonoptimum. The following surgical guidelines can be used to optimize the postoperative hearing results: (1) one should preserve normal stapes mobility by covering the

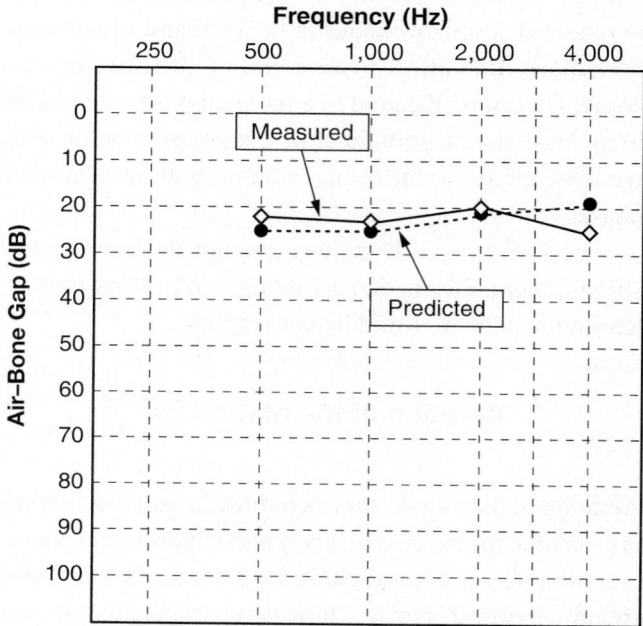

Type IV Tympanoplasty

Figure 3–17 Air–bone gaps after type IV tympanoplasty: the best surgical results are compared with a prediction based on "maximum" acoustic coupling. The predicted and measured results are similar, with an air–bone gap of approximately 20 dB. After Peake and colleagues.[37]

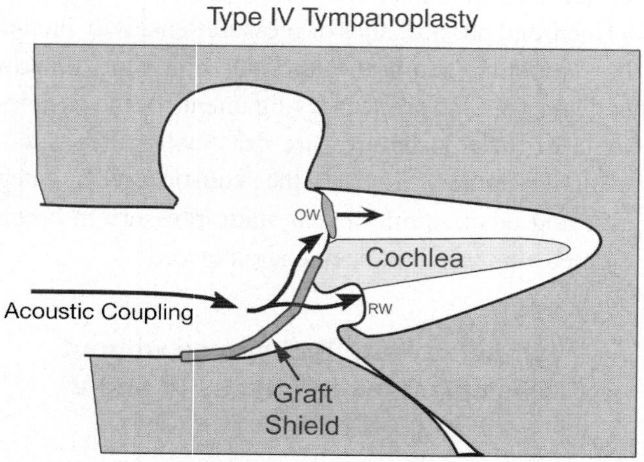

footplate with a thin split-thickness skin graft and not a fascia graft (fascia is much thicker than skin and can increase footplate impedance), (2) one should reinforce the round window fascia graft shield with cartilage or 1-mm-thick Silastic™ (reinforcing the graft shield in this manner increases its stiffness and improves its performance as an acoustic shield), and (3) one should create conditions that promote aeration of the round window niche and preserve mobility of the round window membrane (eg, by preserving all healthy mucosa in the protympanum and hypotympanum).

In a type V tympanoplasty, it is reasonable to assume that the mobility of the fat used to replace the footplate will be greater than that of the normal footplate. Hence, one would predict that the average hearing results for a type V would be better than those for a type IV, especially for low frequencies. This prediction is supported by the available clinical evidence. For example, in a clinical series of 64 cases of type V tympanoplasty, 86% of ears with conditions favorable for round window aeration had an air–bone gap smaller than the 20-dB gap that occurs with an optimum type IV.[96]

Type IV Tympanoplasty

Figure 3–16 Schematic of type IV tympanoplasty. Incoming sound from the ear canal impinges directly on a mobile stapes footplate within the oval window (OW), while the round window (RW) is acoustically protected by a graft shield. With no ossicular coupling, cochlear stimulation depends on acoustic coupling.

Tympanoplasty Techniques with Reconstruction or Preservation of Ossicular Linkage: Types I, II, and III

Type I, II, and III tympanoplasty involve reconstruction of the tympanic membrane and/or the ossicular chain. Besides maintenance of middle ear aeration and static pressure, the postoperative hearing result depends on the efficacies of the reconstructed eardrum and the reconstructed ossicular chain.

Tympanic Membrane Reconstruction

Although the tympanic membrane is responsible for most of the middle ear sound pressure gain, the details of how that gain is achieved are not well understood. Motion of the normal tympanic membrane is complex, especially at frequencies above 1,000 Hz.[22] Clinical observations suggest that surgical techniques that restore or preserve the normal anatomy of the tympanic membrane can lead to good hearing results.[35,36] However, more research is needed to define the optimum acoustic and mechanical properties of reconstructed tympanic membranes. For example:

1. Little is known of the mechanical significance of the arrangements of structural fibers in the tympanic membrane.
2. Although it has been argued that the conical shape of the normal tympanic membrane plays an important role in middle ear function,[7,22] the possible effects of changes in the shape of the tympanic membrane on postoperative hearing results are not understood.
3. Although many existing models of tympanic membrane function have been shown to fit some of the available data,[65] there are wide differences in the structure of these models, and little effort has been made to compare their significant differences and similarities. Further, these models generally have not been applied to reconstructed tympanic membranes. Better understanding of the features of tympanic membrane structure that are critical to its function should lead to improved methods for reconstructing the ear drum.

Ossicular Reconstruction

A wide variety of ossicular grafts and prostheses are in use. However, there are limited scientific data on the opti-mum acoustic and mechanical properties of ossicular prostheses. Factors that can influence the acoustic performance of an ossicular prosthesis include its *stiffness*, *mass*, and *position*; the *tension* imposed by the prosthesis on the drum and annular ligament; and mechanical features associated with *coupling* of the prosthesis to the drum and stapes.[35,36]

In general, the stiffness of a prosthesis will not be a significant factor as long as the stiffness is much greater than that of the stapes footplate cochlear impedance. For clinical purposes, prostheses made of ossicles, cortical bone, and many synthetic materials generally meet this requirement.

Model analysis[87] and some experimental evidence[97] suggest that an increase in ossicular mass does not cause significant detriment in middle ear sound transmission. Shown in Figure 3–18 are model predictions of air–bone gaps resulting from increasing the mass of an ossicle strut, relative to the stapes mass, which is 3 mg. Increases up to 16 times are predicted to cause less than 10-dB conductive loss and only at frequencies greater than 1,000 Hz.

The positioning of the prosthesis appears to be important to its function. Measurements in human temporal bone preparations suggest that the angle between the stapes and a prosthesis should be less than 45 degrees for optimal sound transmission.[98,99] There is also evidence that some variations in positioning produce only small

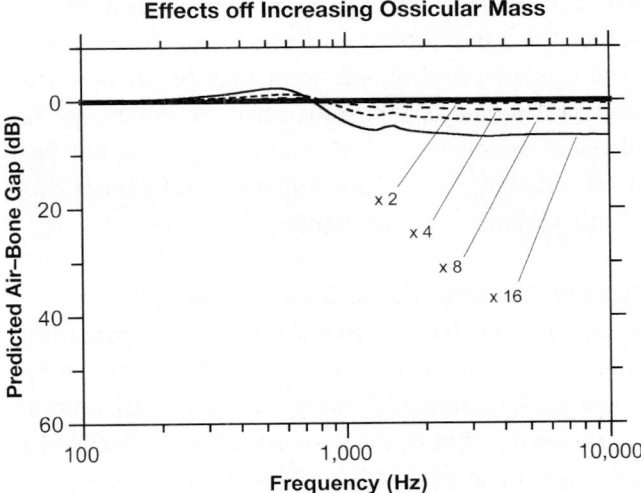

Figure 3–18 Model prediction of the effects of increasing ossicular mass. The mass of an ossicular strut is increased as shown. These increases are relative to the stapes mass, which is 3 mg. Increases up to 16 times are predicted to cause a < 10-dB conductive loss and only at frequencies > 1,000 Hz. After Rosowski and Merchant.[87]

changes. For example, although it is ideal to attach a prosthesis to the manubrium, experimental data show that acceptable results can occur with a prosthesis placed against the posterior-superior quadrant of the tympanic membrane as long as 3 to 4 mm of the prosthesis's diameter contact the drum.[100]

The tension that the prosthesis creates in the middle ear, which is generally a function of prosthesis length, appears critical in determining the hearing result. The mechanical impedance of biologic structures is inherently nonlinear, and measurements such as tympanometry have shown that the tympanic membrane and annular ligament act as linear elements only over the range of small motions (less than 10 micrometers) associated with physiologic sound levels. Larger displacements of the ligament and membrane stiffen these structures. The large static displacements produced by a prosthesis that is too long would stretch the annular ligament and tympanic membrane, resulting in a stiffening of these structures, a reduction in tympano-ossicular motion, and an air–bone gap. Currently, tension cannot be assessed intraoperatively in an objective fashion; a reliable objective test of this tension would be useful to the otosurgeon.

Coupling refers to how well a prosthesis adheres to the footplate or tympanic membrane, and the degree of coupling will determine whether there is slippage in sound transmission at the ends of a prosthesis. Thus, a prosthesis transmits sound effectively only if there is good coupling at both ends. Clinical observations indicate that it is rare to obtain a firm union between a prosthesis and the stapes footplate. Hence, inadequate coupling at the prosthesis-footplate joint may be an important cause of a persistent postoperative air–bone gap. The physical factors that control coupling have not been determined in a quantitative manner, and further study of this parameter is warranted.

Type III Tympanoplasty, Stapes Columella

A classic type III or stapes columella tympanoplasty (Figure 3–19) involves placement of a tympanic membrane graft such as temporalis fascia directly onto the stapes head[91]; that is, the ossicular chain is replaced by the single columella of the stapes. This tympanoplasty is typically performed in conjunction with a canal wall down mastoidectomy. The hearing results after this procedure vary widely, with air–bone gaps ranging from 10 to 60 dB. Large air–bone gaps (40 to 60 dB) occur as a

Type III Tympanoplasty

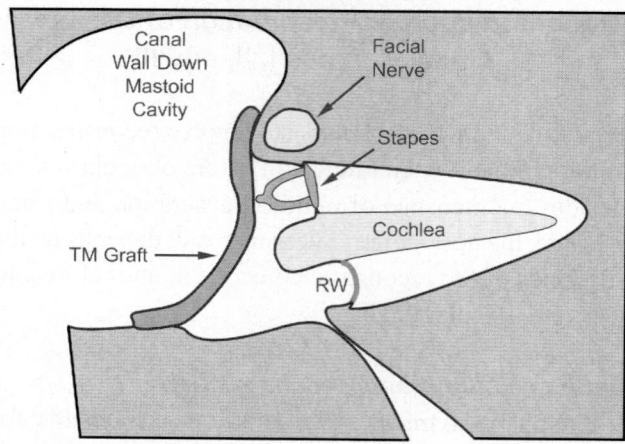

Figure 3–19 Schematic of type III tympanoplasty, stapes columella. A tympanic membrane (TM) graft, usually temporalis fascia, is placed directly onto the stapes head. The procedure is typically performed in conjunction with a canal wall down mastoidectomy. RW = round window.

result of stapes fixation, nonaeration of the middle ear, or both (Figure 3–20). When the stapes is mobile and the middle ear is aerated, the average postoperative air–bone gap is on the order of 20 to 25 dB, suggesting that there is little middle ear sound pressure gain occurring through the reconstruction. The results from experimental and clinical studies of the type III stapes columellar reconstruction have shown that interposing a disk of cartilage between the graft and the stapes head improves hearing in the lower frequencies by 5 to 10 dB.[101] We hypothesize that the cartilage acts to increase the "effective" area of the graft that is coupled to the stapes, which leads to an increase in the middle ear gain of the reconstructed ear.

Canal Wall Up versus Canal Wall Down Mastoidectomy

In a canal wall down mastoidectomy, the bony tympanic annulus and much of the ear canal are removed, and the tympanic membrane graft is placed onto the facial ridge and medial attic wall. This results in a significant reduction in the size of the residual middle ear air space. However, as long as this air space is ≥ 0.4 cc, the resultant loss of sound transmission should be < 10 dB (see above). Since the average volume of the tympanic cavity is 0.5 to 1.0 cc,[27,77] a canal wall down procedure should create no significant acoustic detriment as long as the middle ear is aerated.

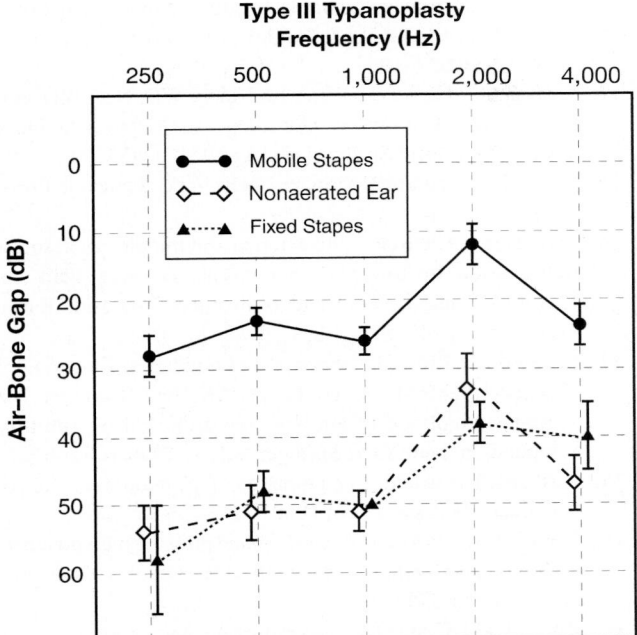

Figure 3–20 Air–bone gaps (mean ± 1 standard error of mean [SEM]) measured in 35 ears after canal wall down mastoidectomy and type III tympanoplasty with temporalis fascia graft onto the stapes head. The results are displayed in three groups: (1) ears with a mobile stapes and an aerated middle ear after surgery (n = 23), (2) ears with a mobile stapes but no aeration of the middle ear postoperatively (n = 10), and (3) ears with an aerated middle ear postoperatively but a fixed stapes footplate (n = 2). The mobility of the stapes was judged at the time of surgery, and aeration of the middle ear was determined on the basis of postoperative computed tomographic scan assessments, pneumatic otoscopy, and visible motion of the graft during Valsalva's maneuver. The best hearing results (air–bone gaps of 15 to 30 dB) are seen in those cases in which the middle ear becomes aerated and the stapes is mobile. Large air–bone gaps of 40 to 60 dB occur as a result of stapes fixation, nonaeration of the middle ear, or both.

A canal wall down procedure also results in the creation of a large air space lateral to the eardrum, that is, the air space within the mastoid bowl including the external auditory canal. This mastoid bowl and ear canal air space generate resonances that can influence middle ear sound transmission favorably or unfavorably.[102] The structure-function relationships between the size and shape of the mastoid cavity and cavity resonances have not been well defined. An improved understanding of this issue may help otosurgeons to configure mastoid cavities in ways that are acoustically beneficial.

Stapedotomy

The output of the middle ear can be quantified by the "volume velocity" of the stapes,[87] where volume veloc-ity is the product of stapes linear velocity and the area of the stapes footplate. After a stapedotomy, the effective area of the footplate is reduced to the area of the prosthesis, thereby reducing the volume velocity produced by a given stapes linear velocity. The reduction in effective footplate area also reduces the area of the cochlear fluid over which the force generated by the stapes is applied. Although the reduced footplate area leads to a local increase in pressure over the surface of the prosthesis, the average pressure at the cochlear entrance is reduced. The reduction in stapes volume velocity and cochlear sound pressure leads to a decrease in ossicular coupling and the development of an air–bone gap. The smaller the area of the stapes prosthesis, the greater the air–bone gap. Model predictions of the relationship between piston diameter and residual air–bone gap after stapedotomy were made using a simple lumped-element model of the middle ear.[87] This analysis suggested that a 0.8-mm piston would cause a 5-dB gap at frequencies of 1,000 Hz and below, a 0.6-mm piston was predicted to cause a 10-dB gap, and a 0.4-mm piston was predicted to cause a 15-dB gap. These predictions are in general agreement with experimental temporal bone data,[103] the results of finite-element modeling data,[104] and clinical observations.[105–107] The predictions made in the simple lumped-element model[87] assumed that the effective vibrating footplate surface area after a stapedotomy is no more than the area of the lower end of the prosthesis. In cases of partial or total stapedectomy with placement of a tissue graft and a stapes prosthesis, the effective vibrating surface may be greater than the area of the prosthesis alone, and the model predictions may overestimate the air–bone gap.

Conclusions Regarding the Contribution of Middle Ear Mechanics to Otologic Practice

Until recently, the history of middle ear surgery has generally progressed with minimal input from basic scientists and engineers who studied the acoustics, mechanics, and physiology of the middle ear. In this chapter, we have made a case for how knowledge of middle ear mechanics can help the clinician to understand important aspects of present-day otologic practice and how close collaboration between clinicians and basic scientists can lead to improvements in an otologist's diagnostic and surgical capabilities. We have pointed out areas in which recent work and new knowledge have produced new guidelines to optimize surgical results (eg, type III and IV tympanoplasty, stapedotomy, some aspects of ossiculoplasty) and have also pointed out areas in which our knowledge is incomplete and more research is needed (eg, tympanic membrane reconstruction, effect of static pressures, some aspects of ossicular reconstruction). Hopefully, some of these latter areas will be better understood by the time the next edition of this book is produced.

ACKNOWLEDGMENT

We thank, Joseph B. Nadol Jr, MD, Michael J. McKenna, MD, Steven D. Rauch, MD, and William T. Peake, ScD, for advice and comments on previous versions of this chapter. The authors' efforts were supported by grants from the National Institute on Deafness and Other Communication Disorders of the National Institutes of Health.

REFERENCES

1. Polizter A. Geschichte der Ohrenheilkunde. Stuggart: F. Enke; 1907–13. (Reprinted, Hildesheim, 1967).

2. Wever EG, Lawrence M. Physiological acoustics. Princeton (NJ): Princeton University Press; 1954.

3. Leicher H, Mittermaier R, Theissing G, editors. Awanglose Abhandlungen aus dem Gebief der Hals-Nasen-Ohren-Heilkunde. Stuttgart: Georg Thieme Verlag; 1960.

4. Hunt FV. Origins in acoustics: the science of sound from antiquity to the age of Newton. New Haven (CT): Yale University Press; 1978.

5. Pappas DG, Kent L. Otology's great moments. Birmingham (UK): Pappas; 2000.

6. Austin DF. Mechanics of hearing. In: Glasscock ME, Shambaugh GE, editors. Surgery of the ear. 4th ed. Philadelphia: WB Saunders; 1990. p. 297–8.

7. Helmholtz HLF. Die Mechanik der Gehörknöchelchen und des Trommelfells. Pflugers Arch Physiol 1868;1:1–60.

8. Yost WA. Fundamentals of hearing. New York: Academic Press; 1994.

9. Stevens SS, Davis H. Hearing. New York: Wiley; 1938.

10. Guinan JJ, Peake WT. Middle ear characteristics of anesthetized cats. J Acoust Soc Am 1967;41:1237–61.

11. Ruggero MA, Rich NC, Shivapuja BG, Temchin AN. Auditory-nerve responses to low-frequency tones: intensity dependence. Auditory Neurosci 1996;2:159–85.

12. Sivian LJ, White SD. On minimum sound audible fields. J Acoust Soc Am 1933;4:288–321.

13. American National Standards Institute. American national standard specifications for audiometers. New York: ANSI; 1970. ANSI-S3.6-1969.

14. Shaw EAG. The external ear. In: Keidel WD, Neff WD, editors. Handbook of sensory physiology. Vol V, Part I: Auditory system. New York: Springer-Verlag; 1974. p. 455–90.

15. Dallos P. The auditory periphery. New York: Academic Press; 1973.

16. Zwislocki J. The role of the external and middle ear in sound transmission. In: Tower DB, editor. The nervous system. Vol 3: Human communication and its disorders. New York: Raven Press; 1975. p. 45–55.

17. Rosowski JJ. Models of external and middle ear function. In: Hawkins HS, McMullen TA, Popper AN, Fay RR, editors. The Springer handbook of auditory research. Vol 6: Auditory computation. New York: Springer-Verlag; 1996. p. 15–61.

18. Kirikae I. The structure and function of the middle ear. Tokyo: University of Tokyo Press; 1960.

19. Puria S, Peake WT, Rosowski JJ. Sound pressure measurements in the cochlear vestibule of human cadaver ears. J Acoust Soc Am 1997;101:2754–70.

20. Kurokawa G, Goode RL. Sound pressure gain produced by the human middle ear. Otolaryngol Head Neck Surg 1995;113:349–55.

21. Aibara R, Welsh J, Puria S, Goode R. Human middle-ear sound transfer function and cochlear input impedance. Hear Res 2001;152:100–9.

22. Tonndorf J, Khanna SM. Tympanic membrane vibrations in human cadaver ears studied by time-averaged holography. J Acoust Soc Am 1972;52:1221–33.

23. Decraemer WF, Khanna SM, Funnell WRJ. Interferometric measurement of the amplitude and phase of tympanic membrane vibrations in cat. Hear Res 1989;38:1–18.

24. Goode RL, Killion M, Nakamura K, Nishihara S. New knowledge about the function of the human middle ear: development of an improved analog model. Am J Otol 1994;15:145–54.

25. Schmitt H. Über die bedeutung der Schalldrucktransformation und der Schallprotektion für die Hörschwelle. Acta Otolaryngol (Stockh) 1958;49:71–80.

26. Terkildsen K. Pathologies and their effect on middle ear function. In: Feldman A, Wilber L, editors. Acoustic impedance and admittance: the measurement of middle-ear function. Baltimore: Williams & Wilkins; 1976. p. 78–102.

27. Whittemore KR, Merchant SN, Rosowski JJ. Acoustic mechanisms: canal wall-up versus canal wall-down mastoidectomy. Otolaryngol Head Neck Surg 1998;118:751–61.

28. Voss SE, Rosowski JJ, Merchant SN, Peake WT. Acoustic responses of the human middle ear. Hear Res 2000;150:43–69.

29. Gopen Q, Rosowski JJ, Merchant SN. Anatomy of the normal cochlear aqueduct with functional implications. Hear Res 1997;107:9–22.

30. Wever EG, Lawrence M. The acoustic pathway to the cochlea. J Acoust Soc Am 1950;22:460–7.

31. Voss SE, Rosowski JJ, Peake WT. Is the pressure difference between the oval and round windows the effective acoustic stimulus for the cochlea? J Acoust Soc Am 1996;100:1602–16.

32. Békésy GV. Experiments in hearing. New York: McGraw-Hill; 1960.

33. Wegel RL, Lane CE. The auditory masking of one pure tone by another and its probable relation to the dynamics of the inner ear. Physiol Rev 1924;23:266–85.

34. Rosen S, Bergman M, Plester D, et al. Presbycusis study of a relatively noise-free population in the Sudan. Ann Otol Rhinol Laryngol 1962;71:727–43.

35. Merchant SN, Ravicz ME, Puria S, et al. Analysis of middle ear mechanics and application to diseased and reconstructed ears. Am J Otol 1997;18:139–54.

36. Merchant SN, Ravicz ME, Voss SE, et al. Toynbee Memorial Lecture 1997. Middle ear mechanics in normal, diseased and reconstructed ears. J Laryngol Otol 1998;112:715–31.

37. Peake WT, Rosowski JJ, Lynch TJ III. Middle ear transmission: acoustic versus ossicular coupling in cat and human. Hear Res 1992;57:245–68.

38. Rosowski JJ. Mechanisms of sound conduction in normal and diseased ears. In: Rosowski JJ, Merchant SN, editors. The function and mechanics of normal, diseased and reconstructed middle ears. The Hague, The Netherlands: Kugler Publications, 2000. p. 137–45.

39. Tonndorf J. Bone conduction hearing. In: Keidel WD, Neff WD, editors. Handbook of sensory physiology. Vol. V, Part III. Berlin: Springer-Verlag; 1974. p. 37–84.

40. Carhart R. The clinical application of bone conduction audiometry. Arch Otol 1950;51:798–808.

41. Carmel PW, Starr A. Acoustic and nonacoustic factors modifying middle ear muscle activity in waking cats. J Neurophysiol 1963;26:598–616.

42. Borg E. A quantitative study of the effect of the acoustic stapedius reflex on sound transmission through the middle ear of man. Acta Otolaryngol (Stockh) 1968;66:461–72.

43. Møller AR. The acoustic middle-ear muscle reflex. In: Keidel WD, Neff WD, editors. Handbook of sensory physiology: auditory system. Vol V, Part I. Berlin: Springer-Verlag; 1974. p. 519–48.

44. Borg E, Zakrisson JE. Stapedius muscle and monaural masking. Acta Otolaryngol (Stockh) 1974;94:385–93.

45. Pang XD, Guinan JJ. Effects of stapedius-muscle contractions on the masking of auditory nerve responses. J Acoust Soc Am 1997;102:3576–86.

46. Borg E, Nilsson R, Engstrom B. Effect of the acoustic reflex on inner ear damage induced by industrial noise. Acta Otolaryngol (Stockh) 1983;96:361–9.

47. Ingelstedt S, Jonson B. Mechanisms of gas exchange in the normal human middle ear. Acta Otolaryngol Suppl (Stockh) 1966; 224:452–61.

48. Marquet J. The incudo-malleal joint. J Laryngol Otol 1981;95: 542–65.

49. Hüttenbrink KB. The mechanics of the middle-ear at static air pressures. Acta Otolaryngol Suppl (Stockh) 1988;451:1–35.

50. Pang XD, Peake WT. How do contractions of the stapedius muscle alter the acoustic properties of the middle ear? In: Allen JB, Hall JL, Hubbard A, et al, editors. Peripheral auditory mechanisms. New York: Springer-Verlag; 1986. p. 36–43.

51. Gyo K, Aritomo H, Goode RL. Measurement of the ossicular vibration ratio in human temporal bones by use of a video measuring system. Acta Otolaryngol (Stockh) 1987;103:87–95.

52. Zwislocki J. Analysis of the middle ear function. Part II. Guinea-pig ear. J Acoust Soc Am 1963;35:1034–40.

53. Møller AR. Experimental study of the acoustic impedance of the middle ear and its transmission properties. Acta Otolaryngol (Stockh) 1965;60:129–49.

54. Khanna SM, Tonndorf J. Tympanic membrane vibrations in cats studied by time-averaged holography. J Acoust Soc Am 1972;51: 1904–20.

55. Nedzelnitsky V. Sound pressures in the basal turn of the cat cochlea. J Acoust Soc Am 1980;68:1676–89.

56. Nuttall AL. Tympanic muscle effects on middle-ear transfer characteristics. J Acoust Soc Am 1974;56:1239–47.

57. McArdle FE, Tonndorf J. Perforations of the tympanic membrane and their effects upon middle ear transmission. Arch Klin Exp Ohren Nasen Kehlkopfheilkd 1968;192:145–62.

58. Bigelow DC, Swanson PB, Saunders JC. The effect of tympanic membrane perforation size on umbo velocity in the rat. Laryngoscope 1996;106:71–6.

59. Wiederhold ML, Zajtchuk JT, Vap JG, Paggi RE . Hearing loss in relation to physical properties of middle ear effusions. Ann Otol Rhinol Laryngol 1980;89 Suppl 68:185–9.

60. Decraemer WF, Khanna SM, Funnell WRJ. Bending of the manubrium in cat under normal sound stimulation. Prog Biomed Optics 1995;2329:74–84.

61. Puria S, Allen JB. Measurements and model of the cat middle ear: evidence of tympanic membrane acoustic delay. J Acoust Soc Am 1998;104:3463–81.

62. Henson OW, Henson MM. The tympanic membrane: highly developed smooth muscle arrays in the annulus fibrosus of mustached bats. J Assoc Res Otolaryngol 2000;1:25–32.

63. Rosowski JJ, Carney LH, Lynch TJ, Peake WT. The effectiveness of external and middle ears in coupling acoustic power into the cochlea. In: Allen JB, Hall JL, Hubbard A, editors. Peripheral auditory mechanisms: proceedings of a conference held at Boston University, Boston, MA, August 13–16, 1985. New York: Springer-Verlag; 1986. p. 3–12.

64. Zwislocki J. Analysis of the middle-ear function. Part I: input impedance. J Acoust Soc Am 1962;34:1514–23.

65. Funnell WRJ, Decraemer WM. On the incorporation of moiré shape measurements in finite-element models of the cat eardrum. J Acoust Soc Am 1996;100:925–32.

66. Rosowski JJ, Davis PJ, Merchant SN, et al. Cadaver middle ears as models for living ears: comparisons of middle ear input immittance. Ann Otol Rhinol Laryngol 1990;99:403–12.

67. Goode RL, Ball G, Nishihara S, Nakamura K. Laser Doppler Vibrometer (LDV)—a new clinical tool for the otologist. Am J Otol 1996;17:813–22.

68. Schuknecht HF. Stapedectomy. Boston: Little, Brown and Co.; 1972.

69. Schuknecht HF. Pathology of the ear. 2nd ed. Philadelphia: Lea & Febiger; 1993.

70. Vincent R, Lopez A, Sperling NM. Malleus-ankylosis: a clinical, audiometric, histologic and surgical study of 123 cases. Am J Otol 1999;20:717–25.

71. Kruger B, Tonndorf J. Middle ear transmission in cats with experimentally induced tympanic membrane perforations. J Acoust Soc Am 1977;61:126–32.

72. Voss SE, Rosowski JJ, Merchant SN, Peake WT. How do tympanic membrane perforations affect human middle-ear sound transmission? Acta Otolaryngol (Stockh) 2001;121:169–73.

73. Voss SE, Rosowski JJ, Merchant SN, Peake WT. Middle-ear function with tympanic membrane perforations I: measurements and mechanisms. J Acoust Soc Am 2001;110:1432–44.

74. Voss SE, Rosowski JJ, Merchant SN, Peake WT. Middle-ear function with tympanic membrane perforations II: a simple model. J Acoust Soc Am 2001;110:1445–52.

75. Molvaer O, Vallersnes F, Kringelbotn M. The size of the middle ear and the mastoid air cell. Acta Otolaryngol (Stockh) 1978;85:24–32.

76. Fria T, Cantekin E, Eichler J. Hearing acuity of children with otitis media. Arch Otolaryngol 1985;111:10–6.

77. Ravicz ME, Merchant SN, Rosowski JJ. Effects of middle-ear fluid on umbo motion in human ears. In: Wada H, Takasaka T, Ikeda K, et al, editors. Recent developments in auditory mechanics. Proceedings of the International Symposium on Recent Developments in Auditory Mechanics. Singapore: World Scientific; 2000. p. 15–21.

78. Lee K, Schuknecht HF. Results of tympanoplasty and mastoidectomy at the Massachusetts Eye and Ear Infirmary. Laryngoscope 1971;81:529–43.

79. Pennington CL. Incus interposition techniques. Ann Otol 1973; 82:518–31.

80. Jackson CG, Glasscock ME, Schwaber MK, et al. Ossicular chain reconstruction: the TORP and PORP in chronic ear disease. Laryngoscope 1983;93:981–8.

81. Brackmann DE, Sheehy JL, Luxford WM. TORPS and PORPS in tympanoplasty: a review of 1042 operations. Otolaryngol Head Neck Surg 1984;92:32–7.

82. Lau T, Tos M. Long-term results of surgery for granulating otitis. Am J Otolaryngol 1986;7:341–5.

83. Ragheb SM, Gantz BJ, McCabe BF. Hearing results after cholesteatoma surgery: the Iowa experience. Laryngoscope 1987;97:1254–63.

84. Colletti V, Fiorino FG, Sittoni V. Minisculptured ossicle grafts versus implants: long term results. Am J Otol 1987;8:553–9.

85. Goldenberg RA. Hydroxylapatite ossicular replacement prostheses: a four year experience. Otolaryngol Head Neck Surg 1992;106:261–9.

86. Liston SL, Levine SC, Margolis RH, Yanz JL. Use of intraoperative auditory brainstem responses to guide prosthesis positioning. Laryngoscope 1991;101:1009–12.

87. Rosowski JJ, Merchant SN. Mechanical and acoustic analysis of middle-ear reconstruction. Am J Otol 1995;16:486–97.

88. Gyo K, Goode RL, Miller C. Effect of middle-ear modification on umbo vibration-human temporal bone experiments with a new vibration measuring system. Arch Otolaryngol Head Neck Surg 1986;112:1262–8.

89. Mach E, J Kessel. Die Function der Trommelhöhle und der Tuba Eustachii. Sitzungsber. Akad Wiss Wein math-nat Cl 1872;66: 329–66.

90. Murakami S, Gyo K, Goode RL. Effect of middle ear pressure change on middle ear mechanics. Acta Otolaryngol (Stockh) 1997;117:390–5.

91. Wullstein H. The restoration of the function of the middle ear, in chronic otitis media. Ann Otol Rhinol Laryngol 1956;65: 1020–41.

92. Gacek RR. Symposium on tympanoplasty. Results of modified type V tympanoplasty. Laryngoscope 1973;83:437–47.

93. Rosowski JJ, Merchant SN, Ravicz ME. Middle ear mechanics of type IV and type V tympanoplasty. I. Model analysis and predictions. Am J Otol 1995;16:555–64.

94. Merchant SN, Rosowski JJ, Ravicz ME. Middle ear mechanics of type IV and type V tympanoplasty. II. Clinical analysis and surgical implications. Am J Otol 1995;16:565–75.

95. Merchant SN, Ravicz ME, Rosowski JJ. Experimental investigation of the mechanics of type IV tympanoplasty. Ann Otol Rhinol Laryngol 1997;106:49–60.

96. Montandon P, Chatelain C. Restoration of hearing with type V tympanoplasty. ORL J Otorhinolaryngol Relat Spec 1991;53: 342–5.

97. Gan RZ, Dyer RK, Wood MW, Dormer KJ. Mass loading on the ossicles and middle ear function. Ann Otol Rhinol Laryngol 2001;110:478–85.

98. Vlaming MSMG, Feenstra L. Studies on the mechanics of the reconstructed human middle ear. Clin Otolaryngol 1986;11: 411–22.

99. Nishihara S, Goode RL. Experimental study of the acoustic properties of incus replacement prostheses in a human temporal bone model. Am J Otol 1994;15:485–94.

100. Goode RL, Nishihara S. Experimental models of ossiculoplasty. In: Monsell E, editor. Ossiculoplasty. Otolaryngol Clin North Am 1994;27:663–75.

101. Mehta RP, Ravicz ME, Rosowski JJ, Merchant SN. Middle-ear mechanics of type III tympanoplasty: basic and clinical studies. Abstracts of 135th Annual Meeting of American Otological Society, Inc, May 10–11, 2002, Boca Raton, FL, p. 22.

102. Goode RL, Friedrichs R, Falk S. Effect on hearing thresholds of surgical modification of the external ear. Ann Otol Rhinol Laryngol 1977;86:441–51.

103. Goode RL, Hato N. A temporal bone model of stapedotomy for otosclerosis. Otolaryngol Head Neck Surg 2000;123:p86–7.

104. Koike T, Wada H, Goode RL. Finite-element method analysis of transfer function of middle ear reconstructed using stapes prosthesis. In: Association for Research in Otolaryngology (ARO) Abstracts of the 24th Midwinter Meeting. Mt. Royal (NJ): Association for Research in Otolaryngology; 2001. p. 221.

105. Smyth GDL, Hassard TH: Eighteen years experience in stapedectomy. The case for the small fenestra operation. Ann Otol Rhinol Laryngol Suppl 1978;49:3–36.

106. Schuknecht HF, Bentkover SH. Partial stapedectomy and piston prosthesis. In: Snow JB Jr, editor. Controversy in otolaryngology. Philadelphia: WB Saunders; 1980. p. 281–91.

107. Teig E, Lindeman HH. Stapedectomy piston diameter: is bigger better? In: Rosowski JJ, Merchant SN, editors. The function and mechanics of normal, diseased and reconstructed middle ears. The Hague, The Netherlands: Kugler Publications; 2000. p. 281–7.

4

Vestibular Physiology and Disorders of the Labyrinth

TIMOTHY E. HULLAR, MD
LLOYD B. MINOR, MD, FACS

The vestibular system collects information about the position and motion of the head. Together with visual and proprioceptive signals, the brain uses this information to coordinate the eyes, head, and body during movement and to give a conscious perception of orientation and motion. Disturbances in this integrative process can lead to dizziness, which is the ninth most common cause of visits to primary care physicians and the most common among patients over 75 years.[1,2] Many of these patients are referred to otologists to determine if a vestibular abnormality accounts for their complaint and to develop a treatment plan. Knowledge of the anatomy and physiology of the vestibular system gives a rational basis for understanding the causes and treatment of many types of dizziness.

In cases of vestibular pathology, the motor reflexes that depend on input from the vestibular system are disturbed. Vestibulo-ocular reflexes are responsible for maintaining the stability of objects on the retina during head movements. Disorders in their physiology can result in nystagmus and/or in impaired eye movements in response to head movements with consequent loss of visual acuity. Nystagmus is a to-and-fro beating of the eyes with slow and fast components. The direction of nystagmus is frequently named in terms of the fast component, although it is the slow component that actually reflects the underlying vestibular imbalance. The fast components are resetting movements that prevent the eye from exceeding its range of motion.

Vestibulospinal reflexes maintain posture with respect to gravity and assist vestibulo-ocular reflexes by producing contraction of neck muscles that compensate for externally applied motion to the neck or body. Disorders of vestibulospinal reflexes can result in tilt of the head, abnormal posture, or ataxia.

This chapter begins with a review of the anatomy and physiology of vestibular pathways, with particular emphasis on those mechanisms important to an understanding of the symptoms and signs seen in vestibular disorders. The highlights of the bedside evaluation of vestibular function, including the history and clinical examination, are then discussed, followed by a review of vestibular tests and an overview of disorders that affect vestibular function. The presentation of these clinical topics emphasizes the basic principles of vestibular physiology, which provide a method for understanding the meaning and significance of many clinical findings.

ANATOMIC ORGANIZATION OF THE VESTIBULAR SYSTEM

Dividing the vestibular system into its peripheral and central parts helps to localize pathologies. The periphery consists of the labyrinth—which includes the horizontal, superior, and posterior semicircular canals as well as the utricle and saccule—and its projections to the brainstem (Figure 4–1). The central vestibular system consists of the lateral, medial, superior, and inferior vestibular nuclei and their projections to the cerebellum, descending spinal cord, and extraocular motor nuclei.

The bony labyrinth of the peripheral vestibular system is hollowed from the dense temporal bone and lined with the membranous labyrinth, which contains structures that sense motion of the head. Afferent nerve fibers in the superior vestibular nerve extend from sensory

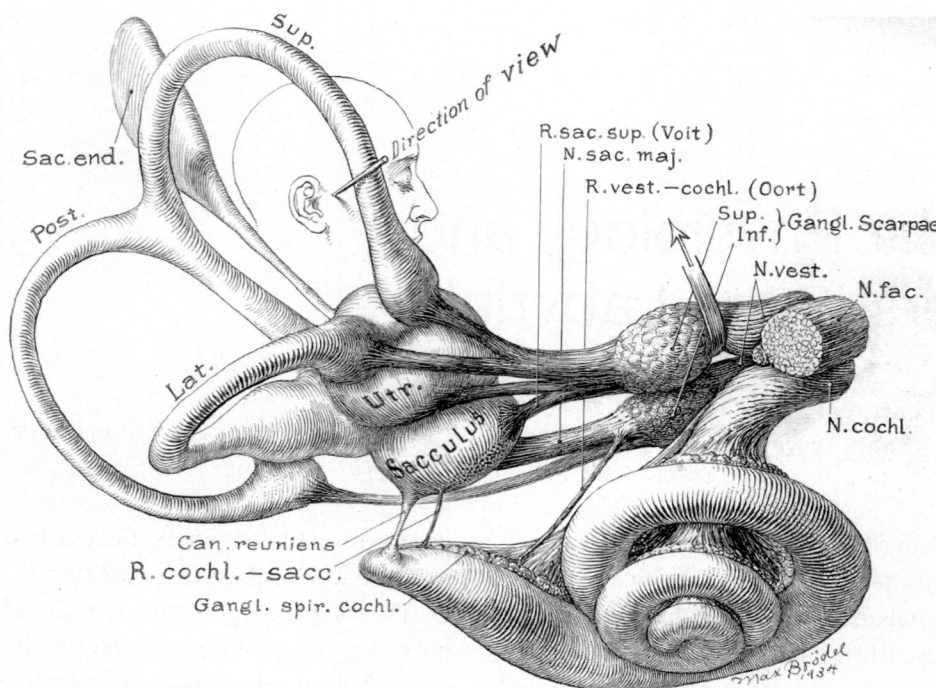

Figure 4–1 Structures of the labyrinth. Structures shown include the utricle (utr.), sacculus, anterior or superior semicircular canal (sup.), posterior semicircular canal (post.), and horizontal or lateral semicircular canal (lat.). The superior vestibular nerve innervates the horizontal and anterior semicircular canals and the utricle. The inferior vestibular nerve innervates the posterior semicircular canal and the saccule. The cell bodies for the vestibular nerves are located in Scarpa's ganglion (Gangl. Scarpae). Drawing from the Brödel Archives, No. 933. Reproduced with permission of the Department of Art as Applied to Medicine, Johns Hopkins University.

structures in the superior and horizontal canals and the utricle to the vestibular nuclei in the brainstem. The inferior vestibular nerve leads from the posterior semicircular canal and the saccule. In humans, each vestibular nerve is made up of about 25,000 neurons.[3] These neurons are bipolar, with cell bodies located in the vestibular nerve near the brainstem in Scarpa's ganglion. In addition to afferents, about 400 to 600 efferent nerves lead from the vestibular nuclei to hair cells and afferent nerves in each labyrinth.[4] The precise role of these efferents in modulating the physiology of vestibular reflexes is unknown.

Information about motion of the head is encoded in the discharge rate of the vestibular nerve afferents. All acceleration can be divided into six components: rotation around an axis lying in each of the three dimensions and linear motion along each of these axes. The semicircular canals serve primarily to measure rotation. Each canal has a synergistic canal on the opposite side lying approximately parallel to it. The horizontal canals act as a pair, while each superior (anterior) canal is paired

with the posterior canal on the opposite side (Figure 4–2). The utricle and saccule sense linear acceleration. These linear forces can arise from translation of the head front to back, side to side, or up and down, as well as from the orientation of the head relative to the pull of gravity.

Each membranous semicircular canal is filled with endolymph, a potassium-rich extracellular fluid, and is bathed in perilymph, which has the approximate composition of cerebrospinal fluid. The ends of the canals open into the vestibule. Near one end of each membranous canal is a widening known as the ampulla, which contains the crista ampullaris and cupula. The crista ampullaris is a saddle-shaped gelatinous structure along one wall of the membranous canal that contains hair cells, the sensory cells of the vestibular system. The cupula acts as a membranous diaphragm, stretching from the crista to the opposite walls of the canal (Figure 4–3). Because the membranous labyrinth is tethered to the skull, the crista and cupula accelerate with the head as it rotates, whereas the inertia of the endolymph causes it to lag behind. The endolymph accumulates with higher pres-

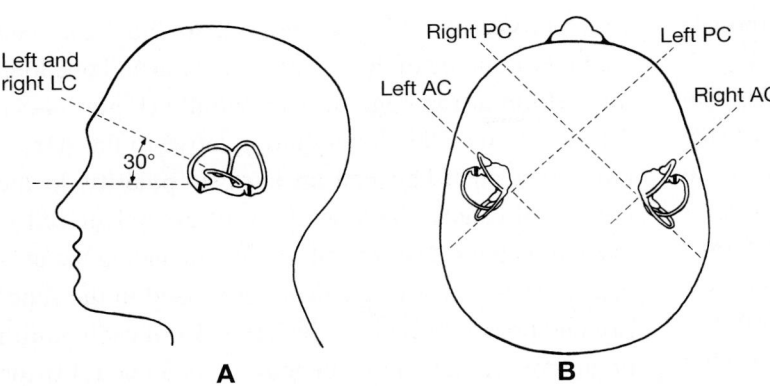

Figure 4–2 Orientation of the semicircular canals. *A*, Horizontal (lateral) semicircular canals. *B*, Anterior (superior) and posterior canals. LC = lateral canal; AC = anterior canal; PC = posterior canal. Relative size of canals exaggerated for clarity. Reproduced with permission from Barber H, Stockwell C. Textbook of electronystagmography. St. Louis: Mosby, 1976.

sure on one side of the cupula than the other, indenting it and bending the hair cells within the crista. When the head ceases to accelerate, the cupula and crista gradually return to their resting positions.

The utricle and saccule, together called the otolith organs, also contain hair cells that bend in response to acceleration of the head. Instead of cristae, however, the sensory epithelium of these organs is covered by flat, kidney-shaped sheets called maculae. One macula is applied horizontally to the ceiling of the utricle, whereas the other hangs sagittally on the wall of the saccule. Each macula is a gelatinous matrix into which hair cells pro-

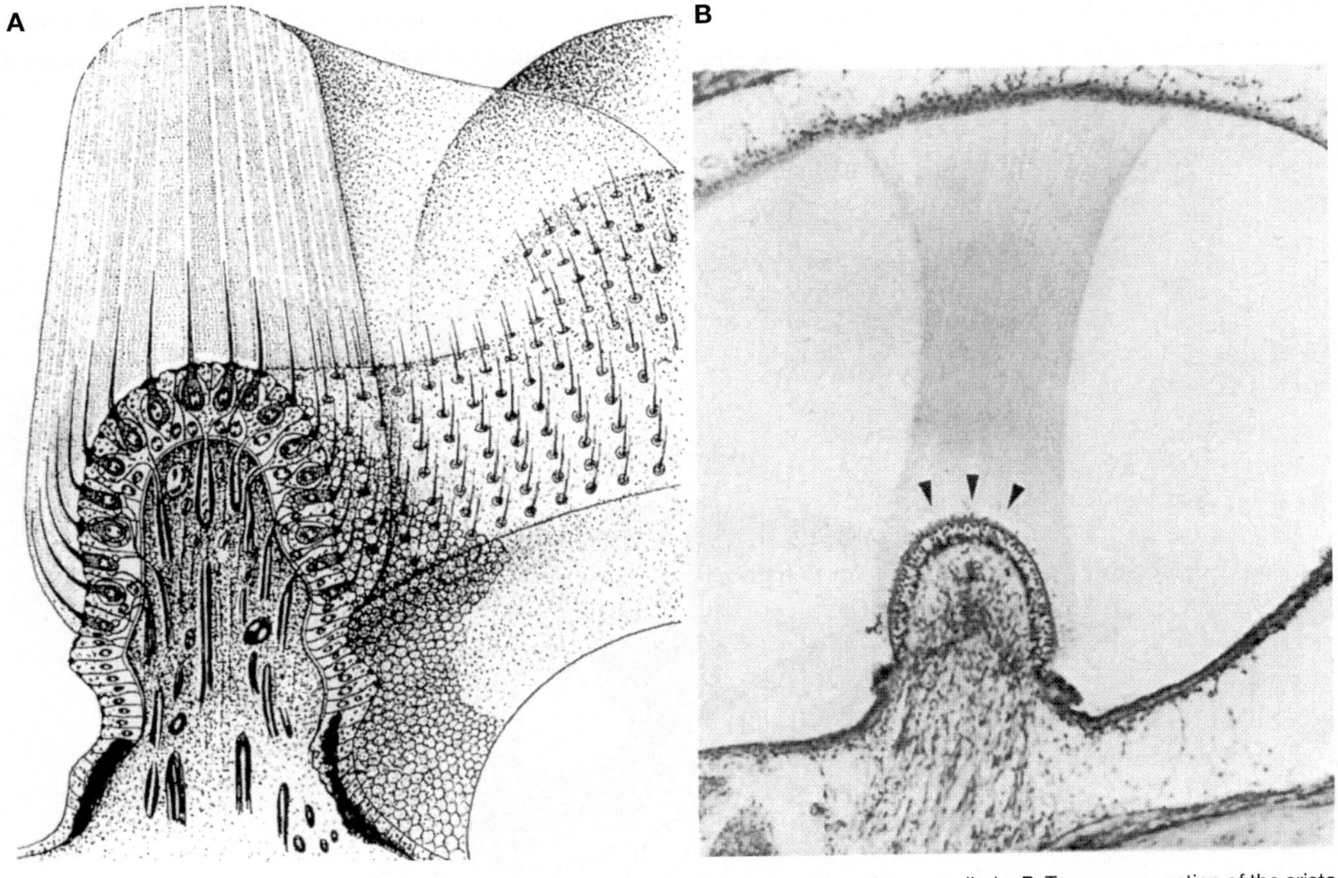

Figure 4–3 Structure of the crista ampullaris and cupula. *A*, Artist's reconstruction of the crista ampullaris. *B*, Transverse section of the crista ampullaris of the monkey. The histologic techniques preserved the attachment of the cupula, which extends from the apex of the crista to the opposite wall of the membranous ampulla. *Arrowheads* indicate subcupular space. *A* reproduced with permission from Wersäll J, Lundquist PG. In: Graybiel A, editor, Second Symposium on the Role of Vestibular Organs in Space Exploration, NASA SP-115. Washington (DC): US Government Printing Office; 1966. *B* reproduced with permission from Igarashi M. In: Graybiel A, editor. Second Symposium on the Role of Vestibular Organs in Space Exploration, NASA SP-115. Washington (DC): US Government Printing Office; 1966.

ject and which is studded with tiny calcium carbonate granules called otoconia.

Whereas the cristae have a specific gravity identical to the surrounding endolymph, the otoconia increase the density of the maculae and render them sensitive to shearing forces parallel to their surfaces caused by gravity or linear motions of the head. Any time the head moves linearly, the heavy maculae lag behind, bending the hair cells embedded in them. The utricle primarily senses lateral tilt and translation of the head, whereas the saccule measures front-to-back tilt and translation as well as motion aligned with the pull of gravity (Figure 4–4).

PHYSIOLOGY OF THE VESTIBULAR SYSTEM

Hair cells located in the sensory epithelia of the semicircular canals and otolith organs are responsible for transforming motion into a modulation in the discharge rate of afferent nerve fibers innervating the vestibular nerve. The hair cells are named after their tufted cilia,

which project into the gelatinous crista. Each hair cell contains a bundle of 50 to 100 stereocilia and one long kinocilium at the edge of each bundle (Figure 4–5). The location of this kinocilium relative to the stereocilia gives each hair cell an intrinsic polarity. In the horizontal canals, the kinocilium of every hair cell is located on the side of the ciliary bundle facing the utricle, whereas this arrangement is reversed in the superior and posterior canals. The hair cells of each otolith organ are arranged in two bands along a central stripe called the striola. The kinocilia of the hair bundles in the utricle are oriented toward the striola and those in the saccule face away.

Displacement of a ciliary bundle toward its kinocilium opens potassium channels along the cilia and depolarizes the hair cell from its resting membrane potential of between –50 and –70 mV. The sensitivity of the hair cell can approach 20 mV of depolarization per micrometer of displacement. This depolarization leads to calcium influx at the basal end of the hair cells and increased

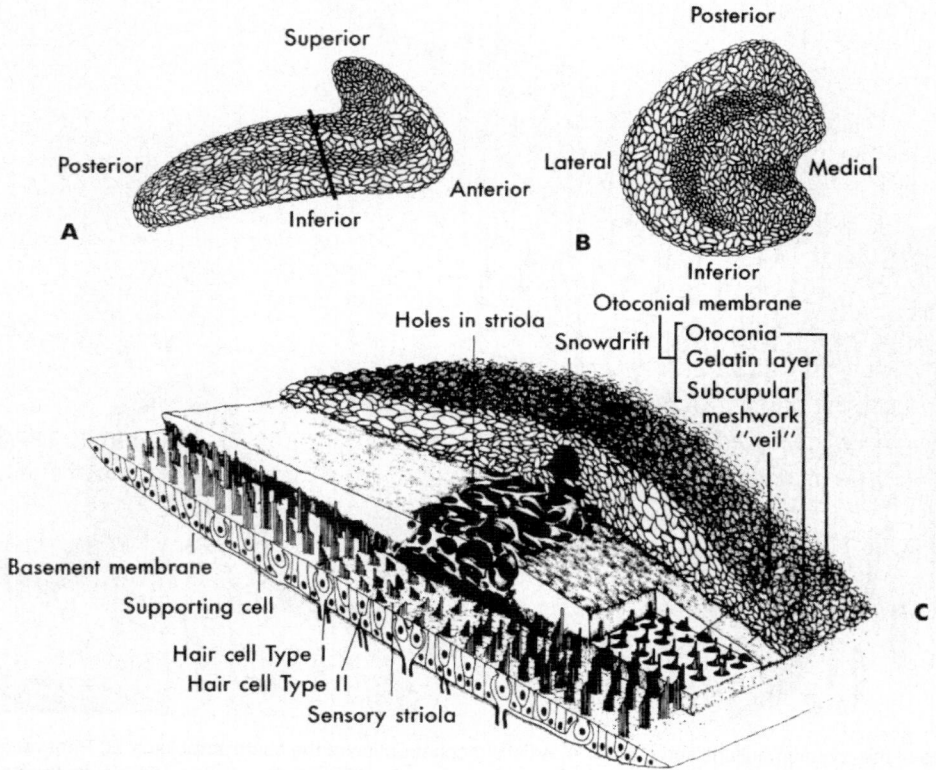

Figure 4–4 Structure of the otolith organs. *A*, Sacculus. *B*, Utriculus. *C*, Composition of otoconial membrane of the saccus in a section taken at the level shown in *A*. Reproduced with permission from Paparella MM, Shumrick DA, editors. Textbook of otolaryngology. Vol 1. Philadelphia: WB Saunders; 1980.

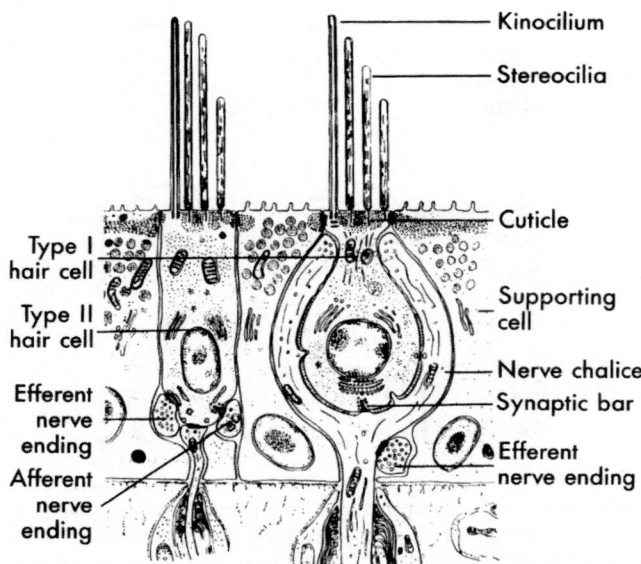

Figure 4–5   Two types of sensory hair cells (types I and II) are found in the mammalian labyrinth. Reproduced with permission from Wersäll J, Bagger-Sjöback D. In: Kornhuber HH, editor. Handbook of sensory physiology. New York: Springer-Verlag; 1974.

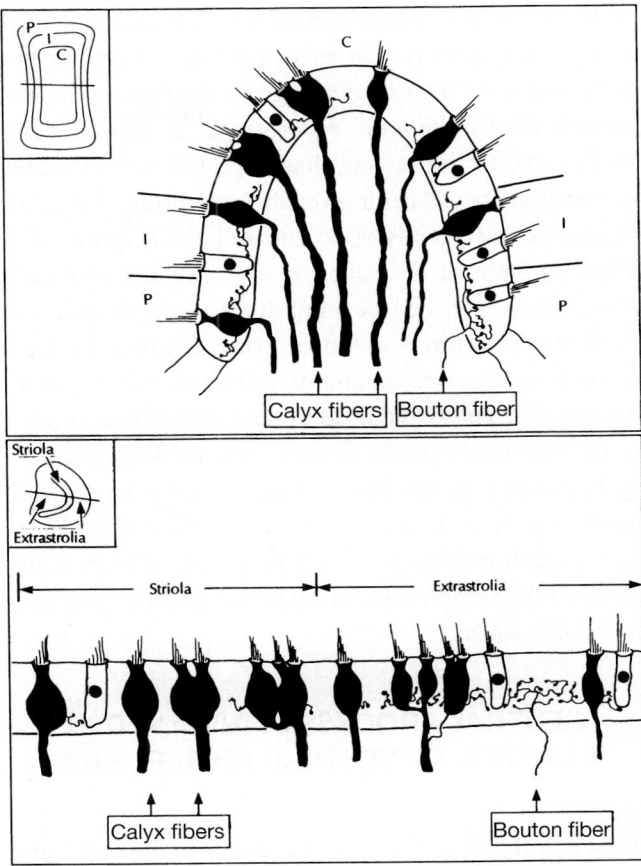

Figure 4–6   Afferent innervation patterns in the mammalian vestibular end-organs. *Top*, The neuroepithelium of the cristae is divided into central (C), intermediate (I), and peripheral (P) zones, shown in plan in the *inset* and in cross-section in the *main panel*. Calyx fibers innervate the central zone, whereas bouton fibers innervate the peripheral zone. Dimorphic fibers are found throughout. *Bottom*, The macula is divided into the striola and the lateral and medial extrastriola (see *inset*). Calyx fibers are found in the striola, bouton fibers in the extrastriola, and dimorphs throughout. Reproduced with permission from Goldberg JM. The vestibular end organs: morphological and physiological diversity of afferents. Curr Opin Neurobiol 1991;1:229–35.

flow of neurotransmitter into the synapse, whereas displacement in the opposite direction hyperpolarizes the cell and reduces neurotransmitter release.

Hair cells in the sensory epithelia of the labyrinth are innervated by vestibular nerve afferents. Almost all vestibular nerve afferents have a spontaneous or resting discharge rate. This resting discharge rate enables the afferents to respond to stimuli that cause inhibition and excitation. Discharge regularity, determined from the spacing between action potentials of the afferent's discharge, has provided a useful marker for many important physiologic processes. Three groups of vestibular nerve afferents have been identified in mammals based on their responses to motion and their innervation profiles within the sensory epithelia of the labyrinth.[5] Bouton-only afferents have terminations exclusively onto type II hair cells in the peripheral zone of the cristae. These afferents are regularly discharging and have low rotational sensitivities. Dimorphic afferents have calyx endings terminating on type I hair cells and bouton endings terminating on type II hair cells (Figure 4–6). Their physiologic properties vary according to the location within the crista. Those dimorphic afferents terminating in the peripheral zone are regularly discharging, whereas those terminating near the central

zone are irregularly discharging with higher rotational sensitivity. There is also a group of afferents that terminate exclusively with calyx endings onto type I hair cells in the central zone. The calyx-only afferents are irregularly discharging and have low rotational sensitivities.

In work done over a century ago, Ewald identified two fundamental principles governing the relationship between the labyrinthine receptors and the vestibular reflexes that they mediate.[6] From experiments performed in pigeons, he noted that fenestration of a semicircular canal followed by mechanical stimulation of the membranous canal led to eye and head movements that were in the plane of that canal.

It was also noted that stimuli that were excitatory led to larger amplitude responses than did similar stimuli that were inhibitory. This larger range for excitatory in comparison with inhibitory responses is, at least in part, attributable to the resting discharge rate of vestibular nerve afferents and central vestibular neurons, which, in mammals, is typically 90 to 100 spikes/s (Figure 4–7). These neurons can be excited up to a firing rate of at least 350 spikes/s but can be inhibited to only 0 spikes/s. Thus, there is a three- to four-fold higher range for excitation in comparison to inhibition. The first observation, motion of the eyes and head in the plane of the affected canal, is termed Ewald's first law (Figure 4–8). The second observation, excitatory responses are larger than inhibitory ones, is referred to as Ewald's second law. These relationships provide a basis for understanding many of the symptoms and signs that occur after injury to the labyrinth.

CENTRAL PROCESSES INVOLVED IN CONTROL OF VESTIBULAR REFLEXES

The central part of the system consists of the vestibular nuclei, which integrate information from vision, pro-

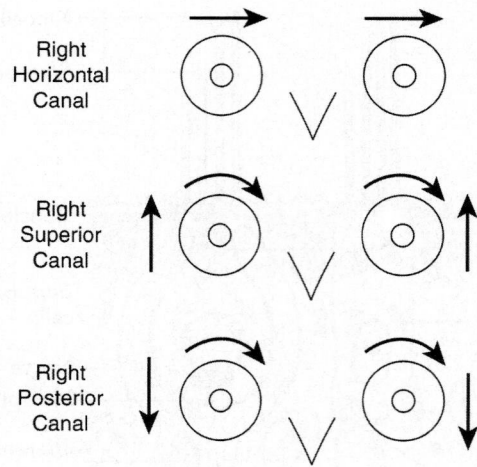

Figure 4–8 Eye movements evoked by excitatory stimulation of individual semicircular canals. The *arrows* depict the motion of the slow-phase components of the nystagmus. Stimulation of the right horizontal canal results in a horizontal nystagmus with leftward slow phases. A vertical-torsional nystagmus is elicited by excitatory stimulation of either the superior or posterior canals. For the right superior canal, the slow-phase components are directed upward and counterclockwise with respect to the patient (superior poles of the eyes moving leftward with intorsion of the right eye and extorsion of the left eye). For the right posterior canal, the slow-phase components are the same for torsion but are directed downward in the vertical plane. Reproduced with permission from Minor LB. Superior canal dehiscence syndrome. Am J Otol 2000;21:9–19.

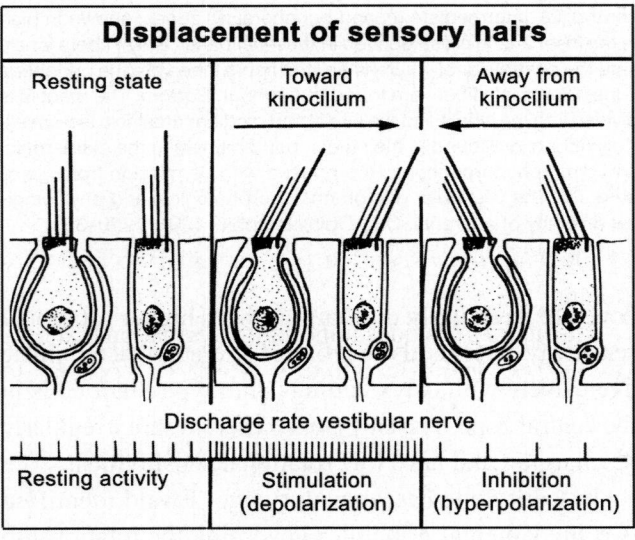

Figure 4–7 Discharge rate of individual vestibular-nerve fibers as a function of the displacement of the cilia. The vestibular nerve afferents fire more frequently when the hair bundles are displaced toward the kinocilia; they fire more slowly when displaced in the opposite direction. Reproduced with permission from Wersäll J, Lundquist P-G. In: Graybiel A, editor. Second Symposium on the Role of Vestibular Organs in Space Exploration, NASA SP-115. Washington (DC): US Government Printing Office; 1966.

prioception via spinal and cervical afferents, and the labyrinth. These nuclei send projections that extend to the oculomotor system, where they help control eye movements, and muscles of the neck and spine, where they steady the head. Central vestibular circuits also include the cerebellum, which is involved in recalibrating the system when necessary.

Vestibular projections to the oculomotor nuclei help maintain a steady image on the retina while the head is turning. The angular vestibulo-ocular reflex (AVOR) is a three-neuron arc consisting of a vestibular afferent neuron, a vestibular interneuron, and an ocular motoneuron. The AVOR is important because it maintains the stability of images on the fovea, thereby facilitating good visual acuity during head movements. The brain interprets stimulation of a particular semicircular canal as motion of the head, and the eyes move reflexively in an equal but opposite amount to compensate. Turning the head to the left, for example, excites the left horizontal semicircular canal, and the eyes track to the right in response. This action leaves the angle of the target relative to the eye unchanged and its image steady on the retina. Similar relationships apply for the vertical canals. The AVOR is the fastest and one of the most exquisitely accurate reflexes in the body. It has a latency of about 7 milliseconds and produces eye movements that typically have < 5% error with respect to head movements. Deficits of the AVOR lead to oscillopsia (the apparent motion of objects that are known to be stationary) during head movements.

To keep an image steady on the retina, tilts and linear movements of the head require compensatory eye motion as well. The linear vestibulo-ocular reflex is responsible for this compensation. Tilting the head side to side evokes ocular counter-rolling, which is torsional movement of the eye about the line of sight that partially compensates for the effect of the rotation. Translational motion in which the head is moved laterally, however, requires the eyes to track with horizontal rotations. The otolith organs cannot distinguish between a tilt and a translational movement, so the system must use other information—such as input from the semicircular canals, the frequency of motion encoded in otolith responses, or visual and proprioceptive cues—to decide how to move the eyes.

PRINCIPLES OF VESTIBULAR ADAPTATION AND COMPENSATION

The vestibular system shows a robust and versatile capacity for adaptive control of reflexes and higher motor behavior.[7] Changes in vestibular receptors with aging or specific pathologic disorders require mechanisms to detect errors and to correct them. Mechanisms of adaptive plasticity are responsible for maintaining the calibration of the AVOR under conditions in which the eye movements required for optimal compensatory function are altered. Such conditions are brought about by optically induced alterations in the motion of images on the retina as occurs with magnifying or miniaturizing spectacles.[8,9] The gain and timing characteristics (phase) of the vestibulo-ocular reflex adapt to meet the demands imposed by the altered viewing conditions.

Recent studies of the AVOR evoked by rapid, high-frequency, high-acceleration head movements have provided evidence of two functional components involved in control of the reflex.[10–13] These rotational stimuli are relevant because they encompass the range of natural

head movements for which the compensatory function of the AVOR is vital.[14] The components differ in their responses with respect to the frequency and velocity of the head movement. The linear component* is responsible for maintaining a constant gain and phase of the reflex across a large range of frequencies, velocities, and accelerations. The nonlinear or phasic component augments responses to higher frequency and velocity rotations and is more highly modifiable following labyrinthine lesions or spectacle-induced adaptation. The linear component is likely to be mediated by regularly discharging afferents,[15] whereas irregularly discharging afferents may provide the inputs for the nonlinear component.

BEDSIDE EVALUATION OF THE VESTIBULAR SYSTEM

History

A seemingly endless number of disorders can result in symptoms of dizziness and dysequilibrium. A patient's history often provides enough information to suspect a vestibular cause for these symptoms. Unsteadiness and light-headedness are nonspecific symptoms that may be caused by hypotension, hypoglycemia, or hyperventilation. Dysequilibrium is a disorder of stance or orientation, the cause of which can lie in the vestibular system; it can lead to changes in posture or gait or be entirely subjective. Two symptoms point directly to problems in the vestibular system: vertigo, which is the illusion of motion—either rotating, tilting, or shifting—and oscillopsia, the perception that stationary objects are moving.

The history provides important information that usually leads to identification of a category or process to which the patient's symptoms are attributable. These symptoms can often be understood in terms of the basic physiologic principles that we have presented. We provide an overview of the key features of the history. A more detailed description of the history can be found in other sources.[16,17] The first step involves asking the patient to describe the problem. If the problem is dizziness, then

---

*The term "linear" refers to the relationship between the response (eye velocity) and the stimulus (head velocity) for head rotations. In this context, "linear" does not refer to otolith-mediated responses.

the patient should be asked to define what dizziness means to him/her. The examiner should be able to answer the following questions from the patient's responses:

- Does the patient have vertigo? Vertigo is an illusory sense of motion. The patient can feel as if the motion is internal or that objects in the surroundings are moving or tilting. The sense of motion can be rotatory, linear, or a change in orientation relative to the vertical. Vertigo indicates a problem within the vestibular system, although the abnormality can be located anywhere within the system.
- Are the symptoms episodic or continuous? Most vestibulopathies cause fluctuating or episodic symptoms, although there may be a persistent sense of dysequilibrium between episodes.
- Do the patient's symptoms reflect a disorder of information processing from the semicircular canals or from the otolith organs? Movement of objects in the visual surround from left to right during an attack of vertigo is usually caused by a nystagmus with slow phases directed from right to left. Abnormal sensations of tilt or sudden drop attacks can be seen with otolith dysfunction.
- Are there underlying medical problems that could cause or exacerbate the patient's symptoms? Thyroid disease, diabetes mellitus, anemia, autoimmune diseases, and hypoperfusion of the brain from postural hypotension or cardiac arrhythmias can lead to dizziness and/or vertigo. A myriad of medications, including those used to treat hypertension, cardiac arrhythmias, and hyperglycemia, can also produce symptoms that mimic peripheral or central vestibular disorders.
- Are there psychogenic disorders that could be responsible for the patient's symptoms? Anxiety disorders, panic syndromes, and agoraphobia can lead to episodic vertigo that mimics a vestibulopathy.
- What brings on the problem? The diagnosis of certain vestibular disorders is strongly suggested from events, stimuli, or movements that trigger symptoms. Benign paroxysmal positional vertigo (BPPV) classically begins on rolling over in bed or tilting the head backward and toward the affected ear. Patients with superior canal dehiscence syndrome experience vertigo and oscillopsia with sound or pressure stimuli.

- What other symptoms are associated with the dizziness or vertigo? Aural fullness and tinnitus can precede an attack of vertigo in patients with Meniere's disease. Dysarthria, diplopia, and paresthesias may accompany the vertigo seen in cases of vertebrobasilar insufficiency. Sweating, dyspnea, and palpitations often accompany panic attacks.

Taking the history of a patient with a complaint related to dizziness should begin in an open-ended fashion, allowing the patient to describe the symptoms with minimal direction from the physician. The process can be facilitated by requesting the patient to complete a questionnaire that asks the patient to describe and respond to queries about symptoms before the first appointment.

Examination

The neurotologic examination specifically evaluates components of vestibular and related oculomotor and postural function to identify abnormalities that are characteristic of pathologic entities. One such approach is presented below in an order that would correspond to the actual examination. The general otolaryngologic examination and assessment of hearing and cranial nerves are a part of the assessment but are not reviewed here.

Inspection for Spontaneous Nystagmus

Spontaneous nystagmus is seen when there is a static imbalance in tonic levels of neural activity in pathways arising from the semicircular canals. A spontaneous nystagmus caused by unilateral vestibular hypofunction is present when the head is still, is dampened by visual fixation, and is increased or only becomes apparent when fixation is eliminated. This latter feature makes it essential to look for spontaneous nystagmus behind Frenzel lenses (magnifying lenses that prevent the patient from using visual fixation to suppress any spontaneous nystagmus). A horizontal-torsional nystagmus is typically observed acutely following unilateral loss of vestibular function. The horizontal component beats toward the "stronger" (intact) ear, and the torsional component involves beating of the superior poles of the eyes toward the intact ear.

The nystagmus should be inspected for dependence on the position of the eye in the orbit. Nystagmus arising from a peripheral lesion and many central lesions is more intense (slow-phase velocity higher) when the eye is deviated in the direction of the quick phase (Figure 4–9).[18]

Skew Deviation and Ocular Tilt Reaction

Skew deviation is the hallmark of an imbalance in tonic levels of activity along pathways mediating otolith-ocular reflexes. It is a vertical misalignment of the eyes that cannot be explained on the basis of an ocular muscle palsy. Patients with skew deviation often complain of vertical diplopia and sometimes torsional diplopia (one image tilted with respect to the other). The alternate cover test is used to detect skew deviation. The examiner covers one eye of the patient with a card and then moves the cover to the patient's other eye while looking for a vertical corrective movement as an index of a vertical misalignment.

The ocular tilt reaction can occur with lesions anywhere along otolith-ocular pathways: labyrinth or vestibular nerve, vestibular nuclei in the medulla, medial longitudinal fasciculus in the pons or caudal midbrain, or interstitial nucleus of Cajal rostral to the oculomotor nucleus. There are three components to the ocular tilt reaction arising from hypofunction of one labyrinth: head tilt toward the lesioned labyrinth, skew deviation with the lower eye being on the side of the lesion, and ocular counter-roll (torsional deviation of the superior poles of the eyes toward the side of the lesion).

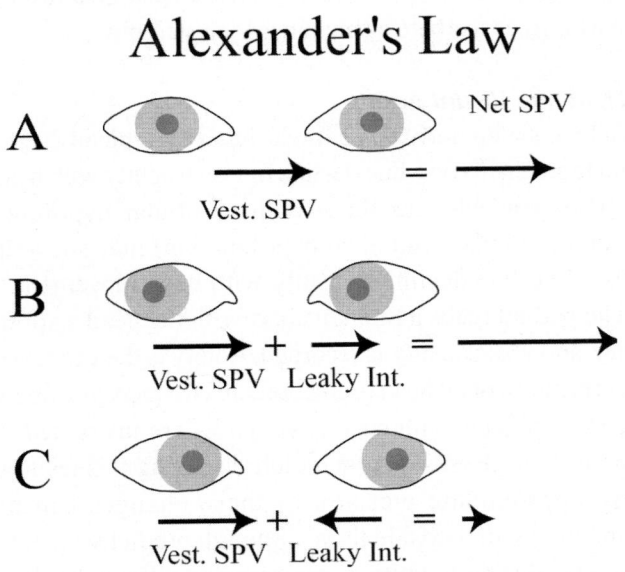

Alexander's Law

Figure 4–9 Alexander's law. After unilateral vestibular loss, a central process (called the "leaky integrator") contributes to eye motion and nystagmus by allowing the eye to drift to center, regardless of its position. The interaction of this motion and the motion of the eye caused by the imbalance in vestibular activity between the two labyrinths cause nystagmus to be more pronounced when looking away from the lesion. In straight-ahead gaze (*A*), the vestibular slow phase alone is manifest. When the eyes look to the direction of the fast phase (right, *B*), the leaky integrator causes the eye to drift to the left. This drift adds to the vestibular slow phase, and the net slow-phase velocity (SPV) increases. When the eyes look to the direction of the slow phase (left, *C*), the leaky integrator causes the eye to drift to the right. This drift subtracts from the vestibular slow phase, and the net SPV decreases. Reproduced with permission from Carey JP, Minor LB. Mixed peripheral and central vestibular disorders. In: Goebel JA, editor. Practical management of the dizzy patient. Philadelphia: Lippincott, Williams, and Wilkins; 2000. p. 237–58.

Head-Shaking Nystagmus

Head-shaking nystagmus (HSN) is a way to look for an imbalance in dynamic vestibular function. With Frenzel lenses in place, the patient is instructed to shake the head vigorously about 30 times horizontally with the chin placed about 30 degrees downward. Head shaking is stopped abruptly, and the examiner looks for any nystagmus. Normal individuals usually have no or occasionally just a beat or two of HSN. With a unilateral loss of labyrinthine function, however, there is usually a vigorous nystagmus with slow-phase components initially directed toward the lesioned side.[19]

The initial phase of HSN arises because there is asymmetry of peripheral inputs during high-velocity head rotations: more activity is generated during rotation toward the intact side than toward the affected side. This asymmetry leads to an accumulation of activity within central "velocity storage" mechanisms during head shaking. Nystagmus following head shaking reflects discharge of that activity. The amplitude and duration of the initial phase of HSN are dependent on the state of the velocity storage mechanism. Because velocity storage is typically ineffective during the immediate period after an acute unilateral vestibular loss, the primary phase of HSN may be absent or attenuated in these circumstances.

Head Thrust Test

Brief, high-acceleration horizontal head thrusts are applied while instructing the patient to look carefully at the examiner's nose. An AVOR of abnormally low amplitude will be evoked in response to head thrusts toward a lesioned or hypoactive labyrinth.[20] A corrective saccade, required to bring the eyes back to the intended point of fixation, is seen in such cases.[21] Corrective saccades observed in head thrust responses from patients with vestibular hypofunction can, with mechanisms of vestibular compensation, occur during the head movement and lead to an eye movement response that appears relatively normal on clinical examination. The sensitivity of the test can be improved by beginning each head movement with the patient's eyes in primary gaze position and moving the head at random intervals and order to the right and left. The test can also be used to detect dysfunction in the vertical canals by delivering the head thrusts in approximately the plane of the left anterior-right posterior or right-anterior-left posterior canals.[22]

Positional Testing

Positional (sustained) and postioning (transient) nystagmus are best observed with the patient wearing Frenzel lenses. Dix-Hallpike positioning for identification of posterior canal BPPV is performed first. The patient sits upright on an examination table. For testing to detect the presence of right posterior canal BPPV, the head is turned 45 degrees, such that the chin is toward the right shoulder. The patient is then brought straight back rapidly into a right head-hanging position. This position is maintained for at least 30 seconds. The nystagmus characteristic of BPPV begins after a latency of 2 to 10 seconds, increases in amplitude over about 10 seconds, and declines in velocity over the next 30 seconds. Posterior canal BPPV results in a vertical-torsional nystagmus. The slow-phase components of the nystagmus are directed downward and toward the uppermost ear. Thus, the fast-phase components of the nystagmus are upward and toward the lower ear. Because of the orientation of pulling directions for the oblique and vertical rectii muscles, the planar characteristics of the nystagmus change with the direction of gaze (when described with respect to an eye-fixed coordinate system): on looking to the dependent ear, it becomes more torsional; on looking to the higher ear, it becomes more vertical.

A horizontal canal variant of BPPV has also been described. In these patients, a strong horizontal nystag-mus builds up and declines over the same time course as for posterior canal BPPV. In some cases, the nystagmus beats toward the dependent ear (geotropic) and in others away from the dependent ear (ageotropic). The standard Dix-Hallpike maneuver may not elicit nystagmus in cases of horizontal canal BPPV. Such a nystagmus can be identified by bringing the patient backward into the supine, head-hanging position and then turning the head left or right ear down. The nystagmus seen with horizontal canal BPPV may last longer than that seen in posterior canal BPPV.

A sustained, usually horizontal, positional nystagmus of low velocity is a common finding in patients with central or peripheral vestibular lesions and may also be present in asymptomatic human subjects.[23] A central lesion is most likely when positional nystagmus is purely vertical or purely torsional or if there is a sustained unidirectional horizontal positional nystagmus of high enough intensity to be observed without Frenzel lenses. Positional testing may also exacerbate a spontaneous nystagmus.

Dynamic Visual Acuity

Subjects with normal vestibular function typically show no more than a one-line decline in visual acuity with head movement, whereas those with vestibular hypofunction (particularly bilateral hypofunction) may show up to a five-line decline in acuity with head movement.[24] The patient reads a Snellen chart with the head stationary, and visual acuity is recorded. Acuity is then checked during horizontal head oscillations at a frequency of about 2 Hz. Subjects with corrective lenses are instructed to wear their glasses or contact lenses during this testing. An approximate measure of these changes can be obtained with bedside tests, although predictive mechanisms during repetitive, sinusoidal oscillations of the head may augment performance during this test and obscure the identification of a deficit.[25]

Other Bedside Tests of Vestibulo-ocular Function

Valsalva's-induced nystagmus should be sought with the patient wearing Frenzel lenses. Craniocervical junction anomalies (eg, Arnold-Chiari malformation), superior canal dehiscence syndrome, and perilymph fistula can produce this sign.

Hyperventilation may induce symptoms in patients with anxiety or phobic disorders but does not usually produce nystagmus. Patients with demyelinating lesions of the vestibular nerve (such as that caused by a tumor, eg, an acoustic neuroma), compression by a small blood vessel, or abnormalities in central structures (multiple sclerosis) may show hyperventilation-induced nystagmus.[26] Hyperventilation reduces P_{CO_2}, which leads to an increase in serum and cerebrospinal fluid (CSF) pH. This relative alkalosis increases the binding of extracellular calcium to albumin and leads to an increase in the discharge rate and conduction in partially demyelinated axons.

Eye movements evoked by sound and/or changes in middle ear pressure should be evaluated, when indicated based on suspicion from the history, by observing the eyes under Frenzel lenses when giving pure tones from 500 to 4,000 dB at intensities of 100 to 110 dB. Next, movement of the tympanic membrane is induced with tragal compression or insufflation through a Siegle's speculum. Tullio's phenomenon is the occurrence of vestibular symptoms and eye movements with sound. Hennebert's sign is the occurrence of these symptoms and signs with motion of the tympanic membrane and ossicular chain. These signs have recently been documented in patients with superior canal dehiscence syndrome.[27,28] The evoked eye movements in this syndrome align with the plane of the affected superior canal.[29] Otic syphilis, Meniere's disease, and perilymph fistula have also been reported to cause these signs, although the specific features of the evoked eye movements have not been well characterized.

Bedside Examination of Vestibulospinal Function

Static imbalance in vestibulospinal reflexes is identified from Romberg's test, tandem walking, stepping tests, and evaluation of pastpointing. Romberg's test is used to assess sway with feet together and tandem in eyes opened and closed condition. Falls during tandem walking are indicative of horizontal canal dysfunction. Fukuda stepping tests (marching in place for 30 seconds with eyes closed) can show excessive turning toward the side of a unilateral vestibular lesion.[30] Pastpointing of the arms to previously seen targets with eyes closed may also be a sign of vestibulospinal imbalance.

Dynamic vestibulospinal function is assessed by observing postural stability during rapid turns or in response to external perturbations imposed by the examiner (ie, a gentle shove forward, backward, or to the side). A complete examination of gait; strength, reflexes, and sensation in the legs; and cerebellar function is essential for the interpretation of postural instability and dysequilibrium.

TESTS OF VESTIBULAR FUNCTION

Quantitative tests of physiologic processes under vestibular control are an important adjunct to the history and clinical examination. Diagnoses are rarely made solely on the basis of findings on these tests. When used in conjunction with a thorough history and examination, these tests can have an important role in directing decisions that have an impact on treatment outcome. Many vestibular disorders are not identified based on a single finding; rather, the diagnosis is established from a characteristic pattern of symptoms, clinical observations, and findings on vestibular tests.

Electronystagmography

Electronystagmography (ENG) refers to the recording of eye movements during various vestibular and oculomotor tests. It remains the most useful laboratory test in the evaluation of patients with complaints of dizziness or balance disturbance. The quantitative information from ENG enables the clinician to monitor progression of or recovery from disorders affecting vestibulo-ocular control.

Techniques for Recording Eye Movements

Three techniques can be used for recording eye movements: electro-oculography (EOG), infrared video image analysis, and magnetic search coil techniques.

Electro-oculography techniques are based on the corneoretinal potential (difference in electrical charge potential between the cornea and the retina) and are the most commonly used methods in clinical ENG laboratories. Movement of the eye relative to surface electrodes on the face produces an electrical signal corresponding to eye position. Horizontal eye movements can typically be resolved to an accuracy of 0.5 degrees, which is not as great as the sensitivity of direct visual inspection by a trained examiner (approximately 0.1 degrees). Clinical examination of small-amplitude eye movements either directly or with the aid of Frenzel lenses or an ophthalmoscope is therefore important for identification of low-amplitude nystagmus. Torsional eye movements cannot be measured with EOG.

Many recent advances have been made in video image analysis techniques, and these methods are used instead of EOG in some clinical laboratories. In principle, infrared video recordings allow eye movements to be recorded in three dimensions and with an accuracy that is comparable to or greater than that achieved with EOG. Although algorithms and procedures are improving, there are still some patients for whom image fitting and analysis do not work properly.

The magnetic search coil technique is based on the principle that changes in voltage are induced in a conductor moving relative to a magnetic field (Faraday's law). As applied to humans, a minute wire is imbedded in a Silastic annulus that is inserted surrounding, but not actually touching, the cornea. Eye movements in three dimensions can be resolved to an accuracy of about 0.02 degrees. The main disadvantage of search coil recordings for general clinical use is the level of expertise required to set up the apparatus, conduct the recording sessions, and analyze the data.

Assessment of Spontaneous and Oculomotor Function

Eye movements are recorded with eyes closed and with eyes opened and while viewing a stationary visual target. Spontaneous nystagmus and the effects of visual fixation on this nystagmus are thereby determined. The patient then looks to the left, right, up, and down so that a positional nystagmus can be detected.

Saccades are assessed by instructing the patient to fixate (eyes moving while keeping the head stationary) on a series of randomly displayed dots or lights at eccentricities of 5 to 30 degrees. Latency, velocity, and accuracy of saccades are analyzed. Smooth pursuit eye movements are recorded while the patient is tracking a target that moves horizontally with a sinusoidal waveform at a low frequency (0.2 to 0.7 Hz) with a position amplitude of 20 degrees in each direction. Optokinetic testing is often performed with the subject surrounded by a visual scene that moves in one direction at velocities of 30 to 60 degrees/s. The optokinetic response is a nystagmus in the plane of motion of the visual scene. The slow-phase abnormalities on optokinetic tests parallel those detected with smooth pursuit testing, whereas abnormalities of the fast components of optokinetic nystagmus are correlated with those detected on saccade testing.

Ocular motility disorders and brainstem and cerebellar abnormalities that affect oculomotor control can be detected with these tests.

Caloric Testing

Evaluation of nystagmus induced by warm or cold water irrigation of the external canals has been used to measure vestibular function since the beginning of the twentieth century. The test allows one labyrinth to be studied independently of the other. The stimuli can be applied relatively easily with techniques that are commonly available.

Bárány proposed that caloric nystagmus was the result of a convective movement of endolymph in the horizontal semicircular canal.[31] The convective flow mechanism is based on warm (44°C) or cold (30°C) water (or air) in the external auditory canal, creating a temperature gradient from one side of the horizontal canal to the other. This temperature gradient results in a density difference within the endolymph of the canal. When the horizontal canal is oriented in the plane of gravity (by elevating the head 30 degrees from the supine position or 60 degrees backward from the upright position), there is a flow of endolymph from the region with more dense fluid to the region with less dense fluid. This convective flow of endolymph leads to a deflection of the cupula and to a change in the discharge rate of vestibular nerve afferents. Endolymph will flow toward the ampulla of the horizontal canal (resulting in an increase in afferent discharge rate) for warm irrigations and away from the ampulla (resulting in a decrease in afferent discharge rate) for cold irrigations. This simple theory accounts for the dependence of the nystagmus direction on temperature and orientation of the head relative to gravity.

Two lines of evidence support the existence of an additional, nonconvective component to the caloric response. First, caloric nystagmus can be elicited in the microgravity environment of orbital spaceflight under conditions in which there is no convection.[32] Second, plugging the horizontal canal provides a method of eliminating the convective component under conditions of 1 g. Caloric nystagmus is still evoked in the squirrel monkey after horizontal canal plugging, and the slow phase is directed toward the ear being cooled. The response is reduced to 30% of that obtained before plugging.[33] A direct effect of temperature on vestibular hair cells and/or afferent nerve fibers is the most likely source of the nonconvective component.

The conventional Fitzgerald-Hallpike technique for caloric stimuli consists of a single temperature irrigation for 60 to 90 seconds.[34] Such stimuli result in a change in temperature in the temporal bone that lasts for 10 to 20 minutes. This prolonged warming or cooling of the temporal bone following a single temperature irrigation makes it necessary to allow at least 10 minutes between successive irrigations. Biphasic caloric irrigations can be used to achieve roughly the same levels of eye velocity as noted with a single temperature irrigation while substantially reducing the duration of the change in the temperature of the temporal bone.[35]

Responses to caloric tests are analyzed by calculating the velocity of each of the slow-phase components of the nystagmus. The maximum response for each irrigation is then determined based on the three to five slow-phase components with the highest velocity. Data are interpreted in terms of unilateral weakness (UW) and directional preponderance (DP) according to formulae described by Jongkees and colleagues,[36] where R and L indicate right and left and W and C indicate warm and cold irrigations; values are velocity of slow-phase responses in degrees per second:

$$\text{Unilateral weakness} = \frac{(RW + RC) - (LW + LC)}{(RW + RC + LW + LC)} \times 100\%$$

$$\text{Directional preponderance} = \frac{(RW + LC) - (LW + RC)}{(RW + LC + LW + RC)} \times 100\%$$

Normative values are established for each laboratory, with a UW greater than 20% and a DP of greater than 25% usually considered significant. Unilateral weakness is a sign of decreased responsiveness of the horizontal canal or the ampullary nerve that provides its innervation. Directional preponderance is commonly seen in patients with spontaneous nystagmus.

ROTATORY TESTS

Head rotation is the "natural" stimulus for the AVOR. Passive, whole-body rotations can be used to deliver con-sistent, reproducible rotational stimuli while eye movements are recorded. Standard clinical tests typically involve low-frequency sinusoidal rotations or steps of head velocity. In cases of unilateral vestibular hypofunction, the stimulus velocity has to reach a peak velocity of 150 to 300 degrees/s to observe an asymmetry between responses for rotations toward in comparison with those away from the side of the lesion. These tests are therefore particularly useful in assessing vestibular function in patients with bilateral vestibular hypofunction and in patients receiving vestibulotoxic medications. The AVOR can also be evaluated from eye movement responses to head-on-body rotations that are actively generated by the patient.[37] Recent evidence suggests that repetitive, predictive rotational stimuli may lead to eye movement responses that arise from extralabyrinthine mechanisms (such as prediction or signals from neck proprioception).[38] Thus, the sensitivity of these tests in the identification of vestibular hypofunction may be lower than for those tests that use passive, unpredictable stimuli.

EVALUATION OF OTOLITH FUNCTION

Subjective Visual Vertical

The perception of the orientation of a laser-projected bar of light relative to the earth-vertical or earth-horizontal planes when subjects are in an otherwise dark room is dependent on vestibular function. The alignment of the subjective visual vertical and subjective visual horizontal has been shown to be tilted toward the lesioned side in cases of unilateral vestibular hypofunction.[39] In acute peripheral vestibular lesions, the tilt of the perception of verticality often initially measures 7 to 12 degrees. In cases of long-standing unilateral vestibular loss, the subjective visual vertical either returns to normal or remains tilted only by 2 to 3 degrees toward the side of the lesion.[40]

Vestibular-Evoked Myogenic Potential Responses

Vestibular-evoked myogenic potential (VEMP) responses are short-latency responses measured from tonically contracting sternocleidomastoid muscles that relax in response to ipsilateral presentation of loud clicks.[41,42] These responses are thought to be of vestibular origin since they disappear after vestibular neurectomy and are still present in patients with absent hearing but intact vestibular function.[43,44] The inferior vestibular nerve has been implicated in the responses because all patients who developed posterior canal BPPV after vestibular neuritis had intact VEMP responses, whereas VEMP responses were absent in most patients after vestibular neuritis who did not develop similar symptoms of posterior canal BPPV.[45]

POSTUROGRAPHY

Techniques for assessment of postural control in patients have developed in an attempt to provide quantitative measurements of processes that maintain upright stance under static and dynamic conditions.[46] These tests have conceptual appeal because they evaluate the sensory systems (vestibular, visual, and somatosensory) that are important for maintaining balance.

The postural tests that are used most commonly include assessment of postural responses to platform movements and determination of effects of manipulations of visual and somatosensory information on balance while standing. Rather than serving as a screening test for establishing a diagnosis in patients with unidentified problems affecting posture and balance, there are specifically defined clinical situations in which computerized postural assessment can have an effect on treatment outcome[47]: (1) planning a course of vestibular rehabilitation and monitoring response to this rehabilitation program in patients with vestibular hypofunction, central nervous system disorders that affect balance, or processes that require a procedure to ablate vestibular function in one ear; (2) determination of the need for procedures that remove CSF (eg, high-volume CSF drainage with lumbar punctures or a shunt) in patients with dysequilibrium or gait disturbances caused by processes that result in abnormal CSF pressure dynamics; and (3) documentation of postural responses when there is suspected malingering, exaggeration of disability for compensation, or conversion disorder.

DISORDERS AFFECTING VESTIBULAR FUNCTION

In this section, we review some of the more common vestibular disorders with an emphasis on their patho-physiology. This brief overview of labyrinthine abnormalities can be supplemented by other sources that address these and other peripheral and central vestibular disturbances in greater detail.

Benign Paroxysmal Positional Vertigo

Benign paroxysmal positional vertigo is the most common cause of vertigo arising from labyrinthine dysfunction.[48] It is characterized by rotatory vertigo brought on when the head is rolled to the side, as when turning over in bed, and backward with a sideways tilt, as when getting out of bed or walking up stairs. In order of frequency, known causes of BPPV include head trauma, middle ear infection, viral labyrinthitis, ear surgery, or bed rest. Half of occurrences have no clear precipitating event. Benign paroxysmal positional vertigo occurs in children and in adults, although the incidence increases with advanced age. Among those cases without a clear cause, the average age of onset was in the sixth decade, with females outnumbering males two to one.[49]

Vertigo typically begins after a latent period—up to 20 seconds after positioning the head—and continues for less than a minute before subsiding. It is commonly provoked by the Dix-Hallpike maneuver, in which a patient is moved rapidly from a sitting to a supine position, head turned sharply to the side and shoulders hanging off the end of the examination table. Symptoms lessen if the head is repeatedly placed in the offending position. Knowledge of the anatomy and physiology of the labyrinth has allowed practitioners to develop a working theory for the cause of these symptoms and exercises to reverse them. Indeed, this sometimes crippling disease can often be completely cured in a single office visit.

In his original description of BPPV, Bárány[50] noted that if a patient's eyes were directed away from the affected ear, they tended to move with a vertical nystagmus (beating upward), whereas if they looked toward the affected ear, they moved with a torsional nystagmus (beating with the superior poles of the eyes directed toward the downward ear). These eye movements are identical to those expected from a stimulation of the posterior semicircular canal,[51] leading this canal to be considered the source of pathology.

The actual mechanism of stimulation of the posterior semicircular canal has been confirmed with the observation of free-floating debris in the canal during surgery on a patient with BPPV,[52] an occurrence that is now termed canalolithiasis. With the head tilted and hanging over the side of the table, free-floating debris in the posterior canal falls away from the cupula, drawing it away from the ampulla as the debris sinks.[53] The brain assumes that this deflection is caused by rotation of the head around the axis of the canal and creates a compensatory motion of the eyes—motion that is seen as nystagmus when a patient with BPPV is placed in the Dix-Hallpike position.

In addition to explaining the direction of nystagmus in BPPV, canalolithiasis also explains its time course: the sludgy debris in the posterior canal takes some time to begin sliding down the wall of the membranous canal after the head assumes a new position and requires about

a minute before coming to rest at the most dependent part of the canal and terminates the episode of vertigo. Repeated motion of the debris may allow some of it to escape through the open end of the canal, causing the signs and symptoms of posterior canal BPPV to wane with serial testing; this process may also explain the resolution of BPPV in some patients.

Several exercises are effective in treating the symptoms of BPPV. Brandt and Daroff treated 67 patients with BPPV by placing their head into the offending position repeatedly until their symptoms ceased.[54] The patients then repeated this exercise at home until 2 days had passed without symptoms. They reported that this cleared up symptoms in 66 of their patients.

Current therapy for BPPV involves repositioning maneuvers that, in cases of canalolithiasis, use gravity

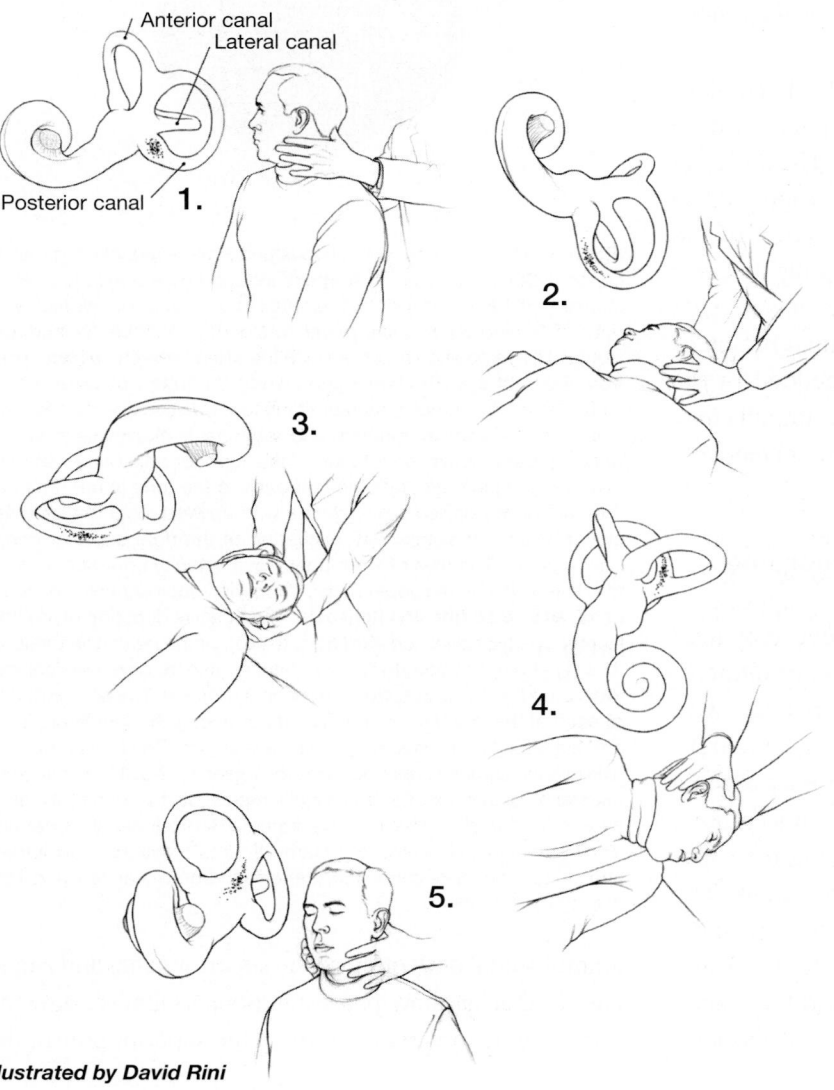

Illustrated by David Rini

Figure 4–10 Canalith repositioning maneuver for treatment of benign paroxysmal positional vertigo (BPPV) affecting the posterior canal. *Panel 1* shows a patient with right posterior canal BPPV. The patient's head is turned to the right at the beginning of the canalith repositioning maneuver. The *inset* shows the location of the debris near the ampulla of the posterior canal. The diagram of the head in each inset shows the orientation from which the labyrinth is viewed. In *panel 2*, the patient is brought into the supine position with the head extended below the level of the gurney. The debris falls toward the common crus as the head is moved backward. In *panel 3*, the head is moved approximately 180 degrees to the left while keeping the neck extended with the head below the level of the gurney. Debris enters the common crus as the head is turned toward the contralateral side. In *panel 4*, the patient's head is further rotated to the left by rolling onto the left side until the patient's head faces down. Debris begins to enter the vestibule. In *panel 5*, the patient is brought back to the upright position. Debris collects in the vestibule. Illustration by David Rini.

to move canalith debris out of the affected semicircular canal and into the vestibule. For posterior canal BPPV, the maneuver developed by Epley[55] and later modified[56] is particularly effective (Figure 4–10). The maneuver begins with placement of the head into the Dix-Hallpike position that evokes vertigo. The posterior canal on the affected side is in the earth-vertical plane with the head in this position. After the initial nystagmus goes away, there is a 180-degree roll of the head (in two 90-degree increments, stopping in each position until any nystagmus resolves) to the position in which the offending ear is up (ie, the nose is pointed at a 45-degree angle toward the ground in this position). The patient is then brought to the sitting upright position. The maneuver is likely to be successful when nystagmus of the same direction continues to be elicited in each of the new positions (as the debris continues to move away from the cupula). The maneuver is repeated until no nystagmus is elicited. This treatment is typically effective in more than 90% of cases in eliminating BPPV.

A lateral canal variant of BPPV has also been identified.[57] The nystagmus typically has a longer duration than that noted with posterior canal BPPV. The direction may beat toward (geotropic) or away from (ageotropic) the downward ear, depending on the location of the debris within the semicircular canal or ampulla. In cases that involve geotropic nystagmus, lying on one side with the affected ear up for about 12 hours eliminates the disorder in most cases. Debris embedded in the cupula or in the canal relatively close to the ampulla may cause ageotropic nystagmus. Repositioning maneuvers may not be effective in these cases.

Superior Canal Dehiscence Syndrome

A syndrome of vertigo and oscillopsia induced by loud noises or by stimuli that change middle ear or intracranial pressure has recently been defined in patients with a dehiscence of bone overlying the superior semicircular canal.[27,28] These patients may also experience chronic dysequilibrium. The dehiscence creates a third mobile window into the inner ear, thereby allowing the superior canal to respond to sound and pressure stimuli. The evoked eye movements in this syndrome align with the affected superior canal (Ewald's first law).[29] Loud sounds, positive pressure in the external auditory canal, and Valsalva's maneuver against pinched nostrils cause

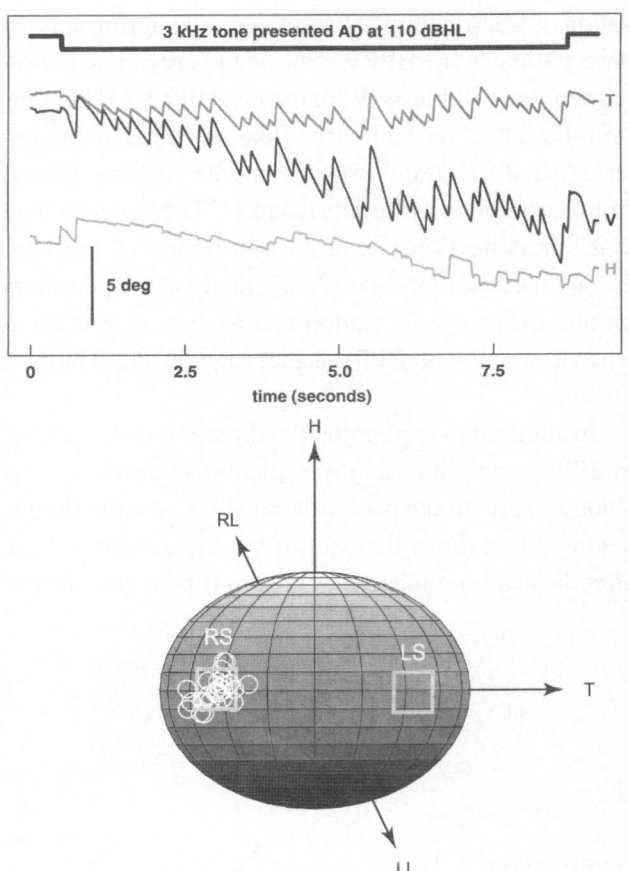

Figure 4–11 Ocular responses to sound in the superior canal dehiscence (SCD) syndrome. Nystagmus induced by a 3-kHz tone at an intensity of 100 dB in the right ear (AD) of a 33-year-old woman with right SCD syndrome. *Upper panel*, torsional (T), vertical (V), and horizontal (H) eye position recorded with the scleral search coil technique from the right eye. The time during which the tone was presented is indicated by the stimulus marker at the top. Positive direction for horizontal is left, vertical is down, and torsional is clockwise (from the patient's perspective, so rotation of the superior pole of the patient's eye is to the patient's right). In response to the tone in her right ear, the patient developed a nystagmus with upward, counterclockwise slow phases consistent with excitation of the right superior canal. *Lower panel*, The axis of slow-phase eye velocity corresponding to the data plotted in the upper panel. The sphere represents the patient's head, as viewed from the right side. The positive direction of the horizontal axis (H) travels upward from the top of the head, the torsional axis (T) straight ahead from the patient's nose, and the vertical axis (obscured by the sphere) from the patient's left ear. The anatomic axis of each of the right superior (RS), left superior (LS), right lateral (RL), and left lateral (LL) semicircular canals is shown. The box around the axis of each superior canal indicates the region (± 2 SD) from the mean orientation of that axis. Each light circle represents the mean eye velocity axis for one slow phase of nystagmus. Reproduced with permission from Minor LB, Cremer PD, Carey JP, and colleagues. Symptoms and signs in superior canal dehiscence syndrome. Ann N Y Acad Sci 2001;942: 259–73.

ampullofugal deflection of the superior canal and a nystagmus that has slow-phase components that are directed upward with torsional motion of the superior pole of the eye away from the affected ear. Conversely, negative pressure in the external canal, Valsalva's maneuver against a closed glottis, and jugular venous compression can cause oppositely directed eye movements (slow-phase components directed downward with torsional motion of the superior pole of the eye toward the affected ear). These eye movement findings have been documented with three-dimensional search coil techniques and can be readily observed on clinical examination (Figure 4–11). Frenzel lenses should be used for this examination because visual fixation can lead to suppression of the evoked eye movements.

Patients with superior canal dehiscence syndrome have abnormally low thresholds for VEMP responses in the affected ear.[58–60] Temporal bone computed tomographic (CT) scans in patients with superior canal dehiscence syndrome reveal an absence of bone overlying the affected canal. It is important to remember, however, that a thin but intact layer of bone can appear as a dehiscence on a CT scan because of partial volume averaging. The

specificity of temporal bone CT in the diagnosis of superior canal dehiscence syndrome can be improved with the use of 0.5-mm collimation scans and projection of images into the plane of the superior canal (Figure 4–12). The diagnosis of this syndrome should not be based exclusively on demonstration of an apparent dehiscence on temporal bone CT.

Many patients are able to control their symptoms by avoiding the sound or pressure stimuli that cause disturbances. For those patients in whom the effects of the syndrome are debilitating, resurfacing or plugging the affected superior canal can be effective in alleviating symptoms.[27,28]

Vestibular Neuritis

The vertigo in vestibular neuritis begins suddenly, may last for days with a gradual resolution, and is frequently

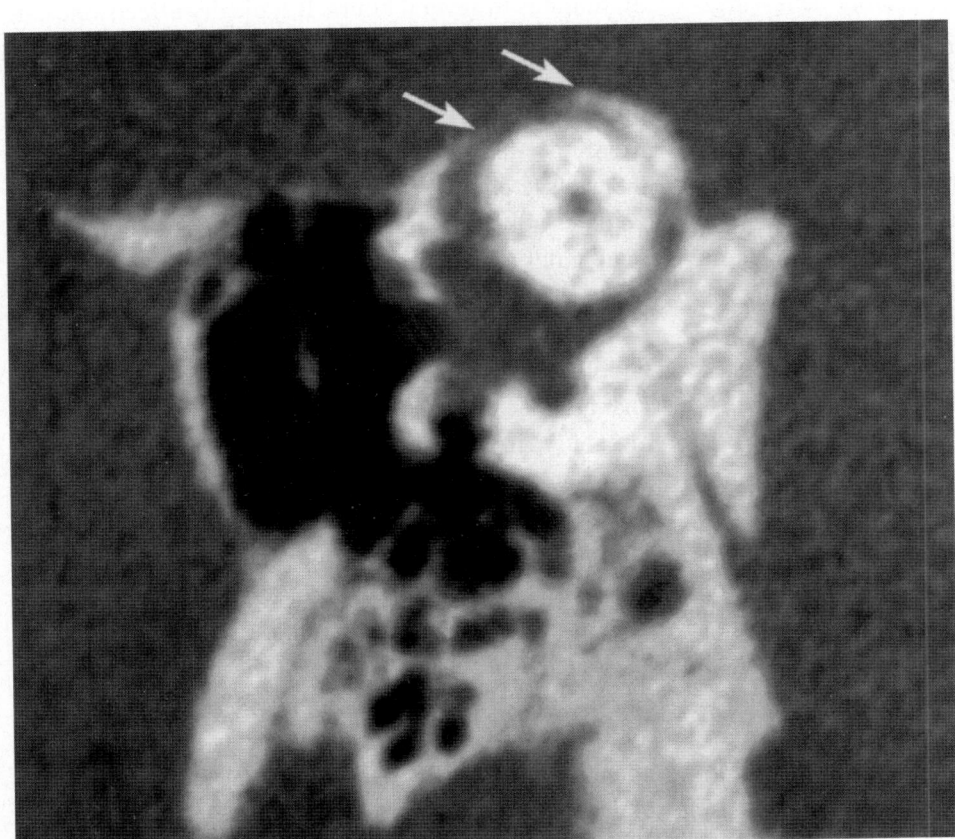

Figure 4–12 Patient's responses shown in Figure 4–12. Temporal bone CT scan from patient with superior canal dehiscence syndrome. Patient's responses shown in Figure 4–9. Projection of the CT image of the right temporal bone into the plane of the superior canal. A dehiscence measuring 3.7 mm in length is noted overlying the superior canal (*arrows*). Reproduced with permission from Minor LB, Cremer PD, Carey JP, and colleagues. Symptoms and signs in superior canal dehiscence syndrome. Ann N Y Acad Sci 2001;942: 259–73.

incapacitating early in its course. In support of an infectious etiology is the occurrence of cases around the same time within households or in association with upper respiratory infections. A vascular etiology has been suspected because the superior division of the vestibular nerve, supplied by anterior vestibular artery, is often affected, but the inferior division, supplied by the posterior vestibular artery, is often spared.

Signs of unilateral vestibular hypofunction are readily apparent early in the course of the illness. These signs include a spontaneous nystagmus with horizontal and torsional slow components that are directed toward the ear with hypofunction and fast components directed oppositely. The horizontal eye velocity of this nystagmus frequently increases in amplitude when patients look in the direction of the fast component.[18] It can be suppressed by looking at a stationary object, whereas the torsional eye velocity (rotation about the line of sight) of the nystagmus is not affected by this maneuver.

It is important that vestibular neuritis be distinguished from infarction and hemorrhage of the cerebellum.[61] Such a stroke involving the inferior cerebellum can lead to swelling of the cerebellum, brainstem compression, and death unless there is prompt neurosurgical intervention. The vertigo and nystagmus in such a lesion of the cerebellum can be similar to that observed in vestibular neuritis. One key distinguishing feature is the degree of postural instability. Patients with cerebellar hemorrhage or infarction are typically unable to walk and are very unstable when standing. Patients with vestibular neuritis, in contrast, are likely to have an unsteady gait, but they can walk. Appropriate imaging such as a magnetic resonance imaging scan of the brain and posterior fossa should be obtained when there is suspicion that the symptoms may arise from an abnormality affecting the cerebellum or brainstem.

Recovery of balance reflexes following vestibular neuritis occurs through three mechanisms: spontaneous return of vestibular function in the affected ear (in about 50% of cases), vestibular adaptation, and substitution of other sensory or motor strategies. Vestibular adaptation involves recalibration of motor responses to diminished signals from a labyrinth. Some examples of substitution strategies include rapid eye movements in response to head movements toward the lesioned labyrinth and use of visual and proprioceptive information to maintain postural stability after loss of vestibular function.

Gentamicin-Induced Vestibulopathy

Whereas vestibular neuritis leads to signs of an unequal level of activity between the two labyrinths, vestibular hypofunction resulting from aminoglycoside toxicity is commonly bilateral and symmetric.[62] Vestibulotoxicity is often noted without accompanying injury to the auditory system and can occur even when serum peak and trough levels are within appropriate ranges.[63] Patients typically do not experience vertigo, although oscillopsia with head movements and dysequilibrium are commonly noted.

Meniere's Disease

Meniere's disease is characterized by episodic vertigo, tinnitus, fluctuating sensorineural hearing loss, and aural fullness (a pressure sensation deep within the ear). In contrast to the vertigo in BPPV, which typically lasts for only seconds during a single episode, the vertigo in an attack of Meniere's disease has a duration that varies from 30 minutes to several hours. It typically affects one ear, although bilateral involvement has been reported in 2 to 78% of cases.[64] An incidence of 15 per 100,000 and a prevalence of 218 per 100,000 have been reported.[65] Meniere's disease typically accounts for about 10% of the visits to clinics specializing in vestibular disorders.[48] Females appear to be affected slightly more commonly than males (1.3:1), and the peak incidence is from ages 40 to 60 years.

Abnormalities in the production and/or resorption of endolymph are thought to underlie the histopathologic changes that are seen in the cochlea and labyrinth of ears affected with Meniere's disease. Most cases are presumed to be idiopathic, although the clinical syndrome can follow infections affecting the inner ear such as mumps or measles, meningitis, and head trauma. Antibodies to a 68-kD protein (heat shock protein 70) have been noted in patients with Meniere's disease but not in age-matched controls, leading to the suggestion that an autoimmune etiology may be involved.[66]

Endolymphatic hydrops, the classic abnormality noted in Meniere's disease, is characterized by dilatation of the endolymphatic spaces with periodic rupture of the membranes that separate endolymphatic from perilymphatic compartments. Although endolymphatic hydrops is a consistent finding in the temporal bones of patients in whom a diagnosis of Meniere's disease had been made, it is not a specific finding as these pathologic changes have been noted in patients with no premorbid symptoms or signs suggestive of Meniere's disease.[67]

Attacks of vertigo are frequently the most disabling symptom in Meniere's disease. The vertigo may be rotatory, in which case semicircular canal dysfunction is suspected, or may consist of a precipitous sensation of being pulled toward one side, as might result from a sudden change in otolith activity. The nystagmus during an episode of vertigo may be "excitatory" with respect to the involved labyrinth (with slow components directed away from the affected ear), although clinical examination between episodes of vertigo may reveal signs of vestibular hypofunction. The hearing loss in Meniere's disease is commonly more severe for the low frequencies.

Low-salt diets and diuretics control episodes of vertigo in most patients. Refractory cases with unilateral involvement can be managed with procedures that ablate vestibular function in the affected ear. Selective sectioning of the vestibular nerve (when there is useful hearing remaining) and labyrinthectomy (when hearing is absent) have been the procedures of choice. More recent studies have demonstrated that vertigo can be controlled in most patients, with a low risk of hearing loss, by injecting gentamicin into the middle ear.[68] Recent studies have shown that a single intratympanic injection of gentamicin is effective in achieving control of vertigo in most cases.[69]

REFERENCES

1. Kroenke K, Arrington ME, Manglesdorff AD. The prevalence of symptoms in medical outpatients and the adequacy of therapy. Arch Intern Med 1990;150:1685–9.
2. Kroenke K, Manglesdorff AD. Common symptoms in ambulatory care: incidence, evaluation, therapy, and outcome. Am J Med 1989;86:262–6.
3. Park JJ, Tang Y, Lopez I, Ishiyama A. Age-related change in the number of neurons in the human vestibular ganglion. J Comp Neurol 2001;431:437–43.
4. Goldberg JM, Fernández C. Efferent vestibular system in the squirrel monkey: anatomical location and influence on afferent activity. J Neurophysiol 1980;43:986–1025.
5. Baird RA, Desmadryl G, Fernández C, Goldberg JM. The vestibular nerve of the chinchilla. II. Relation between afferent response properties and peripheral innervation patterns in the semicircular canals. J Neurophysiol 1988;60:182–203.
6. Ewald JR. Physiologische Untersuchungen uber das Endorgan des Nervus Octavus. Wiesbaden (Germany): Bergmann; 1892.
7. Melvill Jones G. Plasticity in the adult vestibulo-ocular reflex arc. Philos Trans R Soc Lond Biol Sci 1977;278:319–34.
8. Miles FA, Fuller JH. Adaptive plasticity in the vestibulo-ocular responses of the rhesus monkey. Brain Res 1974;80:512–6.
9. Lisberger SG, Pavelko TA. Vestibular signals carried by pathways subserving plasticity of the vestibulo-ocular reflex in monkeys. J Neurosci 1986;6:346–54.
10. Minor LB, Lasker DM, Backous DD, Hullar TE. Horizontal vestibuloocular reflex evoked by high-acceleration rotations in the squirrel monkey. I. Normal responses. J Neurophysiol 1999;82:1254–70.
11. Lasker DM, Backous DD, Lysakowski A, et al. Horizontal vestibuloocular reflex evoked by high-acceleration rotations in the squirrel monkey. II. Responses after canal plugging. J Neurophysiol 1999;82:1271–85.
12. Lasker DM, Hullar TE, Minor LB. Horizontal vestibuloocular reflex evoked by high-acceleration rotations in the squirrel monkey. III. Responses after labyrinthectomy. J Neurophysiol 2000;83:2482–96.
13. Clendaniel RA, Lasker DM, Minor LB. Horizontal vestibuloocular reflex evoked by high-acceleration rotations in the squirrel monkey. IV. Responses after spectacle-induced adaptation. J Neurophysiol 2001;86:1594–611.
14. Grossman GE, Leigh RJ, Abel LA, et al. Frequency and velocity of rotational head perturbations during locomotion. Exp Brain Res 1988;70:470–6.
15. Hullar TE, Minor LB. High-frequency dynamics of regularly discharging canal afferents provide a linear signal for angular vestibuloocular reflexes. J Neurophysiol 1999;82:2000–5.
16. Minor LB, Zee DS. Evaluation of the patient with dizziness. In: Cummings CW, Frederickson JM, Harker LA, et al, editors. Otolaryngology—head and neck surgery. 3rd ed. Chicago: Mosby Year Book; 1998. p. 2623–71.
17. Zee DS, Fletcher WA. Bedside examination. In: Baloh RW, Halmagyi GM, editors. Disorders of the vestibular system. New York: Oxford University Press; 1996. p. 178–90.
18. Robinson DA, Zee DS, Hain TC, et al. Alexander's law: its behavior and origin in the human vestibulo-ocular reflex. Ann Neurol 1984;16:714–22.
19. Hain TC, Fetter M, Zee DS. Head-shaking nystagmus in patients with unilateral peripheral vestibular lesions. Am J Otolaryngol 1987;8:36–47.
20. Halmagyi GM, Curthoys IS, Cremer PD, et al. The human horizontal vestibulo-ocular reflex in response to high-acceleration

stimulation before and after unilateral vestibular neurectomy. Exp Brain Res 1990;81:479–90.

21.   Tian J, Crane BT, Demer JL. Vestibular catch-up saccades in labyrinthine deficiency. Exp Brain Res 2000;131:448–57.

22.   Cremer PD, Halmagyi GM, Aw ST, et al. Semicircular canal plane head impulses detect absent function of individual semicircular canals. Brain 1998;121:699–716.

23.   McAuley JR, Dickman JD, Mustain W, Anand VK. Positional nystagmus in asymptomatic human subjects. Otolaryngol Head Neck Surg 1996;114:545–53.

24.   Kasai T, Zee DS. Eye-head coordination in labyrinthine-defective human beings. Brain Res 1978;144:123–41.

25.   Tian J-R, Shubayev I, Demer JL. Dynamic visual acuity during transient sinusoidal yaw rotation in normal and unilaterally vestibulopathic humans. Exp Brain Res 2001;137:12–25.

26.   Minor LB, Haslwanter T, Straumann D, Zee DS. Hyperventilation-induced nystagmus in patients with vestibular schwannoma. Neurology 1999;53:2158–68.

27.   Minor LB, Solomon D, Zinreich JS, Zee DS. Sound- and/or pressure-induced vertigo due to bone dehiscence of the superior semicircular canal. Arch Otolaryngol Head Neck Surg 1998; 124:249–58.

28.   Minor LB. Superior canal dehiscence syndrome. Am J Otol 2000;21:9–19.

29.   Cremer PD, Minor LB, Carey JP, Della SC. Eye movements in patients with superior canal dehiscence syndrome align with the abnormal canal. Neurology 2000;55:1833–41.

30.   Fukuda T. The stepping test: two phases of the labyrinthine reflex. Acta Otolaryngol (Stockh) 1958;50:95–108.

31.   Bárány R. Untersuchungen uber den vom Vestibularapparat des Ohres reflektorisch ausgelosten rythmischen Nystagmus und seine Begleiterscheinungen. Mschr Ohrenheilkd 1906;40: 193–297.

32.   von Baumgarten R, Benson A, Berthoz A, et al. Effects of rectilinear acceleration and optokinetic and caloric stimulations in space. Science 1984;225:208–12.

33.   Paige GD. Caloric responses after horizontal canal inactivation. Acta Otolaryngol (Stockh) 1985;100:321–7.

34.   Fitzgerald G, Hallpike CS. Studies in human vestibular function: I. Observations on the directional preponderance ("Nystagmusbereitschaft") of caloric nystagmus resulting from cerebral lesions. Brain 1942;65:115–37.

35.   Proctor L, Dix RC. New approach to caloric stimulation of the vestibular receptor. Ann Otol Rhinol Laryngol 1975;84:683–95.

36.   Jongkees LBW, Maas JPM, Philipszoon AJ. Clinical nystagmography: a detailed study of electronystagmography in 341 patients with vertigo. Pract Otorhinolaryngol (Basel) 1962;24: 65–93.

37.   Hoffman DL, O'Leary DP, Munjack DJ. Autorotation test abnormalities of the horizontal and vertical vestibulo-ocular

reflexes in panic disorder. Otolaryngol Head Neck Surg 1994; 110:259–69.

38.   Wiest G, Demer JL, Tian J, et al. Vestibular function in severe bilateral vestibulopathy. J Neurol Neurosurg Psychiatry 2001;71:53–7.

39.   Curthoys IS, Dai MJ, Halmagyi GM. Human ocular torsional position before and after unilateral vestibular neurectomy. Exp Brain Res 1991;85:218–25.

40.   Tabak S, Collewijn H, Boumans LJJM. Deviation of the subjective vertical in long-standing unilateral vestibular loss. Acta Otolaryngol (Stockh) 1997;117:1–6.

41.   Colebatch JG, Halmagyi GM, Skuse NF. Myogenic potentials generated by a click-evoked vestibulocollic reflex. J Neurol Neurosurg Psychiatry 1994;57:190–7.

42.   Ferber-Viart C, Dubreuil C, Duclaux R. Vestibular evoked myogenic potentials in humans: a review. Acta Otolaryngol (Stockh) 1999;119:6–15.

43.   Colebatch JG, Halmagyi GM. Vestibular evoked potentials in human neck muscles before and after unilateral vestibular deafferentation. Neurology 1992;42:1635–6.

44.   Ozeki H, Matsuzaki M, Murofushi T. Vestibular evoked myogenic potentials in patients with bilateral profound hearing loss. ORL J Otorhinolaryngol Relat Spec 1999;61:80–3.

45.   Murofushi T, Halmagyi GM, Yavor RA, Colebatch JG. Absent vestibular evoked myogenic potentials in vestibular neurolabyrinthitis. An indicator of inferior vestibular nerve involvement? Arch Otolaryngol Head Neck Surg 1996;122:845–8.

46.   Nashner LM, Black FO, Wall C III. Adaptation to altered support and visual conditions during stance: patients with vestibular deficits. J Neurosci 1982;2:536–44.

47.   Minor LB. Utility of posturography in management of selected conditions that cause dizziness. Am J Otol 1997;18:113–5.

48.   Nedzelski JM, Barber HO, McIlmoyl L. Diagnosis in a dizziness unit. J Otolaryngol 1986;15:101–4.

49.   Katsarkas A. Paroxysmal positional vertigo: an overview and the deposits repositioning maneuver. Am J Otol 1995;16: 725–30.

50.   Bárány R. Diagnose von Krankheitserscheinungen im Bereiche des Otolithenapparates. Acta Otolaryngol (Stockh) 1921; 2:434.

51.   Cohen B, Suzuki J-I. Eye movements induced by ampullary nerve stimulation. Am J Physiol 1963;204:347–51.

52.   Parnes LS, McClure JA. Free-floating endolymph particles: a new operative finding during posterior semicircular canal occlusion. Laryngoscope 1992;102:988–92.

53.   Epley JM. New dimensions of benign paroxysmal positional vertigo. Otolaryngol Head Neck Surg 1980;88:599–605.

54.   Brandt T, Daroff RB. Physical therapy for benign paroxysmal positional vertigo. Arch Otolaryngol Head Neck Surg 1980;106: 484–5.

55. Epley JM. The canalith repositioning procedure: for treatment of benign paroxysmal positional vertigo. Otolaryngol Head Neck Surg 1992;107:399–404.

56. Herdman SJ, Tusa RJ, Zee DS, et al. Single treatment approaches to benign paroxysmal positional vertigo. Arch Otolaryngol Head Neck Surg 1993;119:450–4.

57. McClure JA. Horizontal canal BPV. J Otolaryngol 1985;14:30–5.

58. Brantberg K, Bergenius J, Tribukait A. Vestibular-evoked myogenic potentials in patients with dehiscence of the superior semicircular canal. Acta Otolaryngol (Stockh) 1999;119:633–40.

59. Watson SRD, Colebatch JG. Vestibular-evoked electromyographic responses in soleus: a comparison between click and galvanic stimulation. Exp Brain Res 1998;119:504–10.

60. Streubel SO, Cremer PD, Carey JP, et al. Vestibular-evoked myogenic potentials in the diagnosis of superior canal dehiscence syndrome. Acta Otolaryngol Suppl (Stockh) 2001;545:41–9.

61. Hotson JR, Baloh RW. Acute vestibular syndrome. N Engl J Med 1998;339:680–5.

62. Minor LB. Gentamicin-induced bilateral vestibular hypofunction. JAMA 1998;279:541–4.

63. Halmagyi GM, Fattore CM, Curthoys IS, Wade S. Gentamicin vestibulotoxicity. Otolaryngol Head Neck Surg 1994;111:571–4.

64. Balkany TJ, Sires B, Arenberg IK. Bilateral aspects of Meniere's disease: an underestimated clinical entity. Otolaryngol Clin North Am 1980;13:603–9.

65. Wladislavosky-Waserman P, Facer GW, Mokri B, Kurland LT. Meniere's disease: a 30-year epidemiologic and clinical study in Rochester, MN. 1951–1980. Laryngoscope 1984;94:1098–102.

66. Rauch SD, San Martin JE, Moscicki RA, Bloch KJ. Serum antibodies against heat shock protein 70 in Meniere's disease. Am J Otol 1995;16:648–52.

67. Rauch SD, Merchant SN, Thedinger BA. Meniere's syndrome and endolymphatic hydrops: double-blind temporal bone study. Ann Otol Rhinol Laryngol 1989;98:873–83.

68. Minor LB. Intratympanic gentamicin for control of vertigo in Meniere's disease: vestibular signs that specify completion of therapy. Am J Otol 1999;20:209–19.

69. Driscoll CLW, Kasperbauer JL, Facer GW, et al. Low-dose intratympanic gentamicin and the treatment of Meniere's disease: preliminary results. Laryngoscope 1997;107:83–9.

5

Neurophysiologic Aspects of Some Auditory Disorders

AAGE R. MØLLER, PHD

Progress in several areas of the hearing sciences has caused an increased interest in the function of the cochlea and the auditory nervous system, and it is now important for the practicing otologist to be familiar with aspects of auditory neurophysiology that earlier only had academic and research-related importance. Cochlear implants are perhaps the most obvious application of auditory neurophysiology in clinical otologic practice. The function of cochlear implants is closely related to the physiology of the auditory system; therefore, patient selection criteria and applications of cochlear implants rely on knowledge of auditory neurophysiology.

Furthermore, it has gradually become evident that the symptoms and signs of some disorders of hearing arise from functional changes in the auditory nervous system caused by the expression of neural plasticity (ie, changes with no detectable morphologic correlates). Neural plasticity is important in the adaptation of the nervous system to changes caused by injury and disease, such as stroke, but it can also have negative effects and cause symptoms and signs of disease. Pain and muscle spasm are widely recognized as symptoms based in the expression of neural plasticity. In the auditory system, tinnitus is the best known symptom related to neural plasticity, but even age-related hearing loss and noise-induced hearing loss have components that are manifestations of auditory nervous system plasticity.

HEARING WITHOUT THE COCHLEA: COCHLEAR AND BRAINSTEM IMPLANTS

There was no remedy for total loss of function of cochlear hair cells before cochlear implants were introduced in the late 1960s.[1] Development of cochlear implants was pioneered by Michelson and House and Urban.[2,3] Simmons and colleagues[4,5] had previously shown that electrical stimulation of the auditory nerve in humans could result in the perception of sound. House did his first implantation in the cochlea of a prosthesis consisting of a single electrode in 1961. These prostheses became available in 1973, and a later version was approved by the US Food and Drug Administration in 1984 for implantation in adults.

The first prostheses that were implanted in patients were primitive compared with presently available cochlear implants, but they could give totally deaf individuals their first sound awareness.[6] An independent evaluation[7] of 13 patients who had undergone cochlear implantation by House found that the cochlear implants improved lipreading and identification of environmental sounds.

These early endeavors were met with great skepticism by auditory physiologists and other professionals. It seemed unbelievable to most auditory physiologists that a wire inserted blindly into the cochlea and fed with electrical signals derived from sounds picked up by a microphone could replace the delicate and very complex functions of the normal cochlea.

Cochlear implants have developed radically during the nearly four decades since House performed his first implantation, and instead of a single channel, modern cochlear implants use several channels,[8] more complex sound processing, and more refined stimulating electrodes.[9] There has been considerable improvement in implant performance over the House single-electrode implant, and it is astonishing what modern cochlear implants can accomplish regarding speech discrimination despite the fact that even the most sophisticated cochlear implants replicate only a few of the complex functions of the normal cochlea.

Despite these major technical developments, the general principles of modern cochlear implants are the same as those of the early House type of implants, namely, electrical stimulation of auditory nerve fibers with electrical signals derived from sound waves picked up by a microphone. The original House cochlear implant stimulated all auditory nerve fibers with the same signal. In contrast, modern cochlear implants provide some frequency separation along the basilar membrane of the cochlea by using several pairs of electrodes. Each electrode pair stimulates different populations of nerve fibers with electrical impulses derived from different frequency bands of the sound reaching the microphone worn by the individual. However, cochlear implants provide only broad frequency separation because sounds within relatively broad frequency bands are applied to each electrode pair. This means that sounds within these broad frequency bands activate large populations of nerve fibers in the same way, differing from the normal cochlea, which provides continuous frequency separation along the basilar membrane and activates auditory nerve fibers accordingly. Thus, cochlear implants stimulate many nerve fibers in very much the same way; therefore, large populations of nerve fibers can be presumed to fire synchronously when activated by cochlear implants.

It is assumed that frequency discrimination and the coding of small changes in sound intensity are essential for speech discrimination. The normal cochlea provides two different codes for the frequency (or the spectrum) of sound: a place code and a temporal code. In other words, the frequency of sound is represented both in the time pattern of the discharge of individual nerve fibers and by which population of nerve fibers is activated. The temporal code is the basis for the temporal hypothesis of frequency discrimination, and the place code is the basis for the place hypothesis of frequency discrimination.

Modern cochlear implants remain relatively crude devices and are liable to similar criticisms as were the pioneering devices. The great success of modern cochlear implants has muted criticism, and there must be a physiologic explanation for this success. The physiologic basis for the speech discrimination achieved with modern cochlear implants is not completely understood, but a review of current knowledge regarding the function of the auditory nervous system can provide some insights. The following section of this chapter discusses the normal function of the cochlea and the features that may explain the ability of cochlear implants to provide speech discrimination.

Normal Function of the Cochlea

The cochlea contains the sensory cells (hair cells*) that transduce sounds into a neural code in individual fibers of the auditory nerve. Such transduction occurs after the frequency selectivity function of the basilar membrane has transformed and filtered the sound according to frequency (or spectrum†).

Each point along the basilar membrane vibrates with its greatest amplitude in response to sound of a specific frequency (or within a narrow spectral range). Low frequencies are represented at the apex of the cochlea and high frequencies near the base. Thus, a frequency scale can be laid out along the basilar membrane. Each point of the basilar membrane is tuned to a specific frequency, and the basilar membrane can be viewed as a continuous spectrum analyzer that separates sounds according to their frequency (or spectrum). As the hair cells of the cochlea are located along the basilar membrane, different populations of hair cells are activated by sounds of different frequencies within the audible spectrum and different inner hair cells are tuned to different frequencies. Since the auditory nerve fibers innervate individual inner hair cells, each auditory nerve fiber becomes tuned to a particular frequency. In other words, the fre-

---

*There are two kinds of hair cells in the cochlea, inner and outer, with different functions. The inner hair cells transform the vibration of the basilar membrane into the discharge pattern of auditory nerve fibers. The outer hair cells participate actively in the micromechanics of the cochlea and amplify the motion of the basilar membrane; this outer hair cell action adds approximately 50 dB to the sensitivity of the cochlea and increases the frequency selectivity of the cochlea for low-intensity sounds, which, in turn, improves the ability to detect soft sounds in noisy environments. The outer hair cells have no known role in transduction of the motion of the basilar membrane into neural activity.

†The term "frequency" is usually used to refer to periodic sounds, such as pure tones, and the term "spectrum" is used to refer to sounds that contain energy over a broader range of frequencies, such as speech sounds.

quency selectivity of the basilar membrane is reflected in the response of individual nerve fibers.

Frequency Selectivity of Auditory Nerve Fibers

The frequency selectivity of individual auditory nerve fibers can be demonstrated in animal experiments by recording from single auditory nerve fibers and determining their response areas with regard to the frequency and the intensity of sound (Figure 5–1). The curve that delimits the response area is known as a "tuning curve." Tuning curves show the thresholds of the nerve fibers as a function of the intensity and frequency of pure tones. The threshold is lowest at a certain frequency known as the fiber's characteristic frequency (CF), that is, the frequency to which the fiber is tuned. Different auditory nerve fibers have different CFs, covering the audible frequency range of the animal in question (Figure 5–2). A nerve fiber's response to a tone that is within its response area (excitatory area) can be decreased

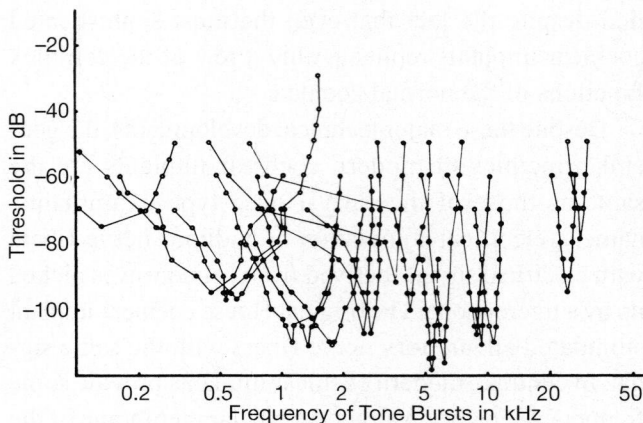

Figure 5–2 A family of auditory nerve tuning curves obtained in a cat. Reproduced with permission from Kiang NYS and colleagues.[73]

(inhibited or suppressed) by a second tone that lies outside its excitatory area. This fact implies that auditory nerve fibers have inhibitory response areas bordering these excitatory response areas (Figure 5–3). This inhibition depends on the micromechanical properties of the cochlea and is referred to as a "two-tone suppression" to distinguish it from inhibition caused by synaptic activity.

The transduction process in the hair cells is sufficiently fast to allow the waveform of the vibration of the basilar membrane to be coded in the discharge pattern of individual auditory nerve fibers (Figure 5–4). Such temporal coding has been demonstrated in experimental animals by recording from auditory nerve fibers for

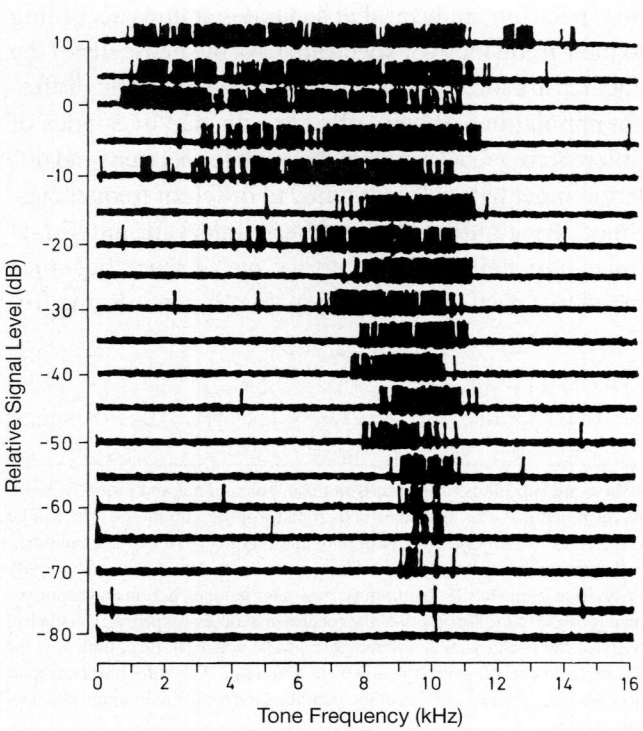

Figure 5–1 Responses of a single auditory nerve fiber in a guinea pig to tones of different frequencies and different intensities. Reproduced with permission from Evans EF.[72]

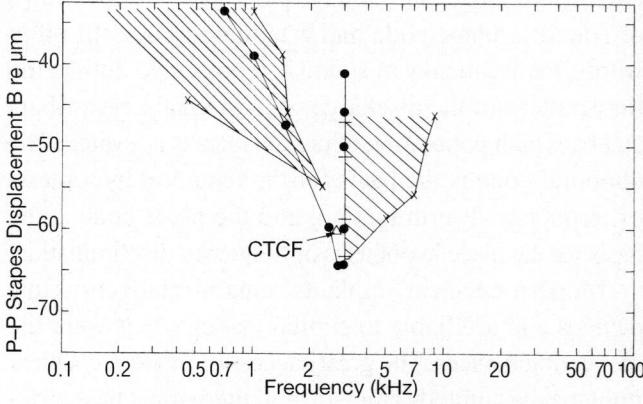

Figure 5–3 Two-tone inhibition in an auditory nerve fiber in a cat. Tones within the shaded areas decrease the response to a tone within the tuning curve (the excitatory response area) (CTCF). Reproduced with permission from Sachs MB and colleagues.[74]

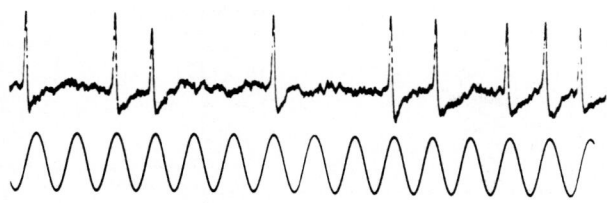

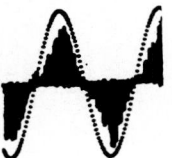

Figure 5–4 Phase-locking in an auditory nerve fiber showing that the probability of a discharge is related to the waveform of the sound. Reproduced with permission from Arthur RM and colleagues.[75]

sounds up to 5 kHz. Since the temporal coding of high-frequency sounds is limited, it is thought that timing information is degraded in the cochlea.[10] The upper cutoff frequency[‡]) for temporal coding has been found to be different in two commonly used experimental animals, the cat and the guinea pig. The cutoff frequency for the cat cochlea is 2.5 kHz,[11] whereas that of the guinea pig cochlea is 1.1 kHz[12]—a considerable difference. It is not known what the frequency limit is for the human cochlea.

Auditory nerve fibers thus communicate two different codes for the frequency of sound to the central auditory nervous system: a place code that is a result of the basilar membrane separating sounds according to their frequencies and a temporal code that reflects the frequency of the vibration of each individual point along the basilar membrane. This coding means that discharges of individual nerve fibers are phase-locked to the frequency of the vibration of individual segments of the basilar membrane.

The place code for frequency is the basis for the place hypothesis for frequency discrimination. The place code is preserved throughout the auditory nervous system in a tonotopic organization that begins in the auditory nerve and includes neurons in the nuclei of the ascending auditory nervous system, which are anatomically organized according to their CF.

Since each point on the basilar membrane acts as a bandpass filter that is centered at a specific frequency, the temporal code in individual nerve fibers communicates information about the waveform and the periodicity of the bandpass-filtered version of sound. Thus, discharges of auditory nerve fibers that respond best to the frequency of the first formant of a vowel are phase-locked to the periodicity of the first formant and communicate the frequency of the first formant to the central nervous system in the form of a temporal code. The temporal code of the discharges of nerve fibers that are tuned to the higher-order formants communicate the frequency of these formants in their discharge pattern (Figure 5–5).

The temporal coding of frequency on which the temporal hypothesis of frequency discrimination is based can be regarded as an "object" code, that is, one that provides information about the properties of sound. Place coding provides (one-dimensional) spatial information. It is possible that these two codes for sound—spatial and object—are processed in different parts of the central nervous system and exemplify stream separation.

Which Code Is the Basis for Frequency Discrimination: Place or Temporal?

Cochlear implants can code the temporal pattern of sound in the evoked discharge pattern of auditory nerve fibers but are much less effective in providing the place representation of the spectrum of sounds. The following discussion therefore focuses on the relative importance of the temporal and place coding for frequency discrimination.

The fact that the frequency (or spectrum) of sound is represented in the auditory nervous system both by a place code and by a temporal code does not mean that these are both necessary for all forms of frequency discrimination. The question of how one (or both) of these two codes is used in sound discrimination has historically been an academic matter. Since the introduction of cochlear implants, this question has assumed practical interest as cochlear implants mainly deliver temporally coded sound, and their ability to provide place-coded frequency information is limited by the number of available channels.

[‡]The cutoff frequency is defined as the frequency at which the reproduction of the waveform of a pure tone in the discharge pattern of an auditory nerve fiber has fallen by 3 dB compared with what it was for low-frequency tones.

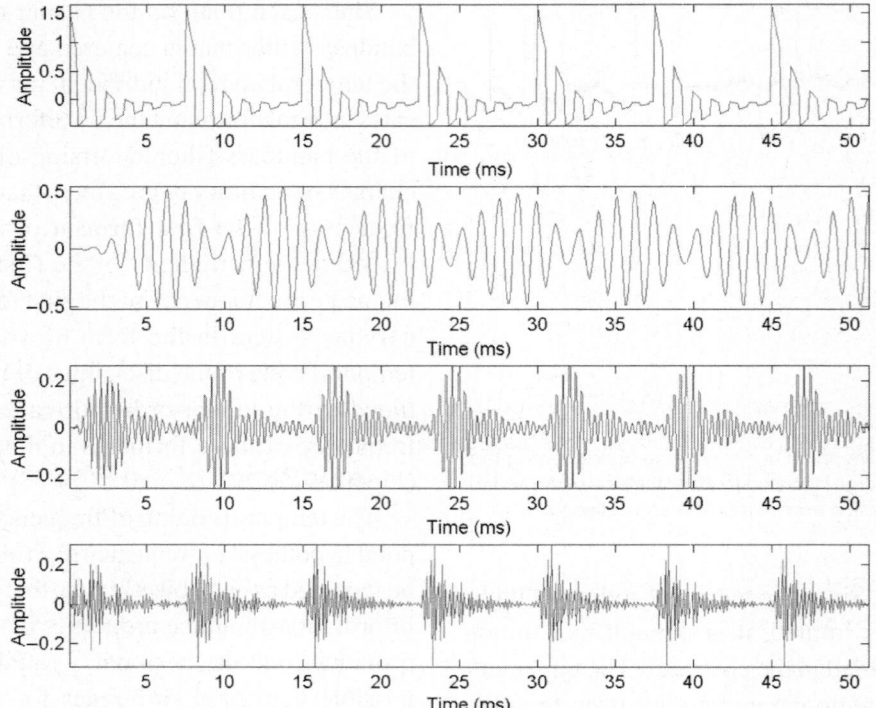

Figure 5–5 Illustration of how the output of bandpass filters that are centered at the formant frequencies of a synthetic vowel resemble damped oscillations, the frequencies of which are equal to the formant frequencies. (The formant frequencies of the synthetic vowel were 500, 1,000, and 1,500 Hz.) Courtesy of Drs. Peter Assmann and Ginger Stickler.

The fact that a tonotopic organization is maintained throughout the auditory nervous system and that individual neurons in the nuclei of the ascending auditory pathways, including those of the cerebral cortex, are specifically tuned with regard to the frequency of audible sound has contributed to the focus on the place hypothesis of frequency discrimination over the temporal hypothesis. The temporal hypothesis has been regarded as less important because of skepticism that temporal coding could be preserved through synaptic transmission and a lack of understanding of how the temporal code may be interpreted in the nervous system.

Experimentation to determine which of the two codes is used for frequency discrimination is hampered by the limited ability to manipulate a sound's time pattern without also changing its spectrum and vice versa. A few psychoacoustic studies in which such manipulations have been done favored the temporal hypothesis for frequency discrimination.[13] Manipulations of speech sounds that remove most of the spectral properties cause little changes in intelligibility.[14] These studies also provided some insight as to how many channels may be necessary to obtain good speech discrimination.

The fact that disorders affecting neural conduction time in the auditory nerve affect speech discrimination more than similar threshold shifts caused by cochlear dysfunction also indicates that timing in the auditory nerve is important for speech discrimination.

Other methods can provide some insight regarding the relative importance of temporal and spectral coding to frequency discrimination. It is known that frequency discrimination is nearly independent of sound intensity, which means that the code (place or temporal) that is the basis for frequency discrimination must also be robust with regard to sound intensity. Further, the neural code used for frequency discrimination must be preserved through the ascending auditory pathways until it is decoded. The place and the temporal codes fulfill these requirements to differing degrees.

It has been shown in many studies that the frequency to which a point of the basilar membrane is tuned depends on the intensity of the sound.[15,16] It has also been shown that the frequency tuning of individual auditory nerve fibers shifts when the intensity of the stimulus sound changes.[17,18] These findings suggest that the place code may not be sufficiently robust to account for the ability to discriminate sound frequency as documented in psychoacoustic studies.[19,20]

Temporal coding is little affected by sound intensity, that is, the shortest interval between nerve impulses in a population of auditory nerve fibers is unaffected by changes in the intensity of the sound. With increased sound intensity, more nerve fibers phase-lock to the sound wave, but the shortest interval is unaffected as it always equals the inverse of the frequency of the vibration of the basilar membrane. Thus, temporal coding is robust with regard to sound intensity.

One reason it has been assumed that temporal coding would be less likely to be the basis for frequency discrimination is that it was thought that synaptic "jitter" would impair transmission of temporal information in the nuclei of the ascending pathways. Studies of directional hearing, however, have shown that a high degree of temporal precision can be preserved through synaptic transmission in the auditory system. Many psychoacoustic studies have shown that humans can detect interaural time differences in the order of 10 microseconds.[21] These results mean that short time intervals must be preserved accurately in neural transmission to the superior olivary complex (SOC), at which point the interaural time difference in the arrival of sound is decoded by neurons serving as coincidence detectors. This transmission of information involves at least two synapses in addition to the synaptic transmission in the hair cells, which proves that auditory temporal information can indeed be preserved through transmission (at least two synapses in addition to that at the hair cells) with a high degree of precision.

The high degree of temporal precision observed in synaptic transmission can be explained by the fact that neurons receive many synaptic inputs. Neurons perform spatial averaging similar to the signal averaging used, for instance, in the recording of evoked potentials to reduce the level of background noise. Experiments using models of neurons have shown that the variability (jitter) of the firing of neurons that receive many synaptic inputs decreases with increasing number of inputs and that the variability of the output of a neuron that receives many inputs is less than that of the inputs.[22] That such a high degree of temporal accuracy can occur in the auditory system has been confirmed by recording the response of neurons in the cochlear nucleus to "click" stimulation.[23]

The other presumed obstacle to the use of temporal coding involves the decoding of the time pattern to recover the periodicity of sound. There is evidence that such decoding can be done by neural circuits similar to those that decode interaural time differences in the arrival of sound.

Importance of the Frequency Selectivity of the Basilar Membrane

The frequency selectivity of the basilar membrane facilitates the temporal coding of sound by separating the spectral components of complex sounds. It would not be possible to code the waveform of a vowel in the discharge pattern of auditory nerve fibers directly, but separating the spectrum of a vowel results in a series of waveforms that are similar to damped sinusoidal oscillations, the frequency of which is (exactly) the frequency of the formants of the vowel in question (see Figure 5–5). This separation makes it possible to code individual formants in separate populations of auditory nerve fibers. The center frequencies of the three filters shown in Figure 5–5 are equal to the formant frequencies of the synthetic vowel, the waveform of which is depicted (500, 1,000, and 1,500 Hz). The output of each of these filters is a damped oscillation, the frequency of which is equal to the respective formant frequencies. The auditory nerve fibers can phase-lock to these damped oscillations as they do to pure tones. It is difficult to imagine that the complete waveform of a vowel could be coded accurately in the temporal pattern of auditory nerve fibers, but it can be seen that the bandpass filtering has reduced the task of communicating the formant frequencies of vowels through temporal coding of the firing of auditory nerve fibers. The cochlear spectral analyzer acts as a series of bandpass filters that separates the spectral components of sound before converting the waveform into a neural code and may therefore be the most important function of the cochlea. This function can be emulated by a bank of relatively few bandpass filters as is done in modern cochlear implants.

How to apply such filtering to cochlear implants is a design question that involves the number of channels necessary to accomplish such spectral separation.[9,14] A similar question does not arise with respect to the normal cochlea because cochlear frequency analysis is continuous; therefore, there are always populations of hair cells (and thus nerve fibers) that are tuned to each of the formants of a vowel.

The size of the population of nerve fibers that is activated by the normal cochlea depends on the spectrum and the intensity of the sound. The discharges of members of populations of nerve fibers that are activated by the same sound are phase-locked to the same waveform, namely, the bandpass-filtered sounds. Thus, the discharges in such a population of nerve fibers are phase-locked to each other.[24] Such phase-locking of neural activity in populations of nerve fibers may be important for the detection of sound[25] and for the coding of complex sounds such as speech.

Other Functions of the Cochlea

The frequency selectivity of the cochlea is emulated by a set of bandpass filters in cochlear implants. However, the excitatory response area of an auditory nerve fiber is bordered by two inhibitory areas (known as two tone inhibition; see above) (see Figure 5–3). These areas of suppression are a function of the cochlea and are thus a feature of normal cochlear function. The sound processors of cochlear implants do not include suppression. The importance of such suppression for sound discrimination is unknown, but it may be assumed that they may sharpen frequency resolution just as lateral inhibition in the visual system enhances contrast.

The cochlea also provides amplitude compression, which is essential for neural coding of sound within the intensity range of hearing. Amplitude compression means that an increase in sound intensity by 10 dB results in an increase in the excitation of hair cells that is (much) less than 10 dB. There are several sources of amplitude compression in the cochlea. One such source is the amplification resulting from action of the outer hair cells. As that amplification is greater for sounds of low intensity than for sounds of high intensity, the amplitude of the vibration of the basilar membrane is compressed. The transduction process in the inner hair cells is another

source of amplitude compression. The acoustic (stapedius) reflex provides some amplitude compression for sounds above approximately 85 dB HL. Amplitude compression can be achieved electronically in cochlear implants.

Auditory Brainstem Implants (Cochlear Nucleus Implants)

Auditory brainstem implants (ABIs) were developed for use in patients whose auditory nerve has been destroyed bilaterally, as may occur with the removal of the vestibular schwannomas of neurofibromatosis 2.[26] Bilateral absence of cochlear nerve function is also found in children with auditory nerve aplasia,[§] and the use of ABIs in such patients has recently been described.[27]

Auditory brainstem implants electrically stimulate the cochlear nucleus, thus bypassing both the cochlea and the auditory nerve. Auditory brainstem implants are placed in the lateral recess of the fourth ventricle, the floor of which is the dorsal surface of the ventral and the dorsal divisions of the cochlear nucleus[29] (see Chapter 33 for additional details of ABI placement).

There are considerable technical obstacles to the implementation of ABIs. Only recently has it been possible to place the electrode array in such a way that stable and constant function is achieved. Ideally, the electrode array should probably be placed on the surface of the ventral cochlear nucleus, but precise positioning of the array is difficult as it is inserted "blindly." Intraoperative recording of auditory evoked potentials is used to check the position of the electrode array.[30] Furthermore, it is not known which orientation of the electrode array on the surface of the cochlear nucleus gives optimal results. It seems logical to presume that the array should be oriented according to the tonotopic organization of the cochlear nucleus; however, the tonotopic organization of the human cochlear nucleus is not well characterized and is likely to be individually variable.

---

§Auditory nerve aplasia is a rare condition that may not always be distinguished from deafness that is caused by cochlear injury. The hearing loss of neural aplasia may mistakenly be diagnosed as a cochlear disorder. A child with auditory aplasia may therefore get a cochlear implant, which will not be of any help.[28]

Normally, each auditory nerve fiber connects to neurons of all three main divisions of the cochlear nucleus—the first manifestation of parallel processing in the auditory system. The fact that ABIs can stimulate only one of the three main divisions of the cochlear nucleus means that they cannot replicate such parallel processing. Thus, there is more work to be done before ABIs are perfected. Nonetheless, although limited, the results with ABIs are encouraging.

Importance of Neural Plasticity in Cochlear Implant Patients

Cochlear implants and ABIs emulate only some of the functions of the cochlea, and the neural activity generated in the auditory nerve differs in many respects from that generated by the normal cochlea.

The sound discrimination achieved with cochlear implants benefits from changes in the way in which the central auditory nervous system processes signals received from the auditory nerve. Neural plasticity allows neural processing to adapt to abnormal situations (eg, cochlear implants) through more or less extensive "rewiring" of parts of the central nervous system. Such reorganization can result from sprouting of axons and from adjusting the efficacy of specific synapses, the latter probably being the most important factor in the adaptation to cochlear implants and ABIs.

Neural plasticity is a form of unconscious learning. The plasticity of the central nervous system is greatest during childhood development, which emphasizes the importance of early implantation. The extensive capability of the adult central nervous system to adapt to abnormal situations has only recently become evident. Neural plasticity can thus be assumed to play an important role in achieving the high degree of speech discrimination seen in implant recipients. Naturally, learning in the normal sense also plays an important role in achieving optimal results with implants.

Although the auditory nervous system can change in response to abnormal situations, adequate stimulation is important for normal development of the nervous system in childhood. This fact again points out the importance of early implantation. The changes needed for good results from ABIs during childhood are therefore more extensive than those needed for adaptation to cochlear implants in postlingually deafened adults.

NEUROPHYSIOLOGIC BASIS FOR CENTRAL AUDITORY DISORDERS[¶]

The symptoms and signs of disorders of the auditory nervous system reflect changes in the neural conduction of the auditory nerve or changes in synaptic efficacy in the central auditory nervous system. Altered function of the auditory nerve causes hearing loss, typically with greater impairment of speech discrimination than seen with similar threshold shifts caused by conductive or cochlear dysfunction and tinnitus. Auditory nuclear injury resulting from destruction of their fibers or cells causes more complex clinical manifestations.

Changes in the function of the auditory nervous system sufficient to cause clinical manifestations can occur despite the absence of any detectable morphologic abnormalities. Thus, neural plasticity can alter organization and function by changing synaptic efficacy, outgrowth of new connections (sprouting), or interruption of normal connections. Recently, plasticity in the auditory nervous system has been implicated in disorders such as tinnitus, hyperacusis, and phonophobia (with involvement of the nonclassic auditory system with activation of limbic structures, especially the amygdala[31,32]). Neural plasticity has also been linked to the hearing loss caused by noise exposure and presbycusis.[33,34] Presbycusis may represent neural plasticity caused by deprivation of auditory input. It is clear that disorders traditionally ascribed solely to cochlear dysfunction (loss of hair cells) may, in fact, emanate from a combination of dysfunction of the cochlea and of the central auditory nervous system.

This section first discusses the neurophysiologic basis for the typical symptoms and signs of disorders of the auditory nerve and the auditory nervous system that are caused by morphologic changes and then discusses

---

[¶]The term "auditory neuropathy" has recently been introduced to describe what were previously referred to as central auditory disorders. It describes a hearing impairment in which patients have normal otoacoustic emissions (indicating normal function of the outer hair cells) but absent or extremely abnormal auditory brainstem response (ABR). Such patients have a greater impairment of speech discrimination than seen in cochlear disorders with the same pure-tone threshold. The word neuropathy means disorders affecting the nervous system, but neurologists commonly use the term neuropathy for describing disorders of peripheral and cranial nerves. The use of the term auditory neuropathy is not yet established; presently, it is a loosely defined term for hearing disorders that are not caused by dysfunction of the cochlea or the sound-conducting apparatus.

disorders that reflect plasticity of the auditory nervous system.

Anatomy and Physiology of the Auditory Nervous System

The ascending auditory nervous system has two parts: classic and nonclassic ascending pathways. Classic ascending pathways are the youngest phylogenetically and are also the best understood with respect to their anatomy and physiology.

Classic Ascending Auditory Nervous System

The first nucleus of the classic ascending auditory pathway (Figure 5–6) is the cochlear nucleus in which the information in all auditory nerve fibers is relayed by synaptic transmission. The cochlear nucleus has three main parts: the anterior ventral cochlear nucleus (AVCN), the posterior ventral cochlear nucleus (PVCN), and the dorsal cochlear nucleus (DCN). The afferent fibers of the auditory nerve fibers bifurcate with one branch terminating in the AVCN; the other branch bifurcates, with one branch terminating in the PVCN and the other in the DCN. Each of the three divisions of the cochlear nucleus connects to the inferior colliculus (ICC) via the three acoustic striae and the lateral lemniscus (LL). Some fibers of the acoustic stria synapse in one or more of the several nuclei of the SOC, whereas some fibers of the LL make synaptic contacts in the dorsal or the ventral nuclei of the LL (DNLL and VNLL). All fibers of the LL make synaptic contacts with neurons in the central nucleus (ICC) of the IC. The ICC projects to the ventral part of the medial geniculate body (MGB) (the thalamic nucleus of the classic auditory system). Neurons in the ventral portion of the MGB project to the primary auditory cortex (AI).

Nonclassic Ascending Auditory System

The nonclassic ascending auditory pathway is thought of as an "adjunct" to the classic pathway. It receives its auditory input through connections with the ICC, the external nucleus of the IC (ICX), and the dorsal cortex of the IC (DC) (Figure 5–7).

Ascending fibers from the ICX and the DC connect to neurons in the medial and dorsal MGB. These neu-

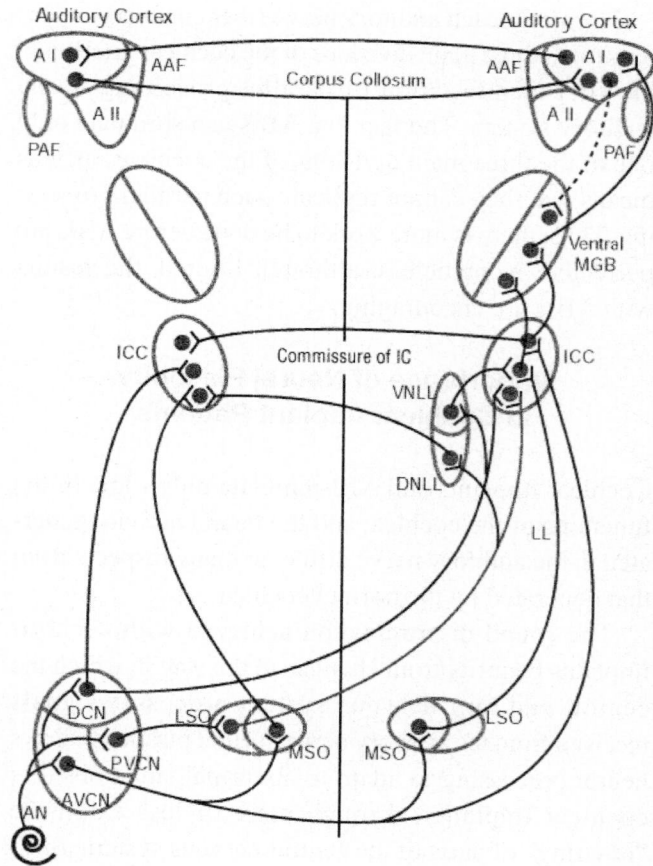

Figure 5–6 Classic ascending auditory pathways. AN = auditory nerve; DCN = dorsal cochlear nucleus; PVCN = posterior ventral cochlear nucleus; AVCN = anterior ventral cochlear nucleus; LSO = lateral superior olivary nucleus; MSO = medial superior olivary nucleus; LL = lateral lemniscus; DNLL = dorsal nucleus of the lateral lemniscus; VNLL = ventral nucleus of the lateral lemniscus; IC = inferior colliculus; ICC = central nucleus of the inferior colliculus; MGB = medial geniculate body; PAF = posterior auditory field; AI = primary auditory field; AII = secondary auditory field; AAF = anterior auditory field. Reproduced with permission from Møller AR.[76]

rons project to association cortex and to structures of the limbic system, such as the ventrobasal division of the amygdala, which is involved in affective reactions such as fear. The ICX and DC also project to motor systems; some of these connections involve the superior colliculus (SC).

Much less is known about the nonclassic pathway than the classic pathway. Whereas the classic ascending auditory system receives input only from the cochlea, the nonclassic auditory system also receives input from other sensory systems. The connections of the somatosensory system to the nonclassic auditory pathways are the best understood.

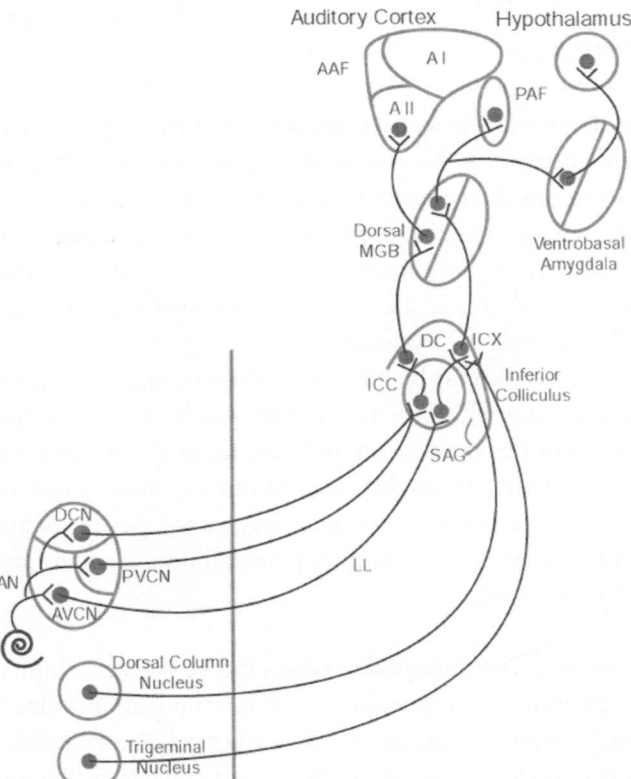

Figure 5–7 Nonclassic ascending auditory pathways. (Superior olivary nuclei are not shown.) AN = auditory nerve; DCN = dorsal cochlear nucleus; PVCN = posterior ventral cochlear nucleus; AVCN = anterior ventral cochlear nucleus; LL = lateral lemniscus; ICC = central nucleus of the inferior colliculus; ICX = external nucleus of the IC; DC = dorsal cortex of the IC; SAG = sagulum; MGB = medial geniculate body; PAF = posterior auditory field; AI = primary auditory field; AII = secondary auditory field; AAF = anterior auditory field. Reproduced with permission from Møller AR.[76]

Thus, the ICX receives input from the somatosensory system (dorsal column nuclei), and the dorsal cortex of the IC sends axons to motor systems. There is also evidence that dorsal column neurons connect to neurons of the cochlear nucleus.[35,36] Some neurons of the trigeminal nucleus also connect to the cochlear nucleus.[37]

The nonclassic auditory system is phylogenetically older than the classic system. Responses recorded from single neurons of the nonclassic ascending pathway show broader tuning and less distinct responses than those of the classic pathway. This difference in response pattern is more pronounced in some studies[38,39] than in others.[40] These differences in response patterns may reflect the fact that different studies used different animal species. There is also some doubt regarding the def-

inition of the border between the ICC, the ICX, and the DC, which means that some recording presumed to be from neurons in the ICX might, in fact, have been from neurons in the ICC. Animal experiments have shown evidence of input, which can be inhibitory or excitatory, from the somatosensory system to the auditory system at the midbrain level.[41]

Disorders of the Auditory Nervous System

Auditory nervous system dysfunction may be caused by tumors, infection, bleeding, stroke, and functional changes of neural plasticity. The most well-recognized disorders are those affecting the auditory nerve, and only recently has it been appreciated that neural plasticity plays an important role in provoking auditory system dysfunction.

Disorders of the Auditory Nerve

Acoustic tumors (vestibular schwannomas) are probably the most common lesions of the auditory nerve that cause auditory nerve dysfunction, but viral infection and vascular compression can also affect auditory nerve function. The symptoms and signs of auditory nerve dysfunction are poor speech discrimination, tinnitus, irregularly shaped pure-tone audiograms (with small dips that can appear at any frequency), elevated acoustic reflexes and/or poor growth of the reflex response above threshold. There is an increased interval between peaks I and III and between I and V on ABR testing. Speech discrimination is typically poorer than that seen in cochlear injuries with similar audiograms.

These manifestations may be caused directly by altered function of the auditory nerve alone or in combination with functional changes of more centrally located auditory nervous system structures, such as those caused by neural plasticity from a change (decrease) in input. Deprivation of input is a strong promoter of neural plasticity; animal experiments have shown that deprivation of input causes auditory hypersensitivity and altered temporal integration.[42,43]

Congenital disorders of the auditory nerve, such as auditory nerve aplasia, may cause severe hearing loss with an absent ABR but with normal otoacoustic emissions. A rare disorder of the cochlea in which the inner hair cells cannot activate auditory nerve fibers in a temporally coherent way demonstrates a similar response to testing.

DECREASED CONDUCTION VELOCITY IN THE AUDITORY NERVE. Injury or disease of nerves and fiber tracts almost universally causes a decrease in conduction velocity. Decreased conduction velocity (prolonged delay) is the most prominent sign of dysfunction of the auditory nerve and is seen with acoustic tumors or stretching of the auditory nerve as may occur during operations in the cerebellopontine angle.[44] Decreased conduction velocity within the auditory nerve can be identified as an increased latency of a response that depends on conduction through the nerve in question (such as the ABR). Auditory brainstem response findings of decreased conduction velocity consist of an increase in the latency of peak II as well as all subsequent peaks. The latency of peak I is normal because it is generated in the peripheral portion of the auditory nerve and is unaffected by neural conduction in the auditory nerve. Similarly, electrocochleographic potentials are unaffected by auditory nerve injury.

TEMPORAL DISPERSION IN INJURED NERVES. With increasing neural injury, conduction in some fibers of the nerve is blocked, and if very severe, all fibers may cease conducting impulses. Impairment of temporal coherence of the auditory nerve is believed to be the cause of the reduced speech discrimination common to auditory nerve injury. Temporal coherence of neural activity is important in auditory nerve fibers because frequency discrimination depends on the temporal coding of sounds. If the arrival time of neural impulses from different parts of the cochlea to the cochlear nucleus is altered (because some auditory nerve fibers conduct more slowly than normal), discrimination of speech is impaired.

The ABR reflects the conduction in the entire auditory nerve but does not provide information regarding individual nerve fiber latencies, which would have greater clinical utility.

ABNORMAL DISCHARGE PATTERN. The discharge pattern of a nerve may be altered, and subsequent to injury, nerve fibers may fire in bursts instead of in their normal continuous pattern. The receiving neuron is likely to respond differently to burst firing even though the average firing rate may be normal. Burst firing can cause synapses that are normally not conducting to open (unmasking of dormant synapses[#]).

INJURED NERVES AS IMPULSE GENERATORS. Injured sensory nerves may become impulse generators and generate neural discharges with an abnormal temporal pattern in the absence of sensory stimulation. Since most auditory nerve fibers have spontaneous activity, such impulse generation entails increased spontaneous activity or an altered pattern of spontaneous activity.

Synapses may be nonconducting (dormant) because the excitatory input is too infrequent to exceed the threshold of the neuron, because temporal summation of excitatory postsynaptic potentials is insufficient to reach threshold, or because inhibitory postsynaptic potentials prevent membrane potential from reaching firing threshold.

EPHAPTIC TRANSMISSION BETWEEN NERVE FIBERS. Injury to their myelin may make direct communication, known as "ephaptic" transmission, between nerve fibers possible. Ephaptic transmission has been implicated in facial and auditory nerve (facial nerve) abnormalities.[25] It can synchronize (lock together) the discharge pattern of many nerve fibers and thus cause the normal spontaneous activity in a population of auditory nerve fibers to become phase-locked, resembling the activity generated in response to sound stimulation. Such neural activity could result in the perception of sound despite the absence of any sound reaching the ear (eg, tinnitus). However, no study has been able to demonstrate the etiologic relevance of ephaptic transmission to specific disorders.

Disorders of the Central Auditory Nervous System (Excluding the Auditory Nerve)

The most common disorders of the central auditory nervous system (excluding the auditory nerve) are tumors, stroke, and hemorrhage. When such disorders are located in the temporal lobe, the auditory cortex may be affected.

#Synapses that are normally not conducting may become conducting in several ways: by a decrease in inhibitory influence, by an increase in the firing rate of the input to excitatory synapses, or by a change in the pattern of input from random firing to burst firing.

Disorders of the brainstem auditory pathways are very rare and usually present with symptoms and signs from many systems. Chemical insults can preferentially affect the nuclei of the auditory system; thus, hyperbilirubinemia seems to affect the cochlear nucleus to a greater degree than other parts of the auditory system. Tumors, strokes, and bleeding all share the feature of causing structural changes, and such changes can be detected by imaging techniques. Specific symptoms and signs are related to the observed morphologic changes.

LESIONS OF THE AUDITORY CORTEX. Tumors or other lesions of the temporal lobe affecting the auditory cortex on the one side have few obvious effects on hearing. Pure-tone thresholds are little affected, and speech discrimination is usually normal bilaterally when tested using standard methods. Therefore, the auditory cortex on the unaffected side must receive input from both ears despite findings from anatomic studies indicating that the auditory pathways are mainly crossed. Although there are uncrossed connections from the cochlear nucleus to the IC, it is assumed that bilateral representation is achieved by connections between the two primary auditory cortices through the corpus callosum. Bilateral representation is, however, not complete, as indicated by the finding that the discrimination of low-redundancy speech)** is impaired when presented to the ear contralateral to the affected side (Figure 5–8).[45,46]

Neural Plasticity as a Cause of Symptoms and Signs

It has become increasingly evident that changes in the central nervous system caused by neural plasticity can give rise to symptoms and signs of disease. Such changes consist of altered synaptic efficacy and the creation or elimination of connections, none of which have detectable morphologic correlates.

Functional changes in the central nervous system caused by neural plasticity may underlie a wide variety of symptoms and signs, most commonly chronic neu-

---

**Examples of low-redundancy speech include speech that is interrupted periodically (eg, 10 interruptions per second), time-compressed speech, and filtered speech (see Korsan-Bengtsen[46]).

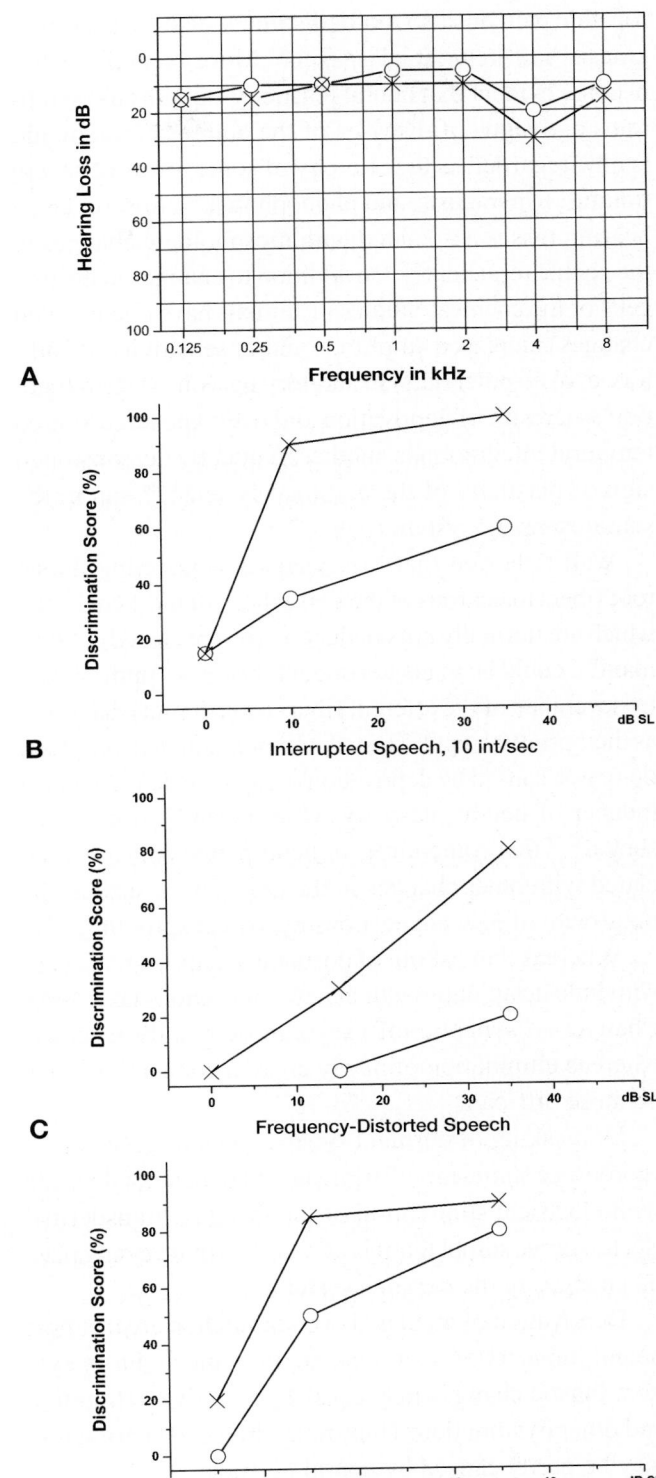

Figure 5–8 Speech discrimination in a patient with an astrocytoma in the left temporal lobe that involves the auditory cortex. *A*, Preoperative pure-tone audiogram; speech discrimination using *B*, interrupted speech; *C*, frequency distorted; and *D*, time-compressed speech. Circles = right ear; crosses = left ear. Reproduced with permission from Møller AR.[77] After Korsan-Bergtsen MAMM.[46]

ropathic pain but also motor disorders such as facial syn-kinesis and hemifacial spasm.[47] More recently, it has become evident that neural plasticity explains the symp-toms and signs of diseases of the auditory system and is now regarded as the etiology of some forms of severe tinnitus, hyperacusis, and phonophobia.[48] Noise-induced hearing loss is associated with morphologic changes in the cochlear nucleus[33,34] in addition to changes in the hair cells of the cochlea. Studies in animals have documented changes (increased amplitude and/or sensitivity of audi-tory evoked potentials) in auditory nervous system func-tion as a result of deprivation and overexposure. Altered temporal integration is another frequently demonstrated sign of plasticity of the auditory system[43,49] and in the somatosensory system (pain).[50]

Wall[51] showed that the synapses connecting dorsal root fibers to neurons of the dorsal horn of the spinal cord, which are normally not conducting (ie, are closed or "dor-mant"), could be made to conduct (become "unmasked") by severance of the afferent fibers (dorsal root) that serve as their primary input. Thus, this expression of neural plas-ticity was caused by deprivation of input, which is a potent inducer of neural plasticity. More recently, it has been shown[52,53] that some forms of neuropathic pain are asso-ciated with other changes in the dorsal horn such as the outgrowth of new connections by axonal sprouting.

Whereas unmasking of dormant synapses may occur with little delay, outgrowth of new connections takes time. Changes in synaptic efficacy can be readily reversed, whereas elimination of newly created connections may be more difficult.

Unmasking of dormant synapses can be reversed by appropriate stimulation. The treatment of neuropathic pain with electrical stimulation of the skin (eg, transdermal electric nerve stimulation) is an example of reversing plas-tic changes in the nervous system.

Deprivation of input and overstimulation are the most potent inducers of neural plasticity in the auditory sys-tem. Plastic changes may cause hyperactivity (tinnitus) and other dysfunction. Thus, noise-induced hearing loss may be partly caused by neural plasticity.[33,34]

Tinnitus, Hyperacusis, Phonophobia, and Other Abnormal Auditory Perceptions.
Tinnitus is a manifestation of hyperactivity that is of particular inter-est to the otologist. There are many forms, and also many causes, of tinnitus. Tinnitus often occurs in con-junction with hearing loss of cochlear origin. The dep-rivation of input to the auditory pathways may promote neural plasticity, hyperactivity, and hypersensitivity,[42] which, in turn, may cause spontaneous neural activity that is perceived as sound. Tinnitus almost always accompanies acoustic neuromas and is a frequent symp-tom of individuals with vascular compression of the auditory nerve. Tinnitus therefore appears to be asso-ciated with injury or irritation of the auditory nerve. How tinnitus develops is not known, but observation of other forms of cranial nerve injury or irritation (such as those caused by close contact with blood vessels) has shown that such injury/irritation can lead to hyperac-tivity of the associated nucleus (eg, for motor systems, hemifacial spasm, and for sensory systems, trigeminal neuralgia).[54]

Hyperacusis often accompanies tinnitus but may also occur without tinnitus. Phonophobia less commonly accompanies tinnitus. Hyperacusis may be the result of hyperactivity and other forms of altered sound process-ing. Since the incidence of tinnitus increases with age, it is thought that it may be a result of progressive dete-rioration of neural systems. The increase in prevalence of tinnitus with age may be specifically affected by the decrease in production of γ-aminobutyric acid (GABA),[55] an inhibitory neurotransmitter that has been implicated in tinnitus. It is known that benzodiazepines, which are $GABA_A$ receptor agonists, can alleviate tinnitus in some individuals.[56]

The abnormal sensation of sound (hyperacusis and phonophobia) that often accompanies severe tinnitus may also be mediated by the nonclassic auditory system. The subcortical connections of the thalamic auditory nucleus of the nonclassic auditory system to limbic structures such as the amygdala[57] may explain why phonophobia and affective reactions often accompany severe tinnitus. Functional imaging studies[32] have shown signs of activation of limbic structures in some individ-uals with tinnitus.

The nonclassic auditory system also receives input from other sensory systems such as the somatosensory system, which may explain why some individuals with tinnitus note changes in their tinnitus when moving their eyes[58-60] or contracting neck muscles (Levine, personal communication).

Activation of the nonclassic auditory system can explain why some individuals with tinnitus perceive sound when touching certain regions of the skin[††] (eg, a patient with severe tinnitus was reported to hear a sound when rubbing his back with a towel).[61]

The abnormal auditory sensations perceived in response to somatosensory stimulation that often accompany tinnitus may be similar to allodynia,[‡‡] which often accompanies neuropathic pain. Allodynia is an example of rerouting of sensory information and probably occurs as a result of unmasking normally dormant synapses. Thus, there are many similarities between severe tinnitus and some forms of neuropathic pain.[48,61]

Many patients with chronic neuropathic pain also experience hyperpathia,[§§] which may be similar to hyperacusis in individuals with tinnitus.

It is not known how the nonclassic auditory nervous system becomes activated in individuals with tinnitus, but it seems likely that the connections between the classic auditory system and the nonclassic auditory system in adult humans, which are normally dormant,[31] may become unmasked after abnormal external or intrinsic events (ie, are a manifestation of neural plasticity). Recently, evidence has been presented[62] that the nonclassic pathways are active in children.

Some of the changes in the function of sensory systems that can be attributed to neural plasticity may have detectable signs in addition to the symptomatic changes in perception of the sensory stimulation. It has been shown in animal experiments that temporal integration is altered after sound deprivation.[43] Overstimulation can also cause altered temporal integration (as demonstrated in experiments with rats that were exposed to loud sounds—4-kHz tones at 104 dB SPL for 30 minutes),[63] similar to the altered temporal integration demonstrated by electrical stimulation of the skin[50] in neuropathic pain.

HEARING LOSS. Hearing loss caused by noise exposure, administration of ototoxic drugs, and aging is associated with loss of (mainly) the outer hair cells of the cochlea.

There is also evidence that such hearing loss is associated with morphologic changes in the cochlear nucleus.[52] Hearing loss from noise exposure can be reduced by prior exposure to noise ("toughening").[64,65] The mechanism remains unknown. It may be that such "use" of hair cells makes them less susceptible to noise injury. Since noise-induced hearing loss is assumed to result from damage to the outer hair cells, the observed reduction in hearing loss from noise exposure could be a result of neural activity in the efferent system (olivocochlear bundle) that controls the mechanical properties of the outer hair cells. Even age-associated hearing loss can be reduced by exposure to sound. Thus, Turner and Willott[66] and Willott and colleagues[67] have shown that exposure to sound of moderate intensity ("augmented acoustic environment") can prevent or delay the progression of hearing loss in animals. The mechanism of this effect of sound exposure is also unknown; it could represent an effect on the outer hair cells, but it could also be mediated by the central auditory nervous system through the olivocochlear bundle affecting the function of the outer hair cells. Finally, presbycusis may have a neural component that can be affected by prior exposure to sound through neural plasticity.

DEFICITS CAUSED BY SOUND DEPRIVATION. It is established knowledge that sound, and probably meaningful sound, is necessary for the normal ontogenetic development of the auditory nervous system. Total congenital deafness from cochlear causes results in functional abnormalities of the auditory nervous system. Lesser degrees of hearing loss may also impair the development of the auditory nervous system and may cause more general deficits in other parts of the central nervous system because of reduced input of information. Hearing loss early in life may thus impair speech development. An important question that has been discussed often in connection with middle ear disorders is how severe does hearing loss need to be to cause noticeable deficits later in life?

Motor Disorders

Motor disorders, such as muscle spasms, may reflect neural plasticity. Evidence has been presented that hemifacial spasm is caused by hyperactivity of the facial motor nucleus, probably caused by plastic changes.[47,68] There is also evidence that synkinesis, which often accompa-

---

[††]Perception of sound from stimulation of the skin is an abnormal situation that may violate the law of specific nerve energies (Johannes Muller, in his monumental *Handbook of Human Physiology*, published in the 1830s), which states that stimulation of a specific sensory nerve will result in a sensation of that sensory modality.

[‡‡]Allodynia is the perception of a painful sensation from what would normally be considered an innocuous stimulation of skin receptors, such as touching the skin.

[§§]Hyperpathia is an exaggerated reaction to mild and moderate pain stimulation.

nies hemifacial spasm, is caused by the opening of dormant connections between motoneurons that supply different muscles of the face.[47] Other studies indicate that facial spasm and synkinesis following facial nerve trauma are also caused by plastic changes in the function of the facial motor nucleus.[69]

Animal experiments have confirmed that repeated stimulation of the facial nerve can lead to spasm of the facial muscles.[70] This phenomenon is similar to the Kindling phenomenon, which was first demonstrated by stimulation of the amygdala of rats[71]; after weeks of daily stimulation for short periods, the rats developed seizures. It has been hypothesized that the spasm of hemifacial spasm is caused by a similar mechanism, and animal experiments have supported this hypothesis.

REFERENCES

1. House WH. A personal perspective on cochlear implants. In: Schindler RA, Merzenich MM, editors. Cochler implants. New York: Raven Press; 1985:13–6.

2. Michelson RP. Stimulation of the human cochlea. Arch Otolaryngol 1971;93:317–23.

3. House WF, Urban J. Long term results of electrode implantation and electrical stimulation of the cochlea in man. Ann Otol Rhinol Laryngol 1973;82:503–10.

4. Simmons FB, Mongeon CJ, Lewis WR, et al. Electrical stimulation of acoustical nerve and inferior colliculus. Arch Otolaryngol 1964;79:559–67.

5. Simmons FB. Electrical stimulation of the auditory nerve in man. Arch Otolaryngol 1966;84:22–76.

6. House WH. Cochlear implants. Ann Otol Rhinol Laryngol 1976;85 Suppl 27:3–91.

7. Bilger RC. Evaluation of subjects presently fitted with implanted auditory protheses. Ann Otol Rhinol Laryngol 1977;86 Suppl 38:1–76.

8. Clark GM, Tong YC, Martin LF, Budby PA. A multiple channel cochlear implant. Acta Otolaryngol (Stockh) 1981;91:173–5.

9. Dorman MF, Loizou PC, Kemp LL, Kirk KI. Word recognition by children listening to speech processed into a small number of channels: data from normal-hearing children and children with cochlear implants. Ear Hear 2000;21:590–6.

10. Kidd RC, Weiss TF. Mechanisms that degrade timing information in the cochlea. Hear Res 1990;49:181–208.

11. Johnson DH. The relationship between spike rate and synchrony in responses of auditory-nerve fibers to single tones. J Acoust Soc Am 1980;68:1115–22.

12. Palmer AR, Russell IJ. Phase-locking in the cochlear nerve of the guinea-pig and its relation to the receptor potential of inner hair cells. Hear Res 1986;24:1–15.

13. Nordmark J. Time and frequency analysis. In: Tobias JV, editor. Foundation of modern auditory theory. Vol 1. New York: Academic Press; 1970:55–83.

14. Shannon RV, Zeng F-G, Kamath V, et al. Speech recognition with primarily temporal cues. Science 1995;270:303–4.

15. Rhode WS. Observations of the vibration of the basilar membrane in squirrel monkeys using the mossbauer technique. J Acoust Soc Am 1971;49:1218–31.

16. Johnstone BM, Patuzzi R, Yates GK. Basilar membrane measurements and the travelling wave. Hear Res 1986;22:147–53.

17. Møller AR. Frequency selectivity of single auditory nerve fibers in response to broadband noise stimuli. J Acoust Soc Am 1977;62:135–42.

18. Møller AR. Frequency selectivity of phase locking of complex sounds in the auditory nerve of the rat. Hear Res 1983;11:267–84.

19. Møller AR. Review of the roles of temporal and place coding of frequency in speech discrimination. Acta Otolaryngol (Stockh) 1999;119:424–30.

20. Zwislocki JJ. What is the cochlear place code for pitch? Acta Otolaryngol (Stockh) 1992;111:256–62.

21. Tobias JV, Zerlin S. Lateralization threshold as a function of stimulus duration. J Acoust Soc Am 1959;31:1591–4.

22. Burkitt AN, Clark GM. Analysis of integrate-and-fire neurons: synchronization of synaptic input and spike output. Neural Computation 1999;11:871–901.

23. Møller AR. Unit responses in the rat cochlear nucleus to repetitive transient sounds. Acta Physiol Scand 1969;75:542–51.

24. Eggermont JJ. Between sound and perception: reviewing the search for a neural code. Hear Res 2001;157:1–42.

25. Møller AR. Pathophysiology of tinnitus. Ann Otol Rhinol Laryngol 1984;93:39–44.

26. Brackmann DE, Hitselberger WE, Nelson RA, et al. Auditory brainstem implant: 1. Issues in surgical implantation. Otolaryngol Head Neck Surg 1993;108:624–33.

27. Colletti V, Fiorino FG, Sacchetto L, et al. Hearing rehabilitation with auditory brainstem implantation in two children with cochlear nerve aplasia. Int J Pediatr Otorhinolaryngol 2001;60:99–111.

28. Maxwell AP, Mason SM, O'Donoghue GM. Cochlear nerve aplasia: its importance in cochlear implantation. Am J Otol 1999;20:335–7.

29. Kuroki A, Møller AR. Microsurgical anatomy around the foramen of Luschka with reference to intraoperative recording of auditory evoked potentials from the cochlear nuclei. J Neurosurg 1995;82:933–9.

30. Waring MD. Intraoperative electrophysiologic monitoring to assist placement of auditory brain stem implant. Ann Otol Rhinol Laryngol Suppl 1995;166:33–6.

31. Møller AR, Møller MB, Yokota M. Some forms of tinnitus may involve the extralemniscal auditory pathway. Laryngoscope 1992;102:1165–71.

32. Lockwood AH, Salvi RJ, Coad ML, et al. The functional neuroanatomy of tinnitus. Evidence for limbic system links and neural plasticity. Neurology 1998;50:114–20.

33. Morest DK, Bohne BA. Noise-induced degeneration in the brain and representation of inner and outer hair cells. Hear Res 1983;9:145–52.

34. Morest DK, Ard MD, Yurgelun-Todd D. Degeneration in the central auditory pathways after acoustic deprivation or overstimulation in the cat. Anat Rec 1979;193:750.

35. Itoh K, Kamiya H, Mitani A, et al. Direct projections from dorsal column nuclei and the spinal trigeminal nuclei to the cochlear nuclei in the cat. Brain Res 1987;400:145–50.

36. Weinberg RJ, Rustioni A. A cuneocochlear pathway in the rat. Neuroscience 1987;20:209–19.

37. Shore SE, Vass Z, Wys NL, Altschuler RA. Trigeminal ganglion innervates the auditory brainstem. J Comp Neurol 2000; 419:271–85.

38. Aitkin L. The auditory midbrain, structure and function in the central auditory pathway. Clifton (NJ): Humana Press; 1986.

39. Rouiller EM, Rodrigues-Dagaeff C, Simm G, et al. Functional organization of the medial division of the medial geniculate body of the cat: tonotopic organization, spatial distribution of response properties and cortical connections. Hear Res 1989;39:127–42.

40. Syka J, Popelar J, Kvasnak E, Astl J. Response properties of neurons in the central nucleus and external and dorsal cortices of the inferior colliculus in guinea pig. J Exp Brain Res 2000; 133:254–66.

41. Szczepaniak WS, Møller AR. Interaction between auditory and somatosensory systems: a study of evoked potentials in the inferior colliculus. Electroencephalogr Clin Neurophysiol 1993;88:508–15.

42. Gerken GM, Saunders SS, Paul RE. Hypersensitivity to electrical stimulation of auditory nuclei follows hearing loss in cats. Hear Res 1984;13:249–60.

43. Gerken GM, Solecki JM, Boettcher FA. Temporal integration of electrical stimulation of auditory nuclei in normal hearing and hearing-impaired cat. Hear Res 1991;53:101–12.

44. Møller AR. Intraoperative neurophysiologic monitoring. Luxembourg: Harwood Academic Publishers; 1995.

45. Bocca E, Calearo C, Cassinari V. A new method for testing hearing in temporal lobe tumours. Acta Otolaryngol (Stockh) 1954; 44:219.

46. Korsan-Bengtsen MAMM. Distorted speech audiometry. Acta Otolaryngol Suppl (Stockh) 1973;310:1–75.

47. Møller AR. Cranial nerve dysfunction syndromes: pathophysiology of microvascular compression. In: Barrow DL, editor. Neurosurgical topics book 13: surgery of cranial nerves of the posterior fossa. Park Ridge (IL): American Association of Neurological Surgeons; 1993:105–29.

48. Møller AR. Similarities between severe tinnitus and chronic pain. J Am Acad Audiol 2000;11:115–24.

49. Szczepaniak WS, Møller AR. Effects of (-)-baclofen, clonazepam, and diazepam on tone exposure-induced hyperexcitability of the inferior colliculus in the rat: possible therapeutic implications for pharmacological management of tinnitus and hyperacusis. Hear Res 1996;97:46–53.

50. Møller AR, Pinkerton T. Temporal integration of pain from electrical stimulation of the skin. Neurol Res 1997;19:481–8.

51. Wall PD. The presence of ineffective synapses and circumstances which unmask them. Philos Trans R Soc Lond B Biol Sci 1977;278:361–72.

52. Woolf C, Thompson S. The induction and maintenance of central sensitization is dependent on N-methyl-D-aspartic acid receptor activation: implications for the treatment of post-injury pain hypersensitivity states. Pain 1991;293–9.

53. Kohama I, Ishikawa K, Koesis JD. Synaptic reorganization in the substantia gelatinosa after peripheral nerve neuroma formation: aberrant innervation of lamina II neurons by beta afferents. J Neurosci 2000;20:1538–49.

54. Møller AR. Vascular compression of cranial nerves. II. Pathophysiology. Neurol Res 1999;21:439–43.

55. Caspary DM, Raza A, Lawhorn A, et al. Immunocytochemical and neurochemical evidence for age-related loss of GABA in the inferior colliculus: implications for neural presbycusis. J Neurosci 1990;10:2363–72.

56. Simpson JJ, Davies E. Recent advances in the pharmacological treatment of tinnitus. Trends Pharmacol Sci 1999;20:12–8.

57. LeDoux JE. Brain mechanisms of emotion and emotional learning. Curr Opin Neurobiol 1992;2:191–7.

58. Cacace AT, Lovely TJ, McFarland DJP, et al. Anomalous cross-modal plasticity following posterior fossa surgery: some speculations on gaze-evoked tinnitus. Hear Res 1994;81:22–32.

59. Cacace AT, Cousins JP, Parnes SM, et al. Cutaneous-evoked tinnitus. II. Review of neuroanatomical, physiological and functional imaging studies. Audiol Neurootol 1999;4:258–68.

60. Cacace AT, Cousins JP, Parnes SM, et al. Cutaneous-evoked tinnitus. I. Phenomenology, psychophysics and functional imaging. Audiol Neurootol 1999;4:247–57.

61. Møller AR. Similarities between chronic pain and tinnitus. Am J Otol 1997;18:577–85.

62. Møller AR, Rollins P. The non-classical auditory system is active in children but not in adults. Neurosci Lett 2002;319:41–4.

63. Szczepaniak WS, Møller AR. Evidence of neuronal plasticity within the inferior colliculus after noise exposure: a study of evoked potentials in the rat. Electroencephalogr Clin Neurophysiol 1996;100:158–64.

64. Canlon B, Borg E, Flock A. Protection against noise trauma by pre-exposure to a low level acoustic stimulus. Hear Res 1988; 34:197–200.

65. Skellett RA, Cullen JKJ, Fallon M, Bobbin RP. Conditioning the auditory system with continuous vs. interrupted noise of equal acoustic energy: is either exposure more protective? Hear Res 1998;116:21–32.

66. Turner JG, Willott JF. Exposure to an augmented acoustic environment alters auditory function in hearing-impaired DBA/2J mice. Hear Res 1998;118:101–13.

67. Willott JF, Turner JG, Sundin VS. Effects of exposure to an augmented acoustic environment on auditory function in mice: roles of hearing loss and age during treatment. Hear Res 2000;142: 79–88.

68. Møller A, Jannetta PJ. On the origin of synkinesis in hemifacial spasm: results of intracranial recordings. J Neurosurg 1984;61:569–76.

69. Brach JS, Van Swearingen JM, Lenert J, Johnson PC. Facial neuromuscular retraining for oral synkinesis. Plast Reconstr Surg 1997;99:1922–31.

70. Sen CN, Møller AR. Signs of hemifacial spasm created by chronic periodic stimulation of the facial nerve in the rat. Exp Neurol 1987;98:336–49.

71. Goddard GV. Amygdaloid stimulation and learning in the rat. J Comp Physiol Psychol 1964;58:23–30.

72. Evans EF. The frequency response and other properties of single fibers in the guinea pig cochlear nerve. J Physiol 1972;226: 263–87.

73. Kiang NYS, Watanabe T, Thomas EC, Clark LF. Discharge patterns of single fibers in the cat's auditory nerve. Cambridge (MA): MIT Press; 1965.

74. Sachs MB, Kiang NYS. Two tone inhibition in auditory nerve fibers. J Acoust Soc Am 1968;43:1120–8.

75. Arthur RM, Pfeiffer RR, Suga N. Properties of "two tone inhibition" in primary auditory neurons. J Physiol (Lond) 1971;212: 593–609.

76. Møller AR. Sensory systems: anatomy and physiology. San Diego: Academic Press; 2002.

77. Møller AR. Hearing: its physiology and pathophysiology. San Diego: Academic Press; 2000.

6

Genetics in Otology and Neurotology

ANIL K. LALWANI, MD
ANAND N. MHATRE, PhD

The success of the human genome project in sequencing of the entire human genome has directly impacted our understanding of otologic and neurotologic disorders. Specifically, we have gained insights into the molecular mechanisms of hearing impairment, vestibular schwannomas, and glomus tumors. In this chapter, the principles of mendelian genetics are reviewed and our understanding of the aforementioned diseases is summarized.[1]

PRINCIPLES OF MENDELIAN GENETICS

Autosomal Dominant Inheritance

In autosomal dominant disorders, the transmission of a rare allele of a gene by a single heterozygous parent is sufficient to generate an affected child (Figure 6–1, A). A heterozygous parent can produce two types of gametes. One gamete carries the mutant form of the gene of interest and the other the normal form. Each of these gametes then has an equal chance of being used in the formation of a zygote. Thus, the chance that an offspring of an autosomal dominant affected parent will itself be affected is 50%. Equal numbers of affected males and females are expected for an autosomal dominant trait, and roughly half of the offspring of an affected individual will be affected. If male-to-male transmission of the trait is observed, the possibility that the trait is X-linked can be eliminated.

If the mutant phenotype is always expressed in individuals carrying the disease allele, then its penetrance is said to be complete; otherwise, it is incomplete. Where penetrance of the affected gene is complete, or 100%, the pattern of its inheritance may be discerned in a relatively straightforward manner. Complete pene-

trance of the dominant allele results in expression of the disease phenotype in all carriers of that allele without skipping generations. However, with incomplete penetrance of the affected gene, the inheritance pattern of the affected trait becomes relatively harder to discern, that is, one cannot easily distinguish between dominant inheritance with reduced penetrance and more complicated modes of inheritance. The failure of the gene to express itself may be owing to a variety of reasons. The most common rationale put forth to explain reduced penetrance is the effect of genetic background. Factors such as genetic redundancy, presence of more than one gene for the performance of a given function, and modifiers affect a variety of genes. Incomplete penetrance can also be seen in traits that are inherited in an autosomal recessive, X-linked recessive, and X-linked dominant manner.

Variable expression of different aspects of syndromes is common. Some aspects may be expressed in a range encompassing mild to severe forms and/or different combinations of associated symptoms may be expressed in different individuals carrying the same mutation within a single pedigree. An example of variable expressivity is seen in families transmitting autosomal dominant Waardenburg's syndrome. Within the same family, some affected members may have dystopia canthorum, white forelock, heterochromia irides, and hearing loss, whereas others with the same mutation may only have dystopia canthorum.

Autosomal Recessive Inheritance

An autosomal recessive trait is characterized by having two unaffected parents who are heterozygous carriers for

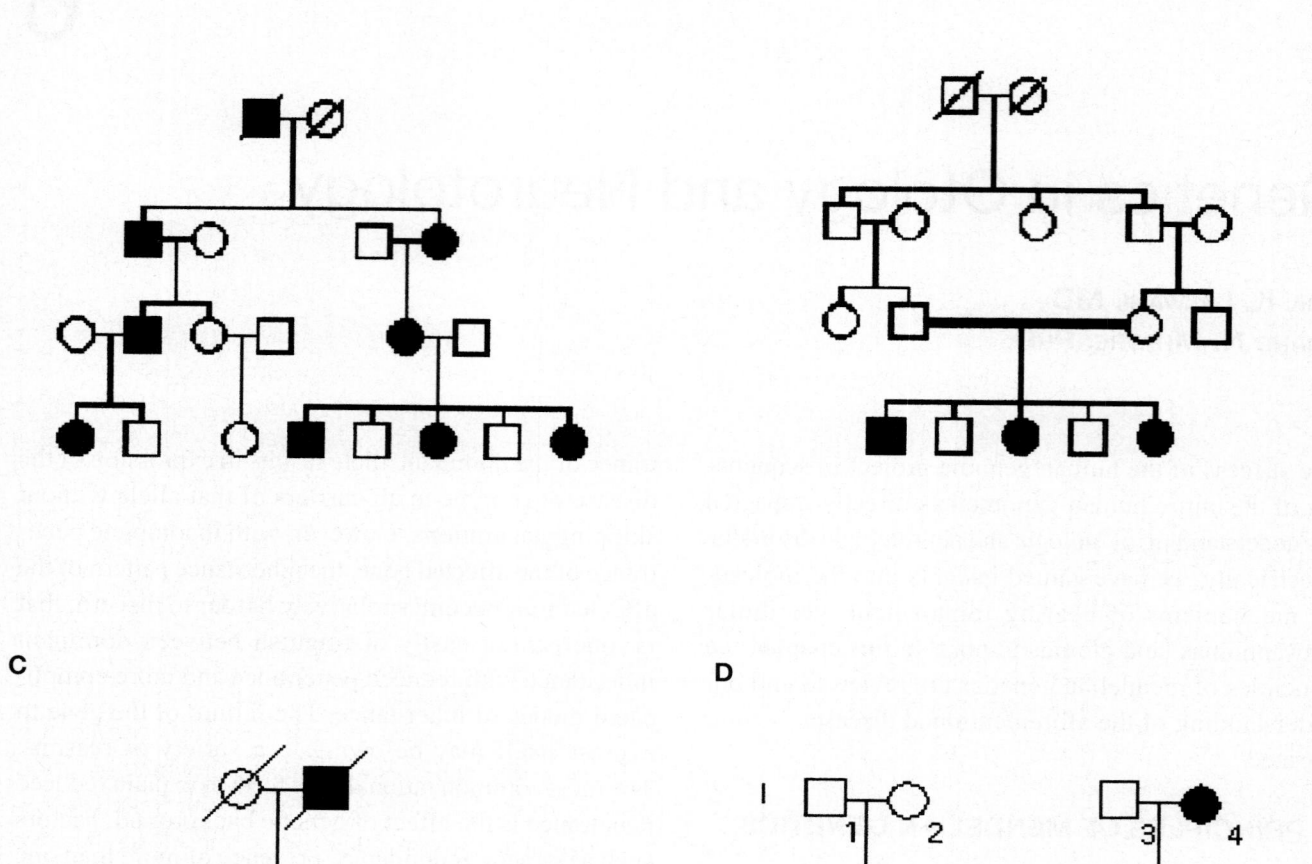

Figure 6–1 Patterns of inheritance. Pedigrees showing autosomal dominant (*A*), autosomal recessive (*B*), X-linked (*C*), and mitochondrial inheritance (*D*). Autosomal dominant inheritance is characterized by vertical transmission in contrast to the horizontal pattern seen in recessive inheritance; transmission of recessive disease is more common in consanguineous mating depicted in the pedigree. In X-linked diseases, the unaffected carrier mothers (depicted as a *dot* in the center of the square or the circle) have affected and unaffected sons, whereas all daughters are unaffected. On the other hand, affected fathers only have unaffected children. Mitochondrial diseases can only be transmitted from the mother as mitochondrial DNA is present only in the egg.

mutant forms of the gene in question but in whom the phenotypic expression of the mutant allele is masked by the normal allele. These heterozygous parents (A/a) can each generate two types of gametes, one carrying the mutant copy of the gene (a) and the other having a normal copy of the gene (A). Of the four possible combinations of these two gamete types from each of the parents, only the offspring that inherits both mutant copies (a/a) will exhibit the trait. Of the three remaining possibilities, all will have a normal hearing phenotype, but two of the three will be heterozygous carriers for the mutant form of the gene, similar to the carrier parents. A typical recessive pedigree with affected members in a single generation (horizontal pattern), showing a consanguineous mating between cousins, is depicted in Figure 6–1, B.

X-Linked Inheritance

In humans, females have 22 pairs of autosomes and a pair of X chromosomes (46XX), and males have 22 autosomes, one X chromosome, and one Y chromosome (46XY). Accordingly, males always receive their Y chromosome from their father and their X chromosome from their mother, whereas females receive one of their X chromosomes from each of their two parents. Because males have one copy of the X chromosome, they are hemizygous for genes on the X chromosome, and the X chromosome is active in all of their nucleated cells. In general, only one of the two X chromosomes carried by a female is active in any one cell, whereas the other is rendered inactive by a natural process known as lyonization. This random inactivation process makes all females who are heterozygous for X-linked traits mosaic at the tissue level, resulting in variable expression of the mutant gene. Diseases that are rarely expressed clinically in heterozygous females are called X-linked recessive. In female tissues, various proportions of cells may exist in which one or the other of two alleles for an X-linked locus is expressed. Occasionally, a carrier female may manifest some symptoms of an X-linked recessive disorder owing to this mosaicism if she, by chance, has an abundance of cells with the mutant allele being expressed. Transmission of an X-linked recessive trait in a pedigree is illustrated in Figure 6–1, C.

VARIATIONS ON MENDELIAN PRINCIPLES

Mendel established the two fundamental principles of genetics: segregation of genes and their independent assortment. These principles refer to processes that occur in the formation of germ cells known as meiosis. Segregation refers to separation of homologous genes, representing the paternal and the maternal contribution to the individual's genotype, into two separate daughter cells. Thus, the diploid genome is reduced to the haploid state in the germ cells. The principle of independent assortment states that segregation of one gene occurs independently of other genes. These principles have served well for analysis and understanding of the inheritance of traits through a single locus. However, a number of variations on these principles do exist, some of which have already been stated implicitly above. These variations and their underlying principles have contributed toward increasing our understanding of the genetic etiology of disease.

Linkage and Recombination

Not all genes assort independently of each other. This variation on the mendelian principle was initially identified by Thomas Morgan through analysis of transmission of selected traits in fruit flies. Experiments showed inheritance of specific pairs of alleles in a combination not present in the parental phenotype. This new combination of alleles was considered to result from crossing over and exchange of genetic material between two homologous chromosomes, known as homologous recombination, yielding the new combination of alleles not present in the original parental chromosomes. Analysis of recombination frequencies between two traits considered to be controlled by genes residing on the same linkage group, that is, the same chromosome, provided two essential concepts that led to the development of the genetic map: genes are arranged in a linear order, and the frequency with which two alleles are inherited together is a function of the relative physical distance to each other. Thus, the closer the two genes, the greater the chance that they will remain linked post meiosis. The relative chromosomal positions of genes may be readily mapped through the application of these principles of linkage and recombination to generate genetic maps. The genetic distance between two linked genes as measured through the frequency of recombinants between the two alleles is measured in centiMorgans (cM); for example, two loci are one cM apart on the genetic map if there is a 1% chance of a recombination between them in meiosis. Thus, genes that are far apart on a chromosome will assort in an apparently independent manner, whereas genes that are close together will tend to remain linked post meiosis.

Mitochondrial Inheritance

Not all genes are equally inherited from both parents. The extranuclear genome is inherited solely through the mother. Male mitochondria are not contributed to newly formed zygotes. This inheritance pattern gives rise to pedigrees in which all of the children of an affected mother may be affected and none of the children of an affected father will be affected (Figure 6–1, D). In practice, the expression of mitochondrially inherited disorders is often variable and may be incompletely penetrant. If all of the mitochondria transmitted by the mother are of the same genotype, it is called homoplasmia; if there are genetic differences between them, it is called heteroplasmia.

Genomic Imprinting

The manifestation of some genetic diseases depends on the sex of the transmitting parent. This occurrence is considered to result from genomic imprinting. This phenomenon runs counter to the teachings of mendelian genetics that emphasize equal contribution from paternal and maternal genes, with the obvious exception of genes on the sex chromosomes. Thus, in certain instances, despite the presence of both the paternal and maternal alleles, only one of the parental alleles is expressed. This differential expression of the parental alleles is detected in certain disease states when inheritance of that disorder is dependent on the sex of the parent who transmits the mutant gene. The gene-specific imprinting is presumed to be the consequence of reversible "epigenetic" modification of the parental allele during gametogenesis, leading to its differential expression. The precise mechanism of imprinting and its evolutionary significance remain unknown. Hypermethylation of the imprinted gene represents one possible mechanism.

Genomic imprinting at the level of a specific gene has been identified in familial cases of nonchromaffin paragangliomas (PGs; benign tumors of the paraganglionic cells, also known as glomus tumors). Although benign, their enlargement can cause deafness and/or facial palsy. Familial PGs have shown an autosomal dominant inheritance with genomic imprinting of the maternal allele. Thus, the transmission of the disease occurs via the affected paternal allele and not the maternal allele.

Multifactorial Inheritance

An expression of a phenotype, the outcome of which is determined by a single gene, is termed a mendelian trait. Its pattern of transmission within a pedigree can be readily discerned in most cases, as described above. On the other hand, most common human diseases and traits show irregular inheritance patterns. These traits are considered to be determined from the action of multiple genes and/or nongenetic factors. A phenotype that is an outcome of both genetic and environmental factors is called a multifactorial, or complex, trait. The low proportion of mendelian traits relative to the number of multifactorial traits in humans is better illustrated by considering the proportion of total number of mendelian traits known (approximately 6,000 according to McKusick's Mendelian Inheritance In Man) to the total number of genes that are estimated to exist (approximately 30,000 to 100,000). It should be emphasized that classification of mendelian traits as being "determined" by single genes is an oversimplification. As more mendelian disorders are identified and their phenotypes investigated, their phenotypic variability and complexity are becoming increasingly clear, and, concomitantly, their distinction from complex or multifactorial traits is becoming increasingly blurred. Phenotype variability or variable expression seen in a single gene disorder such as Waardenburg's syndrome may reflect interaction of that major gene, such as *PAX3*, with "modifier" genes. Identification of these modifier genes has important implications for the understanding and treatment of mendelian disorders with variable expressivity.

The relatively irregular mode of inheritance that characterizes a multifactorial trait is presumed to result from interaction of multiple genes (polygenic). This interaction is apparently distinct from that presumed for mendelian traits. But this distinction may be at a quantitative rather than a qualitative level. For example, instead of a predominant influence or effect of one gene on expression of the phenotype, the multifactorial trait is characterized by a number of genes with equivalent influence or effect. The genetic component of multifactorial traits is referred to by terms such as increased risk, predisposition, or susceptibility. Because of their complexity, the factors that contribute to the multifactorial traits are poorly defined. Several well-studied diseases, such as cardiovascular conditions and diabetes, as well as distinct behavioral disorders, are classified as multifactorial. The influence of nongenetic factors, for example, environmental agents or stochastic processes during development, on a variety of traits is also clearly illustrated in the studies of identical twins.

GENETICS OF HEARING LOSS

Hearing loss is the most common form of sensory impairment in humans. Nearly 10% of the US population or 30 million Americans have significant auditory dysfunction. For some, the hearing loss is present at the beginning of life. The prevalence of permanent, moderate-to-severe sensorineural hearing loss (SNHL) is estimated to be between 1 and 3 per 1,000 live births.[2,3] Prelingual deafness, in contrast to late-onset hearing loss, can be devastating to the child. Significant delays in the acquisition of speech and language, as well as other developmental childhood milestones, can occur without adequate rehabilitation. The predominant etiology of hearing impairment in children has evolved with advances in medical knowledge and therapeutics. Historically, infectious disorders such as otitis media, maternal rubella infections, and bacterial meningitis, as well as environmental factors such as intrauterine teratogenic exposure or ototoxic insult, were the dominant causes of congenital and acquired hearing losses. The introduction of antibiotics, vaccines, and improved knowledge and enhanced awareness about teratogens have led to a decline in hearing loss resulting from infections and environmental agents. Currently, more than half of all childhood hearing impairment is thought to be hereditary. As a result of advances in clinical and basic medical research, significant progress has been made in understanding the causes of hereditary hearing impairment (HHI).

Classification

When SNHL occurs in isolation, it is called nonsyndromic.[4] On the other hand, hearing loss accompanied by other systemic disturbance is termed syndromic. Two-thirds of HHI is nonsyndromic, whereas the remaining one-third is syndromic. Over 1,100 syndromes are associated with otologic manifestations. Nonsyndromic HHI is further classified by the mode of inheritance. The majority of HHI is inherited in an autosomal recessive fashion (80%), with the autosomal dominant mode of inheritance being less common (15 to 18%).[5] Rare modes of transmission include X-linked and mitochondrial transmission, which account for the remaining 2% of hearing impairment.

Auditory Phenotype in Hereditary Hearing Impairment

Clinically, HHI can be described by several characteristics of the hearing loss: severity of hearing impairment, age of onset, type of hearing impairment, frequencies involved, unilateral/bilateral, stable/progressive, and syndromic/nonsyndromic. In general, recessive HHI tends to be more severe than dominantly inherited hearing impairment. Recessive HHI is predominantly congenital or prelingual in onset, whereas dominant HHI is delayed or postlingual. In contrast to the profound hearing loss associated with recessive deafness, autosomal dominant hearing loss is less severe and progresses with age. Many dominant hearing impairments progress at the rate of about 1 dB/year. Recessive deafness usually affects all frequencies equally. Although there are some types that have predominantly low-frequency or flat hearing loss, dominant hearing impairment more commonly affects the high frequencies, mimicking presbycusis. The frequencies involved in syndromic forms of hearing impairment are variable. Nonsyndromic hearing impairment is usually symmetric. In contrast, syndromic HHI can be unilateral or bilateral and symmetric or asymmetric.

Molecular Genetics Of HHI

Rapid progress has been made in the identification of genes responsible for syndromic and nonsyndromic hereditary hearing impairment. In syndromic hearing impairment, more than 100 genes have been identified since 1990, showing a large heterogeneity even in the same type of syndromic hearing impairment, for example, Usher's syndrome type Ia-f with six different genetic loci (Table 6–1). In nonsyndromic hearing impairment, as of 2001, 40 autosomal dominant, 30 autosomal recessive, 6 X-linked, and 2 mitochondrial loci have been mapped on the human genome. In addition, the current count of 18 nonsyndromic genes identified since 1994 will continue to rapidly increase (Table 6–2; Hereditary Hearing Loss Homepage: <http://www.uia.ac.be/dnalab/hhh>).

The identified deafness genes play a variety of different roles in cellular physiology (see Tables 6–1 and 6–2). The responsible genes include cytoskeletal proteins important in maintaining cellular structure, division,

Table 6–1 SYNDROMIC HEREDITARY HEARING IMPAIRMENT GENES

Syndrome/locus	Gene	Function
Alport's	COL4A3	Cytoskeletal protein
	COL4A4	Cytoskeletal protein
	COL4A5	Cytoskeletal protein
Branchio-oto-renal	EYA1	Developmental gene
	BOR2?	
Jervell and Lange-Nielsen	KVLQT1	Delayed rectifier potassium channel
	KCNE1	Delayed rectifier potassium channel
Norrie's	NORRIN	Cell-cell interactions?
Pendred's	PDS	Chloride-iodide transporter
Stickler's	COL2A1	Cytoskeletal protein
	COL11A1	Cytoskeletal protein
	COL11A2	Cytoskeletal protein
Treacher Collins	TCOF1	Nucleolar-cytoplasmic transport
Usher's	MYO7A	Cytoskeletal protein
	USH1C	?
	CDH23	Intercellular adherence protein
	USH2A	Cell adhesion molecule
	USH3	?
	Others	
Waardenburg's type I, III	PAX3	Transcription factor
Waardenburg's type II	MITF	Transcription factor
Waardenburg's type IV	EDNRB	Endothelin-B receptor
	EDN3	Endothelin-B receptor ligand
	SOX10	Transcription factor

and intracellular transport; transcription factors that regulate the expression of other genes; ion channels important in the transport of sodium, potassium, chloride, and iodine; developmental genes that regulate morphogenesis; and proteins involved in intercellular communications such as gap and tight junctions.

Table 6–2 NONSYNDROMIC HEREDITARY HEARING IMPAIRMENT GENES

Locus	Gene	Function
DFNA1	DIAPH1	Cytoskeletal protein
DFNA2	GJB3 (CX31)	Gap junctions
DFNA2	KCNQ4	Potassium channel
DFNA3	GJB2 (CX26)	Gap junctions
DFNA3	GJB6 (CX30)	Gap junctions
DFNA5	DFNA5	Unknown
DFNA6/14	WFS1	Endoplasmic reticulum protein
DFNA8/12	TECTA	Tectorial membrane protein
DFNA9	COCH	Unknown
DFNA10	EYA4	Developmental gene
DFNA11	MYO7A	Cytoskeletal protein
DFNA13	COL11A2	Cytoskeletal protein
DFNA15	POU4F3	Transcription factor
DFNA17	MYH9	Cytoskeletal protein
DFNA22	MYO6	
DFNB1	GJB2 (CX26)	Gap junctions
DFNB2	MYO7A	Cytoskeletal protein
DFNB3	MYO15	Cytoskeletal protein
DFNB4	PDS	Chloride-iodide transporter
DFNB8/10	TMPRSS3	Transmembrane serine protease
DFNB9	OTOF	Trafficking of membrane vesicles
DFNB12	CDH23	Intercellular adherence protein
DFNB16	STRC	Stereocilia protein
DFNB21	TECTA	Tectorial membrane protein
DFNB29	CLDN14	Tight junctions
Unnamed	GJA1 (CX43)	Gap junctions
DFN3	POU3F4	Transcription factor

As a result of progress in the genetics of deafness (and genetics in general), several conventional notions have had to be modified. It is now clear that a single gene may cause syndromic or nonsyndromic forms of deafness or may be associated with autosomal dominant or autosomal recessive mode of inheritance. Identification of myosin 7A as the gene responsible for both syndromic and nonsyndromic deafness has led to the abandonment of the "one gene, one disease" dogma. In addition, pendrin mutations cause both Pendred's syndrome and isolated (nonsyndromic) large vestibular aqueduct (LVA). To muddle things further, different mutations in myosin 7A cause both dominant and recessive forms of nonsyndromic deafness. The same is true for connexin 26: it is associated with both a dominant and a recessive mode of transmission. In addition to the disease-causing gene, the patient's genetic background and the role of other modifier genes in determining the clinical severity is now better appreciated. For example, the severity of Waardenburg's syndrome in a given patient will be determined not only by the mutation in the *PAX3* gene but also by what other genes are present in the remaining genome.

Several of the genes are especially important in clinical otology including connexins, *PDS*, myosins, and mitochondrial gene 12S ribosomal ribonucleic acid (rRNA) and are discussed below.

Connexin 26

The apparent genetic heterogeneity of HHI is contrasted by the predominance of *CX26* as a major cause of inherited and sporadic nonsyndromic deafness. Mutations of *CX26* are responsible for both recessive (*DFNB1*—DFN for deafness, B for recessive) and dominant (*DFNA3*) forms of HHI; it is an important contributor to childhood hearing loss, accounting for nearly 50% of congenital recessive sensorineural hearing impairment. Connexin 26 is a member of a family of proteins that are involved in the formation of gap junctions. Connexins are transmembrane proteins that form channels allowing transport of ions or small molecules between adjacent cells. Each connexin subunit contains three intracellular domains and two extracellular domains, crossing the plasma membrane four times. The second intracellular domain contains the cytoplasmic loop. The other two intracellular domains consist of the N terminus and the C terminus.[6] Six connexin subunits join to form a con-

nexon. A pair of connexons, one in each adjacent cell, comes together to form an intercellular channel. The family of connexin proteins plays an important role in normal hearing as mutations in several members of the family are associated with hearing impairment. To date, mutations in *CX26*, *CX30*, *CX31*, *CX32*, and *CX43* have been implicated in hearing loss (Connexin and Deafness Home Page: <http://www.iro.es/deafness>). Its expression has been shown in the stria vascularis, basement membrane, limbus, and spiral prominence of the human cochlea.[7] One possible biochemical function of connexin 26 has been suggested by studying rat cochlear gap junctions. The organization of gap junctions and information provided by other investigators suggest that they serve as the structural basis for recycling of potassium ions back to the endolymph of the cochlear duct after stimulation of the sensory hair cells.[8,9]

Several studies have demonstrated the prevalence of *CX26* mutations in 50% of individuals with recessive deafness, with a carrier rate as high as 4%.[7,10–15] Currently, more than 60 different mutations have been identified (Connexin and Deafness Home Page: <http://www.iro.es/deafness>). Two single base pair deletions account for nearly half of all mutations in this gene: 35delG and 167delT. The 35delG mutation has been found to be common in several populations and accounts for up to 70% of *CX26* mutant alleles in families from the United Kingdom, France, Italy, Spain, Tunisia, Lebanon, Israel, Australia, Greece, United States, and New Zealand, as well as up to 40% of sporadic cases of congenital deafness in these countries.[12,13,16–20] The 35delG mutation leads to frameshift, early termination of the nascent protein, and a nonfunctional intracellular domain in the protein.[12,16,21] Alternatively, this mutation may lead to an unstable RNA, leading to its early degradation or absence of its translation into protein. Clinically, homozygous patients with the 35delG mutation show a variable phenotype, ranging from mild to profound hearing impairment. However, most patients with the homozygous 35delG mutation show a severe to profound phenotype.

In contrast, the 35delG mutation may be less common in the Japanese populations in which 235delC is the prevalent *CX26* mutation.[22–24] Likewise, in the Ashkenazi Jewish population, the 167delT mutation has been found to be more common than the 35delG mutation, with a carrier rate of 4%.[15]

Of the genes identified to date, *CX26*, because of its small size, the single coding exon, frequency of involvement, and predominance of two mutations, lends itself to mutation screening. However, it is unlikely that screening for the two common mutations will be sufficient to identify the vast majority of *CX26* deafness. We have recently screened 154 individuals with SNHL for mutations in *CX26* by DNA sequencing and identified 34 patients with mutations for an overall incidence of 22% in the study population.[25] Of all *CX26* mutations, the 35delG mutation accounted for 26%. The 35delG mutation was present in a homozygous state in only 4 individuals (each of the two chromosomes harbored the 35delG mutation) and heterozygous in 6 individuals (only one chromosome had the 35delG mutation). Herein lies the fundamental problem with screening for only 35delG: only 4 of 34 individuals (12%) with *CX26* mutations, or 154 individuals in total (3%), had a homozygous mutation that would be required to clearly implicate *CX26* as the causative gene. The identification of a single copy of 35delG mutation does not implicate this gene in deafness and may simply reflect the high carrier rate that is present in the population. In this case, the rate of identifying the cause of childhood SNHL by genetic testing is significantly less than radiologic imaging. The predominance of the two common mutations in a heterozygous state (with a second uncommon *CX26* mutation) has been replicated by others.[26,27] Therefore, genetic testing for 35delG and 167delT mutations only, without sequencing the entire *CX26* gene, is inadequate. Although screening for the two common *CX26* mutations is now available at numerous medical centers and laboratories, its role in the management of children with hearing impairment has yet to be determined.

Pendrin

Mutations in pendrin may be associated with an isolated LVA (the most common radiologic abnormality associated with childhood deafness), as well as Pendred's syndrome. Vaughan Pendred, while he was working in the Ear, Nose, and Throat Department at Newcastle Royal Infirmary, observed the association between deaf-mutism and goiter in two sisters.[28,29] The first sister appeared to be profoundly deaf and developed the goiter at the age of 13 years; the second sister was not completely deaf and also developed a notable thyroid mass at the age of 13. It has been estimated that as much as 10% of all HHI may be attributable to Pendred's syndrome, making it one of the most common syndromic HHI disorders.[30] Goiter

may appear at birth, in childhood, or after puberty. The delay in onset, or sometimes absence, of goiter can make clinical diagnosis of Pendred's syndrome difficult. Patients are usually euthyroid but can be hypothyroid. The elevation of thyrotropin-releasing hormone suggests a compensatory hypothyroidism.[31] The mild organification defect in Pendred's syndrome can be noted by the partial discharge of iodine in the perchlorate challenge test.[32] The perchlorate ion ($ClO4^-$) is a competitor of iodine. When perchlorate is given orally or intravenously following radioactive iodine administration, the perchlorate blocks further uptake of iodine and releases unbound iodine in the thyroid follicular cells. In Pendred's syndrome, in which there is an intrinsic thyroid organification defect, the perchlorate displaces more iodine than in a normal thyroid gland, leading to a greater iodine "discharge" and a decrease in thyroid radioactivity over time. The hearing loss of Pendred's syndrome is usually congenital and profound. However, there are reports of milder or progressive hearing impairments. Hypoplasia of the cochlea and enlargement of the vestibular aqueduct can be associated with Pendred's syndrome as demonstrated by histologic and radiologic studies.[33,34]

Everett and colleagues[35] identified mutations in the *PDS* gene on chromosome 7q31 as the cause of Pendred's syndrome. The gene contains 21 exons. The gene product pendrin encodes a 780-amino acid (86-kD) protein that contains 11 transmembrane domains resembling sulfate transporters.[35] Recent evidence suggests that pendrin functions as a chloride-iodide anion transport protein.[36] In the mouse inner ear, pendrin localizes to the endolymphatic duct and sac, distinct areas in the utricle and saccule, and the external sulcus region within the cochlea, implicating a possible role in endolymph resorption. Van Hauwe and colleagues[37] noted two particularly frequent missense mutations, L236P (707 T to C) and T416P (1246 A to C); subsequently, a third common mutation, E384G (1151 A to G), has also been identified. Although the gene is too large for screening by direct sequencing, identification of common mutations opens the opportunity for screening for these isolated mutations.

PDS mutations are also responsible for nonsyndromic hearing loss associated with LVA. The isolated presence of an LVA is one of the most common forms of inner ear anomaly. Genetic studies of families with LVA disorder identified a recessive nonsyndromic locus, *DFNB4*, that also mapped to the same region as the *PDS* gene.

This led to the evaluation of the *PDS* gene and the subsequent identification of seven *PDS* mutations responsible for LVA with nonsyndromic HHI.[38] Like Pendred's syndrome, different mutations, V480D, V653A, I490L and G497S, have been found to be commonly associated with LVA. In a review of our experience at the University of California at San Francisco, LVA was the most common imaging abnormality detected in children with nonsyndromic SNHL.[39] At least 40% of children with LVA will develop profound SNHL.[40] Patients with LVA are at risk for progressive hearing loss after minor head trauma. Identifying this anomaly influences parent counseling with respect to the dangers of incidental head trauma. In summary, the spectrum of *PDS* mutations and the wide range of phenotypic manifestations show that pendrin is an important participant in ear structural development and in the normal functioning of the inner ear and thyroid. Screening for mutations may play an important role in the diagnosis and management of a child as well as their siblings with hearing impairment.

Myosins

The importance of myosins in inner ear function is manifest in the growing list of unconventional (non–class II) myosin heavy chain genes pathogenically linked to HHI. These disease genes encode the heavy chains in/of myosin VI, VII, and XV. Expression of these unconventional myosins is not limited to the cells and the tissues of the inner ear. Yet the expression of their dysfunction is largely restricted to hearing impairment. In the mouse, myosin VI has been identified as the Snell's waltzer gene; the cochlear and vestibular neurosensory epithelium of Snell's waltzer mice degenerates soon after birth. The role of myosin VI in human deafness remains to be determined. Myosin VII has been linked to both rodent and human deafness. Mutations in the gene encoding myosin VIIA are responsible for mouse shaker 1, human Usher's syndrome type 1, and human nonsyndromic hearing impairment DFNB2 and DFNA11. Shaker 1 mice are deaf and have vestibular defects. Mice that are homozygous for mutant shaker 1 allele display disorganized stereocilia. Myosin XV is the largest of all myosin heavy chains, having a molecular weight of 395 kD. Mutations in myosin XV have been pathogenically linked to DFNB3 in humans and the shaker 2 phenotype in mice.

The unconventional myosins are distributed throughout the mechanosensory hair cells. Moreover, histopathologic study of mouse models of myosin XV dysfunction has been valuable to understanding the consequences of myosin dysfunction on the sensory hair cells. Myosin VI is localized within the actin-rich cuticular plate, as well as in the rootlet actin filaments that descend from the stereocilia into the cuticular plate, suggesting a role in stabilizing the basal attachment of stereocilia.[41,42] Myosin VIIA is localized in the stereocilia and cell body of hair cells.[42] Postulated roles for myosin VIIA include maintaining stereocilia integrity and membrane trafficking in the inner hair cells. On histopathologic evaluation, the inner ears of mouse models of myosin XV dysfunction reveal significantly shortened stereocilia in the sensory hair cells, demonstrating the importance of myosin XV in the maintenance of hair cell structure and thereby its function.

Recently, a mutation in a conventional, or class II, myosin, *MYH9*, has been described. The class II myosins are broadly expressed in skeletal, cardiac, and smooth muscle as well as nonmuscle tissue and consist of a pair of heavy chains, a pair of light chains, and a pair of regulatory light chains.[43] The N-terminal motor domain is the most highly conserved region of the myosin heavy chain and contains the adenosine triphosphate and actin binding sites. The apparent molecular weight of the class II myosin heavy chain is 200 kDa. The myosin that mediates skeletal muscle contraction, also known as the sarcomeric myosin, represents the most well-characterized representative of the class II myosin family. Cardiac and smooth muscle cells also express isoforms of class II myosin, distinct from the sarcomeric myosin that mediates contraction in these muscle cells. Mutation in MYH9, a conventional nonmuscle myosin, was described in an American family with autosomal dominant nonsyndromic hereditary hearing impairment (DFNA17) associated with cochleosaccular degeneration.[44-46] The affected members of the DFNA17 family exhibit progressive, postlingual onset hearing loss, a pattern that is observed in the majority of nonsyndromic autosomal dominant HHI. The cosegregation of the mutant MYH9 with nonsyndromic hearing impairment illustrates a biologically significant role for MYH9 in hearing and an organ-specific pathology associated with the mutant allele.

Two other myosin genes have been predicted to have an important role in hearing. Myosin V is an abundant protein of afferent nerve fibers innervating both inner and outer hair cells.[47] Myosin Iβ has been implicated as an effector of adaptation of the hair cell transduction apparatus.[48] The preponderance of myosins is not surprising given the diversity of actin filament systems in the inner ear.[49]

Aminoglycoside Ototoxicity

To date, there are 326 syndromes, disorders, or peculiar phenotypes associated with mutations in the mitochondrial genome.[50] Twenty-one of these disorders have some involvement with SNHL, indicating that the requirement for a healthy population of mitochondria is very important to the cells involved in normal hearing.[51–54] One of the most striking examples of a mitochondrially inherited trait whose expression is environmentally affected is that for hearing loss caused by hypersensitivity to aminoglycosides.[51] The aminoglycoside hypersensitivity phenotype is the result of a single base transition of A to G at position 1555 in the mitochondrial 12S rRNA. This mutation causes a portion of the 12S rRNA transcript structure to closely resemble the binding site of aminoglycosides to bacterial rRNA. When an aminoglycoside such as streptomycin is administered to patients carrying this mutation, it binds to the mutant 12S rRNA and prevents it from functioning in the translation of mitochondrially transcribed genes, resulting in the loss of mitochondria in cells and perhaps cell death or impairment of normal function. Screening for this mutation prior to initiation of aminoglycoside therapy may reduce the incidence of ototoxicity.

GENETICS OF NEUROFIBROMATOSIS 2

Neurofibromatosis 2 (NF2) is much rarer than NF1, with an incidence estimated between 1 in 33,000 and 1 in 50,000.[55] Inheritance of NF2 is autosomal dominant, and gene penetrance is over 95%. Neurofibromatosis 2 most frequently presents in the second and third decades of life. The mean age of onset of symptoms from vestibular schwannomas in Kanter and colleagues's series was 20.4 years.[56] Vestibular schwannomas comprise approximately 8% of intracranial tumors and account for approximately 80% of cerebellopontine angle tumors.[57] The majority of vestibular schwannomas are sporadic in occurrence and unilateral, presenting in the fifth decade.

Patients with NF2 with bilateral vestibular schwannomas represent 2 to 4% of all vestibular schwannomas.[58,59]

Neurofibromatosis 2 has often been confused with NF1. The conclusive proof that NF1 and NF2 were distinct disease entities did not occur until 1987. Molecular biologic investigations by Barker and colleagues,[60] among others, showed that the gene responsible for NF1 was located near the proximal long arm of chromosome 17. At the same time, under separate investigation, the gene responsible for NF2 was located on chromosome 22 by Rouleau and colleagues.[61]

Neurofibromatosis 2 results from the inheritance of a mutation in the gene on chromosome 22. The incidence of mutation rate within the NF2 gene has been estimated at 6.5×10^{-6}.[55] In approximately 50% of cases, there is no family history, and these patients represent new germline mutations.[62] Chromosome 22 was first thought to be the likely source of the NF2 gene following cytogenetic studies of meningiomas in 1982.[63] The NF2 gene was subsequently mapped to chromosome 22 by both linkage studies and loss of heterozygosity analysis in 1986 and 1987, respectively.[61,64] In 1993, the NF2 gene, designated merlin or schwannomin, was isolated by two groups working independently.[65,66] The NF2 gene is spread over approximately 100 kb on chromosome 22q12.2 and contains 17 exons. The coding sequence of the messenger RNA is 1,785 bp in length and encodes a protein of 595 amino acids.[65,66] The gene product is similar in sequence to a family of proteins including moesin, ezrin, radixin, talin, and members of the protein 4.1 superfamily. These proteins are involved in linking cytoskeletal components with the plasma membrane and are located in actin-rich surface projections such as microvilli. The N-terminal region of the merlin protein is thought to interact with components of the plasma membrane and the C-terminal with the cytoskeleton.

Merlin or schwannomin is predominantly expressed in the cells of the nervous system and in the lens and is predominantly located in membrane ruffles and cellular protrusions.[67,68] It is currently believed that merlin protein overexpression can inhibit cell growth and that it induces cell surface protrusions and elongation of cells.[68,69] In 1994, Tikoo and colleagues[70] tested merlin's ability to function as a tumor suppressor gene. Following introduction of the NF2 protein into v-Ha-Ras-transformed NIH 3T3 cells, they were able to demonstrate the reversal of the malignant phenotype, thus confirming the tumor suppressor properties of merlin. Although the exact function of the NF2 protein is as yet unknown, the evidence available so far suggests that it is involved in cell-cell or cell-matrix interactions and that it is important for cell movement, cell shape, or communication. Loss of function of the merlin protein therefore could result in a loss of contact inhibition and consequently lead to tumorigenesis.

Mutations involving the NF2 gene have been observed in 22 to 59% of patients with sporadic vestibular schwannoma.[71] Welling and colleagues[72] compared the rate of identification of genetic mutations in sporadic vestibular schwannoma versus patients with NF2 and found a significant difference, 66 to 33%, respectively, while noting that different mutational mechanisms may exist in tumorigenesis.[72] To date, more than 200 mutations of the NF2 gene have been identified, including single base substitutions, insertions, and deletions.[73,74] Most mutations lead to truncation of the C-terminal end of the protein; only 13 missense mutations have been identified.[74] NF2 gene defects have been detected in other malignancies including meningiomas, malignant mesotheliomas, melanomas, and breast carcinomas.[64,75–78]

Recent genotype-phenotype correlation studies suggest that mutations in the NF2 gene are associated with variable phenotypic expression. Ruttledge and colleagues[79] found that mutations in the NF2 gene that result in protein truncation are associated with a more severe clinical presentation of NF2 (Wishart), whereas missense and splice site mutations are associated with a milder (Gardner) form of the disease. Similarly, Parry and colleagues[80] have reported that retinal abnormalities were associated with the more disruptive protein truncation mutations of the NF2 gene. Both studies showed intrafamilial variability of phenotypic expression.

Although mutations in the NF2 gene play a dominant role in the biology of vestibular schwannoma, it is also possible that other genetic loci contribute to the development of vestibular schwannoma. In addition, NF2 gene mutations are not uniformly identified in patients with vestibular schwannoma, and published genotype-phenotype correlations are variable, which suggests that other genetic loci may contribute to the genesis of vestibular schwannoma and the ultimate phenotype of affected individuals.[79,80]

The recent identification of the gene responsible for NF2 has significantly advanced our understanding of the molecular pathology and factors responsible for the clinical heterogeneity among patients with NF2. Understanding the function of merlin in tumor formation will lead to the development of novel therapies, which may eventually alleviate the suffering associated with NF2.

GENETICS OF FAMILIAL PARAGANGLIOMAS

With the exception of the genes located on the sex chromosomes (X and Y), we inherit two copies of every gene. In most cases, both the maternal and the paternal copy of the gene are active. Therefore, when inheriting a disease that is transmitted in an autosomal dominant fashion, it usually does not matter which parent passes down the single mutated gene for the child to be affected. However, there are genes in which only the paternal or maternal copy is active or functional and the inactive gene is said to be imprinted. Imprinted genes are normally involved in embryonic growth and behavioral development, but occasionally they also function inappropriately as oncogenes or tumor suppressor genes.

Familial PG is inherited in an autosomal dominant manner with maternal imprinting. Therefore, when an individual inherits the PG gene from the mother (regardless of whether she herself is affected), that child is unaffected and becomes a silent carrier of the mutated gene. On the other hand, when a child inherits the PG gene from the father, the offspring will have PGs regardless of the affected status of the father. Subsequently, the affected/unaffected child harboring the abnormal PG gene will be able to pass the gene to his/her children; he/she will have affected children only if the transmitting parent is a father. This unusual form of incomplete genetic penetrance is caused by sex-specific gene modification during gametogenesis.[81]

Because of the unusual pattern of inheritance outlined above, it is difficult to determine whether every case of "sporadic" PGs is, in fact, sporadic or a hereditary tumor camouflaged as sporadic. In all likelihood, many sporadic tumors are probably familial and the incidence of hereditary tumors considerably higher than just 1 in 10 PGs. Similar to their familial counterparts, sporadic tumors also demonstrate loss of heterozygosity at *PGL1* and *PGL2*. Bikhazi and colleagues[82] demonstrated loss of heterozygosity to be present in 38% of sporadic cases of carotid body tumors and glomus tumors when tested with markers located at *PGL1* and *PGL2*. This indirectly suggests that one-third of sporadic tumors may indeed be inherited. Similar to NF2, sporadic and familial PGs likely have a common genetic etiology.

The quest for the identification of genes responsible for PG has been greatly aided by the human genome project and the availability of large families with inherited PG. This has led to the delineation of at least three different genes associated with PG.

The First Locus: PGL1

Genetic linkage analysis of a large Dutch family with hereditary PG mapped a gene called *PGL1* to the short arm of chromosome 11, 11q22-q23.[83,84] This finding was confirmed in North American families and further localized to 11q23.[85,86] Tumor cells from affected individuals with the *PGL1* mutation revealed preferential loss of maternal DNA from chromosome 11q harboring the *PGL1* gene, providing genetic support for maternal imprinting. The phenomenon where DNA is deleted is termed a loss of heterozygosity.[85,87] This loss of heterozygosity associated with tumor formation strongly suggests that *PGL1* is a tumor suppressor gene. In the tumor suppressor hypothesis, tumor formation requires the loss of both functional copies of a tumor suppressor gene since a single functioning copy of the tumor suppressor gene is sufficient to prevent tumors. The NF2 and retinoblastoma genes are examples of tumor suppressor genes. The loss of function of one tumor suppressor gene by inheritance of a mutated allele and a subsequent random mutation of the second allele results in tumorigenesis.[88] This phenomenon, described by Knudson,[88] is known as the "two-hit" hypothesis. In familial PG, like NF2, the inherited first "hit" predisposes the individual to multicentric tumors owing to multiple random second "hits."

The gene responsible for PGL1 was recently cloned within the large chromosomal span of 11q23 by screening a candidate gene involved in oxygen metabolism located in this area.[89] This gene, known as *SDHD* (for succinate-ubiquinone oxidoreductase subunit D), encodes a small subunit of mitochrondrial cytochrome b (cybS) involved in Krebs cycle aerobic metabolism.[89] Using five families with hereditary PG, single base pair mutations leading to a loss of function of the *SDHD* gene product were identified. A nonsense mutation was found in two families leading to early truncation in the formation of the SDHD protein and consequently the loss of cybS

production. The other three families showed evidence of missense mutations with change of a single amino acid, presumably dramatically altering cybS conformation, rendering it nonfunctional. Interestingly, typical postgametogenesis maternal imprinting was not found since biallelic expression of both the maternal and the paternal gene was found in somatic tissues. It appears that only when the normal maternal allele is later imprinted or lost that the mutated paternal allele encoding the mutated *SDHD* leads to tumor formation owing to a loss of tumor suppressor activity. The discovery of this gene will undoubtedly lead to more efficient efforts in screening family members at risk for heritable PG.

The Second Locus: PGL2

Mapping of another large, unrelated Dutch family with hereditary PGs has revealed a second locus, PGL2, found on the short arm of chromosome 11. This locus at chromosome 11q13 harbors another gene for PG that by genetic mapping is clearly distinct from *PGL1*.[90,91]

The Third Locus: PGL3

A large German family with hereditary PG has revealed a third locus, PGL3.[92] Markers flanking the 11q23 and 11q13 loci associated with *PGL1* and *PGL2* excluded linkage to this area. Inheritance in this family was also autosomal dominant, similar to *PGL1* and *PGL2*, but there was no evidence of maternal imprinting. This family was mapped to chromosome 1q21. Subsequently, as mutations in *SDHD* had been identified as the cause of type 1 PG, Niemann and Muller investigated *SDHC* in this family.[93] They found a G-to-A transition in exon 1 of *SDHC* in all affected members but not in unaffected members. The mutation destroyed the start codon ATG of the gene at nucleotide position 958. In mitochondrial complex II, *SDHA* and *SDHB* constitute the catalytic domains and are anchored in the inner mitochondrial membrane by subunits *SDHC* and *SDHD*. It is quite possible that mutations in the other members of this complex, *SDHA* and *SDHB*, are also associated with PG formation.

Genetic Screening

Rapid advances in molecular genetics and biology have allowed the practicing otolaryngologist insight into the etiology of a rare yet well-described tumor of the head and neck. On evaluation of a patient with a PG, an extended family history should be elicited to identify additional members with evidence of head and neck tumors suspicious for PG. If hereditary PG is suspected, a detailed family pedigree should be obtained and the patient's family should be offered genetic screening. If the pedigree is sufficiently large, it could be determined by genetic linkage analysis if the family's PGs map to either *PGL1* or *PGL2*. Based on the genetic data, individuals harboring the affected chromosome and thus at risk for tumor formation could be identified. Individuals with a transmitted paternal allele who are at risk for PG should be aggressively followed both clinically and radiologically on a regular basis and offered genetic counseling. Those who have inherited the affected gene through maternal transmission should be advised of the clinically silent carrier state and be offered genetic counseling. Those with a noncarrier state can be advised that no increased risk for tumor development is present over the general population.[94]

Alternatively, the DNA extracted from the patient's blood could be directly tested for mutation in *SDHD* using polymerase chain reaction and direct DNA sequencing. If a mutation is identified, the family members could then be tested to see if they too harbor the mutation and therefore are at risk for tumor formation. It is hoped that genetic screening will lead to earlier identification of tumors to reduce the morbidity and mortality associated with its natural history and treatment. Ultimately, identification of the genetic alteration involved in both hereditary and sporadic PGs should lead to opportunities for genetic manipulation of tumor growth.

SUMMARY

A basic understanding of genetics is crucial to the practicing otologist and neuro-otologist. Genetic screening and genetic testing have already permeated into our daily practice. In the very near future, gene-based therapies too will dramatically change how we treat hearing loss and tumors of the temporal bone and cerebellopontine angle.

REFERENCES

1. Lalwani AK, Lynch E, Mhatre AN. Molecular genetics: a brief overview. In: Lalwani A, Grundfast K, editors. Pediatric otology and neurotology. Philadelphia: Lippincot-Raven; 1998. p. 49–86.
2. Brookhouser P. Sensorineural hearing loss in children. Pediatr Clin North Am 1996;43:1195–216.
3. Mehl A, Thomson V. Newborn hearing screening: the great omission. Pediatrics 1998;101:e4.
4. Kheterpal U, Lalwani AK. Nonsyndromic hereditary hearing impairment. In: Lalwani A, Grundfast K, editors. Pediatric otology and neurotology. Philadelphia: Lippincott-Raven; 1998. p. 313–40.
5. Mhatre AN, Lalwani AK. Molecular genetics of deafness. Otolaryngol Clin North Am 1996;29:421–35.
6. Yaeger M, Nicholson BJ. Structural of gap junction intercellular channels. Curr Opin Struct Biol 1996;6:183–92.
7. Kelsell DP, Dunlop J, Stevens HP, et al. Connexin 26 mutations in hereditary non-syndromic sensorineural deafness. Nature 1997;387:80–3.
8. Kikuchi T, Adams JC, Paul DL, Kimura RS. Gap junction systems in the rat vestibular labyrinth: immunohistochemical and ultrastructural analysis. Acta Otolaryngol (Stockh) 1994; 114:520–8.
9. Kikuchi T, Kimura RS, Paul DL, Adams JC. Gap junctions in the rat cochlea: immunohistochemical and ultrastructural analysis. Anat Embryol 1995;191:101–18.
10. Guilford P, Ben Arab S, Blanchard S, et al. A non-syndromic form of neurosensory recessive deafness maps to the pericentromeric region of chromosome 13q. Nat Genet 1994;6:24–8.
11. Van Camp G, Willems PJ, Smith RJH. Nonsyndromic hearing impairment: unparalleled heterogeneity. Am J Hum Genet 1997;60:758–64.
12. Zelante L, Gasparini P, Estivill X, et al. Connexin 26 mutations associated with the most common form of non-syndromic neurosensory autosomal recessive deafness (DFNB1) in Mediterraneans. Hum Mol Genet 1997;6:1605–9.
13. Kelley PM, Harris DJ, Comer BC, et al. Novel mutations in the connexin 26 gene (GJB2) that cause autosomal recessive (DFNB1) hearing loss. Am J Hum Genet 1998;62:792–9.
14. Cohn ES, Kelley PM. Clinical phenotype and mutations in connexin 26 (DFNB1/GJB2), the most common cause of childhood hearing loss. Am J Med Genet 1999;89:130–6.
15. Morell RJ, Kim HJ, Hood LJ, et al. Mutations in the connexin 26 gene (GJB2) among Ashkenazi Jews with nonsyndromic recessive deafness. N Engl J Med 1998;339:1500–5.
16. Denoyelle F, Weil D, Maw MA, et al. Prelingual deafness: high prevalence of a 30delG mutation in the connexin 26 gene. Hum Mol Genet 1997;6:2173–7.
17. Estivill X, Fortina P, Surrey S, et al. Connexin 26 mutations in sporadic and inherited sensorineural deafness. Lancet 1998; 351:394–8.
18. Lench N, Houseman M, Newton V, et al. Connexin 26 mutations in sporadic non-syndromal sensorineural deafness. Lancet 1998;351:415.
19. Antoniadi T, Rabionet R, Kroupis C, et al. High prevalence in the Greek population of the 35delG mutation in the connexin 26 gene causing prelingual deafness. Clin Genet 1999;55:381–2.
20. Sobe T, Vreugde S, Shahin H, et al. The prevalence and expression of inherited connexin 26 mutations associated with nonsyndromic hearing loss in the Israeli population. Hum Genet 2000;106:50–7.

21. Carrasquillo MM, Zlotogora J, Barges S, Chakravarti A. Two different connexin 26 mutations in an inbred kindred segregating non-syndromic recessive deafness: implications for genetic studies in isolated populations. Hum Mol Genet 1997;6: 2163–72.

22. Fuse Y, Doi K, Hasegawa T, et al. Three novel connexin 26 gene mutations in autosomal recessive non-syndromic deafness. Neuroreport 1999;10:1853–7.

23. Abe S, Usami S, Shinkawa H, et al. Prevalent connexin 26 (GJB2) mutations in Japanese. J Med Genet 2000;37:41–3.

24. Kudo T, Ikeda K, Kure S, et al. Novel mutations in the connexin 26 gene (GJB2) responsible for childhood deafness in the Japanese population. Am J Med Genet 2000;90:141–5.

25. Lin D, Goldstein JA, Mhatre AN, et al. Assessment of denaturing high-performance liquid chromatography (DHPLC) in screening for mutations in connexin 26. Hum Mutat 2001; 18(1):42–51.

26. Denoyelle F, Marlin S, Weil D, et al. Clinical features of the prevalent form of childhood deafness, DFNB1, due to a connexin-26 gene defect: implications for genetic counselling. Lancet 1999;353:1298–303.

27. Marlin S, Garabedian EN, Roger G, et al. Connexin 26 gene mutations in congenitally deaf children: pitfalls for genetic counseling. Arch Otolaryngol Head Neck Surg 2001;127:927–33.

28. Pendred V. Deaf mutism and goitre. Lancet 1896;11:532.

29. Smith RE. Pendred's syndrome. A historical note. Guys Hosp Rep 1969;118:519–21.

30. Batsakis JG, Nishiyama RH. Deafness with sporadic goiter: Pendred's syndrome. Arch Otolaryngol 1962;76:401–6.

31. Gomez-Pan A, Evered DC, Hall R. Pituitary-thyroid function in Pendred's syndrome. BMJ 1974;2:152–3.

32. Fraser GR, Morgans ME, Trotter WR. The syndrome of sporadic goiter and congenital deafness. Q J Med 1960;29:279–95.

33. Cremers CW, Admiraal RJ, Huygen PL, et al. Progressive hearing loss, hypoplasia of the cochlea and widened vestibular aqueducts are very common features in Pendred's syndrome. Int J Pediatr Otorhinolaryngol 1998;45:113–23.

34. Phelps PD, Coffey RA, Trembath RC, et al. Radiological malformations of the ear in Pendred's syndrome. Clin Radiol 1998;53:268–73.

35. Everett LA, Glaser B, Beck JC, et al. Pendred's syndrome is caused by mutations in a putative sulphate transporter gene (PDS). Nat Genet 1997;17:411–22.

36. Scott DA, Wang R, Kreman TM, et al. The Pendred's syndrome gene encodes a chloride-iodide transport protein. Nat Genet 1999;21:440–3.

37. Van Hauwe P, Everett LA, Coucke P, et al. Two frequent missense mutations in Pendred's syndrome. Hum Mol Genet 1998;7: 1099–104.

38. Usami S, Abe S, Weston MD, et al. Non-syndromic hearing loss associated with enlarged vestibular aqueduct is caused by PDS mutations. Hum Genet 1999;104:188–92.

39. Scott DA, Wang R, Kreman TM, et al. Functional differences of the PDS gene product are associated with phenotypic variation in patients with Pendred's syndrome and non-syndromic hearing loss (DFNB4). Hum Mol Genet 2000;9:1709–15.

40. Mafong DD, Shin EJ, Lalwani AK. Utility of laboratory evaluation and radiologic imaging in the diagnostic evaluation of children with sensorineural hearing loss. Laryngoscope 2002; 112:1–7.

41. Avraham KB, Hasson T, Sobe T, et al. Characterization of unconventional MYO6, the human homologue of the gene responsible for deafness in Snell's waltzer mice. Hum Mol Genet 1997;6:1225–31.

42. Hasson T, Walsh J, Cable J, et al. Effects of shaker-1 mutations on myosin-VIIa protein and mRNA expression. Cell Motil Cytoskeleton 1997;37:127–38.

43. Sellers JR. Myosins: a diverse superfamily. Biochim Biophys Acta 2000;1496:3–22.

44. Lalwani AK, Linthicum FH, Wilcox ER, et al. A three-generation family with late-onset, progressive hereditary hearing impairment and cochleosaccular degeneration. Audiol Neurootol 1997;2:139–54.

45. Lalwani AK, Luxford WM, Mhatre AN, et al. A new locus for nonsyndromic hereditary hearing impairment (DFNA17) maps to chromosome 22 and represents a gene for cochleosaccular degeneration. Am J Hum Genet 1999;64:318–23.

46. Lalwani AK, Goldstein JA, Kelley MJ, et al. Human nonsyndromic deafness DFNA17 is due to a mutation in nonmuscle myosin MYH9. Am J Hum Genet 2000;67:1121–8.

47. Coling DE, Espreafico EM, Kachar B. Cellular distribution of myosin-V in the guinea pig cochlea. J Neurocytol 1997;26: 113–20.

48. Gillespie PG. Deaf and dizzy mice with mutated myosin motors. Nat Med 1996;2:27–9.

49. Tilney LG, Derosier DJ, Mulroy MJ. The organization of actin filaments in the stereocilia of cochlear hair cells. J Cell Biol 1980;86:244–59.

50. Wallace DC. Mitochondrial DNA mutations in diseases of energy metabolism. J Bioenerg Biomembr 1994;26:241–50.

51. Prezant TR, Agapian JV, Bohlman MC, et al. Mitochondrial ribosomal RNA mutation associated with both antibiotic-induced and non-syndromic deafness. Nat Genet 1993;4: 289–94.

52. van den Ouweland JM, Lemkes HH, Trembath RC, et al. Maternally inherited diabetes and deafness is a distinct subtype of diabetes and associates with a single point mutation in the mitochondrial tRNA(Leu[UUR]) gene. Diabetes 1994;43: 746–51.

53. Ballinger SW, Shoffner JM, Hedaya EV, et al. Maternally transmitted diabetes and deafness associated with a 10.4 kb mitochondrial DNA deletion. Nat Genet 1992;1:11–5.

54. Katagiri H, Asano T, Ishihara H, et al. Mitochondrial diabetes mellitus: prevalence and clinical characterization of diabetes due to mitochondrial tRNA(Leu[UUR]) gene mutation in Japanese patients. Diabetologia 1994;37:504–10.

55. Evans DGR, Huson SM, Donnai D, et al. A genetic study of type 2 neurofibromatosis in the United Kingdom. 1. Prevalence, mutation rate, fitness and confirmation of maternal transmission effect on severity. J Med Genet 1992;29:841–6.

56. Kanter WR, Eldridge R, Fabricant R, et al. Central neurofibromatosis with bilateral acoustic neuroma: genetic, clinical and biochemical distinctions from peripheral neurofibromatosis. Neurology 1980;30:851–9.

57. King TT, Gibson WPR, Morrison AW. Tumors of the VIIIth cranial nerve. Br J Hosp Med 1976;16:259–72.

58. Abaza MM, Makariow EV, Armstrong M, Lalwani AK. Growth rate characteristics of acoustic neuromas associated with neurofibromatosis type 2. Laryngoscope 1996;106:694–9.

59. Lalwani AK, Abaza MM, Makariow EV, Armstrong M. Audiologic presentation of vestibular schwannomas in neurofibromatosis type 2. Am J Otol 1998;19:352–7.

60. Barker D, Wright E, Nguyen L, et al. Gene for von Recklinghausen neurofibromatosis is in the pericentromeric region of chromosome 17. Science 1987;236:1100–2.

61. Rouleau G, Seizinger VR, Ozelius LG, et al. Genetic linkage analysis of bilateral acoustic neurofibromatosis to a DNA marker on chromosome 22. Nature 1987;329:246–8.

62. Evans DG, Huson SM, Donnai D, et al. A genetic study of type 2 neurofibromatosis in the United Kingdom. II. Guidelines for genetic counselling. J Med Genet 1992;29:847–52.

63. Zang KD. Cytological and cytogenetics studies on human meningioma. Cancer Genet Cytogenet 1982;6:249–74.

64. Seizinger BR, Martuza RL, Gusella JF. Loss of genes on chromosome 22 in tumorigenesis of human acoustic neuroma. Nature 1986;322:644–7.

65. Rouleau GA, Merel P, Lutchman M, et al. Alteration in a new gene encoding a putative membrane-organizing protein causes neurofibromatosis type 2. Nature 1993;363:515–21.

66. Trofatter JA, MacCollin MM, Rutter JL, et al. A novel moesin-, ezrin-, radixin-like gene is a candidate for the neurofibromatosis 2 tumor suppressor. Cell 1993;72:791–800.

67. Gonzalez-Agosti C, Xu L, Pinney D, et al. The merlin tumor suppressor localises preferentially in membrane ruffles. Oncogene 1996;13:1239–47.

68. Vaheri A, Carpen O, Heiska L, et al. The ezrin protein family: membrane cytoskeleton interactions and disease associations. Curr Opin Cell Biol 1997;9:659–66.

69. Lutchman M, Rouleau GA. The neurofibromatosis type 2 gene product, schwannomin, suppresses growth of NIH 3T3 cells. Cancer Res 1995;55:2270–74.

70. Tikoo A, Varga M, Ramesh V, et al. An anti-RAS function of neurofibromatosis type 2 gene product. J Biol Chem 1994;269:23389–90.

71. Irving RM, Moffat DA, Hardy DG, et al. Molecular genetic analysis of the mechanism of tumorigenesis in acoustic neuroma. Arch Otolaryngol Head Neck Surg 1993;119:1222–8.

72. Welling DB, Guida M, Goll F, et al. Mutational spectrum in the neurofibromatosis type 2 gene in sporadic and familial schwannomas. Hum Genet 1996;98:189–93.

73. Merel P, Hoang-Xuan K, Sanson M, et al. Predominant occurrence of somatic mutations of the NF2 gene in meningiomas and schwannomas. Genes Chromosomes Cancer 1995;13:211–6.

74. Kluwe L, Mautner VF. A missense mutation in the NF-2 gene results in moderate and mild clinical phenotypes of neurofibromatosis type 2. Hum Genet 1996;97:224–7.

75. Bianchi AB, Hara T, Ramesh V, et al. Mutations in transcript isoforms of the neurofibromatosis 2 gene in multiple human tumour types. Nat Genet 1994;6:185–92.

76. Bianchi AB, Mitsunaga SI, Cheng JQ, et al. High frequency of inactivating mutations in the neurofibromatosis type 2 gene (NF2) in primary malignant mesotheliomas. Proc Natl Acad Sci U S A 1995;92:10854–8.

77. Ruttledge MH, Sarrazin J, Rangaratnam S, et al. Evidence for the complete inactivation of the NF2 gene in the majority of sporadic meningiomas. Nat Genet 1994;6:180–4.

78. Sekido Y, Pass H, Bader S, et al. Neurofibromatosis type II (NF-2) gene is somatically mutated in mesothelioma but not in lung cancer. Cancer Res 1995;55:1227–31.

79. Ruttledge MH, Andermann AA, Phelan CM, et al. Type of mutation in the neurofibromatosis type 2 gene (NF2) frequently determines severity of disease. Am J Hum Genet 1996;59: 331–42.

80. Parry DM, MacCollin MM, Kaiser-Kupfer MI, et al. Germ-like mutations in the neurofibromatosis 2 gene: correlation with disease severity and retinal abnormalities. Am J Hum Genet 1996; 59:529–39.

81. Hall JG. Genomic imprinting: review and relevance to human diseases. Am J Hum Genet 1990;46:857–73.

82. Bikhazi PH, Messina L, Mhatre AN, et al. Molecular pathogenesis in sporadic head and neck paraganglioma. Laryngoscope 2000;110:1346–8.

83. Heutink P, van der Mey AG, Sandkuijl LA, et al. A gene subject to genomic imprinting and responsible for hereditary paragangliomas maps to chromosome 11q23-qter. Hum Mol Genet 1992;1:7–10.

84. Heutink P, van Schothorst EM, van der Mey AG, et al. Further localization of the gene for hereditary paragangliomas and evidence for linkage in unrelated families. Eur J Hum Genet 1994;2:148–58.

85. Baysal BE, Farr JE, Rubinstein WS, et al. Fine mapping of an imprinted gene for familial nonchromaffin paragangliomas, on chromosome 11q23. Am J Hum Genet 1997;60:121–32.

86. Milunsky J, DeStefano AL, Huang XL, et al. Familial paragangliomas: linkage to chromosome 11q23 and clinical implications. Am J Med Genet 1997;72:66–70.

87. Devilee P, van Schothorst EM, Bardoel AF, et al. Allelotype of head and neck paragangliomas: allelic imbalance is confined to the long arm of chromosome 11, the site of the predisposing locus PGL. Genes Chromosomes Cancer 1994;11:71–8.

88. Knudson AG Jr. Genetics of human cancer. J Cell Physiol Suppl 1986;4:7–11.

89. Baysal BE, Ferrell RE, Willett-Brozick JE, et al. Mutations in SDHD, a mitochondrial complex II gene, in hereditary paraganglioma. Science 2000;287:848–51.

90. Mariman EC, van Beersum SE, Cremers CW, et al. Analysis of a second family with hereditary non-chromaffin paragangliomas locates the underlying gene at the proximal region of chromosome 11q. Hum Genet 1993;91:357–61.

91. Mariman EC, van Beersum SE, Cremers CW, et al. Fine mapping of a putatively imprinted gene for familial non-chromaffin paragangliomas to chromosome 11q13.1: evidence for genetic heterogeneity. Hum Genet 1995;95:56–62.

92. Niemann, S, Steinberger D, Muller U. PGL3, a third, not maternally imprinted locus in autosomal dominant paraganglioma. Neurogenetics 1999;2:167–70.

93. Niemann S, Muller U. Mutations in SDHC cause autosomal dominant paraganglioma, type 3. Nat Genet 2000;26:268–70.

94. Bikhazi PH, Roeder E, Attaie A, et al. Familial paragangliomas: the emerging impact of molecular genetics on evaluation and management. Am J Otol 1999;20:639–43.

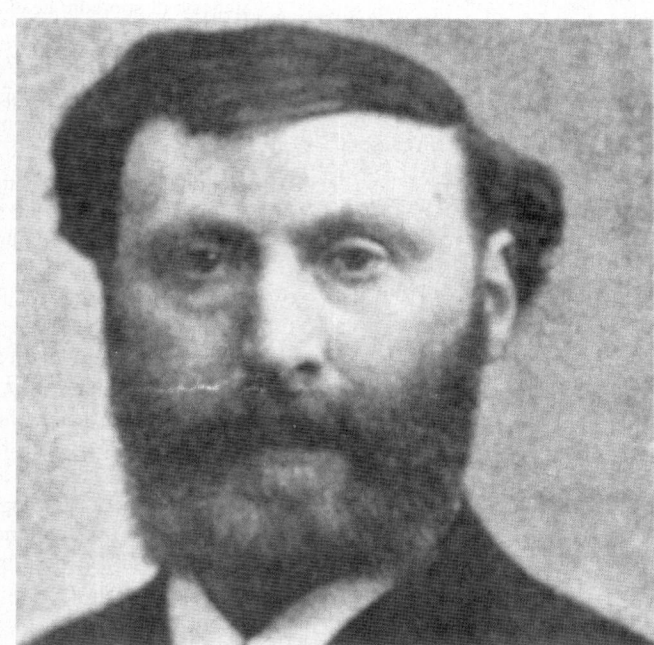

Adam Politzer (1835–1920). Foremost teacher of otologic diagnosis and therapy of the Vienna school.

II

Clinical
Evaluation

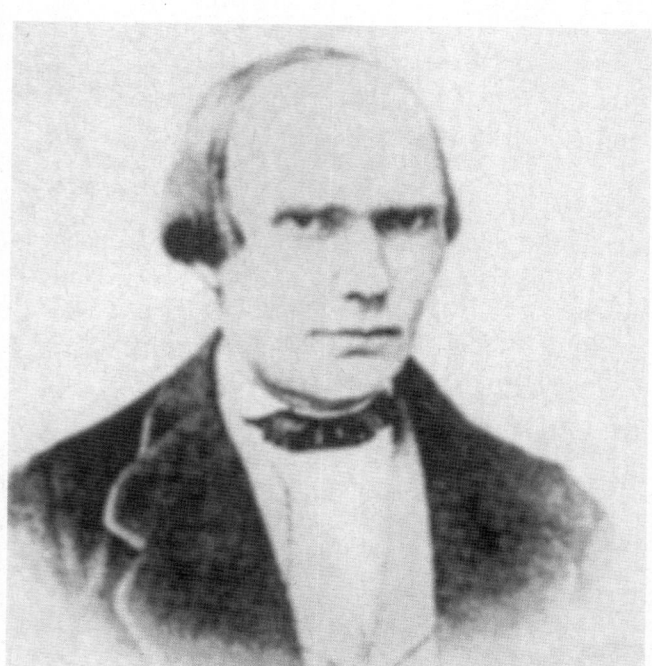

Heinrich Adolph Rinne (1819–1868). In 1855 described the tuning fork test, which is still the best method for diagnosis of conductive versus sensorineural hearing loss. Reproduced with permission from Heck WE. Dr. A. Rinne. Laryngoscope 1962;72:647.

7

Clinical Diagnosis

DAVID S. HAYNES, MD

Establishing a diagnosis in a patient with a hearing or balance disorder always begins with a thorough history and physical examination. In particular, the history is of critical importance in ascertaining an accurate diagnosis and thereby allowing the physician to provide adequate counseling and institute appropriate therapy. This chapter addresses the basic neuro-ototologic history and physical examination techniques that are important in the complete assessment of the patient with a hearing or balance complaint. This chapter also discusses differential diagnosis of otologic and neurotologic disease and provides a brief overview of common disorders.

HISTORY

General

As with any medical disorder, a thorough history and physical examination are essential in the evaluation of the patient with a neurotologic disorder.[1,2] In the assessment of the patient with the primary complaint of vertigo, the physical examination is often unrevealing, leaving the history as the most important diagnostic tool.[3] An assessment form (Figure 7–1) is a commonly employed and useful tool for guiding and documenting the examination. An otologic assessment form is advantageous for several reasons: (1) it allows the initial examination to be focused and directed, (2) it ensures that all critical information is obtained and not inadvertently omitted, and (3) it provides a precise reference for follow-up examinations or surgery. A questionnaire completed by the patient is also very useful in the otologic

evaluation. The questionnaire may be completed on arrival or may be mailed to the patient and completed prior to the office visit. The questionnaire should include all aspects of the patient history including history of present illness, previous evaluation(s), previous medical therapy or surgery, social history, history of trauma, and onset and exacerbation of systems. This history, recorded by the patient, does not supplant but rather complements the standard history performed by the examiner. This questionnaire may also be useful because it is a history taken "by the patient" and can avoid discrepancies regarding onset of symptoms, previous evaluation, or previous surgery, an area of significant import in medical legal cases.

The standard patient history should include history of present illness, past medical history review of symptoms, medications, previous therapy (including medications used and their efficacy or complications), previous surgery, history of trauma, and social history. The history should not concentrate just on symptoms of hearing and balance but on the patient as a whole as many systemic disorders can affect the vestibular or auditory system (Table 7–1).[4] Rheumatologic disorders, diabetes, multiple sclerosis, and thyroid disorders are just a few of the systemic disorders that can cause or exacerbate neurotologic symptoms. Occupational, recreational, and military noise exposure should also be documented.[5]

All current medications should be recorded as well as any past medications that have been employed to treat the patient's current symptoms. A list of potentially ototoxic medications is provided in Table 7–2.[6–9] Aminoglycoside antibiotics, salicylates, furosemide, and other commonly used medications may be directly oto-

MC 4920 (2/97)

Vanderbilt University Medical Center
OTOLARYNGOLOGY
Nashville, TN 37232-5555
(615) 322-6180

OTOLOGY/NEUROTOLOGY
ASSESSMENT FORM

Patient Name: Date:

DOB: AGE:

MR #

Referring Physician:

Dictation: Y   N

Chief Complaint:

HPI:

HEARING	Right	Left	VERTIGO
Duration			Onset
Prog.			Frequency
Tinnitus			Duration
Fullness			Spinning
Otitis			Unsteadiness
Bet. Ear			Nausea
Fluctuation			Positional
Hearing Aid			MRI

Current Medications: Allergies:

Trauma:

Family History

Noise Exposure:

Physical Exam:

Right		Left	
	Normal		
	Perf w/ chol		
	Perf w/o chol		
	Serous OM		
	Acute OM		
AC>BC ; BC>AC	(W)	AC>BC ; BC>AC	

Neurotology Exam
Romberg
Cerebellar
Cranial Nerve
Nystagmus
Dix Hallpike

HEENT:

IMPRESSION: Bruits:

EVALUATION:

Imaging:	Lab Work	Vestibular Testing	TREATMENT
CT	FTA	ENG	
Temporal Bone	ESR	ECoG	
Coronal Sinus	ANA	Rotary Chair	
MRI head w/GAD	RF	Posturography	
w/o GAD	Chol	Vestibular Rehab.	
	SMA-20		
Follow up			
Audiogram			

Figure 7–1   neurotologic assessment form.

Table 7–1 SYSTEMIC DISORDERS AFFECTING THE EAR[4]

Granulomatous/infectious disease	Progressive systemic sclerosis
Langerhans' cell histiocytosis	Bone disease
Eosinophilic granuloma	Paget's disease
Hand-Schüller-Christian disease	Osteogenesis imperfecta
Letterer-Siwe disease	Fibrous dysplasia
Sarcoidosis	Osteopetrosis
Lyme disease	Osteitis fibrosa cystica
Fungal infections	Chronic osteomyelitis
Wegener's granulomatosis	Miscellaneous
Tuberculosis	Acquired immune deficiency syndrome (AIDS)
Autoimmune disease/collagen vascular disease	Mucopolysaccharidoses
Relapsing polychondritis	Polyarteritis nodosa
Systemic lupus erythematosus	Cogan's syndrome
Rheumatoid arthritis	Neoplastic disease
Giant cell arteritis	Leukemia
Sjögren's syndrome	Lymphoma
Polymyositis/dermatomyositis	Paraganglioma
Ankylosing spondylitis	Multiple myeloma
Vogt-Koyanagi-Harada syndrome	Metastatic disease/meningeal carcinomatosis
Behçet's syndrome	
Autoimmune inner ear disease	
Cardiac disorders (arrhythmias)	
Anemia	

toxic. Other medications may lead to a sense of imbalance (antihypertensives, antidepressants) without being directly ototoxic. Somnolence is common with many medications (antihistamines, benzodiazepines) and can exacerbate symptoms of imbalance, especially among elderly patients.[10] Head trauma, even if mild or remote, should be documented.

Auditory System

A history for the patient with hearing loss should include the following:

- Duration, age of onset
- Rate of progression (sudden or gradual)
- Stable or fluctuating
- Unilateral or bilateral
- Prior use of amplification
- Other associated symptoms (ie, tinnitus, vertigo, infections, fullness, otalgia, otorrhea)
- Family history of hearing loss, including previous surgery for hearing loss
- Better-hearing ear

In addition to the standard history, evaluation of a child for hearing loss also requires gestational, perinatal, post-

Table 7–2 AGENTS AND MEDICATIONS THAT CAN CAUSE VESTIBULAR AND AUDITORY OTOTOXICITY[6-9]

Antibiotics
  Aminoglycoside antibiotics
    Primarily cochleotoxic
      Neomycin
      Kanamycin
      Tobramycin
      Dihydrostreptomycin
      Amikacin
    Primarily vestibulotoxic
      Gentamicin
      Streptomycin
  Other
    Erythromycin
    Vancomycin
Antineoplastic agents
  Cisplatin
  Carboplatin
  Nitrogen mustard
  Vincristine
  Vinblastine
Diuretics
  Furosemide
  Ethacrynic acid
  Bumetanide
Anti-inflammatory agents
  Salicylates
  Quinine
  Nonsteroidal anti-inflammatory agents
  Chloroquine
Chelating agents
  Desferoxime
Chemicals
  Mercury
  Gold
  Lead arsenic aniline dyes

natal, and family histories. Parental or other family member concern regarding hearing loss should be addressed. Parents may notice hearing difficulty in their children, but smaller losses may not actually be detected by family members.[11] Approximately 50% of congenital hearing impairment is hereditary, with 60 to 70% of these cases being of autosomal recessive mode of inheritance.[12] A list of some of the causes of hearing loss is provided in Tables 7–3 and 7–4.[13–17] Establishing a definitive etiology may prove difficult. In one large series[18] 31.9% had no obvious etiology; establishing an etiology in unilateral cases was lower (50%) than in bilateral cases (75.4%). Despite multiple diagnostic tests available, the history remains the most important instrument in diagnosing childhood hearing loss.

Tinnitus is a symptom that is defined as any sound perceived by the patient when no external source of the sound exists. It is generally divided into two categories, objective and subjective. Objective tinnitus is infrequent and is audible to the examiner. Subjective tinnitus, much more common than objective tinnitus, is not audible to the examiner. Objective tinnitus may be caused by vascular, neurologic, or eustachian tube disorders. Vascular disorders may cause pulsatile tinnitus by generating turbulent flow in arterial or venous vessels in the neck, cranial vault, or temporal bone. Vascular disorders that may cause objective tinnitus include venous hums, arterial bruits, arteriovenous malformations and shunts, aneurysms, aberrant vessels, and vascular neoplasms.

Neurologic disorders that cause objective tinnitus include palatal myoclonus and idiopathic stapedius and tensor tympani muscle spasm. Palatomyoclonus is an uncommon disorder characterized by an irregular, rapid, clicking sound. The sound is generated when the mucosa of the eustachian tube snaps together as the palatal muscles undergo myoclonic contractions. Middle ear muscle spasms (stapedius, tensor tympani) produce an intermittent, bothersome, fluttering sound in the ear as the muscles contract during spasm. External sounds may accentuate these spasms.

Subjective tinnitus is far more common than objective tinnitus and is generally associated with high-frequency sensorineural hearing loss, typically as a result of noise exposure or aging (presbycusis). Other causes are idiopathic, metabolic, genetic, cardiologic/vascular, neurologic, pharmacologic, dental, psychologic, and otologic factors. Tinnitus associated with symmetric sensorineural hearing loss may not necessitate evaluation beyond a complete audiologic and head and neck examination. Unilateral or pulsatile tinnitus and tinnitus associated with asymmetric sensorineural hearing loss or conductive hearing loss generally necessitates additional investigation by means of imaging or neurophysiologic testing.[2]

Table 7–3 CAUSES OF SENSORINEURAL HEARING LOSS[13–15]	
Infectious disease	Autoimmune disorders
Acute otitis media	Vascular disease
Bacterial (suppurative) labyrinthitis	Neoplasms
Serous labyrinthitis	Meningeal carcinomatosis
Meningitis	Congenital disorders
Syphilis	Perinatal infections
Chronic osteomyelitis	Rubella
Lyme disease	Cytomegalovirus
Viral	Cochlear otosclerosis
Mumps	Migraine-associated hearing loss
Herpes zoster oticus	Metabolic disorders
Trauma	Diabetes
Noise-induced hearing loss	Renal failure
Occupational	Thyroid disorders
Recreational	Mucopolysaccharidoses
Basilar skull fracture	Hematologic disorders
Cochlear concussion	Psychogenic deafness
Barotrauma	Presbycusis
Perilymph fistula	Vasculitis
Drug toxicity	Paget's disease
Neurologic disorders	Multiple sclerosis
Systemic disease (see Table 7–4)	

Table 7–4   CAUSES OF CONDUCTIVE HEARING LOSS[16,17]

Inflammatory or infectious causes	**Neoplasia**
Otitis externa	Paraganglioma
Eustachian tube dysfunction	Facial nerve neuroma
Adhesive middle ear disease	Rhabdomyosarcoma
Acute otitis media	Squamous cell carcinoma
Serous otitis media	Middle ear adenoma
Chronic otitis media	Neurofibroma
Malignant otitis externa	Hemangiopericytoma
Cholesteatoma	Lymphangioma
Tympanosclerosis	Lymphoma
Myringosclerosis	Leukemia
Tympanic membrane perforation	Multiple myeloma
Otomycosis	Pleomorphic adenoma
Aural tuberculosis	Adenoid cystic carcinoma
Syphilis	Hemangioma
Systemic disorders	Basal cell carcinoma
Sarcoidosis	**Congenital abnormalities**
Fibrous dysplasia	Microtia
Mucopolysaccharidosis	Atresia
Wegener's granulomatosis	Branchial cleft cyst
Histiocytosis/eosinophilic granuloma (Langerhans' cell histiocytosis)	Congenital ossicular fixation
Relapsing polychondritis	Otosclerosis
Polyarteritis nodosa	Osteogenesis imperfecta
Keratosis obturans	Treacher Collins syndrome
Cerumen	Pierre Robin syndrome
Trauma	Marfan syndrome
Barotrauma	Mohr syndrome
Basilar skull fracture/temporal bone fracture	Pyle's disease
Hemotympanum	Achondroplasia
Traumatic perforation	Paget's disease
External canal laceration/avulsion	Apert's disease
Miscellaneous	Goldenhar's syndrome
Cerebrospinal fluid effusion	Turner's syndrome
Keloid	Crouzon's disease
External canal osteoma	
External canal exostosis	
Osteopetrosis	

Otalgia is a symptom uncommon among patients with hearing loss unless associated with infection of the external canal, middle ear, or mastoid. If otalgia is present, the following are important points: Is the pain relieved by otorrhea, drops, or antibiotics? Are there any exacerbating features, such as pain with chewing (as occurs in temporomandibular joint dysfunction)? Has there been recent dental work? Do dentures (if present) fit properly? Is there a history of laryngitis or gastric reflux? Is there a history of previous head and neck surgery, including surgery for malignancy? Is it relieved by Valsalva's maneuver? Is there a history of previous ear surgery, including pressure equalizing tube placement? Is there a history of other surgical procedure (ie, cervical laminectomy) or malignancy (thinking of metastases)? Is there a history of recurrent headaches or migraines? Is there a history of trauma? Is there a history of any other head and neck disorder, including recurrent sinusitis or allergies?

If drainage is the primary complaint, the patient should be questioned regarding the presence of otorrhea and its characteristics, such as profuse or scant, purulent, clear, mucoid, bloody, or foul smelling.[19–22] The presence of ear pain and response to antibiotic drops or oral antibiotics are important to note. When otorrhea is present, knowledge of any prior surgical procedure is of undeniable importance.[23] Multiple and bilateral procedures performed over many years and by multiple surgeons can obviously be confusing to patients and examiners. Occasionally, a patient may not remember having ear surgery at all. It is imperative to document the type, approximate date, and side of the procedure. The patient should always be asked which ear is the better-hearing ear regardless of what the physical evaluation, tuning fork test, or audiogram reveals.

Vestibular System

Dysequilibrium is a complex symptom that can result from aberrations of the vestibular system. Unsteadiness, drunkenness, giddiness, wooziness, vertigo, dizziness, a sensation of being off-balance, imbalance, light-headedness, wobbliness, and spinning are some of the terms used to describe vestibular symptoms. In patients age 75 years or older, dizziness is the most common complaint discussed with their physician.[24] Symptoms of vertigo should never be attributed to normal aging; a specific etiology should be identifiable in the majority of cases.[25] The clinician should address the following features of dysequilibrium to support the diagnosis:

- Duration
- Severity
- Progression (improving or worsening)
- Gradual or sudden onset
- Episodic or constant
- If episodic, how long does each episode last? Are there symptoms between episodes?
- Exacerbating or remitting factors
- How is the dysequilibrium described? (primarily differentiate between unsteadiness or true spinning)
- Are symptoms related to head position?
- Are the vestibular symptoms associated with hearing loss, tinnitus, focal neurologic signs, migraine, or nausea and vomiting?
- Is there a history of head and neck trauma or barotrauma?
- Is there a history of chronic ear disease? Is there a history of otorrhea?
- Is there a history of previous ear, head, neck, vascular, cardiac, or intracranial surgery?
- Is the patient able to work, drive, or perform activities of daily living?
- Is there a history of recurrent falling?[26]

All too often the physical examination in the patient with vertigo is unrevealing and vestibular testing inconclusive, leaving the history the most important, if not the only instrument, that can be used to establish a clinical diagnosis. The importance of the history in correctly diagnosing these disorders cannot be overemphasized.

PHYSICAL EXAMINATION

This section will review the general examination of the patient with a hearing and balance disorder, which includes a general examination of the head and neck, ear, nose, and throat. The examination also includes a neurotologic examination that includes cerebellar testing, cranial nerve evaluation, and a limited neurologic examination.

OTOLOGIC EXAMINATION

Auricle

The auricle is inspected for incisions or scarring indicating prior surgery, congenital abnormalities, trauma, infection cellulitis, dermatitis, or neoplasia. A misshapen auricle, preauricular pits, or skin tags may be present and indicate faulty fusion of the auricular hillocks or other congenital abnormalities. Movement of the auricle often causes pain when cellulitis, dermatitis, or external otitis is present.

External Auditory Canal

Although a handheld otoscope is useful as a screening tool, its use is limited by the absence of binocular vision. The operating microscope (Figure 7–2) is always used to examine a pathologic condition of the external canal, tympanic membrane, and middle ear. The patient is reclined and the head is positioned properly to compensate for the natural angle of the canal. As the head is turned slightly away from the examiner, the ear canal is straightened by gently pulling the auricle posteriorly and superiorly. Typically, the largest speculum that can be inserted comfortably into the ear canal is chosen. The examiner may also pull the tragus slightly anteriorly to assist in visualization. Care is taken to insert the speculum only into the cartilaginous canal because

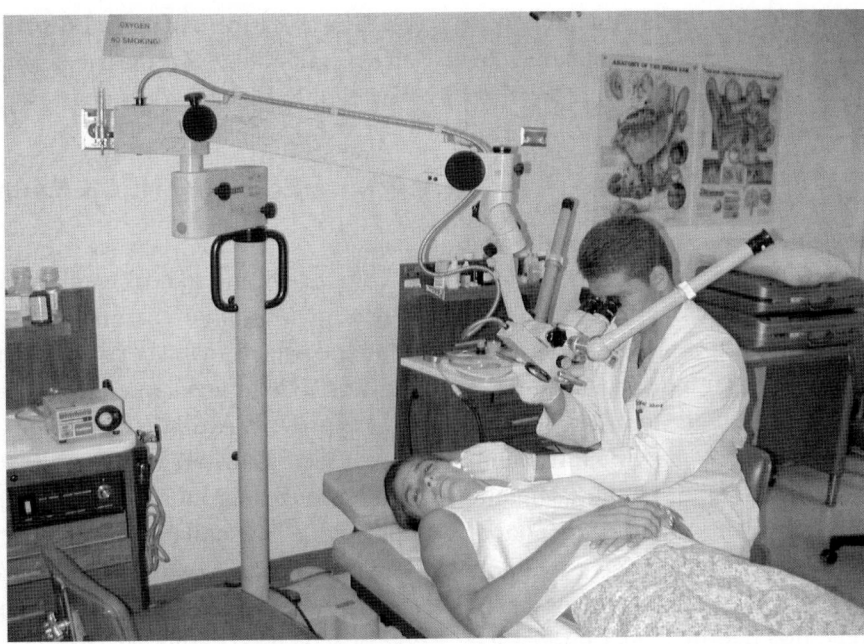

Figure 7–2 Technique of otomicroscopy. Note equipment cabinets on either side of the table to facilitate examination.

deeper penetration near the bony canal can be painful. Both adults and children are informed in advance of the above steps. This simple forewarning facilitates the examination, avoids patient apprehension, and gains trust.

To truly examine the ear, cerumen, desquamated skin, and purulent debris must be completely removed with loops, alligator forceps, curettes, or suction. Cleaning the ear of even a small amount of wax is crucial for proper visualization. Missing an otologic diagnosis because of cerumen or debris is unacceptable. Video-otoscopic examination can be performed easily in the office and may assist in photo-documentation and patient counseling. With video monitors in the patient's direct view, the patient can better appreciate any existing abnormality such as tympanic membrane perforation or retraction or a cholesteatoma. Most patients have never seen their tympanic membranes and appreciate visualizing for themselves any abnormalities that may exist. Video-otoscopic examination can be performed with the 0-degree sinus endoscope usually found in an otolaryngologist's office or with smaller 0-degree otoscopes specifically designed for otoscopic examination.

The external auditory canal is inspected for stenosis, cellulitis, furuncles, cysts, edema, dermatitis, exposed bone, and neoplastic changes. The presence of granulation tissue, purulent or mucoid discharge, or squamous debris is assessed.[21] Bony osteomas or exostoses are confirmed by means of gentle, direct palpation. Aural polyps may be manipulated to determine their site of origin. It is important to differentiate polyps of external ear canal origin from those that arise from the middle ear or tympanic membrane. Polyps protruding directly from the middle ear through a tympanic membrane perforation or, less commonly, directly from the tympanic membrane suggest chronic middle ear disease or cholesteatoma. Removal of aural polyps in the office is not recommended as these lesions indicate more significant disease not amenable to simple removal and may be intimately involved with vital structures such as the ossicular chain and facial nerve.[27,28]

Tympanic Membrane

The tympanic membrane is inspected for retraction, perforation, effusion, myringitis, granulation tissue, cholesteatoma, or other pathologic process. Lateralization or blunting of the tympanic membrane is noted. Mobility of the tympanic membrane is assessed with a handheld otoscope outfitted with a pneumatic bulb, with a Siegle speculum, or by tympanometry. Pneumatic otoscopy is especially useful in assessing middle ear fluid when the examination is inconclusive (ie, no air-fluid level, bubbles, or discoloration is evident). Pneumatic otoscopy is also useful in distinguishing tympanosclerosis from middle ear cholesteatoma and in evaluating atelectatic or retracted areas of the tympanic membrane. A monomeric area of the tympanic membrane must be differentiated from true perforation. A dehiscent jugular bulb or carotid artery, glomus tumor, facial neuroma (tympanic segment), or middle ear adenoma may appear as a vascular mass behind an intact tympanic membrane. A white mass visible medial to the tympanic membrane may represent purulent debris, congenital or acquired cholesteatoma, tympanosclerosis, or a middle ear mass such as a neuroma. Abnormal development of the ossicular chain may also manifest as a middle ear mass.

Occasionally, atelectasis, atrophy, or retraction of the tympanic membrane can be difficult to diagnose. Assessment is best performed with the binocular vision provided by the operating microscope. Pneumatic otoscopy may be of use in certain cases. Positive or negative pressure applied to the tympanic membrane may cause the retracted segment to move, allowing the examiner to assess the extent of retraction or atelectasis. Application of positive or negative pressure may also be useful to distinguish between a monomeric membrane and a tympanic membrane perforation. Serous fluid may be more evident with pneumatic otoscopy as the fluid may shift or may adhere to the tympanic membrane as the drum moves with applied pressure. The extent of retraction, presence of squamous debris or cholesteatoma, otorrhea, associated perforation, and, if possible, the status of the ossicular chain must be assessed to recommend proper therapy.

Examination of the patient who has undergone previous surgery is more difficult owing to altered anatomy and surgical scarring. Determining the type of surgical procedure(s) performed, such as canal wall down or intact canal wall mastoidectomy, can be more difficult in some ears than expected. The presence of endaural, postauricular, or peritragal incisions is noted. Pathology particular to revision ears includes recurrent cholesteatoma, graft failure (perforation, lateralization, blunting, or retraction), and prosthesis extrusion. In canal wall down cavities, assessment of meatal size, dependent or retracted areas, graft failure, otorrhea, recurrent cholesteatoma, and height of the facial ridge is necessary.[19,23,29]

HEAD AND NECK EXAMINATION

A complete head and neck examination is an integral part of the neurotologic examination. Auscultation of the head and neck is mandatory for all patients with pulsatile tinnitus. Bruits are appreciable when turbulent blood flow is present. Auscultation is performed not only over the carotid bifurcation but also over the ear canal, the pre- and postauricular areas, and adjacent areas of the temporal bone. Auscultation of the ear canal may be performed with a Toynbee otoscope, modified electronic stethoscope, or standard stethoscope. Valsalva's maneuver may be used to increase subtle vascular flow abnormalities.[30] Venous flow abnormalities (venous hum) may occasionally be auscultated. They are most often described as a "swooshing type" of sound and are not truly pulsatile. The loudness is generally diminished by reducing venous blood flow with gentle compression of the jugular vein without compression of the carotid artery. Turning the head toward the uninvolved side, deep breathing, or Valsalva's maneuver may objectively or subjectively make the hum louder.

Because otalgia may represent referred pain from the head and neck, the nasopharynx, larynx, oral cavity, and hypopharynx are examined for occult malignancy. Sinusitis, temporomandibular joint abnormalities, eustachian tube obstruction, pharyngitis, and adenotonsillar disease may also cause otalgia. Nasopharyngitis or adenotonsillitis may provoke otalgia secondary to glossopharyngeal nerve (ninth cranial nerve) involvement, as demonstrated by the relatively common incidence of otalgia following tonsillectomy. Laryngeal lesions lead to otalgia secondary to vagus nerve (tenth cranial nerve) involvement. Laryngeal carcinoma may present solely with otalgia, underlining the importance of a complete head and neck evaluation.

Unfortunately, no reliable clinical test of eustachian tube function exists. The presence of tympanic membrane retraction, middle ear effusion, adenoidal hypertrophy or infection, and nasal disease and the ability to perform Valsalva's maneuver may give some indication of eustachian tube function. Furthermore, the status of the contralateral ear may provide some insight as to the status of eustachian tube function.[13]

The neck and parotid are palpated for masses, especially when signs of partial or total facial paralysis are evident. Funduscopic examination is performed as a routine part of the neurotologic examination, particularly when increased intracranial pressure is suspected or if pulsatile tinnitus is a complaint. Pulsatile tinnitus may be a sign of benign intracranial hypertension.[31] Benign intracranial hypertension is a syndrome characterized by headache and elevated cerebrospinal fluid (CSF) pressure without ventricular dilation and with normal CSF composition. The physical examination in these patients is normal except for papilledema and occasional sixth nerve palsy.[32]

Tuning Fork Tests

A tuning fork examination comprises a part of the routine neurotologic examination and may be performed easily at the bedside or in the office. Even though most patients with otologic symptomatology are likely to undergo formal audiometric testing, tuning fork testing remains a mandatory component of the neurotologic evaluation.

To perform a Weber's test, a vibrating tuning fork (512 Hz) is placed on the forehead, nasal dorsum, central incisors of the maxilla, or mandibular symphysis to conduct the tone directly to the cochlea. It is important to strike the tuning fork on a soft surface to prevent the development of high-frequency overtones, as may occur when striking the fork on a hard surface. A patient who hears the tone more clearly in one ear is said to have lateralized to that ear. If the sound does not lateralize, then the test is reported as midline or normal. As a rule, sound lateralizing to one ear implies either an ipsilateral conductive loss (typically 3 to 5 dB with a 512-Hz fork) or a contralateral sensorineural loss. Patients with a unilateral conductive hearing loss are sometimes hesitant to acknowledge hearing a tone louder in the "bad" ear. Although a Weber's test is a reliable and trusted test, its acoustic basis is unclear. It has been proposed that sound reflection caused by impedance mismatch accounts for test results.[33] The exact mechanism, however, may still require further explanation.[34]

The Rinne test is performed, ideally with a 512-tuning fork, by placing the vibrating fork against the mastoid process (bone conduction) and comparing its loudness with that of the tuning fork placed just outside the canal (air conduction). If the patient perceives the tone as being louder at the ear canal level, air conduction is said to be greater than bone conduction (AC > BC — a "positive" Rinne), consistent with either ipsilateral normal hearing or a sensorineural hearing loss. If the tone is louder when the tuning fork is placed on the mastoid tip, bone conduction is said to be greater than air conduction (BC > AC — a "negative" Rinne) and implies a conductive hearing loss in the tested ear. The positive/negative Rinne terminology is sometimes confusing as a positive test is a normal result. The author prefers to describe the test results as AC > BC, AC = BC, or BC > AC. BC > AC (a negative Rinne) with a 512-Hz tuning fork indicates a conductive hearing loss of 20 dB or worse. In otosclerosis, Rinne testing with a broad spectrum of tuning forks (eg, 256-, 512-, 1,024-Hz forks) can give some idea as to the severity of the conductive hearing loss. In early otosclerosis, which tends to have an "upward-sloping" conductive component, the Rinne test will be negative for only the lower-frequency forks. As the otosclerotic fixation of the stapes footplate becomes more complete and the conductive loss "flattens," the Rinne test will be negative with all tuning fork frequencies.[35] The importance of both the Weber's and Rinne tests in the bedside and office examinations cannot be overemphasized as they may confirm or refute audiometric test results; therefore, these tests are critical in otologic diagnosis.[36,37]

Vestibular Evaluation

Nystagmus is an involuntary rapid eye movement that may occur as a result of vestibular, optokinetic, or pursuit system dysfunction.[38] A disturbance of one of these systems leads to a drift of the eyes during attempts at visual fixation (slow phase or slow component of nystagmus). A corrective phase of the eyes (quick phase or quick component) attempts to reset the drift. Constant velocity drifts create a repetitive, quick corrective response, resulting in nystagmus. A peripheral vestibular abnormality resulting in unilateral hypofunction leads to a drift of the eyes directed toward the side of the lesion, and the subsequent fast, corrective phase is directed contralaterally. By convention, the direction of the nystagmus is designated by the fast phase of nystagmus.

Nystagmus is classified as either spontaneous or evoked. Nystagmus is described on physical examination in terms of direction (right-beating or left-beating, geotrophic or ageotrophic), plane (horizontal, rotary, or vertical), and intensity (first, second, or third degree). First-degree nystagmus is the least intense and occurs when gaze is in the direction of the fast component of nystagmus. Second-degree nystagmus occurs with gaze in the direction of the fast component as well as midline. Third-degree nystagmus occurs in all directions of gaze, including the slow phase, indicating the most severe form of nystagmus. Nystagmus may also be described as direction fixed (beating in the same direction despite different head positions) or direction changing (beating in different directions with associated different head positions).

Frenzel lenses are magnifying (20 diopter) lenses incorporated into glasses that are used to aid the examiner in visualizing nystagmus and to prevent the patient from visual fixation, which may lead to suppression of nystagmus.

Fistula Test

The fistula test is performed by applying positive and negative pressure to the tympanic membrane using a pneumatic otoscope; nystagmus and vertigo with applied pressure constitute a positive fistula test. Examiner visualization of nystagmus can be supplemented with electronystagmographic recording. Hennebert's sign is a positive fistula test in an ear with an intact tympanic membrane and without evidence of middle ear disease.[39,40] In the presence of a fistula, or vestibulofibrosis,[40] the applied pressure causes deviation of the cupula, resulting in nystagmus and vertigo. A positive fistula test can be seen in oval or round window fistulae, post-stapedectomy perilymph leaks, horizontal canal fistulae, Meniere's disease, labyrinthitis, or syphilis.[39,40] Nystagmus that occurs with tragal compression or a Valsalva's maneuver may be caused by superior semicircular canal dehiscence syndrome.[41]

Dix-Hallpike Maneuver

The Dix-Hallpike maneuver (Hallpike testing, the Nylèn-Bárány maneuver) may be performed routinely on all patients complaining of vertigo or may be limited to those patients who have positional vertigo, that is, vertigo provoked by certain head positions such as looking up or rolling over in bed. As for other aspects of the physical examination, this test and why it is being performed are briefly explained to the patient before the test is performed. The test, which is performed on a table or a chair capable of reclining completely flat, begins with the patient sitting up and positioned so that when reclined, the head extends beyond the edge of the table (Figure 7–3). The patient is then rapidly brought to the supine position, with the head turned to the side and hanging slightly (Figure 7–4). The presence of nystagmus and subjective complaints of vertigo are noted. The patient is returned to the sitting position, the test is repeated, and the response is noted. Finally, the test is repeated with the head turned to the opposite side. The abnormal ear is the one that, when placed in the "down" or lowermost position, elicits vertigo and nystagmus.

Head Shaking Nystagmus Testing

In this test, the patient's head, with the chin inclined down 30 degrees, is rotated abruptly by the examiner (or by the patient), and the patient is examined for nystagmus (see also Chapter 4).[43] A normal response comprises no, or a few beats, of nystagmus. With a unilateral loss of labyrinthine function, nystagmus is visualized, the slow phase of which is initially directed toward the dysfunctional labyrinth and which then reverses and is directed toward the opposite (uninvolved) side.

TESTS OF NEUROLOGIC FUNCTION

Cranial Nerve Examination

The neurotologic examination includes a full evaluation of the cranial nerves. In general, tests of smell and visual

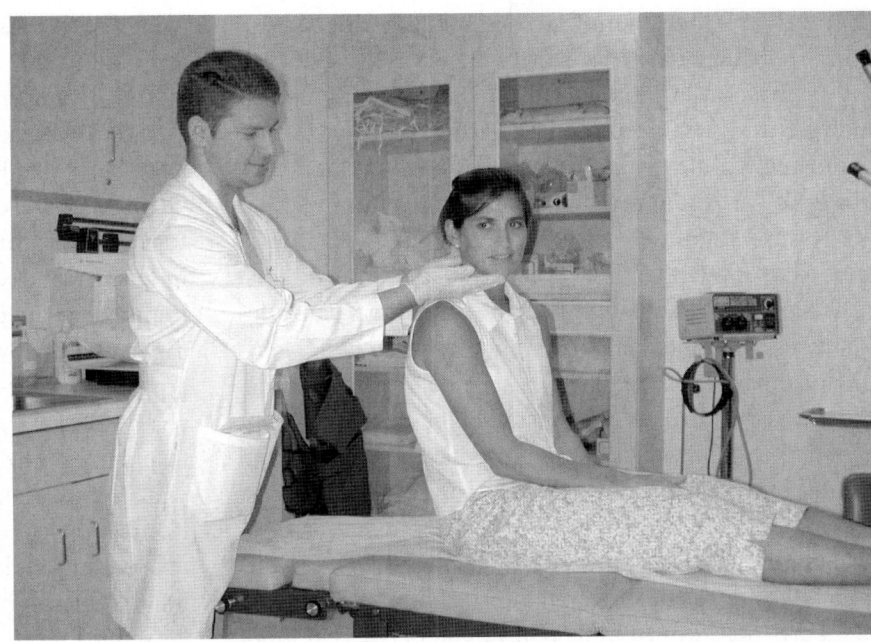

Figure 7–3   Dix-Hallpike examination testing the right ear.

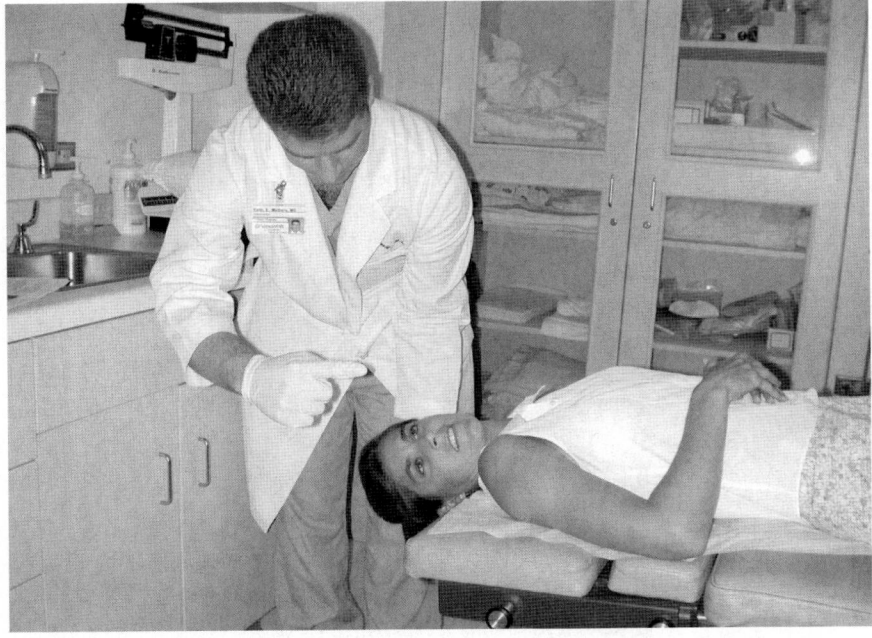

Figure 7–4   Dix-Hallpike examination of the right ear.

acuity are not usually performed unless indicated clinically. Cranial nerves III through XII are assessed systematically as part of the routine neurotologic examination. The reader is referred elsewhere for a full description of the cranial nerve examination.[2,44]

Cerebellar Function

Cerebellar testing is included in the neurotologic examination when there is a complaint of vertigo or dysequilibrium. Cerebellar disease may manifest with ataxia, dysmetria, hyperdysmetria, or dysdiadochokinesia. Poor coordination with repetitive finger-to-nose testing or rapid alternating head movements (dysmetria) may be a sign of cerebellar dysfunction. Uncoordinated heel-to-toe testing or tandem gait (ataxia) is also a sign of cerebellar dysfunction. Patients tend to deviate toward the side of an uncompensated vestibular lesion during gait testing. When moving a limb against resistance, a patient should be able to compensate adequately when the resistance is suddenly removed. Failure to compensate adequately is termed hyperdysmetria. Fine motor control may be tested by having the patient flip his/her hands over, rapidly alternating the palm and the back of the hand side up. Failure to perform this test adequately is termed dysdiadochokinesia.

Romberg's test (Figure 7–5) is a test of vestibulospinal tract function. Romberg's test and gait assessment are measures of both central and peripheral input to the limb and spinal muscles. This test is performed with the patient standing erect with feet together both with eyes open and with eyes closed. Consistent falling to one side is an abnormal test; there is a tendency to fall to the side of an uncompensated, unilateral vestibular lesion. The sharpened Romberg's test (Figure 7–6), thought to be more sensitive than the standard Romberg's test, is performed by having the patient stand with the feet aligned in tandem and arms folded to the chest. Fukuda[45] testing is performed by having the patient march in place (30 to 50 steps) with eyes closed and arms extended. The arms tend to deviate to, or the patient may turn excessively toward the side of, a vestibular lesion. Vestibulospinal testing depends on integration of proprioceptive, visual, and vestibular inputs. Closing the eyes during Romberg's test eliminates visual input, and Romberg's test on a 6-inch foam mat eliminates proprioceptive input, rendering the patient solely dependent on vestibular input for orientation.[46]

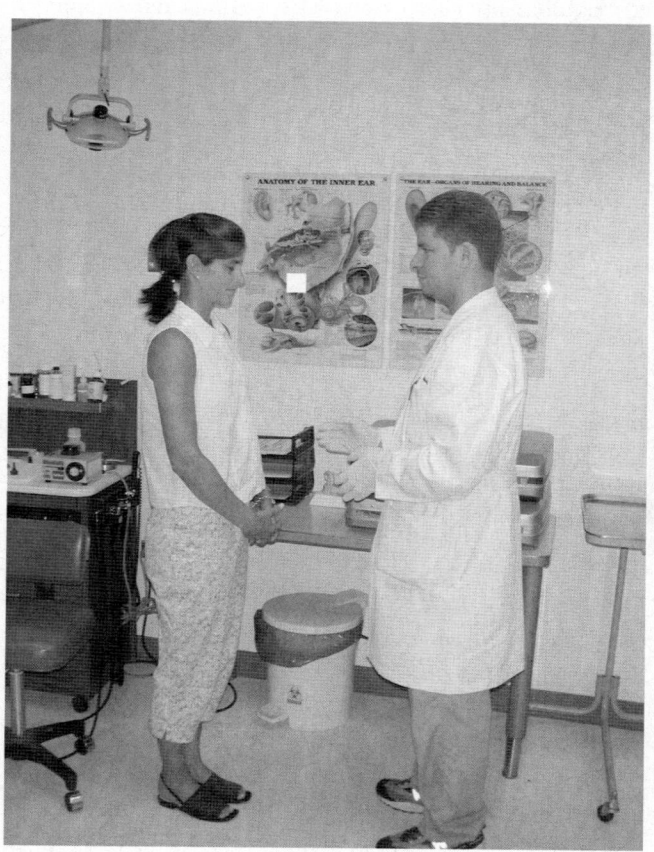

Figure 7–5 Romberg's test.

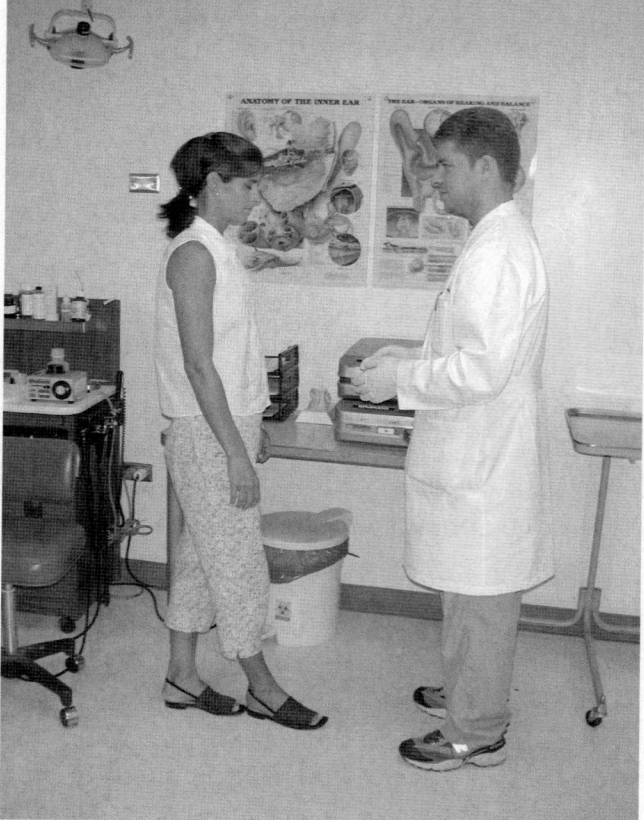

Figure 7–6 Sharpened Romberg's test.

Table 7–5   DISORDERS OF THE VESTIBULAR SYSTEM
Benign paroxysmal positional vertigo
Labyrinthitis
Meniere's disease
Vestibular neuronitis
Drug toxicity (ototoxicity)
Cerebellopontine angle tumors
Metabolic disorders
Perilymph fistula
Trauma
Systemic disorders (see table)
Autoimmune inner ear disease
Central disorders
Vertebral basilar insufficiency
Presyncope
Multiple sclerosis
Trauma
Familial ataxia
Arnold-Chiari malformation
Communicating hydrocephalus
Migraine
Central nervous system lesion or tumor
Cerebellar degeneration
Parkinson's disease
Nutritional disorders (vitamin B_{12} deficiency)

Table 7–6   AAO-HNS COMMITTEE OF HEARING AND EQUILIBRIUM DIAGNOSIS OF MÉNIÈRE'S DISEASE
Certain Meniere's disease
Definite Meniere's disease plus histologic confirmation
Definite Meniere's disease
Two or more definitive spontaneous episodes of vertigo 20 minutes or longer
Audiometrically documented hearing loss on at least one occasion
Tinnitus or aural fullness in the treated ear
Other causes excluded
Probable Meniere's disease
One definitive episode of vertigo
Audiometrically documented hearing loss on at least one occasion
Tinnitus or aural fullness in the treated ear
Other causes excluded
Possible Meniere's disease
Episodic vertigo of the Meniere type without hearing loss, or
Sensorineural hearing loss, fluctuating or fixed, with dysequilibrium but without definitive episodes
Other causes excluded

DIAGNOSIS OF OTOLOGIC DISEASE

The previous section discussed the otologic/neuro-otologic history and physical examination and their importance in establishing a clinical diagnosis. A brief overview of common otologic and neurotologic diagnoses is presented in the following section.

Disorders of the Auditory and Vestibular System

Meniere's Disease

Meniere's disease is a clinical disorder classified as idiopathic endolymphatic hydrops. The diagnosis of Meniere's disease can only be made with certainty after death by demonstrating endolymphatic hydrops on temporal bone histopathologic examination. During life, the diagnosis is suggested by a low-tone, fluctuating sensorineural hearing loss, tinnitus, aural fullness, and episodic vertigo. Frequently encountered in otology and neurotology practices, Meniere's disease is infrequently diagnosed in multidisciplinary balance clinics.[47]

The American Academy of Otolaryngology-Head and Neck Surgery (AAO-HNS) Committee on Hearing and Equilibrium elaborated on the definition of Meniere's disease for the purposes of diagnosis and reporting.[48] The Committee delineated four levels of certainty in the diagnosis of Meniere's disease, which are reproduced in Table 7–6.

The vertigo of Meniere's disease is characteristically a true spinning vertigo; it is incapacitating and severe and constitutes the most distressing symptom.[49] Variants of Meniere's disease include Lermoyez[50] attacks, in which the hearing loss and tinnitus improve with the attack of vertigo, and the otolithic crises of Tumarkin,[51] in which vestibular dysfunction manifests not as spinning vertigo but as a sudden severe fall or "drop attack." The terms cochlear Meniere's disease (hearing loss, tinnitus, and aural fullness, without vertigo) and vestibular Meniere's disease (the vestibular symptoms of Meniere's with no auditory symptoms) are occasionally used to describe patients who do not have the full spectrum of symptoms of Meniere's disease. The AAO-HNS Committee on Hearing and Equilibrium[52] recommended abandoning these terms in the absence of documentation that they are based on the same pathologic disorder (ie, endolymphatic hydrops). For the purposes of diagnosis and reporting treatment results, the classification of Meniere's disease in Table 7–6 should be used.

Benign Paroxysmal Positional Vertigo

Benign paroxysmal positional vertigo (BPPV) is a disorder frequently seen in neurotologic practice and stems from loose otoconia in the posterior[53,54] (most commonly), horizontal,[55–57] or superior semicircular canals. Intense vertigo is provoked by head position changes, such as rolling over in bed, lying down, or looking up. Hallpike testing can make the diagnosis and determine the involved side in posterior canal BPPV.[58] The nystagmus of BPPV is pathognomonic: it has a several (2- to 10-) second latency, is geotropic (beating toward the ground) and horizontal-rotary, lasts no more than 30 seconds before abating, and fatigues with repetition of the Hallpike maneuver. A modified Hallpike maneuver is used to test for horizontal canal BPPV. In this test, the patient lies supine and the head is rapidly rotated to one side (without extension beyond the table edge); the head is returned to the supine position and is then turned to the contralateral ear. The evoked nystagmus is horizontal, geotrophic, or ageotrophic and is less likely to fatigue.[59] Superior canal BPPV is uncommon and may be elicited by standard Hallpike testing.

Vestibular Neuritis

Inflammation and edema of the vestibular nerve confined in the bony internal auditory canal (IAC) leading to dysfunction of the nerve (vertigo) is termed vestibular neuritis.[60] Isolated atrophy of the vestibular nerve with little end-organ degeneration can be seen on histopathologic examination and is thought to reflect a viral etiology. The vertigo is abrupt in onset, is described as a severe, spinning sensation, and is usually accompanied by nausea and vomiting. Few other otologic symptoms are present except, occasionally, aural fullness. The acute phase lasts 48 to 72 hours and is followed by a period of dysequilibrium and a sensation of unsteadiness that usually lasts 4 to 6 weeks but may persist for several months. The variability of time to recovery depends on the extent of the damage to the vestibular nerve and of compensation for the vestibular injury.[61]

Perilymph Fistula

Inner ear fistulae include labyrinthine fistulae, perilymph fistulae, and intramembranous communications. Although all are considered inner ear fistulae, each represents a distinct clinical entity. A perilymph fistula is a leak of perilymph fluid into the middle ear or mastoid, although actual visualization of fluid, even with microscopic examination, is unusual. Precipitating insults include surgery, blunt trauma, penetrating trauma, barotrauma, infection, cholesteatoma, or sudden changes in CSF pressure as can occur with straining, sneezing, or Valsalva's maneuver. Congenital ear abnormalities may predispose to perilymph leaks. Spontaneous perilymph fistulae are believed to be infrequent.[62] The clinical picture of perilymph fistulae is variable, with symptoms ranging from mild to incapacitating. Vertigo, or more often unsteadiness, is the most common symptom. Hearing loss, tinnitus, or aural fullness may be present. A thorough history inquiring about activities such as trauma, scuba diving, flying, and straining is critical in the diagnosis of this disorder as the symptoms are vague and coincident with other vestibular disorders. A fistula test should be performed in a patient suspected of having a perilymph fistula (see above).

Another type of inner ear fistula is defined as an abnormal communication between the endolymphatic space and the perilymphatic space. This type of fistula is usually referred to as an intramembranous communication or a cochlear membrane tear and is theorized to be an etiology of (idiopathic) sudden sensorineural hearing loss.

The term labyrinthine fistula is used to describe an inner ear fistula that typically involves the semicircular canals. The usual etiologies are trauma and infection. Erosion of the horizontal canal (or less frequently the posterior or superior canals) from cholesteatoma or granulation tissue may lead to a labyrinthine fistula if the integrity of the bony labyrinth is violated. Inflammatory hypertrophy of the perilymphatic tissues prevents the flow of perilymph through the fistula; however, surgical disruption of the barrier precipitates the flow of perilymph. A patient known to have cholesteatoma in whom dysequilibrium develops is considered to have labyrinthine fistula until proven otherwise.

Metabolic Disorders

Metabolic disorders such as diabetes mellitus, thyroid dysfunction, and hyperlipoproteinemia may cause disorders of hearing and balance.[63] neurotologic symptoms may also arise from hormonal imbalance occurring with estrogen replacement therapy, oral contraceptive use, and the premenstrual or perimenopausal periods. The effects of these disorders on the cochlea and vestibular labyrinth are variable. The diagnosis of these disorders as a cause of auditory-vestibular symptoms may be elusive for some are rare, and those that are more common (eg, diabetes mellitus) do not consistently generate auditory-vestibular symptoms.

Aminoglycoside Ototoxicity

Aminoglycoside antibiotics can be toxic to the auditory and vestibular end-organs.[6,64] These medications can cause degeneration of the hair cells of the cochlea, the cristae of the semicircular canals, and the maculae of the utricle and the saccule. Some aminoglycoside antibiotics are relatively cochleotoxic, causing hearing loss (eg, neomycin), whereas others are relatively vestibulotoxic (eg, gentamicin). Because the toxic effects are bilateral, in vestibulotoxicity, the primary symptom is severe unsteadiness without vertigo. Oscillopsia, the perception that stationary objects are moving, and gait disturbances are common. Improvement in dysequilibrium is generally slow, requiring months to years. Romberg's test may be abnormal (positive), and there may be associated sensorineural hearing loss and tinnitus. As some patients develop ototoxicity after a small aminoglycoside dose or in the face of normal peak and trough drug levels, a genetic predisposition has been postulated. Two different mitochondrial mutations, in the same mitochondrial 12S ribosomal ribonucleic acid gene, have been shown to be responsible for the genetic susceptibility.[65]

Cerebellopontine Angle Tumors

Benign cerebellopontine angle tumors (eg, vestibular schwannomas and meningiomas) underlie unilateral (or asymmetric) sensorineural hearing loss, tinnitus, and dysequilibrium. Even small tumors may cause considerable symptomatology when they exert pressure on the seventh and eighth cranial nerves in the IAC. Other less common symptoms include facial weakness or paralysis, fifth cranial nerve involvement (facial numbness and decreased corneal reflex), and pain or headache. Despite compression and destruction of the vestibular nerves, imbalance is a relatively uncommon presenting symptom; the gradual progression of vestibular dysfunction allows for compensation of the deficit. Dysequilibrium, if present, is mild; true spinning vertigo is rare. Large tumors may be associated with dysequilibrium, ataxia, nausea, vomiting, and headache, indicative of brainstem, cerebellar, or fourth ventricular compression or increased intracranial pressure.

Sensorineural Hearing Loss

There is a myriad of etiologies for sensorineural hearing loss.[14] Presbycusis and noise-induced hearing loss are by far the most common. Other causes of sensorineural hearing loss are listed in Tables 7–1 and 7–3. The diagnosis of both common and uncommon causes ultimately depends on a thorough history and physical examination.

Noise-Induced Hearing Loss

Hearing loss affects approximately 28 million people in the United States, with 10 million attributed at least in part to noise exposure. Sound loud enough to damage the inner ear can produce hearing loss not reversible by any known medical or surgical therapy. Sound levels of 75 dB or less, even after long exposure, are unlikely to cause any permanent hearing loss. Sound levels above 85 dB, with exposure of at least 8 hours per day, will generally produce a permanent hearing loss.[5]

Labyrinthitis

Inflammation of the labyrinth is known as labyrinthitis.[66] Bacterial (suppurative) labyrinthitis takes a more fulminant course than nonsuppurative, serous labyrinthitis and manifests in the sudden onset of profound hearing loss and fulminant vertigo that lasts several days and is usually associated with nausea and vomiting. Unsteadiness, as in vestibular neuritis, may last for several months. However, unlike vestibular neuritis, there are usually associated cochlear symptoms, for example, hearing loss, fullness, otalgia, and tinnitus. Serous labyrinthitis is an inflammatory process within the labyrinth without associated infection. A viral labyrinthitis may be suspected in a patient presenting with the acute onset of vertigo and sensorineural hearing loss in the absence of any other precipitating circumstance. Other causes of labyrinthitis include contamination of perilymph with bacterial or inflammatory toxins, blood, or surgery (eg, stapedectomy). Evidence of acute otitis media, cholesteatoma, or chronic ear disease may be present, but the ear examination is normal in the majority of cases. Nystagmus may be present and beats away from the affected ear. Nonotolaryngologists typically refer to a wide variety of otologic disorders that cause vertigo as labyrinthitis; otolaryngologists usually reserve the term for the specific entities as described above.

Sudden Sensorineural Hearing Loss

Sudden sensorineural hearing loss is defined as a loss of at least 30 dB in at least three contiguous frequencies over a period of no more than 3 days.[67] Viral, vascular, and inflammatory processes, as well as abnormal endolymph/perilymph fluid mechanics, have been proposed as possible etiologies for idiopathic sudden sensorineural hearing loss. Hearing loss is generally the only symptom, but vertigo and aural fullness may accompany the hearing loss. High-dose prednisone appears to be an effective treatment.[67]

Conductive Hearing Loss

Twenty to 30% of the 28 million people with hearing loss in the United States are estimated to have conductive hearing loss.[16] Patients with conductive hearing losses are generally younger than patients with sensorineural loss and have no cognitive or other sensory deficits.[68] Etiologies of conductive hearing loss are listed in Table 7–4.

Systemic Disorders Affecting the Ear and Temporal Bone

Systemic disorders (see Table 7–1) can directly or indirectly affect hearing and balance. These diagnoses may be elusive as many of the disorders are uncommon.[4] Also, some of the more common disorders (eg, diabetes mellitus) do not consistently affect hearing and balance.

Eustachian Tube Dysfunction

Eustachian tube dysfunction is a common disorder generally described as ear fullness or pressure with an intermittent "popping sensation." The type of eustachian tube dysfunction encountered most frequently entails inadequate eustachian tube opening. Inflammatory processes, mucosal edema, allergic rhinitis, rhinosinusitis, and tumors of the nasopharynx can lead to eustachian tube dysfunction. Disorders such as cleft palate, with tensor veli palatini muscle dysfunction, can cause eustachian tube dysfunction. Hearing loss, mild aural fullness, and, rarely, tinnitus are associated symptoms. The fullness may be alleviated with Valsalva's maneuver. The physical examination in these patients varies depending on the disease process. Typically, the tympanic membrane is normal; however, tympanic membrane abnormalities ranging from atelectasis to retraction to cholesteatoma may be seen. In more chronic or severe cases of dysfunction, there may be an associated serous effusion.

Far less commonly encountered than inadequate eustachian tube dysfunction is a patulous (or open) eustachian tube. A history of autophony (abnormally hearing one's voice or breathing) in the problematic ear suggests a patulous eustachian tube. Surprisingly, the symptoms of a blocked eustachian tube and a patulous eustachian tube are markedly similar, contributing to the difficulty of making the correct diagnosis. Aural fullness may be more bothersome in patients with patulous eustachian tube, who generally do not have allergic rhinitis or sinusitis. On examination, the tympanic membrane is normal, although in some cases, one can see lateral and medial excursions of the drum with respiration. The symptoms of a patulous tube may be alleviated by maneuvers that close the tube, such as bending over, which, in effect, creates edema of the tissues of the tube orifice.

Otosyphilis

Otosyphilis is mentioned here because this disease continues to present a diagnostic challenge.[69] The diagnosis is suggested in patients with cochleovestibular dysfunction and positive serologic testing (eg, fluorescent treponemal antibody absorption or microhemagglutination-*Treponema palladium* [MHA-TP]). The manifestation(s) of syphilitic cochleovestibular dysfunction are extremely variable.[69,70] Hearing loss, which may be fluctuant, is the most common symptom (bilateral in 82% of the cases), followed by vertigo in 42%. Approximately one-fourth of patients with otosyphilis have symptoms consistent with endolymphatic hydrops.[71]

Migraine-Related Vertigo

Migraine is a neurologic disorder characterized by headache and other neurologic symptoms that affects 6 to 18% of adults in the United States. Migraine is a frequent but often overlooked cause of episodic vertigo. In practices that treat patients with headaches, dysequilibrium or episodic vertigo has been reported in 33 to 72% of cases.[72,73] Both true vertigo and nonvertiginous dizziness can occur. Interestingly, in the majority of patients, the vertigo is unassociated with their headache.[74]

Superior Canal Dehiscence Syndrome

Sound- or pressure-induced vertigo caused by dehiscence of the superior semicircular canal has been described.[41,42,75] Patients with this disorder develop vertical-torsional eye movements aligned with the plane of the superior canal in response to loud sounds or maneuvers that change middle ear or intracranial pressure. The diagnosis is made by observing vertical-torsional nystagmus with the slow phase directed upward and away from the suspect ear following positive tragal pressure, Valsalva's maneuver, or a loud (110-dB) sound. Ultra-high resolution computed tomographic scanning of the temporal bones may demonstrate thinning or dehiscence of the bone of the superior canal.

CONCLUSION

Despite the wide array of electrophysiologic and radiographic modalities that are used in the diagnosis of otologic disease, the history and physical examination remain the most important and most informative aspects of a thorough patient evaluation. Numerous conditions may be diagnosed on the basis of history alone, and a thorough history and complete physical examination promote efficient diagnosis and treatment of all otologic and neurotologic complaints, potentially minimizing expensive tests and unnecessary interventions. We have provided an extensive discussion of the key points of the history and physical examination for disorders of the ear, in addition to an overview of many of the pathologic conditions encountered in clinical practice.

REFERENCES

1. Glasscock ME, Haynes DS, Storper IS, Bohrer P. Otology and neurotology. In: Adkins RB, Scott HW, editors. Surgical care of the elderly. 2nd ed. Philadelphia: Lippincott-Raven; 1998. p. 193–200.
2. Strasnick B, Haynes DS. Otologic history and physical examination of the ear. In: Canalis RF, Lambert PR, editors. The ear: comprehensive otology. Philadelphia: Lippincott Williams and Wilkins; 2000. p. 157–66.
3. Bojrab DI, Bhansali SA. Objective evaluation of a patient with vertigo. In: Canalis RF, Lambert PR, editors. The ear: comprehensive otology. Philadelphia: Lippincott Williams and Wilkins; 2000. p. 181–96.
4. Nadol JB, Merchant SN. Systemic disease manifestations in the middle ear and temporal bone. In: Cummings CW, Harker LA, Krause CJ, et al, editors. Otolaryngology-head and neck surgery. Vol 3. St. Louis: Mosby; 1998. p. 3088–107.
5. Noise and hearing loss: consensus conference. JAMA 1990;263:3185–90.
6. Roland JT, Cohen NL. Vestibular and auditory ototoxicity. In: Cummings CW, Harker LA, Krause CJ, et al, editors. Otolaryngology-head and neck surgery. Vol 3. St. Louis: Mosby; 1998. p. 3186–95.
7. Van Der Hulst RJAM, Dreschler W, Urbanus NAM. High-frequency audiometry in prospective clinical research of ototoxicity due to platinum derivatives. Ann Otol Rhinol Laryngol 1988;97:133–7.
8. Rybak LP. Ototoxicity of loop diuretics. Otolaryngol Clin North Am 1993;26:829–43.
9. Jung TK, Rhee CK, Lee CS, et al. Ototoxicity of salicylate, nonsteroidal anti-inflamatory drugs and quinine. Otolaryngol Clin North Am 1993;26:791–809.
10. Hart CW. Clinical evaluation of the dizzy patient. In: Hughes GB, Pensak ML, editors. Clinical otology. New York: Thieme; 1997. p. 169–74.
11. Brody R, Rosenfeld RM, Goldsmith AJ, Madell JR. Parents cannot detect mild hearing loss in children. Otolaryngol Head Neck Surg 1999;121:681–6.
12. Grundfast KM, Lalwani AK. Practical approach to diagnosis and management of hereditary hearing impairment (HHI). Ear Nose Throat J 1992;71:479–93.
13. Bauer CA, Jenkins HA. Otologic symptoms and syndromes. In: Cummings CW, Harker LA, Krause CJ, et al, editors. Otolaryngology-head and neck surgery. Vol 3. St. Louis: Mosby; 1998. p. 2547–58.
14. Arts A. Differential diagnosis of sensorineural hearing loss. In: Cummings CW, Harker LA, Krause CJ, et al, editors. Otolaryngology-head and neck surgery. Vol 3. St. Louis: Mosby; 1998. p. 2908–28.
15. Okumura T, Takahashi H, Takagi A, Mitamura K. Sensorineural hearing loss in patients with large vestibular aqueduct. Laryngoscope 1995;105:289–93.
16. Backous D, Niparko J. Evaluation and surgical management of conductive hearing loss. In: Cummings CW, Harker LA, Krause CJ, et al, editors. Otolaryngology-head and neck surgery. Vol 3. St. Louis: Mosby; 1998. p. 2894–907.
17. Scholtz AW, Fish JH, Kammen-Jolly K, et al. Goldenhar's syndrome: congenital hearing deficit of conductive or sensorineural origin? Temporal bone histopathologic study. Otol Neurootol 2001;22:501–5.
18. Billings KR, Kenna MA. Causes of pediatric sensorineural hearing loss. Arch Otolaryngol Head Neck Surg 1999;125:517–21.

19. Glasscock ME, Haynes DS, Storper IS, Bohrer PS. Surgery for chronic ear disease. In: Hughes GB, Pensak ML, editors. Clinical otology. New York: Thieme; 1997. p. 215–32.

20. Myer CM. Post tympanostomy tube otorrhea. Ear Nose Throat J 2001;80(6 Suppl):4–7.

21. Roland PS. Chronic external otitis. Ear Nose Throat J 2001; 80(6 Suppl):2–6.

22. Pappas DG, Hoffman RA, Cohen NL, Pappas DG. Spontaneous temporal bone cerebrospinal fluid leak. Amn J Otolaryngol 1992;13:534–9.

23. Haynes DS. Surgery for chronic ear disease. Ear Nose Throat J 2001;80(6 Suppl):8–11.

24. Kroenke K, Arrington ME, Manglesdorff AD. The prevalence of symptoms in medical outpatients and the adequacy of therapy. Arch Intern Med 1990;150:1685–9.

25. Sloane PD, Baloh RW, Honrubia V. The vestibular system in the elderly: clinical implications. Am J Otolaryngol 1989;10: 422–9.

26. Herdman SJ, Blatt P, Schubert MC, Tusa RJ. Falls in patients with vestibular deficits.Am J Otolaryngol 2000;21:847–51.

27. Novick NL. Fundamentals of dermatologic diagnosis and therapy. In: Lucente FE, Lawson W, Novick NL, editors. The external ear. Philadelphia: WB Saunders; 1995. p. 25–39.

28. Lucente FE. Techniques of examination. In: Lucente FE, Lawson W, Norvick NL, editors. The external ear. Philadelphia: WB Saunders; 1995. p. 18–24.

29. Jackson CG, Glasscock ME, Nissen AJ, et al. Open mastoid procedures: contemporary indications and surgical technique. Laryngoscope 1995;95:1037–43.

30. Bluestone CD, Klein JO. Methods of examination: clinical examination. In: Bluestone CD, Stool SE, Kenna MA, editors. Pediatric otolaryngology. 3rd ed. Philadelphia: WB Saunders; 1996. p. 150–64.

31. Sismanis A. Pulsatile tinnitus. A 15 year experience. Am J Otolaryngol 1998;19:472.

32. Soler D, Cox T, Bullock P, et al. Diagnosis and management of benign intracranial hypertension. Arch Dis Child 1998;78:89.

33. Blakeley BW, Siddique S. A qualitative explanation of the Weber's test. Otolaryngol Head Neck Surg 1999;120:1–4.

34. Sichel JY, Eliashar R, Dano I. Explaining the Weber's test. Otolaryngol Head Neck Surg 2000;122:465–6.

35. Glasscock ME, Shambaugh GE. Surgery of the ear. 4th ed. Philadelphia: WB Saunders; 1991.

36. Capper JW, Slack RW, Maw AR. Tuning fork tests in children. J Laryngol Otol 1987;101:780–3.

37. Sheehy JL, Gardner G Jr, Hambley WM. Tuning fork tests in modern otology. Arch Otolaryngol 1971;94:132–8.

38. Minor LB, Zee DS. Evaluation of the patient with dizziness. In: Cummings CW, Harker LA, Krause CJ, et al, editors. Otolaryngology-head and neck surgery. Vol 3. St. Louis: Mosby; 1998. p. 2623–71.

39. Hennebert C. A new syndrome in hereditary syphilis of the labyrinth. Presse Med Belg Brux 1911;63:467.

40. Nadol JB. Positive Hennebert's sign in Meniere's disease. Arch Otolaryngol Head Neck Surg 1977;103:524–30.

41. Minor LB. The superior canal dehiscence syndrome. Am J Otolaryngol 2000;2:9–19.

42. Minor LB, Solomon D, Zinreich JS, Zee DS. Sound- and/or pressure-induced vertigo due to bone dehiscence of the superior semicircular canal. Arch Otolaryngol Head Neck Surg 1998;124: 249–58.

43. Hain TC, Fetter M, Zee DS. Head-shaking nystagmus in patients with unilateral peripheral lesions. Am J Otolaryngol 1987;8: 36–47.

44. Burton MJ, Niparko JK. Evaluation of the cranial nerves. In: Hughes GB, Pensak ML, editors. Clinical otology. New York: Thieme; 1997. p. 131–46.

45. Fukuda T. The stepping test-two phases of the labyrinthine reflex. Acta Otolaryngol (Stockh) 1958;50:95.

46. Lambert PR. History and physical examination of a patient with dizziness. In: Canalis RF, Lambert PR, editors. The ear: comprehensive otology. Philadelphia: Lippincott Williams and Wilkins; 2000. p. 167–79.

47. Bath AP, Walsh RM, Ranalli P, et al. Experience from a multidisciplinary "dizzy" clinic. Am J Otolaryngol 2000;21:92–7.

48. Committee on Hearing and Equilibrium. Committee on Hearing and Equilibrium guidelines for the diagnosis and evaluation of therapy in Meniere's disease. Otolaryngol Head Neck Surg 1995;113:181–5.

49. Schuknecht HF, Brackman DE, Glasscock ME, Jenkins H. Difficult decisions: Meniere's disease. Oper Tech Otolaryngol Head Neck Surg 1991;2:47–53.

50. Lermoyez M. Le vertige qui fait entendre (angiospasme labyrinthique) Presse Med 1919;27:1.

51. Tumarkin A. The otolithic catastrophe: a new syndrome. BMJ 1936;2:175.

52. Pearson BW, Brackmann DE. Committee on Hearing and Equilibrium guidelines for reporting treatment results in Meniere's disease. Otolaryngol Head Neck Surg 1985;93:579.

53. Herdman SJ, Tusa RJ, Zee DS, et al. Single treatment approaches to benign paroxysmal positional vertigo. Arch Otolaryngol Head Neck Surg 1993;119:450–4.

54. Epley JM. The canalith repositioning procedure: for treatment of benign paroxysmal positional vertigo. Otolaryngol Head Neck Surg 1992;107:399–404.

55. Baloh RW, Jacobson K, Honrubia V. Horizontal semicircular canal variant of benign positional vertigo. Neurology 1993;43: 2542–9.

56. McClure J. Horizontal canal BPV. J Otolaryngol 1985;14:30–5.

57. Lempert T, Tiel-Wilk K. A positional maneuver for treatment of horizontal-canal benign positional vertigo. Laryngoscope 1996;106:476–8.

58. Dix MR, Hallpike CS. The pathology, symptomatology and diagnosis of certain common disorders of the vestibular system. Ann Otol Rhinol Laryngol 1952;61:987–1016.

59. Schessel DA, Minor LA, Nedzelski J. Meniere's disease and other peripheral disorders. In: Cummings CW, Harker LA, Krause CJ, et al, editors. Otolaryngology-head and neck surgery. Vol 3. St. Louis: Mosby; 1998. p. 2672–705.

60. Schuknecht HF, Kitamura K. Vestibular neuritis. Ann Otol Rhinol Laryngol Suppl 1981;78:1–19.

61. Glasscock ME, Haynes DS. Evaluation and treatment of the patient with vertigo. Volta Rev 1998;99:129–40.

62. Friedland DR, Wackym PA. A critical appraisal of spontaneous perilymphatic fistulas of the inner ear. Am J Otolaryngol 1999;20:261–79.

63. Rybak L. Metabolic disorders of the vestibular system. Otolaryngol Head Neck Surg 1995;112:128–32.

64. Langman AW. Neomycin ototoxicity. Otolaryngol Head Neck Surg 1994;110:441–4.

65. Rosaria AMS, Casano MS, Johnson DF, et al. Inherited susceptibility to aminoglycoside ototoxicity: genetic heterogeneity and clinical implications. Am J Otolaryngol 1999;20:151–6.

66. Wilson WR, Veltri RW, Laird N, Sprinkle PM. Viral and epidemiologic studies of idiopathic sudden hearing loss. Otolaryngol Head Neck Surg 1983;91:653.

67. Wilson WR, Byl FM, Laird N. The efficacy of steroids in the treatment of idiopathic sudden hearing loss: a double-blind clinical study. Arch Otolaryngol 1980;106:772–6.

68. Stewart MG, Coker NJ, Jenkins HA, et al. Outcomes and quality of life in conductive hearing loss. Otolaryngol Head Neck Surg 2000;123:527–32.

69. Gleich LL, Linstrom CJ, Kimmelman CP. Otosyphilis: a diagnostic and therapeutic dilemma. Laryngoscope 1992;102:1255–9.

70. Birdsall HH, Baughn RE, Jenkins HA. The diagnostic dilemma of otosyphilis. Arch Otolaryngol Head Neck Surg 1990;116:617–21.

71. Steckleberg JM, McDonald TJ. Otologic involvement in late syphilis. Laryngoscope 1984;94:753–7.

72. Selby G, Lance JW. Observations on 500 cases of migraine and allied vascular headache. J Neurol Neurosurg Psychiatry 1960;23:23–32.

73. Kayan A, Hood JD. Neuro-otological manifestations of migraine. Brain 1984;107:1123–42.

74. Johnson GD. Medical management of migraine-related dizziness and vertigo. Laryngoscope 1998;108 Suppl:1–20.

75. Ostrowski VB, Byskosh A, Hain TC. Tullio phenomenon with dehiscence of the superior semicircular canal. Otol Neurootol 2001;22:61–5.

8

Audiologic Evaluation of Otologic/Neurotologic Disease

Brad A. Stach, PhD

AUDIOLOGIC CONTRIBUTION TO DIAGNOSIS

The process and strategies used to evaluate hearing have their greatest utility in the audiologic diagnosis of communication disorders resulting from hearing loss. Nevertheless, the results of the audiologic evaluation can be useful in the otologic/neurotologic diagnosis of ear disease. Patterns of results on measures of pure-tone thresholds, speech recognition, acoustic reflexes, otoacoustic emissions (OAEs), and auditory evoked potentials may indicate the need for additional diagnostic testing or may serve to corroborate clinical otologic findings. They may also serve as a useful means of quantifying post-treatment outcome.

Audiometric measures evaluate auditory system function. The extent to which a disease process interferes with function will dictate their usefulness in the diagnostic process. Should the condition not interfere measurably with function, the audiologic outcomes will be of little utility diagnostically. In contrast, if function is affected, the results on these audiometric measures may serve a useful diagnostic purpose and may help to quantify the impact of the disorder.

The value of audiometric test results in the diagnostic process varies with the nature of the disorder. For example, a middle ear disorder is readily identifiable with immittance measures and OAEs, whereas a brainstem disorder might elude audiologic diagnosis if the influence on function is too subtle. The value of audiometric test results in the diagnostic process also depends on the sensitivity of other diagnostic measures. For example, the increasing sensitivity of imaging techniques, capable of detecting ever smaller lesions, has reduced the utility of the auditory brainstem response (ABR) in the diagnosis of disorders of the eighth nerve and has relegated to audiometric measures the role of screening for, rather than identifying, specific lesions.

Regardless, the audiologic evaluation of otologic/neurotologic disease plays an important role in the diagnosis and management of patients. Whether for the purposes of corroboration, identification, or quantification, audiometric outcomes are often valuable components of the clinical evaluation. This chapter provides an overview of hearing and its disorders, audiometric measures and audiologic approaches, and anticipated measurement outcomes as a function of the type of hearing disorder.

OVERVIEW OF HEARING

The auditory system is characterized by high sensitivity, sharp frequency tuning, rapid temporal processing, and wide dynamic range. It is sensitive enough to perceive acoustic signals with pressure wave amplitudes of very small magnitude. It is very finely tuned to an extent that it is capable of resolving frequencies with precise acuity. It is capable of processing rapidly varying acoustic signals ranging in magnitude to significant proportion.

The physical processing of acoustic information occurs in the outer, middle, and inner ears. Physiologic processing begins primarily in the cochlea and continues, via the eighth cranial nerve, to the central auditory nervous system. Psychological processing begins primarily in the brainstem and pons and continues to the auditory cortex and beyond.

The outer ear serves to collect and resonate sound and assist in sound localization, and functions as a protective mechanism for the middle ear. The auricles serve mainly to collect sound waves and funnel them to the external auditory canal. The auricles are important for sound localization in the vertical plane and for protection of the ear canal. The auricles also serve as resonators, enhancing sounds around 4,500 Hz. The external auditory canal directs sound to the tympanic membrane. It serves as a resonator, enhancing sounds around 2,700 Hz. It also serves to protect the tympanic membrane by its narrow opening. The tympanic membrane is set into motion by acoustic pressure waves striking its surface. The membrane vibrates with a magnitude proportional to the intensity of the sound wave at a speed proportional to its frequency.

The middle ear structures function as an impedance matching device, providing a bridge between the airborne pressure waves striking the tympanic membrane and the fluidborne traveling waves of the cochlea. In this way, the middle ear acts as an impedance matching transformer. Briefly, the ease or difficulty of energy flow is different through air than it is through fluid. Pressure waves propagating through air are substantively reflected by a fluid-filled space because of the difference in energy flow through the two media. The different impedances of these two media must be matched or the functional gap between them bridged. The ossicular chain serves this purpose. Air pressure waves vibrate the tympanic membrane, which, in turn, vibrates the ossicles and sets the fluid of the cochlea into motion. If the middle ear did not exist, the air pressure waves would have to set the fluid of the cochlea into motion directly, and a substantial amount of energy would be lost in the process. Perhaps the best way to understand this concept is to consider the fact that the fish auditory system does not require a middle ear. Because the sounds that fish hear are propagated through water, the energy waves travel as fluid motion and set the inner ear fluids into motion directly. Little loss of energy results. However, the sounds perceived by humans consist of air borne energy waves and must be transformed into mechanical energy before being converted to hydraulic energy. The mechanical energy of the middle ear serves as an efficient energy converter from air to fluid, a task the middle ear is designed to accomplish in several ways. First, there is a substantial difference in surface area between the tympanic membrane and the oval window. This difference serves much the same purpose as the head of a nail. Pressure applied on the large end results in substantially greater pressure at the narrow end. The ossicles also act as a lever, pivoting around the incudomalleal joint, which contributes to an increase in vibrational amplitude at the stapes.

The auditory labyrinth, or cochlea, consists of fluid-filled membranous channels within a spiral canal that encircles a bony central core. Here sound waves, transformed into mechanical energy by the middle ear, set the fluid of the cochlea into motion in a manner determined by their intensity and frequency. Waves of fluid motion impinge on the membranous labyrinth and set off a chain of events that result in the generation of neural impulses within the eighth cranial nerve. As the stapes vibrates in and out of the oval window, the fluid in the cochlea is set into a wavelike motion. This motion is referred to as the traveling wave, which proceeds down the course of the cochlear partition, growing in magnitude until it reaches a certain point of maximum displacement. For higher frequencies, the point of maximum displacement occurs closer to the oval window, nearer the basal end of the cochlea. For lower frequencies, it occurs farther from the oval window, at the apical end of the cochlea. The basilar membrane is maximally displaced as the traveling wave reaches its point of maximum energy. At the point of maximal displacement of the basilar membrane, the inner hair cells are stimulated, sending neural impulses to the auditory nerve.

The traveling wave by itself does not explain the extraordinary sensitivity and frequency selectivity of the cochlea. Rather, an active process in the cochlea intervenes to turn the basilar membrane displacement by the traveling wave into a sensitive, sharply tuned response at the inner hair cell. The mechanism for this active process is increasingly well understood. The exquisite tuning of cochlear nerve fibers, the existence of OAEs, and the motility of outer hair cells has led to the very compelling implication of outer hair cell contribution to hearing sensitivity. In brief, the sensitivity of the inner hair cells to low-intensity sound is controlled by the outer hair cells. Outer hair cells, the cilia of which are embedded in the tectorial membrane, are mostly innervated by efferent neurons. Low-intensity sound excites or inhibits the outer hair cells, causing them to change shape and to influence tectorial membrane function in a manner that affects the inner hair cells, enhancing their sensitivity. When the inner hair cells are stimulated, neurotransmitters activate neuronal endings of the cochlear branch of the eighth nerve.

The auditory nervous system is primarily an afferent system that transmits neural signals from the cochlea to the auditory cortex. The auditory system is functionally crossed so that information from the right ear is transmitted primarily to the left cortex and vice versa. The auditory system also has an efferent component, which has multiple functions, including regulation of the outer hair cells and a general inhibitory action throughout the central auditory nervous system.

Nerve fibers leave the cochlea in an orderly (tonotopic) manner and synapse in the lower brainstem. From that point on, the system becomes richly complex, with multiple crossing pathways and ample opportunity for efferent and intersensory-modality interaction. Nerve fibers from the inner hair cells exit the organ of Corti through the osseous spiral lamina, beyond which their cell bodies cluster to form the spiral ganglion in the modiolus. The nerve fibers exit the modiolus in an orderly manner, with fibers from the most apical turn of the cochlea in the center of the nerve bundle and fibers from the basal end joining on the outside of the bundle. In this way, the frequency arrangement of the cochlea is preserved anatomically, with low frequencies from the apex in the middle and high frequencies from the base on the outside. This tonotopic organization is preserved throughout the primary auditory pathways to the cortex.

The eighth nerve codes auditory information in several ways. In general, intensity is coded in the rate of neural discharge. Frequency is coded in the place of neural discharge by fibers that are arranged tonotopically. Additionally, frequency may be coded in the temporal aspects of the discharge patterns of neuronal firing.

Eighth nerve fibers have an obligatory synapse at the cochlear nucleus on the ipsilateral side of the brainstem. Fibers entering the cochlear nucleus bifurcate, with one fiber synapsing in the primary auditory portion of the nucleus and the other synapsing in portions of the nucleus that spawn secondary or parallel pathways. From the cochlear nucleus, approximately three-quarters of the nerve fibers cross over to the contralateral side of the brainstem. Some fibers terminate on the medial nucleus of the trapezoid body and some on the medial superior olive. Others proceed to nuclei beyond the superior olivary complex. Of those on the ipsilateral side of the brainstem, some terminate in the medial superior olive, some at the lateral superior olive, and others at higher level nuclei. From the superior olivary complex, neurons proceed to the lateral lemniscus, the inferior colliculus, and the medial geniculate body. Nerve fibers may synapse in any of these nuclei or proceed beyond. Also, at each of these nuclei, some fibers cross over from the contralateral side of the brain. From the medial geniculate body, nerve fibers course in the auditory radiations to the primary auditory cortex.

The rudimentary processing of sound begins in the lower brainstem. For example, initial processing for sound localization occurs at the superior olivary complex, where small interaural timing and intensity differences are detected. As another example, the acoustic stapedial reflex occurs at the level of the cochlear nucleus, with sound of sufficient loudness, resulting in stapedius muscle contraction and stiffening of the ossicular chain.

Processing of speech information occurs throughout the central auditory system and in most humans is predominantly represented in the left temporal lobe. Speech that is detected by the right ear proceeds through the dominant, contralateral auditory channels to the left temporal lobe. Speech that is detected by the left ear proceeds through the dominant, contralateral channel to the right cortex and then via the corpus callosum to the left auditory cortex. Thus, in most humans, the right ear is dominant for the processing of speech information.

The ability to hear relies on this very sophisticated series of structures that process sound. The pressure waves of sound are collected by the pinna and funneled to the tympanic membrane by the external auditory canal. The tympanic membrane vibrates in response to the sound, which sets the ossicular chain into motion. The mechanical movement of the ossicular chain then sets the fluids of the cochlea in motion, causing the hair cells on the basilar membrane to be stimulated. These hair cells send neural impulses through the eighth cranial nerve to the auditory brainstem. From the brainstem, networks of neurons act on the neural stimulation, sending signals to the auditory cortex.

NATURE AND IMPACT OF HEARING DISORDERS

A hearing disorder is classified as (a) a hearing sensitivity loss, (b) a suprathreshold hearing disorder, or (c) a functional hearing loss. Hearing sensitivity loss is the most common form of hearing disorder. It is characterized by a reduction in the sensitivity of the auditory mechanism so that sounds need to be of higher intensity than normal before they are perceived. Suprathreshold disorders result in reduced ability to hear or perceive sounds properly at intensity levels above threshold. Functional hearing loss is the exaggeration or fabrication of a hearing loss.

Hearing Sensitivity Loss

Hearing sensitivity loss is caused by an abnormal reduction of sound being delivered to the brain by a disordered ear. This reduction of sound can result from any number of factors that affect the auditory mechanism. When sound is not conducted well through a disordered outer or middle ear, the result is a conductive hearing loss. When the sensory or neural mechanisms within the cochlea are absent or not functioning, the result is a sensorineural hearing loss. When structures of both the conductive mechanism and the cochlea are disordered, the result is referred to as a mixed hearing loss. A sensorineural hearing loss can also be caused by a disorder of the eighth nerve or auditory brainstem. Such disorders are usually referred to separately as retrocochlear disorders because their diagnosis, treatment, and impact on hearing ability can differ substantially from a sensorineural hearing loss of cochlear origin.

Conductive Hearing Loss

A conductive hearing loss is caused by an abnormal reduction or attenuation of sound as it travels through the conductive mechanisms of the outer and middle ear. A conductive hearing loss or the conductive component of a hearing loss is quantified by comparing the air- and bone-conduction thresholds on an audiogram. Air-conduction thresholds represent hearing sensitivity as measured through the outer, middle, and inner ears. Bone-conduction thresholds represent hearing sensitivity as measured primarily through the inner ear. Thus, if air-conduction thresholds are poorer than bone-conduction thresholds, it can be assumed that the attenuation of sound is occurring at the level of the outer or middle ears. The size of the conductive component is usually referred to as the air–bone gap. The audiometric con-

figuration of a conductive hearing loss varies from low frequency to flat to high frequency, depending on the physical obstruction of the structures of the conductive mechanism. In general, any disorder that adds mass to the conductive system predominantly affects the higher audiometric frequencies. Any disorder that adds or reduces stiffness to the system predominantly affects the lower audiometric frequencies. Any disorder that changes both mass and stiffness affects a broad range of audiometric frequencies.

Because a conductive hearing loss acts primarily as an attenuator of sound, it has little or no impact on suprathreshold hearing. That is, once sound is of sufficient intensity, the ear acts as it normally would at suprathreshold intensities. Thus, perception and growth of loudness, ability to discriminate loudness and pitch changes, and speech recognition ability are all normal once the conductive hearing loss is overcome by raising the intensity of the signal.

Although readily amenable to otologic treatment, there can be a more insidious effect of conductive hearing loss. Some children with chronic otitis media with effusion experience inconsistent auditory input during their formative years and do not develop appropriate suprathreshold auditory and listening skills.[1-4] Such children may be at risk for later learning and achievement problems.

Sensorineural Hearing Loss

A sensorineural hearing loss is caused by a failure in the cochlear transduction of sound from mechanical energy in the middle ear to neural impulses in the eighth nerve. When a structure of this sensorineural mechanism is in some way damaged, its ability to transduce mechanical energy into electrical energy is reduced, resulting in a number of changes in cochlear processing, including a reduction in the sensitivity of the cochlear receptor cells, in the frequency-resolving ability of the cochlea, and in the dynamic range of the hearing mechanism.

A sensorineural hearing loss is most often characterized clinically by its effect on cochlear sensitivity and thus the audiogram. If the outer and middle ears are functioning properly, then air-conduction thresholds accurately represent the sensitivity of the cochlea and are equal to bone-conduction thresholds. The audiometric configuration of a sensorineural hearing loss varies from low frequency to flat to high frequency depending on the location of hair cell loss or other damage along the basilar membrane.

A sensorineural hearing loss has at least three fundamentally important effects on hearing: a reduction in cochlear sensitivity, in frequency resolution, and in the dynamic range of the hearing mechanism. In many ways, the reduction in hearing sensitivity can be thought of as having the same effect as a conductive hearing loss in terms of reducing the audibility of speech. That is, a conductive hearing loss and a sensorineural hearing loss of the same degree and configuration will have the same effect on the audibility of speech sounds. The difference between the two types of hearing loss becomes manifest at suprathreshold levels.

One of the consequences of sensorineural hearing loss is recruitment (abnormal loudness growth). Loudness grows more rapidly than normal at intensity levels just above threshold in an ear with sensorineural hearing loss. This recruitment results in a reduced dynamic range from the threshold level to the discomfort level.

Reduction in frequency resolution and in dynamic range affects the perception of speech. In most sensorineural hearing losses, this effect on speech understanding is predictable from the audiogram and is poorer than would be expected from a conductive hearing loss of similar magnitude. In the extreme, the reduction in frequency resolution and dynamic range can severely limit the usefulness of residual hearing.

Mixed Hearing Loss

A hearing loss comprising both sensorineural and conductive components is termed a mixed hearing loss. A mixed hearing loss indicates that a disordered outer or middle ear attenuates the sound delivered to an impaired cochlea. Bone-conduction thresholds reflect the degree and configuration of the sensorineural component of the hearing loss. Air-conduction thresholds reflect both the sensorineural loss and the additional conductive component.

Retrocochlear Hearing Loss

A retrocochlear hearing loss is caused by a change in neural structure and function of some component of the peripheral or central auditory nervous system. As a rule of thumb, the more peripheral a lesion, the greater its impact on hearing sensitivity and on auditory function in general—sometimes referred to as the "bottleneck" principle. Conversely, the more central the lesion, the more subtle its impact. One might conceptualize this principle by thinking of the nervous system as a large tree. If one of its many branches were damaged, overall growth of the tree would be affected only subtly. Damage to its trunk, however, would impact the entire tree significantly. A well-placed tumor on the auditory nerve can substantially impact hearing, whereas a lesion in the midbrain is likely to have a more subtle effect.

Perhaps the best illustration of the bottleneck principle comes from reports of cases with lesions that effectively disconnect the cochlea from the brainstem. These cases manifest severe or profound hearing loss and very poor speech recognition despite normal cochlear function, as indicated by normal OAEs or eighth nerve action potentials. In cases involving lesions of the cerebellopontine angle secondary to tumor,[5] multiple sclerosis,[6] and miliary tuberculosis,[7] the results have shown how a lesion strategically placed at the bottleneck can substantially affect hearing ability. The bottleneck in the case of the auditory system is, of course, the eighth nerve as it enters the auditory brainstem.

One specific auditory nervous system disorder identified recently is auditory neuropathy,[8,9] a term used to describe a condition in which cochlear function and eighth nerve function are abnormal. It is distinguishable from disorders caused by space-occupying lesions in that imaging results of the nerve and brainstem are normal. Nevertheless, auditory neuropathy is a disorder that exemplifies the consequences of a disorder at the level of the bottleneck.

If the bottleneck is unaffected, then lesions at higher levels will have effects on auditory processing ability that are more subtle. These effects tend to become increasingly subtle as the lesions are located more centrally in the system. For example, whereas a lesion at the bottleneck can cause a substantial hearing sensitivity loss, a brainstem lesion often results in only a mild low-frequency sensitivity loss,[10] and a temporal lobe lesion is unlikely to affect hearing sensitivity at all. Similarly, speech recognition of words presented in quiet can be very poor in the case of a lesion at the periphery but will be unaffected by a lesion at the level of the temporal lobe.

A retrocochlear lesion, then, may or may not affect auditory sensitivity, depending on many factors, including lesion size, location, and impact. A tumor of the eighth cranial nerve can cause a substantial sensorineural hearing loss, depending on how much pressure it places on the nerve, the damage that it causes to the nerve, or the extent to which it interrupts blood supply to the cochlea. A temporal lobe tumor, however, is quite unlikely to result in any change in hearing sensitivity.

Suprathreshold Hearing Disorder

Although there is a tendency to think of hearing impairment as the sensitivity loss that can be measured on an audiogram, there are other types of hearing impairment that may or may not be accompanied by sensitivity loss. These other impairments result from disease, damage, or decline of the auditory nervous system in adults or delayed or disordered auditory nervous system development in children.

A disordered auditory nervous system, regardless of cause, will have functional consequences that can vary from subclinical to a substantial, easily measurable auditory deficit. When impairment is caused by an active, measurable disease process, such as a tumor or other space-occupying lesion, or from damage caused by trauma or stroke, it is often referred to as a retrocochlear disorder. When impairment is caused by a developmental disorder or delay or from diffuse changes such as aging, it is often referred to as an auditory processing disorder. The consequences of both types of disorders can be remarkably similar from an audiologic perspective, but the disorders are treated differently because of the consequences of diagnosis and the likelihood of a significant residual communication disorder.

Retrocochlear Disorder

In addition to possible hearing sensitivity loss, retrocochlear disease can cause a more subtle hearing disorder that is often noted in measures of suprathreshold function such as speech recognition ability. In general, hearing loss from a retrocochlear disorder is distinguishable from cochlear or conductive hearing loss by the extent to which it can adversely affect speech perception. Conductive loss impacts speech perception only by attenuating sound. Cochlear hearing loss adds dis-

tortion, but it is often minimal and predictable. A retrocochlear disorder can cause severe distortion of incoming speech signals in a manner that limits the usefulness of hearing.

In addition to speech recognition deficits, other suprathreshold abnormalities can occur. Loudness growth can be abnormal in patients with a retrocochlear disorder. Instead of the abnormally rapid growth of loudness characteristic of cochlear hearing loss, retrocochlear disorder can actually result in decruitment, an abnormally slow growth in loudness with increasing intensity. A retrocochlear disorder can also result in abnormal auditory adaptation. The normal auditory system tends to adapt to ongoing sound, especially at near-threshold levels, so that, as adaptation occurs, an audible signal becomes inaudible. At higher intensity levels, ongoing sound tends to remain audible without adaptation. However, in an ear with retrocochlear disorder, the audibility may diminish rapidly owing to excessive auditory adaptation, even at higher intensity levels.

The impact of a retrocochlear disorder often depends on the level in the auditory nervous system at which the disorder is located. A disorder of the eighth nerve is likely to have a significant impact on hearing sensitivity and on speech perception. A disorder of the brainstem may spare hearing sensitivity and negatively influence only hearing of speech in noisy or other complex acoustic environments.

Auditory Processing Disorder

Auditory processing disorders are most common in children and in aging adults. These disorders are characterized by poor suprathreshold hearing. A primary sign of auditory processing disorder is hearing ability that seems to be disproportionate to the degree of hearing sensitivity loss. The most common symptom is difficulty extracting a signal of interest from a background of noise. Patients simply have difficulty hearing in noise. Another common symptom is difficulty localizing a sound source, especially in the presence of background noise. These symptoms are not unlike those of patients with peripheral hearing sensitivity loss, but they are usually out of proportion to what might be expected from the degree of loss. It should be no surprise that an auditory disorder, regardless of its locus, would result in similar perceived difficulties. Perhaps the distinguishing feature for patients with an auditory processing disorder is the inability to extract sounds of interest in noisy environments despite an ability to perceive the sounds with adequate loudness. These patients also exhibit difficulty on various tasks related to spatial hearing.

Functional Hearing Loss

Functional hearing loss is the exaggeration or feigning of hearing impairment. Many terms have been used to describe this type of hearing "impairment," including nonorganic hearing loss, pseudohypacusis, malingering, factitious hearing loss, and so on. Since there may be some organicity to the hearing loss, it is probably best considered as an exaggerated hearing loss or a functional overlay to an organic loss. The term functional hearing loss is the term most commonly used to describe such outcomes.

In many cases of functional hearing loss, particularly in adults, an organic hearing sensitivity loss exists but is willfully exaggerated,[11] usually for compensation. In other cases, often secondary to trauma of some kind, the entire hearing loss is willfully feigned.

Adults and children feign hearing loss for different reasons. Adults usually seek secondary emotional or financial gain. Thus, an employee may apply for worker's compensation for hearing loss secondary to excessive sound exposure in the workplace; alternatively, an individual discharged from the military may seek compensation for hearing loss from excessive noise exposure. Although most patients have legitimate concerns and provide honest results, a small percentage try to exaggerate hearing loss in the mistaken notion that they will receive greater compensation. There are also those who have had an accident or altercation and are involved in a lawsuit against an insurance company, for example. Occasionally, such a person will think that feigning a hearing loss will lead to a greater monetary award.

Children with functional hearing loss often are using hearing impairment as an excuse for poor performance in school or to gain attention. The idea may have emerged from watching a classmate or sibling receive special treatment for having a hearing impairment. It may also be secondary to a bout of otitis media and the consequent parental attention paid to the episode.

AUDIOLOGIC ASSESSMENT TOOLS

Behavioral Measures

Pure-Tone Audiometry

Pure-tone audiometry is used to establish hearing threshold sensitivity at discrete frequencies across a range important for human communication. Threshold levels are plotted on an audiogram to show how threshold sensitivity varies across the frequency range. The complete pure-tone audiogram consists of air- and bone-conduction threshold curves for each ear.

The pure-tone audiogram is based on audiometric zero, or average normal hearing, across a defined frequency range. By definition, 0 dB HL is the average intensity level at which threshold of sensitivity is measured in normal-hearing individuals. For clinical purposes, the standard deviation is considered to be 5 dB, so that 95% of the normal population will have thresholds varying from −10 to +10 dB HL. Based on the pure-tone audiogram, then, hearing loss is often classified as minimal (15 to 25 dB), mild (25 to 40 dB), moderate (40 to 55 dB), moderately severe (55 to 70 dB), severe (70 to 90 dB), or profound (more than 90 dB). Although hearing loss in the minimal range may or may not result in impairment or handicap, it is incorrect to consider thresholds in this range to be within normal limits. The pure-tone audiogram is also used to describe the shape of loss or the audiometric contour or configuration. The audiogram also provides a measure of interaural symmetry or the extent to which hearing sensitivity is the same in both ears or better in one than the other. In addition, the combination of air- and bone-conduction audiometry is used to determine type of hearing loss.

Speech Audiometry

Speech audiometric measures are used routinely in an audiologic evaluation to measure threshold for speech, cross-check pure-tone sensitivity, quantify suprathreshold hearing, and assist in differential diagnosis.

For clinical purposes, speech audiometric measures fall into one of three categories: speech recognition threshold, word recognition score, and sensitized speech measures. In a typical clinical situation, a speech threshold (awareness or recognition) will be determined early as a cross-check for the validity of pure-tone thresholds.[12] Following completion of pure-tone audiometry, word recognition scores will be obtained as estimates of suprathreshold speech understanding in quiet. Finally, either as part of a comprehensive audiologic evaluation or as part of an expanded speech audiometric battery, sensitized speech measures will be obtained to assess processing at the level of the central auditory nervous system.

The most common way to describe suprathreshold hearing ability is with word recognition measures. Word recognition testing, also referred to as speech discrimination, word discrimination, and phonetically balanced (PB) word testing, is an assessment of a patient's ability to identify and repeat single-syllable words presented at some suprathreshold level. Speech recognition ability is usually measured with monosyllabic word tests. A number of tests have been developed over the years.[13–15] Most use single-syllable words in lists of 25 or 50. Lists are usually developed to resemble, to some degree, the phonetic content of speech in a particular language. Word lists are presented to patients at suprathreshold levels, and the patients are instructed to repeat the words. Speech recognition is expressed as a percentage of correct identification of words presented.

The goal of word recognition testing is to estimate the patient's maximum ability or score. To obtain a maximum score, lists of words or sentences are presented at several intensity levels, extending from just above the speech threshold to the upper level of comfortable listening. In this way, a performance versus intensity (PI) function is generated for each ear. The shape of this function often has important diagnostic significance. In most cases, the PI function rises systematically as speech intensity is increased to an asymptotic level representing the best speech understanding that can be achieved in the test ear. In some cases, however, there is a paradoxical rollover effect in which the function declines substantially as speech intensity increases beyond the level producing the maximal performance score. In other words, as speech intensity increases, performance rises to a maximum level and then declines or "rolls over" sharply as intensity continues to increase. This rollover effect is commonly observed when the site of the hearing loss is retrocochlear, in the auditory nerve or the auditory pathways in the brainstem.[16,17] The use of PI functions is a way of sensitizing speech by challenging the auditory system at high intensity levels. Because of its ease of admin-

istration, many audiologists use it routinely as a screening measure for retrocochlear disorders. The most efficacious clinical strategy is to present a word list simply at the highest intensity level and terminate testing if the score is sufficient to rule out rollover.

Interpretation of word recognition measures is based on the predictable relation of maximum word recognition scores to degree of hearing loss.[18,19] If the maximum score falls within a given range for a given degree of hearing loss, then the results are considered to be within expectation for a cochlear hearing loss. If the score is poorer than expected, then word recognition ability is considered to be abnormal for the degree of hearing loss and consistent with retrocochlear disorder. Table 8–1 can be used to determine whether a score exceeds expectations based on the degree of hearing loss. The number represents the lowest maximum score that 95% of individuals with cochlear hearing loss will obtain on a specified measure. Any score below this number for a given hearing loss is considered to be abnormal.

Other techniques for measuring suprathreshold hearing involve sensitizing speech in some way to more effectively challenge the auditory system. Such measures

Table 8–1 LOWER LIMITS OF MAXIMUM WORD RECOGNITION FOR TWO SPEECH AUDIOMETRIC MEASURES AS A FUNCTION OF COCHLEAR HEARING SENSITIVITY LOSS FOR THE NU-6 TEST[18] OR FOR THE PAL PB-50 TEST[19]			
PTA (dB)	NU-6 (%)	PTA2 (dB)	PAL PB-50
0	100	0	90
5	96	5	84
10	96	10	78
15	92	15	74
20	88	20	69
25	80	25	63
30	76	30	58
35	68	35	53
40	64	40	48
45	56	45	42
50	48	50	37
55	44	55	32
60	36	60	26
65	32	65	21
70	28	70	16
		75	12
		80	8
		85	4

PTA = pure-tone average of thousands at 500, 1,000, and 2,000 Hz;
PTF2 = pure-tone average of thousands at 1,000, 2,000, and 4,000 Hz;
NU-6 = Northwestern University Auditory Test No. 6;
PAL = psychoacoustics laboratory; PB = phonetically balanced.

include low-pass filtered speech,[20–22] time-compressed speech,[23,24] and the presentation of speech in noise or competition.[25] Another effective approach for assessing suprathreshold hearing is the use of dichotic tests.[26–30] In the dichotic paradigm, two different speech targets are presented simultaneously to the two ears. The pattern of results can reveal auditory processing deficits, especially those caused by disorders of the temporal lobe and corpus callosum.

Speech audiometric measures can be useful in differentiating whether a hearing disorder is caused by changes in the outer or middle ear, cochlea, or auditory peripheral or central nervous systems. A summary is presented in Table 8–2. In the case of a cochlear disorder, word recognition ability is usually predictable from the degree and slope of the audiogram. Although there are some exceptions, such as hearing loss caused by endolymphatic hydrops, word recognition ability and performance on other forms of speech audiometric measures are highly correlated with degree of hearing impairment in certain frequency regions. When performance is poorer than expected, the likely culprit is a disorder of the eighth nerve or central auditory nervous system structures. Thus, unusually poor performance on speech audiometric tests lends a measure of suspicion about the site of the disorder causing the hearing impairment.

Speech audiometric measures are also used to measure suprathreshold hearing. As neural impulses travel from the cochlea through the eighth nerve to the auditory brainstem and cortex, the number and complexity of neural pathways expand progressively. The system, in its vastness of pathways, includes a certain level of redundancy or excess capacity of processing ability. Such redundancy serves many useful purposes, but it also makes the function of the auditory nervous system somewhat impervious to examination. For example, a patient can have a rather substantial lesion of the auditory brainstem or auditory cortex and still have normal hearing and normal word recognition ability. Accordingly, sensitized speech audiometric measures must be used to assess auditory nervous system function and dysfunction.

Other Behavioral Measures

A number of other behavioral measures can be used for various purposes in the audiologic evaluation. Some of the early strategies designed to differentiate cochlear from retrocochlear disorder were based primarily on measures of auditory adaptation and recruitment. They are seldom used in modern practice and will be described only briefly here.

One of the consequences of cochlear hearing loss is recruitment, or abnormal loudness growth. That is, loudness grows more rapidly than normal at intensity levels just above threshold in an ear with cochlear site of disorder. Clinically, this means that if recruitment is present, then the site of disorder is cochlear rather than retrocochlear. One effective way to measure recruitment is with the alternate binaural loudness balance (ABLB) test.[31] The ABLB was designed for use in patients with unilateral hearing loss and was shown to be reasonably effective in identifying a cochlear site of lesion.[32,33] Another strategy involved measuring the difference limen for intensity. An indirect method that was used clinically for a number of years is the short increment sensitivity index (SISI).[34–37] It, too, was shown to be effective in identifying cochlear hearing loss.

Another consequence of retrocochlear hearing loss is abnormal auditory adaptation. The normal auditory system tends to adapt to ongoing sound, especially at near-threshold levels, so that, as adaptation occurs, an audible signal becomes inaudible. At higher intensity levels, ongoing sound tends to remain audible without adaptation. However, in an ear with retrocochlear disorder, the audibility may diminish rapidly owing to excessive auditory adaptation even at higher intensity levels. Two popular behavioral measures of adaptation in the past were the tone decay test (TDT)[38–40] and diagnostic Békésy audiometry.[41,42] These tests were designed to assess the patient's ability to perceive sustained tones. Although popular for a time, the

Table 8–2 EXPECTED PATTERNS OF ABNORMALITY ON SPEECH AUDIOMETRIC TESTS AS A FUNCTION OF SITE OF DISORDER					
Site	WRS max	WRS PI	SC max	SC PI	Dichotic
Cochlea	–	–	–	–	–
Eighth nerve	++	++	++	++	–
Brainstem	–	+	++	++	–
Temporal lobe	–	–	+	+	++

Tests include maximum word recognition scores presented in quiet (WRS max), performance-intensity function of word recognition scores in quiet (WRS PI), maximum score on sentence identification in competition (SC max), performance-intensity function of sentence identification in competition (SC PI), and score on a dichotic measure. Predicted performance on these measures would be –, normal or predictable from the degree of hearing sensitivity loss; +, sometimes abnormal, depending on the site, size, and extent of influence of the lesion; or ++, usually abnormal.

tests were not particularly sensitive to eighth nerve disorder or specific to cochlear disorder.[43–46]

All of these measures—ABLB, SISI, TDT, and Békésy audiometry—were useful in the diagnosis of retrocochlear site in the days when tumors or other disorders had to reach a substantial size before they could be diagnosed radiographically. As imaging and radiographic techniques improved, smaller lesions that had less functional impact on the auditory system could be visualized and the utility of the classic test battery diminished. Today these measures are mostly of historical interest, although they can occasionally be useful in evaluating patients with severe hearing loss.

One behavioral diagnostic measure that has withstood the test of time is a measure of lower brainstem function known as the masking level difference (MLD). Abnormal performance on the MLD is consistent with brainstem disorder.[47–50] The MLD measures binaural release from masking owing to interaural phase relationships. The binaural auditory system is an exquisite detector of differences in timing of sound reaching the two ears and thus helps in localizing low-frequency sounds, which reach the ears at different points in time. The MLD is based on the concept of binaural release from masking, which occurs as a result of processing by the brainstem at the level of the superior olivary complex. The concept can be described as follows: if identical low-frequency tones are presented in phase to both ears and noise is added to both ears to mask the tones, when the phase of the tone delivered to one earphone is reversed, the tone becomes audible again.

The MLD test is designed to measure binaural release from masking. To carry out the MLD test, a 500-Hz interrupted tone is split and presented in phase to both ears. Narrow-band noise is also presented, at a fixed level of 60 dB HL. Using a tracking procedure, threshold for the in-phase tones is determined in the presence of the noise. Then the phase of one of the tones is reversed, and threshold is tracked again. The MLD is the difference in threshold between the in-phase and the out-of-phase conditions. For a 500-Hz tone, the MLD should be greater than 7 dB and is usually around 12 dB.

A number of behavioral measures are used to identify patients who are feigning hearing loss and to try to quantify the degree of any underlying organic disor-

der.[51] Two that have withstood the test of time are the Stenger and Lombard tests.

The Stenger test is designed to identify functional hearing loss in patients with unilateral or significantly asymmetric hearing loss. If the hearing loss is feigned or exaggerated, the Stenger test can detect the functional component. The test is based on the principle that tones presented to both ears will be perceived only in the ear in which the tone is louder if an ear difference exists. To carry out the test, either speech or pure-tone stimuli are presented simultaneously to both ears. Initially, the signal is presented to the good ear at a comfortable, audible level of about 20-dB sensation level and to the poorer ear at 20 dB below the level of the good ear. The patient will respond because he/she will hear the signal presented to the good ear. Testing proceeds by increasing the intensity level of the signal presented to the poorer ear. If the loss in the poorer ear is organic, the patient will continue to respond to the signal being presented to the good ear (ie, a negative Stenger). If the loss is functional, the patient will stop responding when the loudness of the signal in the poorer ear exceeds that in the good ear because the signal will be heard only in the poorer ear owing to the Stenger principle. Because an audible signal is still being presented to the good ear, it becomes clear that the patient is not cooperating. This result is a positive Stenger, indicative of functional hearing loss.

The Lombard test is used in the patient with suspected bilateral functional hearing loss. It is based on the principle that a patient's vocal effort will be raised in the presence of background noise. The test involves the sudden presentation of noise to a patient reading aloud and an assessment of any change in vocal intensity. Thus, the Lombard test, along with other behavioral measures, can be used to identify the presence of functional hearing loss.

The audiologic goal in cases of functional hearing loss is to establish a valid and reliable behavioral audiogram that indicates the true extent of the hearing loss. Should behavioral measures fail, auditory evoked potentials are used to predict hearing sensitivity.

Pure-tone audiometry, speech audiometry, and the other procedures noted above constitute the basic behavioral measures available to quantify hearing impairment and determine the type and site of auditory disorder.

Electroacoustic and Electrophysiologic Measures

Immittance Audiometry

Immittance audiometry is one of the most powerful tools available for the evaluation of auditory disorder.[52] It serves at least three functions in audiologic assessment: (1) it is sensitive in detecting middle ear disorder, (2) it can be useful in differentiating a cochlear from a retrocochlear disorder, and (3) it is helpful in estimating the degree of peripheral hearing sensitivity and is often used as a cross-check to pure-tone audiometry in pediatric assessment. As a result of its comprehensive value, immittance audiometry is a routine component of the audiologic evaluation and is often the first assessment administered in the test battery.

Immittance is a physical characteristic of all mechanical vibratory systems. In very general terms, it is a measure of how readily a system can be set into vibration by a driving force. The ease with which energy will flow through the vibrating system is called its admittance. The reciprocal concept, the extent to which the system resists the flow of energy through it, is called its impedance. If a vibrating system can be forced into motion with little applied force, the admittance is high and the impedance is low. On the other hand, if the system resists being set into motion until the driving force is relatively high, then the admittance of the system is low and the impedance is high. Immittance is a term that is meant to encompass both of these concepts.

Immittance audiometry can be thought of as a way to assess the manner in which energy flows through the outer and middle ears to the cochlea. If the middle ear system is normal, energy will flow in a predictable way. If it is not, then energy will flow either too well (high admittance) or not well enough (high impedance).

Immittance is measured by delivering a pure-tone signal of a constant sound pressure level into the ear canal through a mechanical probe that is seated at the entrance of the ear canal. The signal, which is referred to by convention as the probe tone, is a 220-Hz pure tone that is delivered at 85 dB SPL. The sound pressure level of the probe tone is monitored by an immittance meter, and any change is noted as a change in energy flow through the middle ear system.

Three immittance measures are generally used in the clinical assessment of middle ear function: tympanometry, static immittance, and acoustic reflex thresholds.

Tympanometry measures how the acoustic immittance of the middle ear vibratory system changes as air pressure is varied in the external ear canal. Transmission of sound through the middle ear mechanism is maximal when air pressure is equal on both sides of the tympanic membrane. For a normal ear, maximum transmission occurs at or near atmospheric pressure. The clinical value of tympanometry is that middle ear disorder modifies the shape of the tympanogram in predictable ways. Various tympanometric patterns are related to various auditory disorders. The conventional classification system designates three tympanogram types: A, B, and C.[53] The characteristically normal shape, with its peak at atmospheric pressure (0 daPa), is designated Type A.

If the middle ear space is filled with fluid (eg, as in otitis media with effusion), then the tympanogram loses its sharp peak and becomes relatively flat or only slightly rounded; this pattern is caused by the mass added to the ossicular chain by the fluid. This shape is designated Type B.

In eustachian tube dysfunction, oxygen becomes trapped in the middle ear and is absorbed by the mucosal lining, resulting in a reduction of air pressure in the middle ear space relative to the pressure in the external ear canal. This pressure differential draws the tympanic membrane medially. The effect on the tympanogram is to move the sharp peak away from 0 daPa and into the negative air pressure region, reflecting the fact that the maximum energy flow occurs when the pressure in the ear canal is negative, this matching that in the middle ear space. This tympanogram, which is normal in shape but peaks at a substantially negative air pressure, is designated Type C.

Anything that causes the ossicular chain to become stiffer than normal can result in a reduction in energy flow through the middle ear. The added stiffness simply attenuates the peak of the tympanogram. The shape will remain normal Type A, but the entire tympanogram will become shallower. Such a tympanogram is designated Type A_s to indicate that the shape is normal, with the peak at or near 0 daPa of air pressure but with significant reduction in the height of the peak. The subscript "s" denotes stiffness or shallowness. The disorder most commonly associated with a Type A_s tympanogram is otosclerosis.

Anything that causes the ossicular chain to lose stiffness can result in too much energy flow through the middle ear. For example, in ossicular discontinuity (effectively detaching the tympanic membrane from the cochlea), the tympanogram retains its normal shape, but the peak is much greater than normal. With the heavy load of the cochlear fluid system removed from the chain, the tympanic membrane responds more freely to forced vibration. The energy flow through the middle ear is greatly enhanced, resulting in a very deep tympanogram. This shape is designated A_d to indicate that the shape of the tympanogram is normal, with the peak at or near 0 daPa of air pressure, but the height is significantly increased. The subscript "d" denotes deep or discontinuity.

In contrast to the dynamic measure of middle ear function represented by the tympanogram, static immittance refers to the isolated contribution of the middle ear to the overall acoustic immittance of the auditory system. It can be thought of as simply the absolute height of the tympanogram at its peak. The static immittance is measured by comparing the probe-tone sound pressure level or immittance when the air pressure is at 0 daPa, or at the air pressure corresponding to the peak, with the immittance when the air pressure is raised to positive 200 daPa. Values lying below 0.3 cc or above 1.6 cc are strong evidence of middle ear disorder. This information is useful in deciding whether a Type A tympanogram is normal, shallow, or deep. For example, if the tympanogram is Type A and the static immittance is 0.2, then the tympanogram can be considered shallow and indicative of increased stiffness of the middle ear mechanism. Unfortunately, the range of normal static immittance is so large that many of the milder forms of middle ear disorder will fall within the normal boundaries. Thus, the test lacks transitivity in that only one outcome is meaningful. That is, if the static immittance falls outside the normal range, it is safe to predict middle ear disorder. But values within the normal range do not necessarily exclude the possibility of middle ear disorder.

A number of other strategies for tympanometric assessment have emerged over the years in an effort to more accurately and sensitively measure middle ear function.[54,55] Measures of multifrequency tympanometry,[56] multicomponent analysis,[57] otoreflectance,[58] and other methods can be used for this purpose. The clinical challenge resulting from these sensitive measures of function is often one of understanding the relation of measurement outcome to active ear disease. Because they are so sensitive, such measures are prone to false-positive identification of meaningful otologic conditions.

The third measure of the typical immittance battery is the acoustic stapedial reflex. The stapedius muscle is attached, via its tendon, to the head of the stapes. When the muscle contracts, the tendon exerts tension on the stapes, stiffens the ossicular chain, and reduces low-frequency energy transmission through the middle ear. The result of this reduced energy transmission is an increase in probe-tone SPL in the external ear canal. Therefore, when the stapedius muscle contracts in response to high-intensity sounds, a slight change in immittance can be detected by the circuitry of the immittance instrument.

Both stapedius muscles contract in response to sound delivered to one ear. Therefore, ipsilateral (uncrossed) and contralateral (crossed) reflexes are recorded with sound presented to each ear. For example, when a signal of sufficient magnitude is presented to the right ear, a stapedius reflex will occur in both the right (ipsilateral or uncrossed) and the left (contralateral or crossed) ears. These are called the right uncrossed and right crossed reflexes, respectively. When a signal is presented to the left ear and a reflex is measured in that ear, it is referred to as a left uncrossed reflex. When a signal is presented to the left ear and a reflex is measured in the right ear, it is referred to as a left crossed reflex.

The threshold is the most common measure of the acoustic stapedial reflex and is defined as the lowest intensity level at which a middle ear immittance change can be detected in response to sound. In patients with normal hearing and normal middle ear function, reflex thresholds for pure tones will be reached at levels ranging from 70 to 100 dB HL. The average threshold level is approximately 85 dB. These levels are constant across the frequency range from 500 to 4,000 Hz. Threshold measures are useful for at least two purposes: differential assessment of auditory disorder and prediction of hearing sensitivity.

Several methods have been developed for using acoustic reflex thresholds to predict hearing sensitivity. One method that has gained some popularity is the sensitivity prediction by the acoustic reflex (SPAR) test.[59,60] The SPAR test is based on the well-documented difference between acoustic reflex thresholds to pure tones versus broad-band noise (BBN) and on the change in BBN thresholds, but not pure-tone thresholds, as a result of sensorineural hearing loss. That is, thresholds to BBN signals are lower than thresholds to pure-tone signals.

However, sensorineural hearing loss has a differential effect on the two signals, raising the threshold to BBN signals but not to pure-tone signals. The SPAR test capitalizes on this effect to provide a general prediction of the presence or absence of hearing loss.

To compute the SPAR value, the BBN threshold is subtracted from the average reflex threshold to pure tones of 500, 1,000, and 2,000 Hz. The magnitude of this difference will vary according to the specific equipment used to carry out the measures. A correction factor is then applied to yield a SPAR value of 20 in normal-hearing subjects. If a patient's SPAR value is less than 15, there is a high probability of a sensorineural hearing loss.

Use of the SPAR or other techniques based on acoustic reflex thresholds is effective only in predicting general degree of hearing loss. Clinical application of such techniques appears to be most effective when used to predict presence or absence of a sensorineural hearing loss. Prediction of hearing sensitivity by acoustic reflex thresholds can be very valuable in testing a child on whom behavioral thresholds cannot be obtained and for sensitivity prediction in the case of a patient who is feigning hearing loss.

Reflex threshold measurement has been valuable in both the assessment of middle ear function and the differentiation of cochlear from retrocochlear disorder.[61–63] In terms of the latter, whereas reflex thresholds occur at reduced sensation levels in ears with cochlear hearing loss, they are typically elevated or absent in ears having an eighth nerve disorder. Similarly, reflex thresholds are often abnormal in patients with a brainstem disorder. Comparison of crossed and uncrossed thresholds has also been found to be helpful in differentiating eighth nerve from brainstem disorders.[64]

Auditory Evoked Potentials

An auditory evoked potential is a waveform that reflects the electrophysiologic function of a specific portion of the central auditory nervous system in response to sound. For audiologic purposes, it is convenient to group the auditory evoked potentials into categories based loosely on the latency ranges over which the potentials are observed. The earliest of the evoked potentials, occurring within the first 5 msec following signal presentation, is the electrocochleogram (ECoG) and reflects activity of the cochlea and eighth nerve.

The most frequently used evoked potential is the auditory brainstem response (ABR), which occurs within the first 10 msec following signal onset. The ABR reflects neural activity from the eighth nerve to the midbrain. The middle latency response (MLR) occurs within the first 50 msec following signal onset and reflects activity at or near the auditory cortex. The late latency response (LLR) occurs within the first 250 msec following signal onset and reflects activity of the primary-auditory and association areas of the cerebral cortex.

Diagnostic assessment is usually conducted with the ABR, MLR, and LLR. The ABR is highly sensitive to disorders of the eighth nerve and auditory brainstem and is often used in conjunction with imaging and radiologic measures to assist in the diagnosis of acoustic tumors and brainstem disorders.[65–70] Surgical monitoring of evoked potentials is usually carried out with ECoG, ABR, and/or direct-nerve recordings.[71,72] These evoked potentials are monitored during eighth nerve tumor removal surgery in an effort to preserve hearing.

The ECoG is a response composed mainly of the compound action potential that occurs at the distal portion of the eighth nerve. A click stimulus is used to elicit this response. The rapid onset of the click provides a stimulus that is sufficient to cause the fibers of the eighth nerve to fire in synchrony. This synchronous discharge of nerve fibers results in the action potential. There are two other, smaller components of the ECoG. One is referred to as the cochlear microphonic, which is a response from the cochlea that mimics the input stimulus. The other is the summating potential, which is a direct current response that reflects the envelope of the input stimulus.

The ECoG is best recorded as a near-field response, with an electrode close to the source. Unlike the ABR, MLR, and LLR, which can readily be recorded as far-field responses with remote electrodes, it is more difficult to record the ECoG from surface electrodes. Thus, the best recordings of the ECoG are made from an electrode that is placed through the tympanic membrane and onto the promontory of the cochlea or from an electrode in the ear canal placed near the tympanic membrane.

The ABR occurs within the first 10 msec following signal onset and consists of a series of five positive peaks or waves. The ABR has properties that make it very useful clinically. First, the response can be recorded from surface electrodes. Second, the waves are robust and can be recorded easily in patients with adequate hearing and normal auditory nervous system function. Third, the response is immune to the influences of the patient's state so that it can be recorded in patients who are sleeping or sedated. Fourth, the latencies of the various waves are quite stable within and across individuals so that they serve as a sensitive measure of brainstem integrity. In addition, the time intervals between peaks are prolonged by auditory disorders central to the cochlea, which makes the ABR useful for differentiating cochlear from retrocochlear sites of disorder.

The ABR is generated by the auditory nerve and by structures in the auditory brainstem. Wave I originates in the distal or peripheral portion of the eighth nerve near the point at which the nerve fibers leave the cochlea. Wave II originates from the proximal portion of the nerve near the brainstem. Wave III has contribution from this proximal portion of the nerve and from the cochlear nucleus. Waves IV and V have contributions from the cochlear nucleus, superior olivary complex, and lateral lemniscus.

The MLR is characterized by two successive positive peaks: the first (Pa) at about 25 to 35 msec and the second (Pb) at about 40 to 60 msec following stimulus presentation. The MLR is probably generated by some combination of projections to the primary auditory cortex and the cortical area itself. Although the MLR is the most difficult auditory evoked potential to record clinically, it is sometimes used diagnostically and as an aid in the identification of auditory processing disorder.

The LLR is characterized by a negative peak (N1) at a latency of about 90 msec followed by a positive peak (P2) at about 180 msec following stimulus presentation. This potential is greatly affected by subject state. It is best recorded when the patient is awake and carefully attending to the sounds being presented. There is an important developmental effect on the LLR during the first 8 to 10 years of age. In older children or adults, however, it is robust and relatively easy to record. In children or adults with relatively normal hearing sensitivity, abnormality or absence of the LLR is associated with auditory processing disorder.

Otoacoustic Emissions

Otoacoustic emissions are low-intensity sounds that are generated by the cochlea and are carried by the middle ear into the ear canal.[73,74] Otoacoustic emissions are probably not essential to hearing but rather are the by-product of active processing by the outer hair cells. Of clinical interest is that OAEs are present when outer hair cells are healthy and absent when outer hair cells are damaged. Thus, OAEs reveal, with exquisite sensitivity, the integrity of outer hair cell function.

There are two broad categories of OAEs: spontaneous and evoked. Spontaneous OAEs are narrow-band signals that occur in the ear canal without the introduction of an eliciting signal. Spontaneous OAEs are present in over half of all normal-hearing ears and absent in all ears at frequencies at which sensorineural hearing loss exceeds approximately 30 dB. It appears that spontaneous OAEs originate from outer hair cells corresponding to that portion of the basilar membrane tuned to their frequency.

A sensitive, low-noise microphone housed in a probe is used to record spontaneous OAEs. The probe is secured in the external auditory canal with a flexible cuff. Signals detected by the microphone are routed to a spectrum analyzer, which is a device that provides real-time frequency analysis of the signal. Usually, the frequency range of interest is swept several times, and the results are signal-averaged to reduce background noise. Spontaneous OAEs, when they occur, appear as peaks of energy along the frequency spectrum.

Because spontaneous OAEs are absent in many ears with normal hearing, clinical applications have not been forthcoming. Efforts to relate spontaneous OAEs to tinnitus have revealed a relationship in some but not many subjects who have both. Other clinical applications await development.

Evoked OAEs occur during and after the presentation of a stimulus. That is, an evoked OAE is elicited by a stimulus. Evoked OAEs bear a close resemblance to the eliciting signal; thus, the term echo has been employed to describe them. There are several classes of evoked OAEs, two of which have proven to be useful clinically: transient evoked OAEs (TEOAEs) and distortion-product otoacoustic emissions (DPOAEs).[75,76]

Transient evoked OAEs are elicited with transient signals or clicks. Series of click stimuli are presented, usually at an intensity level of about 80 to 85 dB SPL. Output from the microphone is signal-averaged, usually within a time window of 20 msec. In a typical clinical paradigm, alternating samples of the emission are placed into separate memory locations so that the final result provides two traces of the response for comparison purposes.

Transient evoked OAEs begin about 4 msec following stimulus presentation and persist for about 10 msec. Because a click is a broad-spectrum signal, the echo is similarly broad in spectrum as well. By convention, these waveforms are subjected to spectral analysis, the results of which are often shown in a graph depicting the amplitude-versus-frequency components of the emission. One important aspect of TEOAE analysis is the reproducibility of the response. This similarity or reproducibility of successive samples of a response is expressed as a percentage, with 100% being identical. If the magnitude of the emission exceeds the magnitude of the noise, and if the reproducibility of the emission exceeds a predetermined level, then the emission is said to be present. If an emission is present, it is likely that the outer hair cells are functioning in the frequency region of the emission.

Distortion-product OAEs occur as a result of nonlinear processes in the cochlea. When two tones are presented to the cochlea, distortion occurs in the form of other tones that are not present in the two-tone eliciting signals. These distortions are combination tones or harmonics that are related to the eliciting tones in a predictable mathematical way. The two tones used to elicit the DPOAE are, by convention, designated f_1 and f_2. The most robust distortion product occurs at the frequency represented by the equation $2f_1 - f_2$. As with TEOAEs, a probe is used to deliver the tone pairs and to record the response. Pairs of tones are presented across the frequency range to elicit distortion products from approximately 1,000 to 6,000 Hz. The tone pairs that are presented are at a fixed frequency and intensity relationship. Typically, the pairs are presented from low frequency to high frequency. As each pair is presented, measurements are made at the $2f_1 - f_2$ frequency to determine the amplitude of the DPOAE and also at a nearby frequency to provide an estimate of the noise floor at that moment in time.

Distortion-product OAEs are typically depicted as the amplitude of the distortion product as a function of frequency of the f_2 tone. If the amplitude exceeds the background noise, the emission is said to be present. If an emission is present, it is likely that the outer hair cells are functioning in the frequency region of the f_2 tone.

The results of TEOAE and DPOAE testing provide a measure of the integrity of outer hair cell function. Both approaches have been successfully applied clinically as objective indicators of cochlear function.

DIFFERENTIAL DIAGNOSIS AND MEASUREMENT OUTCOME

Functional outcomes of structural changes in the auditory system are reasonably predictable from the battery of assessment tools described. Table 8–3 summarizes the probable outcomes as a function of disorder sites.

Outer and Middle Ear Disorders

Audiologic determination of the nature of the outer and middle ear disorder relates to the consequence that a disorder has on the function of the outer and middle ear structures. For example, excessive cerumen in the ear canal may or may not impede the transduction of sound to the tympanic membrane. Similarly, tympanosclerosis may or may not reduce the functioning of the tympanic membrane. The first goal is to determine whether

Table 8–3 EXPECTED OUTCOMES ON AUDIOMETRIC MEASURES AS A FUNCTION OF SITE OF DISORDER

Measure	Cochlea	VIIIth Nerve	Brainstem	Temporal Lobe
Otoacoustic emissions	++	+	–	–
Pure-tone audiometry	++	+	+	–
Word recognition scores	–	++	+	–
Acoustic reflexes	–	++	+	–
Auditory brainstem response	–	++	++	–
Dichotic speech measures	–	–	+	++

Predicted performance on these measures would be –, normal or predictable from the degree of hearing sensitivity loss; +, sometimes abnormal, depending on the site, size, and extent of influence of the lesion; or ++, usually abnormal.

these structural changes result in a disorder in function.

The second goal of the evaluation is to determine whether and how much this disorder in function is causing a hearing loss. In some circumstances, a structural change in the outer and middle ear can result in outer or middle ear disorder without causing a measurable loss of hearing. For example, a tympanic membrane can be perforated without causing a significant conductive hearing loss. On the other hand, a similar perforation located elsewhere on the tympanic membrane can result in a substantial conductive hearing loss. Similarly, eustachian tube dysfunction, resulting in significant negative pressure in the middle ear space, may result in hearing loss in one case but not in another.

In cases of outer and middle ear disorder, the pure-tone audiogram will often be an important metric by which the outcome of the treatment is judged. That is, the pretreatment audiogram will be compared with the post-treatment audiogram to evaluate the success of the treatment.

Immittance audiometry is used to evaluate outer and middle ear function, and pure-tone audiometry is used to evaluate the degree of conductive component caused by the presence of middle ear disorder. In most cases, rudimentary speech audiometry will be carried out as a cross-check of pure-tone thresholds and as a gross assessment of suprathreshold word recognition ability.

Immittance Audiometry

The first step in the evaluation process is immittance audiometry. Because it is the most sensitive indicator of middle ear function, a full battery of tympanometry, static immittance, and acoustic reflex thresholds is indicated. The results will provide information indicating whether a disorder is caused by

- an increase in the mass of the middle ear mechanism,
- an increase or decrease in the stiffness of the middle ear system,
- the presence of a perforation of the tympanic membrane, or
- significant negative pressure in the middle ear space.

If all immittance results are normal, any hearing loss measured by pure-tone audiometry can be attributed to sensorineural hearing loss. If immittance results indicate the presence of a middle ear disorder, pure-tone audiom-

etry by air and bone conduction must be carried out to assess the degree of conductive component of the hearing loss attributable to the middle ear disorder.

Immittance results vary with the nature of the disorder. The pattern of results consistent with an increase in the mass of the middle ear system—for example, otitis media with effusion and cholesteatoma—comprises a Type B tympanogram, excessively low static immittance, and absent reflexes recorded in the disordered ear (in the case of right ear disorder, right uncrossed and left crossed acoustic reflexes would be absent).

An increase in the stiffness of the middle ear system (eg, otosclerosis) demonstrates a pattern of results characterized by a Type $_A$s tympanogram, relatively low static immittance, and absent acoustic reflexes in the probe ear.

Excessive immittance of the middle ear system, exemplified by ossicular disarticulation, manifests a pattern of results characterized by a Type A_d tympanogram, excessively high static immittance, and absent acoustic reflexes in the probe ear (if the left ear is affected, then the left uncrossed and right crossed will be absent).

A perforation of the tympanic membrane yields another pattern of immittance findings, characterized by an inability to measure a tympanogram, excessive volume, and unmeasurable acoustic reflexes from the affected probe ear (in the case of right ear disorder, the right uncrossed and left crossed reflexes would be absent).

The pattern of results consistent with significant negative pressure in the middle ear space, secondary to eustachian tube dysfunction, is composed of a Type C tympanogram (peak at < -200 daPa), normal static immittance, and absent acoustic reflexes in the probe ear.

Pure-Tone Audiometry

Pure-tone audiometry is used to quantify the degree to which a middle ear disorder contributes to a hearing sensitivity loss. If immittance audiometry shows any abnormality in outer or middle ear function, then complete air- and bone-conduction audiometry is indicated for both ears to determine the degree of conductive hearing loss.

It is important to carry out both air- and bone-conduction testing to quantify the extent of the conductive component. It is important to test both ears because the presence of a conductive hearing loss mandates the use of masking in the nontest ear, and that ear cannot be properly masked without knowledge of its air- and bone-conduction thresholds.

Generally, a middle ear disorder manifests as an air–bone gap on the audiogram. A disorder that adds mass to the system influences the higher frequencies; a disorder that adds or subtracts stiffness affects the lower frequencies. Although the presence of a middle ear disorder is correlated with conductive hearing loss, the correlation is not perfect. The measurement of air- and bone-conduction thresholds is not as sensitive to a middle ear disorder as immittance audiometry or other measures. As a consequence, a middle ear disorder can exist without an air–bone gap. Nevertheless, a middle ear disorder is likely to result in some degree of conductive hearing loss, and pure-tone audiometry can serve as a useful quantification of pre- and post-treatment function.

Speech Audiometry

In cases of outer and middle ear disorder, the most important component of speech audiometry is determination of the speech recognition threshold as a cross-check of the accuracy of pure-tone thresholds. Many audiologists prefer to establish the speech threshold before carrying out pure-tone audiometry so that they have a benchmark for the level at which pure-tone thresholds should occur. Although this is good practice in general, it is particularly useful in the assessment of young children. Speech thresholds can also be established by bone conduction, permitting the quantification of an air–bone gap to speech signals.

Assessment of word recognition is also often carried out, although more as a matter of routine than importance. Conductive hearing loss has a predictable influence on word recognition scores, and if such testing is of value, it is usually only to confirm this expectation.

In conductive hearing loss caused by a middle ear disorder, the effect on speech recognition will be negligible except to elevate the speech threshold by the degree of hearing loss in the ear with the disorder. Suprathreshold speech recognition is not affected by the hearing loss, except to shift the intensity level at which maximum performance is reached by the amount of the air–bone gap.

Auditory Evoked Potentials

Auditory evoked potentials are affected only by conductive hearing loss to the extent that attenuation of the eliciting signals influences waveform interpretation. For example, ABR waveform latencies become longer and earlier waves become less identifiable as intensity level is reduced. A 30-dB conductive hearing loss causes an ABR waveform elicited at 90 dB nHL to resemble a waveform elicited at 60 dB in an otherwise normal ear. Absolute latencies are delayed, but in a predictable manner. Interwave intervals are unaffected. So long as the amount of the air–bone gap is considered, interpretation of the ABR should not be affected.

Otoacoustic Emissions

Otoacoustic emissions are likely to be absent in cases of middle ear disorder.[77–81] Their presence or absence depends both on an adequate signal reaching the cochlea and on the ability of the middle ear to transduce the emission into the ear canal. Thus, if the middle ear disorder is causing a conductive hearing loss of a magnitude sufficient to block the elicitation of a measurable echo, no emission will be recorded. Similarly, if the cochlea generates an emission but the middle ear mechanism does not convey a sufficient response to the ear canal, no emission will be recorded. In routine clinical assessment, the distinction is probably unimportant. Efforts to elicit OAEs with bone-conduction stimulation may clarify the contributing factor in some cases, but the clinical relevance remains unclear.

As is usually the case with OAEs, the absence of OAEs lends little to the diagnostic process other than corroboration of other findings. The presence of a response, however, may provide useful information about the severity of a disorder.

Cochlear Disorders

Audiologic contribution to the assessment of a cochlear disorder is directed at answering the following questions:

- Is there a hearing loss and what is its extent?
- Is the loss solely cochlear or is there also a conductive component?
- Is the loss truly cochlear or is it retrocochlear?
- Is the loss fluctuating or stable?
- Could the loss be attributed to a treatable condition such as endolymphatic hydrops?

The first goal is to determine whether a middle ear disorder is contributing to the problem. The second goal is to determine the degree and type of hearing loss. The third goal is to scrutinize the audiologic findings for any evidence of a retrocochlear disorder. Immittance audiometry is used to evaluate outer and middle ear function, indicate the presence of cochlear hearing loss, and assess the integrity of eighth nerve and lower auditory brainstem function. Pure-tone audiometry is used to evaluate the degree and type of hearing loss. Speech audiometry is used as a cross-check of pure-tone thresholds and as an estimate of suprathreshold word recognition ability.

Immittance Audiometry

In cochlear hearing loss, the tympanogram is normal, static immittance is normal, and acoustic reflex thresholds are consistent with the degree of sensorineural hearing loss. If immittance audiometry suggests the presence of a middle ear disorder, then any cochlear loss is likely to have a superimposed conductive component that must be quantified by pure-tone audiometry. If immittance audiometry is consistent with normal middle ear function but acoustic reflexes are elevated above what would be expected for the degree of sensorineural hearing loss, then suspicion is raised for the possibility of retrocochlear disorder.

Again, the typical immittance pattern associated with a cochlear disorder includes a normal tympanogram, normal static immittance, and normal reflex thresholds.[82] Reflex thresholds are only normal, however, as long as the sensitivity loss by air conduction does not exceed 50 dB HL. Above this level, the reflex threshold is usually elevated in proportion to the degree of loss. Once a behavioral threshold exceeds 70 dB, the absence of a reflex is an equivocal finding because it can be attributed to the degree of peripheral hearing loss and to a retrocochlear disorder.

In ears with cochlear hearing loss, acoustic reflex thresholds are present at reduced sensation levels.[82,83] In normal-hearing ears, behavioral thresholds to pure tones are, by definition, at or around 0 dB HL. Acoustic reflex thresholds occur at or around 85 dB HL, or at a sensation level of 85 dB. In a patient with a sensorineural hearing loss of 40 dB, reflex thresholds still occur at around 85 dB HL, or at a sensation level of 45 dB. This reduced sensation level of the acoustic reflex threshold is characteristic of cochlear hearing loss.

Ears with cochlear hearing loss also show reduced SPARs. That is, the sensitivity prediction by acoustic reflexes is at or below 15 dB, indicative of the presence of cochlear hearing loss.[60]

Pure-Tone Audiometry

Pure-tone audiometry is used to quantify the degree of sensorineural hearing loss caused by the cochlear disorder. If all immittance measures are normal, then air-conduction testing must be completed on both ears. Bone conduction is not necessary because outer and middle ear function are normal, and air-conducted signals can properly evaluate the sensitivity of the cochlea. If all immittance measures are not normal, then air- and bone-conduction thresholds must be obtained for both ears to assess the possibility of the presence of a mixed hearing loss. In either case, both ears must be tested because the use of masking is likely to be necessary and cannot be properly carried out without knowledge of the air- and bone-conduction thresholds of the nontest ear.

Pure-tone audiometry is also important in assessing the symmetry of the hearing loss. If a sensorineural hearing loss is asymmetric, in the absence of another explanation, suspicion is raised for the presence of a retrocochlear disorder.

The hearing loss configuration may provide additional clinical evidence for the cause of the auditory disorder. Characteristic configurations are associated with noise-induced hearing loss, congenital hearing loss, and Meniere's disease and provide some clinical insight as to the nature of the hearing loss.

There are other ways in which pure-tone audiometry can be useful in the otologic diagnosis of cochlear disorder. For those that are dynamic and may be treatable at various stages, the results of pure-tone audiometry can be used as both partial evidence of the presence of the disorder and as a means for assessing benefit from the treatment regimen.

Speech Audiometry

Speech audiometry is used in two ways in the assessment of a cochlear disorder. First, speech reception thresholds are used as a cross-check of the validity of pure-tone thresholds in an effort to ensure the organicity of the disorder. Second, word recognition and other suprathreshold measures are used to assess whether the cochlear hearing loss has the expected effect on speech recognition. That is, in most cases, suprathreshold speech recognition ability is predictable from the degree and configuration of a sensorineural hearing loss if the loss is cochlear.[19] Therefore, if word recognition scores are appropriate for the degree of hearing loss, then the results are consistent with a cochlear site of disorder. If scores are poorer than would be expected from the degree of hearing loss, then suspicion is aroused that the disorder may be retrocochlear.

If a sensorineural hearing loss is caused by a cochlear disorder, the speech threshold is elevated in that ear to a degree predictable by the pure-tone average of audiometric thresholds obtained at 500, 1,000, and 2,000 Hz. Suprathreshold word recognition scores are predictable from the degree of hearing sensitivity loss. Sensitized speech measures are normal or predictable from the degree of loss, and dichotic measures are normal. One exception is that in endolymphatic hydrops, the cochlear disorder causes so much distortion that word recognition scores are poorer than predicted from degree of hearing loss.[84]

Auditory Evoked Potentials

Auditory evoked potentials can be used for several purposes in the assessment of a cochlear disorder.

First, if there is suspicion that the disorder might be retrocochlear, the ABR can be used in an effort to differentiate a cochlear from a retrocochlear site. Cochlear hearing loss has a predictable influence on ABR waveform latency and morphology. Once that influence is accounted for, ABR results will be consistent with the degree and configuration of the cochlear hearing loss. If the high-frequency pure-tone average of 1,000, 2,000, and 4,000 Hz exceeds 70 dB, the absence of a response is equivocal because it can be explained equally by the degree of cochlear hearing loss and by retrocochlear disorder.[85]

Second, if there is suspicion that the hearing loss is exaggerated, evoked potentials can be used to predict the degree of organic hearing loss. Typically, ABR thresholds to click stimuli are used to predict high-frequency hearing, and late-latency or other evoked potentials are used to predict lower frequency thresholds.[86]

Third, ECoG measures have been used successfully to assist in the diagnosis of Meniere's disease,[87,88] as the ratio of the action potential to the summating potential amplitude has been shown to be abnormal in a substan-

tial proportion of cases. Recent modifications of this strategy have demonstrated that AP latencies to condensation and rarefaction clicks are significantly different in patients with Meniere's disease when compared to the negligible polarity differences seen in patients with normal hearing or other forms of cochlear hearing loss.[89,90]

Otoacoustic Emissions

Otoacoustic emissions can be used in the assessment of sensorineural hearing loss as a means of verifying that there is a cochlear component to the disorder. For example, if the cochlea is disordered, OAEs are expected to be abnormal or absent.[91] Although this finding does not preclude the presence of a retrocochlear disorder, it does implicate the cochlea. Conversely, if OAEs are normal in the presence of a sensorineural hearing loss, a retrocochlear site of disorder is implicated.[7,92]

Otoacoustic emission measures have also been used effectively to monitor cochlear function, particularly in patients undergoing treatment with potentially ototoxic medications.[93–95] For example, it is not uncommon for DPOAEs to be used to monitor outer hair cell function in an attempt to detect ototoxicity during chemotherapy. The exquisite sensitivity of DPOAEs to change in cochlear function across a focused frequency range enables detection of the onset of ototoxic effects before they can be identified with the pure-tone audiogram.

Retrocochlear Disorders

Audiologic contribution to the assessment of a retrocochlear disorder is directed at answering the following questions:

- Is there a hearing loss, and what is its extent?
- Is the loss unilateral or asymmetric?
- Is speech understanding asymmetric or poorer than predicted from the hearing loss?
- Are acoustic reflexes normal or elevated?
- Is there other evidence of a retrocochlear disorder?

One goal of the audiologic evaluation is to determine the degree and type of hearing loss. Another goal is to scrutinize the audiologic findings for any evidence of retrocochlear disorder. Often a third goal is to assess the integrity of the eighth nerve and auditory brainstem with electrophysiologic measures.

On most audiologic measures, there are indicators that can alert the otologist to the possibility of retrocochlear disorder. Acoustic reflex thresholds, symmetry of hearing sensitivity, configuration of hearing sensitivity, and measures of speech recognition all provide clues as to the nature of the disorder.

Prior to the advent of sophisticated imaging and radiographic techniques, specialized audiologic assessment was an integral part of the differential diagnosis of auditory nervous system disorders. Behavioral measures of differential sensitivity to loudness, loudness growth, and auditory adaptation were designed to assist in the diagnostic process. Then, for a number of years in the late 1970s and early 1980s, auditory evoked potentials were used as a very sensitive technique for assisting in the diagnosis of neurologic disorders.[65,67,70] For a time, these measures of neurologic function were thought to be even more sensitive than radiographic techniques in the detection of lesions. However, progress in imaging and radiographic assessment of structural changes has advanced to a point where functional measures such as the ABR have lost some of their utility and thus importance. That is, imaging studies have permitted the visualization of ever smaller lesions in the brain. Sometimes the lesions are of a small enough size or are in such a location that they result in little or no measurable functional consequence. Thus, measures of function, such as behavioral measures and the ABR, may not detect their presence.[96-98] Regardless, auditory evoked potentials, particularly the ABR, remain valuable indicators of eighth nerve and auditory brainstem function. Although not as often as in the past, auditory evoked potentials are still used to assess neural function as a supplement to the assessment of structure provided by magnetic resonance imaging and other imaging studies.

The diagnostic use of OAEs has begun to reveal distinctions between the primary influences of retrocochlear disease on auditory nervous system function and the secondary influences of retrocochlear disease on cochlear function.[92,99,100] For example, in some vestibular schwannomas, audiologic outcomes reflect a primary effect on nerve function in a pattern of results that includes abnormal acoustic reflexes, abnormal auditory adaptation, disproportionately poor speech recognition, rollover of the speech function, abnormal ABR, and preserved OAEs.

In other vestibular schwannomas, audiologic outcomes reflect what appears to be a secondary influence of the tumor on cochlear function, presumably owing to an interruption in cochlear blood supply. In such cases, the results may be more consistent with cochlear hearing loss than retrocochlear loss, including the absence of OAEs. The distinction is probably important in appreciating the relative value of audiologic measures in the diagnostic process.

Immittance audiometry is used to evaluate outer and middle ear function and to assess the integrity of the seventh and eighth cranial nerve and lower auditory brainstem function. Pure-tone audiometry is used to evaluate the extent of any hearing asymmetry. Speech audiometry is used as a cross-check of pure-tone thresholds, an estimate of suprathreshold speech recognition ability, a measure of hearing symmetry, and an assessment of any abnormality of hearing under adverse listening conditions. Electroacoustic and electrophysiologic measures are used in an effort to assess the integrity of the cochlea, eighth nerve, and auditory brainstem.

Immittance Measures

Acoustic reflex threshold or suprathreshold patterns can be helpful in differentiating cochlear from retrocochlear disorders. Immittance audiometry can also be important in assessing middle ear function in cases of suspected retrocochlear disorder because a middle ear disorder and any resultant conductive hearing loss can affect interpretation of other audiometric measures.

If the disorder is retrocochlear, the typical immittance pattern is characterized by normal tympanometry, normal static immittance, and abnormal elevation of reflex threshold, or absence of a reflex response, whenever the reflex-eliciting signal is delivered to the suspect ear in either the crossed or the uncrossed mode.[62,64] For example, with a right-sided vestibular schwannoma, the tympanograms and static immittance would be normal. Abnormal elevation of reflex thresholds would be observed for the right uncrossed and the right-to-left crossed reflex responses. A retrocochlear disorder can also result in acoustic reflex decay, reflecting abnormal auditory adaptation.[62,101-103] Abnormal decay occurs when a reflex contraction is not sustained to continuous stimulation at suprathreshold levels.

A key to differentiating elevated reflex thresholds from a retrocochlear versus a cochlear disorder is the audiometric level at the test frequency. As stated previously, in cochlear hearing loss, reflex thresholds are not elevated until the audiometric loss exceeds 50 dB HL, and even above this level, the degree of elevation is proportional to the audiometric level. In the case of retrocochlear disorder, however, the elevation is more than would be predicted from the audiometric level. The reflex threshold may be elevated by 20 to 25 dB even though the audiometric level shows no more than a 5- or 10-dB loss. If the audiometric loss exceeds 70 to 75 dB, then the absence of the acoustic reflex is ambiguous. The abnormality could be attributed either to retrocochlear disorder or to cochlear loss.

For diagnostic interpretation, acoustic reflex measures are probably best understood if viewed in the context of a three-part reflex arc: (1) the sensory or input portion (afferent), (2) the central nervous system portion that transmits neural information (central), and (3) the motor or output portion (efferent).[104,105]

An afferent abnormality occurs as the result of a disordered sensory system in one ear. An example of a pure afferent effect is a profound unilateral sensorineural hearing loss on the right or a vestibular schwannoma of the right eighth nerve. Both reflexes with signal presented to the right ear (right uncrossed and right-to-left crossed) would be absent.

An efferent abnormality occurs as the result of a disordered motor system or middle ear in one ear. An example of a pure efferent effect is a right facial nerve paralysis. Both reflexes measured by the probe in the right ear (right uncrossed and left-to-right crossed) would be absent.

A central pathway abnormality occurs as the result of a brainstem disorder. An example of a pure central effect is multiple sclerosis that affects the crossing fibers of the central auditory nervous system. In this situation, one or both of the crossed acoustic reflexes would be elevated or absent in the presence of normal uncrossed reflex thresholds.

Disorders of the eighth nerve, then, often result in afferent abnormalities.[64,101,105,106] Brainstem disorders can result in afferent, efferent, or central pathway abnormalities,[105,107–109] depending on the effect of the lesion.

Pure-Tone Audiometry

Pure-tone audiometry is useful in assessing the symmetry of hearing loss. Asymmetric sensorineural hearing loss,

in the absence of another explanation, raises suspicion for the presence of retrocochlear disorder.

Certain audiometric configurations have been attributed to various retrocochlear disorders. Although any configuration can occur, progressive asymmetric high-frequency hearing loss has been associated with eighth nerve disorders.[110] Similarly, low-frequency hearing loss has been associated with brainstem disorders.[10,111] Although hearing loss is usually insidious in neurologic disorders, it is not uncommon for a sudden hearing loss to be associated with a retrocochlear lesion.[112,113]

Although asymmetric hearing loss is a common finding in retrocochlear disorders, so is normal hearing.[113–117] As diagnosis has improved generally, reports have increased of normal hearing sensitivity in patients with eighth nerve disorder.

Speech Audiometry

Measurement of speech recognition is important in screening for a retrocochlear disorder. In most cochlear hearing losses, speech recognition ability is predictable from the degree of loss and the configuration of the audiogram. That is, given a hearing sensitivity loss of a known severity and configuration, the ability to recognize speech is roughly equivalent among individuals and nearly equivalent between ears within an individual. Expectations of speech recognition ability, then, lie within a certain predictable range for a given cochlear hearing loss. In many retrocochlear hearing losses, however, speech recognition ability is poorer than would be expected from the audiogram. Thus, if performance on speech recognition measures falls below that expected, suspicion is aroused that the hearing loss is caused by a retrocochlear rather than a cochlear disorder.[19]

If a sensorineural hearing loss is caused by an eighth nerve disorder, the speech threshold will be elevated in that ear to a degree predictable by the pure-tone average. Suprathreshold word recognition ability is likely to be substantially affected.[44,118] Maximum scores are likely to be poorer than predicted from the degree of hearing loss, and rollover of the PI function is likely to occur.[16,17,119,120] Speech-in-competition measures are also likely to be depressed.[25,121,122] Abnormal results will occur in the same, or ipsilateral, ear in which the lesion occurs. Dichotic measures will be normal.

If a hearing disorder occurs as a result of a brainstem lesion, the speech threshold will be predictable from the pure-tone average. Suprathreshold word recognition ability is likely to be affected substantially.[121,123] Word recognition scores in quiet may be normal or depressed or may show rollover. Speech-in-competition measures are likely to be depressed in the ear ipsilateral to the lesion. Dichotic measures will likely be normal.

If a hearing disorder occurs as the result of a temporal lobe lesion, hearing sensitivity is unlikely to be affected, and the speech threshold and word recognition scores are likely to be normal. Sensitized speech measures may or may not be abnormal in the ear contralateral to the lesion.[20–22,24] Dichotic measures are the most likely of all to show a deficit because of the temporal lobe lesion.[26,28,124,125]

Auditory Evoked Potentials

If a retrocochlear disorder is suspected, and if audiometric indicators heighten suspicion, it is customary to assess the integrity of the auditory nervous system directly with the ABR. The ABR is a sensitive indicator of the integrity of eighth nerve and auditory brainstem function.[66,126,127] If it is abnormal, there is a very high likelihood of a retrocochlear disorder.

In recent years, imaging techniques have improved to the point that structural changes in the nervous system can sometimes be identified before those changes have a functional influence. Thus, the presence of a normal ABR does not rule out the presence of a neurologic disease process.[128] It simply indicates that the process is without apparent functional consequence. The presence of an abnormal ABR, however, remains a strong indicator of neurologic disorder and is useful in the diagnosis of retrocochlear disease.[96,129,130]

The ABR component waves, especially waves I, III, and V, are easily recorded and are very reliable in terms of their latency. As a general rule, wave I occurs at about 2 msec following signal presentation, wave III at 4 msec, and wave V at 6 msec. Although these absolute numbers vary among clinics, the latencies are quite stable across individuals. In most adults, the I–V interpeak interval is approximately 4 msec, with a standard deviation of about 0.2 msec. Thus, 95% of the adult population has I–V interpeak intervals of 4.4 msec or less. If the I–V interval exceeds this amount, it is considered abnormal.

These latency measures are reasonably consistent across the population. In newborns, they are prolonged compared with adult values, but in a predictable way. Once a child reaches 18 months, normal adult latency values can be expected and will continue throughout life. Because of the consistency of latencies within an individual over time and across individuals in the population, assessment of latency is relied on as an indicator of integrity of the eighth nerve and auditory brainstem.[131]

The decision about whether an ABR is normal is usually based on the following considerations:

- interaural latency difference in I–V interpeak interval
- I–V interpeak interval
- interaural difference in wave V latency
- absolute latency of wave V
- interaural differences in V/I amplitude ratio
- V/I amplitude ratio
- selective loss of late waves
- grossly degraded waveform morphology

Again, the ABR is used to assess the integrity of the eighth nerve and auditory brainstem in patients who are suspected of having a vestibular schwannoma or other neurologic disorder. In interpreting ABRs, the consistency of the response across individuals is exploited to ask whether the measured latencies compare well between ears and with the population in general.

The MLR and LLR are less useful than the ABR in identifying discrete lesions.[132,133] Sometimes a vestibular schwannoma that affects the ABR will also affect the MLR. Also, sometimes a cerebral vascular accident or other discrete insult to the brain results in an abnormality in the MLR.[134,135] However, these measures are probably more useful as indicators of generalized disorders of auditory processing ability rather than in the diagnosis of a specific disease process. For example, MLRs and LLRs have been found to be abnormal in patients with multiple sclerosis.[133,136] Although neither response has proven to be particularly useful in helping to diagnose this disorder, the fact that MLR and LLR abnormalities occur has proven to be valuable in describing the resultant auditory disorders. That is, patients with neurologic disorders often have auditory complaints that cannot be measured on an audiogram or with simple speech audiometric measures. The MLR and LLR are sometimes helpful in quantifying such auditory complaints.

Otoacoustic Emissions

Otoacoustic emissions can be used in the assessment of a retrocochlear disorder, although the results are often equivocal. If a hearing loss is caused by a retrocochlear disorder through an effect on eighth nerve function, OAEs may be normal despite the hearing loss.[7,137] In such cases, outer hair cell function is considered normal, and the hearing loss can be attributable to the neurologic disease process. That is, the loss is caused by neural disorder, and the cochlea is functioning normally. In some cases, however, a retrocochlear disorder can affect cochlear function, presumably by interrupting its blood supply, resulting in a hearing loss and abnormality of OAEs.[92,99,100] Thus, in the presence of hearing loss and normal middle ear function, the absence of OAEs indicates either a cochlear or a retrocochlear disorder. On the other hand, the preservation of OAEs in the presence of a hearing loss suggests that the disorder is retrocochlear.

One other aspect of OAEs that may be interesting from a diagnostic perspective is that the amplitude of a TEOAE is suppressed to a certain extent by stimulation of the contralateral ear. This contralateral suppression is a small but consistent effect that occurs when broad-spectrum noise is presented to one ear and transient emissions are recorded from the other.[138,139] The effect is mediated by the medial olivocochlear system, which is part of the auditory system's complex efferent mechanism. In some cases of peripheral and central auditory disorder, contralateral suppression is absent,[140] so that the TEOAE is unaffected by stimulation of the contralateral ear. Contralateral suppression is emerging as a promising tool in the assessment of auditory nervous system function.

Suprathreshold Processing Disorders

Over the past two decades, techniques that were once used to assist in the diagnosis of neurologic disease have been adapted for use in the assessment of communication impairment that occurs as a result of a central auditory processing disorder. Sensitized speech audiometric measures are now commonly used to evaluate auditory processing ability. A typical battery of tests might include

• the assessment of speech recognition across a range of signal intensities,

• the assessment of speech recognition in the presence of competing speech signals, and

• the measurement of dichotic listening—the ability to process two different signals presented simultaneously to both ears.

The results of such an assessment provide an estimate of central auditory processing ability and a more complete profile of a patient's auditory abilities and impairments. Such information is often useful in providing guidance regarding appropriate amplification strategies or other rehabilitation approaches.

Many patients with an auditory processing disorder are elderly and consequently have some degree of cochlear hearing loss. Outcomes of assessment with immittance audiometry, pure-tone audiometry, and OAEs do not differ substantially in these patients from those seen in patients with purely peripheral deficits. The differences that do exist are most readily identified by speech audiometry and, to a lesser extent, auditory evoked potentials.

Immittance Measures

Immittance audiometry can be expected to show normal middle ear function and reflex results consistent with normal hearing sensitivity or cochlear hearing loss. Tympanograms, static immittance, and acoustic reflex thresholds are normal or are abnormal consistent with the degree of sensorineural hearing loss. A cochlear hearing loss also causes an elevation of the acoustic reflex thresholds to noise stimuli relative to pure-tone stimuli, resulting in a reduced SPAR value.

Pure-Tone Audiometry

In the absence of a middle ear disorder, pure-tone audiometry demonstrates normal hearing sensitivity or sensorineural hearing loss. There is some evidence of a low-frequency sensorineural component to the hearing loss in patients with an auditory processing disorder.

Speech Audiometry

Speech audiometric deficits in patients with auditory processing disorders can be categorized as (a) deficits in hearing in noise (or competition), (b) difficulty processing in the temporal domain, (c) binaural hearing deficits, and (d) disordered spatial hearing.

One of the most common indicators of auditory processing disorder is an inability to extract signals of interest from a background of noise. This inability can be measured directly with a number of different speech audiometric techniques. The results show that patients with auditory processing disorders have considerable difficulty identifying speech in the presence of competition.[25,141–146] In general, the more meaningful or speech-like the competition, the more interfering will be its influence on perception.[147,148]

Much of the early work in this area focused on monaural perception of speech targets in a background of competition presented to the same ear. Other studies have shown deficits in patients with auditory processing disorders when competition is presented to the opposite ear or when both targets and competition are presented to both ears in a soundfield.[149]

Impairment in processing in the time domain is also a common sign in auditory processing disorders.[150–155] Temporal processing deficits have been identified on the basis of a number of measures, including time compression of speech, duration pattern discrimination, duration difference limens, and gap detection. Deficits in temporal processing are often considered the underlying cause of and primary contributor to many of the other measurable deficits associated with auditory processing disorders.

Most individuals with intact auditory nervous systems are able to identify different signals presented simultaneously to both ears and demonstrate a slight right ear advantage in dichotic listening ability for linguistic signals. In a patient with an auditory processing disorder, particularly one caused by impairment of the corpus callosum and auditory cortex, dichotic deficits, characterized by substantial reduction in left ear performance, are often seen.[30,156,157]

As stated earlier, the auditory system is exquisitely sensitive to differences in the timing of sound reaching the two ears. This sensitivity helps localize low-frequency sounds, which reach the ears at different points in time. One way of assessing how sensitive the ears are to these timing or phase cues is by measuring binaural release from masking. Abnormal binaural release from masking is a sign of auditory processing disorder

and occurs as a result of impairment in the lower auditory brainstem.[4,47,50]

A different kind of binaural processing deficit is referred to as binaural interference. Normally, binaural hearing provides an advantage over monaural hearing. This "binaural advantage" has been noted in judgments of loudness, speech recognition, and evoked potential amplitudes. In contrast, with binaural interference, binaural performance is actually poorer than the best monaural performance. In such cases, performance on a perceptual task with both ears can actually be poorer than performance with the better ear in cases of asymmetric perceptual ability.[158] It appears that the poorer ear actually reduces binaural performance below the better monaural performance. Binaural interference has been reported in elderly individuals and in patients with multiple sclerosis.[158,159]

The ability to locate acoustic stimuli in space generally requires auditory system integration of sound from both ears. Some patients with auditory disorders have difficulty locating the directional source of a sound. Disorders of the auditory nervous system have been associated with deficits in the ability to localize the source of a sound in a soundfield or to lateralize the perception of a sound within the head.[154,160–162]

Auditory Evoked Potentials

In auditory processing disorders, the ABR may be abnormal if the disorder is secondary to nervous system disruption in the lower brainstem. More commonly, however, the ABR is normal. Abnormal MLR and LLR have been associated with auditory processing disorders secondary to diffuse changes in brain function.[163] Usually, however, conventionally measured evoked potentials are normal. Assessment with topographic brain mapping has revealed abnormalities in patients with auditory processing disorders.[164]

Otoacoustic Emissions

In an auditory processing disorder, OAEs are either normal or abnormal consistent with the degree of hearing sensitivity loss. However, in some cases of auditory processing disorder, contralateral suppression of OAEs is absent.

Illustrative Cases

Middle Ear Disorder

Case 1 is a 28-year-old woman with bilateral otosclerosis who developed hearing problems during pregnancy. She describes her problem as a muffling of other people's voices. She also reports bilateral tinnitus that bothers her at night. There is a family history of otosclerosis on her mother's side.

The results of immittance audiometry, as shown in Figure 8–1, A, are consistent with a middle ear disorder, characterized by a Type A$_s$ tympanogram, low static immittance, and bilaterally absent crossed and uncrossed acoustic reflexes. This pattern of results suggests an increase in the stiffness of the middle ear mechanism and is often associated with fixation of the ossicular chain.

Pure-tone audiometric results are shown in Figure 8–1, B. The patient has a moderate, bilaterally symmetric, conductive hearing loss. Typical for otosclerosis, the patient also has an apparent bone-conduction hearing loss at around 2,000 Hz in both ears—the so-called Carhart's notch. Carhart's notch actually reflects the elimination of the middle ear contribution to bone-conducted hearing rather than a loss in cochlear sensitivity.[165]

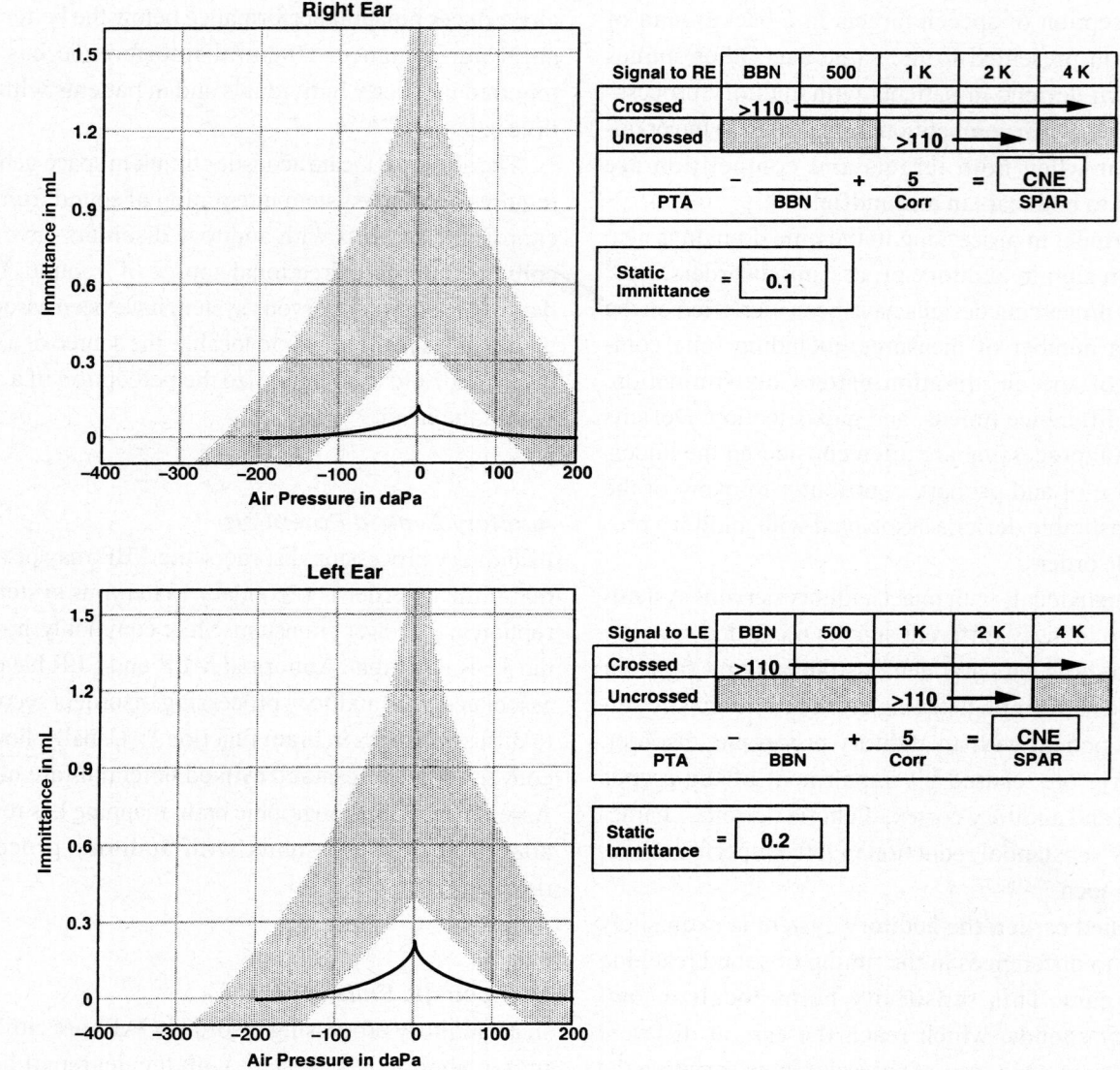

Figure 8–1 Audiometric results of a 28-year-old woman with otosclerosis. Immittance measures (*A*) are consistent with an increase in the stiffness of the middle ear mechanism. BBN = broad-band noise; CNE = could not evaluate; PTA = pure-tone average; SPAR = sensitivity prediction by the acoustic reflex.

Illustration continued on following page

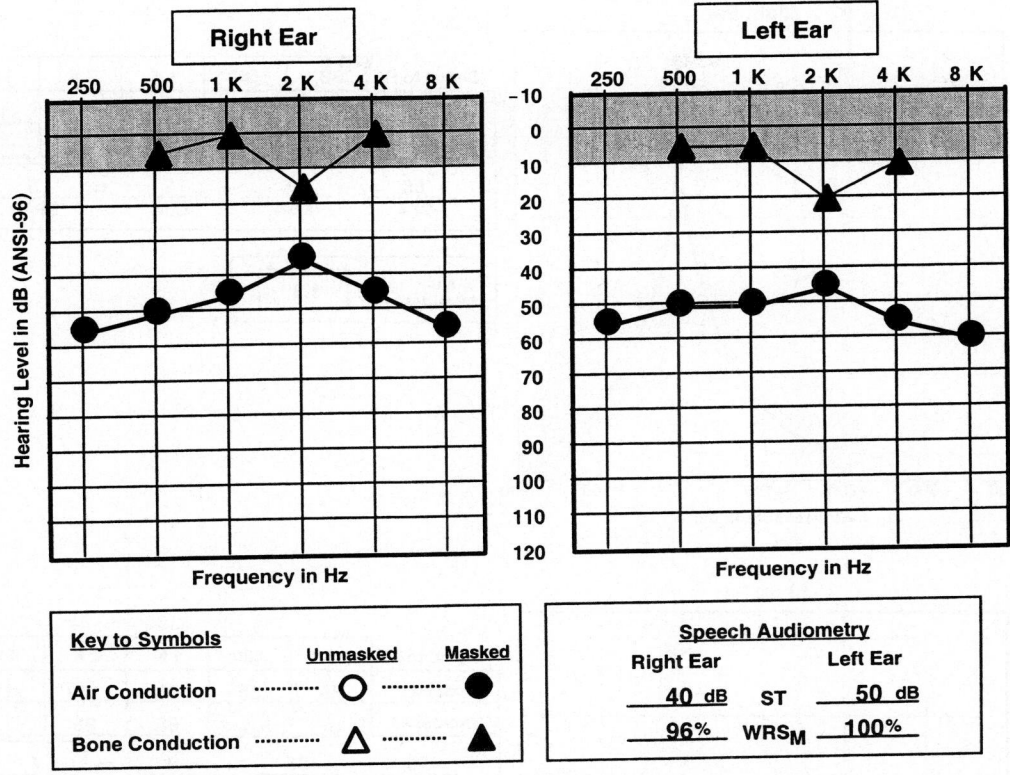

Figure 8–1 Continued. Pure-tone audiometric results (*B*) show a moderate conductive hearing loss bilaterally. Speech thresholds (ST) are consistent with pure-tone thresholds, and word recognition scores are consistent with conductive hearing loss. WRS$_M$ = maximum word recognition score.

Speech audiometric results show speech thresholds consistent with pure-tone thresholds. Suprathreshold speech recognition ability is normal once the effect of the hearing loss is overcome by presenting speech at higher intensity levels. Word recognition scores are 100% bilaterally.

Cochlear Disorder

Case 2 is a 60-year-old man with bilateral sensorineural hearing loss of cochlear origin, secondary to ototoxicity. The patient recently finished a round of chemotherapy that included cisplatin.

Immittance audiometry (Figure 8–2, A) is consistent with normal middle ear function bilaterally, characterized by Type A tympanograms, normal static immittance, and normal crossed and uncrossed acoustic reflex thresholds. The SPAR results (below 15 dB) predict a sensorineural hearing loss.

Pure-tone audiometry is shown in Figure 8–2, B, and shows a bilaterally symmetric, high-frequency sensorineural hearing loss, progressing from mild levels at 2,000 Hz to profound at 8,000 Hz. Further doses of

chemotherapy would be expected to begin to affect the remaining high-frequency hearing and progress downward toward the low frequencies.

Speech audiometric results are consistent with the degree and configuration of cochlear hearing loss. Speech thresholds match the pure-tone thresholds, and word recognition scores, although reduced, are consistent with this degree of hearing loss. Maximum word recognition scores are 100% for the right ear and 92% for the left ear.

Case 3 is a 38-year-old man with unilateral sensorineural hearing loss secondary to endolymphatic hydrops. Two weeks prior to evaluation, the patient experienced fluctuating hearing loss, aural fullness, tinnitus, and an episode of severe vertigo. After multiple attacks, the hearing loss has persisted. A diagnosis of Meniere's disease was made following otologic examination.

Immittance audiometry (Figure 8–3, A) is consistent with normal middle ear function bilaterally, characterized by a Type A tympanogram, normal static immittance, and normal crossed and uncrossed reflex thresholds.

Pure-tone audiometry is shown in Figure 8–3, B. The results show a moderate, rising (upward-sloping),

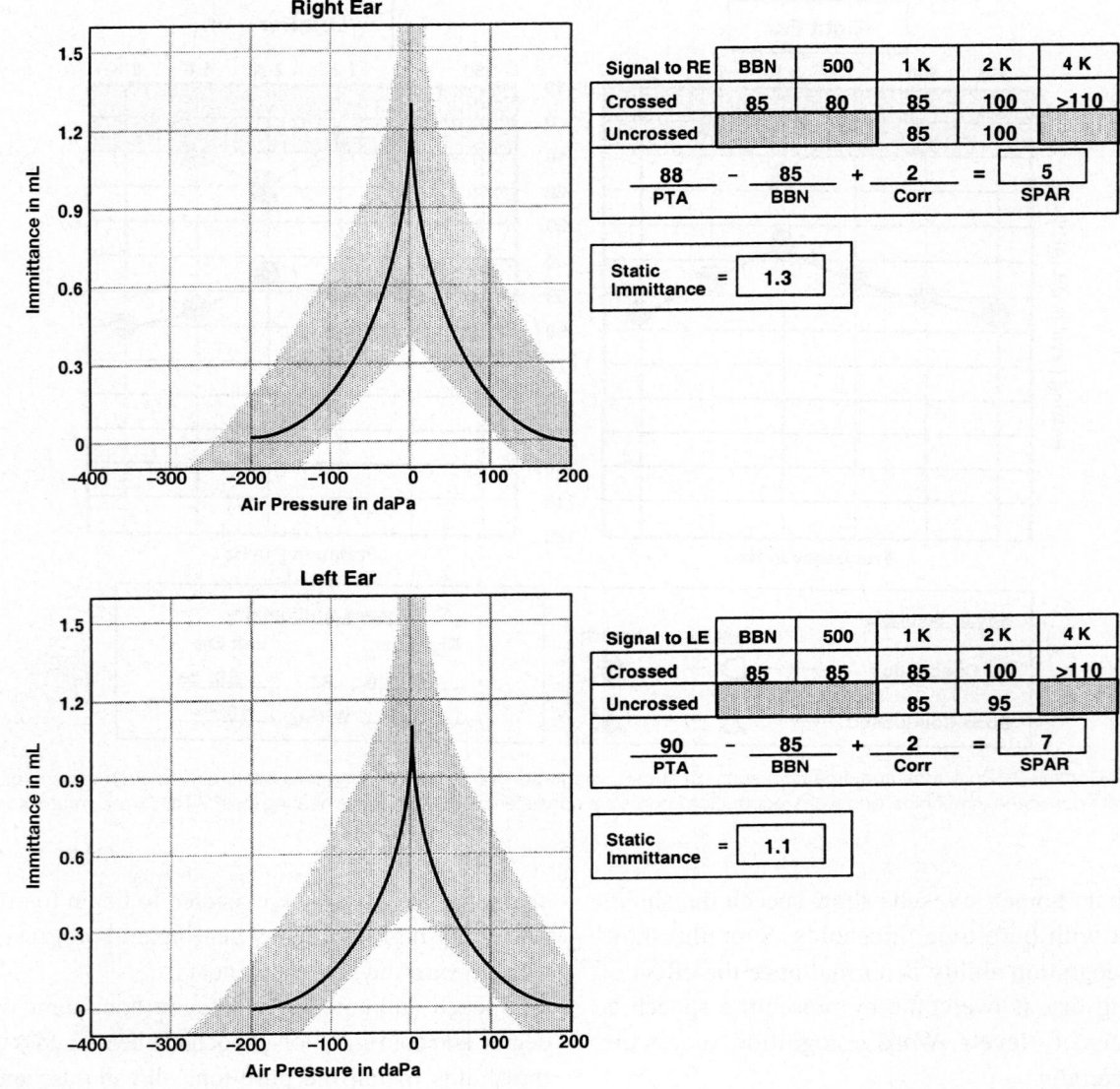

Figure 8–2 Audiometric results of a 60-year-old man with cochlear hearing loss caused by ototoxicity. Immittance measures (*A*) are consistent with normal middle ear function. The sensitivity prediction by the acoustic reflex (SPAR) predicts the presence of hearing loss. BBN = broad-band noise; PTA = pure-tone average.

Illustration continued on following page

sensorineural hearing loss in the left ear and normal hearing sensitivity on the right.

Speech audiometric results are normal for the right ear. On the left, however, although speech thresholds agree with the pure-tone thresholds, suprathreshold speech recognition scores are very poor for the left ear. This performance is significantly reduced from what would normally be expected for a cochlear hearing loss. These results are atypical for cochlear hearing losses other than Meniere's disease.

Auditory brainstem response results showed absolute and interpeak latencies that are normal and symmetric, supporting the diagnosis of cochlear disorder.

Eighth Nerve Disorder

Case 4 is a 54-year-old woman with a 4-month history of left tinnitus caused by a left vestibular schwannoma. Her health and hearing histories are otherwise unremarkable.

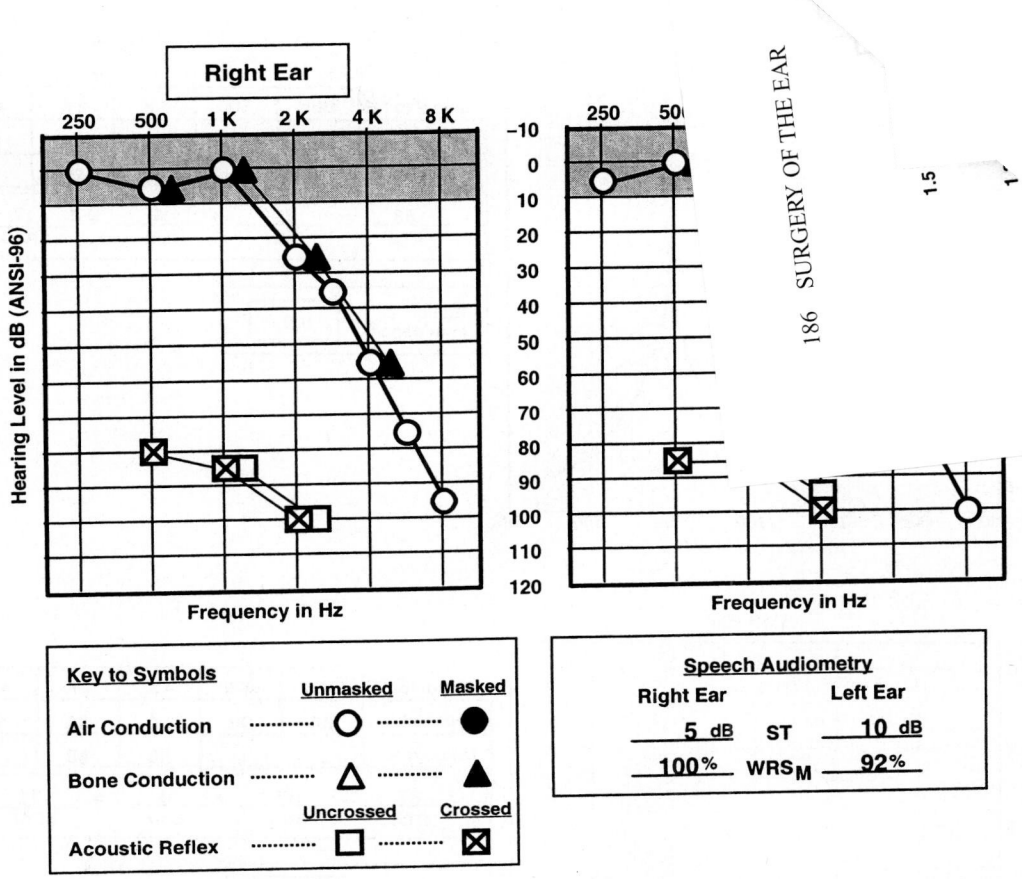

2B

Figure 8–2 Continued. Pure-tone audiometric results (*B*) show a high-frequency, sensorineural hearing loss bilaterally. Speech thresholds (ST) are consistent with pure-tone thresholds, and word recognition scores are consistent with the degree and configuration of the cochlear hearing loss. WRS$_M$ = maximum word recognition score.

Immittance audiometry (Figure 8–4, A) is consistent with normal middle ear function bilaterally, characterized by a Type A tympanogram, normal static immittance, and normal right crossed and right uncrossed reflex thresholds. Left crossed and left uncrossed reflexes are absent, consistent with an afferent abnormality on the left—the vestibular schwannoma.

Pure-tone audiometric results are shown in Figure 8–4, B. The patient has normal hearing sensitivity in the right ear and a mild, relatively flat sensorineural hearing loss in the left.

Speech audiometric results, shown in Figure 8–4, C, are normal in the right ear but abnormal in the left. Although maximum speech recognition scores are normal at lower intensity levels, the PI function demonstrates significant rollover or poorer performance at higher intensity levels, consistent with a retrocochlear site of lesion.

The ABR results are normal on the right ear. Left ear results show delayed latency of wave V and prolonged interpeak intervals. These results are also consistent with a retrocochlear site of disorder.

Cerebellopontine Angle Disorder

Case 5 is a 28-year-old female with a unilateral hearing loss of unusual etiology, central nervous system miliary tuberculosis.[7] Four weeks prior to evaluation, the patient noted that she could not use the telephone with her left ear. She also reported a "heaviness" on the left side of her head. She denied having tinnitus or dizziness. Her hearing history was otherwise unremarkable. There was no family history of hearing loss or history of other risk factors for hearing loss. The results of a neurotologic evaluation, including otoscopic examination, were normal. Significantly, the patient had a long history of tuberculosis and had recently begun medical therapy for miliary tuberculosis involving her nervous system.

Immittance audiometry indicated normal middle ear function bilaterally, characterized by Type A tym-

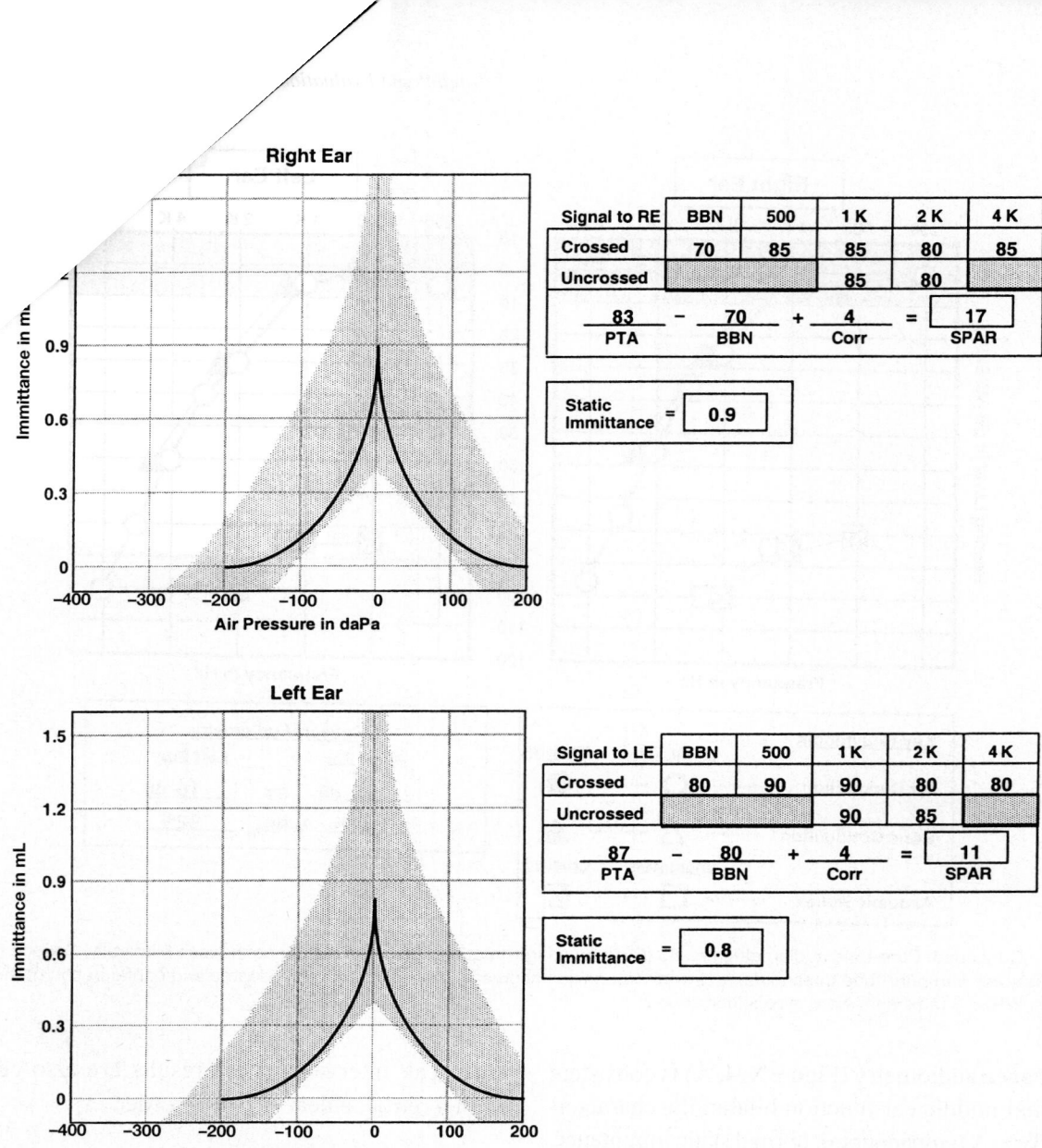

Right Ear

Signal to RE	BBN	500	1 K	2 K	4 K
Crossed	70	85	85	80	85
Uncrossed			85	80	

$$\frac{83}{\text{PTA}} - \frac{70}{\text{BBN}} + \frac{4}{\text{Corr}} = \boxed{\frac{17}{\text{SPAR}}}$$

Static Immittance = $\boxed{0.9}$

Left Ear

Signal to LE	BBN	500	1 K	2 K	4 K
Crossed	80	90	90	80	80
Uncrossed			90	85	

$$\frac{87}{\text{PTA}} - \frac{80}{\text{BBN}} + \frac{4}{\text{Corr}} = \boxed{\frac{11}{\text{SPAR}}}$$

Static Immittance = $\boxed{0.8}$

3A

Figure 8–3 Audiometric results of a 38-year-old man with cochlear hearing loss caused by endolymphatic hydrops. Immittance measures (A) are consistent with normal middle ear function. The sensitivity prediction by the acoustic reflex (SPARs) test predicts the presence of hearing loss in the left ear. BBN = broad-band noise; PTA = pure-tone average.

Illustration continued on following page

panograms, normal static immittance, and normal right crossed and right uncrossed reflex thresholds. However, crossed and uncrossed acoustic reflexes were absent when the eliciting signal was presented to the left ear (Figure 8–5, A). This reflex pattern is consistent with a left afferent abnormality, either a significant cochlear or retrocochlear disorder, on that side.

Pure-tone results are shown in Figure 8–5, B. Left ear results revealed a profound hearing loss. Hearing sensitivity could be measured only at 250 and 500 Hz at 105 and 110 dB HL, respectively. No responses were obtained at any other frequencies, and no responses were obtained to bone-conducted signals at equipment limits. The speech awareness threshold was 105 dB HL. Word recognition ability could not be measured. Right ear results showed normal hearing sensitivity from 250 to 4,000 Hz and a minimal sensitivity loss at 6,000 and 8,000 Hz. The word recognition score was 100% at 80 dB HL.

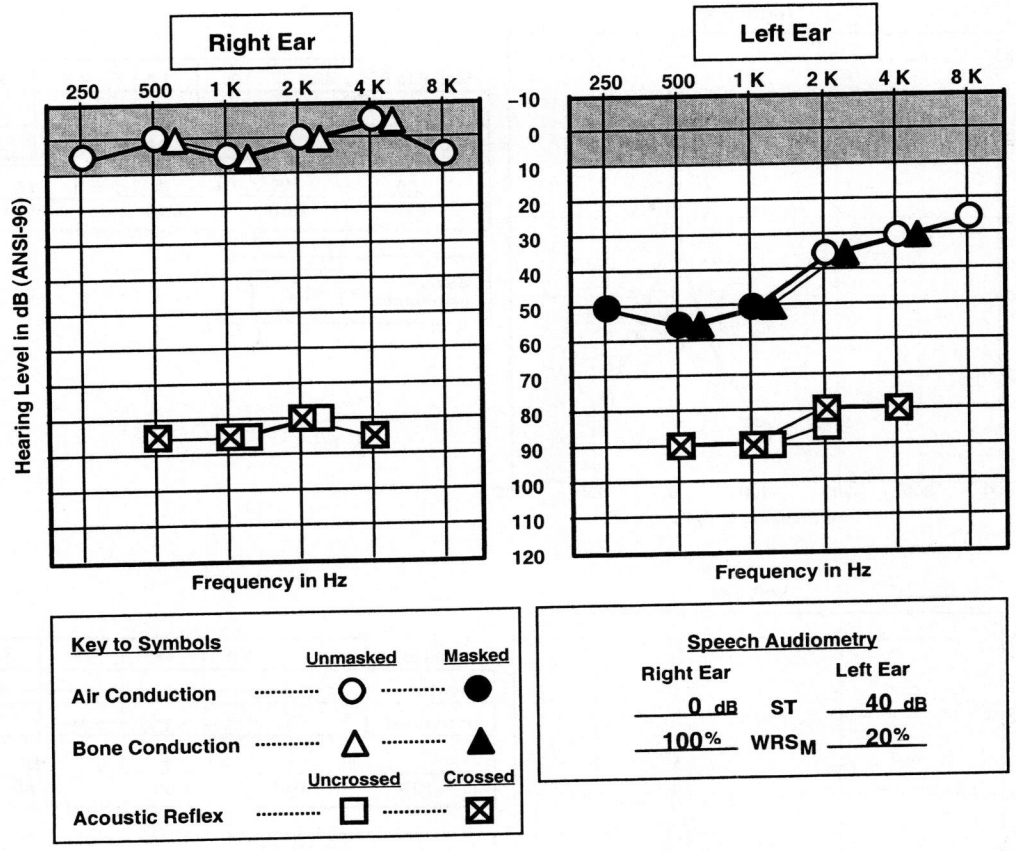

3B

Figure 8–3 Continued. Pure-tone audiometric results (*B*) show normal hearing sensitivity on the right ear and a moderate, rising sensorineural hearing loss on the left. The word recognition score on the left ear is poorer than would be expected from the degree and configuration of the cochlear hearing loss. BBN = broad-band noise; PTA = pure-tone average; ST = speech threshold; WRS$_M$ = maximum word recognition score.

As a matter of routine clinical procedure in the evaluation of a unilateral hearing loss, a Stenger test was carried out to assess the organicity of the hearing loss. The result of a speech Stenger test was negative for functional hearing loss on the left. As a further indication of the organic nature of the loss, a shadow curve was noted on the left audiogram at expected levels for insert earphones when the right ear was not masked.

Distortion-product OAEs were measured to assess cochlear function. Distortion-product OAE amplitudes as a function of f$_2$ frequency are plotted in Figure 8–5, C. The results showed substantive emissions across the frequency range for both the right and left ears. These results are consistent with normal cochlear outer hair cell function in both ears and suggest that, despite the presence of a profound hearing loss on the left, cochlear function, or at least outer hair cell function, was normal.

Auditory brainstem results are shown in Figure 8–5, D. Right ear responses were well formed, with component peaks at normal absolute and interpeak latencies. Left ear results were abnormal; only component wave I was observable. The absolute latency of wave I was 1.5 msec in both ears. The presence of wave I on the left is consistent with the OAE results, indicating near-normal cochlear function. The absence of later waves suggests a site of lesion at the proximal end of the eighth nerve or low auditory brainstem.

Audiologic and otologic findings were consistent with a left retrocochlear disorder, characterized by a profound hearing loss, absent acoustic reflexes, normal OAEs, and the presence of only wave I of the ABR. Imaging studies revealed the presence of multiple punctate lesions, one of which was extra-axial and located in the left cerebellopontine angle.

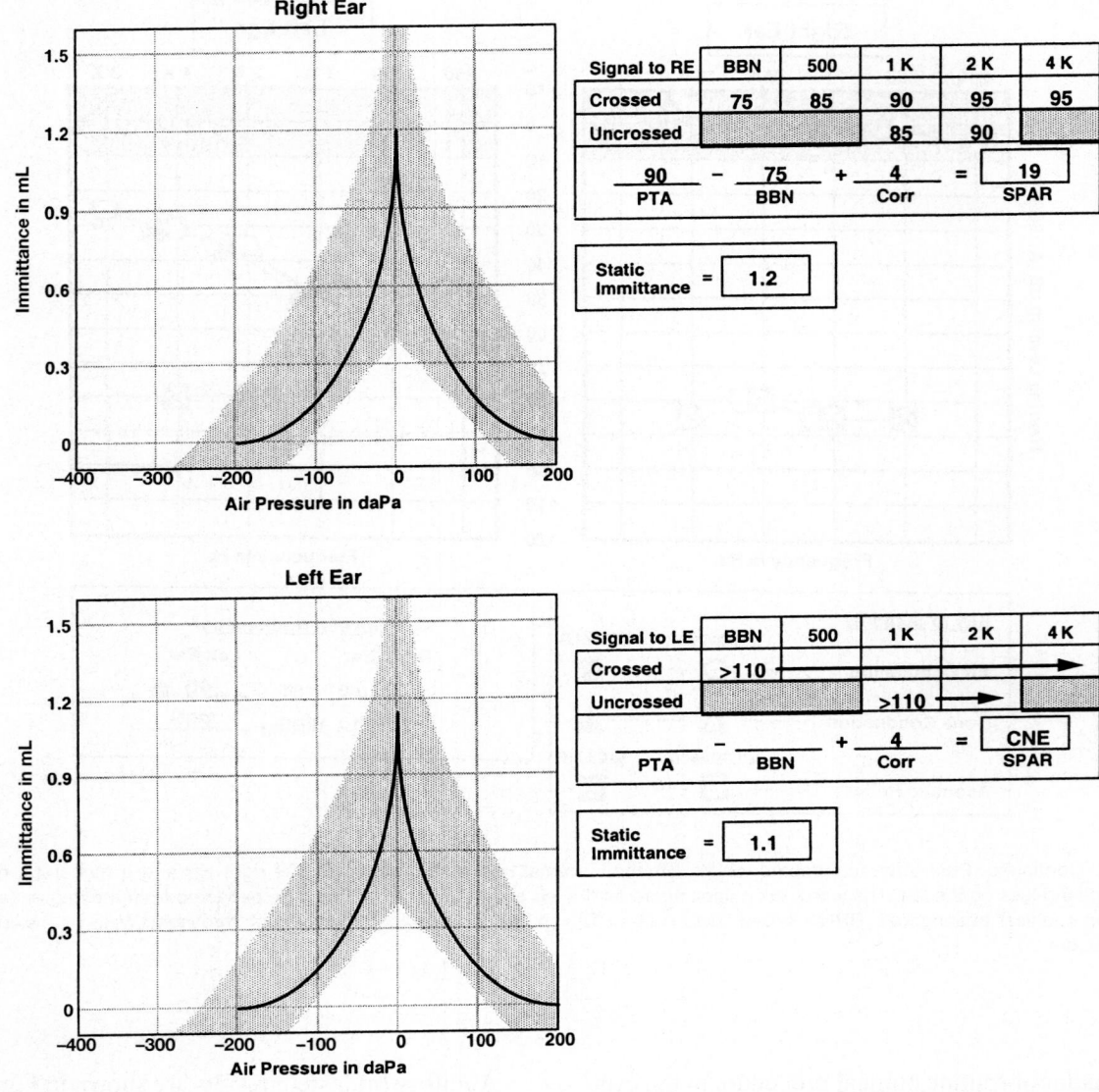

Right Ear

Signal to RE	BBN	500	1 K	2 K	4 K
Crossed	75	85	90	95	95
Uncrossed			85	90	

$$\underset{\text{PTA}}{90} - \underset{\text{BBN}}{75} + \underset{\text{Corr}}{4} = \underset{\text{SPAR}}{19}$$

Static Immittance = 1.2

Left Ear

Signal to LE	BBN	500	1 K	2 K	4 K
Crossed	>110 →				→
Uncrossed			>110 →		

$$\underset{\text{PTA}}{} - \underset{\text{BBN}}{} + \underset{\text{Corr}}{4} = \underset{\text{SPAR}}{\text{CNE}}$$

Static Immittance = 1.1

4A

Figure 8–4   Audiometric results of a 54-year-old woman with a left vestibular schwannoma. Immittance measures (*A*) are consistent with normal middle ear function. Left crossed and left uncrossed reflexes are absent, consistent with a left afferent disorder. BBN = broad-band noise; PTA = pure-tone average; SPAR = sensitivity prediction by the acoustic reflex.

Illustration continued on following page

Brainstem Disorder

Case 6 is a 42-year-old woman with auditory complaints secondary to multiple sclerosis. Two years prior to her evaluation, she experienced an episode of diplopia, accompanied by tingling and weakness in her left leg. These symptoms gradually subsided, only to reappear in a slightly more severe form a year later. Ultimately, she was diagnosed as having multiple sclerosis. Among a variety of complaints, she had vague hearing difficulty, particularly in the presence of background noise.

Immittance audiometry (Figure 8–6, A) is consistent with normal middle ear function, characterized by a Type A tympanogram, normal static immittance, and normal right and left uncrossed reflex thresholds. How-

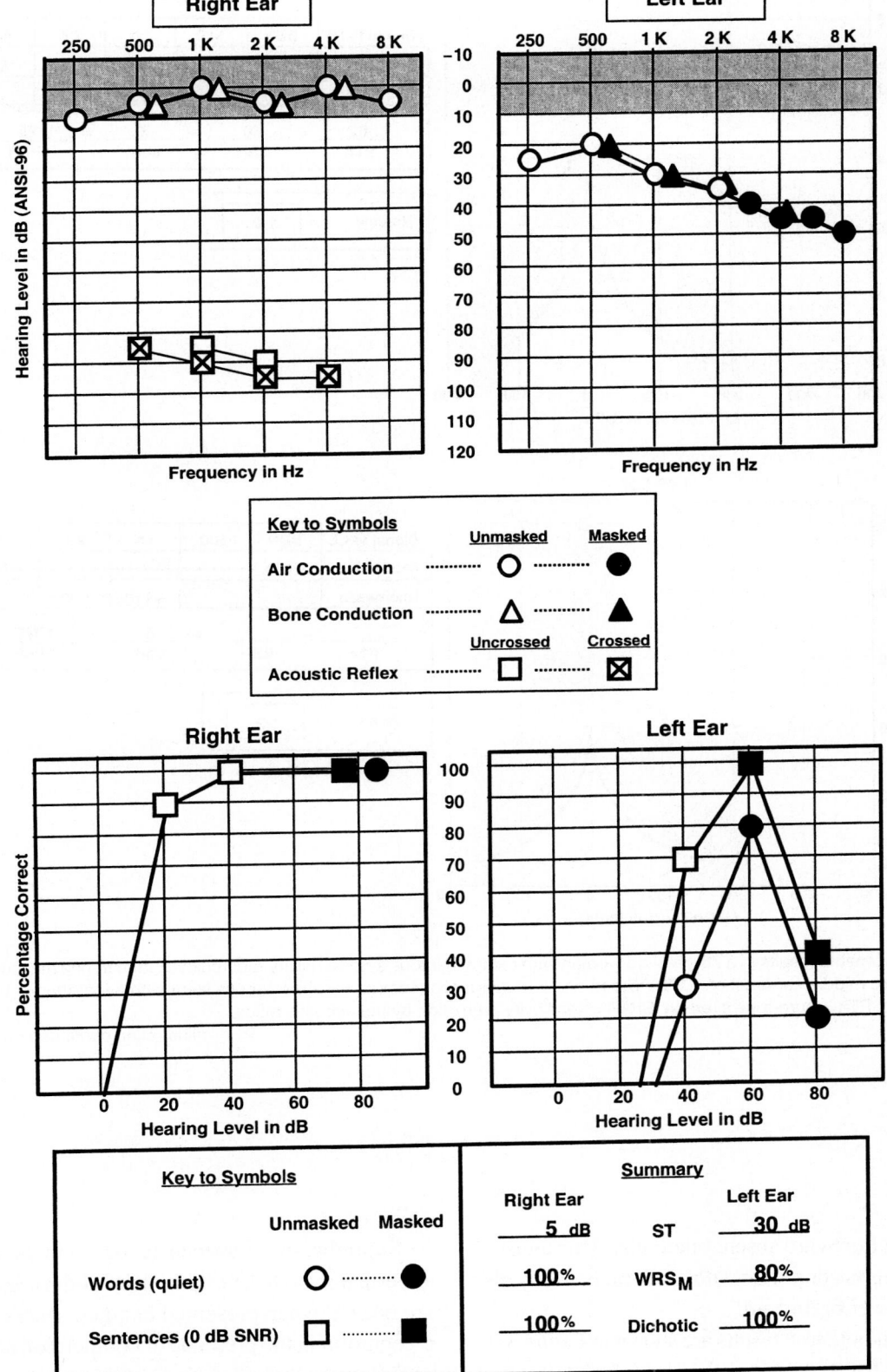

4B

4C

Figure 8–4 Continued. Audiometric results of a 54-year-old woman with a left vestibular schwannoma. Pure-tone audiometric results (*B*) show normal hearing sensitivity on the right ear and a mild, relatively flat sensorineural hearing loss on the left. Speech audiometric results (*C*) show rollover of the performance intensity function on the left. SNR = signal-to-noise ratio; ST = speech threshold; WRS_M = maximum word recognition score.

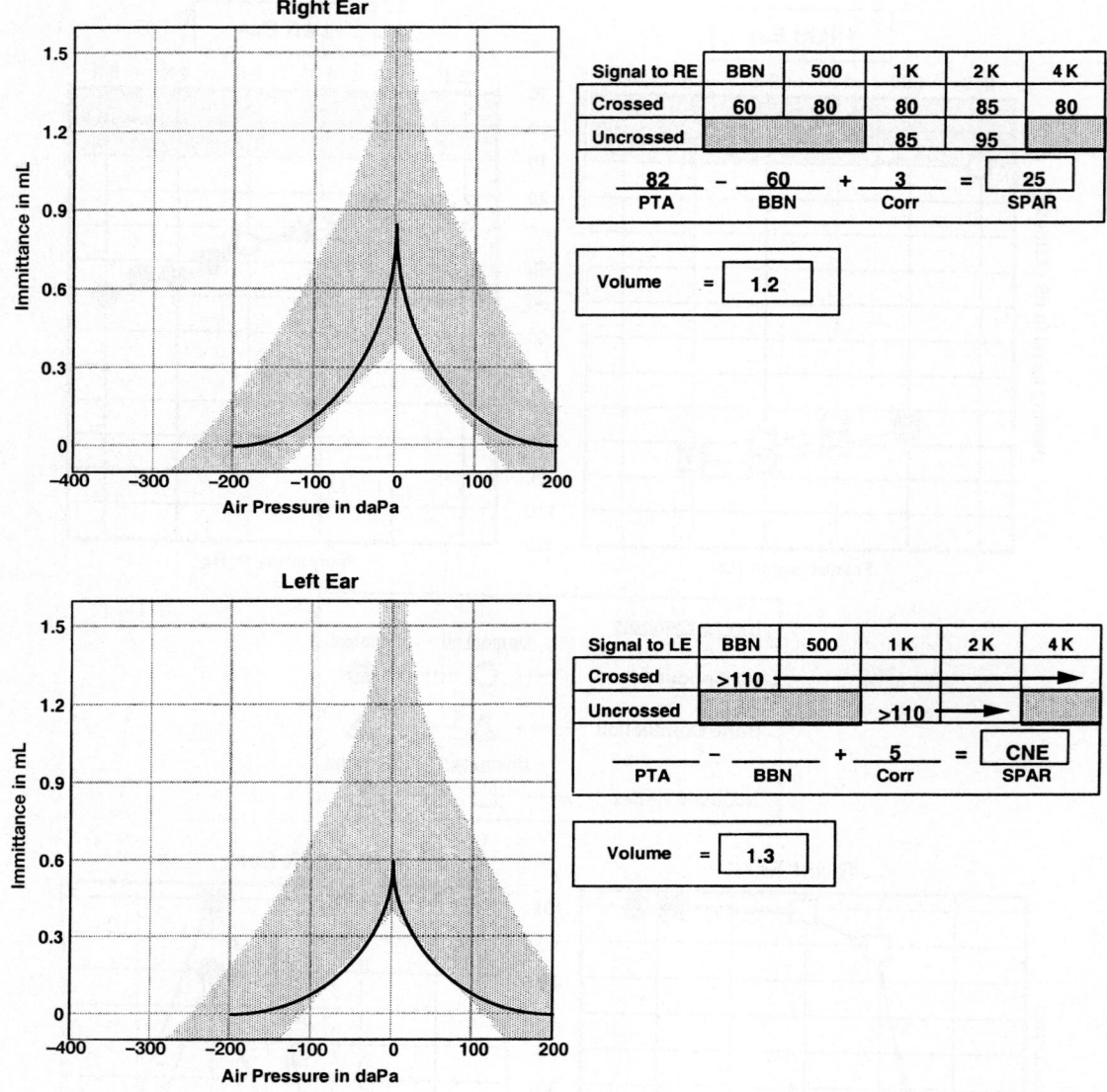

Right Ear

Signal to RE	BBN	500	1 K	2 K	4 K
Crossed	60	80	80	85	80
Uncrossed				85	95

$$\frac{82}{PTA} - \frac{60}{BBN} + \frac{3}{Corr} = \boxed{\frac{25}{SPAR}}$$

Volume = 1.2

Left Ear

Signal to LE	BBN	500	1 K	2 K	4 K
Crossed	>110 →				→
Uncrossed			>110 →		

$$\frac{}{PTA} - \frac{}{BBN} + \frac{5}{Corr} = \boxed{\frac{CNE}{SPAR}}$$

Volume = 1.3

5A

Figure 8–5 Audiometric results in a 28-year-old woman with central nervous system miliary tuberculosis. Immittance measures (*A*) are consistent with normal middle ear function. Left crossed and left uncrossed reflexes are absent, consistent with a left afferent disorder. BBN = broad-band noise; PTA = pure-tone average; SPAR = sensitivity prediction by the acoustic reflex.

Illustration continued on following page

ever, crossed reflexes are absent bilaterally. This unusual pattern of results is consistent with a central pathway disorder of the lower brainstem.

Pure-tone audiometric results are shown in Figure 8–6, B. The patient has a mild low-frequency sensorineural hearing loss bilaterally, a finding that is not uncommon in brainstem disorder.[10,111]

Suprathreshold speech recognition performance is abnormal in both ears. Although word recognition scores are normal when presented in quiet, scores on sentence recognition in the presence of competition are abnormal, as shown in Figure 8–6, C. Dichotic scores were normal. Auditory evoked potentials are also consistent with an abnormality in brainstem function. On the left, no waves

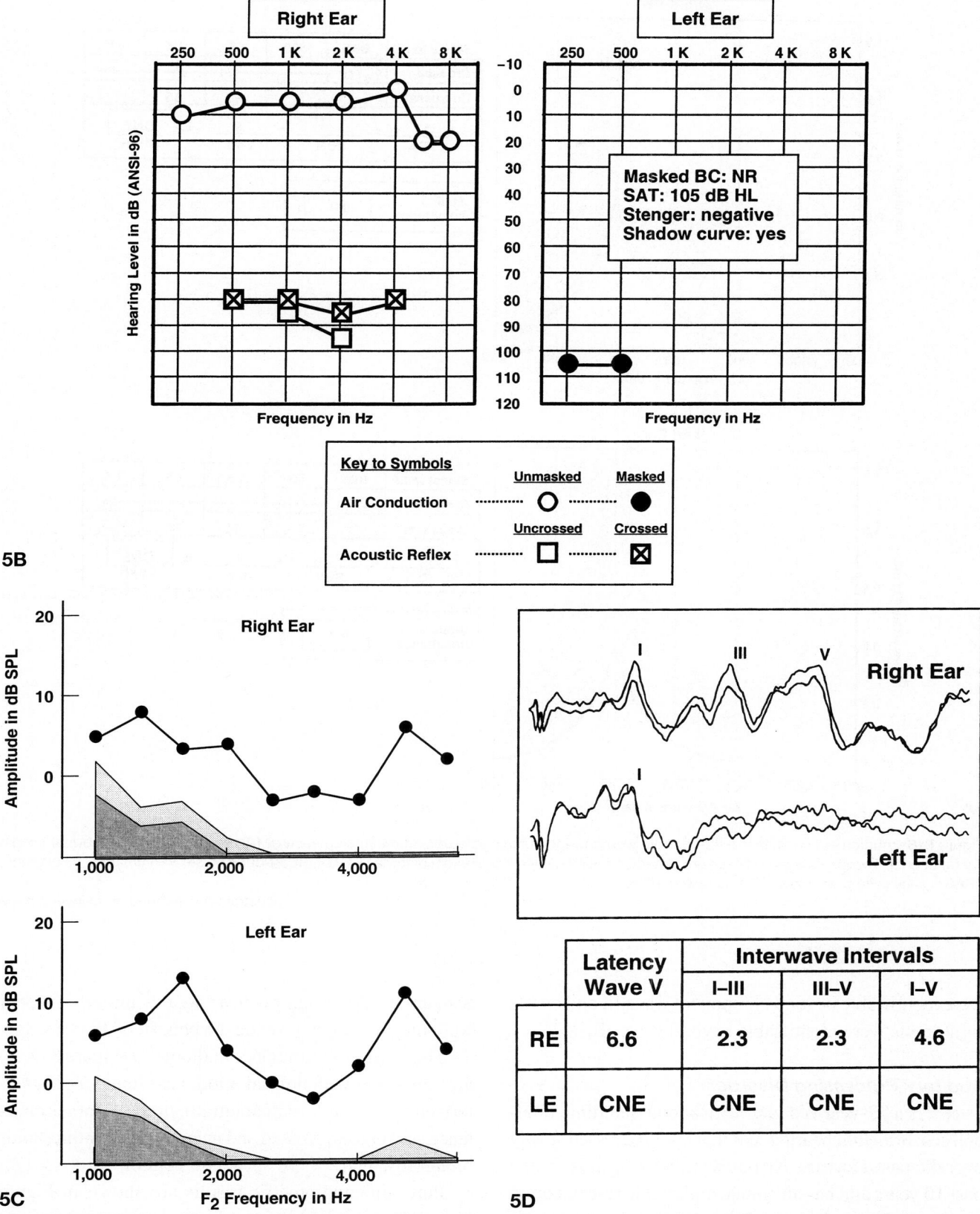

Figure 8–5 Continued. Pure-tone audiometric results (*B*) show normal hearing in the right ear and a profound sensorineural hearing loss on the left. Distortion-product otoacoustic emissions (*C*) are consistent with normal cochlear function bilaterally. Auditory brainstem response results (*D*) are normal for the right ear, but only wave I can be detected on the left. BC = bone conduction; SAT = speech awareness threshold; NR = no response.

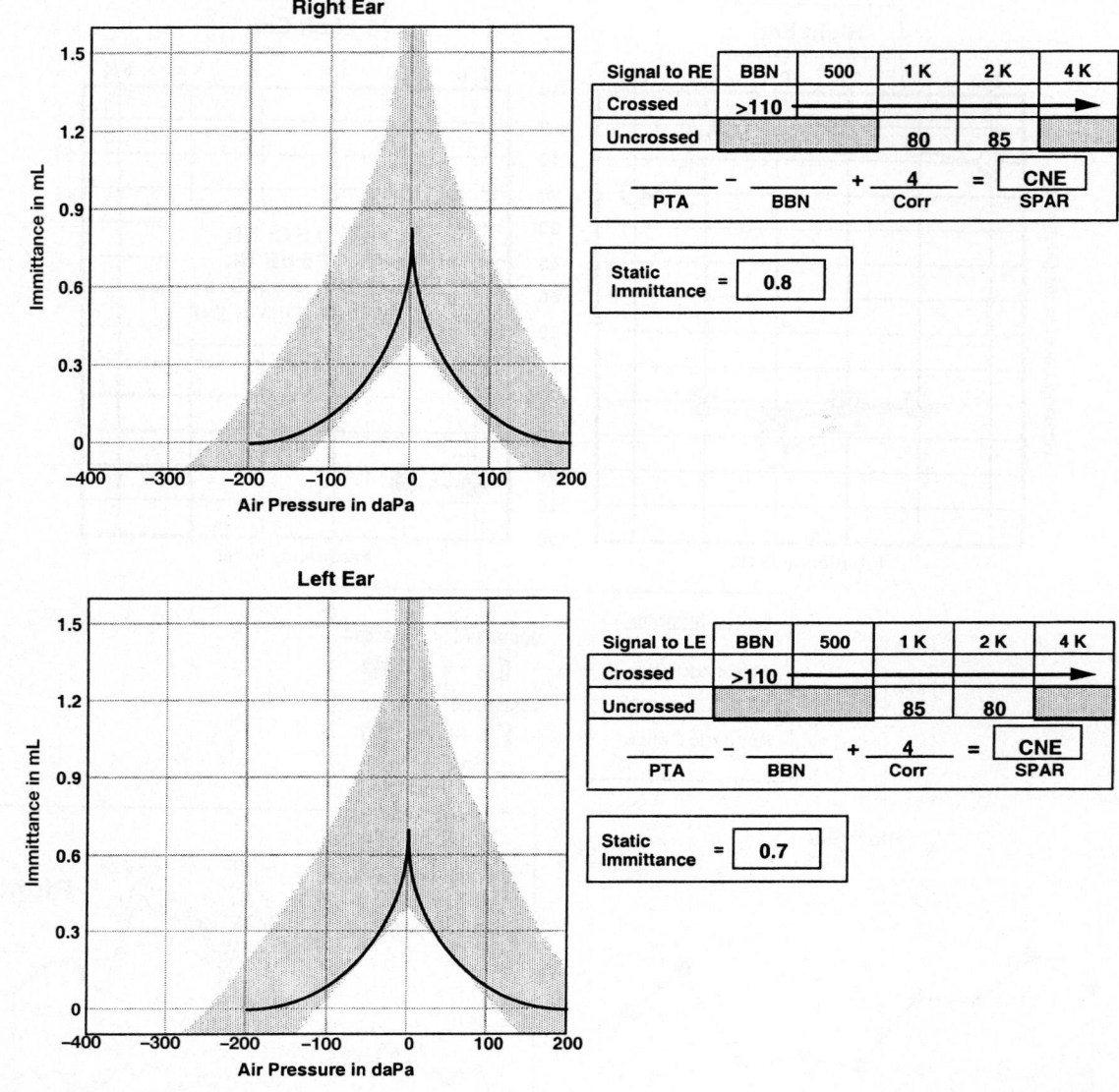

Figure 8–6 Audiometric results in a 42-year-old woman with multiple sclerosis. Immittance measures (*A*) are consistent with normal middle ear function. However, crossed reflexes are absent, consistent with a brainstem disorder. BBN = broad-band noise; PTA = pure-tone average; SPAR = sensitivity prediction by the acoustic reflex.

Illustration continued on following page

were identifiable beyond component wave II, and on the right, none were identifiable beyond wave III.

Auditory Processing Disorder

Case 7 is a 72-year-old man with a long-standing, bilateral sensorineural hearing loss that has progressed slowly over the past 15 years. He has worn hearing aids for the past 10 years and has an annual audiologic re-evaluation each year. His major complaints relate to communicating with his grandchildren and trying to hear in noisy restaurants. Although his hearing aids initially worked well, they no longer provide the benefit of 10 years ago.

The results of immittance audiometry (Figure 8–7, A) are consistent with normal middle ear function, characterized by a Type A tympanogram, normal static immittance, and normal crossed and uncrossed reflex thresholds bilaterally.

Pure-tone audiometric results are shown in Figure 8–7, B. The patient has a moderate, bilaterally symmetric, sensorineural hearing loss. Hearing sensitivity is

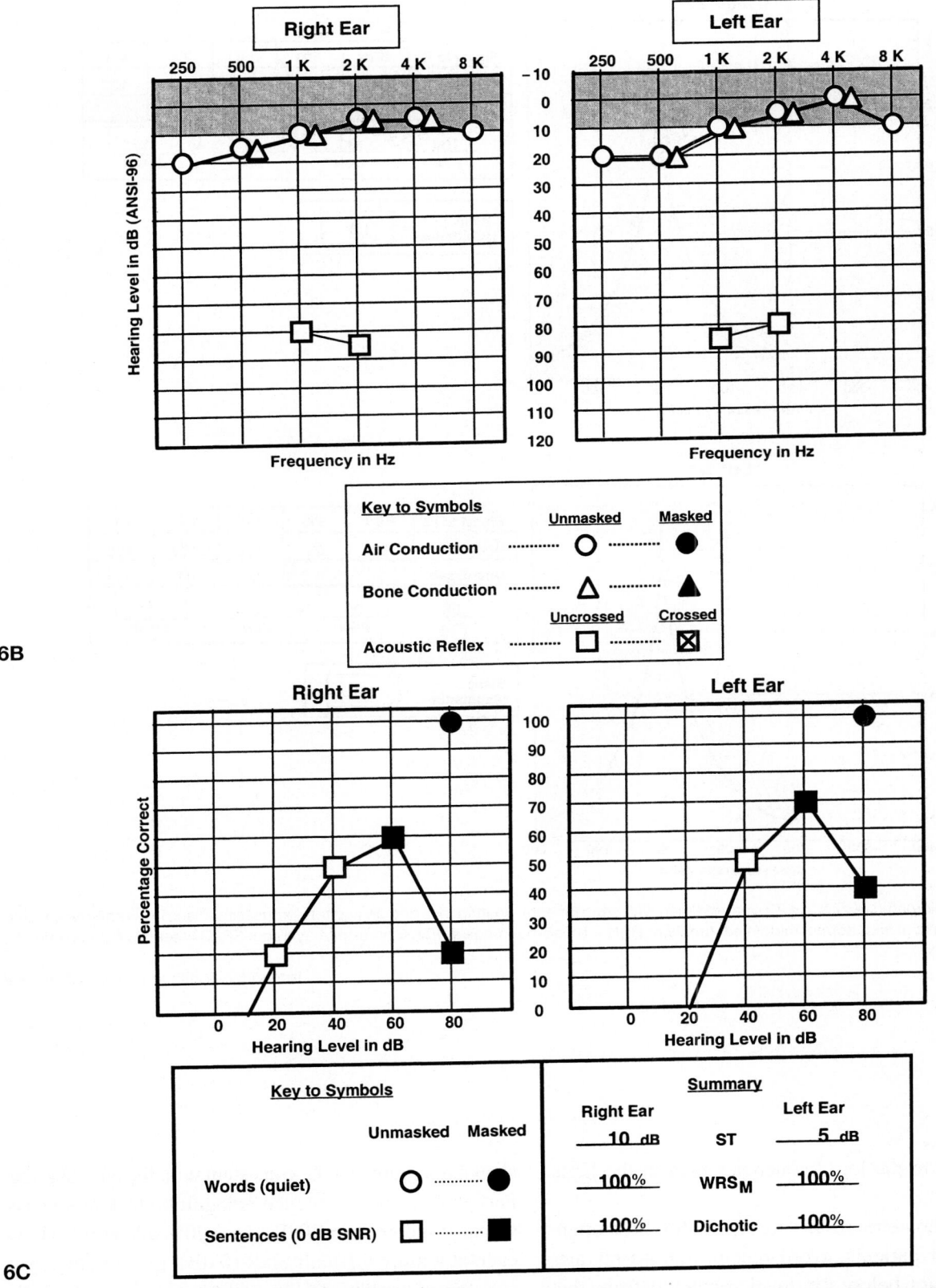

6B

6C

Figure 8–6 Continued. Pure-tone audiometric results (*B*) show a mild low-frequency sensorineural hearing loss bilaterally. Speech audiometric results (*C*) show reduced maximum performance and rollover of the performance-intensity function on a measure of sentence recognition in competition. SNR = signal-to-noise ratio; ST = speech threshold; WRS$_M$ = maximum word recognition score.

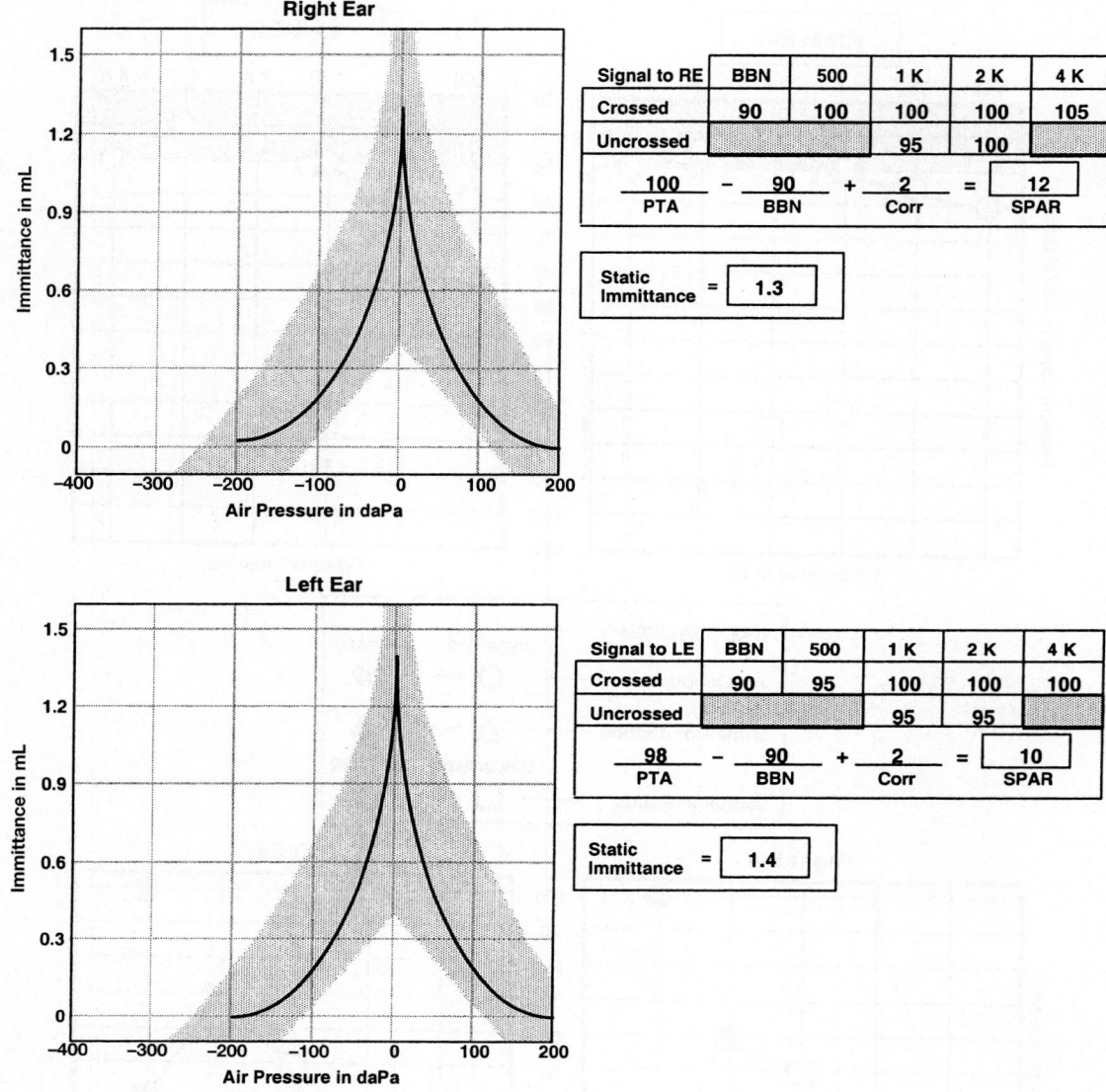

Right Ear

Signal to RE	BBN	500	1 K	2 K	4 K
Crossed	90	100	100	100	105
Uncrossed			95	100	

$$\underset{\text{PTA}}{100} - \underset{\text{BBN}}{90} + \underset{\text{Corr}}{2} = \underset{\text{SPAR}}{12}$$

Static Immittance = 1.3

Left Ear

Signal to LE	BBN	500	1 K	2 K	4 K
Crossed	90	95	100	100	100
Uncrossed			95	95	

$$\underset{\text{PTA}}{98} - \underset{\text{BBN}}{90} + \underset{\text{Corr}}{2} = \underset{\text{SPAR}}{10}$$

Static Immittance = 1.4

7A

Figure 8–7   Audiometric results in a 72-year-old man with sensorineural hearing loss and an auditory processing disorder. Immittance measures (A) are consistent with normal middle ear function. BBN = broad-band noise; PTA = pure-tone average; SPAR = sensitivity prediction by the acoustic reflex.

Illustration continued on following page

slightly better in the low frequencies than in the high frequencies.

Speech audiometric results are typical for those often found in older patients. Word recognition scores are reduced, but not below the level predicted from the degree of hearing loss. However, speech recognition in the presence of competition is substantially reduced, as shown in Figure 8–7, C, consistent with the patient's age. Performance on a sentence recognition task at an easy signal-to-noise ratio (SNR) was 100% bilaterally. However, at a more difficult SNR (0 dB), performance was substantially reduced. In addition to these monotic deficits, he also shows evidence of a dichotic deficit, with reduced performance in the left ear.

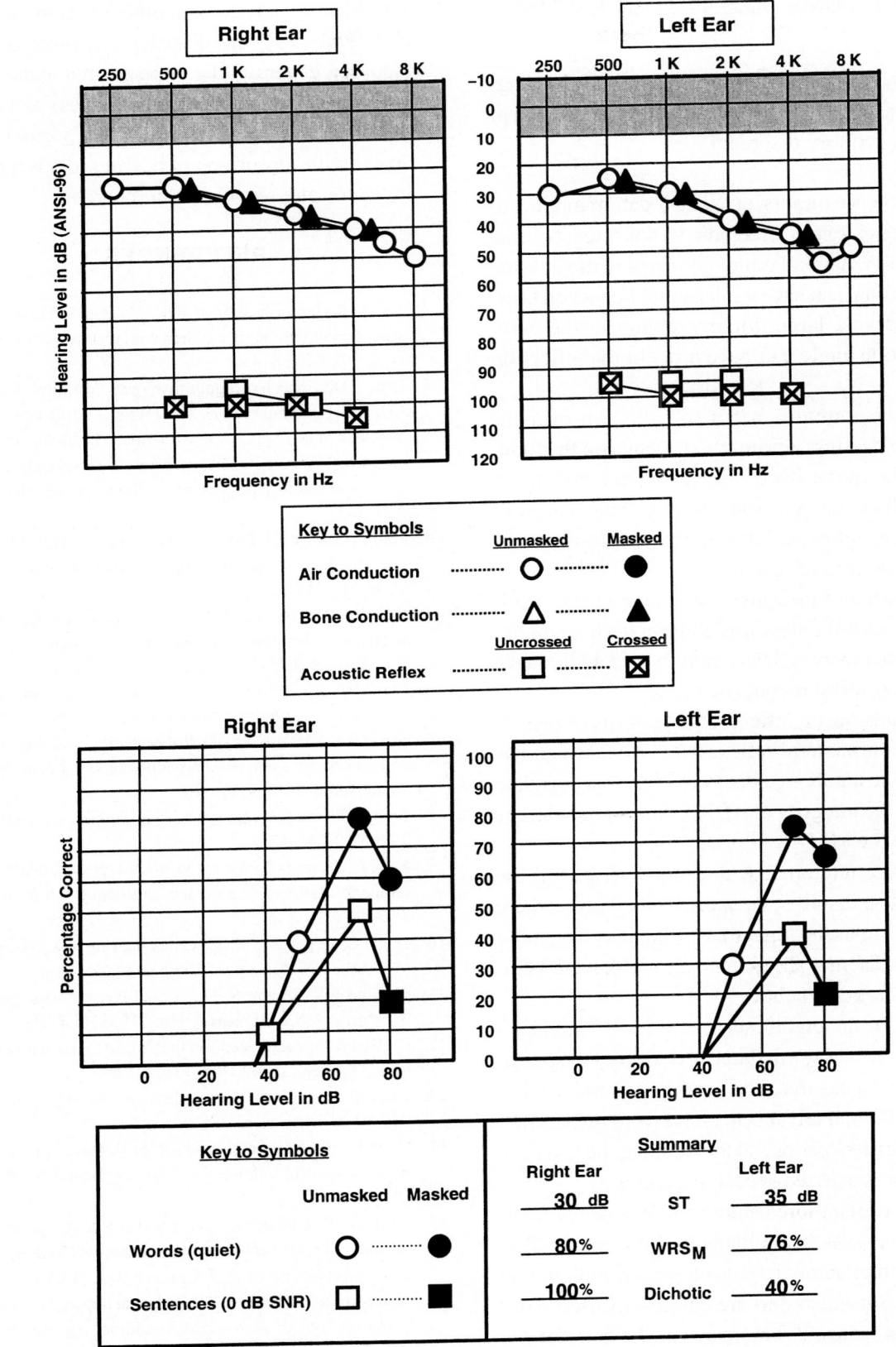

Figure 8–7 Continued. Pure-tone audiometric results (*B*) show a bilaterally symmetric, moderate sensorineural hearing loss. Speech audiometric results (*C*) show reduced word recognition in quiet, consistent with the degree and configuration of the cochlear hearing loss. Sentence recognition in competition and dichotic performance are substantially reduced. SNR = signal-to-noise threshold; ST = speech threshold; WRS_M = maximum word recognition score.

SUMMARY: SOME DIAGNOSTIC LESSONS

Following, by way of summary, are some of the diagnostic lessons learned from the audiologic evaluation of patients with auditory disorder:

1. In eighth nerve tumors, size and location interact to dictate the extent to which the tumor impacts hearing function. A small tumor confined to the internal auditory canal can have a substantial impact on hearing, whereas a large tumor growing in the cerebellopontine angle can have a negligible effect on hearing.

2. Eighth nerve tumors seem to have two primary effects on hearing: a primary influence on the function of the nerve itself and secondary effects on cochlear function. Accordingly, audiologic outcomes can reflect a retrocochlear pattern, cochlear pattern, or mixed pattern of results.

3. With immittance measures, tympanometry by itself is seldom useful unless it is abnormal. In combination with acoustic reflexes, immittance audiometry can be a powerful diagnostic tool.

4. Regarding acoustic reflexes, the patterns of ipsilateral and contralateral reflexes are critical to understanding the nature of a disorder. Reflexes correlate well with the integrity of ABR wave III and with the results on the MLD.

5. In pure-tone audiometry, the more peripheral the retrocochlear disorder, the more likely it is that there is a significant sensorineural hearing loss. The more central the disorder, the more likely it is that the influence on hearing is subtle.

6. Disorders of the eighth nerve and lower brainstem are likely to show ipsilateral deficits on speech audiometric measures. The more peripheral the disorder, the more likely it is to affect word recognition scores. The more peripheral the disorder, the less need there is for sensitized speech measures.

7. Disorders of the more central portions of the auditory nervous system are likely to show both ipsilateral and contralateral deficits on speech audiometric measures. Such disorders are unlikely to affect word recognition scores. The more central the disorder, the more need there is for sensitized speech measures to reveal its influence.

8. The ABR correlates with other measures in peripheral nervous system disorder. The more central the disorder, generally the more normal is the ABR.

9. If abnormal, OAEs are largely useless as a diagnostic tool. In contrast, the presence of normal OAEs in an ear with sensorineural hearing loss is a powerful indicator of a retrocochlear disorder.

REFERENCES

1. Jerger S, Jerger J, Alford BR, Abrams S. Development of speech intelligibility in children with recurrent otitis media. Ear Hear 1983;4:138–45.
2. Brown DP. Speech recognition in recurrent otitis media: results in a set of identical twins. J Am Acad Audiol 1994;5:1–6.
3. Schilder AGM, Snik AFM, Straatman H, van den Broek P. The effect of otitis media with effusion at preschool age on some aspects of auditory perception at school age. Ear Hear 1994;15:224–31.
4. Hall JW, Grose JH, Pillsbury HC. Long-term effects of chronic otitis media on binaural hearing in children. Arch Otolaryngol 1995;121:847–52.
5. Cacace AT, Parnes SM, Lovely TJ, Kalathia A. The disconnected ear: phenomenological effects of a large acoustic tumor. Ear Hear 1994;15:287–98.
6. Stach BA, Delgado-Vilches G. Sudden hearing loss in multiple sclerosis: case report. J Am Acad Audiol 1993;4:370–5.
7. Stach BA, Westerberg BD, Roberson JB. Auditory disorder in central nervous system miliary tuberculosis: a case report. J Am Acad Audiol 1998;9:305–10.
8. Starr A, Picton TW, Sininger Y, et al. Auditory neuropathy. Brain 1996;119:741–53.
9. Starr A, Sininger Y, Winter M, et al. Transient deafness due to temperature-sensitive auditory neuropathy. Ear Hear 1998;19:169–79.
10. Jerger S, Jerger J. Low frequency hearing loss in central auditory disorders. Am J Otol 1980;2:1–4.
11. Gelfand SA, Silman S. Functional hearing loss and its relationship to resolved hearing levels. Ear Hear 1985;6:151–8.
12. Carhart R. Speech reception in relation to pattern of pure tone loss. J Speech Disord 1946;11:97–108.
13. Egan JP. Articulation testing methods. Laryngoscope 1948;58:955–91.
14. Hirsh IJ, Davis H, Silverman SR, et al. Development of materials for speech audiometry. J Speech Hear Disord 1952;17:321–37.
15. Tillman TW, Carhart R. An expanded test for speech discrimination utilizing CNC monosyllabic words (Northwestern University Test No. 6). Brooks Air Force Base (TX): USAF School of Aerospace Medicine; 1966. Technical Report, SAM-TR-66-55 USAF School of Aerospace Medicine, Aerospace Medical Division (AFSC).
16. Jerger J, Jerger S. Diagnostic significance of PB word functions. Arch Otolaryngol 1971;93:573–80.

17. Dirks DD, Kamm C, Bower D, Betsworth A. Use of performance-intensity functions for diagnosis. J Speech Hear Disord 1977;42:408–15.

18. Dubno JR, Lee FS, Klein AJ, et al. Confidence limits for maximum word-recognition scores. J Speech Hear Res 1995;38:490–502.

19. Yellin MW, Jerger J, Fifer RC. Norms for disproportionate loss of speech intelligibility. Ear Hear 1989;10:231–4.

20. Bocca E, Calearo C, Cassinari V. A new method for testing hearing in temporal lobe tumours. Acta Otolaryngol (Stockh) 1954;44:219–21.

21. Jerger J. Observations on auditory behavior in lesions of the central auditory pathways. Arch Otolaryngol 1960;71:797–806.

22. Lynn GW, Gilroy J. Evaluation of central auditory dysfunction in patients with neurological disorders. In: Keith RW, editor. Central auditory dysfunction. New York: Grune & Stratton; 1977. p. 177–222.

23. Calearo C, Antonelli AR. Audiometric findings in brain stem lesions. Acta Otolaryngol (Stockh) 1968;66:305–19.

24. Kurdziel S, Noffsinger D, Olsen W. Performance by cortical lesion patients on 40 and 60% time-compressed materials. J Am Audiol Soc 1976;2:3–7.

25. Jerger J, Hayes D. Diagnostic speech audiometry. Arch Otolaryngol 1977;103:216–22.

26. Kimura D. Some effects of temporal lobe damage on auditory perception. Can J Psychol 1961;15:157–65.

27. Berlin CI, Lowe-Bell SS, Jannetta PJ, Kline DG. Central auditory deficits of temporal lobectomy. Arch Otolaryngol 1972;96:4–10.

28. Musiek FE. Results of three dichotic speech tests on subjects with intracranial lesions. Ear Hear 1983;4:318–23.

29. Fifer RC, Jerger JF, Berlin CI, et al. Development of a dichotic sentence identification test for hearing-impaired adults. Ear Hear 1983;4:300–5.

30. Jerger J, Chmiel R, Allen J, Wilson A. Effects of age and gender on dichotic sentence identification. Ear Hear 1994;15:274–86.

31. Fowler EP. A method for the early detection of otosclerosis: a study of sounds well above threshold. Arch Otolaryngol 1936;24:731–41.

32. Dix MR, Hallpike CS, Hood JD. Observations upon the loudness recruitment phenomenon, with especial reference to the differential diagnosis of disorders of the internal ear and VIII nerve. Proc R Soc Med 1948;41:516–26.

33. Jerger J. Recruitment and allied phenomena in differential diagnosis. J Auditory Res 1961;2:145–51.

34. Lüscher E, Zwislocki J. A simple method for indirect monaural determination of the recruitment phenomenon (difference limen in intensity in different types of deafness). Acta Otolaryngol Suppl (Stockh) 1949;78:156–72.

35. Jerger J. A difference limen test and its diagnostic significance. Laryngoscope 1952;62:1316–32.

36. Jerger J, Shedd J, Harford E. On the detection of extremely small changes in sound intensity. Arch Otolaryngol 1959;69:200–11.

37. Thompson GA. Modified SISI technique for selected cases with suspected acoustic neurinoma. J Speech Hear Disord 1963;28:299–302.

38. Carhart R. Clinical determination of abnormal auditory adaptation. Arch Otolaryngol 1957;65:32–9.

39. Olsen WO, Noffsinger D. Comparison of one new and three old tests of auditory adaptation. Arch Otolaryngol 1974;96:231–47.

40. Jerger J, Jerger S. A simplified tone decay test. Arch Otolaryngol 1975;101:403–7.

41. Békésy G. A new audiometer. Acta Otolaryngol (Stockh) 1947;35:411–22.

42. Jerger J. Békésy audiometry in analysis of auditory disorders. J Speech Hear Res 1960;3:275–87.

43. Sanders JW, Josey AF, Glasscock ME. Audiologic evaluation in cochlear and eighth-nerve disorders. Arch Otolaryngol 1974;100:283–93.

44. Johnson EW. Auditory test results in 500 cases of acoustic neuroma. Arch Otolaryngol 1977;103:152–8.

45. Jerger S, Jerger J. Evaluation of diagnostic audiometric tests. Audiology 1983;22:144–61.

46. Turner RG, Shepard NT, Frazer GJ. Clinical performance of audiological and related diagnostic tests. Ear Hear 1984;5:187–94.

47. Noffsinger D, Kurdziel S, Applebaum EL. Value of special auditory tests in the lateromedial inferior pontine syndrome. Ann Otol 1975;84:384–90.

48. Olsen WO, Noffsinger D. Masking level differences for cochlear and brain stem lesions. Ann Otol 1976;85:820–5.

49. Lynn GE, Gilroy J, Taylor PC, Leiser RP. Binaural masking-level differences in neurological disorders. Arch Otolaryngol 1981;107:357–62.

50. Hannley M, Jerger JF, Rivera VM. Relationships among auditory brain stem responses, masking level differences and the acoustic reflex in multiple sclerosis. Audiology 1983;22:20–33.

51. Silman S, Silverman CA. Functional hearing impairment. In: Silman S, Silverman CA, editors. Auditory diagnosis: principles and applications. San Diego: Singular Publishing Group; 1997. p. 137–57.

52. Stach BA, Jerger JF. Immittance measures in auditory disorders. In: Jacobson JT, Northern JL, editors. Diagnostic audiology. Austin (TX): Pro-Ed; 1990. p. 113–40.

53. Jerger J. Clinical experience with impedance audiometry. Arch Otolaryngol 1970;92:311–24.

54. Shanks JE, Shelton C. Basic principles and clinical applications of tympanometry. Otolaryngol Clin North Am 1991;24:299–328.

55. Hunter LL, Margolis RH. Effects of tympanic membrane abnormalities on auditory function. J Am Acad Audiol 1997;8:431–46.

56. Vanhuyse VJ, Creten WL, Van Camp KJ. On the W-notching of tympanograms. Scand Audiol 1975;4:45–50.

57. Shahnaz N, Polka L. Standard and multifrequency tympanometry in normal and otosclerotic ears. Ear Hear 1997;18:326–41.

58. Voss SE, Allen JB. Measurement of acoustic impedance and reflectance in the human ear canal. J Acoust Soc Am 1994;95:372–84.

59. Niemeyer W, Sesterhenn G. Calculating the hearing threshold from the stapedius reflex threshold for different sound stimuli. Audiology 1974;13:421–7.

60. Jerger J, Burney P, Mauldin L. Predicting hearing loss from the acoustic reflex. J Speech Hear Disord 1974;39:11–22.

61. Anderson H, Barr B, Wedenberg E. Early diagnosis of VIIIth-nerve tumours by acoustic reflex tests. Acta Otolaryngol (Stockh) 1970;262:232–7.

62. Jerger J, Harford E, Clemis J, Alford B. The acoustic reflex in eighth nerve disorder. Arch Otolaryngol 1974;99:409–13.

63. Mangham CA, Lindeman RC, Dawson WR. Stapedius reflex quantification in acoustic tumor patients. Laryngoscope 1980; 90:242–50.

64. Jerger S, Jerger J. Diagnostic value of crossed vs. uncrossed acoustic reflexes. Eighth nerve and brainstem disorders. Arch Otolaryngol 1977;103:445–53.

65. Starr A, Achor J. Auditory brain stem responses in neurological disease. Arch Neurol 1975;32:761–8.

66. Selters WA, Brackmann DE. Acoustic tumor detection with brain stem electric response audiometry. Arch Otolaryngol 1977;103:181–7.

67. Stockard JJ, Stockard JE, Sharbrough FW. Detection and localization of occult lesions with brainstem auditory responses. Mayo Clinic Proc 1977;52:761–9.

68. Clemis JD, McGee T. Brain stem electric response audiometry in the differential diagnosis of acoustic tumors. Laryngoscope 1979;89:31–42.

69. Eggermont JJ, Don M, Brackmann DE. Electocochleography and auditory brainstem electric responses in patients with pontine angle tumors. Ann Otol Rhinol Laryngol Suppl 1980;75: 1–19.

70. Musiek FE, Sach E, Geurkink NA, Weider DJ. Auditory brainstem response and eighth nerve lesions: a review and presentation of cases. Ear Hear 1980;1:297–301.

71. Grundy BI, Lina A, Procopio PT, Jannetta PJ. Reversible evoked potential changes with retraction of the eighth cranial nerve. Anesth Analg 1981;60:835–8.

72. Moller AR, Jannetta PJ. Monitoring auditory functions during the cranial nerve microvascular decompression operations by direct recording from the eighth nerve. J Neurosurg 1983;59: 493–9.

73. Kemp DT. Stimulated acoustic emissions from within the human auditory system. J Acoust Soc Am 1978;64:1386–91.

74. Probst R. Otoacoustic emissions: an overview. Adv Otorhinolarygnol 1990;44:1–91.

75. Harris F, Probst R. Reporting click-evoked and distortion-product otoacoustic emission results with respect to the pure tone audiogram. Ear Hear 1991;12:399–405.

76. Probst R, Harris FP. Transiently evoked and distortion-product otoacoustic emissions: comparison of results from normally hearing and hearing-impaired human ears. Otolaryngol Head Neck Surg 1993;119:858–60.

77. Owens JJ, McCoy MJ, Lonsbury-Martin BL, Martin GK. Influence of otitis media on evoked otoacoustic emissions in children. Semin Hear 1992;13:53–66.

78. Owens JJ, McCoy MJ, Lonsbury-Martin BL, Martin GK. Otoacoustic emissions in children with normal ears, middle-ear dysfunction, and ventilating tubes. Am J Otol 1993;14: 34–40.

79. Lonsbury-Martin BL, Martin GK, McCoy MJ, Whitehead ML. Testing young children with otoacoustic emissions: middle-ear influences. Am J Otol 1994;15(Suppl 1):13–20.

80. Trine MB, Hirsch JE, Margolis RH. The effect of middle ear pressure on transient evoked otoacoustic emissions. Ear Hear 1993;14:401–7.

81. Margolis RH, Trine MB. Influence of middle-ear disease on otoacoustic emissions. In: Robinette MS, Glattke TJ, editors. Otoacoustic emissions: clinical applications. New York: Thieme Medical Publishers; 1997. p. 130–50.

82. Jerger J, Jerger S, Mauldin L. Studies in impedance audiometry. I. Normal and sensorineural ears. Arch Otolaryngol 1972; 96:513–23.

83. Metz O. Threshold of reflex contractions of muscles of middle ear and recruitment of loudness. Arch Otolaryngol 1952;55: 536–43.

84. Bess FH. Clinical assessment of speech recognition. In: Konkle DF, Rintelmann WF, editors. Principles of speech audiometry. Baltimore: University Park Press; 1983. p. 127–201.

85. Jerger J, Mauldin L. Prediction of sensorineural hearing level from the brainstem evoked response. Arch Otolaryngol 1978; 104:456–61.

86. Stach BA, Jerger J, Oliver TA. Auditory evoked potential testing strategies. In: Jacobson JT, editor. Principles and applications in auditory evoked potentials. Needham Heights (MA): Allyn & Bacon; 1993. p. 541–60.

87. Portmann M, Aran JM. Electrocochleography. Laryngoscope 1971;81:899–910.

88. Gibson WR, Moffat DA, Ramsden RT. Clinical electrocochleography in the diagnosis and management of Meniere's disorder. Audiology 1977;16:389–401.

89. Margolis RH, Rieks D, Fournier EM, Levine SC. Tympanic electrocochleography for diagnosis of Meniere's disease. Arch Otolaryngol Head Neck Surg 1995;121:44–55.

90. Orchik DJ, Ge NN, Shea JJ. Action potential latency shift by rarefaction and condensation clicks in Meniere's disease. J Am Acad Audiol 1998;9:121–6.

91. Probst R, Lonsbury-Martin BL, Martin GK, Coats AC. Otoacoustic emissions in ears with hearing loss. Am J Otol 1987;8: 73–81.

92. Robinette MS. EOAE contributions in the evaluation of cochlear versus retrocochlear disorders. Semin Hear 1999;20:13–28.

93. Balkany TJ, Telischi FF, Lonsbury-Martin BL, Martin GK. Otoacoustic emissions in clinical practice. Am J Otol 1994;15 Suppl 1:29–38.

94. Zorowka PG, Schmitt HJ, Gutjahr P. Evoked otoacoustic emissions and pure tone threshold audiometry in patients receiving cisplatinum therapy. Int J Pediatr Otorhinolaryngol 1993;25: 73–80.

95. Ozturan O, Jerger J, Lew H, Lynch GR. Monitoring of cisplatin ototoxicity by distortion-product otoacoustic emissions. Auris Nasus Larynx 1996;23:147–51.

96. Chandrasekhar SS, Brackmann DE, Devgan KK. Utility of auditory brainstem response audiometry in diagnosis of acoustic neuromas. Am J Otol 1995;16:63–7.

97. Gordon ML, Cohen NL. Efficacy of auditory brainstem response as a screening test for small acoustic neuromas. Am J Otol 1995; 16:136–9.

98. Ruckenstein MJ, Cueva RA, Morrison DH, Press G. A prospective study of ABR and MRI in the screening for vestibular schwannomas. Am J Otol 1996;17:317–20.

99. Durrant JD, Kamerer DB, Chen D. Combined OAE and ABR studies in acoustic tumor patients. In: Hoehmann D, editor. ECoG, OAE and intraoperative monitoring. Amsterdam: Kugler; 1993. p. 231–9.

100. Telischi FF, Roth J, Stagner BB, et al. Patterns of evoked otoacoustic emissions associated with acoustic neuromas. Laryngoscope 1995;105:675–82.

101. Anderson H, Barr B, Wedenberg E. Intra-aural reflexes in retrocochlear lesions. In: Hamberger C, Wersall J, editors. Nobel Symposium 10: disorders of the skull base region. Stockholm: Almquist & Wiskell; 1969. p. 49–55.

102. Olsen WO, Noffsinger D, Kurdziel S. Acoustic reflex and reflex decay. Occurrence in patients with cochlear and eighth nerve lesions. Arch Otolaryngol 1975;101:622–5.

103. Olsen WO, Stach BA, Kurdziel SA. Acoustic reflex decay in 10 seconds and in 5 seconds for Meniere's disease patients and for VIIIth nerve patients. Ear Hear 1981;2:180–1.

104. Stach BA, Jerger JF. Acoustic reflex averaging. Ear Hear 1984; 5:289–96.

105. Stach BA, Jerger JF. Acoustic reflex patterns in peripheral and central auditory system disease. Semin Hear 1987;8:369–77.

106. Sanders JW, Josey AF, Glasscock ME, Jackson CG. The acoustic reflex test in cochlear and eighth nerve pathology ears. Laryngoscope 1981;91:787–93.

107. Bosatra A, Russolo M, Poli P. Modifications of the stapedius muscle reflex under spontaneous and experimental brain-stem impairment. Acta Otolaryngol (Stockh) 1975;80:61–6.

108. Greisen O, Rasmussen PE. Stapedius muscle reflexes and otoneurological examinations in brain-stem tumors. Acta Otolaryngol (Stockh) 1970;70:366–70.

109. Jerger J, Oliver TA, Rivera V, Stach BA. Abnormalities of the acoustic reflex in multiple sclerosis. Am J Otolaryngol 1986;7: 163–76.

110. Jerger S, Jerger J. Auditory disorders: a manual for clinical evaluation. Boston: Little, Brown; 1981.

111. Stach BA, Delgado-Vilches G, Smith-Farach S. Hearing loss in multiple sclerosis. Semin Hear 1990;11:221–30.

112. Pensak ML, Glasscock ME, Josey AF, et al. Sudden hearing loss and cerebellopontine angle tumors. Laryngoscope 1985;95: 1188–93.

113. Selesnick SH, Jackler RK. Atypical hearing loss in acoustic neuroma patients. Laryngoscope 1993;103:437–41.

114. Musiek FE, Josey AF, Glasscock ME. Auditory brain stem responses—interwave measurements in acoustic neuromas. Ear Hear 1986;7:100–5.

115. Roland PS, Glasscock ME, Bojrab DI, et al. Normal hearing in patients with acoustic neuromas. South Med J 1987;80:166–9.

116. Saleh EA, Aristegui M. Naguib MB, et al. Normal hearing in acoustic neuroma patients: a critical evaluation. Am J Otol 1996; 17:127–32.

117. Lustig LR, Rifkin S, Jackler RK, Pitts LH. Acoustic neuromas presenting with normal and symmetrical hearing: factors associated with diagnosis and outcome. Am J Otol 1998;19:212–8.

118. Olsen WO, Noffsinger D, Kurdziel S. Speech discrimination in quiet and in white noise by patients with peripheral and central lesions. Acta Otolaryngol (Stockh) 1975;80:375–82.

119. Bess FH, Josey AF, Humes LE. Performance intensity functions in cochlear and eighth nerve disorders. Am J Otol 1979;1: 27–31.

120. Meyer DH, Mishler ET. Rollover measurements with the Auditec NU-6 word lists. J Speech Hear Disord 1985;50: 356–60.

121. Jerger J, Jerger S. Clinical validity of central auditory tests. Scand Audiol 1975;4:147–63.

122. Russolo M, Poli P. Lateralization, impedance, auditory brain stem response and synthetic sentence audiometry in brain stem disorders. Audiology 1983;22:50–62.

123. Jerger JF, Jerger SW. Auditory findings in brainstem disorders. Arch Otolaryngol 1974;99:342–9.

124. Hurley R, Musiek FE. Effectiveness of three central auditory processing (CAP) tests in identifying cerebral lesions. J Am Acad Audiol 1997;8:257–62.

125. Sparks R, Goodglass H, Nickel B. Ipsilateral versus contralateral extinction in dichotic listening resulting from hemisphere lesions. Cortex 1970;6:249–60.

126. Josey AF, Glasscock ME, Musiek FE. Correlation of ABR and medical imaging in patients with cerebellopontine angle tumors. Am J Otol 1988;9:12–6.

127. Josey AF, Jackson CG, Glasscock ME. Brainstem evoked response audiometry in confirmed eighth nerve tumors. Am J Otolaryngol 1980;1:285–9.

128. Telian SA, Kileny PR, Niparko JK, et al. Normal auditory brainstem response in patients with acoustic neuroma. Laryngoscope 1989;99:10–4.

129. Don M, Masuda A, Nelson R, Brackmann D. Successful detection of small acoustic tumors using the stacked derived-band auditory brain stem response amplitude. Am J Otol 1997;18: 608–21.

130. Stanton SG, Cashman MZ. Auditory brainstem response. A comparison of different interpretation strategies for detection of cerebellopontine angle tumors. Scand Audiol 1996;25:109–20.

131. Musiek FE, Lee WW. The auditory brain stem response in patients with brain stem or cochlear pathology. Ear Hear 1995; 16:631–6.

132. Harker L, Backoff P. Middle latency electric auditory response in patients with acoustic neuroma. Otolaryngol Head Neck Surg 1981;89:131–6.

133. Stach BA, Hudson M. Middle and late auditory evoked potentials in multiple sclerosis. Semin Hear 1990;11:265–75.

134. Kileny P, Paccioretti D, Wilson AF. Effects of cortical lesions on middle-latency auditory evoked responses (MLR). Electroencephalogr Clin Neurophysiol 1987;66:108–20.

135. Kraus N, Özdamar Ö, Hier D, Stein L. Auditory middle latency responses (MLRs) in patients with cortical lesions. Electroencephalogr Clin Neurophysiol 1982;54:275–87.

136. Robinson K, Rudge P. Abnormalities of the auditory evoked potentials in patients with multiple sclerosis. Brain 1977;100: 19–40.

137. Kileny PR, Edwards BM, Disher MJ, Telian SA. Hearing improvement after resection of cerebellopontine angle meningioma: case study of the preoperative role of transient otoacoustic emissions. J Am Acad Audiol 1998;9:1–6.

138. Collet L, Kemp DT, Veuillet E, et al. Effect of contralateral auditory stimuli on active cochlear micro-mechanical properties in human subjects. Hear Res 1990;43:251–62.

139. Berlin CI, Hood LJ, Wen H, et al. Contralateral suppression of non-linear click-evoked otoacoustic emissions. Hear Res 1993; 71:1–11.

140. Berlin CI, Hood LJ, Hurley A, Wen H. Contralateral suppression of otoacoustic emissions: an index of the function of the medial olivocochlear system. Otolaryngol Head Neck Surg 1994;110:3–21.

141. Goetzinger C, Proud G, Dirks D, Embrey J. A study of hearing in advanced age. Arch Otolaryngol 1961;73:662–74.

142. Helfer KS, Wilber LA. Hearing loss, aging, and speech perception in reverberation and noise. J Speech Hear Res 1990;33: 149–55.

143. Jerger J. Audiological findings in aging. Adv Otorhinolaryngol 1973;20:115–24.

144. Konig E. Audiological tests in presbycusis. Int Audiol 1969;8: 240–59.

145. Orchik D, Burgess J. Synthetic sentence identification as a function of age of the listener. J Am Audiol Soc 1977;3:42–6.

146. Wiley TL, Cruickshanks KJ, Nondahl DM, et al. Aging and word recognition in competing message. J Am Acad Audiol 1998;9:191–8.

147. Stuart A, Phillips DP. Word recognition in continuous and interrupted broadband noise by young normal-hearing, older normal-hearing, and presbyacusic listeners. Ear Hear 1996;17: 478–89.

148. Sperry JL, Wiley TL, Chial MR. Word recognition performance in various background competitors. J Am Acad Audiol 1997;8:71–80.

149. Jerger J, Jordan C. Age-related asymmetry on a cued-listening task. Ear Hear 1992;4:272–7.

150. Fitzgibbons PJ, Gordon-Salant S. Auditory temporal processing in elderly listeners. J Am Acad Audiol 1996;7:183–9.

151. Konkle D, Beasley D, Bess F. Intelligibility of time-altered speech in relation to chronological aging. J Speech Hear Res 1977;20:108–15.

152. McCroskey R, Kasten R. Temporal factors and the aging auditory system. Ear Hear 1992;3:124–7.

153. Price PJ, Simon HJ. Perception of temporal differences in speech by "normal-hearing" adults: effect of age and intensity. J Acoust Soc Am 1984;76:405–10.

154. Cranford JL, Romereim B. Precedence effect and speech understanding in elderly listeners. J Am Acad Audiol 1992;3: 405–9.

155. Phillips SL, Gordon-Salant S, Fitzgibbons PJ, Yeni-Komshian GH. Auditory duration discrimination in young and elderly listeners with normal hearing. J Am Acad Audiol 1994;5:210–5.

156. Wilson RH, Jaffe MS. Interactions of age, ear, and stimulus complexity on dichotic digit recognition. J Am Acad Audiol 1996;7: 358–64.

157. Jerger J, Stach BA, Johnson K, et al. Patterns of abnormality in dichotic listening in the elderly. In: Jensen JH, editor. Proceedings of the 14th Danavox Symposium on Presbyacusis and Other Age Relate Aspects. Odense (Denmark): Danavox; 1990. p. 143–50.

158. Jerger J, Silman S, Lew HL, Chmiel R. Case studies in binaural interference: converging evidence from behavioral and electrophysiologic measures. J Am Acad Audiol 1993;4:122–31.

159. Silman S. Binaural interference in multiple sclerosis: case study. J Am Acad Audiol 1995;6:193–6.

160. Hausler R, Colburn S, Marr E. Sound localization in subjects with impaired hearing: spatial-discrimination and interaural-discrimination tests. Acta Otolaryngol Suppl (Stockh) 1983;400: 1–62.

161. Stephens SDG. Auditory temporal summation in patients with central nervous system lesions. In: Stephens SDG, editor. Disorders of auditory function. London: Academic Press; 1976. p. 243–52.

162. Cranford JL, Boose M, Moore CA. Tests of precedence effect in sound localization reveal abnormalities in multiple sclerosis. Ear Hear 1990;11:282–8.

163. Stach BA. Central auditory disorders. In: Lalwani AK, Grundfast KM, editors. Pediatric otology and neurotology. Philadelphia: Lippincott-Raven Publishers; 1998. p. 387–96.

164. Jerger J, Alford B, Lew H, et al. Dichotic listening, event-related potentials, and interhemispheric transfer in the elderly. Ear Hear 1995;16:482–98.

165. Carhart R. Clinical application of bone conduction. Arch Otolaryngol 1950;51:798–807.

9

Vestibular Testing

Dennis I. Bojrab, MD
B. Maya Kato, MD

Vestibular testing is an important tool in the management of the patient with dizziness. The bedside evaluation of the dizzy patient, with a careful history and a thorough neurotologic examination, is crucial for making an accurate clinical diagnosis. We do not believe that vestibular testing is to be used as a "stand alone" diagnostic test battery for patients with dizziness. Accurate testing may aid in establishing a diagnosis, determining the side or site of the lesion, staging of the illness, following the patient's condition with and without treatment over the course of the illness, and selecting treatment options for the patient. We therefore recommend a thorough understanding of how these tests are performed and interpreted and how we can use this information in the clinical setting.

Although bedside and office examinations provide information about the status of the vestibular system, major limitations are the inability to quantify responses and to monitor the course of the illness or the results of medical and surgical management of the dizzy patient. The uses of the vestibular laboratory are cited in Table 9–1. Current technologies available for assessing the vestibular system include electronystagmography (ENG), rotation testing, and dynamic posturography. The first two modalities evaluate the vestibular system by testing vestibulo-ocular interactions or the vestibulo-ocular reflex (VOR). Dynamic posturography is a test of postural stability and reveals information about the vestibulospinal reflex (VSR). We discuss how each of these tests are performed and what information each test provides and provide guidelines for their use in various clinical situations.

ELECTRONYSTAGMOGRAPHY

Electronystagmography is the most common method of laboratory evaluation of the vestibular system. The examination consists of a battery of tests that are collectively referred to as the ENG. Electronystagmography monitors eye movements using electro-oculography. The vestibular and ocular systems are connected through the VOR; thus, patients with peripheral and/or central balance disorders often exhibit abnormal eye movements that can be measured and recorded. Electronystagmography assesses whether labyrinthine dysfunction is present and what degree of dysfunction exists and is unique among the vestibular tests in that it can provide specific information about each ear separately (ie, it lateralizes dysfunction).

Eye Movement Recording Equipment

A variety of eye movement recording equipment is currently available. In performing the ENG, the patient's eye movements are measured relative to head position, which can be achieved in a number of ways: measuring elec-

Table 9–1 USES OF VESTIBULAR LABORATORY
Aid in establishing diagnosis
Location — central versus peripheral lesion
Lateralization
Documentation
Assist in devising treatment plan
Aid in long-term management

tric potentials, measuring magnetic potentials, using video cameras, or using infrared technology.

Corneoretinal Potential

The most commonly used technology depends on the fact that there is a steady DC potential, termed the corneoretinal potential (CRP), between the cornea and the retina (Figure 9–1). These potentials create an electric field at the front of the head that rotates as the eyes rotate. The CRP is generated by the metabolic activity of the retinal pigment epithelium. The retina is negatively charged relative to the cornea; thus, an electrical potential can be measured between the two by means of skin surface electrodes. When the eyes are looking straight ahead (primary gaze), the average potential measured at the cornea is about 1 mV. As the eyes move, the potential changes, relative to the skin electrodes. Thus, differences in electric potential are measured and reflect movement of the eyes. Rotation of this electric field produces a roughly linear change in the voltage between electrodes attached to the skin on either side of the eyes. Horizontal eye position is monitored by electrodes

placed on the temples; vertical eye position is monitored by electrodes placed above and below one eye. Of note, it is difficult to detect torsional nystagmus with traditional electro-oculography because rotation of the eye about the axis of the pupil does not effect a change in the CRP.

ELECTRONYSTAGMOGRAPHIC TRACING

Electronystagmography results are recorded on an electrocardiogram strip in which time is plotted on the horizontal axis and eye movements are recorded on the vertical axis. By convention, rightward eye movement is recorded as an upward deflection, and leftward eye motion is shown as a downward deflection. When ENG testing was first developed, the data from the strip tracing were hand-calculated into meaningful results. The recent development of computerized ENG analysis has been a substantial enhancement and permits efficient storage and easy retrieval of eye movement data and eliminates the cutting and pasting of strip chart recordings. In addition, computerized ENG allows rapid and sophisticated analysis of saccade, tracking, and caloric tests—analyses that could not be done on strip chart recordings.

Video-oculography and Others

Other techniques have been developed to record eye motion but are not available in all ENG laboratories. These alternative methods of evaluating eye movement include videonystagmography (VNG), magnetic scleral search coil devices, and infrared recording devices.

One current trend in many vestibular laboratories is toward the use of video-recorded nystagmography. *Videonystagmography* is a computer-based system for eye movement testing (Figure 9–2). This technique records eye movements with digital video technology using infrared illumination and a high-technology goggle. The images are then displayed on a computer monitor. The computer software records and analyzes the data. These images may then be recorded on videotape. The VNG technique determines eye position by locating the pupil and tracking its center; the internal computer program plots, measures, and analyzes the eye movement similar to traditional ENG.

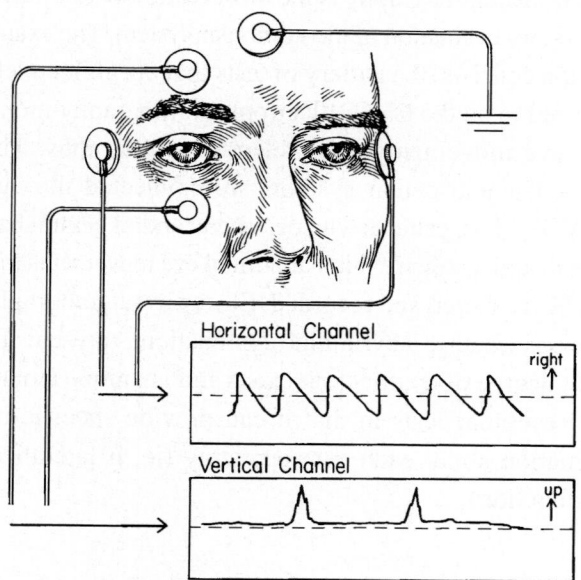

Figure 9–1 Electro-oculography (EOG). The cornea is relatively positively charged in comparison to the retina; thus, an electric potential exists between the two. Electrodes are placed around the eyes, and rotation of the eye brings the cornea closer to one electrode and the negatively charged retina closer to the other. The relative voltage difference provides the basis for EOG. By convention, rightward movement of the eye is recorded as an upward deflection on the electronystagmographic tracing.

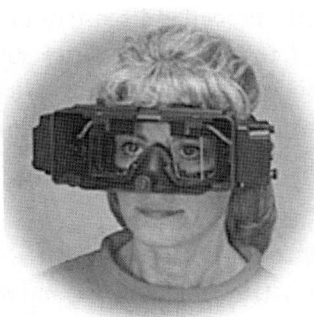

Figure 9–2 Videonystagmography equipment. The goggles contain video cameras that allow the patient's eye movements to be recorded for later viewing and analysis. Direct visualization of the eyes allows for superior documentation of torsional nystagmus, when compared with traditional electro-oculography-based systems.

The VNG technique permits visualization and recording of eye movements — helpful for later study and for teaching personnel and patients. This capacity is especially important in evaluating patients with benign paroxysmal positional vertigo (BPPV) — one of the more common vestibular abnormalities encountered. Videonystamographic tracings are clean with no drift, which improves the accuracy of analysis and interpretation. This technique is easier and quicker than using electrodes and only one calibration is necessary, eliminating the cost of accessories. There are limitations to the VNG that are noteworthy. Test equipment is more expensive, some patients with significant claustrophobia may not tolerate the sensation of confinement, and patients with ptosis, pupil-obscuring eyelashes, or other eye abnormalities may be difficult to test.

The *magnetic search coil technique* places the patient in a cage controlling a magnetic field. The patient wears a soft contact lens in which a wire coil is embedded. Eye movement effects a change in the magnetic field, which is recorded. The advantage of this method is that it gives very high-resolution data for all types of eye movements, including torsional nystagmus. Its disadvantages are the slight discomfort to the patient (owing to the lens) and the very high cost of the equipment. This procedure has yet to gain widespread acceptance and is rarely used.

Infrared oculography is based on the differing reflectance properties of the iris compared to the sclera and the fact that the photocells of the eye remain stationary while the edge of the iris moves with the eye. As a result, the light sensed by the photocells differs according to eye position. The advantage of this technique is that a direct estimate of the eye position as a function of time can be calculated. The disadvantages of this technique include the bulk of the equipment, which limits visual stimulation somewhat, and the interference with eyelid motion (eg, blink), which makes vertical recording difficult at times.[1]

ROUTINE COMPONENTS OF ELECTRONYSTAGMOGRAPHY

The ENG test battery usually consists of three groups of tests. By convention, the tests are performed in a systematic fashion to assess the oculomotor and vestibular systems and their corresponding interaction. Test procedures are designed to test each function and to detect the presence of "pathologic" (spontaneous, gaze, positional, and positioning) nystagmus.

The first group of tests investigates *visual-oculomotor function* and evaluates nonvestibular eye movements. The saccade test detects disorders of the saccadic control system; the tracking test and the optokinetic test both detect disorders of the pursuit control system.

The second group of tests looks for the *presence of abnormal eye movements* and whether they change with altered head position. The gaze test evaluates limitations of eye movement, gaze stability, ocular flutter, spontaneous nystagmus, and latent nystagmus. The positional test determines whether various head positions cause or modify nystagmus. The Dix-Hallpike positioning maneuver test for BPPV.

The third group assesses *vestibulo-oculomotor function*. The bithermal caloric test, involving four irrigations, is the most indispensable test of the ENG battery and primarily detects dysfunction of the labyrinth or vestibular nerve (ie, the "peripheral" vestibular system).

Tests of Visual-Oculomotor Function

Visual and vestibular inputs are both important in gaze stabilization during motion. A variety of oculomotor testing paradigms are used to test the central oculomotor control system. Three eye movements assessed as part of the ENG are saccades, smooth pursuit, and optokinetic nystagmus. The three oculomotor systems interact with vestibular reflexes to modulate visual input relevant to the task at hand. The saccade test detects disorders of the saccade control system, and the tracking test and the optokinetic test assess disorders of the pursuit control system.

Saccade (Calibration) Test

The saccade control system generates all voluntary and involuntary fast eye movements. The saccade test is performed at the beginning of the test, while calibrating eye movements. The purpose of the saccade system is to rapidly capture interesting visual targets in the periphery of the visual field onto the fovea. This quick foveating eye movement is a saccade. It is the fastest type of eye movement, sometimes with peak velocities as high as 700 degrees/second and an average velocity of 200 degrees/second.

Horizontal eye movements are first calibrated by having the patient capture an image at a known distance that requires a 20-degree angle of visual excursion. Eye movements are calibrated in both the vertical and horizontal planes. Once calibrated, the patient's saccade function is tested; the testing paradigm may be performed differently in various laboratories. In one version of the test, the patient's horizontal eye movements are monitored with fixation on a computer-controlled visual target that jumps back and forth in the horizontal plane in random sequence. The complete sequence consists of 80 target jumps (40 to the right and 40 to the left), with amplitudes ranging from 5 to 25 degrees. After testing, the computer deletes invalid eye movement data and calculates three values for each saccade: peak velocity, accuracy, and latency.

Abnormally slow-*velocity* saccades are seen in many degenerative and metabolic diseases of the central nervous system (CNS); internuclear ophthalmoplegia; disturbances in the cerebral hemispheres, the superior colliculus, the oculomotor neurons, or the extraocular muscles; drug intoxication; or drowsy or inattentive patients. Abnormally fast-velocity saccades may occur with orbital tumors and myasthenia gravis.[2] The cerebellum plays an important role in determining the accuracy of saccadic movements. Inaccurate saccades, or ocular dysmetria, are classified as hypermetria (overshooting the target) or hypometria (undershooting) and may be seen with cerebellar disease or brainstem disorders. Saccadic latency abnormalities may be seen in patients with abnormal vision, Parkinson's disease, Huntington's chorea, Alzheimer's disease, and focal hemispheric lesions.[3]

Pursuit and Optokinetic Tests

Two tests of pursuit, the tracking test and the optokinetic test, are typically performed as part of the ENG. Pursuit tracking, or the smooth pursuit system, allows continuous foveation of moving objects and works with the saccade system to maintain foveation when the target is moving. The smooth pursuit system is used to track targets at slower speeds and operates when the eyes move within the orbit and the head is still. The VOR is used when the target is moving at faster speeds and the head is moving.

The *smooth pursuit system* has neural pathways from the fovea to several cortical and subcortical pathways. The pursuit tracking test can be performed simply with a pendulum swinging back and forth, producing a sinusoidal moving target. In a computer-generated version of the test, the patient's horizontal eye movements are monitored while following a computer-controlled visual target that moves back and forth (at frequencies from 0.2 to 0.7 Hz) in the horizontal plane, following a sinusoidal waveform. After testing, the computer deletes invalid eye movement data; it then deletes interpolated saccades, differentiates the eye position signal, calculates the gain of eye velocity with respect to target velocity separately for rightward and leftward tracking at each target frequency, and plots these data. Normal individuals are able to follow the target smoothly in both directions at all target frequencies. Deficits in smooth pursuit may result from age, medication, visual problems, attention deficit, or lesions of the brainstem, cerebellum, and occipitoparietal junction.

Figure 9–3 shows the results of the tracking test in a patient with a unilateral pursuit defect. The patient was unable to follow the rightward-moving target smoothly and instead approximated its motion using successive saccades, producing a stair-step pattern on the eye movement tracing. Tracking of leftward-moving targets was normal. These findings indicate an asymmetric central nervous system (CNS) lesion involving the pursuit control system.

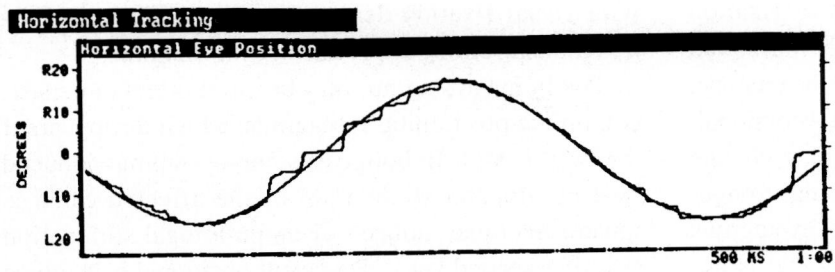

Figure 9-3 The results of the tracking test in a patient with a unilateral pursuit defect. The patient was unable to follow the rightward-moving target smoothly and instead approximated its motion using successive saccades, producing a stair-step pattern on the eye movement tracing. Tracking of leftward-moving targets was normal. This patient's abnormality indicates an asymmetric central nervous system lesion involving the pursuit eye movement control system.

Optokinetic function is a phylogenetically older system that is found in animals lacking well-developed foveae. The optokinetic pathways are subcortical, involving the accessory optic system. In humans, there is an overlap in function by neurons in the cortical and subcortical visual systems. The smooth pursuit system dominates the operation of the overall pursuit system. The optokinetic system differs from smooth pursuit in that optokinetic eye movements follow a moving object until the eye position becomes relatively eccentric. Optokinetic nystagmus consists of an involuntary pursuit of a repetitive image (slow phase) that is followed by a quick saccade that recenters the eyes (fast component). The conduct of the optokinetic test varies according to testing laboratory. In one version, the patient's horizontal eye movements are monitored while following a series of visual targets that move to the right and then to the left. This stimulus evokes a nystagmus with the slow phase in the direction of target motion, periodically interrupted by fast phases in the opposite direction. The optokinetic test, like the tracking test, is a test of eye pursuit pathways, and the results of the tracking and optokinetic tests show concordance with tasks of similar difficulty. In normal individuals, the slow-phase eye velocities approximately match target velocities for both rightward- and leftward-moving targets. Figure 9-4 shows the results of the optokinetic test for a patient whose optokinetic nystagmus was defective for rightward-moving targets and normal for leftward-moving targets.

Abnormal Eye Movements

Gaze Test

This test is valuable in the detection of nystagmus that occurs without vestibular stimulation. It may reveal disorders, vestibular and nonvestibular, of CNS origin, congenital nystagmus, or a spontaneous nystagmus of peripheral vestibular origin. The test differentiates gaze-evoked, dysconjugate, rebound, and spontaneous nystagmus.

The gaze test is performed by recording eye movements first in the primary position and then while fixating on a target 30 degrees to the right, left, above, and below the center position. Each position should be held for at least 30 seconds. Some examiners also attempt to monitor eye movements in these gaze positions (with visual fixation denied), but the tracing is often difficult to interpret. Young, normal individuals rarely have any nystagmus while fixating at any of these gaze positions, but many elderly individuals demonstrate end-point nystagmus. This nystagmus is always faint, with a centripetal slow phase, and generally is of equal intensity on right and left gaze.

Spontaneous vestibular nystagmus occurs when there is an imbalance in the tonic input from the vestibular apparatus. It is typically seen with unilateral vestibular lesions and usually beats away from the side of the injured labyrinth or nerve. Frequently, it is better appre-

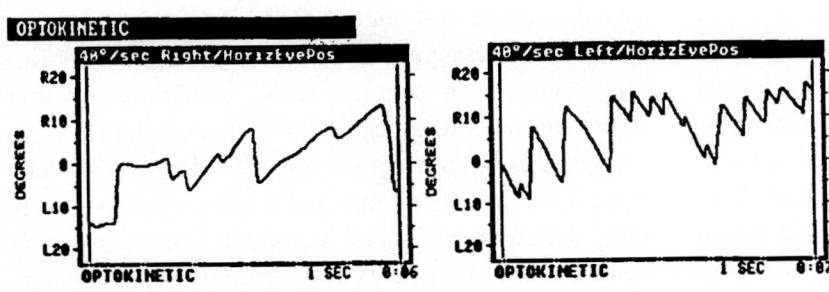

Figure 9-4 Optokinetic test for a patient whose optokinetic system was defective for rightward-moving targets and normal for leftward-moving targets.

ciated during the positional test with visual fixation denied, and it manifests on ENG as a purely horizontal nystagmus because the ENG is insensitive to the torsional component; however, it is actually horizontal-torsional. The intensity of spontaneous nystagmus may change with a change in the direction of the gaze, being stronger when looking toward the direction of the nystagmus (Alexander's law). Spontaneous nystagmus that is not diminished (or increases) with visual fixation (failure of fixation suppression) suggests a central lesion. Upbeat nystagmus usually is a result of medullary lesions that involve the vertical vestibular pathways. Other types of central nystagmus seen in the gaze test are described by Leigh and Zee,[4] and ENG tracings of many of these are illustrated by Barber and Stockwell.[5]

Gaze-evoked nystagmus (nystagmus exposed by gazing away from the primary position) may be a side effect of a variety of medications, including anticonvulsants, sedatives, and alcohol. It can also occur in such diverse conditions as myasthenia gravis, multiple sclerosis, and cerebellar atrophy. Dysconjugate gaze nystagmus is commonly present with medial longitudinal fasciculus lesions, such as internuclear ophthalmoplegia.

Positional Test

The purpose of the positional test is to determine if different head positions induce or modify vestibular nystagmus. Nystagmus induced by positional testing is referred to as positional nystagmus (or static positional nystagmus) to differentiate it from the paroxysmal or positioning nystagmus of the Dix-Hallpike maneuver. During the positional tests, the patient's eye movements are monitored while the head is in at least four positions: sitting, supine, head right (right ear down), and head left (left ear down). If nystagmus appears or is modified in either of the latter two positions, the patient is tested again while lying on that side to determine if the effect is caused by neck rotation. Eye movements are monitored in each position for about 20 seconds, both with visual fixation (eyes open and fixating on a visual target at center gaze) and with visual fixation denied. Most examiners deny fixation simply by asking patients to close their eyes, but eye closure may inhibit nystagmus. A better method is to monitor eye movements with eyes open in total darkness. The examiner usually asks the patient to perform a mental task, such as mental arithmetic, when testing

with visual fixation denied to maintain mental alertness, thus avoiding suppression of nystagmus.

Positional nystagmus may be intermittent or persistent, unlike positioning nystagmus, which disappears if the head is still. In both cases, the nystagmus induced by ampullopetal stimulation of the affected canal is greater than that induced by ampullofugal stimulation (Ewald's second law).[6] Persistent positional nystagmus is sustained as long as the head position is maintained and may reflect the effect of changing otolithic influences. As with positioning nystagmus, the terms geotropic (beating toward the ground) and ageotropic may be used to describe the direction of the nystagmus. The nystagmus may be direction fixed (beating to the same direction in different head positions) or direction changing (changing direction with differing head positions). Both of these types of nystagmus occur most commonly with peripheral vestibular disorders, but they may also occur with central lesions. Peripheral vestibular nystagmus is eliminated or diminished with visual fixation. Thus, positional nystagmus is a valuable indicator of vestibular system dysfunction. Other signs and clinical data must be used to localize the lesion.

The most common abnormality seen in the positional test is spontaneous nystagmus. Spontaneous nystagmus has been defined as nystagmus that is unmodulated by changes in head position and has been distinguished from positional nystagmus, which is modulated by head position changes, but this distinction does not appear to be clinically useful. In fact, tonic horizontal-torsional vestibular nystagmus is occasionally modulated by a change from the sitting to the supine position and is often modulated by changes from the right-ear-down, to the supine, and to the left-ear-down positions. In some cases, the nystagmus even changes in direction, for example, from strongly right-beating in the right-ear-down position, to more weakly right-beating in the supine position, to left-beating in the left-ear-down position. Spontaneous nystagmus may be suppressed by visual fixation, and often suppression is so strong that spontaneous nystagmus is abolished by fixation. Poor fixation suppression is an indication of CNS dysfunction in the pathways responsible for VOR cancellation.

Spontaneous nystagmus is a reflection of tonic left-right vestibular asymmetry and is typically seen shortly after unilateral peripheral vestibular lesion, in which case, the fast phase beats away from the side of lesion.

Occasionally, spontaneous nystagmus is seen in the absence of a recent unilateral peripheral lesion, in which case, it provides evidence of, but does not localize, a vestibular lesion.

When a persistent nystagmus is seen, it is important to extend the observation period to at least 2 minutes; certain types of direction-changing nystagmus, for example (acquired) periodic alternating nystagmus, reverse direction every 2 minutes. Periodic alternating nystagmus is usually caused by a CNS lesion.[4]

Positioning Test

Many patients complain of vertigo or dizziness that occurs with head movement, that is, positioning nystagmus. The terminology can be confusing because positioning nystagmus is seen in patients with BPPV. The purpose of the positioning test is to see if the positioning maneuver induces nystagmus at the completion of the motion. This nystagmus differs from positional nystagmus, discussed above, in which different head positions, not head movement, elicit nystagmus.

The most frequently employed test for positioning nystagmus is the *Dix-Hallpike maneuver* (Figure 9–5). In this test, the patient is subjected to two brisk movements, both beginning with the patient in the sitting position. The patient's head is first turned 45 degrees toward one side, and then the patient is briskly brought backward to assume the supine position with the head (still turned) hanging over the end of the examining

table. The examiner holds the patient's head in position for at least 20 seconds and looks for nystagmus. The duration and direction of any nystagmus are noted. Next the patient is returned to the sitting position and eye movements are observed for any nystagmus. If nystagmus was elicited with the initial positioning maneuver, the same maneuver is repeated to assess the fatigability of the response. The maneuver is then performed with the patient's head turned 45 degrees to the other side.

During the backward movement, the Dix-Hallpike maneuver normally induces a few beats of nystagmus; however, after the head is in the hanging position, normal individuals do not have nystagmus. Patients with BPPV display a burst of intense nystagmus—paroxysmal positional nystagmus—the hallmark of the disorder. Paroxysmal positional nystagmus can be readily appreciated by visual observation with the patient's eyes open or, better yet, with the patient wearing Frenzel lenses in a darkened room. The examiner sees primarily the torsional component of the nystagmus, with a counter-clockwise fast phase when the right ear is involved and clockwise fast phase with left ear involvement. Electronystagmography is useful in documenting the response (Figure 9–6). Electronystagmography is insensitive to the torsional component of the nystagmus but does record the horizontal and vertical components. The horizontal component generally has the fast phase away from the undermost ear, and the vertical component invariably has an upbeating fast phase.[7] The ENG tracing seems paradoxical in comparison with the clinically observed tor-

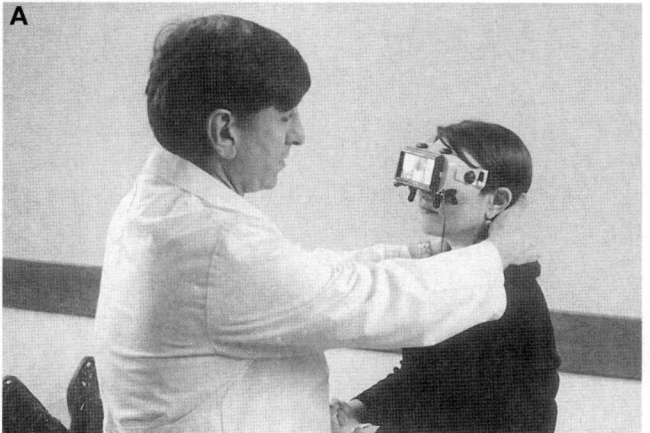
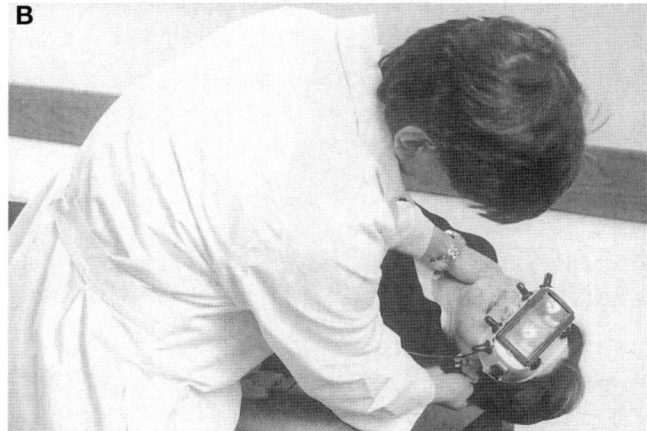

Figure 9–5   Dix-Hallpike maneuver. The patient's head is first turned to the left. The patient is then rapidly brought into the head-hanging position. Patients with benign paroxysmal positional vertigo typically demonstrate a geotropic, torsional nystagmus with the affected ear down. Frenzel's lenses are used to prevent fixation-suppression. The test is repeated on the opposite side.

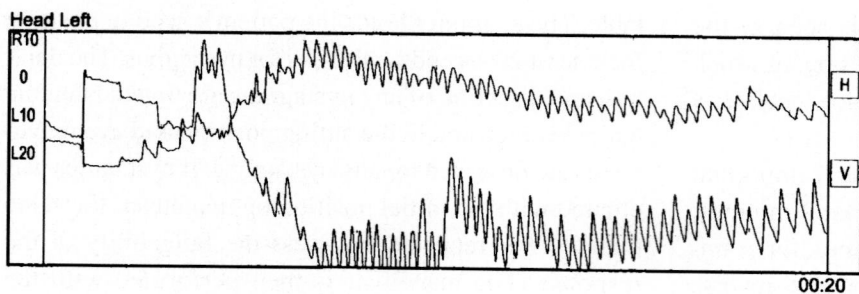

Figure 9–6 Electronystagmographic tracing demonstrates horizontal and vertical components of the torsional nystagmus seen in benign paroxysmal positional vertigo.

sional nystagmus that appears to beat toward the ground; however, this paradox occurs because the torsional component of the nystagmus cannot be recorded with standard ENG, and the main vector of the recorded nystagmus is directed away from the ground. Paroxysmal positional nystagmus changes somewhat with the direction of the patient's gaze.[8] The rotary component is more prominent during gaze toward the undermost ear, whereas the vertical component is more prominent during gaze toward the uppermost ear.

Positioning nystagmus has four distinctive features[9]:

1. It has a delayed onset. Usually, there is an interval of at least a few (2 to 20) seconds after the patient reaches the head-hanging position before the nystagmus begins.
2. It is always transient, that is, it rapidly builds in intensity (crescendos), slowly abates (decrescendos), and finally disappears (within 45 seconds) as the head remains in position.

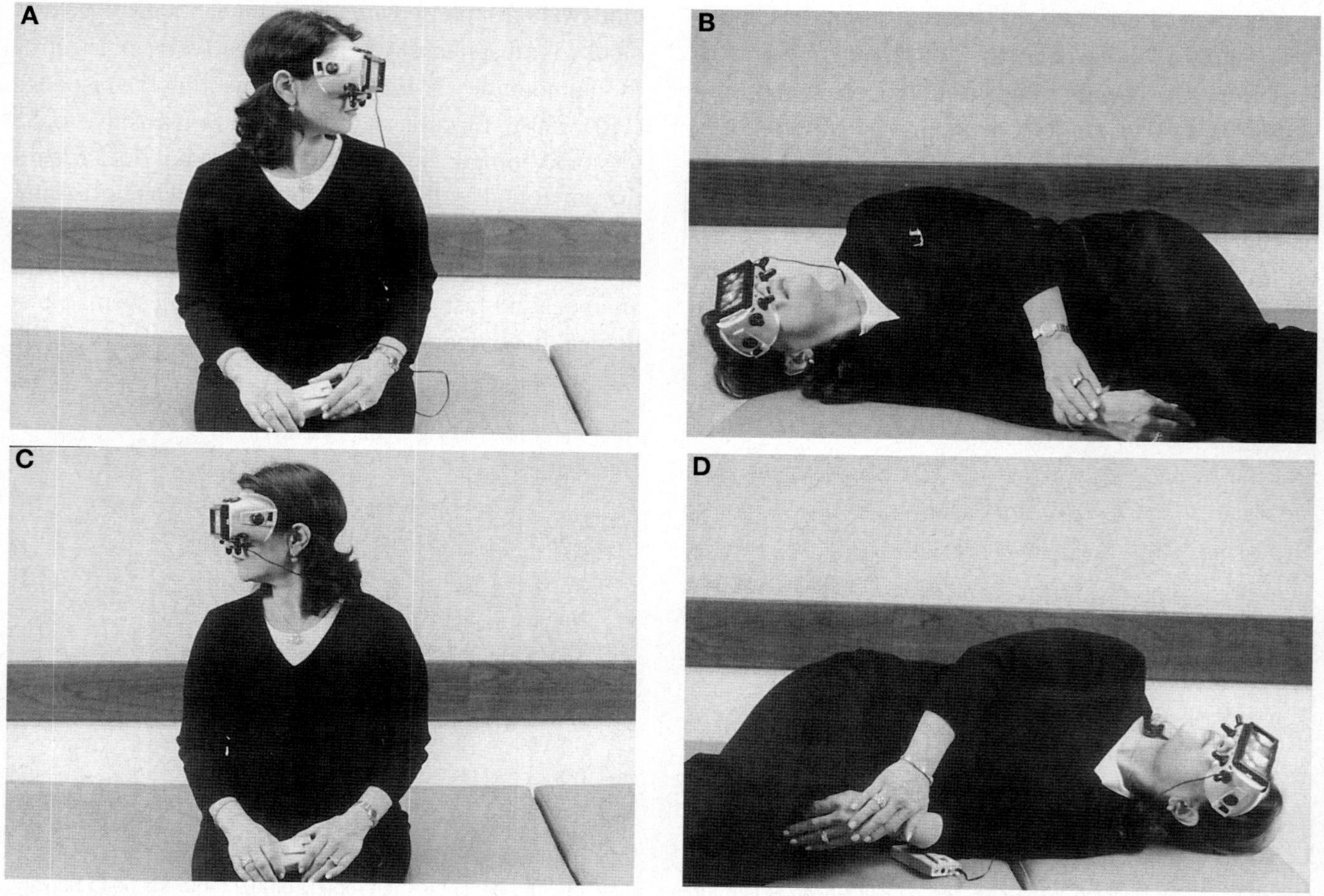

Figure 9–7 Bojrab-Calvert maneuver for benign paroxysmal positional vertigo. This positioning maneuver is useful in assessing positioning nystagmus in elderly or other individuals who cannot tolerate the neck extension position used in the Dix-Hallpike maneuver.

3. It is always accompanied by vertigo, usually intense, which follows the same time course as the nystagmus.

4. It is usually fatigable, that is, it progressively diminishes in intensity with repetition of the Dix-Hallpike maneuver.

The Dix-Hallpike maneuver occasionally provokes other types of nystagmus, for example, downbeat nystagmus, which is exacerbated when the patient is moved to the head-hanging position. If downbeat nystagmus is mild, it may be missed during the gaze or positional tests and be observed for the first time with the Dix-Hallpike maneuver. It generally is not accompanied by vertigo. Rarely, other types of nystagmus, generally of CNS origin, are provoked by the Dix-Hallpike maneuver.

One limitation of the Dix-Hallpike maneuver is that it cannot be performed on patients with cervical spine disease that limits neck extension or back disorders that prohibit rapid positioning of the patient into the head-hanging position. In those patients, a sidelying *Bojrab-Calvert maneuver* may be employed. The senior author has been using this technique for over 14 years as his primary technique in elderly patients or patients with significant cervical neck disease. This maneuver allows the same positioning of the posterior semicircular canal as with the Dix-Hallpike maneuver, without the head hanging.

The Bojrab-Calvert maneuver (Figure 9–7) begins with the patient in the sitting position, facing the examiner. The head is turned 45 degrees to the right so that the pinna is perpendicular to the table surface. The examiner holds the head in that position as the patient is briskly lowered onto his/her shoulder with the head resting on the table. This position is held for at least 20 seconds, while eye movements are monitored. The patient is then returned to the sitting position. If nystagmus was elicited, the examiner repeats the same maneuver to determine if the nystagmus is fatigable. The maneuver is performed with the contralateral side. As with the Dix-Hallpike maneuver, the ear that is dependent when nystagmus is elicited is thought to be the diseased side.

Lateral semicircular canal BPPV can be detected with the Dix-Hallpike maneuver; however, a more effective maneuver involves placing the patient in the supine position, turning the head quickly to the right-ear-down position, and holding it there for at least 30 seconds (or, if nystagmus is provoked, for up to several minutes). The patient's head is then returned slowly to the supine position; lastly, the head is turned quickly into the left-ear-down position and held there for at least 30 seconds (or, if nystagmus is provoked, for up to several minutes). In patients with lateral canal BPPV, this maneuver provokes horizontal nystagmus, as described by Baloh and colleagues.[10] The nystagmus of lateral canal BPPV is (1) geotropic (right-beating in the right-ear-down position and left-beating in the left-ear-down position) and often followed by an ageotropic secondary nystagmus; (2) stronger when the ear presumed to be diseased is undermost; (3) transient (although more persistent than the response of posterior canal BPPV); (4) accompanied by vertigo, usually intense, which follows the same time course as the response; (5) not delayed in onset; and (6) not fatigable.

Tests of Vestibulo-oculomotor Function

Bithermal Caloric Test

The bithermal caloric test has proven highly sensitive to unilateral lesions of the peripheral vestibular system because it allows the examiner to stimulate each ear separately. Other vestibular test procedures, such as rotation testing and posturography, stimulate both labyrinths simultaneously, thereby permitting the masking of abnormal responses from one labyrinth by normal responses from the opposite ear.

The bithermal (Hallpike) caloric test tests the integrity of the lateral semicircular canals and their afferent pathways. The patient is placed in the supine position with the head elevated 30 degrees, thereby placing the lateral semicircular canal in the vertical plane (Figure 9–8). Testing should be done with the patient wearing Frenzel goggles to prevent fixation-suppression. Asking the patient to engage in mental tasks can also be helpful in releasing the nystagmus.

Caloric testing uses a nonphysiologic stimulus (temperature) to induce fluid flow in the lateral semicircular canal. Each ear is irrigated twice: once with air (or water) at 7 degrees above body temperature and then with air (or water) at 7 degrees below body temperature. The caloric stimulus causes the endolymph to circulate, resulting, after a short latency period, in a brief (1 to 2 minutes) burst of nystagmus. In a healthy patient, irrigation with a warm stimulus provokes nystagmus with

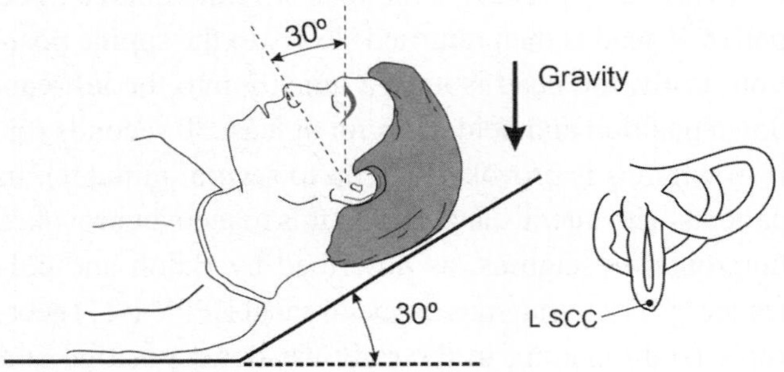

Figure 9–8 Caloric testing may be performed with air or water. The correct position places the patient in the reclined position, 30 degrees elevated from the table, which places the horizontal canal in the vertical plane.

the fast phase directed toward the stimulated ear; irrigation with a cool stimulus evokes nystagmus with the fast phase directed away from the stimulated ear (cold, opposite; warm, the same).

The caloric data are analyzed, and five characteristics of the calorically induced nystagmus are calculated: duration, latency, amplitude, frequency, and velocity. Of these parameters, the most important variable is the peak slow-phase eye velocity. In normal individuals, the slow-phase eye velocity should be equally strong in both directions. Comparing the peak slow-phase eye velocity of the cool and warm caloric responses of the right ear with those of the left ear allows the examiner to determine whether a unilateral vestibular weakness exists. To assess the function of each labyrinth, the caloric responses of the two ears are compared. Because both ears receive the same stimuli, they should demonstrate equal caloric responses.

Caloric stimuli are uncalibrated, that is, stimulus strength varies from person to person depending on the size and shape of the external ear canal and other uncontrollable variables. However, the basic assumption of the caloric test is that, for a given individual, the two ears receive equal caloric stimuli. If both ears are normal, they should produce responses of approximately equal intensity. Therefore, the intensity of the caloric responses of the two ears is compared by evaluating the peak slow-phase eye velocities using the following formula:

$$\frac{(RW + RC) - (LW + LC)}{RW + RC + LW + LC} \times 100\% = UW$$

where RW, RC, LW, and LC are peak slow-phase eye velocities of the responses to right warm, right cool,

left warm, and left cool responses, respectively, and UW is unilateral weakness. In general, a unilateral caloric weakness (CW) of greater than 20% indicates peripheral vestibular dysfunction on the side of the weaker response.[11]

Patients with labyrinthine hypofunction may demonstrate reduced or absent caloric responses to the initial bithermal stimuli. In this case, the test is repeated with ice water (approximately 0°C) irrigations. However, one should keep in mind that the absence of a caloric response does not always imply absent peripheral function as the stimulus levels are below the level within which the VOR generally functions.[12]

Various patterns of ENG abnormalities can be seen with vestibular system dysfunction. For example, a patient with an acute, unilateral peripheral vestibular lesion often demonstrates spontaneous nystagmus and a unilateral caloric weakness (Figure 9–9).[13] The presence of spontaneous nystagmus may affect the results of the caloric test, creating a bias that resets the caloric baseline (Figure 9–10). Spontaneous nystagmus is not diagnostic of a recent peripheral vestibular lesion. Figure 9–11 shows data for a patient with spontaneous nystagmus but without caloric weakness. Such a finding is nonlocalizing as the nystagmus can be associated with numerous entities, including recovery from a previously compensated peripheral vestibular lesion or a central peripheral vestibular lesion.

Whereas the bithermal caloric test is highly sensitive to unilateral peripheral vestibular dysfunction, it is relatively insensitive to bilateral dysfunction because the caloric stimulus is uncalibrated. Even though the stimulus at the entrance to the external ear canal is the same for everyone, the stimulus reaching the inner ear shows great interindividual variability owing to differences in the size and shape of the ear canal and the status of the middle ear. Therefore, the range of normal absolute response intensities is extremely wide, and bilateral caloric weaknesses must be severe to fall below them. The usual rule of thumb is that a bilateral weakness exists if the caloric responses (warm response plus cool response) of both ears fall below 12 degrees/second, per side. A bilateral weakness usually indicates bilateral peripheral vestibular dysfunction.[5] Bilateral weaknesses can be of CNS origin but are usually accompanied by other signs of CNS dysfunction.

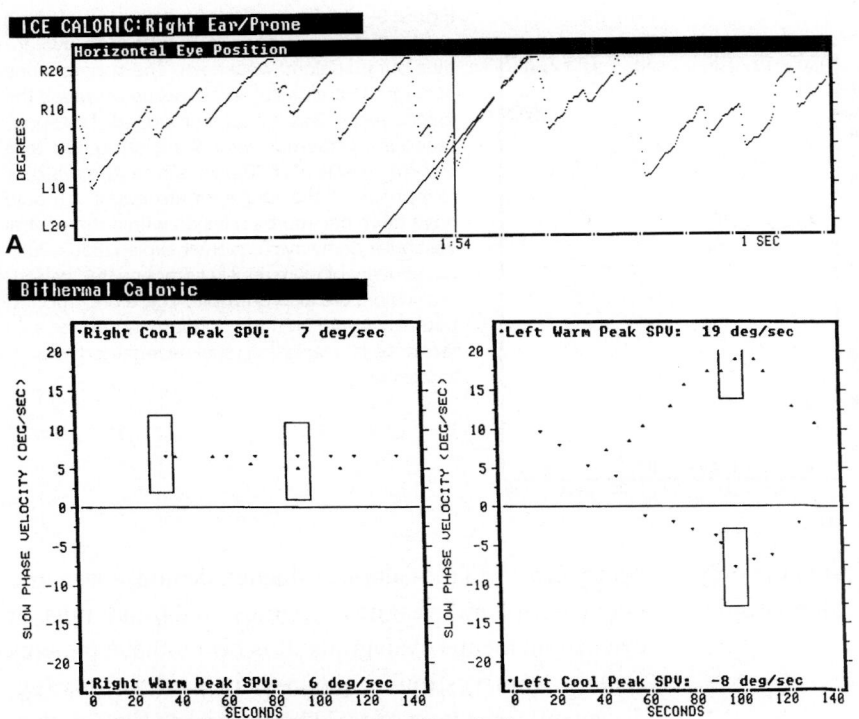

Figure 9–9 Electronystagmographic data from a patient with an acute, left vestibular lesion. A reduction in the tonic resting input from the damaged ear causes a slow drift of the eyes toward the injured side, with a corrective saccade in the opposite direction. The caloric testing shows reduced responses to both warm and cold air in the left ear.

Indications

Although ENG essentially replicates portions of the physical examination, it is an important part of the evaluation of many patients with complaints of dizziness or balance disturbance. Electronystagmographic testing has a number of advantages: (1) the results of the test are quantified, and there are well-defined normal limits; (2) the bithermal caloric test cannot be done as accurately without the precise stimulus control and response quantification provided by ENG; (3) because ENG provides accurate documentation of results, it can be used to follow the patient with known vestibular disease; (4) standardized documentation is helpful in medical-legal

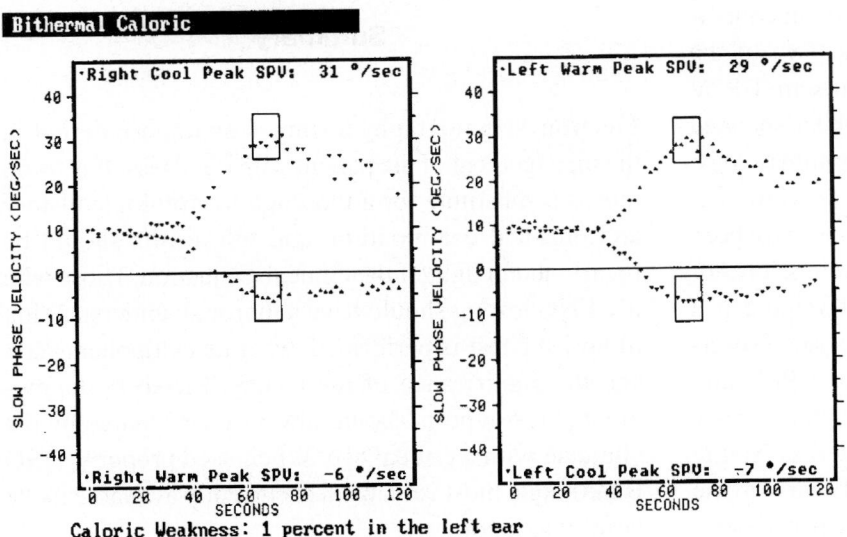

Figure 9–10 Electronystagmographic data 3 days after an acute unilateral vestibular lesion. The patient has spontaneous nystagmus that creates a bias; caloric responses were symmetric about a new baseline corresponding to the slow-phase velocity of this nystagmus. It would be difficult to distinguish between the effects of this bias and a unilateral caloric weakness on the basis of peak slow-phase velocities if only one irrigation temperature were used in the test. When both warm and cool irrigations are used, responses are elicited in both directions, and the sum of the two peak responses is used as the measure of response strength of a particular ear. This cancels the effect of the bias and allows a valid comparison to be made between the two ears.

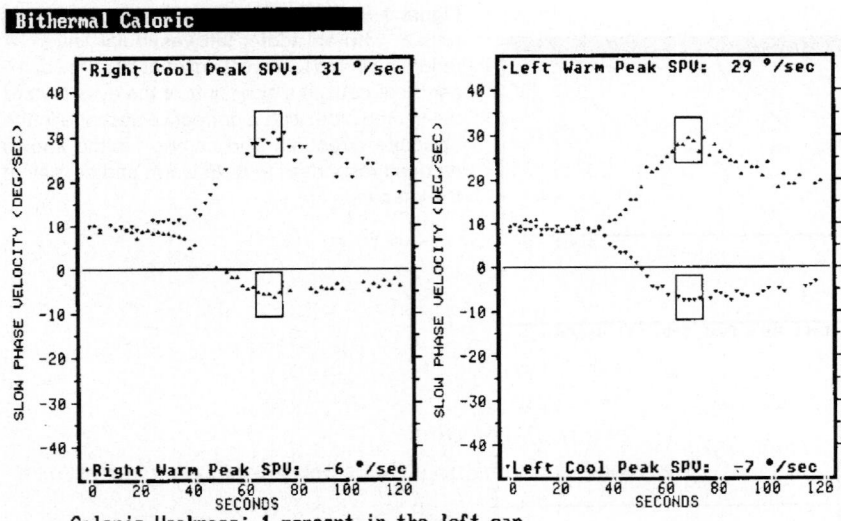

Bithermal Caloric

Caloric Weakness: 1 percent in the left ear

Figure 9–11 Electronystagmographic data for a patient with spontaneous, left-beating nystagmus but no caloric weakness. The spontaneous nystagmus creates a new baseline on which the caloric responses are superimposed. The spontaneous nystagmus cannot be attributed to a recent vestibular lesion since the caloric responses of the two ears are equal. It could have been caused by a lesion within the central vestibular pathways, but other explanations, such as recovery of a previously compensated peripheral lesion, are also possible. Therefore, spontaneous nystagmus that cannot be attributed to a recent vestibular lesion must be regarded as nonlocalizing.

and workers' compensation cases; and (5) it is the only test that assesses each ear separately and can give side-of-lesion localizing information.

Limitations

Electronystagmography testing has its limitations. It is important to recognize that ENG tests only the lateral semicircular canal and provides little information about the status of the posterior or superior semicircular canals, utricle, or saccule. Traditional ENG testing using electro-oculography is also relatively insensitive to torsional nystagmus because rotational movement of the eye about the axis of the pupil does not move the cornea with respect to any of the skin electrodes. However, this limitation is easily overcome using VNG.

The results of ENG testing may fluctuate in concordance with the patient's disease process. Two of the more common illnesses seen in our patients are BPPV and Meniere's disease. Both illnesses can be associated with a normal ENG despite "classic" symptomatology. For example, on the day of testing a patient with complaints consistent with BPPV, the response may have been fatigued or the disease may have gone into remission. For that patient, the test results may be normal or indicate a unilateral vestibular weakness on the suspect side. Nevertheless, we maintain clinical suspicion of BPPV and ask the patient to return for retesting on a particularly "dizzy day." Similarly, the patient suspected as having Meniere's disease may have a normal ENG early in the course of the illness, and only later, on a particularly

"dizzy day," will the caloric evaluation demonstrate a unilateral peripheral weakness, gaze-evoked nystagmus, or even spontaneous nystagmus. It is best to have patients abstain from vestibular suppressant medications (eg, diazepam) for at least 48 to 72 hours prior to ENG as they can also cause a "false-negative" test.

Some patients may present with dizziness not related to vestibular system dysfunction, for example, syncope or presyncope, vertebral-basilar insufficiency, migraine-associated dizziness, multiple sclerosis, ocular dizziness, motion sickness syndrome, or cardiovascular disease. In these patients, a unilateral weakness found on ENG does not necessarily implicate vestibular dysfunction as the cause of their symptoms. The ENG finding may be incidental and must be considered in light of the clinical history and physical examination.

Summary

Electronystagmography testing is an important tool in the management of the patient with dizziness. It is by no means a substitute for a thorough neurotologic history and physical examination, and the results should be interpreted in light of the clinical evaluation. Those who use ENG testing should have a thorough understanding of how the test is performed, what its components are, and the significance of the results. Electronystagmographic test reports should always be evaluated by the clinician with a critical eye. When used properly, ENG is the single most valuable test currently available in the vestibular laboratory.

ROTATIONAL TESTS

Rotational tests have been used to evaluate vestibular function for nearly a century. They provide another method of testing for vestibular disorders that affect the VOR. Rotational tests can be classified as either passive rotational tests, in which the patient's body is rotated without any movement between the head and body, or as active rotational tests, in which the patient rotates his or her own head back and forth while the body remains stationary.

Rotary Chair Test

The rotary chair test (RCT) has proven to be the most useful of the rotational tests.[14,15] It is a passive rotational test in which the patient is seated in a chair so that the axis of rotation is vertical and passes through the center of the head, thus stimulating only the lateral semicircular canals. The base of the chair is bolted to a computer-controlled servomotor that determines the frequency of chair rotation. The patient's head is positioned so that the lateral semicircular canals are in the plane of rotation and is firmly restrained so that it exactly follows body and chair motion (Figure 9–12). Horizontal eye movements are monitored using electro-oculography as in ENG testing.

Testing Paradigms

Rotary chair testing can be performed using various testing paradigms, but the one typically employed is slow harmonic acceleration. In this paradigm, the patient is oscillated in a sinusoidal fashion about a vertical axis at

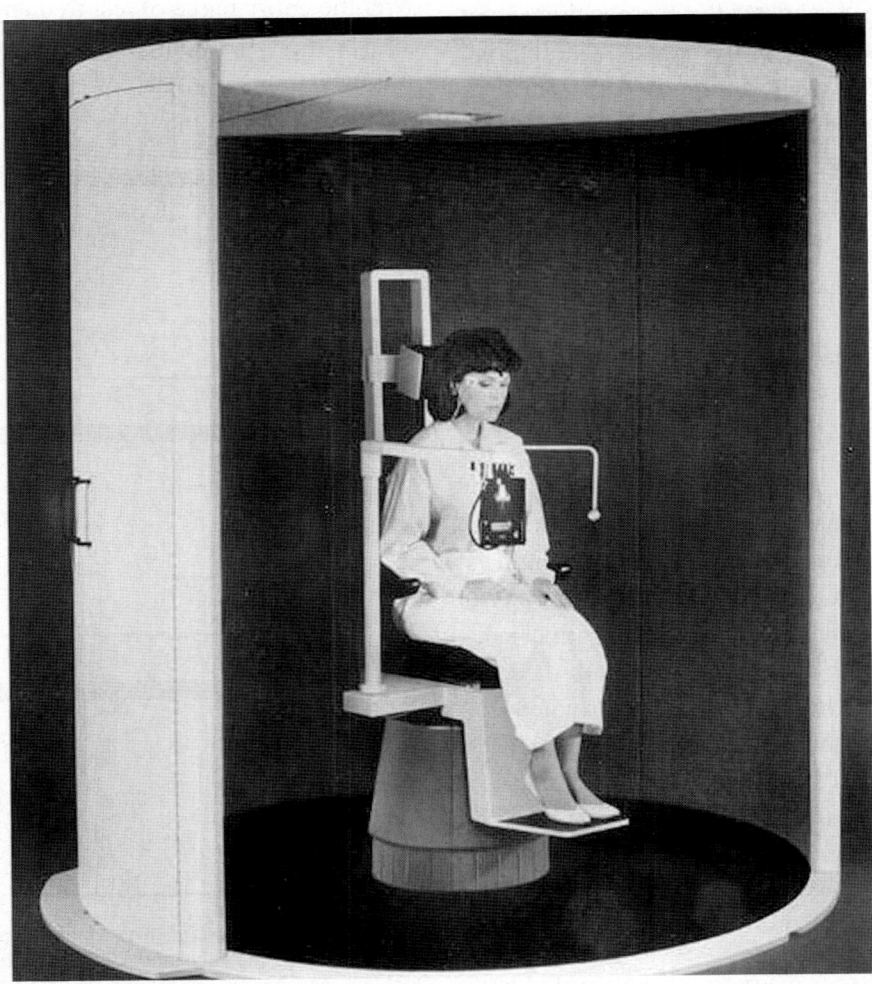

Figure 9–12 Rotational chair testing equipment. The patient is seated in a chair so that the horizontal semicircular canals are in the plane of rotation. Electro-oculography is used to monitor eye movements.

various test frequencies (ranging from 0.01 to 01.28 Hz). The exact test protocol varies somewhat among laboratories, but oscillation frequencies of 0.01, 0.02, 0.04, 0.08, 0.16, 0.32, and 0.64 Hz, with peak angular velocities of 50 degrees/second at each frequency, are usually used. The patient undergoes multiple cycles of oscillation at each frequency; the oscillations are gradually increased, and the chair is rotated in a sinusoidal harmonic acceleration paradigm. The stimulus level delivered by the rotary chair is much greater than that delivered in caloric testing, which delivers a stimulus equivalent only to frequencies between 0.002 and 0.004 Hz.

Components of Rotary Chair Testing

Rotary chair testing stimulation generates right-beating nystagmus when the patient is moving rightward and left-beating nystagmus when moving to the left. After testing, the computer differentiates the eye position signal and removes the fast phase of nystagmus, yielding the slow-phase eye velocity. The computer then compares the head velocity and slow-phase eye velocity and calculates three measurements, phase, gain, and symmetry, for each of the test frequencies.

GAIN. Gain is defined as the slow eye velocity divided by the head velocity. It is used as an indicator of overall responsiveness of the system. Clinically, a reduction in gain is used to help determine the overall level of function reduction in patients with bilateral vestibular disease.

PHASE ANGLE. The phase angle measures the temporal relationship between eye and head velocities and is measured in degrees. Of the three parameters, phase angle has the greatest clinical significance. In normal individuals, movement of the head to the right results in deviation of the eyes to the left. If the patient is rotated at a low frequency for a prolonged period of time, eye movement actually precedes the head movement. Increased phase lead implies peripheral vestibular system dysfunction, whereas decreased phase lead may suggest a cerebellar lesion.

SYMMETRY. Symmetry is the ratio of rightward to leftward slow-phase eye velocity. This parameter gives information as to whether any bias is present in the sys-

tem, favoring one direction over the other. Asymmetry may result from a peripheral vestibular weakness on the side of the larger slow-phase component or an excitatory lesion of the contralateral labyrinth.

The relationship between head and eye movement during several cycles of sinusoidal oscillation for a normal individual is shown in Figure 9–13. The purpose of the VOR is to produce eye movements that compensate for head movements, and the eye velocity is approximately 180 degrees out of phase with head velocity. When a normal individual is oscillated at low frequencies, slow-phase eye velocities exhibit progressively lower gains and are no longer exactly opposite in phase.[16] Instead, they display progressively larger phase leads, that is, changes in slow-phase eye velocity occur more and more in advance of head velocity. Figure 9–14 shows graphic plots of phase, gain, and symmetry data for a normal individual over the entire range of test frequencies.

The slow harmonic acceleration test shows abnormalities primarily at the lowest and at the highest oscil-

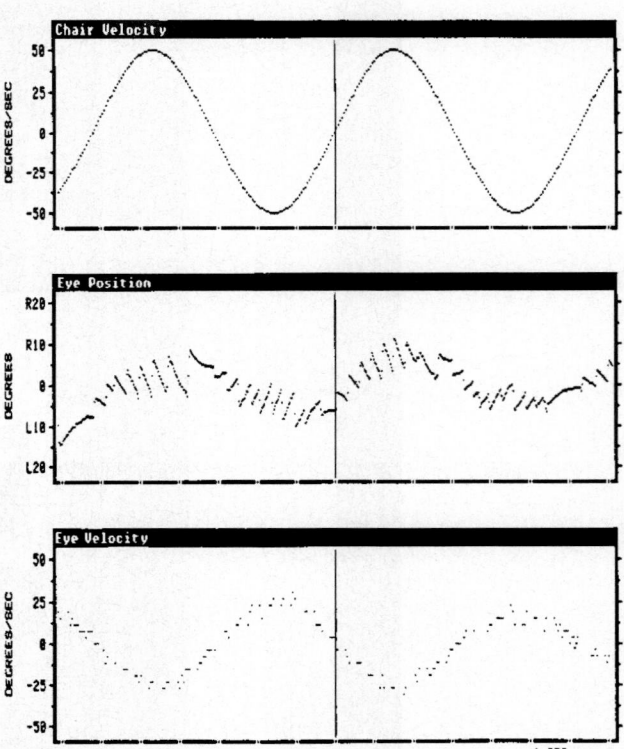

Figure 9–13 Rotary chair test data from a normal individual. The oscillation frequency in this example was 0.16 Hz, near the middle of the test frequency range. Eye movements are 180 degrees out of phase with head movement. The patient had nystagmus with leftward slow phases when their head was moving rightward and nystagmus with rightward slow phases when their head was moving leftward.

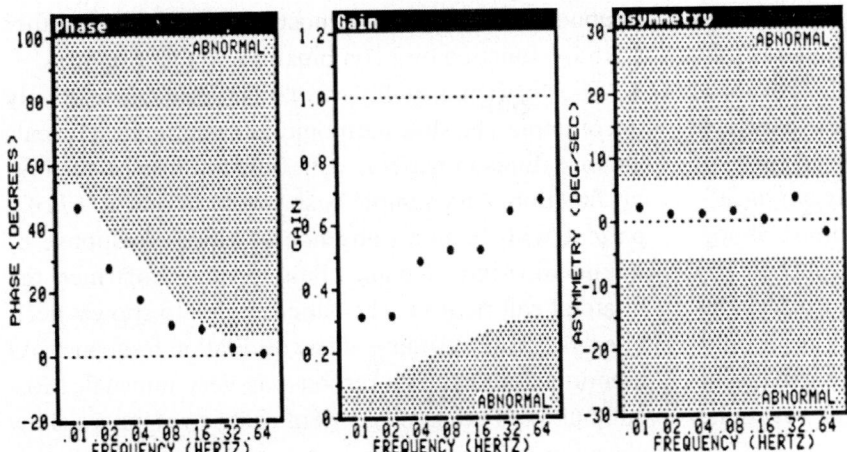

Figure 9–14 Phase, gain, and asymmetry values in relation to oscillation frequency from a normal individual. Note that eye velocity signal is inverted during the analysis so that a phase angle of 180 degrees is expressed as a phase angle of 0 degrees. Phase leads become progressively larger and gains become progressively lower as oscillation frequency decreases. Symmetry values are approximately zero at all frequencies.

lation frequencies. Low frequencies reveal abnormal phase leads and gain reductions. High frequencies reveal asymmetries.

In our experience, abnormalities seen on RCT can be classified into four categories: (1) vestibular habituation and asymmetry, (2) vestibular habituation, (3) vestibular deficit, and (4) vestibular asymmetry.

Vestibular habituation and asymmetry—abnormal low-frequency phase leads and high-frequency asymmetry (with the asymmetry always toward the side of the lesion)—is most often seen in patients with acute unilateral peripheral dysfunction. These patients demonstrate the most severe abnormalities. Figure 9–15 shows test results in a patient who underwent the slow harmonic acceleration test shortly after the sudden onset of severe vertigo. Electronystagmography, performed at the same time as RCT, showed left-beating spontaneous nystagmus as well as right reduced caloric responses.

At the lower oscillation frequencies, this patient displayed progressively greater than normal phase leads, which are thought to be caused by a loss of velocity storage normally provided by the central vestibular system to enhance the low-frequency response of the vestibulo-ocular system.[17,18] Loss of velocity storage seems to represent habituation to the strong tonic asymmetry produced by the unilateral peripheral vestibular lesion.[18] Loss of velocity storage is not an exclusive feature of unilateral peripheral vestibular lesions as it is also seen in a variety of vestibular disorders, both peripheral and central, and has also been observed in normal individuals who have undergone prolonged rotation.[19]

This patient also had a rightward asymmetry, that is, nystagmus with rightward slow phases was stronger than nystagmus with leftward slow phases. At low oscillation frequencies, the asymmetry was about equal to the slow-phase velocities of the patient's spontaneous nys-

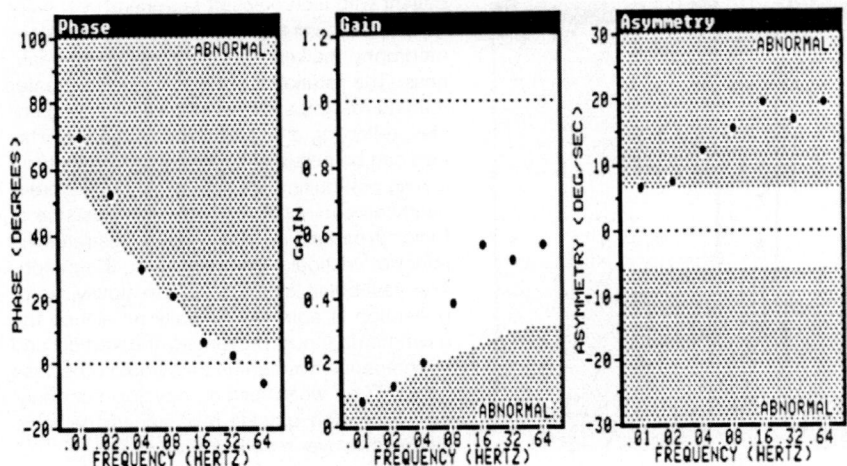

Figure 9–15 Phase, gain, and asymmetry values in relation to oscillation frequency for a patient with an acute right peripheral vestibular lesion. At lower oscillation frequencies, this patient shows progressively greater than normal phase leads. The patient also has a rightward asymmetry. This response pattern — abnormal low-frequency phase leads and high-frequency asymmetry — is routinely observed in patients with acute unilateral vestibular loss. The asymmetry is always toward the side of the loss.

tagmus with eyes closed, but at higher frequencies, the asymmetry was greater than could be accounted for by this bias. This additional asymmetry is thought to be attributable to either saturation of inhibitory responses of the intact labyrinth during rotation toward the side of the lesion or an asymmetric loss of velocity storage.[20]

Vestibular habituation is the most common abnormality found on RCT and consists solely of abnormally large phase leads at the lower oscillation frequencies. This abnormality is often seen in patients with a chronic, unilateral peripheral vestibular lesion. An example is seen in Figure 9–16 from a patient with a right vestibular schwannoma.

This response pattern—abnormal low-frequency phase leads—is by far the most common abnormality seen in the slow sinusoidal rotation test. Stockwell reported abnormal low-frequency phase leads as the sole abnormality on the slow harmonic acceleration test in 109 of 305 patients with dizziness.[21] Twenty-seven of these patients (8 with a diagnosis of unilateral Meniere's disease and the rest with a variety of diagnoses) showed no abnormality on ENG. Fifty-five of the 305 patients showed evidence of a chronic unilateral peripheral vestibular lesion, that is, a significant unilateral caloric weakness without significant spontaneous nystagmus, and most were diagnosed as having either Meniere's disease or a vestibular schwannoma. The reduction in vestibular caloric response in these patients was nearly always greater than 50%. Patients with a unilateral caloric weakness of less than 50% generally did not have abnormal phase leads. The remaining 27 patients showed a variety

of abnormalities on ENG, mostly consistent with either CNS dysfunction or a combination of abnormalities.

The third abnormality, vestibular deficit, is relatively uncommon. The slow harmonic acceleration test reveals abnormalities in patients with bilateral loss of vestibular function. An example is shown in Figure 9–17 of a patient with bilateral absence of caloric response of unknown origin. Rotary chair testing confirmed the bilateral caloric loss. The patient failed to show a definite nystagmus response at any oscillation frequency. As mentioned above, this response is very unusual. Most patients with bilaterally absent caloric responses show absent or reduced response gains at the lower oscillation frequencies but normal gains at the highest frequencies. An example is shown in Figure 9–18 of a patient who developed unsteadiness following a course of gentamicin therapy and showed a bilateral absence of caloric response. Baloh and colleagues reported that RCT often demonstrates normal vestibular function at high frequencies even when ice water irrigations have failed to provoke a response from either ear.[22] In these cases, the results of caloric and rotation tests are not contradictory because the caloric response is a response to a low-frequency stimulus and therefore should be similar to responses to low-frequency rotational stimuli. However, in other cases, RCT shows normal response gains at all frequencies, despite absent caloric responses, indicating a false-positive caloric test result.[23] Clearly, the slow harmonic acceleration test is the procedure of choice in evaluating patients suspected of having bilateral loss of vestibular function because the caloric test, even with ice

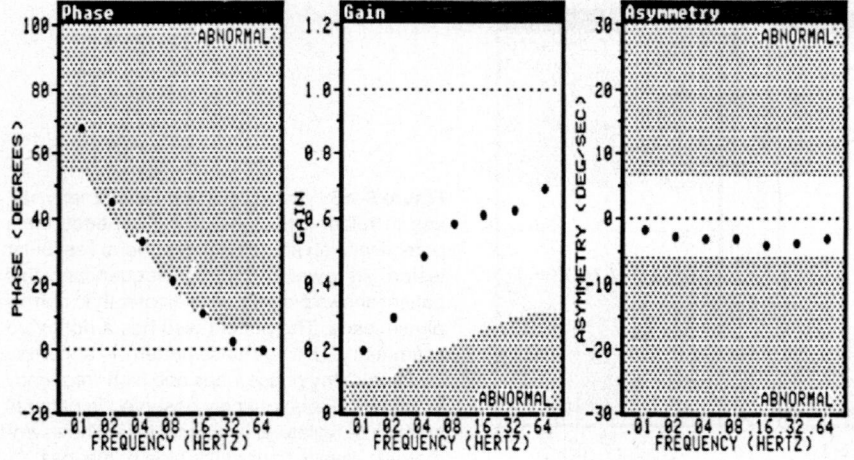

Figure 9–16 Phase, gain, and asymmetry values in relation to oscillation frequency for a patient with a chronic left peripheral vestibular lesion (vestibular schwannoma). Electronystagmography showed a severe right caloric weakness. The rotational chair test shows greater than normal phase leads at lower test frequencies, reflecting a loss of velocity storage. This loss can be persistent, remaining for years following vestibular malfunction, although there is nearly always some recovery. The absence of tonic asymmetry in this individual illustrates the effect of vestibular compensation. If a peripheral vestibular lesion develops slowly, compensation is able to gradually rebalance the asymmetric input, preventing the vertigo and spontaneous nystagmus that would otherwise occur. Even when lesions develop suddenly, compensation quickly rebalances the tonic asymmetry over a period of days.

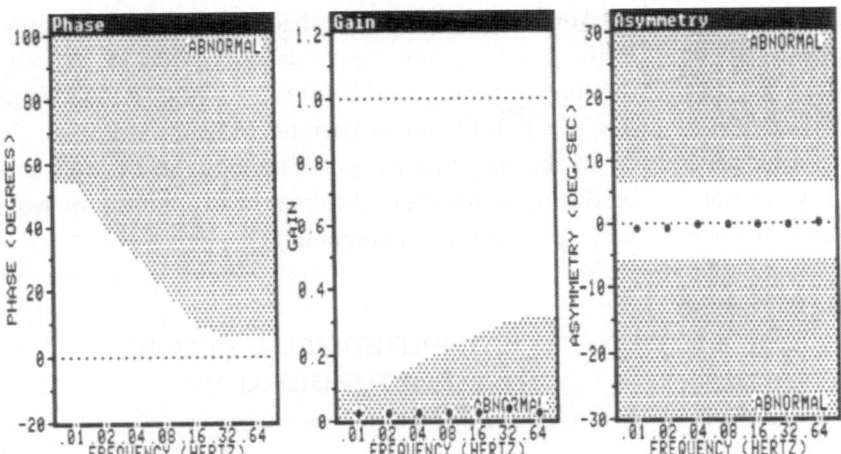

Figure 9–17 Phase, gain, and asymmetry values in relation to oscillation frequency for a patient with bilateral absence of caloric responses, showing absent responses at all oscillation frequencies. Phase values were not plotted owing to low response gains.

water, does not define the extent of the loss and sometimes yields false-positive results.

The final abnormality is vestibular asymmetry, which is characterized by an asymmetry at high frequencies. It is similar to the high-frequency asymmetry seen in patients with acute unilateral peripheral lesions, which we have attributed to low firing rates of central vestibular neurons. However, these patients have chronic complaints and do not show the spontaneous nystagmus and low-frequency phase leads of patients with acute peripheral lesions. We suspect that vestibular asymmetry reflects a central vestibular disorder because several patients have shown clear concomitant evidence of CNS dysfunction, but we do not have enough numbers to justify making a firm statement regarding the clinical significance of this finding.

Clinical Indications for Rotational Chair Testing

Rotational chair testing stimulates both peripheral vestibular systems simultaneously; however, it may be helpful in determining the site of lesion in certain disorders. Shepard makes some suggestions as to when chair testing may be helpful in patient evaluation.[24] First, when the ENG is normal and oculomotor results are either normal or observed abnormalities would not invalidate rotational chair results, RCT is used to expand the assessment of peripheral system dysfunction and status of compensation. Second, when the ENG suggests a well-compensated state, despite the presence of a clinically significant unilateral caloric weakness and active symptomatology, RCT is used to expand the investigation of compensation in a patient with a known lesion site and complaints suggesting poor compensation. Third, when

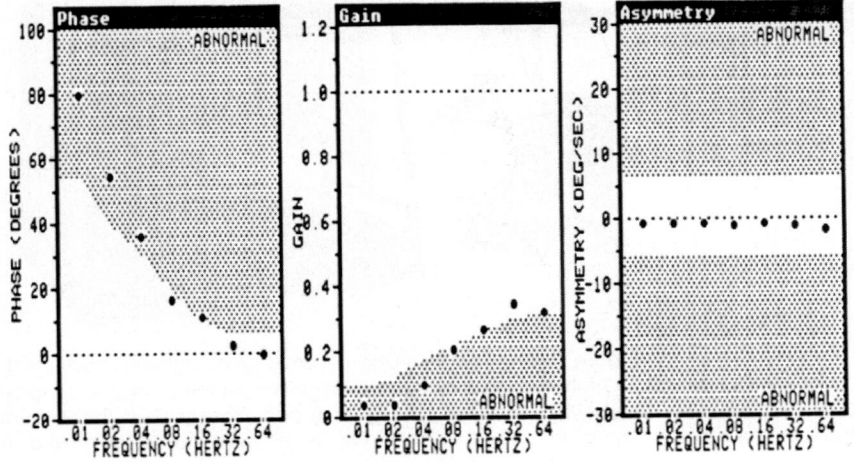

Figure 9–18 Phase, gain, and asymmetry values in relation to oscillation frequencies for a patient with bilateral absence of caloric responses, showing normal response gains at the higher frequencies.

the caloric irrigations are below 12 degrees/second bilaterally, when caloric irrigations cannot be performed, or when results in the two ears may not be compared reliably because of anatomic variability, RCT is used to verify the presence, and define the extent, of a bilateral weakness or to investigate further the relative responsiveness of the peripheral vestibular apparatus in each ear when caloric studies are unreliable or unavailable. Lastly, RTC may be beneficial when a baseline measure is needed to follow the natural history of the patient's disorder (eg, possible early Meniere's disease) or to assess the effectiveness of a particular treatment (such as chemical ablation).

Vestibular Autorotational Testing

Vestibular autorotational testing is an active rotation test in which the patient actively shakes his/her head from side to side with increasing frequency. An angular sensor is fixed to a headband which is worn by the patient, and the eyes are evaluated with electro-oculography (Figure 9–19).

Advantages of VAT over the other tests include portability of testing equipment, relatively brief (18 seconds) duration of the test, and ability to test high-frequency (2 to 6 kHz) oscillations (when the VOR is active).

At the present time, as the methodology is not standardized, the results of different head autorotation tests may not be directly comparable.

COMPUTERIZED DYNAMIC POSTUROGRAPHY

Posturography is a quantitative balance test that assesses standing balance function under a variety of conditions. It is based on a computerized testing device, called the Equitest™ (manufactured by Neurocom International, Inc, Portland, Oregon) (Figure 9–20). This device consists of a platform that is capable of moving back and forth and tilting in the pitch plane about an axis co-linear with the patient's ankle joints. During the test, the patient stands independently on the platform, wearing a harness for safety and facing a visual screen that is

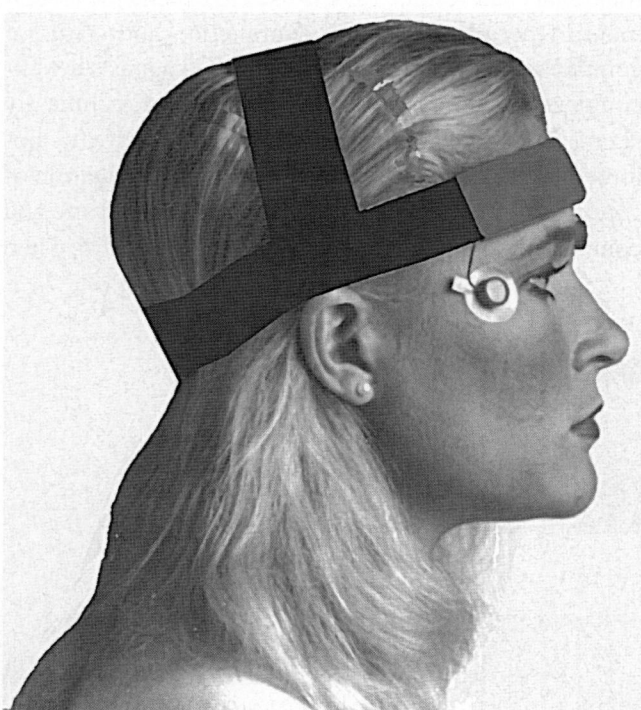

Figure 9–19 Vestibular autorotational equipment. A portable computer is connected to an instrumented head strap containing a head velocity sensor. Active head oscillations are performed by the subject at frequencies from 2 to 6 Hz.

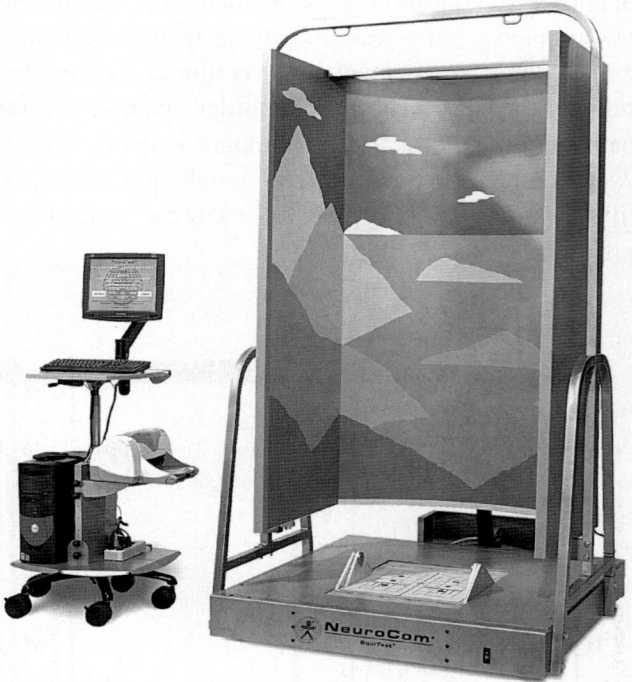

Figure 9–20 Computerized dynamic posturography equipment. The subject stands on a computer-driven platform containing a force plate. Various testing paradigms are performed in which the platform and/or the visual surround can be either stationary or moved. A safety harness is worn at all times.

capable of tilting about the same axis as the platform. As the patient sways on the platform, a built-in force plate measures the changes in the position of the patient's center of gravity. These data are transmitted to the computer, which calculates the angle of the body sway in the pitch plane.

Posturography consists of two tests: the sensory organization test and the movement coordination test. Of the two, the sensory organization test is the more useful in the evaluation of patients with dizziness because it is designed primarily to test vestibular function. In the sensory organization test, the patient's postural stability is evaluated under six conditions in which either visual or proprioceptive cues (or both) are denied. Normally, individuals maintain their balance by integrating visual and somatosensory cues. The visual cues can be disrupted in one of two ways: visual input can be denied (by blindfolding) or visual cues can be disrupted by sway-referencing the surroundings. Normal subjects ignore inaccurate sway-referenced visual input, relying on other information to maintain balance.[25,26]

The six test conditions in the sensory organization test are as follows:

1. Support fixed, eyes open, visual fixed
2. Support fixed, eyes closed, visual fixed
3. Support fixed, eyes open, visual sway-referenced
4. Support swayed, eyes open, visual fixed
5. Support swayed, eyes closed, visual fixed
6. Support swayed, eyes open, visual sway-referenced

The patient is subjected to each test condition three times, and an equilibrium score is calculated for each condition. The equilibrium score compares the patient's sway in the anteroposterior direction, compared to the theoretical limits of anteroposterior sway. A score of 100% implies little sway, and lower scores correspond to greater amounts of sway. The differences in scores for the six conditions are then analyzed to determine the specific nature of the patient's balance disorder. Of particular interest is the vestibular ratio, which compares conditions 1 and 5 and delineates the reduction in stability when visual and somatosensory inputs are disrupted. Although healthy subjects sway a little in condition 5, those with vestibular disease score poorer than average. An example of such a posturography test is shown in Figure 9–21.

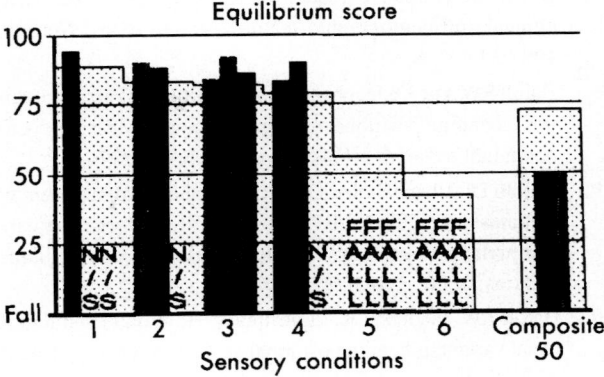

Figure 9–21 Posturography test of a patient with total bilateral loss of vestibular function owing to ototoxicity. He has normal postural stability when tested under conditions 1 through 4 but marked instability on conditions 5 and 6, in which he had to rely solely on vestibular cues. This type of result may be seen in patients with acute unilateral peripheral vestibular lesions. Only rarely is it seen in patients with chronic unilateral vestibular dysfunction.

Posturography may be helpful in evaluating patients with balance disorders in whom the history and physical examination do not suggest any apparent etiology. In this regard, it is occasionally ordered for patients with vague symptoms of dizziness and unsteadiness, without vertigo. It can also be used to detect malingerers, who will tend to overexaggerate their symptoms, and demonstrates results that are inconsistent with those seen in patients with true vestibular dysfunction. More than a diagnostic tool, it can also be used to evaluate how patients with known balance problems are progressing in terms of compensation and return to health.

REFERENCES

1. Stockwell CW. Vestibular testing: past, present, future. Br J Audiol 1997;31:387–98.
2. Bhansali SA, Honrubia V. Current status of electronystagmography testing. Otolaryngol Head Neck Surg 1999;120: 419–26.
3. Baloh RW, Honrubia V. Clinical neurophysiology of the vestibular system. Philadelphia: FA Davis; 1990.
4. Leigh RJ, Zee DS. The neurology of eye movements. Philadelphia: FA Davis; 1991.
5. Barber HO, Stockwell CW. Manual of electronystagmography. 2nd ed. St. Louis: CV Mosby; 1980.
6. Baloh RW, Honrubia V, Konrad HR. Ewald's second law reevaluated. Acta Otolaryngol (Stockh) 1977;83:474–9.

7. Baloh RW, Honrubia V, Jacobson K. Benign positional vertigo: clinical and oculographic features in 240 cases. Neurology 1987;37:371–8.

8. Baloh RW, Yue O, Jacobson KM, Honrubia V. Persistent direction-changing positional nystagmus: another variant of benign positional nystagmus? Neurology 1995;45:1297–301.

9. Bojrab DI, Bhansali SA. Objective evaluation of a patient with dizziness. In: Canalis RF, Lambert PR, editors. The ear — comprehensive otology. Philadelphia: Lippincott, Williams & Wilkins; 2000. p. 181–96.

10. Baloh RW, Jacobson K, Honrubia V. Horizontal semicircular canal variant of benign positional vertigo. Neurology 1993;43:2542–9.

11. Jacobson GP, Newman CW, Peterson EL. Interpretation and usefulness of caloric testing. In: Jacobson GP, Newman CW, Kartush JM, editor. Handbook of balance function testing. San Diego: Singular; 1997. p. 193–234.

12. Bojrab DI, Bhansali SA, Battista RA. Peripheral vestibular discorders. In: Jackler RK, Brackman DE, editors. Neurotology. St. Louis: Mosby-Year Book; 1994. p. 629–50.

13. Bojrab DI, Stockwell CW. Electronystagmography and rotation tests. In: Jackler RK, Brackman DE, editors. Neurotology. St. Louis: Mosby-Year Book; 1994. p. 219–28.

14. Bhansali SA, Stockwell CW, Bojrab DI. Oscillopsia in patients with loss of vestibular function. Otolaryngol Head Neck Surg 1993;109:120–5.

15. Stockwell CW, Bojrab DI. Background and technique of rotational testing. In: Jacobson GP, Newman CW, Kartush JM, editors. Handbook of balance function testing. St. Louis: Mosby-Year Book; 1993. p. 237–48.

16. Stockwell CW, Bojrab DI. Interpretation and usefulness of rotational testing. In: Jacobson GP, Newman CW, Kartush JM,

editors. Handbook of balance function testing. St. Louis: Mosby-Year Book; 1993. p. 249–58.

17. Raphan T, Matsuo V, Cohen B. Velocity storage in the vestibulo-ocular reflex arc (VOR). Exp Brain Res 1979;35:229–48.

18. Honrubia V, Jenkins HA, Balon RW, et al. Vestibulo-ocular reflexes in peripheral labyrinthine lesions: I. Unilateral dysfunction. Am J Otolaryngol 1984;5:15–26.

19. Baloh RW, Henn V, Jager J. Habituation of the human vestibulo-ocular reflex by low frequency harmonic acceleration. Am J Otolaryngol 1982;3:235–41.

20. Honrubia V, Jenkins HA, Balon RW, et al. Evaluation of rotatory vestibular tests in peripheral labyrinthine lesions. In: Honrubia V, Brazier MAB, editors. Nystagmus and vertigo. Clinical approaches to the patient with dizziness. New York: Academic Press; 1982. p. 57–78.

21. Stockwell CW. Vestibular function testing: 4-year update. In: Cummings CW, Harker, Kralee, et al, editors. Otolaryngology-head and neck surgery: update II. St. Louis: Mosby-Year Book; 1989. p. 39–53.

22. Baloh RW, Honrubia V, Yee RD, et al. Changes in the human vestibulo-ocular reflex after loss of peripheral sensitivity. Ann Neurol 1984;16:222–8.

23. Baloh RW, Sills AW, Honrubia V. Impulsive and sinusoidal rotatory testing: a comparison with results of caloric testing. Laryngoscope 1979;89:646–54.

24. Shepard NT. Rotational chair testing. In: Goebel JA, editor. Practical management of the dizzy patient. Philadelphia: Lippincott Williams and Wilkins; 2001. p. 129–41.

25. Nashner LM. Computerized dynamic posturography. In: Goebel JA, editor. Practical management of the dizzy patient. Philadelphia: Lippincott Williams and Wilkins; 2001. p. 143–70.

26. Stockwell CW. Posturography. Otolaryngol Head Neck Surg 1981;89:333–5.

10

Endoscopic Diagnosis of Eustachian Tube Dysfunction

Dennis S. Poe, MD, FACS

The eustachian tube is a dynamic conduit between the middle ear and the nasopharynx with secretory, ciliary, and dilatory functions. The eustachian tube serves to regulate air pressure in the middle ear and mastoid system, clear material from the middle ear, and prevent reflux of material or sound from the nasopharynx. The eustachian tube in the normal adult measures approximately 31 to 38 mm in length.[1]

The anatomy of the eustachian tube will be defined in this chapter from the perspective of the endoscopic surgeon approaching the tube from the nasopharyngeal orifice. Proximal refers to the nasopharynx and distal refers toward the middle ear. When viewing a cross-section of the tubal lumen, there are superior and inferior halves and anterolateral and posteromedial halves.

The distal one-third is, in effect, a bony, funnel-shaped extension of the middle ear that becomes narrowest at the isthmus, the smallest aperture in the entire tube. The bony portion, lined with a thin layer of cuboidal respiratory epithelium,[2] is a fixed conduit, and is normally patent.[3]

The proximal two-thirds of the eustachian tube are called the pharyngeal portion and are composed of a cartilaginous skeleton to which is attached a complex arrangement of peritubal muscles capable of a wide range of dynamic movements. The lumen is lined by respiratory epithelium that is taller, more columnar, and more ciliated inferiorly than the cuboidal epithelium in the superior one half. A submucosal layer of lymphatics and fat adds to the lining's thickness within the tubal lumen. The cartilaginous portion is normally closed in the resting state. Muscular contractions initiate rotational movements of the cartilaginous framework and create tension in the anterolateral wall to produce active dilation of the lumen and transient opening. It is believed that intermittent brief dilation of the tube is the principal mechanism for equilibration of middle ear pressure with the ambient atmosphere.[4] Fluid and secretions in the middle ear are cleared by a combination of muscular pumping action associated with the tubal closing process[2] and by mucociliary activity.[5] Reflux of nasopharyngeal secretions into the middle ear is limited or prevented by the closed position of the resting pharyngeal eustachian tube and by the trapped volume of gas in the middle ear and mastoid bone, which creates a "gas cushion." Reflux of the sounds of breathing and vocalization is also blocked by the closed resting position of the pharyngeal eustachian tube.[5]

Endoscopy of the human eustachian tube has significantly increased our understanding of the functional processes in normal and pathologic tubes. Initial work done by the insertion of microfiberoptic instruments into the tubal lumen yielded only limited information since the bony isthmus is only about 1.0 to 1.5 mm in horizontal diameter and 2 to 3 mm in vertical diameter.[6] To pass through the narrow isthmus, endoscope diameters must be restricted to 1 mm or less, which sufficiently compromises image resolution. Gross structures within the middle ear, such as ossicles, may be visualized, whereas fine details of movements cannot be appreciated. Direct contact of the endoscope lens with secretions and mucosal folds obscures visualization within the lumen and most reports have only been able to describe gross observations such as the presence of lesions or degree of patency.[7–10]

Large-diameter (3–4 mm) fiberoptic nasopharyngoscopes or rigid Hopkins rod endoscopes have been used for more detailed studies of the tubal lumen. The endoscope may be carefully positioned in the nasopharyngeal orifice with the view directed superiorly and laterally into the lumen, allowing for observation of most of the pharyngeal portion of the tube as it rotates into the dilated position during the opening sequence. Careful observation of tubal dynamics has become possible with high-resolution optics, and avoidance of direct contact with the mucosa prevents interference with the dilating mechanism and limits problems with fogging of the lens. Video recordings can be made and replayed in slow motion for meticulous analysis of the dilation process and study of normal physiology and pathophysiology.[11,12]

Eustachian tube endoscopy generally yields views distally well into the "valve" area during the time of maximal active dilation. We define the valve as the segment of the cartilaginous tube that is closed at rest and opens during the dilatory sequence. The valve is immediately proximal to the bony–cartilaginous junction that is, in turn, just proximal to the bony isthmus. The opening process can be seen endoscopically as the tube progressively dilates from the nasopharyngeal orifice up toward the isthmus, generally moving the lumen into full view of the endoscope. We have studied normal subjects and patients with tubal dysfunction using these techniques to establish some observed patterns of normal dynamic physiology and pathophysiology.

TECHNIQUE OF EUSTACHIAN TUBE VIDEO ENDOSCOPY

Patients are examined in the sitting position in an office setting. Topical spray anesthetic and decongestant, lidocaine 4% topical mixed with equal parts of phenylephrine hydrochloride 0.5% solution, is applied to both nasal cavities while the patient sniffs. Endoscopes are introduced into the nasal cavity and advanced up to the nasopharyngeal orifice of the eustachian tube, just posterior to the inferior turbinate and identified by the torus torbaris. It is easy to pass by the torus and examine the fossa of Rosenmüller, believing it to be the eustachian tube orifice.

The endoscopes that are used are usually either a 4-mm-diameter steerable flexible fiberoptic nasopharyngoscope EMF-P3 (Olympus, Tokyo, Japan) or a 4-mm-diameter, 30-degree view angle, Hopkins Rod rigid sinus surgery endoscope (Karl Storz, Culver City, Calif.).

The rod endoscopes have high-resolution images, but the fiberoptic endoscopes are easier to pass and can be steered deeper into the eustachian tube lumen if desired.

The 30-degree rigid endoscope is introduced with the view angle looking directly laterally and passed along the nasal floor, following the inferior turbinate until reaching the nasopharyngeal orifice and eustachian tube. Once at the orifice, the endoscope is rotated slightly to look superiorly toward the long axis of the eustachian tube. If the rigid endoscope will not easily pass through a narrow nasal cavity, then a flexible fiberoptic endoscope can usually be admitted. The optimal fiberoptic view is most commonly obtained by introducing the endoscope along the floor of the contralateral nasal cavity and passing the tip behind the vomer. This brings the tip into the proper angle to view up the long axis of the eustachian tube when it dilates. Occasionally, the lumen may be successfully viewed with a fiberoptic scope from the ipsilateral nasal cavity.

The endoscopes are used with a charge-coupled device (CCD) camera in place, and images are viewed on a video monitor. Video recordings are made with an s-VHS video recorder.

The patient is asked to vocalize "K-K-K" repeatedly to isolate the action of the levator veli palatini (LVP) from the tensor veli palatini (TVP). The "Ks" stimulate palatal elevation and posteromedial rotation of the medial cartilaginous lamina and posteromedial wall of the eustachian tube. Swallows are done to induce normal physiologic tubal dilations, and forced yawns are performed to cause maximal sustained dilation.

The procedure is repeated from the contralateral eustachian tube orifice. Lastly, a fiberoptic endoscope is passed through the nasal cavity into the hypopharynx to inspect the larynx for any evidence of laryngopharyngeal reflux (LPR) of gastric contents.

The video of tubal dilations is then reviewed and analyzed in normal time, slow motion, and even stepping through single frames that are captured at a rate of 30 frames per second.

ENDOSCOPY OF THE NORMAL EUSTACHIAN TUBE

Thirty normal subjects underwent endoscopy to study the normal dilation process.[11,12] Normal dilation and opening were observed to have four consistent sequential phases during a normal swallow (Figures 10–1 to 10–3):

1. The soft palate elevated with simultaneous medial rotation of the posteromedial wall. The lateral pharyngeal wall also medialized, causing transient constriction of the nasopharyngeal orifice despite the medial rotation of the eustachian tube medial wall. One hypothesis for this contrary movement could be to provide momentary protection of the eustachian tube against reflux at the initiation of swallow.
2. The palate remained elevated, and the posteromedial wall remained medially rotated as the lateral pharyngeal wall displaced laterally to begin the dilation of the nasopharyngeal orifice.
3. The TVP began to contract, causing dilation of the lumen to propagate from the nasopharyngeal orifice toward the bony isthmus. The dilation occurred by displacement of the anterolateral tubal wall laterally and away from the already contracted and medially rotated posteromedial wall.
4. Tubal opening occurred as the functional valve of the cartilaginous tube dilated into a roughly rounded aperture. The convex bulge seen in the resting anterolateral valve wall became visibly flattened to produce the final opening.
5. Closure of the tube began with closure of the valve area and propagated proximally toward the nasopharyngeal orifice. This distal to proximal closure has been hypothesized to have a pumping action that may protect against reflux.[4]

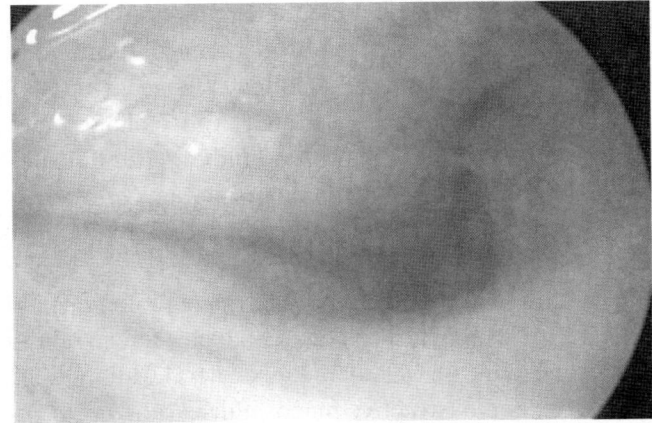

Figure 10–2 Normal eustachian tube from Figure 10–1 during swallow. The palate is elevated, medial cartilaginous lamina is rotated medially, and lateral wall nearly dilated open.

Relaxation of the posteromedial wall, lateral pharyngeal wall, and palate occurred in variable order or even simultaneously.

The thin mucosa and subcutaneous tissues of the normal eustachian tubes permitted visualization of the muscular contractions of the LVP and TVP muscles. Even the ripples of distinct individual fiber contractions were often appreciated.

ENDOSCOPY OF THE DYSFUNCTIONAL EUSTACHIAN TUBE

Forty patients with 58 ears suspected of eustachian tube dysfunction were studied using the above techniques. Each patient had otomicroscopic examinations that

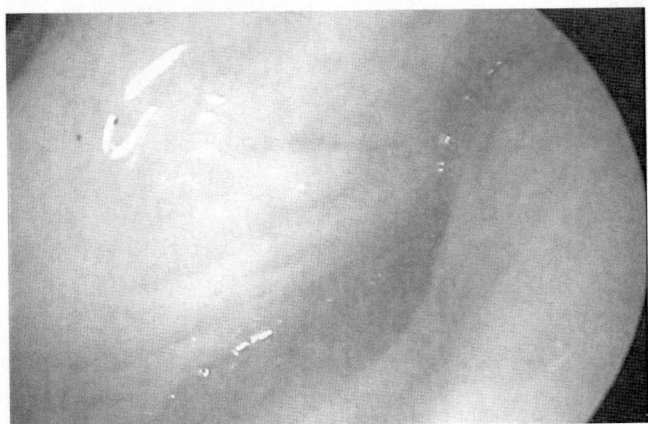

Figure 10–1 Normal resting left eustachian tube. A 4-mm rigid endoscopic view of the left eustachian tube and pharyngeal orifice.

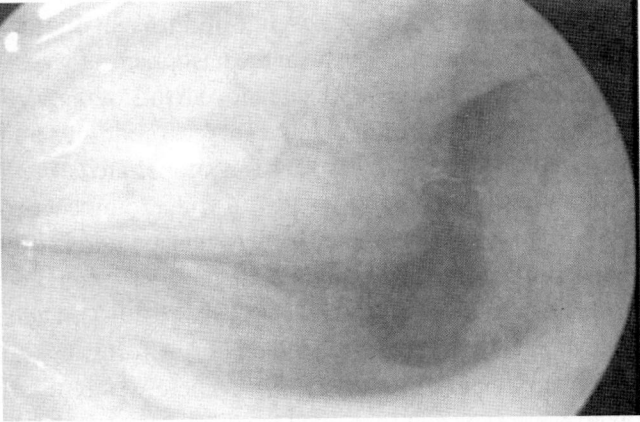

Figure 10–3 Normal eustachian tube from Figures 10–1 and 10–2 during swallow. The tube is fully dilated.

demonstrated tympanic membrane retraction or atelectasis, otitis media with effusion, or chronic otitis media.[12] Dynamic analyses with slow-motion video techniques of all 58 eustachian tubes revealed significant pathology and compromise of tubal dilation. A study of 22 clinically normal eustachian tubes in comparison found only some mild degree of pathology in 7 tubes (32%) on video analysis.

The following is a summary of the pathologic findings in the 58 clinically dysfunctional eustachian tubes: mucosal edema, 48 (83%); reduced lateral wall motion, 43 (74%); and obstructive mucosal disease, 15 (26%).

All 58 had significantly compromised tubal dilation, which was judged to be moderate opening ability, 26 (45%); minimal opening, 21 (36%); and no opening, 11 (19%).

The components of the pharyngeal eustachian tube can be classified as the cartilaginous skeleton, tubal muscles, soft tissue of the submucosa, and epithelium of the lumen. The generally accepted engineering principle that states that "Anything that can go wrong will go wrong" evidently also applies to the moving parts of the eustachian tube. Defects were observed in all of the different components of the pharyngeal tube.

Edema of the mucosa and submucosa was often responsible for decreased luminal diameter and decreased ability to dilate the tube (Figures 10–4 to 10–6). When dilation was thus compromised, considerable muscular effort was noted, working against the increased bulk of the periluminal soft tissues, and it was presumed that muscular function was probably normal.

There were cases in which there was a distinct reduction in muscular function in either the LVP or TVP, even in the absence of tissue edema. In some cases, the TVP showed disorganization or absence of the usual dilatory wave that should progress from the nasopharyngeal orifice toward the isthmus. Muscle movements of the TVP were sometimes minimal or occurred randomly and appeared to fasciculate. Two cases demonstrated excessively strong contractions of the TVP with prominent ripples producing longitudinal ridges that paradoxically reduced the lumen diameter just as the TVP attempted to lateralize the posterolateral wall (Figure 10–7). There were three tubes in which a good dilatory effort was seen in the proximal half of the tube, but there was reduced dilatory effort or failure to open the distal valve area. Two cases demonstrated an unusual double contraction of the

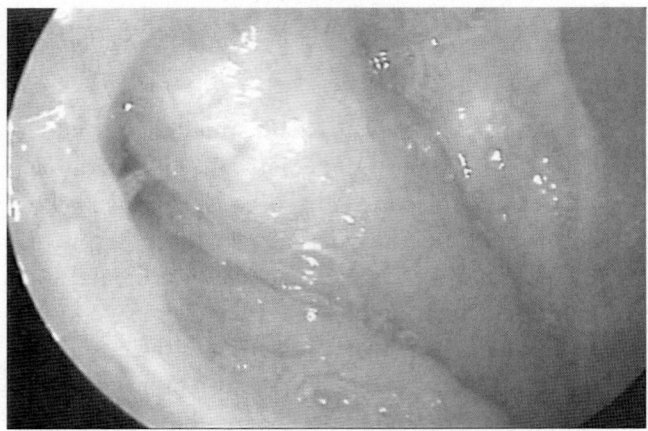

Figure 10–4   Right eustachian tube in patient with acute otitis media with effusion during upper respiratory infection. The mucosa is diffusely edematous and hypersecretory.

LVP and palate during the time that the TVP was attempting to dilate the tube. In another case, the LVP paradoxically relaxed just at the time that the TVP began to contract. These three cases demonstrated a failure of coordination between the LVP and TVP that resulted in failure of dilation of the tube.

Mucosal edema within the tube most commonly was uniformly distributed along the length of the eustachian tube and tended to be most prominent in the inferior half of the tube's cross-sectional diameter. Mucosal swelling was sometimes accompanied with erythema, mucoid secretions, or purulent drainage. Several tubes demonstrated severe edema with bulbous projections into the

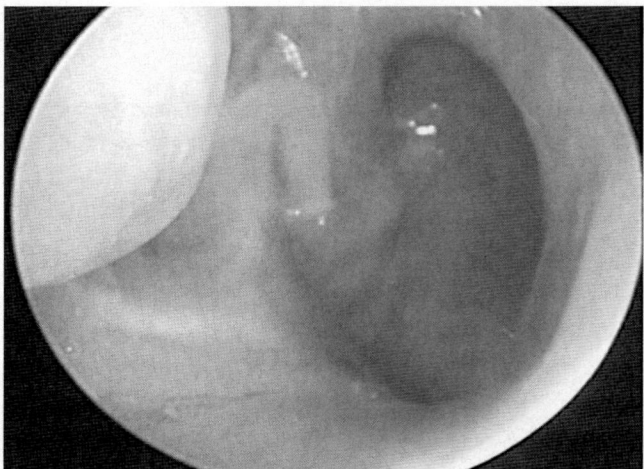

Figure 10–5   Right eustachian tube in a patient with acute otitis media with effusion during pneumonia. Purulent nasal secretions drain over the eustachian tube orifice, which has diffuse edema.

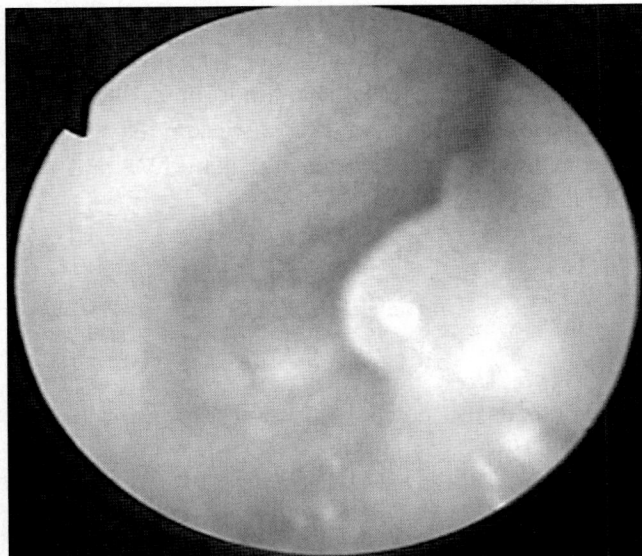

Figure 10–6 Fiberoptic examination of right eustachian tube in a patient with severe allergic rhinitis and diffuse bulbous edematous mucosal changes.

lumen resembling polyps. These tubes were generally unable to dilate open at all.

There was one patient who had adenoid hypertrophy that was not obstructing the nasopharyngeal orifice at rest. During swallowing, however, the adenoid was pressed into the tubal orifice and forced the posterior cushion (posteromedial wall) to completely cover and par-

doxically obstruct the nasopharyngeal orifice at the time when it should be dilating.

A distinct yellow discoloration of the tubal lumen was seen in 11 (19%) tubes and was thought to be caused by mucosal atrophy from chronic disease, as is often seen in the sinuses.

During this study, a suspicion arose that LPR may be responsible for mucosal edema in some cases. The last 10 consecutive patients underwent examination of the hypopharynx and larynx by flexible nasopharyngoscopy. Seven of these 10 patients (70%) demonstrated significant evidence of LPR with erythema or edema in the vocal cords, arytenoids, and aryepiglottic folds. Two of these patients reported routinely sleeping in the lateral decubitus position on the same side as their dysfunctional tube. All of these patients gave a history consistent with reflux on careful questioning.

There was no correlation between the severity of middle ear pathology and the severity or type of eustachian tube pathology. It appeared that changes in the tympanic membrane and middle ear took on an independent pathophysiologic process once eustachian tube dysfunction had passed some critical point.

There were six patulous tubes, and all of them demonstrated a consistent concavity in the superior cross-sectional half of the anterolateral wall within the valve area. Normal tubes have a convexity in this location that flattens during the final stage of the dilation process (Figure 10–8).

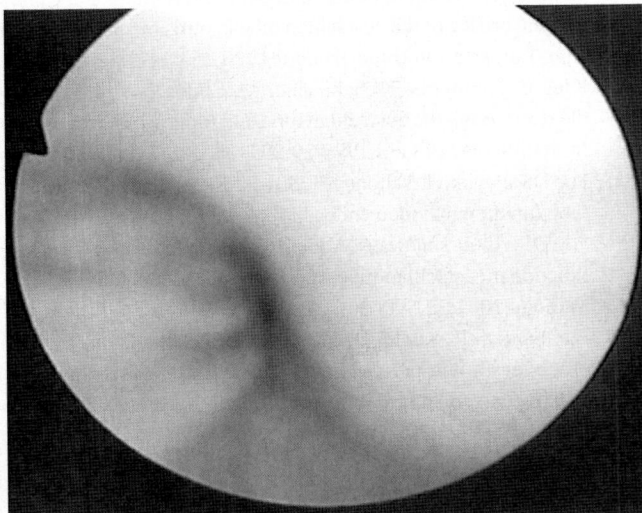

Figure 10–7 Fiberoptic examination of the right eustachian tube in a patient with tympanic membrane retraction and chronic negative middle ear pressure. Bulky hypercontraction of the lateral wall shows prominent ripples of the tensor veli palatini muscle blocking the lumen during swallow.

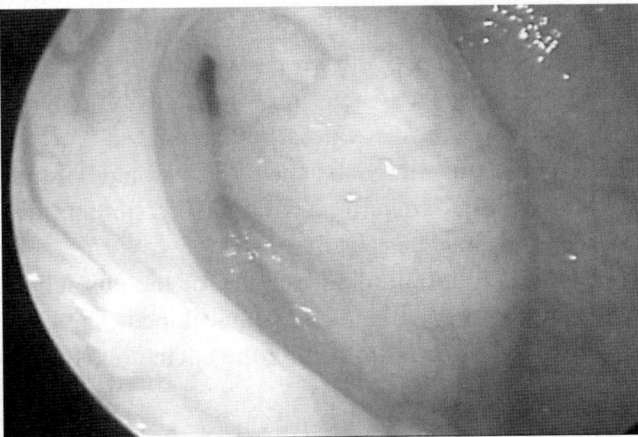

Figure 10–8 A 4-mm rigid endoscopic view of the right resting patulous eustachian tube. The superior aspect of the eustachian tube has concavity in the lateral wall and persistent lumenal patency in distinction from normal tubes, which have a prominent convexity and are closed at rest.

Dilation of the eustachian tube appeared to require a coordinated action and proper functioning of both LVP and TVP. The action of the LVP is to medially rotate the medial cartilaginous lamina within the posteromedial wall of the tube. This contraction should be sustained throughout the remainder of the dilatory phase and may serve as a scaffold against which the TVP can efficiently contract. The TVP runs longitudinally along the anterolateral wall of the tube and is considered to be the active dilator of the tube. Some fibers of TVP stretch from the scaphoid process of the sphenoid bone to the hamulus and other fibers insert directly on the membranous lateral wall of the tube. The fibers inserting on the lateral wall may be referred to as the dilator tubae muscle.[5,13] A weakness in either the LVP or the TVP or a failure of coordination between these muscles is apparently sufficient to cause clinically significant eustachian tube dysfunction.

Eustachian tube dysfunction appears to result from failure of any of the components of the cartilaginous pharyngeal tube. Mucosal edema may be caused by inflammatory disease, infection, allergy, or reflux from the nasopharynx (including LPR). Medical treatment should be directed toward the underlying etiology of edema whenever possible, and middle ear ventilation with tympanostomy tubes is generally recommended when medical treatment is inadequate. The persistence of mucosal edema despite maximal medical treatment and dissatisfaction with tympanostomy tubes may be considered an indication for tubal surgery. Primary muscular disorders including weakness or lack of coordination between the LVP and the TVP may benefit from medical treatment or speech therapy eustachian tube exercises. Intratubal surgery may help some patients failing these conservative measures. Primary anatomic obstruction appears to be quite rare, and such cases should be studied individually to determine what medical or surgical interventions may be effective.

Endoscopic intraluminal surgery of the eustachian tube is now being performed and developed. The principle of the surgery is to debulk the edematous tissues in the posteromedial wall to allow for easier dilation of the tube as the TVP contracts. Cases involving muscular dysfunction may also have a portion of the medial cartilaginous lamina debulked to weaken the spring of the cartilaginous skeleton and facilitate LVP and TVP contraction.

REFERENCES

1. Proctor B. Anatomy of the eustachian tube. Arch Otolaryngol 1973;97:2.
2. Honjo I, Hayashi M, Ito S, et al. Pumping and clearance function of the eustachian tube. Am J Otolaryngol 1985;6:241.
3. Hopf J, Linnarz M, Gundlach P, et al. Die Mikroendoskopie der Eustachischen Rohre und des Mittelhres. Indikationen und klinischer Einsatzpunkt. Laryngorhinootologie 1991;70:391–4.
4. Honjo I. Eustachian tube and middle ear diseases. Tokyo: Springer-Verlag; 1988.
5. Bluestone CD, Klein JO. Otitis media, atelectatis, and eustachian tube dysfunction. In: Bluestone CD, Stool SE, Kenna MA, editors. Pediatric otolaryngology. 3rd ed. Philadelphia: WB Saunders; 1996.
6. Schuknecht HF, Gulya AJ. Anatomy of the temporal bone with surgical implications. Philadelphia: Lea & Febiger; 1986.
7. Chays A, Cohen JM, Magnan J. La microfibroendoscopie tubo-tympanique. Techn Chirug 1995;24:773–4.
8. Kimura H, Yamaguchi H, Cheng SS, et al. Direct observation of the tympanic cavity by the superfine fiberscope. Nippon Jibiinkoka Gakkai Kaiho 1989;92:233–8.
9. Takahashi H, Honjo I, Fujita A. Endoscopic findings at the pharyngeal orifice of the eustachian tube in otitis media with effusion. Eur Arch Otorhinolaryngol 1996;253(1–2):42–4.
10. Klug C, Fabinyi B, Tschabitscher M. Endoscopy of the middle ear through the eustachian tube: anatomic possiblilites and limitations. Am J Otol 1999;20:299–303.
11. Poe DS, Pyykko I, Valtonen H, Silvola J. Analysis of eustachian tube function by video endoscopy. Am J Otol 2000;21:602–7.
12. Poe DS, Abou-Halawa A, Abdel-Razek O. Analysis of the dysfunctional eustachian tube by video endoscopy. Otolog Neurotology 2001;22:590–5.
13. Barsoumian R, Kuehn D, Moon JB, et al. An anatomic study of the tensor veli palatini and dilatator tubae muscles in relation to eustachian tube and velar function. Cleft Palate Craniofac J 1998;35:101–10.

11

Imaging of the Temporal Bone

GALDINO E. VALVASSORI, MD

Diagnostic imaging techniques have been revolutionized by the use of the computer for data storage, analysis, and display and by the introduction of a nonradiography imaging system. Four techniques are applied to study the temporal bone and central auditory-vestibular pathways: conventional radiography, computed tomography (CT), magnetic resonance (MR), and angiography.

CONVENTIONAL RADIOGRAPHY

Today, use of conventional radiography is limited to the evaluation of mastoid pneumatization and to the assessment of the position and integrity of the cochlear implant electrodes. Only three projections are of practical interest today: the lateral or Schüller, the frontal or transorbital, and the oblique or Stenvers. The other special projections have historical significance but no practical application.

Lateral or Schüller Projection

The Schüller projection is a lateral view of the mastoid obtained with the sagittal plane of the skull parallel to the tabletop and with a 30-degree cephalocaudad angulation of the x-ray beam (Figure 11–1). Proper centering is obtained by placing the external auditory canal of the side to be examined 1 cm above the center of the film or of the tabletop. The anterior plate of the lateral sinus casts an almost vertical line superimposed on the air cells. At its upper extremity, this line joins the tegmen plate, which slopes gently forward and downward. The more

medial portion of the superior petrous ridge, from the arcuate eminence to the apex, has been displaced downward by the angulation of the x-ray beam and casts a line that extends forward and downward, crossing the epitympanic area and, more anteriorly, the neck of the mandibular condyle. Above this line, the upper portion of the attic with the head of the malleus is usually visible. Finally, the temporomandibular joint is outlined.

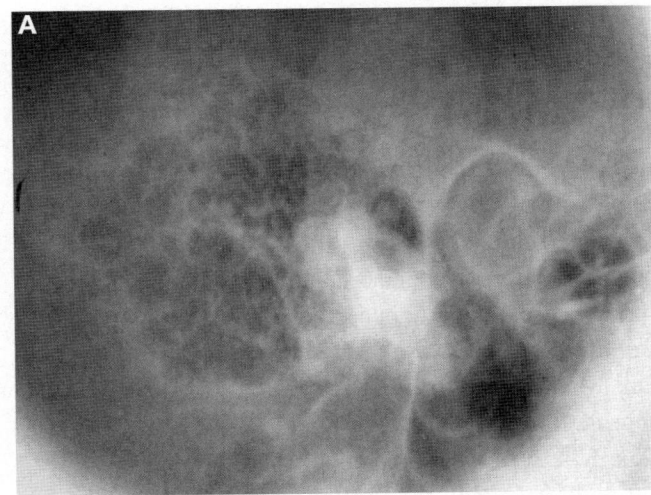

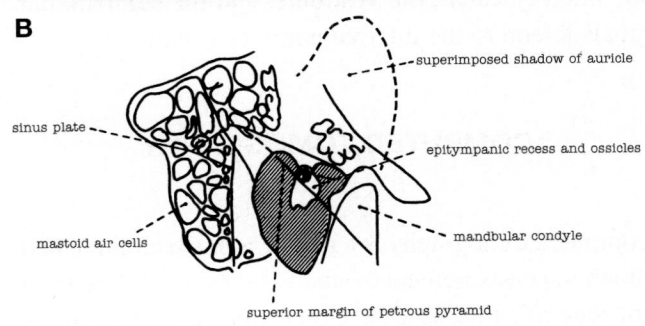

Figure 11–1 Schüller's projection.

Frontal or Transorbital Projection

The view can be obtained with the patient facing to or away from the film. The patient's head is flexed on the chin until the orbitomeatal line is perpendicular to the tabletop (Figure 11–2). For better detail, each side should be filmed separately. The petrous apex is outlined clearly but foreshortened because of its obliquity to the film. The internal auditory canal is visualized in its full length as a horizontal band of radiolucency extending through the petrous pyramid. At the medial end of the canal, the free margin of the posterior wall casts a well-defined and smooth margin concave medially. Lateral to the internal auditory canal, the radiolucence of the vestibule and superior and horizontal semicircular canals are usually detectable. The apical and middle coils of the cochlea are superimposed on the lateral portion of the internal auditory canal, whereas the basilar turn is visible underneath the canal and vestibule.

Oblique or Stenvers Projection

The patient is positioned facing the film with the head slightly flexed and rotated 45 degrees toward the side opposite to the one under examination. The lateral rim of the orbit of the side under investigation should lie in close contact with the tabletop. The x-ray beam is angulated 14 degrees caudad (Figure 11–3). The petrous apex is visualized in its full length lateral to the orbital rim. The porus of the internal auditory canal seen on face appears as an oval-shaped radiolucency open medially and limited laterally by the free margin of the posterior canal wall. Lateral to the porus, the internal auditory canal appears foreshortened. The structures of the labyrinth are usually recognizable: the cochlea underneath the internal auditory canal, the vestibule, and the semicircular canals lateral to the internal auditory canal.

COMPUTED TOMOGRAPHY

Computed tomography is a radiographic technique that allows the measurement of small absorption differentials not recognizable by direct recording on x-ray films. The scan is initiated at a chosen level, and the x-ray tube,

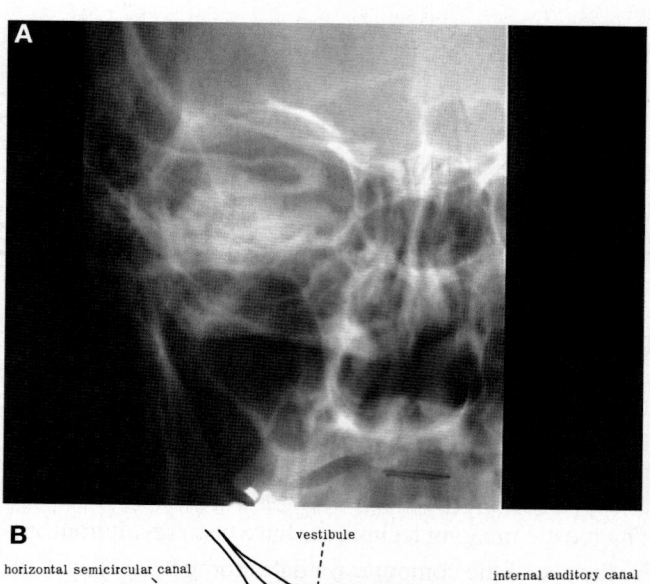

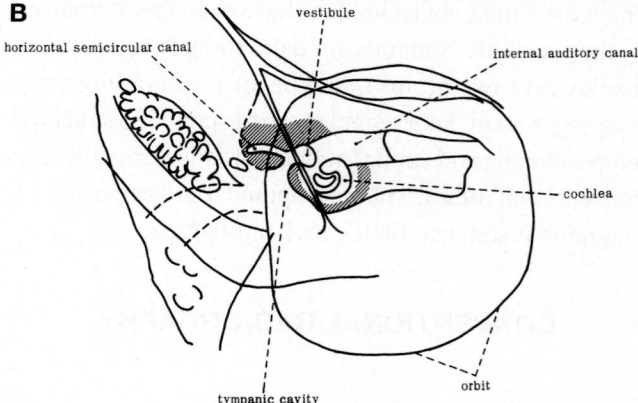

Figure 11–2 Transorbital projection.

collimated to a thin or pencil beam, rotates around the patient. The transmitted x-rays are picked up by detectors, arrayed along the circumference of the tube trajectory, converted into electronic currents, amplified, and transmitted to the computer for storage and processing. The computer analyzes the data and develops an image on a dot matrix in which the brightness of each point is proportional to the attenuation coefficient.

Recently, conventional CT has been replaced by helical or spiral CT that allows rapid acquisition of the volumetric data of the part of the body under examination. Images are acquired at an angled plane of section and then reconstructed by interpolating the volumetric data set as two-dimensional or high-quality three-dimensional reformation. The continuous acquisition of images is made possible by replacing the former electric tubing of the gantry with a slip-ring design, which allows con-

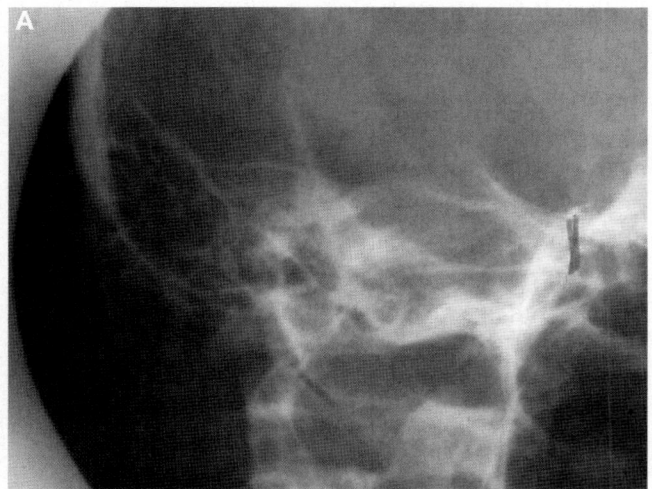

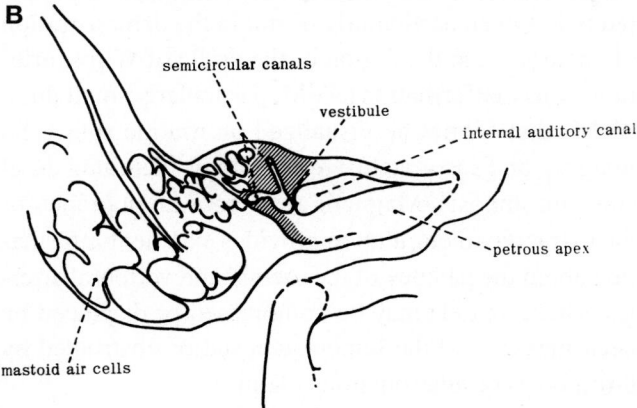

Figure 11–3 Stenvers projection.

tinuous rotation of the source-detector assembly and by the use of high heat capacity x-ray tubes. The advantage of spiral CT includes elimination of respiratory misregistration, decrease of motion artifact, and an obvious improvement in patient comfort owing to the shortening of the examination time. This is particularly important in children, whether they have been administered anesthesia or simple sedation, and in older patients, who have difficulty in overextending the head. Reconstruction of axial data in other planes produces satisfactory images provided that a collimation as small as 1 or 0.5 mm is used. A scanning time of less than 1 minute is sufficient to cover the mastoid and petrous portions of the temporal bone. New multidetector scanners will further decrease the scanning time. The CT images provide exquisite bony details and excellent demonstration of soft tissue density within the air spaces of the mastoid, external auditory canal, and middle ear but very limited identification of the type of substance producing the abnormal density. For instance, the density of a cholesteatoma is identical to that of a tumor or granulation tissue and even of fluid. The study is often repeated after intravenous infusion or bolus injection of contrast material, which produces an increased intensity or enhancement of several anatomic structures and pathologic processes. An enhancement study is mandatory whenever a vascular anomaly, a tumor, or an otogenic abscess is suspected.

MAGNETIC RESONANCE IMAGING

Magnetic resonance is an imaging modality capable of producing cross-section images of the human body in any plane without exposing the patient to ionizing radiation. Unlike CT and other radiographic techniques, in which the obtained pictures are related to the differential absorption of the x-ray beam by tissue, MR images are obtained by the interaction of hydrogen nuclei or protons of the human body, high magnetic field, and radiofrequency pulses. The strength of the MR signal to be converted into imaging data depends on the concentration of the hydrogen nuclei and on two magnetic relaxation times, T_1 and T_2, which are tissue specific.

One of the characteristics and advantages of MR is the possibility of changing the appearance and therefore the information of the images by changing the relative contribution of the T_1 and T_2 relaxation times. This is accomplished by varying the time between successive pulses (TR or repetition time) and the time the emitted signal or echo is measured after the pulse (TE or echo time).

The MR imaging technique has undergone multiple changes and refinement to increase definition of the images and to decrease the acquisition time. First, the use of surface coils placed adjacent to the area of interest has increased the signal-to-noise ratio and consequently improves the image. Shorter acquisitions have been obtained by shortening the TR, using pulses with flip angles smaller than 90 degrees (gradient echo imaging), by reducing the number of phase-encoded steps, and by increasing the data collected per excitation. The latter technique, known as fast spin echo (FSE), uses multiple echos (4 to 16 for excitation), therefore reducing the number of excitations necessary for forming an image.

Arteries usually appear in the MR images as areas of signal void because the stimulated protons of the circulating blood have moved out of the section before the emitted signal can be detected. Veins may instead be bright because of the slower circulation. Air, cortical bone, and calcification also appear as dark areas of low signal because they contain few free protons.

Pathologic processes are demonstrated by MR whenever the hydrogen density and relaxation times of the pathologic tissues are different from those of the normal tissues.

The intravenous injection of ferromagnetic contrast agents has improved the recognition and differentiation of pathologic processes. Because the contrast material does not penetrate the intact blood barrier, normal brain does not enhance except for structures, such as the pituitary gland and several cranial nerves, that lack a complete blood-brain barrier. Enhancement of brain lesions occurs whenever the blood-brain barrier is disrupted, provided that there is sufficient blood flow to the lesions. Extra-axial lesions, such as meningiomas and schwannomas, lack a blood-brain barrier and therefore undergo a strong enhancement.

ANGIOGRAPHY

Angiography is seldom required for the diagnosis of vascular tumors or anomalies within or adjacent to the temporal bone. Angiography, however, is mandatory for identifying the feeding vessels of a lesion, usually a glomus, whenever embolization or surgical ligation is contemplated. Subtraction is necessary to delineate the vascular mass and feeding vessels, which are otherwise obscured by the density of the surrounding temporal bone. The injection should be performed in the common carotid artery to visualize both internal and external carotid circulation. A vertebral arteriogram may also be performed.

Gradient echo techniques and flow-encoded gradients have enabled the development of magnetic resonance angiography. Time of flight angiography is a gradient echo technique in which the stationary tissues within the imaging plane are saturated with the magnetic field so that they will not produce a signal. Blood flowing within the same plane is unsaturated and will be the only tissue to produce a signal. Phase contrast angiography is acquired differently. Instead of saturating the stationary tissues with radiofrequency pulses, a bipolar gradient of magnetization is applied to the entire slice, first with a positive value and then with a negative value. In the stationary tissues, the two opposite gradients cancel each other. In the flowing blood, however, the two opposite gradients cannot cancel each other because the blood will have moved to a different plane in the region before the inverse gradient is applied.

The obtained slices are reconstructed into three-dimensional images, which can be rotated in different planes to separate vessels and eliminate superimposition. Magnetic resonance imaging of the intracranial vasculature has been particularly useful in the demonstration of aneurysms in the region of the circle of Willis, arteriovenous malformation (AVM; particularly small dural AVMs that cannot be visualized on routine spin echo images), and vaso-occlusive pathology, including dural sinus thrombosis. Magnetic resonance angiography of the extracranial circulation provides excellent information about the patency of the carotid and vertebral arteries. These vessels may be compressed or displaced by neck masses and the lumen stenosed or obstructed by thrombosis or atheromatous plaques.

The introduction of ultra-fast CT has opened the possibility of obtaining excellent angiographic images. In CT angiography, the continuous acquisition of the images allows the following of the rapidly intravenously injected bolus of contrast through the arteries and veins of the area under investigation. The reconstructed images can be rotated in the plane that best demonstrates the vessels.

COMPUTED TOMOGRAPHY PROJECTIONS

The CT study of the temporal bones should always include at least two projections. The use of a single projection may lead to serious mistakes because the structures parallel to the plane of the section are not visualized. For instance, in the axial sections, the floor and the superior wall of the external auditory canal cannot be seen; therefore, pathologic processes involving these structures cannot be assessed. The same is true for the anterior and posterior walls of the canal in the coronal sections.

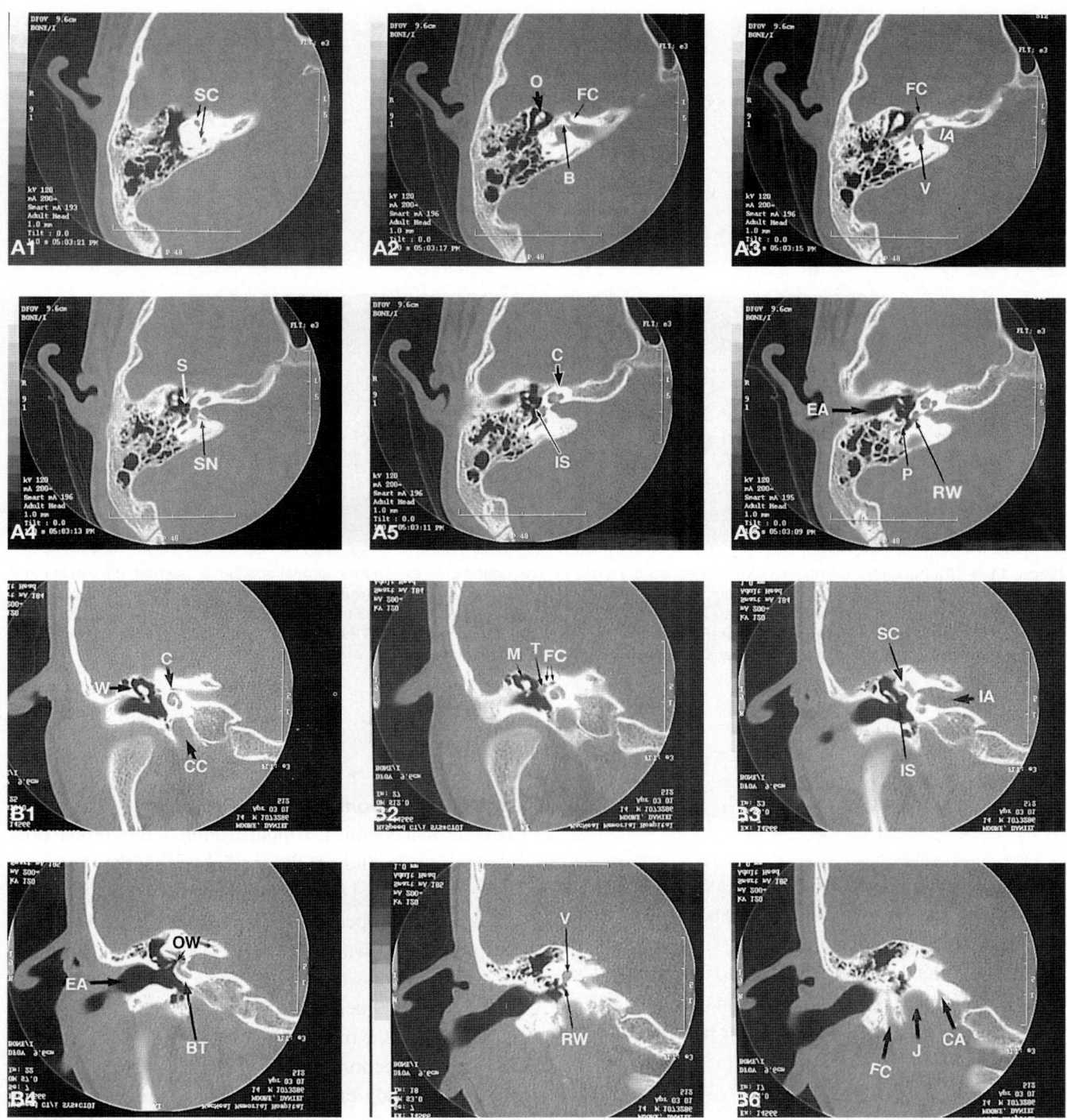

Figure 11–4 Computed tomography sections of a normal right ear: *A*, axial; *B*, coronal. BT = basal turn cochlea; C = cochlea; CA = cochlear aqueduct; CC = carotid canal; CR = common crus; EA = external auditory canal; FC = facial canal; HS = horizontal semicircular canal; IA = internal auditory canal; IS = incudostapedial joint; J = jugular fossa; M = malleus; O = ossicles; OW = oval window; PE = pyramidal eminence; PS = posterior semicircular canal; RW = round window; S = stapes; SC = superior semicircular canal; SN = singular nerve canal; T = tensor tympani canal; V = vestibule; VA = vestibular aqueduct; W = lateral wall attic.

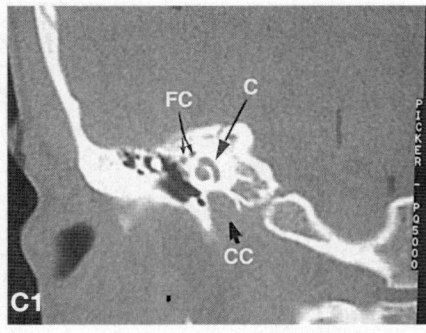
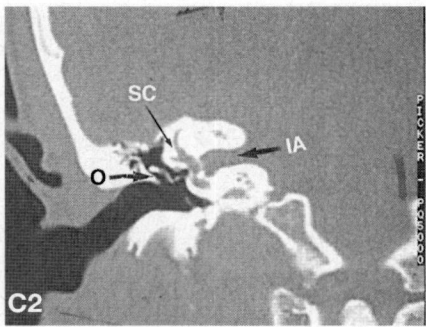
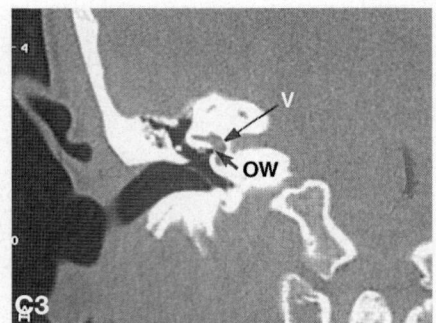

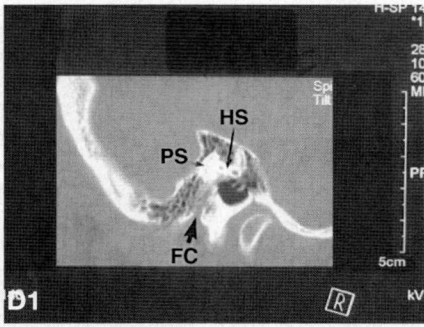
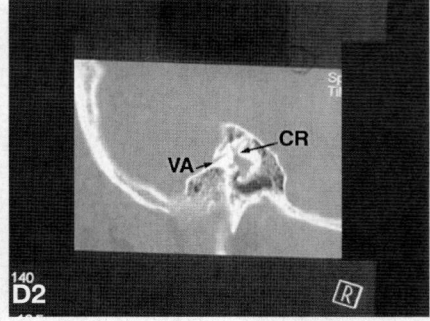

Figure 11–4 (Continued) Computed tomography sections of a normal right ear: *C*, 20-degree coronal oblique; *D*, sagittal. BT = basal turn cochlea; C = cochlea; CA = cochlear aqueduct; CC = carotid canal; CR = common crus; EA = external auditory canal; FC = facial canal; HS = horizontal semicircular canal; IA = internal auditory canal; IS = incudostapedial joint; J = jugular fossa; M = malleus; O = ossicles; OW = oval window; PE = pyramidal eminence; PS = posterior semicircular canal; RW = round window; S = stapes; SC = superior semicircular canal; SN = singular nerve canal; T = tensor tympani canal; V = vestibule; VA = vestibular aqueduct; W = lateral wall attic.

Axial Projection

This is the basic projection because axial or horizontal sections are the easiest to obtain. The patient lies supine on the table with the plane extending from the tragus to the inferior orbital rim perpendicular to the tabletop. Usually, 12 sections at 1.5-mm increments are sufficient to cover the temporal bone, except for the mastoid processes (Figure 11–4, A).

Coronal Projection

Coronal sections are obtained with the patient either supine or prone and the head overextended. The gantry of the scanner is often tilted to compensate for an incomplete extension of the head. Again, 12 sections at 1.5-mm increments are usually sufficient to cover the area of interest (Figure 11–4, B).

20-Degree Coronal Oblique Projection

This coronal oblique is a modification of the coronal projection for the study of the medial wall of the tympanic cavity. The medial or labyrinthine wall of the middle ear forms an angle open posteriorly of 15 to 25 degrees with the midsagittal plane of the skull. The patient is first positioned as for the coronal projection, and the head is then rotated 20 degrees toward the side under examination so that the medial wall becomes perpendicular to the plane of section. This projection is particularly useful for the study of the oval window, promontory, and tympanic segment of the facial canal (Figure 11–4, C).

Sagittal Projection

The direct sagittal projection can be performed in only a limited number of patients with flexible necks. However, satisfactory reformatted images can be obtained with spiral CT from the volumetric data acquired in the axial projection. The sagittal projection is particularly useful for the study of the mastoid segment of the facial canal and of the vestibular aqueduct (Figure 11–4, D).

MAGNETIC RESONANCE STUDY OF THE TEMPORAL BONE

The MR examination is performed with the patient supine and the line extending from the tragus to the inferior orbital rim perpendicular to the tabletop. Different projections are obtained by changing the orientation of the magnetic field gradients without moving the patient's head. Because the cortical or nondiploic bone and air emit a very weak signal, the normal mastoid, external auditory canal, and middle ear appear in the MR images as dark areas without any pattern or structure. The petrous pyramids are equally dark except for the signal received from the fluid within the internal auditory canal, cochlea, vestibule, and semicircular canals. A white cast of these structures is therefore visible within the dark areas of the pyramids (Figure 11–5).

Fluid and tissue caused by trauma, infection, and tumors within the mastoid, external auditory canal, and middle ear are readily identified by MR images as areas of abnormally high signal intensity. Magnetic resonance is more sensitive than CT in the early identification of pathologic changes in the temporal bone. However, the exact location, extent, and involvement of structures, such as the ossicles, scutum, and labyrinthine capsule, cannot be determined by MR imaging because all of the landmarks within the temporal bone are absent, except for the lumen of the inner ear structures. For this reason, CT remains the study of choice for the assessment of middle ear pathology, If the lesion extends outside the confines of the temporal bone, both intracranially and extracranially, MR defines involvement more precisely than CT. This is particularly true for glomus tumors because involvement of the jugular vein and carotid artery may be demonstrated, thus avoiding the need for more invasive vascular studies.

The images obtained in this chapter were obtained with a superconducting magnet and a magnetic field of 15,000 gauss or 1.5 tesla. The stronger the magnetic field, the higher the signal-to-noise ratio. Therefore, the structures that can be imaged are smaller, and the sections that can be obtained are thinner.

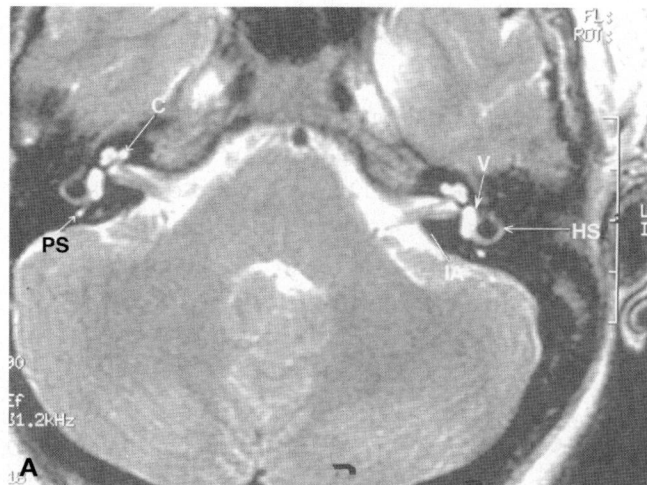

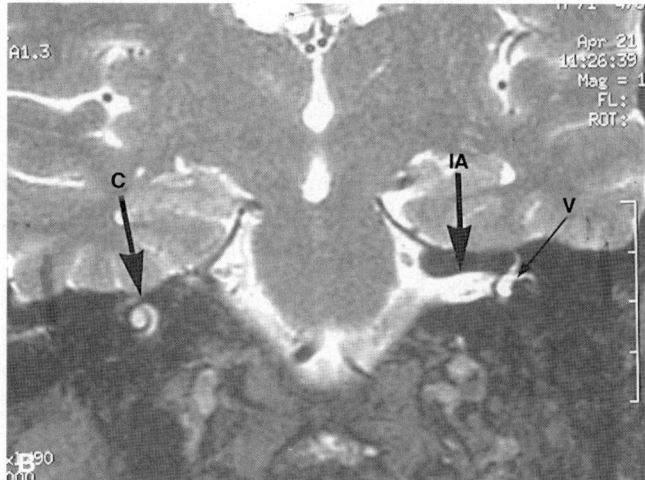

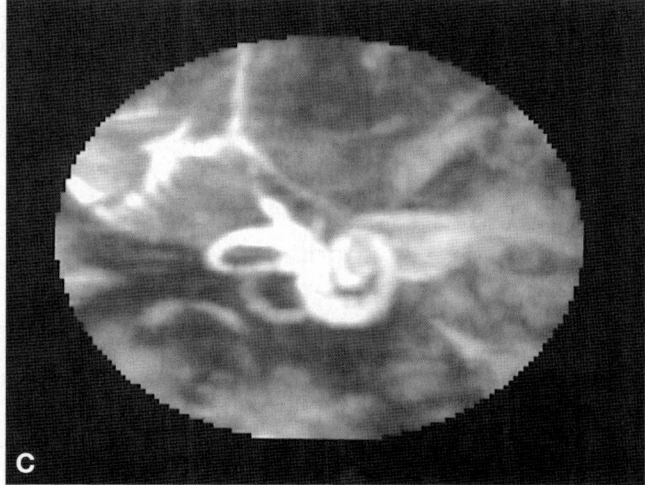

Figure 11–5 Magnetic resonance images of the normal temporal bone: *A*, fast spin-echo (FSE) axial; *B*, FSE coronal; *C*, three-dimensional reconstruction of the inner ear structures. C = cochlea; HS = horizontal semicircular canal; IA = internal auditory canal; PS = posterior semicircular canal; V = vestibule.

DEVELOPMENTAL VARIATIONS

Developmental variations in the size and position of several components of the temporal bone are quite common. These variations should be recognized by the radiologist rather than mistaken for pathologic processes but, above all, should be known to the otologists as they develop their surgical plans.

Mastoid

The development of the mastoid varies from person to person, as well as in degree, from side to side of the same individual. In some mastoids, the pneumatization is limited to a single antral cell; in others, it may extend into the mastoid tip and squama of the temporal bone and even invade the adjacent zygoma and occipital bone. The nonpneumatized mastoid process may be made up of solid bone or contain spongy diploic spaces filled with fatty marrow. The fatty marrow produces a high signal in the T_1 sequence, which decreases in T_2 and should not be confused with fluid or other pathologic processes that usually have a high signal in the T_2 sequence.

Lateral Sinus

The lateral sigmoid sinus forms a shallow indentation on the posterior aspect of the mastoid. Occasionally, the sinus courses more anteriorly and produces a deep groove in the mastoid, best seen in the axial sections. In some cases, only a thin bony plate separates the sinus from the external auditory canal (Figure 11–6).

Tegmen

The tegmen of the mastoid and attic usually passes in a horizontal plane slightly lower than the arcuate eminence produced by the top of the superior semicircular canal. A depression of the tegmental plate is not unusual, particularly in a patient with congenital atresia. As best seen in the coronal sections, the floor of the middle cranial fossa deepens to form a groove lateral to the attic and labyrinth (Figure 11–7). The low-lying dura may cover the roof of the external auditory canal and, when the canal is not developed, dips laterally to the mesotympanum.

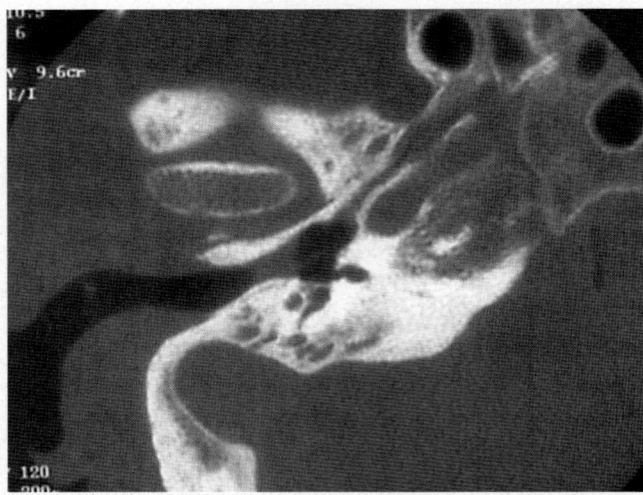

Figure 11–6 Anterior lateral sinus: axial computed tomography of right ear.

Jugular Fossa

There is tremendous variation in the size of the jugular fossa and jugular bulb. The variation occurs not only from patient to patient but also from side to side on the same patient. The size of the jugular fossa is not a criterion for pathologic process. A normal jugular fossa may produce only a slight indentation on the undersurface of the petrous bone or may extend upward as high as the superior petrous ridge posterior to the labyrinth and internal auditory canal (Figure 8, A and B). In these instances, the jugular bulb projects so high that it blocks access to

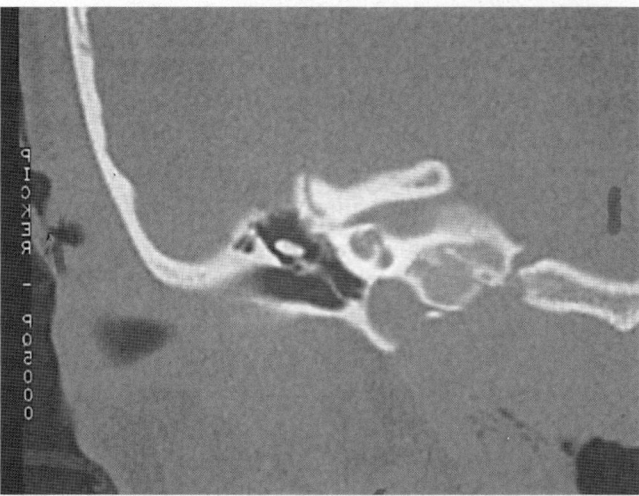

Figure 11–7 Low dura: coronal computed tomography scan of right ear.

the internal auditory canal by the translabyrinthine route in acoustic neuroma surgery. Often the high venous structure is not the jugular bulb itself but rather a diverticulum arising from the jugular bulb. At times, the jugular bulb projects into the hypo- and mesotympanum. There may be a bony cover over the jugular bulb, or the vein may lie exposed in the middle ear in contact with the inner surface of the tympanic membrane. Such a high jugular bulb appears otoscopically as a blue mass that can be misdiagnosed as a glomus tumor.

The MR appearance of a high jugular bulb may be misread as showing a glomus tumor because of the area of mixed signal within the bulb produced by turbulent flow. However, whereas a glomus contains multiple punctate areas of signal void within a mass of medium or high signal, in a high jugular bulb, linear streaks of high and low signal are seen within the lumen of the bulb,

usually paralleling its walls because of variations in flow velocity (Figure 11–8, C).

Carotid Artery

Minor variations in the intratemporal course of the internal carotid arteries are not uncommon but are of no clinical significance. In some cases, the internal carotid artery may take an ectopic course through the middle ear. This anomaly should be recognized prior to surgery to avoid tragic consequences. The proximal portion of the carotid artery, which is always seen in the coronal sections below the cochlea, is absent. The anomalous carotid artery enters the temporal bone through an enlarged tympanic canaliculus or an opening in the floor of the posterior portion of the hypotympanum. The artery extends through the entire length of the middle ear cavity and then passes through a defect in the anterior wall of the middle ear to regain its normal position in the petrous apex.

Arachnoid Granulations

Arachnoid granulations are villous structures that herniate through a small defect in the dura and drain cerebrospinal fluid from the subarachnoid space into the venous system.

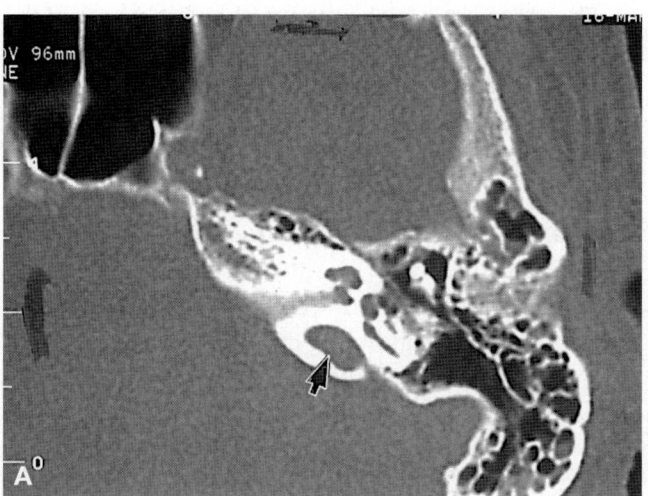

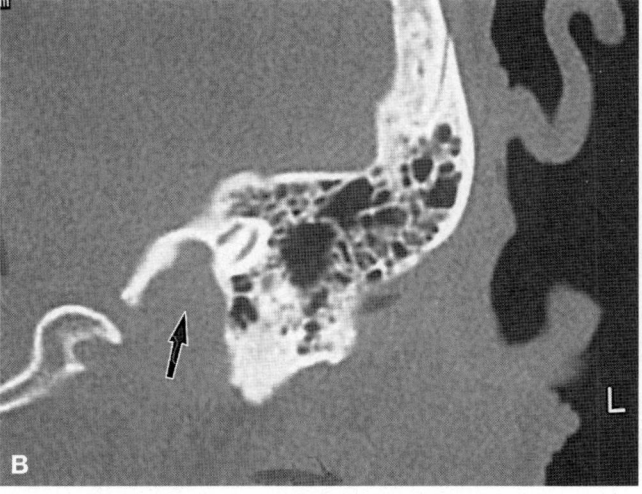

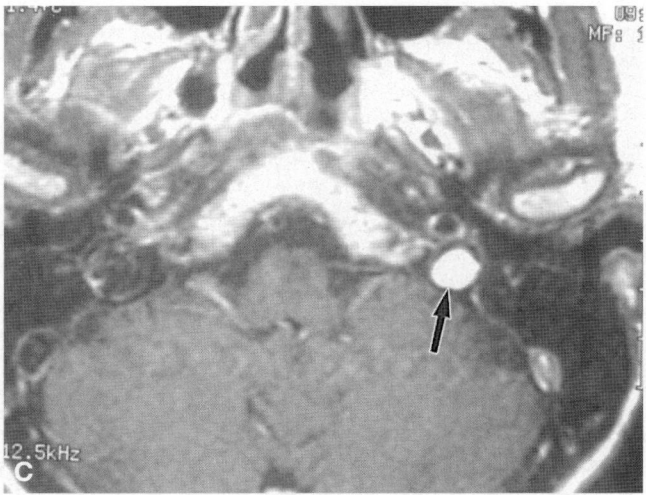

Figure 11–8 High jugular bulb (*arrows*): *A,* axial, and *B,* coronal computed tomography sections; *C,* magnetic resonance T$_1$ image postcontrast.

A variable number of arachnoid granulations do not reach the venous target but come in contact with the intracranial surface of the middle ear and, less frequently, of the posterior surface of the temporal bone. Over a long period of time, the pulsation of the cerebrospinal fluid may produce small areas of bony resorption and erosion.

Arachnoid lesions become clinically significant when they open into the adjacent air spaces (attic, mastoid cells) as they may lead to a spontaneous cerebrospinal otorrhea and, if the mastoid and middle ear cavity are infected, to intracranial complications.

Petrous Apex

The petrous apex may be significantly pneumatized or be made up of compact or diploic bone. In the MR study, the signal intensity of the apex varies with its bony texture: high or bright in the T_1 images when diploic, low or dark when highly pneumatized or compact. Often the bony texture of the two petrous apices of the same person is different, resulting in one apex being brighter than the other (Figure 11–9).

PATHOLOGIC CONDITIONS

The major categories of pathologic conditions that may involve the temporal bone and adjacent base of the skull are congenital malformations, traumatic effects, inflammatory processes, neoplastic conditions, and otodystrophies. The otolaryngologist should learn as much as possible about the nature and extent of the pathologic process before deciding how to treat the patient and, if surgery is indicated, how to approach the lesion.

Congenital Anomalies of the Temporal Bone

A proper imaging assessment is essential in all patients with congenital anomalies of the temporal bone. Otoscopy is of little value in atresia and aplasia of the external auditory canal. Audiometry is often unrealiable in young children. The study should demonstrate the status of the anatomic structures of the ear, the development and course of the facial nerve canal, the position of the sigmoid sinus and jugular bulb, and the course of the carotid canal. Such information is of value for the otologist in determining the proper treatment for conductive and sensorineural hearing losses.

The CT examination is the study of choice, and the examination should always consist of axial and coronal sections. Sagittal images should be added whenever the vestibular aqueduct and mastoid segment of the facial canal are under investigation.

Anomalies of the Sound-Conducting System
A good CT study provides the surgeon with the following basic information, which is needed in the decision about the feasibility of corrective surgery and in determining which type of surgery is indicated:

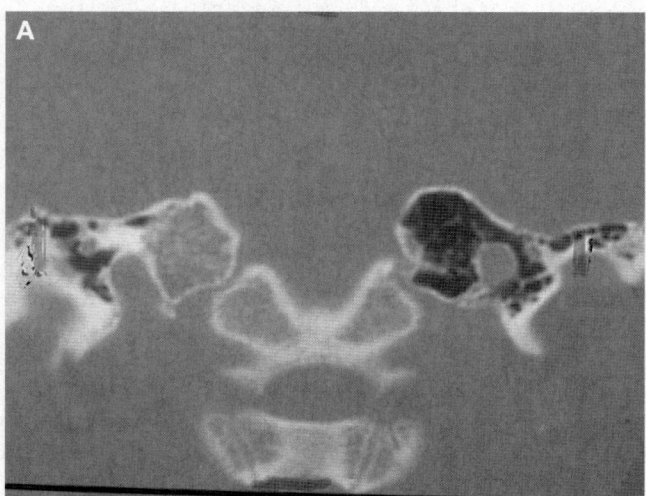 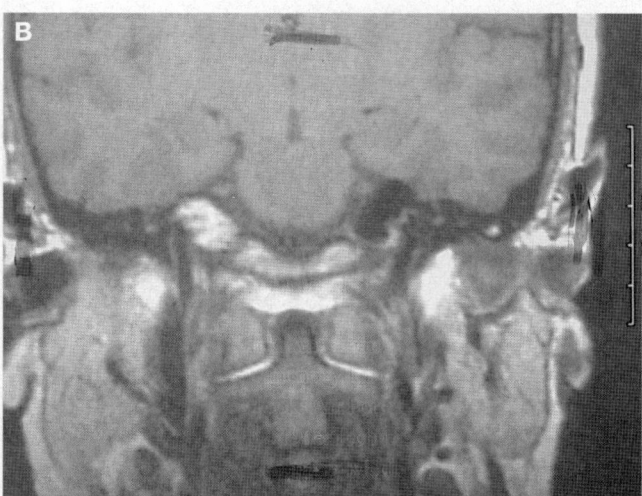

Figure 11–9 Asymmetric pneumatization of the petrous apices: *A*, coronal computed tomography scan; *B*, magnetic resonance coronal T_1 image.

1. The degree and type of abnormality of the tympanic bone. These abnormalities range from a relatively minor deformity to complete agenesis of the external auditory canal (Figures 11–10 and 11–11).
2. The degree and position of the pneumatization of the mastoid air cells and mastoid antrum.
3. The development and aeration of the middle ear cavity.
4. The status of the ossicular chain, the size and shape of the ossicles, and the presence of fusion or fixation (see Figure 11–10 and 11–11).
5. The patency of the labyrinthine windows (see Figure 11–11).
6. The course of the facial nerve canal.
7. The development of the inner ear structures. Defects in the otic capsule, including the modiolus and spiral lamina, are visualized by high-definition spiral CT.
8. The relationship of the meninges to the mastoid tegmen and superior petrous ridge. The middle cranial fossa often forms a deep groove lateral to the labyrinth, which results in a low-lying dura over the mastoid and external auditory canal.

Anomalies of the Inner Ear

With advances in cochlear implants for profound sensorineural deafness, the assessment of the inner ear

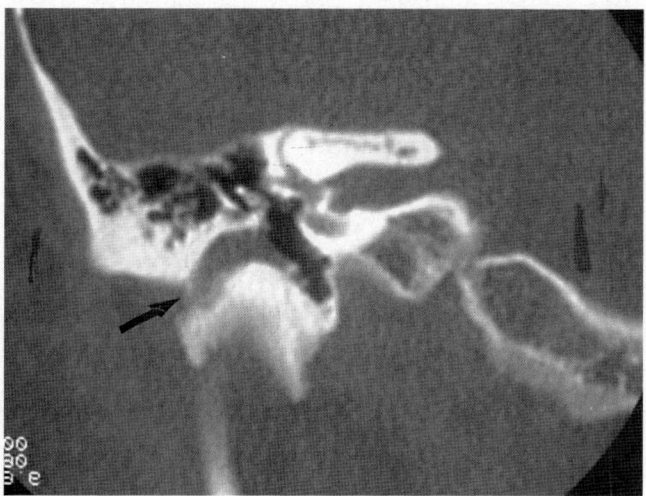

Figure 11–10 Atresia of the external auditory canal: coronal computed tomography scan. The external auditory canal is stenotic and closed at its lateral end by a thin bony plate (*arrow*). The middle ear cavity is aerated and normal in size, but the incus is deformed, with a short and stubby long process.

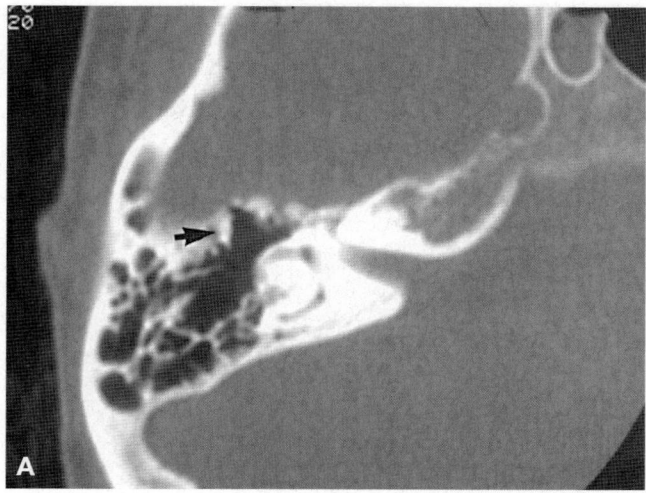

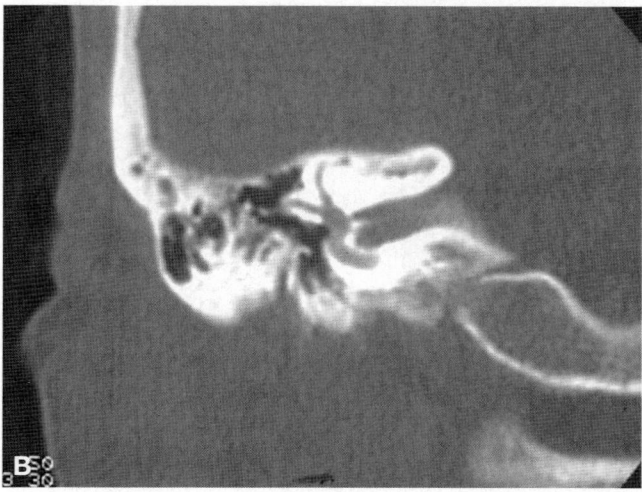

Figure 11–11 Agenesis of the external auditory canal: *A*, axial; *B*, coronal computed tomography scans. The external auditory canal is not developed; the middle ear cavity is aerated but smaller than normal. The malleus and incus are hypoplastic and fixed to the lateral attic wall (*short arrow*). The course of the facial canal, inner ear structures, and oval window are normal.

structures has become essential. Of course, only defects in the otic capsule are visible by imaging. Abnormal development of the membranous labyrinth is not detectable by the present imaging techniques. Anomalies of the otic capsule involve a single structure or the entire capsule and may range from a minor hypoplasia of a single structure to complete agenesis of the inner ear structures (Michel's anomaly). A common deformity of the labyrinthine capsule is Mondini's type, which is characterized by an abnormal development of the cochlea associated with dilatation of the vestibular aqueduct and vestibule (Figure 11–12). The semicircular canals are often malformed and usually hypoplastic.

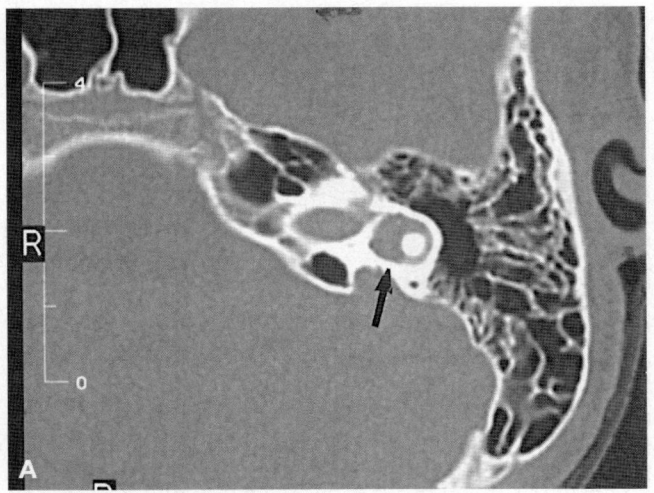

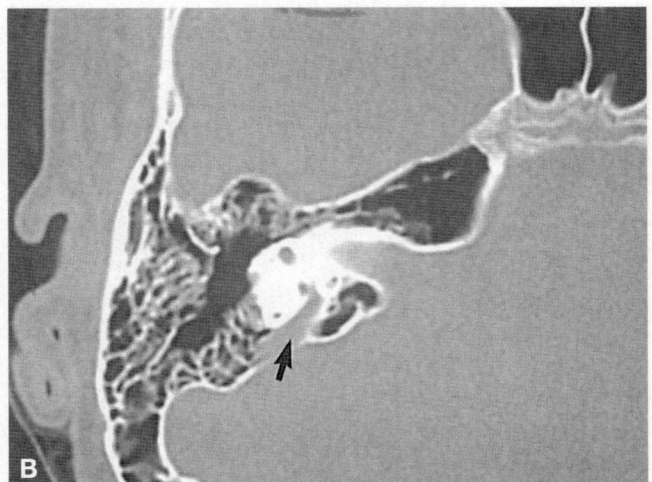

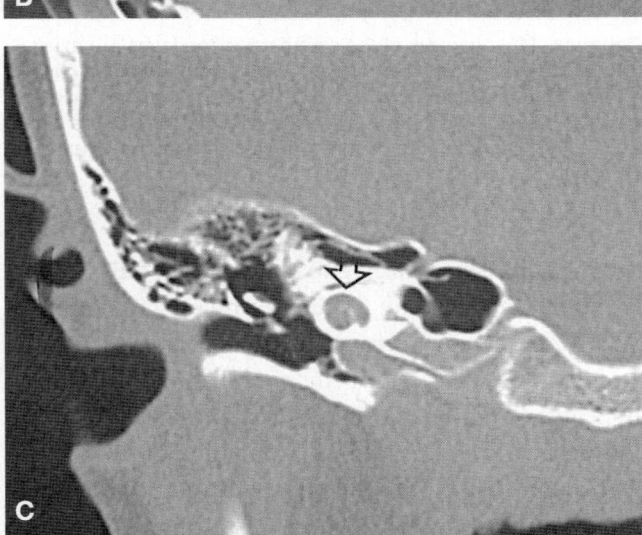

Imaging Assessment for Cochlear Implantation

Candidates for cochlear implants require an imaging study to determine the feasibility of the procedure. The otologic surgeon must know if the mastoid and middle ear are large enough to obtain access to the promontory and round window. If an intracochlear implant is contemplated, the surgeon should know if there is a patent round window and cochlear lumen. If the cochlea is obliterated by bone, the cochlea must be drilled or an extracochlear device used. Marked hypoplasia of the cochlea and internal auditory canal (Figure 11–13) is often

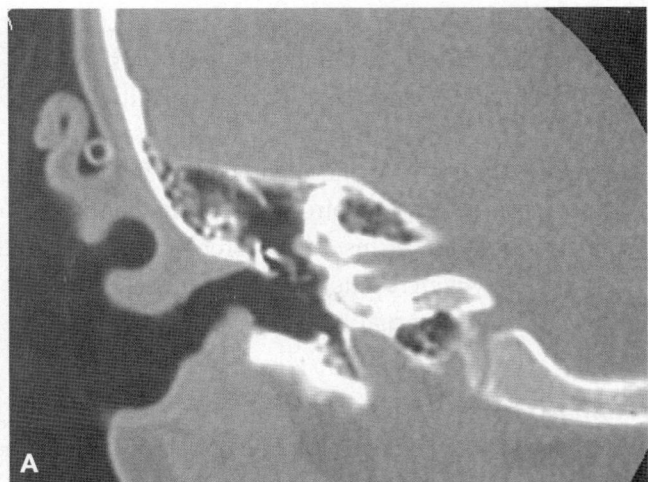

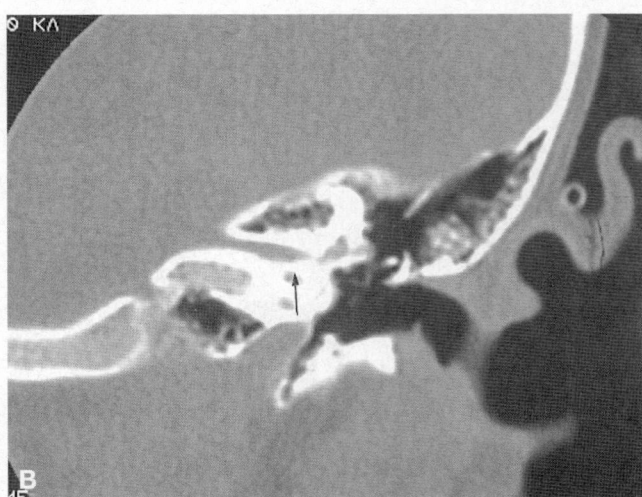

Figure 11–12 Mondini defect: *A* and *B*, axial, and *C*, coronal computed tomography scans. The cochlea (*open arrow*) is normal in size, but the bony partition between the cochlea coils is absent or hypoplastic. The vestibular aqueduct (*short arrow*) is enlarged and the vestibule (*long arrow*) is dilated.

Figure 11–13 Hypoplasia of the internal auditory canal: coronal computed tomography scans. *A*, right; *B*, left. The upper compartment of the left internal auditory canal is normal, but the lower compartment is absent or markedly hypoplastic as shown by the position of the falciform crest (*arrow*). Compare with the normal right side.

indicative of a lack of development of the acoustic nerve, which will make an implant infeasible. Magnetic resonance is indicated to establish the presence and status of the acoustic nerve, rule out fibrous obliteration of the cochlear lumen that cannot be seen by CT, and exclude the presence of central pathology affecting the auditory pathways. A postoperative transorbital or Schüller view should be obtained to determine the position of the electrodes and the integrity of the implanted wires. The latter cannot be established by tomographic techniques because the wires are visualized in several contiguous sections; therefore, the continuity cannot be demonstrated. These views will be used as a baseline for follow-up studies.

Anomalies of the Facial Nerve

Anomalies of the facial canal involve the size and course of the canal. There may be complete or partial agenesis of the facial nerve canal with total paralysis. Occasionally, the facial nerve canal may be unusually narrow and hypoplastic. In these cases, intermittent episodes of facial paresis may occur. The horizontal segment of the facial canal is at times displaced inferiorly to cover the oval window. Anomalies in the course of the mastoid segment are common in congenital atresia of the external auditory canal. The facial canal is usually rotated later-

ally. The rotation varies from a minor obliquity to a true horizontal course.

Temporal Bone Trauma

Imaging studies of the temporal bone following head trauma are indicated when there is cerebrospinal fluid otorrhea or rhinorrhea, hearing loss, or facial nerve paralysis.

The CT study should always include axial and, if possible, direct coronal sections. Lateral reconstructed images may be required in selected patients with longitudinal fractures or facial nerve paralysis. In patients with unconsciousness or neurologic findings, the CT study should be extended to the entire brain to rule out the possibility of intracranial hemorrhage. In addition, a series of scans obtained after intrathecal injection of metrizamide is often useful in demonstration of the site of leak in patients with cerebrospinal fluid rhinorrhea or otorrhea.

Temporal bone fractures are divided into longitudinal and transverse lesions, depending on the direction of the fracture line. Longitudinal fractures occur more frequently than transverse fractures in a ratio of 5 to 1. This classification, however, is somewhat arbitrary because most fractures follow a serpiginous tract in the temporal bone.

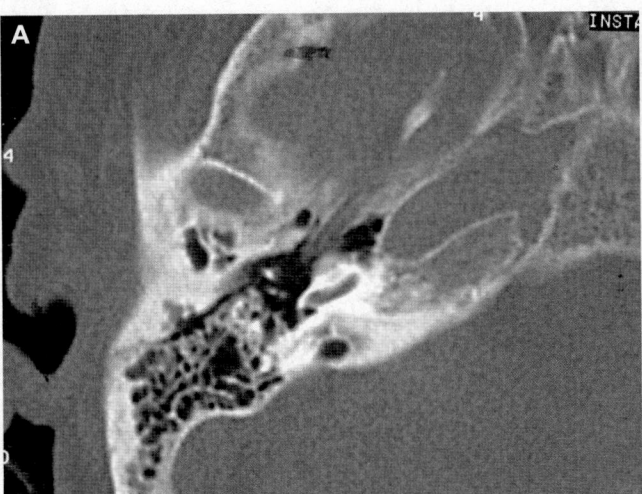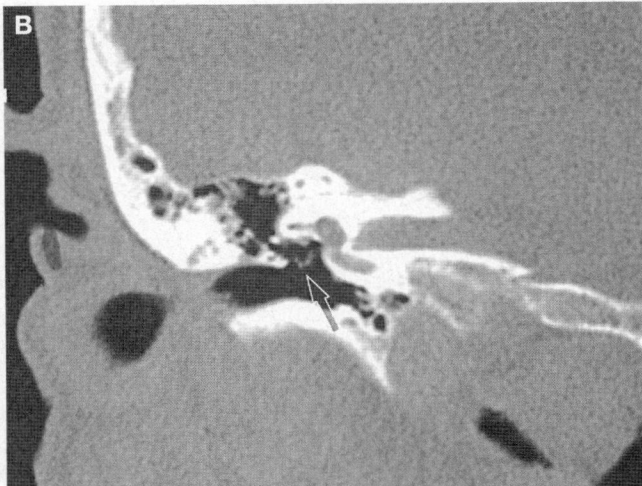

Figure 11–14 Longitudinal fracture of the right temporal bone: *A*, axial, and *B*, coronal computed tomography scans. The mastoid fracture extends to the superior canal wall and to the lateral wall of the attic. The ossicular chain is disrupted at the incudostapedial joint (*arrow*).

The typical longitudinal fracture involves the temporal squama and extends into the mastoid. The fracture usually reaches the external auditory canal and passes medially into the epitympanum, where it produces a disruption of the ossicular chain. From the epitympanum, the fracture extends into the petrosa and follows an intralabyrinthine or extralabyrinthine course. An intralabyrinthine course of the fracture is rare because the labyrinthine bone is quite resistant to trauma. Extralabyrinthine extension occurs either anterior or posterior to the labyrinth. Anterior extension is more common (Figure 11–14).

A transverse fracture of the temporal bone typically crosses the petrous pyramid at a right angle to the longitudinal axis of the pyramid. The fracture usually follows the line of least resistance and runs from the dome of the jugular fossa through the labyrinth to the superior petrous ridge (Figure 11–15).

The fracture line disappears at certain levels only to reappear a few millimeters distant. This apparent gap is not caused by interruption of the fracture but rather by the fact that the plane of the fracture line changes course and becomes invisible in some of the sections.

Longitudinal fractures are best demonstrated in the axial and sagittal sections and transverse fractures in the coronal and 20-degree coronal oblique sections.

Traumatic disruption of the ossicular chain is most common in patients with longitudinal fractures but may occur even in the absence of an actual fracture. Dislocation of the malleus is rare because of its firm attachment to the tympanic membrane and the strong anterior malleal ligament. The incus is most commonly dislocated because its attachment to the malleus and stapes is easily torn (Figure 11–16). Fractures and dislocations of the footplate of the stapes are not directly recognizable but may be identified by the presence of air within the vestibule.

Labyrinthine Concussion and Bleeding

Bleeding within the lumen of the inner ear structures may occur after trauma (Figure 11–17). If a fracture crosses the inner ear, the detection of blood is of academic value since the patient has an irreversible total deafness and vestibular paralysis or both. If bleeding occurs by concussion without actual fracture, MR may be indicated

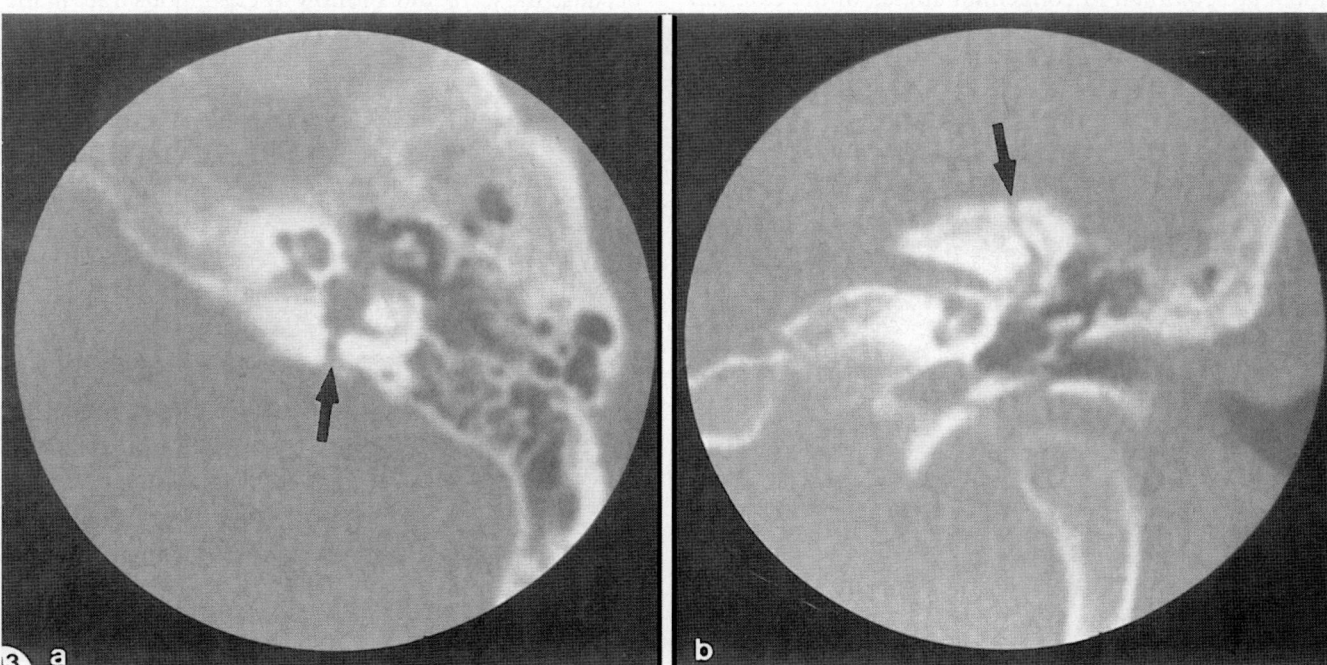

Figure 11–15   Transverse fracture with facial paralysis: *A*, axial; and *B*, coronal computed tomography scans. The fracture splits the vestibule and involves the facial canal anterior to the oval window (*arrow*).

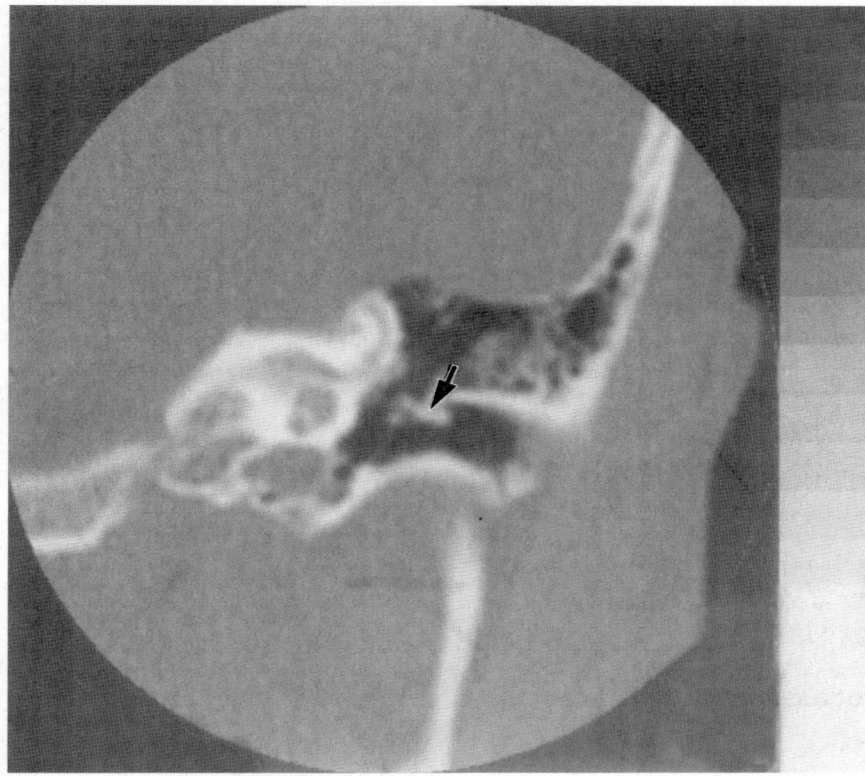

Figure 11–16 Traumatic dislocation of the incus: coronal computed tomography scan. The body of the incus is displaced into the external auditory canal (*arrow*).

to confirm the diagnosis. The study should be performed at least 2 days after the injury to allow the transformation of deoxyhemoglobin into methemoglobin, which has a bright signal in both T_1 and T_2 images. Intracranial bleeding in the region of the cochlear nuclei and auditory pathway may also cause transient or irreversible deafness. Spontaneous intralabyrinthine hemorrhage has also been observed in patients with sickle cell disease owing to vaso-occlusive crisis.

Traumatic Facial Paralysis

Facial paralysis occurs immediately or after a period of a few hours or days following trauma. Immediate onset of facial paralysis is the result of bisection of the facial nerve by the fracture. Delayed facial paralysis is caused by fracture of the facial canal and post-traumatic edema of the nerve. Facial paralysis occurs in approximately 25% of the longitudinal fractures and is of the delayed and often transient type in 50% of the cases. Facial paralysis is observed in 50% of the transverse fractures and is almost always of the immediate and permanent type

(see Figure 11–15). In some cases, the site of involvement of the facial canal cannot be visualized in the CT sections. However, by evaluation of the course of the fracture line, the site of the lesion can be determined.

Meningocele and Meningoencephalocele

Meningocele and meningoencephalocele are usually post-traumatic owing to a tegmental fracture or iatrogenic following mastoid surgery and are rarely spontaneous. The brain and meninges herniate through the defect in the tegmen into the mastoid antrum or into the attic. The constant pulsation of the cerebrospinal fluid is transmitted through the walls at the meningocele to cause gradual resorption of the surrounding bony walls. Computed tomography demonstrates the defect in the tegmen and the adjacent soft tissue mass (Figure 11–18, A). An MR study is performed whenever the nature of the soft tissue mass is unclear. Or MR, a meningocele has a signal identical to cerebrospinal fluid, an encephalocele to brain (Figure 11–18, B).

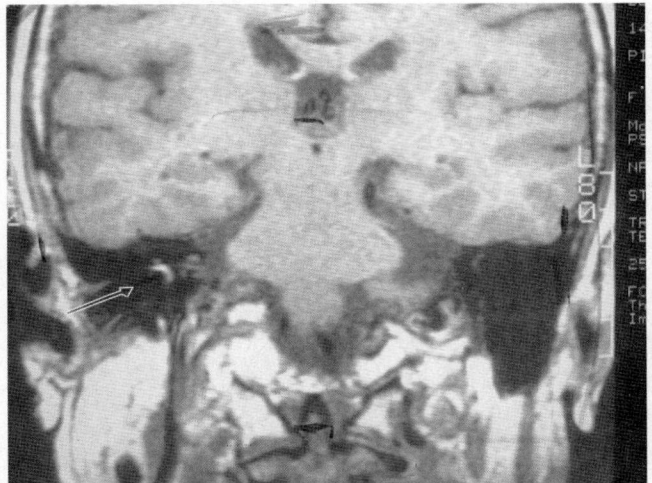

Figure 11–17   Labyrinthine concussion with bleeding: magnetic resonance coronal T₁ image; no contrast. Note the high signal within the vestibule and semicircular canals produced by blood (*arrow*).

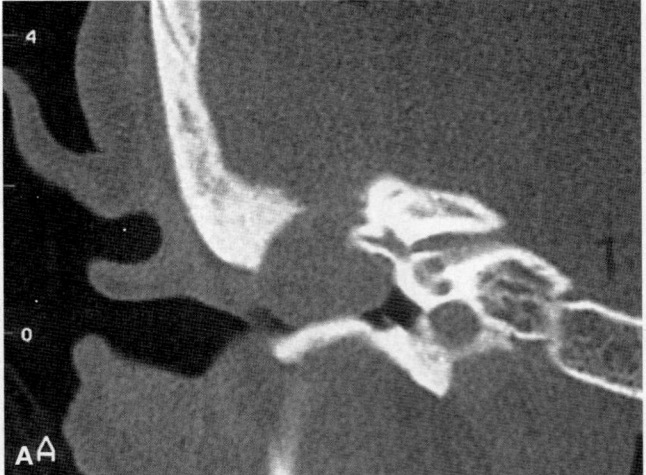

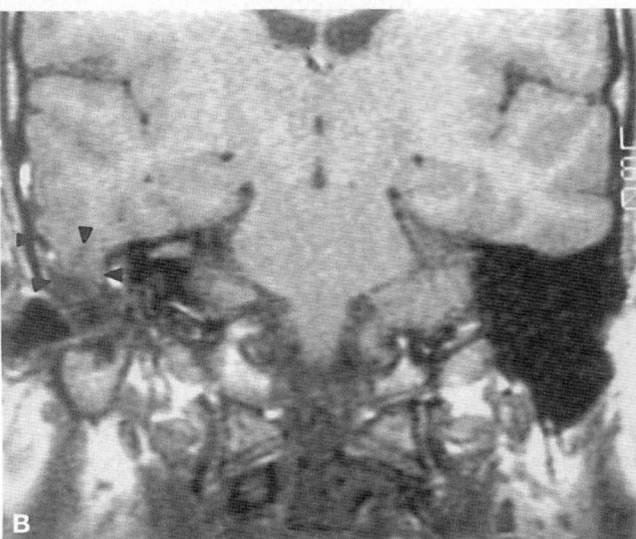

Figure 11–18   Meningoencephalocele: *A*, coronal computed tomography scan; *B*, magnetic resonance (MR) T₁ image. A large well-defined soft tissue mass protrudes into the right external auditory canal through a wide defect in the tegmen. The MR image confirms that the mass is a meningoencephalocele (*arrowheads*).

Inflammatory Process and Cholesteatomas

Acute Otomastoiditis

Acute otitis media with mastoiditis is a clinical diagnosis. In the early stage, the process is characterized by a nonspecific diffuse and homogeneous opacification of the middle ear and mastoid air cells (Figure 11–19). If the infection is not arrested by proper treatment, necrosis of the cell walls develops, which leads to the formation of areas of coalescence and abscesses. The coalescent infection may perforate the mastoid cortex and produce a variety of subperiosteal abscesses. If the tegmen or sinus plate is dehiscent or eroded, intracranial complications develop, such as epidural and brain abscesses, sigmoid sinus thrombosis, and perisinus abscesses (Figure 11–20).

Whenever an intracranial complication is suspected, a CT or MR study with contrast should be obtained to confirm the intracranial involvement and demonstrate the site and extent of the process (Figure 11–21).

Chronic Otomastoiditis

Two types of chronic ear disease are recognizable: chronic infection and tubotympanic disease. Chronic infection is the result of an infection by a low-virulence organism or of an acute infection with incomplete resolution. The typical radiographic findings consist of thickening of the mastoid trabeculae, inhomogeneous

clouding of the air cells, and, if no perforation is present, inhomogeneous opacity of the middle ear cavity (Figure 11–22). The involved air cells become constricted at first and later are completely obliterated. The lumen of the residual air cells, antrum, and middle ear is usually filled with granulation tissue and fluid. Erosion of the long process of the incus may occur.

Tubotympanic disease is the result of a faulty aeration of the middle ear caused by eustachian tube malfunction or obstruction by mucositis. The CT sections demonstrate opacity of the middle ear and mastoid and

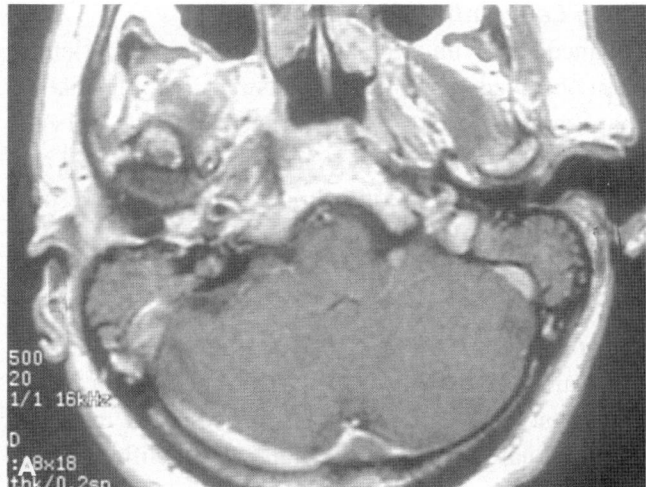

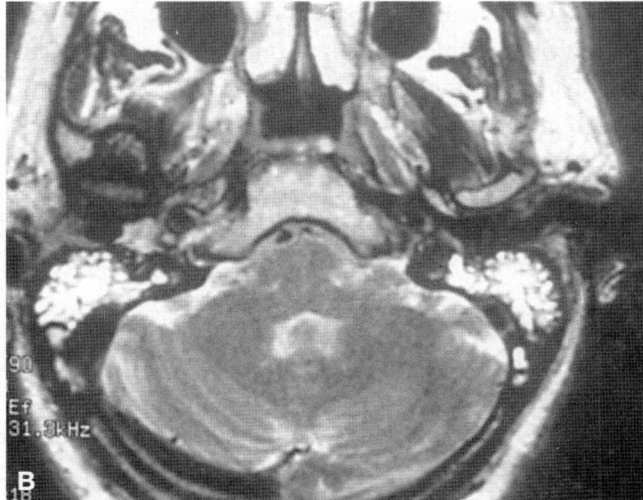

Figure 11–19 Acute otomastoiditis: magnetic resonance images. *A*, T$_1$; *B*, T$_2$. In the T$_1$ image, the mastoid air cells are filled by a medium (pus) of higher signal intensity than clear fluid, which becomes bright in T$_2$.

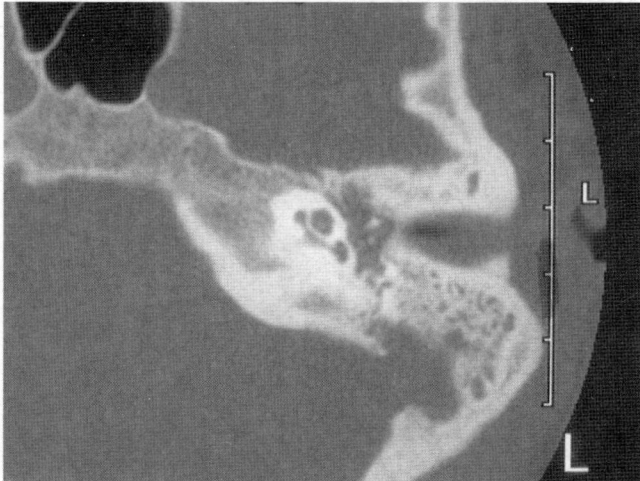

Figure 11–20 Acute mastoiditis with perisinus abscess and sigmoid sinus thrombosis. The axial computed tomography scan shows a coalescent cavity in the left mastoid with erosion of the sinus plate. Note the clouding of the left middle ear cavity and swelling of the external auditory canal skin. L = left.

The infection begins as an external otitis but spreads to involve the surrounding walls of the external canal. The process often extends into the middle ear and mastoid. The infection usually breaks through the floor of the external canal at the bony and cartilaginous junction and spreads along the undersurface of the temporal bone to

contraction of the middle ear space caused by retraction of the tympanic membrane on the promontory. Tympanosclerotic plaques are not uncommon and, if large enough, appear as linear calcifications in the tympanic membrane and mucosa over the promontory or as partially calcified masses in the attic, often surrounding and fixing the ossicles.

Malignant Necrotizing External Otitis

Malignant external otitis is an acute osteomyelitis of the temporal bone that occurs in diabetic, immunosuppressed patients and is caused by the *Pseudomonas* bacterium.

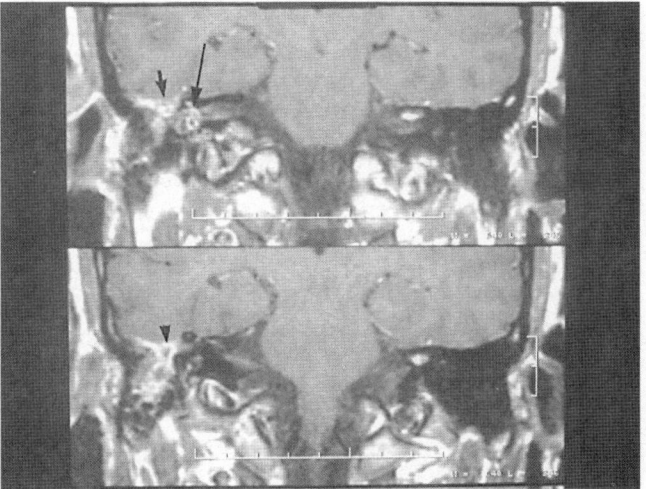

Figure 11–21 Subacute mastoiditis with complications: magnetic resonance coronal T$_1$ image postcontrast. Enhancing granulation tissue and an abscess fill the right mastoid. The tegmen is partially eroded with formation of an epidural abscess (*arrowhead*). Note the thickening and enhancement of the adjacent meninges (*short arrow*) and the enhancement of the inner ear structures caused by an acute labyrinthitis (*long arrow*).

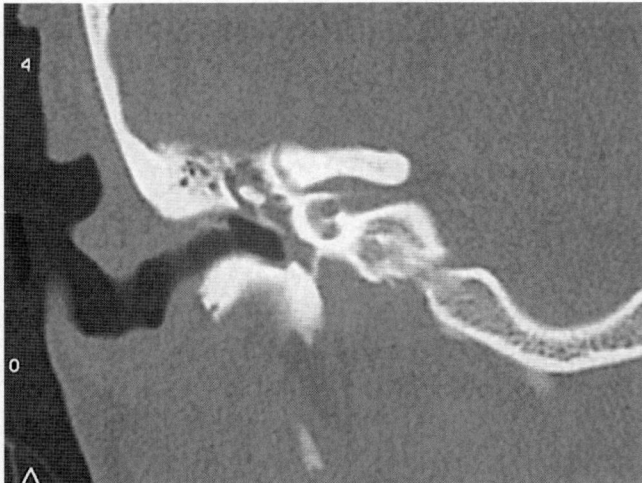

Figure 11–22   Chronic otitis media: coronal computed tomography scan. The middle ear cavity is opacified, and the tympanic membrane is thickened and retracted.

involve the facial nerve at the stylomastoid foramen. Further medial extension involves the jugular fossa and cranial nerves IX, X, XI, and XII. Anterior spread of the infection affects the temporomandibular joint. Computed tomography is excellent for demonstrating involvement of the external auditory canal, middle ear, and petrous pyramid, but MR becomes the study of choice when the infection spreads to the facial nerve and outside the confines of the temporal bone.

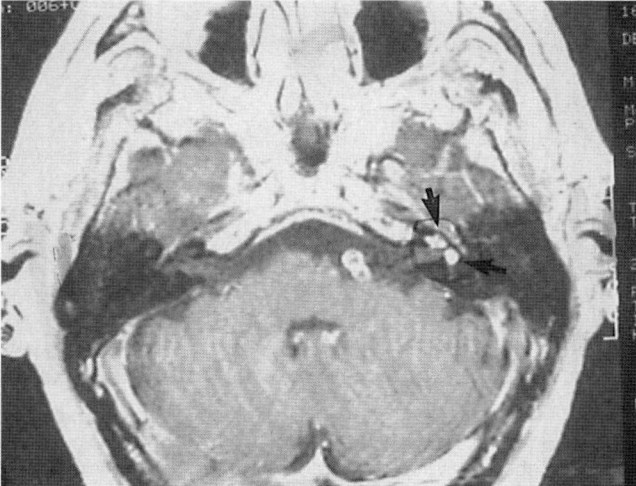

Figure 11–23   Acute labyrinthitis: axial magnetic resonance T_1 image postcontrast showing prominent enhancement of the left cochlea and vestibule (*arrow*).

Acute Labyrinthitis

Enhancement within the lumen of the bony labyrinth is often observed in MR images obtained after injection of contrast material in patients with acute bacterial and viral labyrinthitis and sudden deafness (see Figures 11–21 and 11–23). Enhancement of the inner structures is presumably caused by damage of the capillaries' endothelium, which leads to a disruption of the labyrinth-blood barrier.

Chronic Labyrinthitis

This varies from a localized reaction caused by a fistula of the bony labyrinth to a diffuse process. The lumen of the inner ear is partially or totally filled with granulation and fibrous tissues. Osteitis of the bony labyrinth occurs, which leads to a partial or complete bony obliteration of the lumen. Whereas bony obliteration of the inner ear is readily identified by CT, fibrous obliteration is recognizable only by MR imaging. In the T_2 images, the high signal seen within the normal inner ear structures is absent, therefore making the involved structures no longer recognizable.

Facial Neuritis

Moderate bilateral enhancement of the normal facial nerve, particularly in the region of its anterior genu, is often observed in MR studies obtained after injection of contrast material.

Asymmetric enhancement of the facial nerve more prominent on the paralyzed side is common in patients with Bell's palsy and Ramsey Hunt syndrome. The enhancement varies in intensity with the stage of the process. It is usually more prominent in the early stage and gradually decreases whether the paralysis has resolved or not. In Bell's palsy, the involvement is segmental and usually confined to the anterior genu and adjacent labyrinthine and tympanic segments. Involvement of the mastoid segment is more rare. In Ramsey Hunt syndrome, the involvement by the herpes zoster virus is more consistent and very often extends to the nerve within the internal auditory canal (Figure 11–24).

Cholesteatoma

Cholesteatomas are congenital or acquired epidermoid cysts. Congenital cholesteatomas arise from epithelial

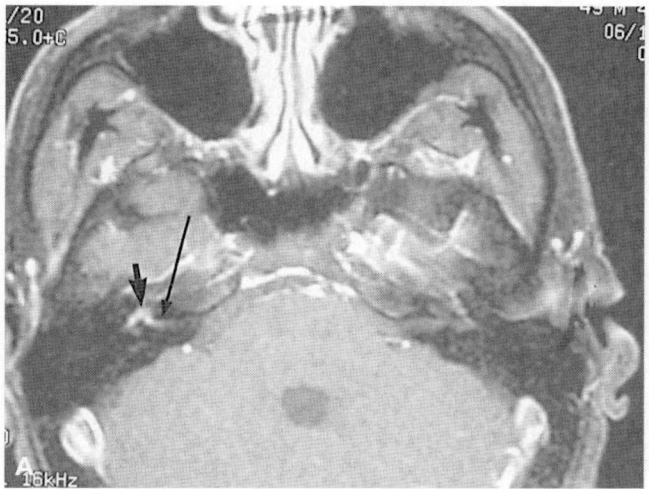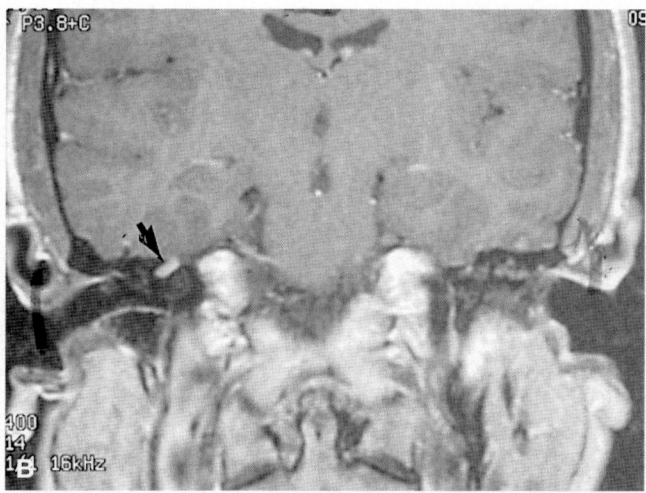

Figure 11–24 Facial neuritis (Ramsey Hunt syndrome): *A*, axial; *B*, coronal magnetic resonance T$_1$ image postcontrast. The anterior genu, labyrinthine, and proximal tympanic segments of the right facial nerve are enhanced (*short arrows*). The enhancement extends to the facial nerve within the internal auditory canal (*long arrow*).

tissue rests within or adjacent to the temporal bone. Acquired cholesteatomas originate in the middle ear from the stratified squamous epithelium of the tympanic membrane or metaplasia of the middle ear mucosa. Another distinct form of cholesteatoma arises in the external auditory canal.

Acquired Cholesteatoma

Cholesteatomas appear as soft tissue masses in the mesotympanum or epitympanum. If the middle ear is aerated,

the entire soft tissue mass is well outlined. When fluid or inflammatory tissue fills the middle ear, the contour of the cholesteatoma is obscured, and it may be difficult to determine its actual size. Characteristic bone changes occur in cholesteatomas that help in diagnosing the lesion and in establishing the site of origin and extension of the process.

Cholesteatomas associated with a perforation of the pars flaccida of the tympanic membrane produce erosion of the anterior portion of the lateral wall of the attic (Figure 11–25) and of the anterior tympanic spine. The

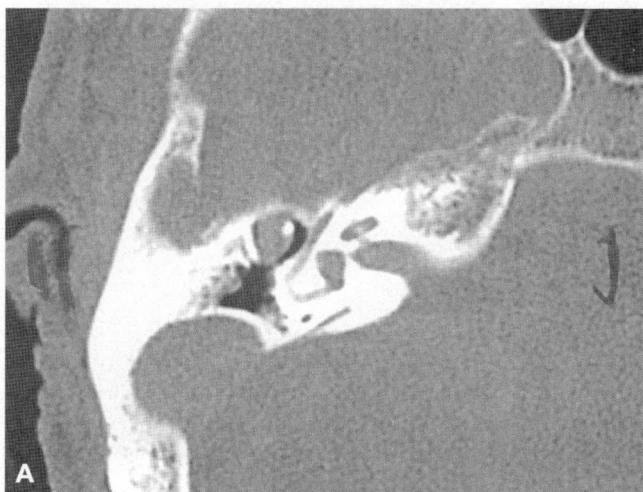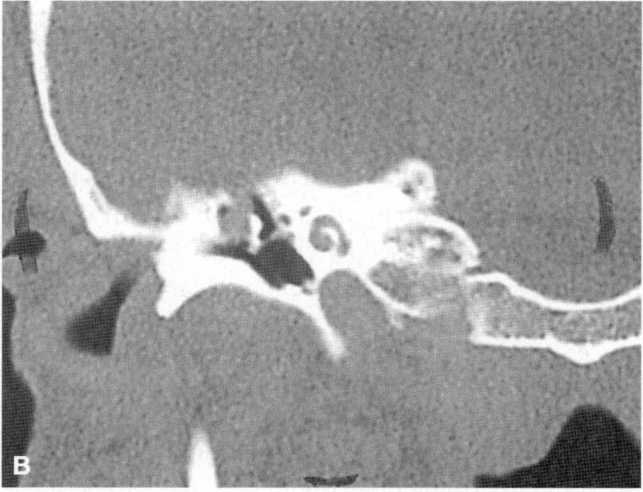

Figure 11–25 Attic cholesteatoma (pars flaccida perforation): *A*, axial; *B*, coronal computed tomography scans. The anterior portion of the lateral wall of the attic is eroded by a soft tissue mass extending into the attic lateral to the ossicles, which appear partially eroded and displaced medialward.

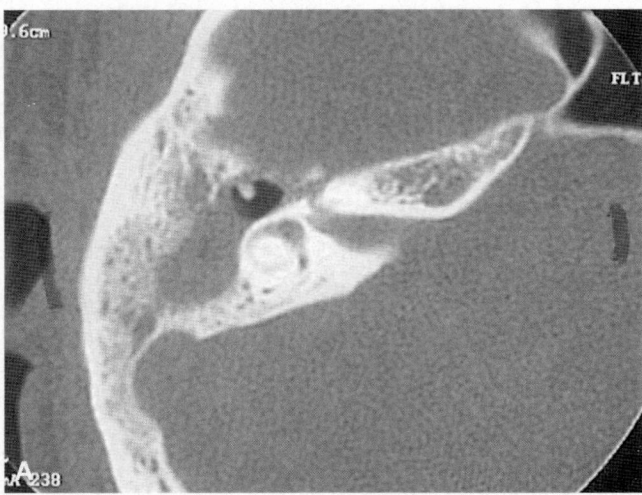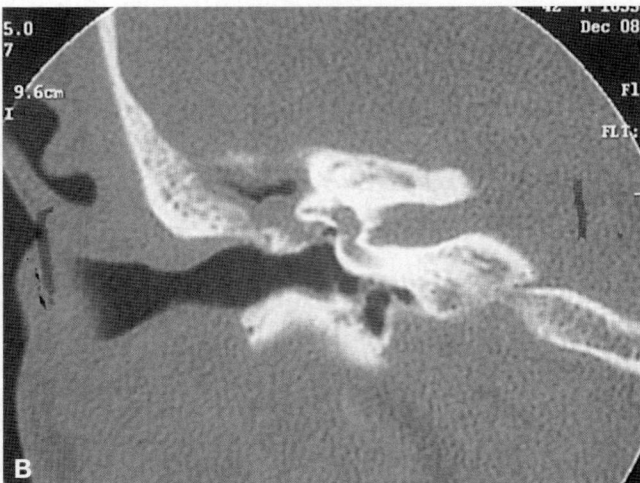

Figure 11–26 Cholesteatoma, pars tensa perforation type: *A*, axial; *B*, coronal computed tomography scans. The posterior portion of the lateral wall of the attic is eroded by a soft tissue mass filling the posterosuperior quadrant of the middle ear cavity and the posterior portion of the attic. The cholesteatoma widens the aditus and passes into the mastoid antrum, which appears enlarged because of erosion of the periantral air cells.

lesion extends laterally to the ossicles, which may be displaced medially. Cholesteatomas associated with a perforation of the pars tensa of the membrane, usually a posterosuperior margin perforation, erode the posterior portion of the lateral wall of the attic and the adjacent posterosuperior wall of the external auditory canal. These lesions extend medial to the ossicles, which are often displaced laterally. The long process of the incus and the stapes superstructure are usually eroded. Further growth of the cholesteatoma produces enlargement of the attic, aditus, and mastoid antrum (see Figure 11–26, A and B) and formation of a cavity in the mastoid as a result of erosion of the cell walls. Involvement of the medial wall of the middle ear cavity leads to the formation of a labyrinthine fistula. The ampullated limb of the horizontal semicircular canal is the most common site of a fistula. Horizontal and coronal CT sections show thinning or absence of the bone covering the lateral end of the canal and flattening of the medial wall of the epitympanic recess caused by erosion of the normal protuberance of the horizontal semicircular canal (Figure 11–27).

Congenital Cholesteatoma

Congenital cholesteatomas histologically are epidermoid tumors originating from embryonic epidermoid rests located anywhere in the temporal bone or adjacent epidural and meningeal spaces.

The clinical symptoms of congenital cholesteatoma depend on the site and size of the lesion. Middle ear congenital cholesteatomas appear as whitish globular masses lying medial to an intact tympanic membrane. There is usually no history of antecedent inflammatory ear disease. Occasionally, there is an associated serous otitis media.

The CT study shows a well-defined soft tissue mass within the middle ear (Figure 11–28). If the cholesteatoma involves the entire middle ear space or if there is

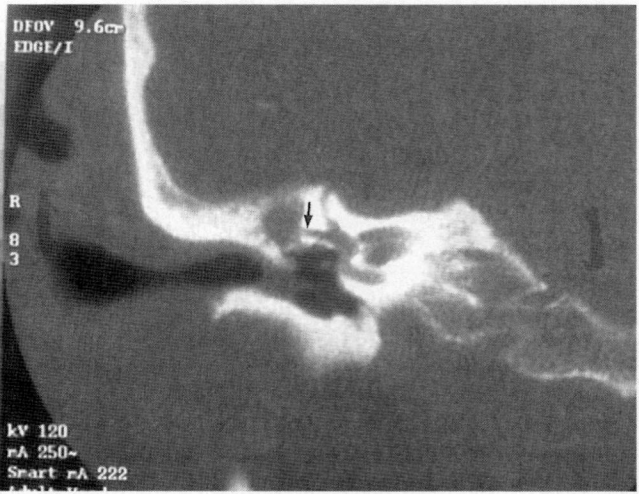

Figure 11–27 Cholesteatoma with fistula of the horizontal semicircular canal: coronal computed tomography scan. The cholesteatoma fills the attic and erodes the capsule of the lateral end of the horizontal semicircular canal (*arrow*).

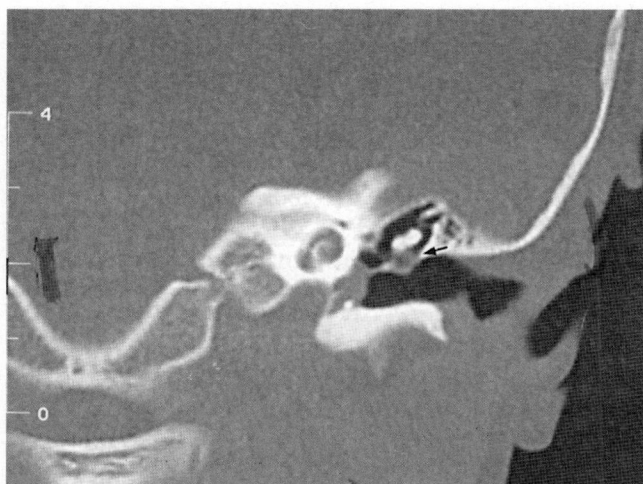

Figure 11–28   Congenital cholesteatoma: coronal computed tomography scan. The tympanic membrane is intact, but two soft tissue masses are seen in the middle ear cavity: a larger in the inferior mesotympanum and a smaller (*arrow*) lateral to the malleus neck.

accompanying serous otitis media, the entire tympanic cavity appears cloudy, and the tympanic membrane bulges laterally. The cholesteatoma mass may erode portions of the ossicular chain.

The inferior margin of the lateral epitympanic wall, which is typically eroded in acquired cholesteatoma, is intact in congenital lesions. However, the lateral epitympanic wall is often eroded from within when the congenital lesion extends into the epitympanum.

Epidermoid Cyst or Congenital Cholesteatoma of the Petrous Pyramid

The findings depend on whether the cholesteatoma arises from within the petrous apex or from the adjacent epidural or meningeal spaces.

When the cholesteatoma arises from within the petrous apex, CT shows an expansile, cystic lesion in the apex. The involved area of the pyramid is expanded, and the superior petrous ridge is usually elevated and thinned out. As the lesion expands, the internal auditory canal and the labyrinth become eroded. Large cholesterol granuloma cysts in the petrous pyramid have often been misdiagnosed as epidermoid cysts because they produce similar CT findings. The two lesions can be differentiated by MR. Epidermoid cysts appear as areas of fairly low signal intensity in the T_1 images and of high intensity in the T_2 images.

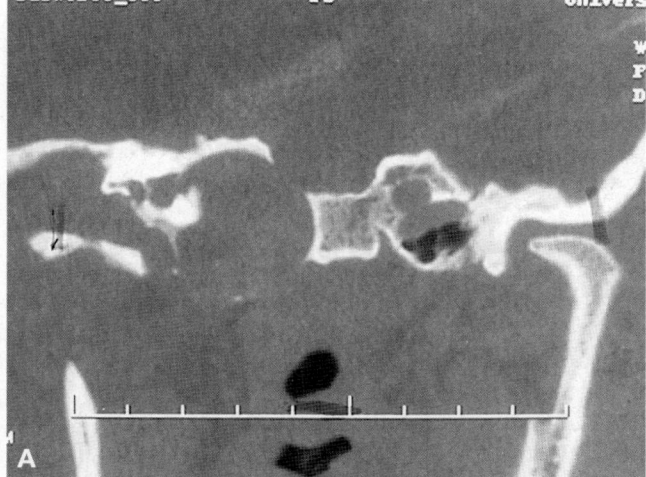

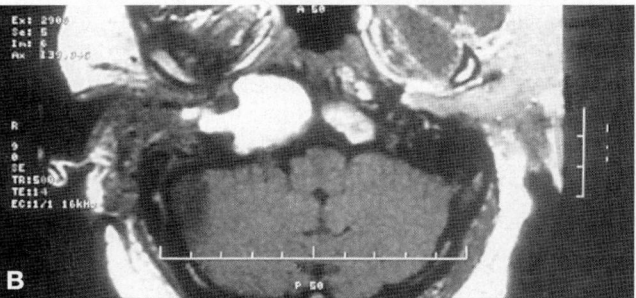

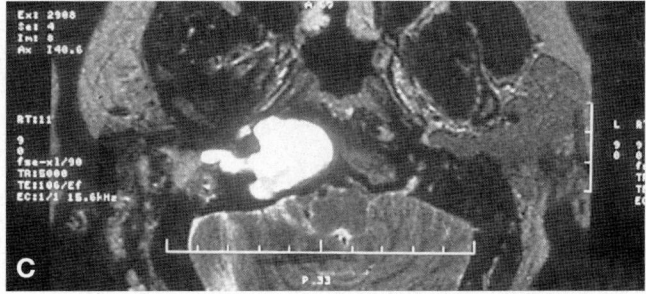

Figure 11–29   Recurrent cholesterol granuloma: *A*, coronal computed tomography scan; *B*, T_1; *C*, T_2 axial magnetic resonance image. An expansile lesion involves the right petrous apex and extends into the internal auditory canal. The mass has a characteristic high signal in both T_1 and T_2 sequences.

Cholesterol granuloma cysts are instead bright in both sequences because of short T_1 and long T_2 relaxation times (Figure 11–29). Dark areas, produced by deposits of hemosiderin, are often observed within the bright mass.

Cholesteatomas arising from the epidural or meningeal spaces on the superior aspect of the pyramid cause a scooped-out defect of the adjacent aspect of the pyramid. The defect is caused by erosion of the pyramid from without, and there is no bony rim, as in lesions that arise from within the pyramid.

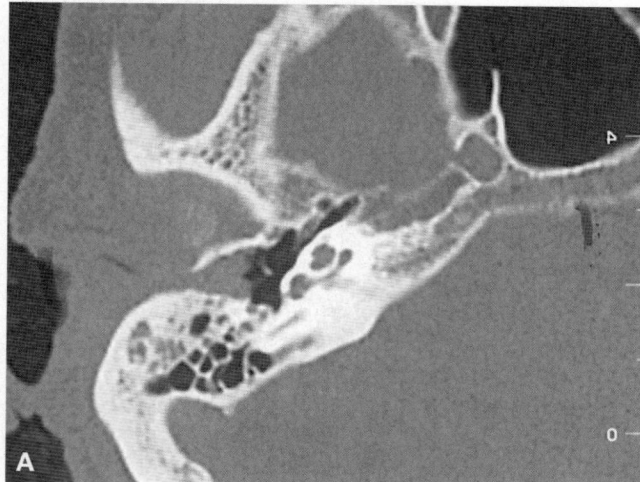

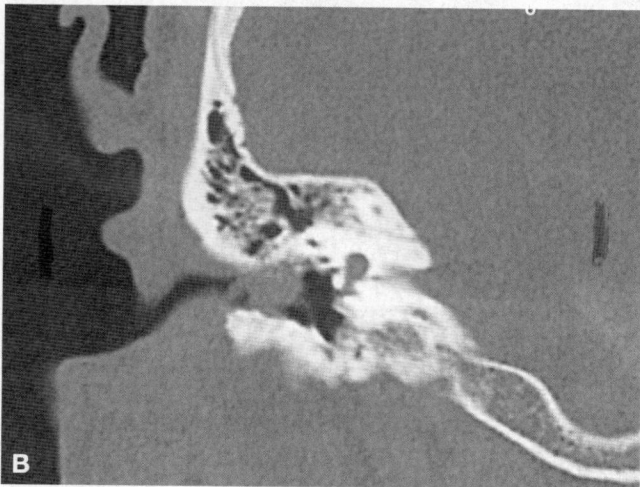

Figure 11–30 External auditory canal cholesteatoma: *A*, axial; *B*, coronal computed tomography scans. The canal is stenotic in the region of the isthmus, and a moderately expansile soft tissue mass fills the lumen of the bony segment of the canal.

localized accumulations of desquamated debris that occur on the floor of the bony canal.

When the external canal cholesteatoma is large and reaches the annulus, the lesion erodes into the middle ear and attic.

Neoplastic Conditions

Neoplastic conditions involving the temporal bone can be divided into five major groups, as follows:

1. Histologically benign tumors with a benign course
2. Histologically benign tumors with a possible malignant clinical course because of the large destruction in the base of the skull and intracranial extension by the growing tumor mass
3. Primary malignant processes
4. Malignant tumors arising in structures adjacent to the petrous bone and involving it by direct extension
5. Metastatic lesions

The first group includes conditions usually involving the external auditory canal, such as osteomas (Figure 11–31), fibromas, and lipomas. The second group includes neuromas (from the seventh to the twelfth cranial nerve), glomus tumors, and meningiomas. These lesions deserve special attention not only because of their relative frequency but above all because of the funda-

Cholesteatomas of the External Auditory Canal

There are two types of cholesteatoma of the external auditory canal. The first type, keratosis obliterans, is caused by osteomas, stenosis of the canal, or hard masses of cerumen. Blockage of the external canal for a long period permits epithelial debris to accumulate in the canal and enlarge the bony contour of the external canal (Figure 11–30).

The other type of cholesteatoma of the external canal is called invasive keratitis, and it is characterized by

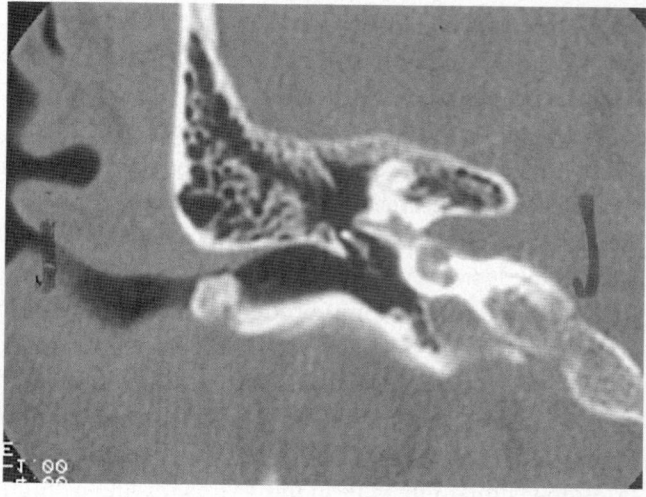

Figure 11–31 Osteoma: coronal computed tomography scan. A bony mass obstructs the right external auditory canal at the isthmus.

mental role played by imaging in their diagnosis. Carcinomas are the most common primary malignant tumors of the temporal bone. Carcinomas usually arise in the external auditory canal, where they produce a partial or total destruction of the canal walls. The lesion may spread into the mastoid, involving the facial canal, or extend into the middle ear cavity, from there involving the jugular fossa and petrous pyramid. Owing to their tendency to infiltrate rather than destroy, carcinomas produce a typical mottled or moth-eaten appearance of the involved bone. Sarcomas usually occur in young children and account for destructive lesions of the petrous pyramid. Sarcomas may arise in the eustachian tube and spread by retrograde extension to the ear.

Involvement of the temporal bone by direct extension may occur in malignant neoplasms arising in adjacent structures, such as the parotid gland and nasopharynx.

Metastatic lesions to the temporal bone have been observed in carcinomas of the breast, prostate, and lungs (Figure 11–32).

Glomus Tumors or Chemodectomas

Chemodectomas or paragangliomas arise from paraganglionic glomus tissues (chemoreceptors). The four common sites are the jugular fossa (glomus jugulare tumors), middle ear (glomus tympanicum tumors), carotid artery bifurcation (carotid body tumors), and

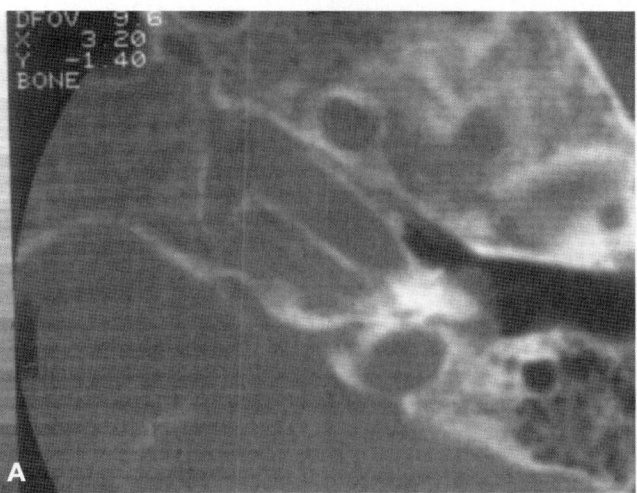

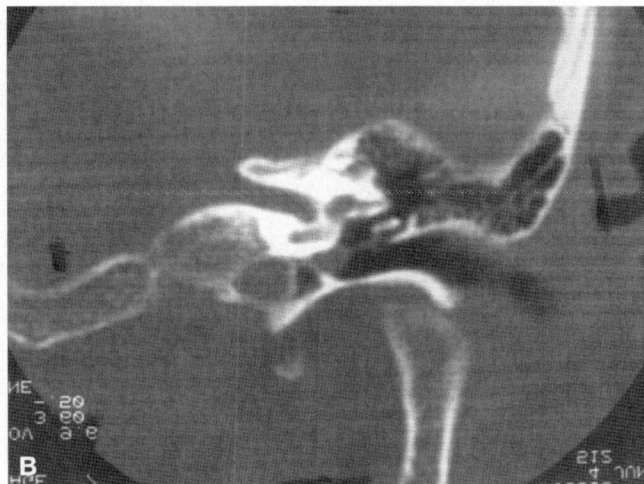

Figure 11–33 Glomus tympanicum: *A*, axial; *B*, coronal computed tomography scan. A well-defined soft tissue mass is seen in the lower portion of the middle ear cavity adjacent to the promontory.

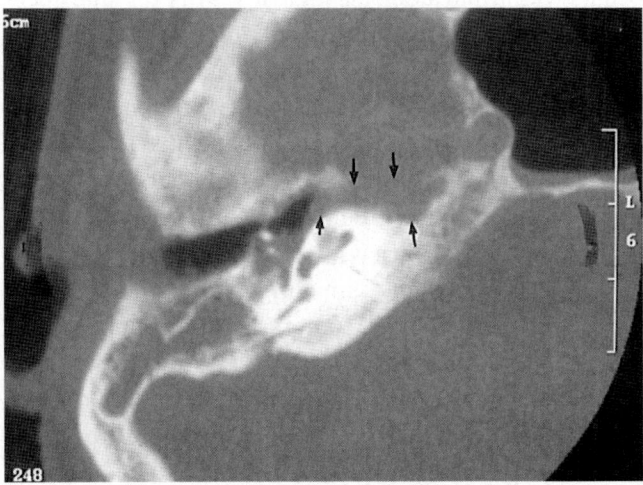

Figure 11–32 Metastatic lesion from carcinoma of the breast: axial computed tomography scan showing a destructive lesion involving the anterior aspect of the right petrous pyramid and extending into the middle ear cavity (*arrows*).

inferior ganglion (ganglion nodosum) of the vagus nerve (glomus vagale). Only the first two are considered in this chapter.

GLOMUS TYMPANICUM TUMORS. Glomus tympanicum tumors arise in the middle ear cavity over the promontory from glomus tissue located in the adventitia of vessels along the tympanic branch (Jacobson's nerve) of the glossopharyngeal nerve and auricular branch (Arnold's nerve) of the vagus nerve. Axial and coronal CT sections demonstrate a well-defined and enhancing soft tissue

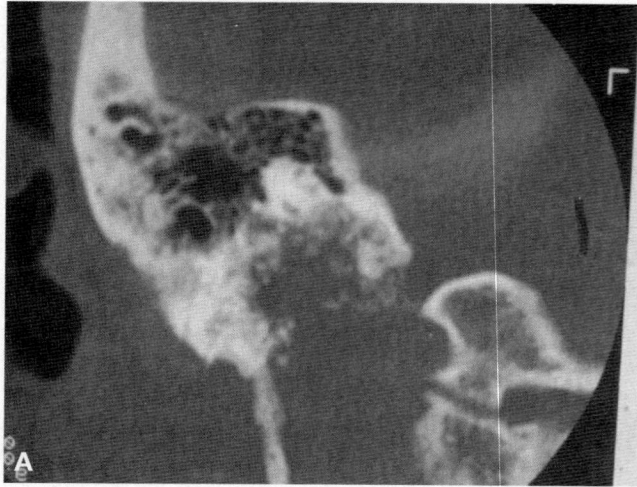

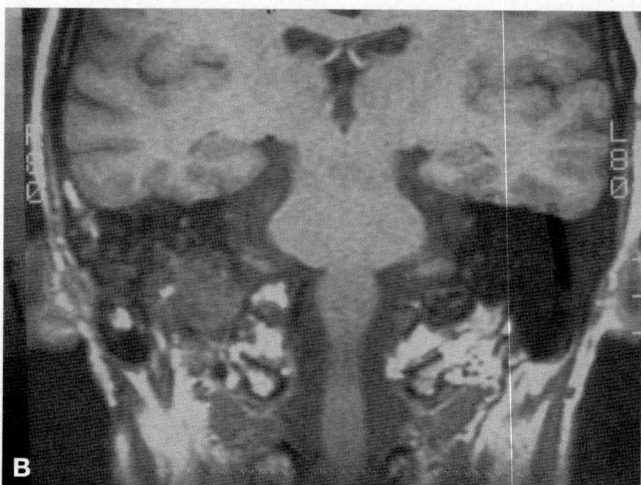

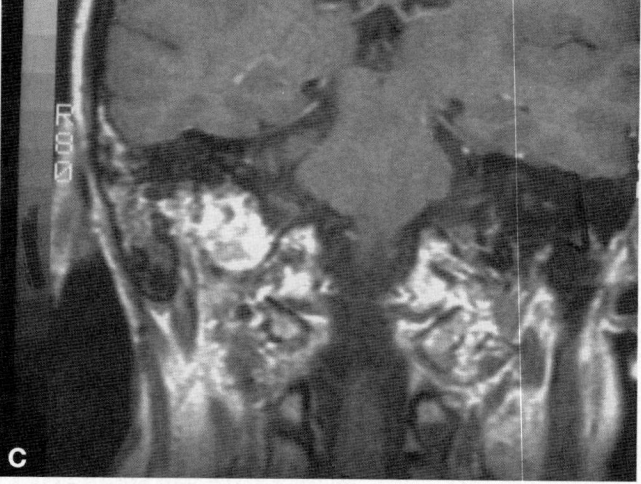

Figure 11–34 Glomus jugulare: *A*, coronal computed tomography scan; *B* and *C*, coronal magnetic resonance (MR) T₁ image prior to and after injection of contrast. The right jugular fossa appears enlarged and its contour eroded. The MR images demonstrate a mass of medium intensity, which enhances with contrast. Note the areas of signal void within the mass produced by blood vessels.

mass of variable size in the lower portion of the middle ear cavity and adjacent to the promontory (Figure 11–33). The hypotympanic floor and jugular fossa are usually intact. As the tumor enlarges, it may fill the entire middle ear cavity, causing a lateral bulge of the tympanic membrane and a smooth indentation of the promontory, and extend posteriorly into the mastoid and inferiorly into the hypotympanic air cells and jugular fossa.

Glomus Jugulare Tumors.   Glomus jugulare tumors arise from glomera of the chemoreceptor system located in the jugular fossa and jugular bulb. The jugular fossa is usually enlarged, with erosion of its cortical outline (Figure 11–34, A) and of the bony septum separating it from the outer opening of the carotid canal. Asymmetry of the jugular fossa and a large jugular fossa without cortical erosion are common anatomic variations of no clinical significance. As the floor of the hypotympanum is eroded, the tumor extends into the middle ear cavity and from there into the external auditory canal. Lateral extension of the lesion into the mastoid often leads to erosion of the facial canal and involvement of the facial nerve. Medial extension first produces undermining of the posteroinferior aspect of the petrous pyramid and then actual destruction of the perilabyrinthine bone and petrous apex. The resistant otic capsule is seldom involved, although the cochlea is often skeletonized by the erosion of the surrounding bone. Intracranial involvement is often observed in large tumors, although the lesion usually remains extradural. Extracranial extension occurs within and along the jugular vein. A CT study performed following a bolus injection of contrast material is excellent for diagnosing the tumor and establishing the extent of the lesion. Both soft tissue and bone parameters of each image should be studied. Intracranial and extracranial soft tissue pathology is, of course, best seen in low-window images, but bone details are best seen in high-definition images with extended scale.

Magnetic resonance imaging is of utmost importance in glomus jugulare tumors. The tumor appears as a mass of medium signal intensity in the T₁ sequence, which becomes brighter in T₂ and enhances after injection of contrast. Multiple punctated areas of no signal produced by blood vessels are observed within the tumor mass (Figure 11–34, B and C). Intracranial and extracranial involvement can be defined more precisely with MR imaging than with CT. Involvement of the jugular vein and carotid artery is readily demonstrated because these vascular structures are clearly visible in the MR images, thus avoiding the need for more invasive vascular studies.

Vestibular Schwannomas

Vestibular schwannomas (acoustic neuromas) account for approximately 10% of the cases of unilateral sensorineural hearing and vestibular loss of unknown origin. Most of the tumors arise from the vestibular nerve within the internal auditory canal. Magnetic resonance imaging is, at present, the study of choice for the assessment of the cerebellopontine angle. The format of examination varies with the clinical symptomatology.

A limited study of the internal auditory canal is performed whenever the patient is referred because of unilateral sensorineural hearing loss, either sudden or progressive. The examination consists of 2-mm contiguous coronal T_1 and axial fast spin echo images of the internal auditory canals obtained prior to the injection of contrast. If a tumor is clearly outlined in the fast spin echo images, as a filling defect within the brightness of the cerebrospinal fluid (Figure 11–35, A), the study is terminated. Otherwise, an injection of contrast is performed, and T_1 images are obtained in the axial and coronal planes. These sections will show tumors as

small as 2 mm (Figure 11–35, B). Vestibular schwannomas should be differentiated from facial neuromas arising within the internal auditory canal, which usually extend into the fallopian canal (Figure 11–36). A complete study of the internal auditory canals and brain is performed in patients with bilateral sensorineural hearing loss to rule out neurofibromatosis and other central nervous system pathology and in patients with vertigo and abnormal vestibular findings, whether or not they are associated with sensorineural hearing loss and whenever the sensorineural hearing loss is associated with other neurologic findings. Before the injection of contrast, this examination includes 3-mm fast spin echo axial images of the posterior cranial fossa and internal auditory canals, 2-mm T_1 coronal sections of the internal auditory canals, and 5-mm fluid-attenuated inversion recovery axial sections of the brain, which are particularly useful to rule out a demyelinating process. After injection of contrast, 2-mm T_1 coronal images of the internal auditory canals and 5-mm axial sections of the brain are obtained.

The limited study is offered at approximately 50% of the cost of the complete examination. Fat suppression images should always be obtained after injection of contrast if the patient had previous surgery for the removal of an acoustic tumor since that fat-containing graft used to plug the surgical tract may obscure the enhancing tumor mass.

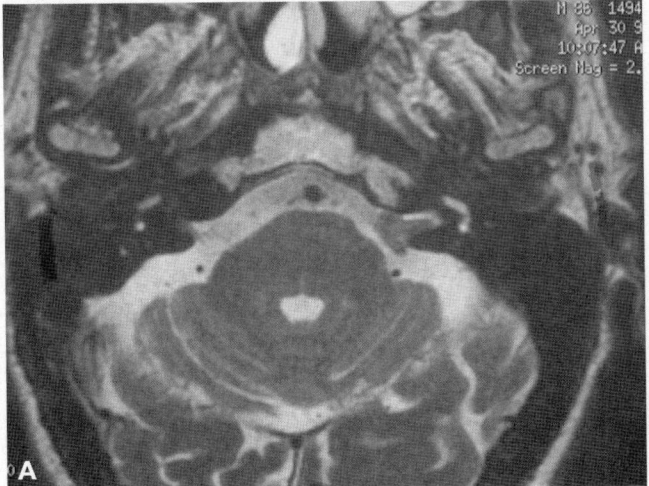 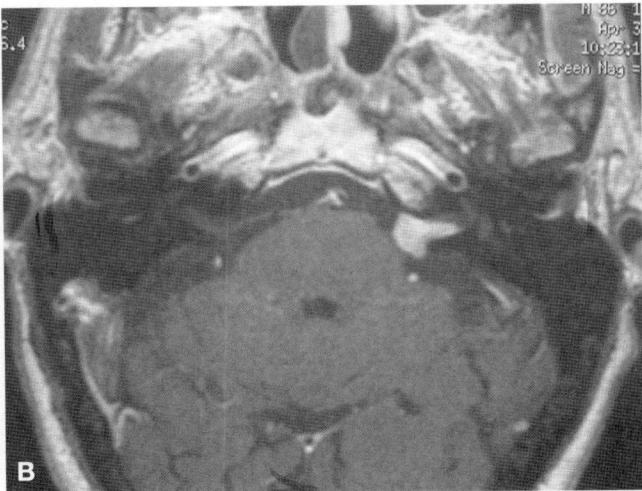

Figure 11–35 Vestibular schwannoma; magnetic resonance images: *A*, fast spin echo (FSE); *B*, T_1 postcontrast. The tumor mass is well seen in the FSE image as a filling defect within the bright cerebrospinal fluid (*A*). The size of the tumor mass is more clearly defined in the postcontrast image (*B*).

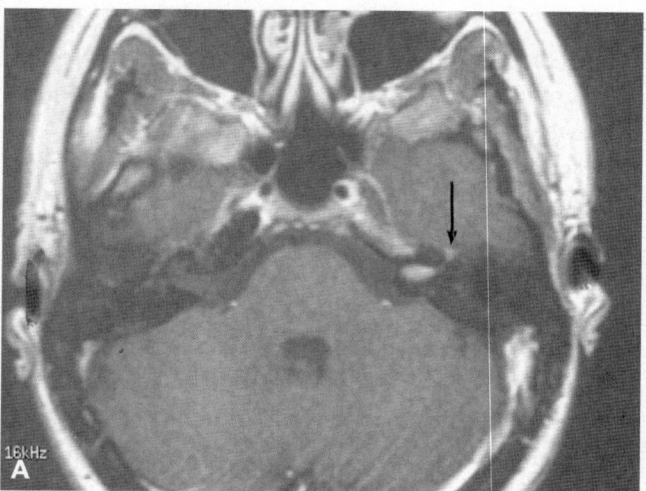
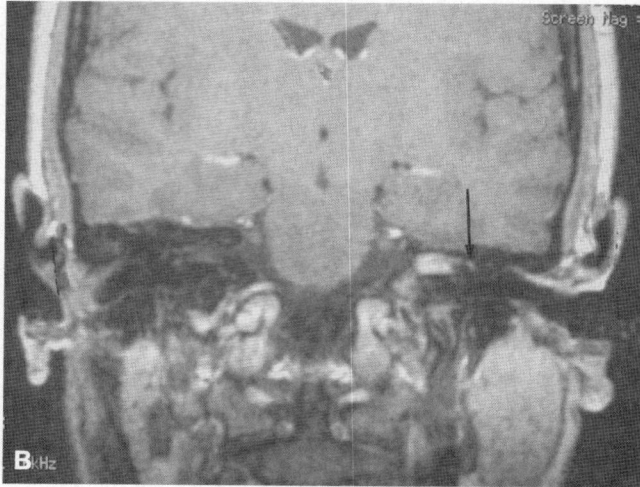

Figure 11–36 Facial schwannoma; magnetic resonance images: *A*, axial; *B*, coronal T$_1$ after contrast. The tumor fills the left internal auditory canal and extends into the facial canal (*arrow*).

A CT study should be performed only if MRI is not available or if the patient cannot undergo an MRI study because of an implanted medical device, such as a pacemaker.

First, the CT study allows a precise assessment of the internal auditory canals. Because the internal auditory canals in the normal individual vary in size from 2 to 12 mm, whereas the two canals of any person are almost identical, both sides should always be examined for comparison purposes. Enlargement of 2 mm or more and shortening of the posterior wall by at least 3 mm in comparison with the canal of the normal-hearing side are usually indicative of a space-occupying lesion.

Enlargement of 1 to 2 mm and shortening of the posterior wall by 2 to 3 mm are only suggestive of a lesion. The examination then consists of a two-step procedure that can be performed in one outpatient visit. First, the intravenous infusion of contrast material is performed. If a tumor is recognized, the study is completed with 1.5-mm sections (Figure 11–37). The infusion study allows the demonstration of extracanalicular tumors as small as 8 mm. Smaller lesions and intracanalicular lesions are usually not visualized. If the infusion study is negative, a spinal puncture is immediately performed, and 3 cc of air or gas (CO_2 or O_2) are injected in the subarachnoid space. By proper positioning, the gas is then moved into the cerebellopontine cistern under examination. When a tumor is present, the gas outlines the medial contour of the mass and reveals a complete or partial block of the internal auditory canal (Figure 11–38). By this technique, intracanalicular tumors, as small as 2 to 3 mm, are clearly identified. The

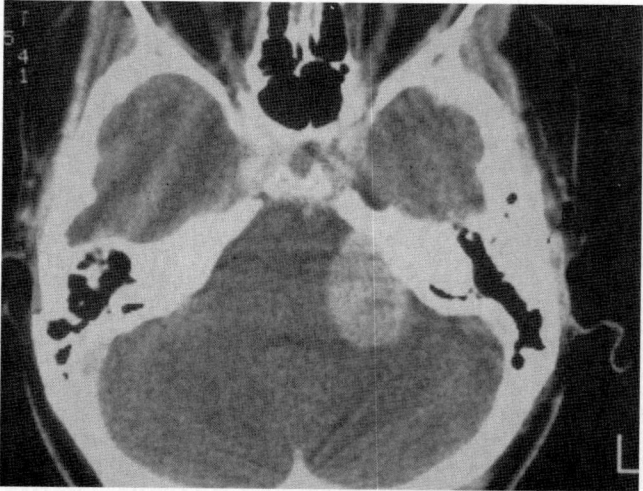

Figure 11–37 Vestibular schwannoma: axial computed tomography postcontrast. A large tumor extends from the left internal auditory canal into the cerebellopontine cistern. The mass compresses the brainstem and the fourth ventricle.

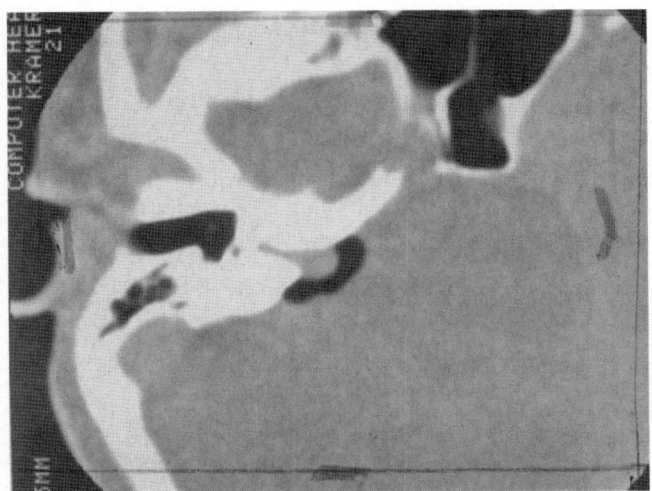

Figure 11–38 Right vestibular schwannoma: computed tomography pneumocisternogram. The air outlines the convex medial aspect of the tumor, which protrudes from the internal auditory canal into the adjacent cerebellopontine cistern.

air is then moved to the opposite side, and the scan is repeated using the same modalities.

Labyrinthine Schwannomas

In the past, small schwannomas have been found within the vestibule and cochlea during postmortem dissection of the temporal bone. These lesions are usually not rec-

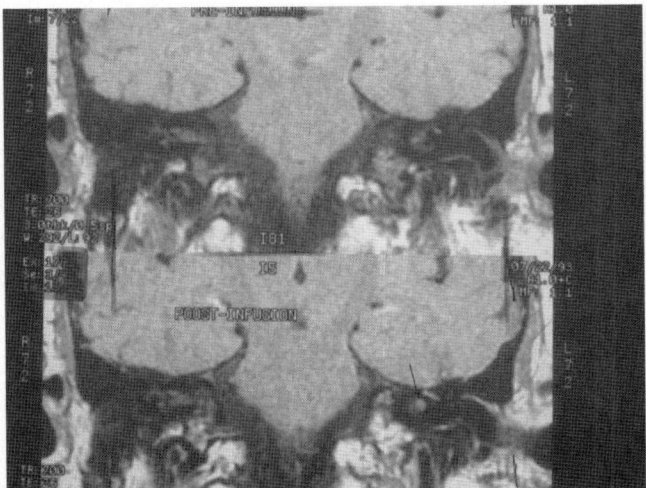

Figure 11–39 Cochlear schwannoma: magnetic resonance image coronal T$_1$, before (*top*) and after (*bottom*) contrast. A 2-mm enhancing mass is seen within the cochlea (*arrow*). The internal auditory canal is normal.

ognizable by CT but are well demonstrated as small enhanced masses in MR examinations performed after injection of contrast material (Figure 11–39).

Meningiomas

Meningiomas are the second most common tumor of the cerebellopontine angle and usually arise outside the internal auditory canal, although they may extend within the medial portion of the canal. Meningiomas limited to the internal auditory canal are rare and mimic, both

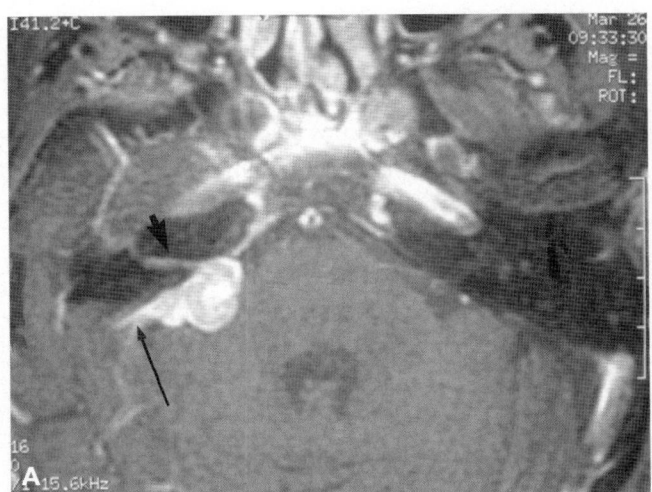

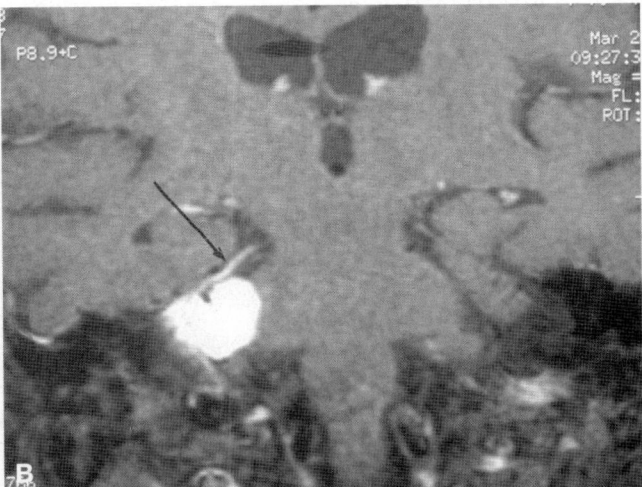

Figure 11–40 Meningioma right cerebellopontine cistern. An unevenly enhancing mass is seen in the right cerebellopontine cistern. The tumor extends into but does not fill the internal auditory canal (*short arrow*). Note the extension of the tumor en plaque (*long arrow*). A, axial; B, coronal T$_1$ images, peak contrast.

clinically and by imaging, vestibular schwannomas. Meningiomas grow as a solid mass or en plaque and may cause hyperostosis or erosion of the adjacent bone structures. Magnetic response images obtained after injection of contrast show enhancement of the tumor and in 10% of cases small areas of signal void caused by calcifications within the mass (Figure 11–40). En plaque lesions appear as areas of enhancing meningeal thickening and are often associated with mass-like tumors producing a so-called "tail" sign, which is helpful but not specific for the diagnosis of meningiomas (Figure 11–40).

Hemangiomas

Small hemangiomas or AVMs limited to the lumen of the internal auditory canal are rare. They appear in the precontrast images as an area of high signal intensity caused by slow flow, which becomes larger following the injection of contrast. The mass has a nonhomogeneous intensity and may contain signal void areas caused by calcifications. Large hemangiomas involve the bone of the petrosa and may extend within the internal auditory canal. This lesion is characterized by a mass of medium intensity in the T_1 precontrast images, which contains multiple spicules of signal void caused by calcifications. The tumor becomes bright after injection of contrast but maintains the same nonhomogeneous intensity.

Lipomas

Lipomas may occur within the cerebellopontine cistern or the internal auditory canal. In the five cases the author has seen, the lipoma was located at the fundus of the internal auditory canal. The diagnosis is made by obtaining T_1 and T_2 precontrast images or by fat suppression images whenever a bright mass is seen on postcontrast T_1-weighted images.

Epidermoid Cysts

Epidermoid cysts usually occur in the cerebellopontine cistern and rarely within the internal auditory canal. The MR study shows a nonenhancing mass of low signal in the T_1 images that becomes bright in the T_2-weighted images.

Aneurysm

An aneurysm within the internal auditory canal is extremely rare. The lesion appears on T_1- and T_2-weighted MR images as a small mass of high signal presumably caused by thrombosis or slow flow. Following the injection of contrast, the lesion becomes slightly larger. Aneurysms within the cerebellopontine cistern may compress the acoustic or facial nerves and mimic the symptomatology of a schwannoma (Figure 11–41). The

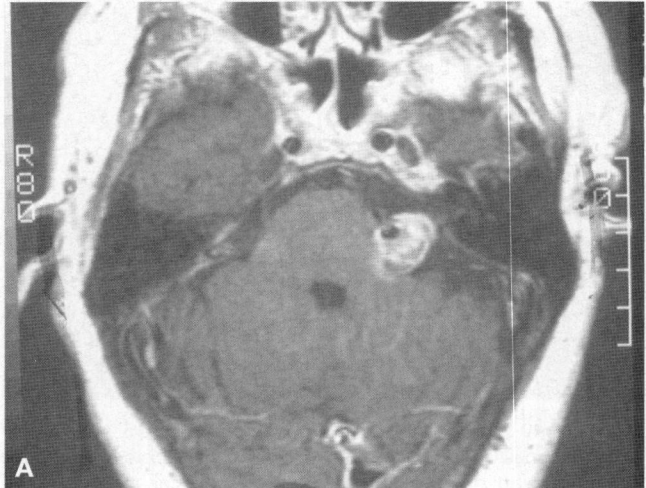 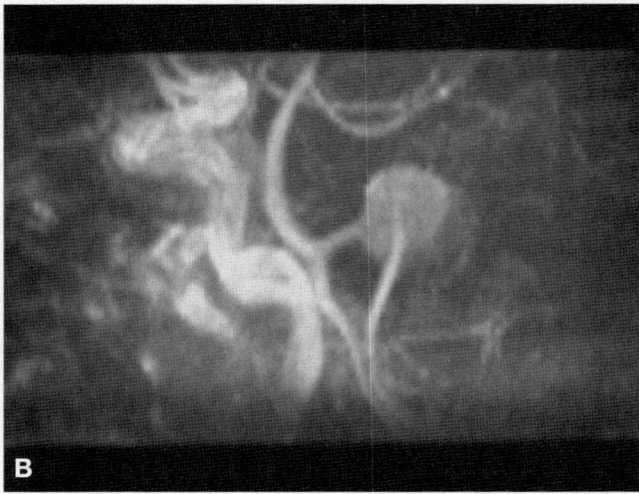

Figure 11–41 Cerebellopontine cistern aneurysm. In the axial magnetic resonance (MR) T_1 image obtained after contrast (*A*), the clotted aneurysm appears as a mass of nonhomogeneous high signal. The area of signal void within it is the patent lumen. The MR angiogram (*B*) confirms the presence of an aneurysm arising from the left vertebral artery.

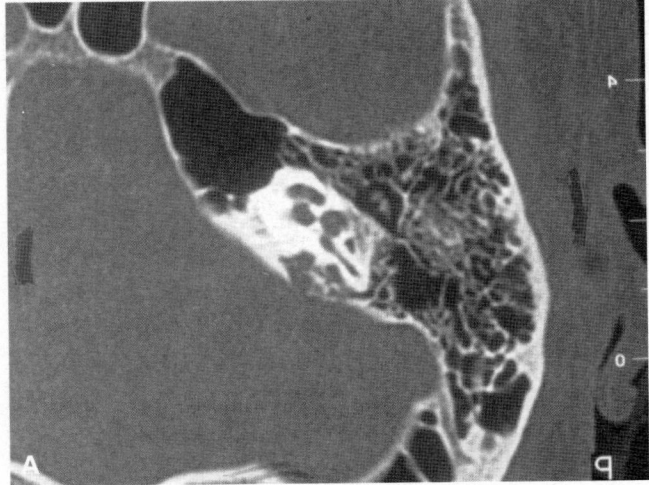

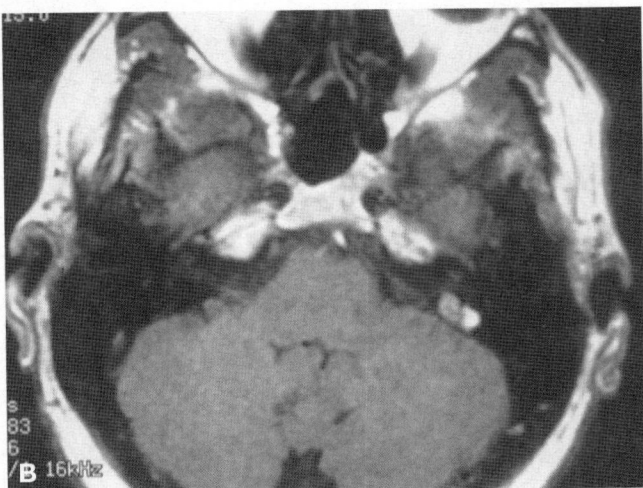

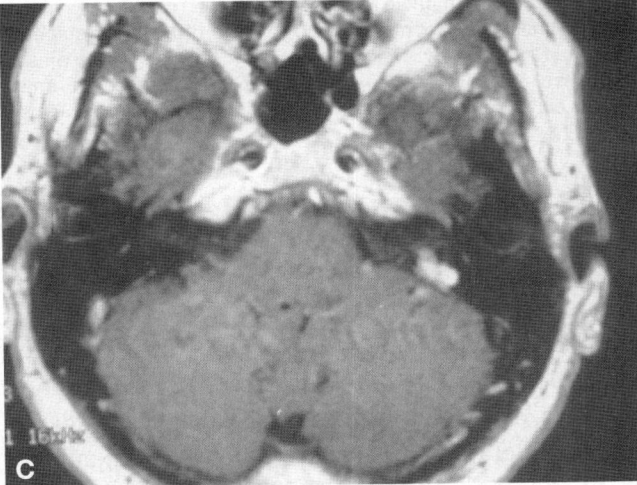

Figure 11–42 Endolymphatic sac tumor: *A*, axial computed tomography scan; *B* and *C*, axial magnetic resonance image before and after contrast. The posterior aspect of the left petrous pyramid is eroded in the region of the endolymphatic sac. The tumor mass has a heterogeneous appearance before contrast (*B*). The solid portion of the tumor enhances with contrast (*C*).

MR images obtained prior to injection of contrast reveal a mass of nonhomogeneous high signal intensity produced by the clot. If the lumen of the aneurysm is partially patent, the flowing blood will appear as an area of signal void (Figure 11–41, A).

Endolymphatic Sac Tumors

Endolymphatic sac tumors are locally aggressive papillary adenomatous tumors. They are often associated with von Hippel-Lindau disease, a genetic multisystem neoplastic disorder. At first, endolymphatic sac tumors involve the adjacent dura and endolymphatic duct. From there the lesion extends to the vestibule, semicircular canals, mastoid, and middle ear cavity, where it appears through an intact tympanic membrane as a bluish mass, often confused with a glomus tumor. Continuous growth leads to complete replacement by tumor of the mastoid and petrous pyramid. Axial CT images initially show a localized area of erosion of the posterior aspect of the petrous pyramid in the region of the endolymphatic sac (Figure 11–42, A). As the lesion enlarges, destruction of the petrous pyramid is observed with involvement of the inner ear structure. In the T_1 MR images, the tumor has a heterogeneous appearance, with areas of high signal caused by cysts filled with blood or high proteinaceous fluid and multiple small areas of signal void caused by calcifications and blood vessels (Figure 11–42, B). Following administration of contrast, the solid portion of the mass undergoes a nonhomogeneous enhancement (Figure 11–42C).

Otodystrophies

Otosclerosis
The diagnosis of fenestral otosclerosis is usually suspected by the otologist on the basis of the clinical history and audiometric tests. A CT study may be performed in these cases to confirm the diagnosis and rule out other possible causes of conductive hearing impairment. The examination consists of axial and 20-degree coronal oblique sections at 1-mm increments. The CT findings vary from loss of definition of the margin of the oval window (owing to demineralization) to narrowing and finally complete obliteration of the oval window opening and niche (Figure 11–43, A and C).

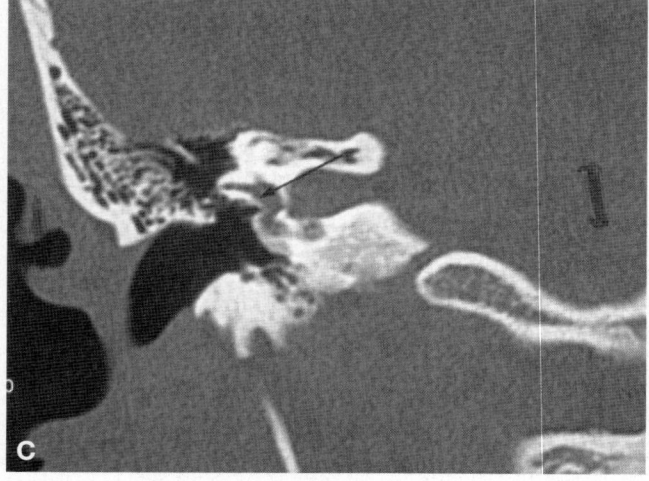

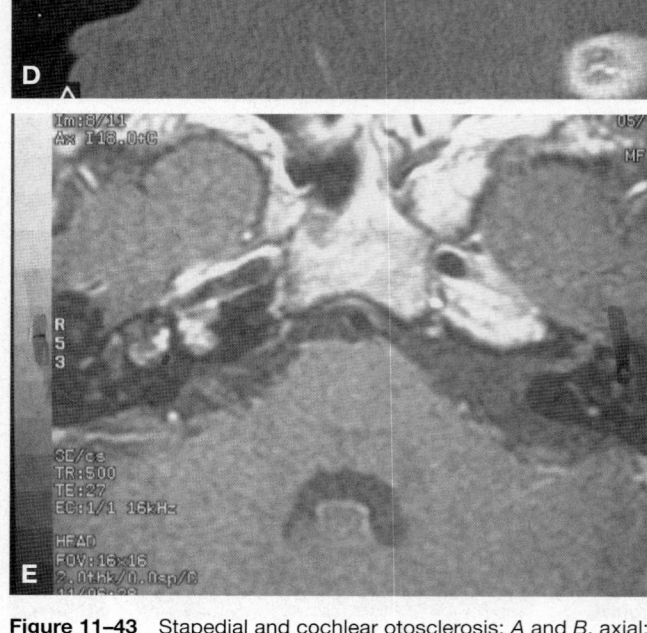

Figure 11–43 Stapedial and cochlear otosclerosis: *A* and *B*, axial; *C* and *D*, coronal computed tomography; *E*, axial magnetic resonance (MR) T$_1$ image after contrast. The footplate of the right stapes is thickened (*A* and *C*, *arrows*). Severe spongiotic changes are present throughout the cochlear capsule (*B* and *D*, *arrows*). The MR image reveals enhancement of the active and vascular foci of otosclerosis.

Computed tomography is extremely helpful in evaluating postsurgical cases in which an initial hearing improvement is subsequently lost and in determining the cause of post-stapedectomy vertigo. The CT study may disclose protrusion of the prosthesis into the vestibule, separation of the lateral end of the strut from the incus, dislocation of the medial end of the prosthesis, and reobliteration of the oval window with fixation of the strut (Figure 11–44). Cochlear otosclerosis occurs by progressive enlargement of the perifenestral foci or as single or multiple foci in other locations of the cochlear and labyrinthine capsules. The diagnosis of cochlear otosclerosis is suspected by the otologist on

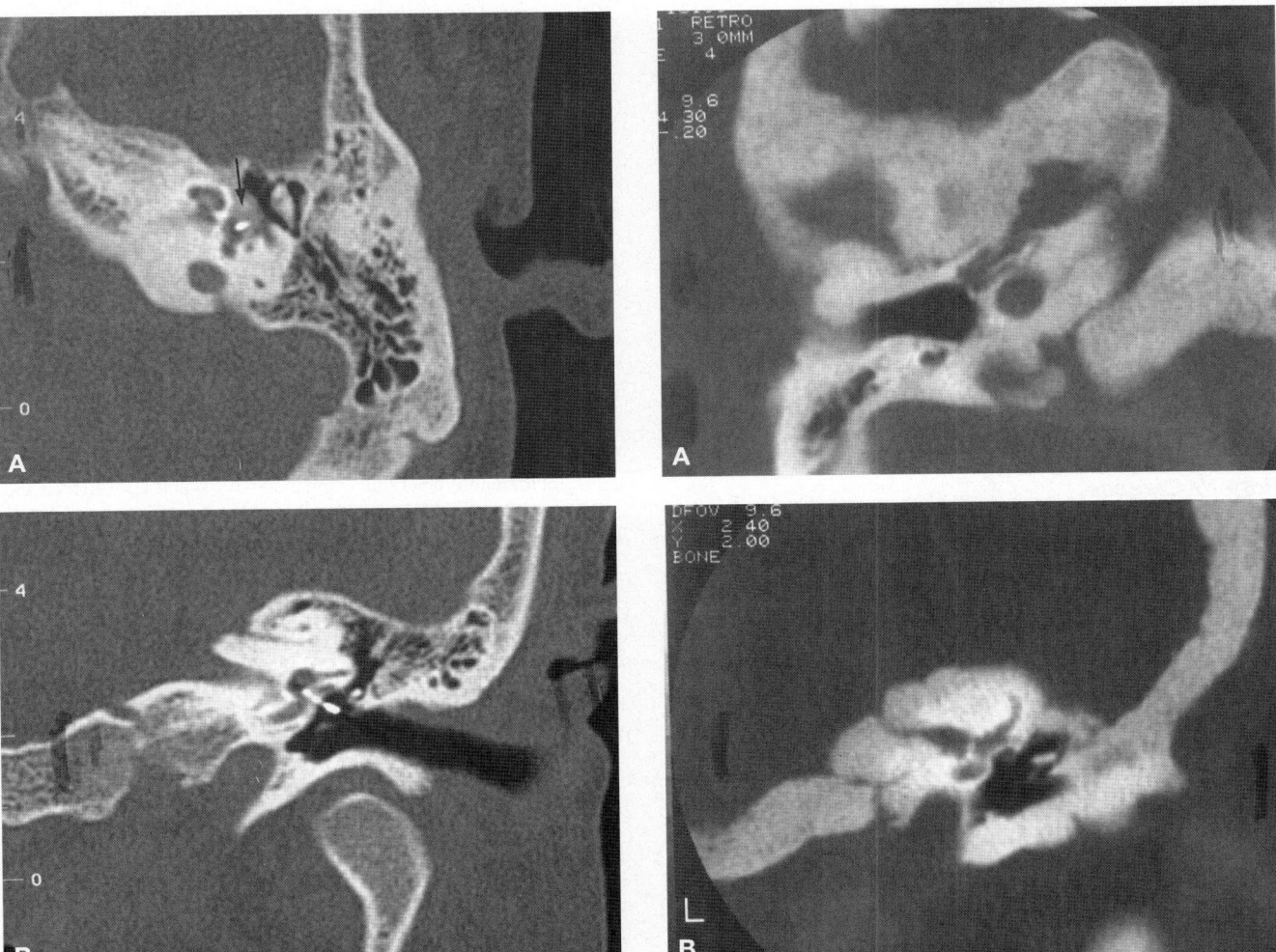

Figure 11–44   Recurrent fenestral otosclerosis after stapedectomy: *A*, axial; *B*, coronal computed tomography scan. A metallic piston extends from the long process of the incus to the oval window, which appears reclosed. The medial end of the piston is in a good position but is fixed by the large focus obliterating the oval window niche (*arrow*). Otospongiotic changes are noted in the cochlear capsule.

Figure 11–45   Fibrous dysplasia: *A*, axial; *B*, coronal computed tomography. There is diffuse thickening and sclerosis of the temporal bone with narrowing of the external and internal auditory canals.

the basis of the audiometric configuration, clinical history, and clinical findings, such as Schwartze's sign, but further confirmation by a proper imaging study is required. The CT examination consists of axial and coronal or 20-degree coronal oblique sections at 1-mm increments. The normal cochlear capsule appears as a sharply defined, homogeneously dense, although not homogeneously thick, bony shell outlining the lumen of the cochlea. Otosclerotic changes range from small and isolated foci of decreased density to diffuse de-

mineralization of a large area of the capsule with complete dissolution of its contour. A typical sign of cochlear otosclerosis is the formation of a double-ring effect caused by confluent spongiotic foci within the thickness of the capsule (see Figure 11–43, B and D). The band of intracapsular demineralization is in some cases limited to a segment of the capsule, but in others it follows almost the entire contour of the cochlea. A more precise and quantitative assessment of the involvement is accomplished by CT densitometric readings. Using the smallest cursor, the contour of the cochlear capsule is scanned, and 31 densitometric readings are obtained. A profile of the density of the capsule is obtained by plotting the densitometric values versus the 31 points where the reading are made. The obtained densitometric curve is then compared to the densitometric profile of the normal capsule that was previously determined.

In several patients with a positive Schwartze's sign and severe spongiotic change in the CT study, MR images obtained after injection of contrast show enhancement within the demineralized foci (see Figure 11–43, E). Presumably, the blushing is produced by pooling of contrast within the numerous blood vessels and lacunae found in active spongiotic foci.

Paget's Disease

Paget's disease can affect the calvarium and the base of the skull, including the petrous pyramids. When the disease process extends into the otic capsule, there will be mixed or sensorineural hearing loss that is progressive.

The haversian bone of the petrosa is affected first, with spread of the disease from the apex laterally. At first, because of severe demineralization of the petrosa, the labyrinthine capsule becomes more prominent than normal. Involvement of the otic capsule begins at the periosteal surface. Slow demineralization occurs, which first produces thinning and finally complete dissolution of the capsule. This results in a washed-out appearance of the entire petrous bone characteristic of Paget's disease.

Fibrous Dysplasia

In the base of the skull, the lesions are the result of abnormal proliferation of fibrous tissue intermixed with trabeculae of woven bone within the medullary cavity. These changes lead to increased density and thickening of the affected areas (Figure 11–45). Involvement by fibrous dysplasia is usually unilateral, which leads to asymmetry (see Figure). In the temporal bone, the squama becomes thickened and the pneumatic system obliterated. The external auditory canal is often stenosed by new bone formation (Figure 11–45, A). As the petrous pyramid becomes thickened and dense, the outline of the labyrinthine capsule becomes poorly distinguishable from the surrounding bone. Further progression may lead to narrowing of the internal auditory canal (Figure 11–45, B) and obliteration of the lumen of the labyrinth.

REFERENCES

1. Valvassori GE, Buckingham RA. Tomography and cross sections of the ear. Philadelphia: Georg Thieme Verlag; 1975.
2. Valvassori GE, Dobben GD. CT densitometry of the cochlear capsule in otosclerosis. AJNR Am J Neuroradiol 1985;6:661–7.
3. Seltzer S, Mark AS. Contrast enhancement of the labyrinth on MR scans in patients with sudden hearing loss and vertigo: evidence of labyrinthine disease. AJNR Am J Neuroradiol 1991;12:13–6.
4. Rodgers GK, Applegate L, De La Cruz A, et al. Magnetic resonance angiography: analysis of vascular lesions of the temporal bone and skull base. Am J Otol 1993;14:56–62.
5. Casselman JW, Kuhweide R, Ampe W, et al. Pathology of the membranous labyrinth: comparison of T1- and T2-weighted and gadolinium-enhanced spin-echo and 3DFT-CIS imaging. AJNR Am J Neuroradiol 1993;14:59–69.
6. Casselman JW, Kuhweide R, Deimling M, et al. Constructive interference in steady state-3DFT MR imaging of the inner ear and cerebellopontine angle. AJNR Am J Neuroradiol 1993;14:47–57.
7. Valvassori GE, Carter BL, Mafee MF. Imaging of the head and neck. Stuttgart: Georg Thieme Verlag; 1995.
8. Harnsberger HR, Dahlen RT, Shelton C, et al. Advanced techniques in magnetic resonance imaging in the evaluation of the large endolymphatic duct and sac syndrome. Laryngoscope 1995;105:1037–42.
9. Valvassori GE. The internal auditory canal revisited. Otolaryngol Clin North Am 1995;28:431–51.
10. Mukherji SK, Albernaz VS, Lo WW, et al. Papillary endolymphatic sac tumors: CT, MR imaging and angiographic findings in 20 patients. Radiology 1997;202:801–8.
11. Fitzgerald DC, Mark AS. Sudden hearing loss: frequency of abnormal findings on contrast-enhanced MRI studies. AJNR Am J Neuroradiol 1998;19:1433–6.
12. Antonelli PJ, Garside JA, Mancuso AA, et al. Computed tomography and the diagnosis of coalescent mastoiditis. Otolaryngol Head Neck Surg 1999;120:350–4.
13. Stone JA, Castillo M, Neelon B, Mukherji SK. Evaluation of CSF leaks: high resolution CT compared with contrast-enhanced CT and radionuclide cisternography. AJNR Am J Neuroradiol 1999;20:706–12.
14. Bamiou DE, Phelps P, Sirimanna T. Temporal bone computed tomography findings in bilateral sensorineural hearing loss. Arch Dis Child 2000;82:257–60.
15. Dubrulle F, Ernst O, Vincent C, et al. Cochlear fossa enhancement at MR evaluation of vestibular schwannoma: correlation with success at hearing preservation surgery. Radiology 2000;215:458–62.
16. Schmalbrock P, Chakeres DW, Monroe W, et al. Assessment of internal auditory canal tumors: a comparison of contrast-enhanced T1 weighted and steady-state T2 weighted gradient echo MR imaging. AJNR Am J Neuroradiol 1999;20:1207–13.

17. Davidson HC, Harnsberger R, Lemmerling MM, et al. MR evaluation of vestibulocochlear anomalies associated with large endolymphatic duct and sac. AJNR Am J Neuroradiol 1999;20: 1435–41.

18. Gjuric M, Koester M, Paulus W. Cavernous hemangioma of the internal auditory canal arising from the inferior vestibular nerve: case report and review of the literature. Am J Otol 2000;21:110–4.

19. Booth TN, Vezina LG, Karcher G, Dubovsky EC. Imaging and clinical evaluation of isolated atresia of the oval window. A JNR Am J Neuroradiol 2000;21:171–4.

20. Sedwick JD, Gajewski BJ, Prevatt AR, Antonelli PJ. Magnetic resonance imaging in the search for retrocochlear pathology. Otolaryngol Head Neck Surg 2001;124:652–5.

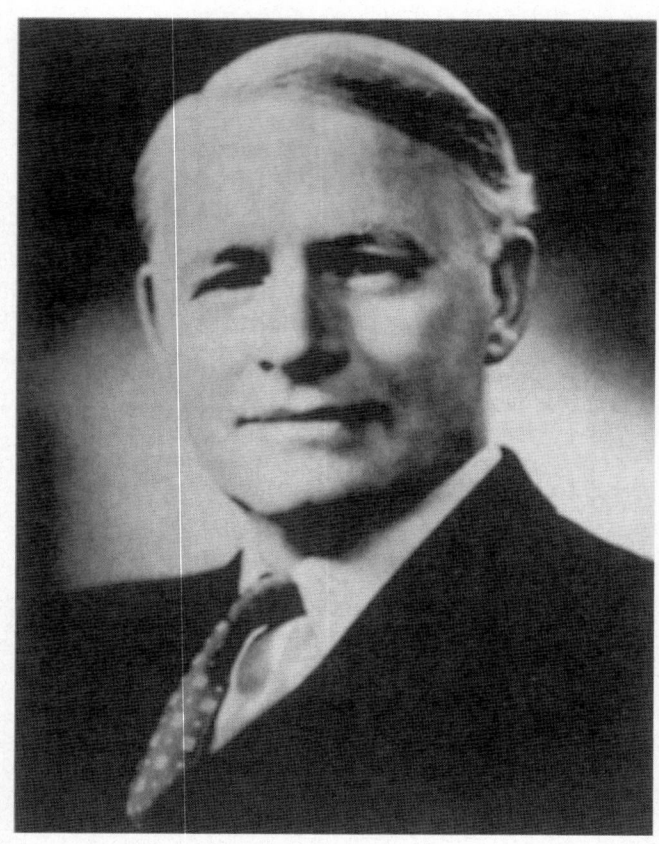

Carl Olaf Nylén (1892–1978). In 1921 introduced the (monocular) otomicroscope for ear surgery.

III

Fundamentals of Otologic/ Neurotologic Surgery

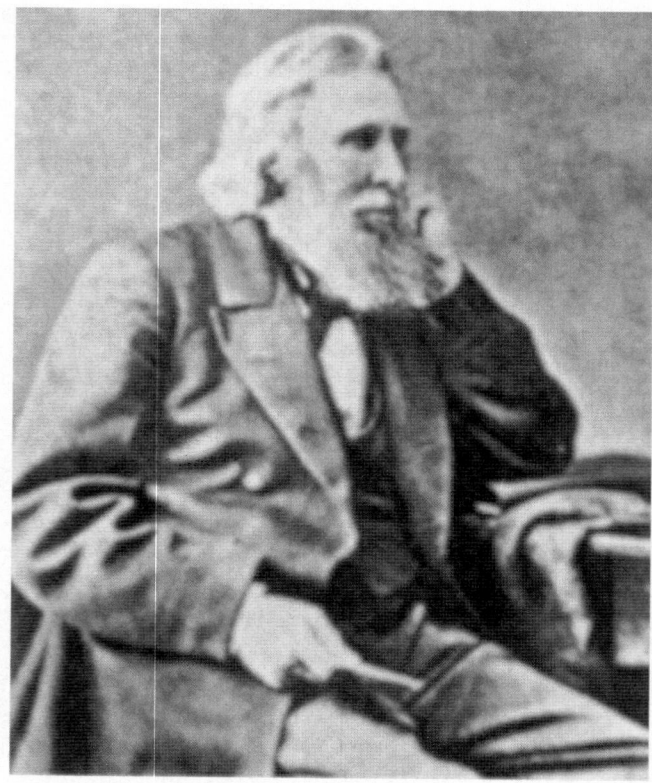

Sir William Wilde (1815–1876). Described the postauricular incision for the management of acute subperiosteal mastoid abscess.

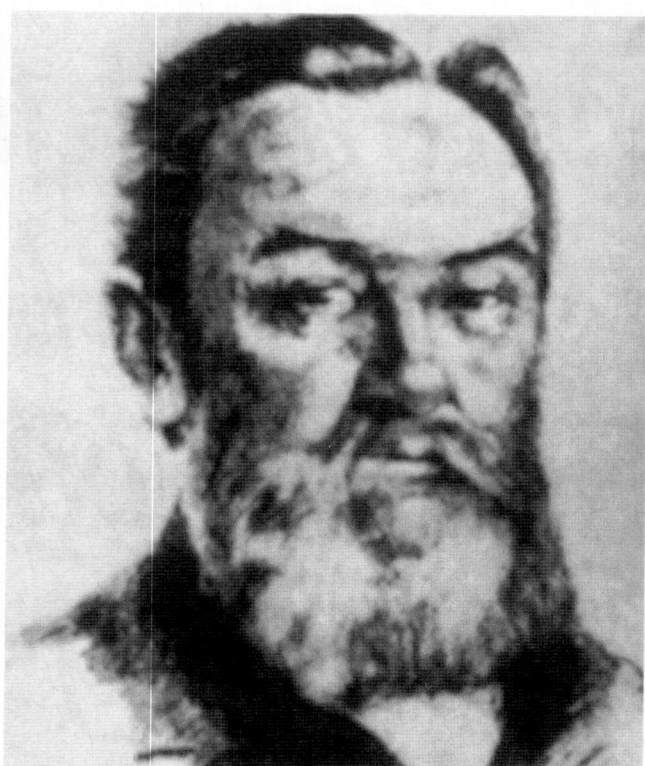

Johannes Kessel (1837–1907). First performed endaural radical mastoidectomy, described by his chief resident in 1892. In 1878 performed the first stapes mobilization and in 1879 described sound protection for the round window.

12

Principles of Temporal Bone and Skull Base Surgery

C. Gary Jackson, MD, FACS

The specific elements of surgical disease management are detailed throughout this text. A thoughtful and comprehensive appreciation of the fundamentals of temporal bone surgery in general, however, affords a basis on which specific treatment principles can be successfully optimized. The elements of disease management within the temporal bone are sufficiently unique to warrant special attention. The basic principles applicable to all of surgery apply to surgery of the temporal bone, but for unknown reasons (perhaps the bony anatomy or the microscopic demands of the exercise), they become inexplicably perverted. Such perversion can compromise the final result.

The compulsive application of each and every fundamental element and principle of surgery maximizes the capacity of the procedure to produce a successful outcome. Anything less underwrites mediocrity.

What follows is an overview of the fundamental principles of temporal bone surgery on which the details of the management of specific diseases is based.

FUNDAMENTALS

Anesthesia

The technological revolution that has propelled surgery and diagnosis has equally affected the anesthetic management of the neurotologic patient. Enormous advances in pharmacology, drug delivery systems, monitoring, and the understanding of physiology have afforded unprecedented levels of intraoperative patient control. It is apparent that what is done or not done (and how) has

a major impact on what happens at the surgical field. Anesthesia is a form of critical care. A thoughtful cooperation between the otologic surgeon and the anesthesiologist must precede the procedure and continue well beyond the procedure itself.

Preoperative Preparation: General

Managed care has impacted all aspects of the surgical process, particularly preoperative preparation. The majority of the routine procedures of preoperative preparation for temporal bone surgery patients must be compulsively executed, despite managed care. Microsurgery should be bloodless. Medications that complicate microsurgical hemostasis should be suspended at least 2 weeks prior to surgery. Pretreatment of brain edema associated with major neurotologic procedures may require the preoperative application of corticosteroid therapy, and selecting an agent that minimizes mineralocorticoid effect is best. Anticonvulsants may be indicated. There is no place for extended preoperative antibiotic prophylaxis.

Cooperative interaction among consultants should be accomplished well in advance of surgery. The expertise of internal medicine, cardiology, neurosurgery, and others is liberally employed, particularly in neurotologic procedures. Outpatient preparation for inpatient events ensures successful management of perioperative details, shares the workload, builds relationships, and strengthens the team's experiential base.

For neurotologic procedures, postsurgical rehabilitation (eg, swallowing/speech therapy and vestibular rehabilitation) is best introduced and taught preoperatively.

Managed care has changed the preoperative routine aspects for patients undergoing temporal bone surgery. Early morning admission is the rule, and the necessary negotiation of transportation details has enhanced patient anxiety. The anesthesiologist is a consultant, with whom a comprehensive preoperative consultation is mandated and should occur well prior to the morning of surgery. Similarly, patients should be informed of parking lot locations, how to get to the admissions office, etc, well in advance of the day of surgery. Preregistration is helpful in avoiding the last-minute scurrying for insurance cards, "pre-certs," and form completion the morning of surgery. Patients living locally can negotiate a 5:30 am arrival; out-of-town patients must be accommodated. All patients undergoing neurotologic procedures and those traveling long distances are provided with locally convenient accommodations for the eve of surgery. Creative solutions to this dilemma continue to evolve, including hospitality suites, hotels, and suites.

Informed consent should be accomplished in advance of the morning of surgery, preferably with the family present, at a time immediately proximate to the procedure. In a quiet environment, operative details, treatment options, reasonable expectations, and potential risks and complications can be related effectively. Both the patient and the family must know what to expect of the postoperative course, what special requirements will be necessary, and what will be expected of them both. The patient's family is an important component of the process. Who is to come? Where are they to go? Where are they to wait? How long will the surgery take? Questions such as these must be answered to their satisfaction. The family is informed when the surgery has begun, is telephoned hourly intraoperatively, and is updated immediately postoperatively and then regularly thereafter.

Presurgical anxiety can be profoundly detrimental. Preoperative sedation has been inappropriately minimized. Compassion and humanity render the preclusion of this detail because of its inconvenience unjustified. Creativity and insistence on the part of the surgeon will ensure that this important prerequisite to surgery does not become a managed care casualty.

Neuromuscular blockade has become customary to anesthesia. The widespread application of intraoperative facial nerve neural integrity monitoring (FNNIM) in otologic procedures and of more comprehensive monitoring of cranial nerves in neurotologic procedures imposes special challenges as we ask anesthesia to facilitate this important electrophysiologic surveillance. Neuromuscular blockade must not be used at all, must be absent at the time of surgery, or must be promptly reversed as a necessary prerequisite to neural integrity monitoring (see Chapter 14).

Techniques

Modern anesthesia has evolved to a level of safety in which the efficient application of a diversity of new agents ensures the maintenance of a still surgical field and hemodynamic and ventilatory support, without compromising microsurgical hemostasis or constituting a postsurgical liability. Most otologic surgeons prefer general anesthesia for the vast majority of mastoid and neurotologic procedures. Many otologic surgeons, however, still choose local anesthesia for middle ear procedures. The advantages of local anesthesia include the ability to test hearing intraoperatively, the capacity to be immediately aware of unintended consequences, and a truncated postsurgical emergence. Some surgeons also claim improved hemostasis with local anesthetic use. Local anesthesia should always be augmented by sedation adequate to induce a state of calm and induce amnesia while avoiding respiratory suppression or hemodynamic alteration. Modern neuroleptics do not conflict with injectable anesthetic agents. A suitable local anesthetic can usually be identified so that the same agents can be used with epinephrine. Today most surgeons use an anesthesiologist (or a nurse anesthetist) to control drug administration and monitor the patient. In the absence of surgical stimulation, suppression of physiology may be significant and delayed. Emergence should be monitored in a postanesthetic surgical recovery (PASR) area; the patient should not be sent back to the hospital room or to an outpatient suite.

Local Anesthesia for Postauricular and External Auditory Canal Incisions

The sensory innervation of the ear emanates from the auriculotemporal nerve to the tympanic membrane and auricle, the greater auricular nerve to the auricle and canal, and Arnold's nerve to the posterior canal and mastoid (Figure 12–1; see also Chapter 2). These nerves can be blocked by local anesthetic infiltration of the anterior canal wall at the bony-cartilaginous junction, the incisura terminalis continuing on to the auricle, behind the auricle over the mastoid process (Figure 12–2), the skin of the floor of the canal, and the periosteum along the anterior surface of the mastoid process (superficial enough to avoid the stylomastoid foramen).

The temporal bone itself is sensitive only in its outer periosteum and minimally so in its medial mucosal lining (ie, in the mastoid cavity, antrum, epitympanum, and tympanum). Thus, sufficient analgesia can be obtained for mastoidectomy solely with the infiltration of local anesthetic as outlined (with sedation).

Local Anesthesia for Transcanal Surgery

Stapedectomy and other middle ear procedures may be done using local anesthesia; however, neural integrity monitoring is confounded.

When infiltration anesthesia is employed, safety guidelines must be assiduously attended. The medical history (for the patient and the family) with respect to the tolerance of local anesthetic agents should be ascertained to identify hypersensitivity reactions or hereditary idiosyncratic responses. Such reactions can occur, may be unpredictable, and precipitate a horrendous hemodynamic sequence, beginning with arrhythmia, continuing with hypertension, pulmonary edema, ventricular fibrillation, and cardiac arrest, and ending in death!

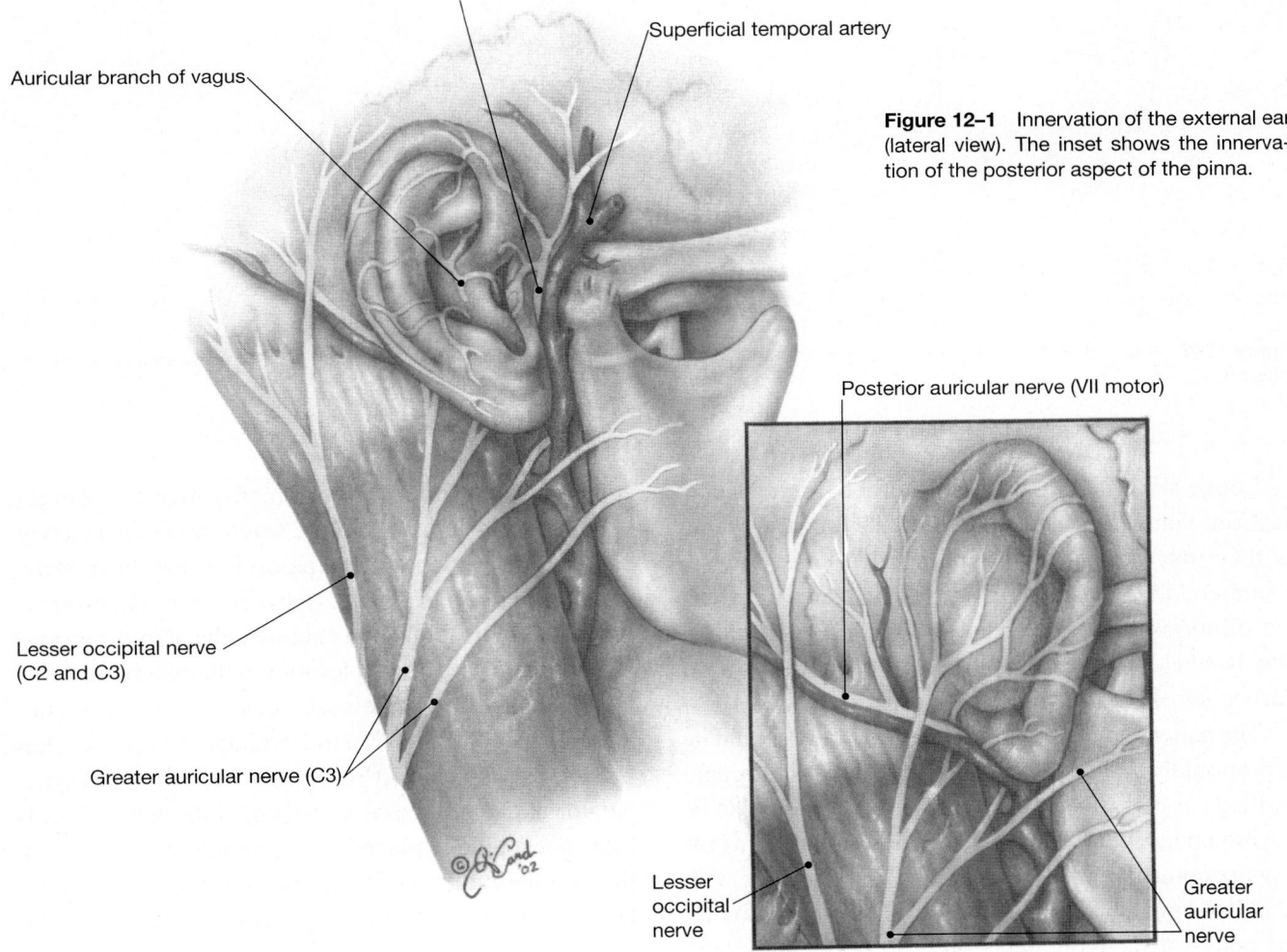

Auricular branch of vagus

Superficial temporal artery

Figure 12–1 Innervation of the external ear (lateral view). The inset shows the innervation of the posterior aspect of the pinna.

Lesser occipital nerve (C2 and C3)

Greater auricular nerve (C3)

Posterior auricular nerve (VII motor)

Lesser occipital nerve

Greater auricular nerve

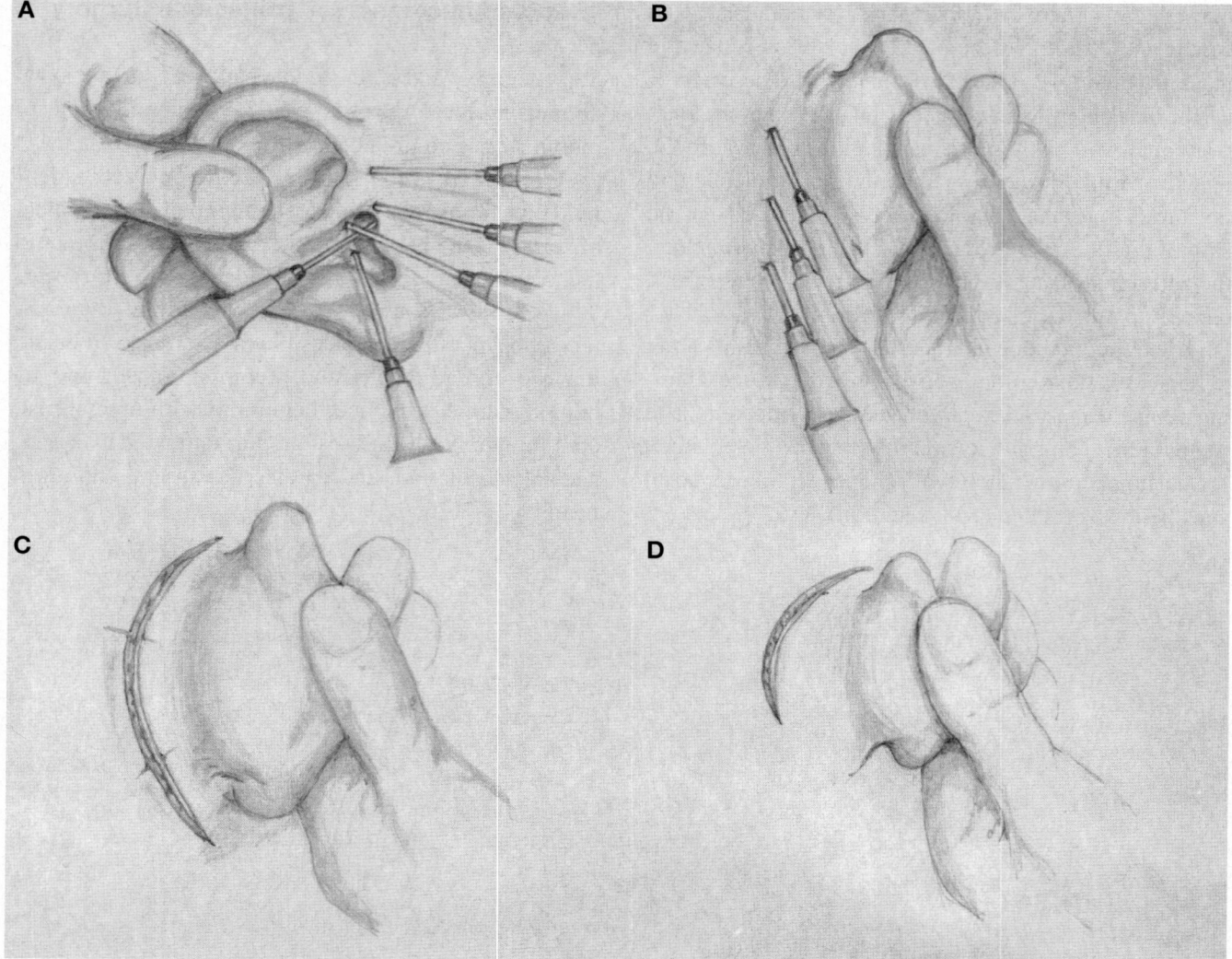

Figure 12–2   *A* and *B*, Points of injection for local anesthesia. *C*, Postauricular incision in adult. *D*, Infant's mastoid process and line for incision.

Loose solutions of drugs (eg, lidocaine and epinephrine) must never be allowed on the operating table as they may be confused, with terrible consequence. Commercially prepared solutions of lidocaine with varied dilutions of epinephrine are available in sealed, clearly labeled dental carpules. Their use, or that of similarly controlled systems, is strongly encouraged.

The patient undergoing middle ear surgery should be appropriately sedated, attended, and monitored. If tragal cartilage or perichondrium is required, the tragus can be infiltrated independently. For canal incisions (eg, as for a tympanomeatal flap), a solution of 2% lidocaine with 1:50,000 epinephrine is infiltrated at, or just medial to, the bony-cartilaginous junction posteriorly, anteriorly,

superiorly, and inferiorly. A small-gauge (27-gauge) needle should be used and the solution injected slowly as rapid infiltration may be painful or may form blebs that compromise exposure. Between the tympanosquamous and tympanomastoid sutures, the skin is particularly prone to excessive elevation with injection.

Adequate time for hemostatic, as well as anesthetic, effect must be allowed (10 to 12 minutes). Once the flap is elevated, discomfort may arise from the mesotympanum and its mucosa. Gelfoam™ impregnated with local anesthetic is placed in the middle ear to remedy this problem; in positioning the Gelfoam, it is important to remain alert to the potential of facial nerve exposure.

General Anesthesia

The majority of modern neurotologic surgery uses general anesthesia, the objectives of which are as follows:

- Maintenance of a still field
- Maintenance of hemodynamic stability and respiratory efficiency
- Maintenance of cerebral perfusion and oxygenation
- Facilitation of electrophysiologic monitoring
- Facilitation of surgical exposure and successful surgery
- Prevention of increased intracranial pressure
- Provision of a smooth, rapid emergence
- Provision of continuation of all of the above in the PASR/intensive care unit
- Facilitation of postoperative airway management

There are special challenges for general anesthesia presented by modern otologic surgery. To facilitate electrophysiologic monitoring, or even for those surgeons who wish to "watch the face" in mastoid surgery, neuromuscular blockade is precluded. In anesthesiology circles, this ban constitutes a challenge, and the solution(s) selected should allow for all of the listed objectives to be achieved. In particular, the choice(s) should be consistent with microsurgical demands for hemostasis. "Balanced techniques" employing narcotics tend to inhibit hemostasis and are more prone to postoperative nausea and delayed emergence.

Nitrous oxide is an efficient anesthetic; however, its tendency to escape into the surgical field complicates otologic surgery, particularly regarding tympanic membrane graft placement. Several viable alternatives exist.

Osmotic diuretics such as mannitol remove free water from the brain, reducing brain volume and obviating excessive retraction. Dosages of 0.5 to 4 g/kg achieve the desired effect, which has a duration of 20 minutes to 5 hours. Ideally, mannitol is used for its short-term effects, and it should be infused slowly and used with caution. Paradoxical swelling may occur, and patients with diminished cardiac reserve can experience heart failure.

Ventricular drains may be required if hydrocephalus is present. More commonly, lumbar drainage is appropriate for the drainage of cerebrospinal fluid (CSF) intra- or postoperatively. Pre- and intraoperative CSF drainage

decisions must be carefully weighed, particularly with posterior fossa lesions in which herniation is a risk. Should lumbar drainage be required, it is placed after induction of general anesthesia yet prior to preparing and draping (or at case conclusion if mass effect is a problem). Remaining clamped, CSF drainage can occur as indicated. Appropriate release of CSF surgically is best; for example, in the translabyrinthine approach to vestibular schwannomas, opening the cochlear aqueduct releases CSF and allows the brain to fall away, enhancing exposure, as long as there is no obstruction to CSF flow.

When increased intracranial pressure (ICP) is a problem, hyperventilation, so as to have the pCO_2 approach 25 mm Hg, may be required. Decreased pCO_2 induces vasoconstriction and a consequent restriction of cardiovascular volume. Head elevation, in the absence of venous obstruction, promotes brain relaxation.

Extensive hemodynamic monitoring (arterial lines, central venous pressure lines, Swan-Ganz catheters) should be established peripherally and contralateral to the side of surgery. As we work on, in, and around the major venous drainage of the head, use of the contralateral internal jugular vein, or even the subclavian vein, jeopardizes the venous drainage of the neuraxis.

neurotologic procedures consume hours in a microsurgical confine in which dead space and indirect fluid loss are minimal. The risk of overhydration must be avoided.

Neurotologic tumors, notably paragangliomas, are biochemically totipotent, elaborating vasoactive amines, neurohormones, and parahormones, which can seriously compromise and complicate general anesthesia induction and maintenance. Secretory status must be determined preoperatively and anticipated during tumor manipulation. Cranial nerve manipulation can provoke dangerous hemodynamic conditions.

Tension pneumocephalus, air embolism, internal carotid artery interruption, blood transfusion and/or coagulopathy, postoperative airway management, patient positioning, and elevated ICP are problems peculiar to anesthesia for neurotologic procedures with which the team must be familiar.

Nausea and vomiting frequently occur postoperatively in otologic and neurotologic patients. Unpleasantness notwithstanding, nausea and vomiting can compromise the surgical outcome or neurotologic safety and must be avoided. Droperidol is very effective but in the neurotologic patient may prolong emergence and obscure baseline neurologic status. The development of ondansetron hydrochloride and dolasetron mesylate has been a major contribution to the intra- and postoperative management of postoperative nausea and vomiting.

Summary

What transpires on the other side of the anesthesia drape or in the administration of local anesthetic has a direct effect on what happens in the surgical field. What happens or does not happen during the preoperative period has a direct effect on the outcome of the surgical procedure.

SPATIAL ORGANIZATION

Within the operating theater, the patient is the center of attention. The orientation of the patient in the operating room (OR) relative to the surgeon, other team members, equipment, and visitors (observers) must ensure maximum efficiency and use of all resources to manage all planned and unintended consequences of the procedure. Space at the head, in or near the surgical field,

is limited. All avenues must be cleared for the surgical access. Figure 12–3 defines the author's version of this organization.

Operating Room Table

The patient lies supine on an electrically operated OR table as close to the edge of the side of surgery as possible, with the head at the foot of the table; this positioning allows the sitting surgeon's knees to fit beneath the operating table in all positions. After securely strapping the patient into position, testing is done to ensure secure mobility in all directions. The head is placed directly on the padding of the OR table (or on sheets to accommodate large shoulders). The head is turned away from the surgeon, placing the operative site "up." The head must not be moved once positioned; rather, the head is rotated with the OR table. Head holders are not used, with the exception of the Mayfield head clamp, which is used in suboccipital procedures. The anesthesiology team is positioned at the foot of the bed, away from the endotracheal tube. The remote control for the OR table also is positioned at the foot of the bed, on the surgeon's side, to allow easy access to OR circulating nurses, who are

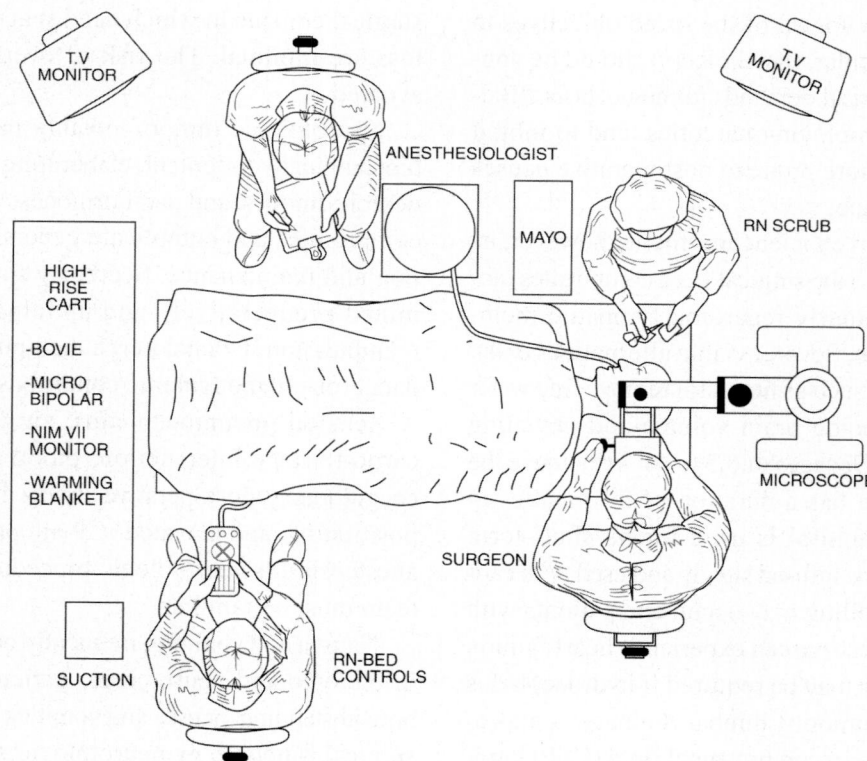

Figure 12–3 Preferred spatial orientation of the operating room.

stationed there to move the bed as directed. Liberal padding helps avoid pressure-related complications.

Surgeon

The surgeon sits at the head end of the table at the operative site—for middle cranial fossa surgery, at the head of the table, and at the side for all other surgeries. Chair height is adjusted to surgeon comfort. The chair is sturdily backed for support; stools are avoided.

Assistants

The nurse surgical assistant (scrub) is positioned at the table opposite the surgeon. She/he may stand or sit. Foot pedals (for the BOVIE®, bipolar cautery, and drill) are placed at the feet of the scrub for her/his control. The only controls the surgeon operates are for instruments such as the laser and the CUSA® (Cavitron Ultrasonic Aspirator). A Mayo stand is situated at the front of the scrub and is highly organized, holding only the more commonly employed instruments. A "back table" for solutions, drapes, gowns, and the less frequently employed instruments stands at the back of the scrub.

The scrub must be actively involved in the procedure. Television monitors are positioned in the room corners so as to be clearly visible. A small "nurse-monitor" is placed on the stand of the microscope within the viewing range of the nurse. Commands and expected responses are rigidly uniform (eg, only "on" means on, only "off" means off).

Microscope

The microscope is positioned at the table head and aseptically isolated with special drapes.

Anesthesiologist/Anesthetist

The anesthesia team and their monitoring equipment are positioned at the table foot on the same side as the scrub yet isolated from the scrub, Mayo stand, and surgical field. Electrophysiologic monitoring outputs, intravenous and other lines, and catheters exit the patient/table to the anesthesia side for access.

The position of the endotracheal tube is verified and secured to the mouth edge secured additionally to the patient's chest and is directed to the bed foot. The dead space of long connectors must be accounted for from a ventilatory standpoint. The anesthesia personnel administer anesthesia, nothing else; they have no additional room or surgical responsibilities.

Monitor/Control Boxes

Control boxes and monitors (eg, BOVIE, bipolar cautery, dynamic compression stockings, irrigators, monitors, etc) are stacked at the foot of the table to allow access to both front and back panels. Control panels face the anesthesia team, the surgeon, and the scrub. Back panels are situated for easy access for battery changes. Settings are rigid and altered only by the surgeon and/or the anesthesiologist.

Supplies

Related instrumentation, sutures, gloves, prostheses, implants, and commonly used appurtenances are stored in the room for prompt access.

Video recording/broadcast and photo-documentation equipment is stored in the room. Patient confidentiality must be ensured.

Observers

Observer access is restricted. The aseptic environment provides safe entry to two observers. An observer apparatus is fitted to the microscope for direct vision while multiple high-quality images are provided for staff as well as observer involvement. Should the proximity of an observer become necessarily less than "remote," as occurs commonly in middle cranial fossa surgeries, in addition to the mandatory surgeon's attire, the observer should be gowned and gloved with hands on the chest or "mummified" (Figure 12–4).

For groups, closed-circuit television broadcast of the procedure "live" to a remote room is appropriate. Sound for dialogue is useful.

INFECTION CONTROL

The ear, like all other parts of the aerodigestive tract in which otolaryngologists operate, is colonized with bac-

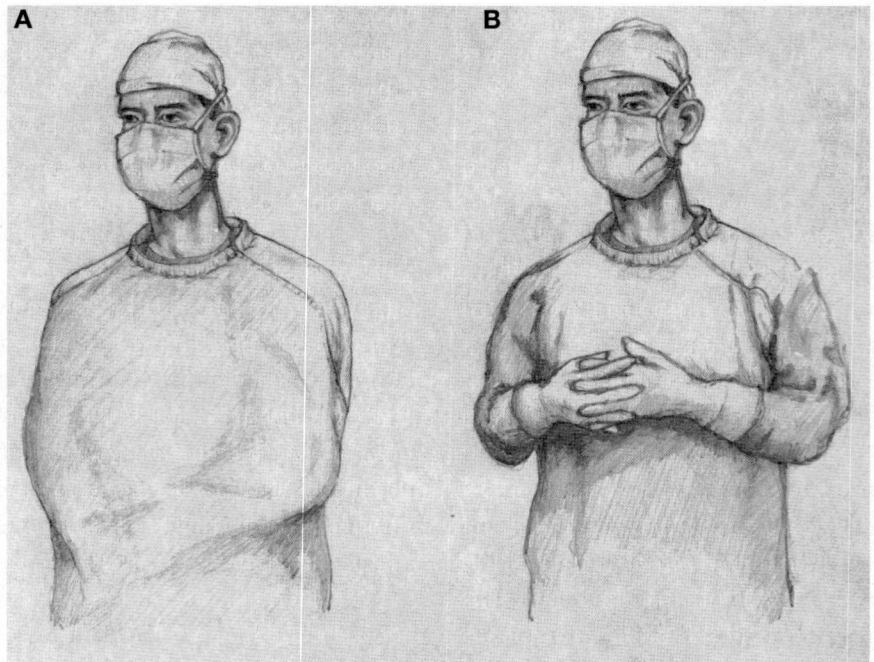

Figure 12–4 *A*, mummified observer. *B*, Surgeon's gloved hands must never be dropped to side or placed under the arms but should be held in front of the chest.

teria. Otologists routinely operate in surgical fields that are considered contaminated. Neurotologic surgery, on the other hand, exploits the ear as an avenue to the surgical target. Accordingly, even this kind of surgery is considered clean-contaminated. Clean fields simply do not exist. The above notwithstanding, wound colonization does not necessarily translate into, or relate to, wound infection. Furthermore, wound infection is not necessarily caused by colonizing bacteria. The host–bacterium interaction is poorly understood. Colony count is important; that is, there is a threshold colony count beyond which host defense mechanisms are overwhelmed and infection occurs. Infection is the direct enemy of surgical success. In addition, the emergence of resistant strains threatens more than surgical success. Infection is to be avoided. In otology, aseptic techniques must be compulsively and rigidly meticulous. Any casual attitude toward aseptic technique that otolaryngologists might have acquired through instrumentation of the oropharynx and related structures must be altered.

The temporal bone surgeon must be absolutely convinced that meticulous aseptic technique is necessary. In otology of the modern era, infection rates are low (1% or so), but even a single infection can have catastrophic

consequences. Poststapedectomy infection, or wound infection, with or without CSF leak, and meningitis following endolymphatic sac surgery, labyrinthectomy, vestibular schwannoma removal, or vestibular nerve section may have life-threatening consequences and are to be avoided. There is no excuse for careless or faulty aseptic technique. No prophylactic umbrella exists under which inadequate asepsis can be tolerated.

The most significant threats to asepsis are people and objects in the OR suite that interact with the surgeon, the scrub, or the surgical field. Observers, particularly those unfamiliar with aseptic technique, must be instructed and then watched by all. Mummification is efficient. The entire OR team must be constantly vigilant.

Modern OR teams know aseptic technique. If a potential break is observed by one, even if based only on a suspicion, it must be acknowledged by all and the situation corrected. Be safe, not sorry. The scrub nurse is regarded as the captain of the aseptic technique guard.

The operating microscope must be draped prior to entry into the sterile field. The surgeon should set all objectives, interpupillary distances, etc, prior to draping. After the face and nose have contacted the scope, reaching up to adjust with a gloved hand courts contamination. The otologic drill and cord must be sterilizable, and, like all other appurtenances running off the table, should not be adjusted below table level by the sterile team.

In neurotologic surgery, it is often necessary to prepare and exclude a field for later intervention. Abdominal fat graft donor sites or free flap donor sites must be prepared and draped for later access. These areas must be respected throughout the case and not disturbed. Violation precludes safe surgery.

If two teams are working simultaneously on separate activities, their interactions must be monitored carefully. Attention to aseptic technique must be heightened; the instruments and personnel of the two sites should not commingle.

The handling of free grafts and prosthetic implants must be particularly assiduous. Free grafts should be harvested and implants delivered to the field immediately proximate to their intended time of application, not left out, risking contamination.

Surgical Preparation

Preparation of the surgical field is compulsive in design to limit colonization of the wound by normal skin contaminants. This preparation must account for the copious irrigation used in temporal bone surgery and limit the contamination of the field by capillary action from the surrounding nonsterile areas. The preparation begins with an antibacterial solution shampoo on the eve of surgery.

In the OR, sufficient hair is shaved to permit isolation of the surgical field. For a postauricular incision, the area shaved extends to about 1 inch around the auricle; far more hair is shaved for neurotologic surgeries (Figure 12–5), whereas no shaving is necessary for transcanal approaches.

After the skin is defatted and adhesive placed to ensure adherence, plastic drapes are applied to the periphery of the shaved area, which is then scrubbed with povidone-iodine soap, and the canal is filled with povidone-iodine solution. A superficial antiseptic preparatory solution is then painted on.

A sterile, nonabsorbent, self-adhering aperture barrier drape is applied, through which the auricle and postauricular region are exposed (Figure 12–6). For neurotologic procedures, a wide-field adhesive drape is positioned and cut out as the incision and exposure evolves. An irrigation collecting system to collect runoff is advisable. The surgical field is thus excluded, and a watertight barrier is established between skin and field. If the drapes do not stick, begin again.

Long drapes then cover the body and table over which all cords and tubing are passed. The sterile team does not venture outside the surgical field (upper chest level).

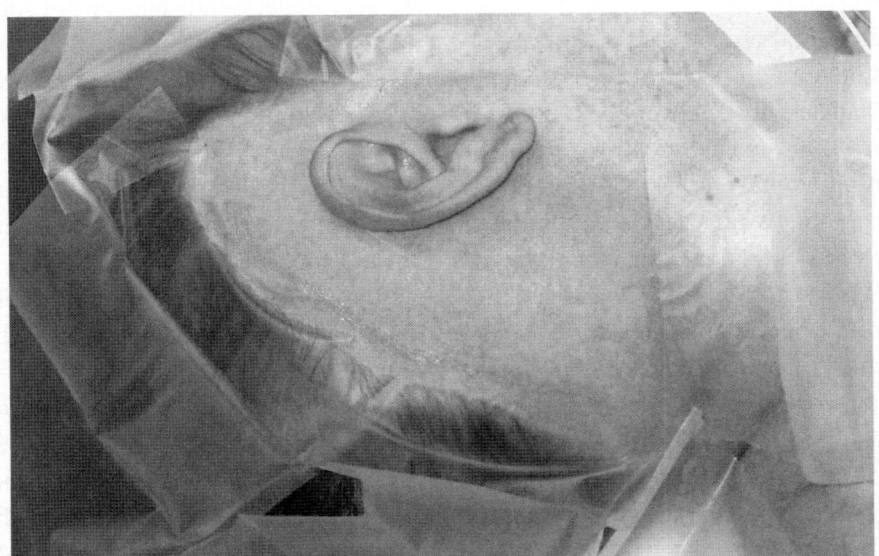

Figure 12–5   Right ear, surgical position. The extent of hair removal and draping for a neurotologic procedure is illustrated.

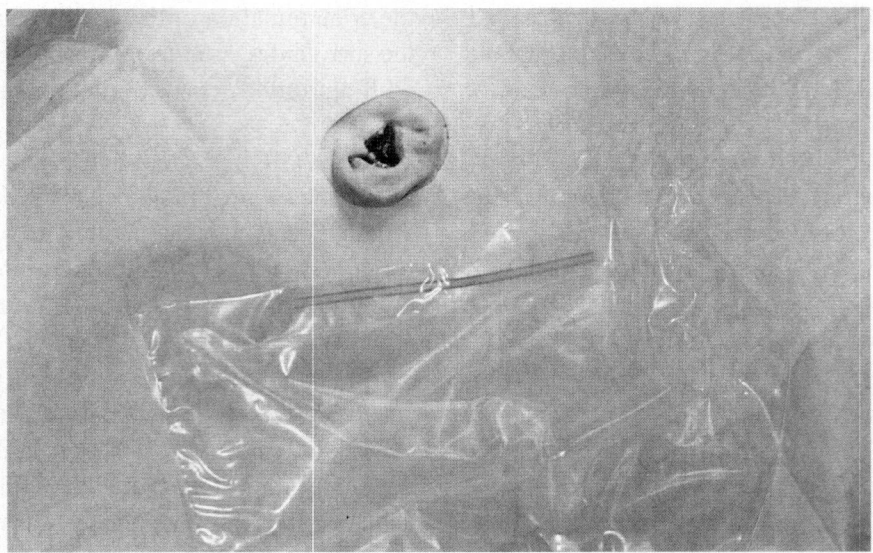

Figure 12–6 Right ear, surgical position. The auricle and postauricle regions are accessible through the barrier drape.

Antimicrobial Prophylaxis

For over 50 years, surgeons have sought improved surgical results and freedom from infectious complication under an umbrella of antimicrobial prophylaxis. The existence of such an umbrella via the application of prophylactic antibiotics is entirely contentious. Antimicrobial prophylaxis decidedly will not cover or excuse faulty tissue manipulation or aseptic technique that lacks integrity.

The aim of antimicrobial prophylaxis is not to sterilize a surgical field but rather to control colony counts so that the host mechanisms are not overwhelmed. Colonization of surgical wounds occurs in over 90%. With aseptic technique, antimicrobial prophylaxis is proposed to limit this colonization. Its efficacy is contentious, particularly in the clean-contaminated wounds of neurotologic surgery. When antimicrobial prophylaxis is used, there is a definitive period during which it is considered effective—within 4 hours of the incision. Therefore, if antimicrobial prophylaxis is to be effective, it should be given parenterally in the OR just prior to making the incision and at regular dosing intervals throughout the procedure. This is particularly important in lengthy neurotologic operations. Extension of antimicrobial prophylaxis to 4 hours prior to incision or more than 24 hours postoperatively is contraindicated.

Antimicrobial prophylaxis should not be "shotgun" but should be directed against the most likely infecting organism, not all organisms present. For example, in chronic otitis media, despite the presence of gram-negative species, gram-positive species, especially *Staphylococcus*, are the usual cause of infection. Antimicrobial prophylaxis should be directed against the latter, not the former, and no more than a first-generation cephalosporin is needed.

As a general rule, data do not support the use of prophylactic antibiotics in middle ear or mastoid surgery. No advantage for antimicrobial prophylaxis has been recorded in surgical success (graft take or hearing results) or reduction in wound infection. The draining ear is a problem. Intuitively, one expects that a draining ear going into surgery would have a higher incidence of failure and infection than a dry ear. This is the case, yet antimicrobial prophylaxis has not altered it. The draining ear is an indication for antimicrobial prophylaxis, but no protocol has, as yet, been proven to be effective.

Unanticipated contamination of a clean environment by the contaminated "chronic ear" is an indication for antimicrobial prophylaxis as illustrated by the following: stapes subluxation in surgery for chronic otitis media; inadvertent violation of the labyrinth, such as uncovering a fistula caused by cholesteatoma, in surgery for chronic otitis media; and CSF leakage or violation of the intracranial cavity in chronic otitis media surgery. Similarly, antimicrobial prophylaxis is indicated in high-risk patients, such as diabetics, the immunocompromised, the elderly, and those receiving implantable devices such as cochlear implants.

Antimicrobial prophylaxis is warranted in neurotologic surgery. The author prefers a combination of parenteral gram-positive coverage (eg, ceftriaxone) given prior to incision and every 12 hours thereafter (for no longer than 24 hours postoperatively) and intraoperative antibiotic irrigation of the field (eg, with gentamicin genitourinary irrigant). In mastoid surgery, there is ample opportunity and indication for this form of antimicrobial prophylaxis, but no established protocol exists. Issues of ototoxicity and related liability exposure impede research and progress.

Antimicrobial prophylaxis provides no magical protection against faulty technique, nor is it a means by which enhanced outcomes can be achieved. The otologic surgeon should not feel medicolegally compelled to use antimicrobial prophylaxis.

Surgical Technique

Healthy, vital tissue is a major component of the host defense mechanisms against infection. Poor tissue handling, with its attendant devitalization, disallows adequate resistance to infection. When tissue is crushed, devascularized, or otherwise traumatized, it becomes vulnerable. Where retained debris, foreign bodies, sequestered bone, bone dust, or inadequate surgery exists, infection is likely. Antimicrobial prophylaxis will not alleviate the liability that accompanies such disrespect for tissue.

Bad surgeons are made, not born. Poor habits translate into poor results. Like antiseptic technique, there is no substitute for meticulous handling of tissue in accordance with the guidelines that have withstood the test of time.

HEMOSTASIS

One fundamental of all surgery is the maintenance of hemostasis. Paradoxically, in microsurgery, where visualization in a bloodless field is an absolute "must," beginning microsurgeons disavow all of the principles they learned from more general surgical exercises. The precision demanded in microsurgery is regularly confounded by poor hemostasis. Special tactics are required

for microsurgical-grade hemostasis and constitute a basic principle, the mastery of which is obligatory.

Infiltration

Local anesthetic with epinephrine infiltration of incision lines is a fundamental component of microsurgical hemostasis. Commercial dental carpules, self-contained and conspicuously labeled, containing 2% lidocaine with varying concentrations of epinephrine are available. These carpules cannot be autoclaved or gas sterilized, so one must make sure that they are bathed in an antiseptic solution for sufficient time prior to use. Expiration dates should be ascertained. As the scrub hands the syringe to the surgeon, the contents of the carpule are announced for all, especially the anesthesiology team, to hear. Via a 27-gauge needle, the skin and subcutaneous tissues are infiltrated. The typical postauricular incision requires approximately 2.5 carpules; in mastoid surgery, injections are made in the external auditory canal, the line of the postauricular incision, and the tragus.

For maximum hemostatic effect, infiltration should be done 10 to 12 minutes prior to the incision. The maximal duration of effect is about 45 minutes. The epinephrine concentration is usually 1:100,000, although a 1:50,000 solution can be used for transcanal incisions. Microsurgical requirements for hemostasis are maximized by this approach, and the size of the field mandates only small amounts. Concentrations greater than 1:50,000 are not necessary. The anesthesiology team must be aware of the concentration and quantity of solution injected. Anesthetic agents minimizing cardiac irritability should be used. Minor heart rate responses are common in children.

When general anesthesia is used, the "carrier" of the hemostatic agent epinephrine is lidocaine. Epinephrine enhances the duration of the anesthetic effect of the lidocaine. Should the chronic ear patient emerge from anesthesia and exhibit a facial paralysis, the possibility of anesthetic effect should be considered for at least 6 hours postoperatively before alternate diagnoses are entertained and reoperation executed.

Topical

The topical application of epinephrine can control modest bleeding. There are several circumstances for which such topical hemostasis may be useful: prior to tympanic membrane graft placement; when dissecting diseased middle ear mucosa or granulation tissue, which bleeds and thus confuses important anatomic relationships; and prior to stapes manipulation; and prior to fistula dissection.

Gelfoam soaked in 1:1,000 epinephrine (as bottled) so that the bioabsorbable sponge is "sloppy wet" can be used as a topical "applicator." It is placed over the area requiring hemostasis and left in place for 5 to 12 minutes while surgical attention is directed to another task. Patience is rewarded by a remarkably bloodless field on removal of the Gelfoam. Minimum cardiac hemodynamic alteration is observed.

Bleeding from bone is a challenge unique to the temporal bone surgeon. Bone wax is a sealant that can be applied to bleeding bone for hemostasis. Applied with a blunt instrument, it can be distributed under a Cottonoid® or placed in a small defect. It is relatively inert but must be regarded as a foreign body and used in infected fields with caution and moderation. Beware of underlying anatomy; for example, avoid compacting bone wax onto an exposed facial nerve.

A diamond bur can be used to achieve hemostasis in bone. Contrary to popular misconception, the diamond bur does not achieve hemostasis by cautery or heat; rather, it pushes bone dust into vascular channels and thus occludes them. Copious irrigation prevents thermal injury to vital regional anatomy.

Defects in the lateral venous sinus can be dangerous as well as exciting. The temporal bone surgeon is sure to encounter this structure in his/her surgical career. Its management in the time of inadvertent instrumentation is critical and should be predetermined as an anticipated event. Continuity of venous return from the head, particularly on the usually dominant right side, is crucial and must be maintained. "Packing it off" is an option only in the most extreme cases. Should the integrity of the lateral venous sinus be violated, immediately occlude the rent with the gloved finger. This prevents air embolism and gives the surgeon an opportunity to reconstitute his/her composure and gather necessary instrumentation. When all is ready, with a large-bore suction handy, the finger is removed and immediately the defect is covered with a patty of wet Gelfoam larger in size than the defect. The patty is then covered by a still larger Cottonoid. Suction and pressure on the Cottonoid for 4 to 5 minutes almost always seal the defect while maintaining the integrity of the flow within the lateral venous sinus.

Electrocautery

Monopolar electrocautery is a helpful tool in macroscopic surgical procedures; however, its spread of tissue desiccation precludes its successful application in the microsurgery world. On the other hand, microbipolar electrocautery (MBPE) is essential to the neurotologic world. It allows exquisitely precise hemostasis by electrocautery while minimizing collateral tissue damage; that is, it can be used to control confounding bleeding on and around vital anatomic structures without causing injury, jeopardizing ultimate functional outcome, or generating complications. It is truly a microsurgical tool. Tips are rarely larger than 1 mm, and smaller tips are commonly in use. Situations in which MBPE is ideal include obtaining hemostasis on dura, exposed lateral venous sinus, the facial nerve, middle ear mucosa/granulation tissue/tumors, canal flaps, and the internal auditory canal.

Power settings vary widely according to manufacturer and model. Prior to application on vital tissue, the instrument should be tested on peripheral tissue. As a general principle, the power setting used for bipolar electrocautery is too high for MBPE systems and should be reduced; for example, the equivalent to a setting of "30" with a macrobipolar electrocautery is approximately 20 to 25 for the MBPE.

A bloodless field is essential to microsurgery—not desirable, *essential*. Should any or all of the above methodologies be ineffective, begin again. This time, wait longer by the clock. Minutes spent achieving hemostasis save minutes to the exponent in the overall procedure and avoid the anguish of an unsuccessful outcome.

EXPOSURE

To be effective, the surgeon, quite simply, must see what he/she is doing. The microsurgeon must resist a paradoxical tendency, perhaps because of the light and magnification provided by the microscope, "to lose sight of the forest for the trees." The vital anatomy of the temporal bone is so compact that exclusion of relationships by viewing only a micro-area owing to poor exposure courts inefficiency as well as complication. Furthermore, the "deep dark hole" of the temporal bone remains exactly that if inadequate exposure prevents the light of the wonderful contemporary light sources from illuminating the field. Ledges, overhangs, and contracted exposure limit the microsurgeon. Complication is a by-product of poor exposure borne of timid surgery or restricted access. "I couldn't have injured the facial nerve; I never saw it!" is the lament of violation of this most vital element of the foundations of surgery.

Microscope

Otolaryngology, in general, and otology, in particular, have led all of surgery into the microscopic era. The advantages of variable magnification have propelled the microscope beyond the fixed-magnification loupe as the optic of choice. Multiple manufacturers of high-grade optics produce instruments of high quality adaptable to each surgeon's unique preferences for otologic and neurotologic surgery.

The operating microscope used can be as complicated as the surgeon desires, but utilitarian necessities are quite simple: high-quality optics with variable magnification, excellent source of illumination, objectives that provide adequate focal distances, a capacity for photo-video-documentation, and adjustable accommodation to interpupillary distances and ocular variations.

Surgeons are not born microscope friendly; skills are learned, and the curve is steeper for some than for others. The microscope must be adapted to the surgeon to satisfy his/her maximum visualization and positions of comfort. Spending hours hunched over a surgical field accommodating to an inappropriate objective focal distance invites poor surgical outcomes and back/neck disease over one's career. The surgeon should sit comfortably in a high-back chair viewing the field through an objective lens affording the necessary focal length; the surgeon should be able to adjust chair/table height, objective lens, etc, to his/her needs. The interpupillary distance should be known and set and the oculars adjusted to the proper diopter setting. The use of eyeglasses must be predetermined. The fields should remain par focal throughout all magnifications. The microscope should be freely moveable on its mounting (floor or ceiling) to allow all adjustment. It should not be locked down to be rendered immobile. Experienced microsurgeons have their equipment so counterbalanced that minor adjustments can be made with the nose, obviating the time and inefficiency of removing one's hands from the surgical task. Video-/photo-documentation is necessary, and equipment should be of the size and placement so as not to interfere with the precise counterbalancing mentioned (Figure 12–7).

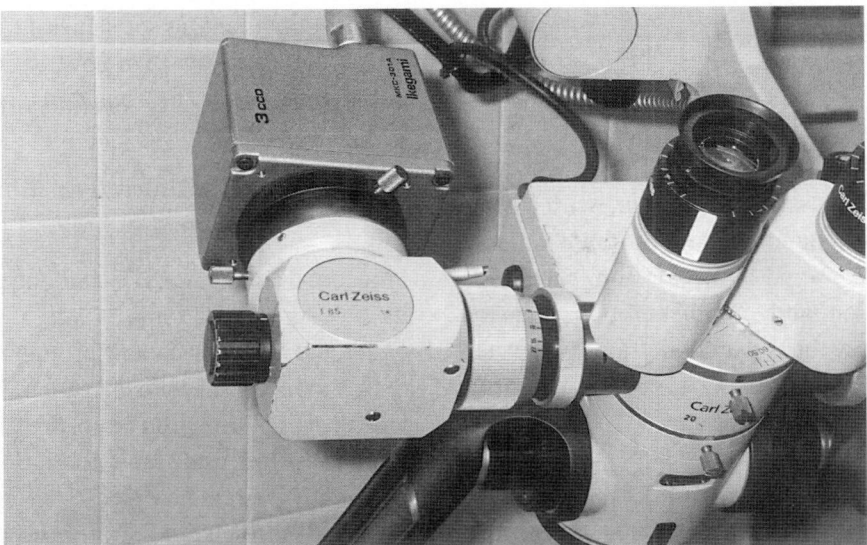

Figure 12–7 The video camera should be mounted on the operating microscope so as not to interfere with counterbalancing.

The operating microscope, shrouded with disposable drapes, is included in the surgical field. The objective lens is covered by plastic to avoid fouling of the lens with bone dust, blood, and other debris. It is always amazing that we spend $100,000 on a microscope and then cover its lens with a scrap of plastic of considerably less value! After the heavy bone work has been completed, the plastic lens cover should be removed to maximize visualization. The microscope is delicate and should not be kicked or bumped by visitors or staff. It survives longer if it is not rolled from room to room; it should be stored covered and proximate to its point of use.

Use the lowest magnification possible to achieve the operative task under way. Broad fields enhance awareness of surrounding and proximate important anatomy so unique to the temporal bone. High magnification should be reserved for those tasks that require this extraordinary level of visualization, for example, dissecting cholesteatoma from the facial nerve or the oval window. Low magnification generates perspective; high magnification slows progress. Use of the microscope is recommended for all operative aspects save incision and closure. One will be more likely to identify an anatomic variant or surgical abnormality using the microscope than with the naked eye. Furthermore, the surgeon's eyes and face are protected from the noxious contaminates generated within the field in this area of prion diseases, acquired immune deficiency syndrome, and hepatitis.

Exposure of important anatomic structures protects them.

INCISIONS

The major routes of access to otologic and neurotologic disease include the tympanomeatal incision, postauricular incision, middle cranial fossa incision, suboccipital craniotomy incision, and lateral skull base incision. The author does not use the endaural incision. These incisions are detailed elsewhere in this text; only basic elements are described in this chapter.

Tympanomeatal Incision

The tympanomeatal incision allows access to the middle ear for exploration, ossicular reconstruction, middle ear mass excision, perilymph fistula repair, etc. It is occasionally used for tympanoplasty. This approach was originally described by Lempert and later popularized by Rosen for use in stapes operations.

Following anesthetic and hemostatic solution local infiltration and cleansing of the external auditory canal with povidone-iodine solution and saline, the canal is dilated by progressively larger ear specula until the nontraumatic maximum snugness is achieved. Fit should be snug to aid in hemostasis. A speculum holder is advised to free the surgeon to use both hands in the surgical procedure.

With "12 o'clock" being superior, the incision begins at "6 o'clock" (a millimeter or so from the inferior annulus), gently curves to just medial to the speculum lip (8 mm to 1 cm) at "9 o'clock" back down to about 2 mm, and ends above the lateral process of the malleus (Figure 12–8). A right-angled Beaver™ blade (#1) is used to make this incision and to medially elevate the flap. A sickle knife elevates the annulus from the tympanic sulcus, and the middle ear is entered. Suctioning of the flap or the tympanic membrane should be avoided as it risks devascularization and perforation. The chorda tympani nerve is identified and gently reflected. In children with congenital aural atresia, beware of large chorda tympani nerves as they may transmit facial nerve motor fibers. The chorda tympani nerve that is obstructing or traumatized should be transected as taste liability is thus reduced. The scutum (posterior-superior canal wall) can be curetted or microdrilled to expose the posterior-superior quadrant, as for stapes surgery. Curetting must reveal the entire oval window, entire stapedius tendon, and facial nerve to be considered adequate.

Postauricular Incision

Freedom from the woes of handling the ear speculum and its exposure limitations, as well as the improved safety of general anesthesia, have promoted the popularization of this incision. The postauricular (Wilde) incision provides particularly good exposure of the mastoid and its process as well as the hidden anterior sulcus of the external auditory canal.

The skin incision follows the postauricular crease and begins at the top of the auricle at least 1 cm posterior to the fold, not in it (Figure 12–9). It extends behind

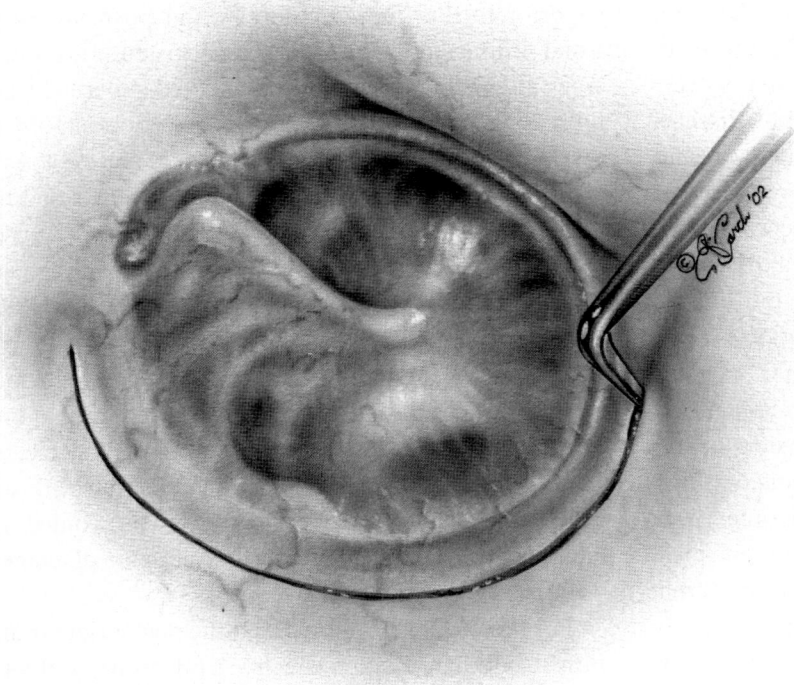

Figure 12–8   The tympanomeatal incision.

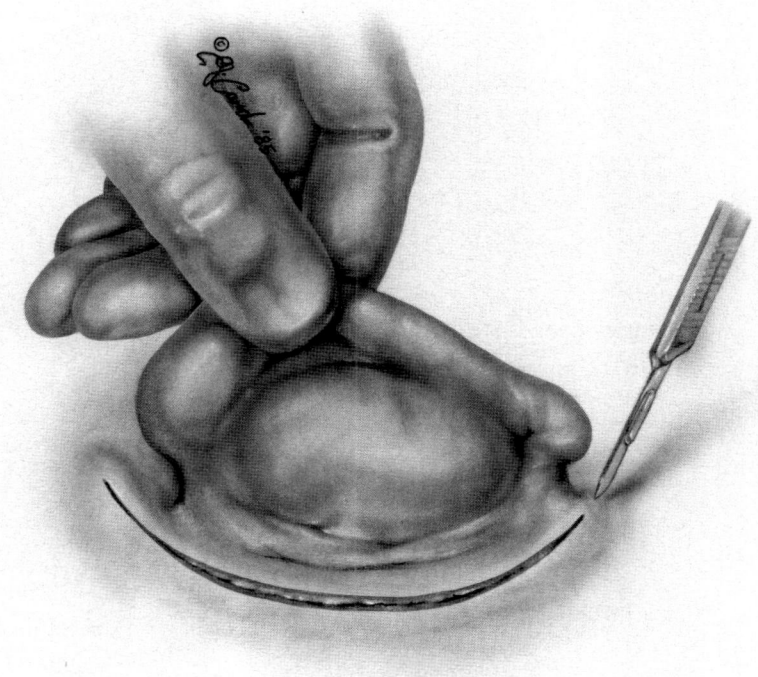

Figure 12–9   The postauricular incision.

the ear and ends over the mastoid tip. In children less than 2 years old, the mastoid tip has not formed; thus, the facial nerve is subcutaneous and vulnerable. Therefore, in infants, the incision is altered to be more posterior or "horizontal." An anteriorly based flap is created by dissecting between the skin and superficial soft tissue overlying the mastoid. The superficial areolar tissue overlying the temporalis muscle is very loose and easily accessible by gently pulling the ear laterally. Sharp or blunt dissection accesses the temporalis fascia for harvesting graft material. Should this be unnecessary, the dissection is simply carried to the margin of the posterior-superior canal.

Soft tissue overlying the mastoid is incised and elevated to expose the bone. A curvilinear incision can be used, but the author prefers a "T"-shaped incision (Figure 12–10). With a cutting cautery, the horizontal incision is carried to bone along the linea temporalis and then an inferior limb is created, which bisects the superior limb and extends inferiorly over the mastoid tip. Prior to making these incisions, it is useful to palpate to be sure that the dura and the lateral venous sinus are covered with bone, a mandatory maneuver in revision surgery. In revision surgery, the soft tissue incisions are placed superior to the linea temporalis and posterior to the usual midmastoid location. The periosteum is elevated from the lateral surface of the mastoid superiorly, posteriorly, and anteriorly. Anterior elevation should not elevate external auditory canal wall skin so as not to risk stenosis. The spine of Henle is a good anterior limit. Alternatively, the canal skin, as demarcated by canal incisions, can be elevated and extracted from the canal should this be intended. Inadvertent canal wall skin tears can be everted and closed, depending on severity, with or without canal stenting. The mastoid process should be completely exposed, as should the root of the zygoma. The ear, periosteal flap with the temporalis muscle, and tip soft tissue are held in the desired position with self-retaining retractors. Excessive force is to be avoided. The facial nerve monitor may educate retractor placement. Bone work can now begin.

For translabyrinthine surgery, the postauricular incision is modified since the mastoidectomy defect is broader superiorly and posteriorly, extending well above the linea temporalis and posterior to the lateral venous

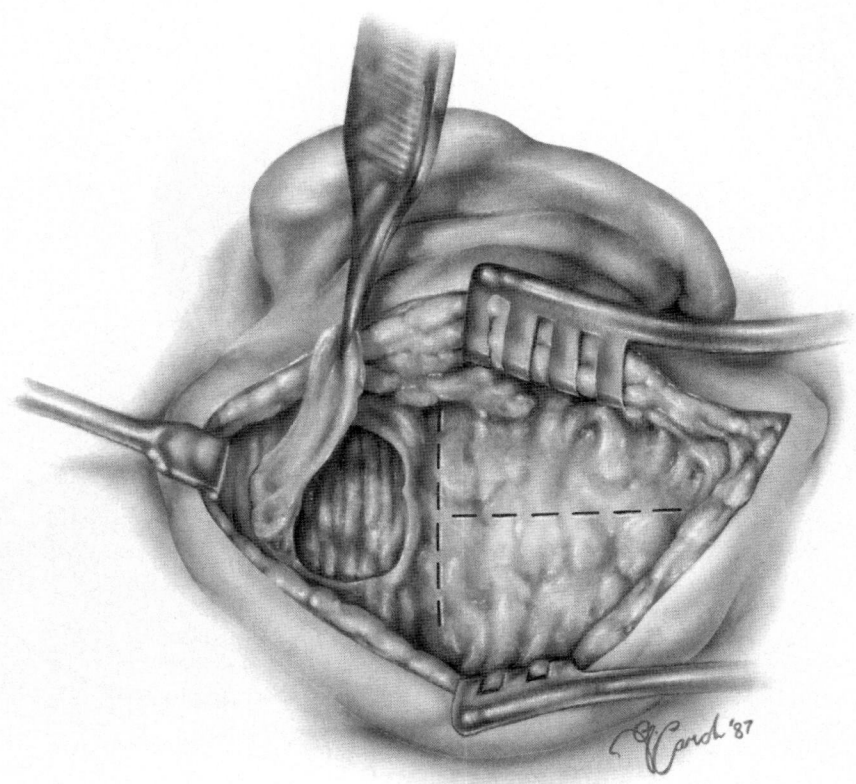

Figure 12–10 The "T-shaped" musculoperiosteal incision.

sinus. As the CSF barrier is violated, the closure must be watertight. Neither the skin nor the periosteal incisions can overlie the mastoid defect. Furthermore, the skin and the periosteal incisions must be imbricated (overlapping or stepped).

After infiltration with local anesthetic/epinephrine solution, the line of the incision is "tattooed" with methylene blue to provide proper alignment for closure. The incision begins some 3 cm above the ear, gently curves two or three fingerbreadths (4 to 5 cm) behind the postauricular crease, and extends 1.5 cm inferior to the mastoid tip. The external auditory canal marks the anterior extent of the incision. The resulting flap is broad-based to optimize its vascular supply and viability (Figure 12–11).

Subsequent to establishing hemostasis, an anteriorly based skin flap is elevated and retracted laterally with double-prong skin hooks. The periosteal incision is imbricated (inset) approximately 1.5 cm from the skin incision and carried down to bone. The periosteal flap is then anteriorly elevated, taking care not to violate the external auditory canal, a potential point of CSF egress. The flap is not extended as far anteriorly as for otologic surgery to avoid creating a dead space in which CSF

might accumulate. The flap is gently retracted over a folded sponge by dura "fish hook" rubber band retractors; kinking the flap is to be avoided. All wound surfaces should be kept moist for the duration of the procedure. For large and inferiorly extending tumors, the inferior limb should extend posterior and inferior to the mastoid process in anticipation of the potential need to perform a facial-hypoglossal nerve anastomosis.

Middle Cranial Fossa Incision

The middle cranial fossa approach has regained popularity. The old version, consisting of a vertical incision through temporalis muscle, was efficient but resulted in temporal wasting and suboptimal postsurgical cosmesis. Contemporary incisions allow mobilization of the intact temporalis muscle with far superior cosmetic outcomes. Furthermore, today's craniotomy is larger as the limits of the exposure continue to be expanded.

Before any hair is shaved, the anterior hairline is marked so as to prohibit incisions beyond it. Since the plane of the internal auditory canal approximates that of the external auditory canal and the root of the zygoma,

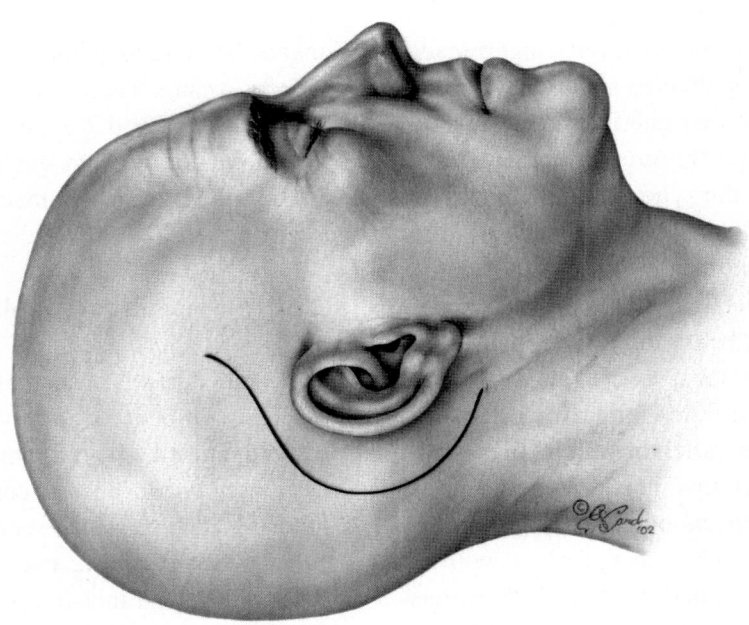

Figure 12–11 The postauricular incision as modified for use in translabyrinthine surgery.

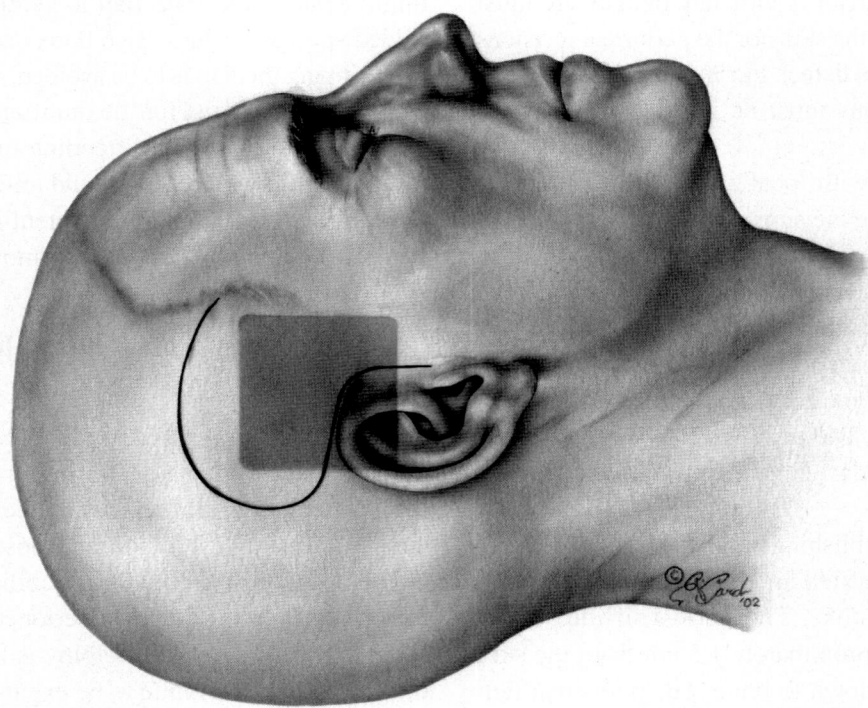

Figure 12–12 The middle fossa incision.

the incision is based at the zygoma, one fingerbreadth anterior to the tragus. It is directed superiorly, curving posterior to the auricle and then anterior-superiorly in the form of a question mark (?) (Figure 12–12). The top of the incision is 8 cm from the zygoma, and the anterior-superior limb is created as far anterior as possible to allow for inferior reflection of the flap. At the zygoma, care is taken to preserve the superficial temporal vessels. The incision should not extend below the zygoma to preserve the frontalis branch of the facial nerve.

Temporalis fascia is harvested for grafting. The temporalis muscle is incised parallel to the skin incision yet well inside it (imbricated); this incision is best located within the most distal aspects of the muscle to allow secure closure. The periosteum is then elevated, with the temporalis muscle pedicled anterior-inferiorly. Free muscle graft can be harvested from its undersurface. The root of the zygoma must be precisely identified; "close" does not count here. The craniotomy should lie 40% poste-

rior and 60% anterior to the root of the zygoma and measure 5 cm square. Therefore, the squamous craniotomy is outlined to extend 2 cm posterior and 3 cm anterior to the root of the zygoma and to measure 5 cm in height. The flap should be gently retracted and maintained as discussed above.

Suboccipital Incision

For the suboccipital incision, the patient is placed in a modified park-bench position with the head secured in Mayfield pinions. The old semisitting position has been largely abandoned. The most common procedures that use a suboccipital approach are acoustic neuroma resection, vestibular nerve section, and vascular decompression.

An "S"-shaped incision is outlined over the subocciput (Figure 12–13). The cephalad aspect of the "S" reaches no higher than the upper one-third of the auricle while its inferior extent is confined to the hairline and

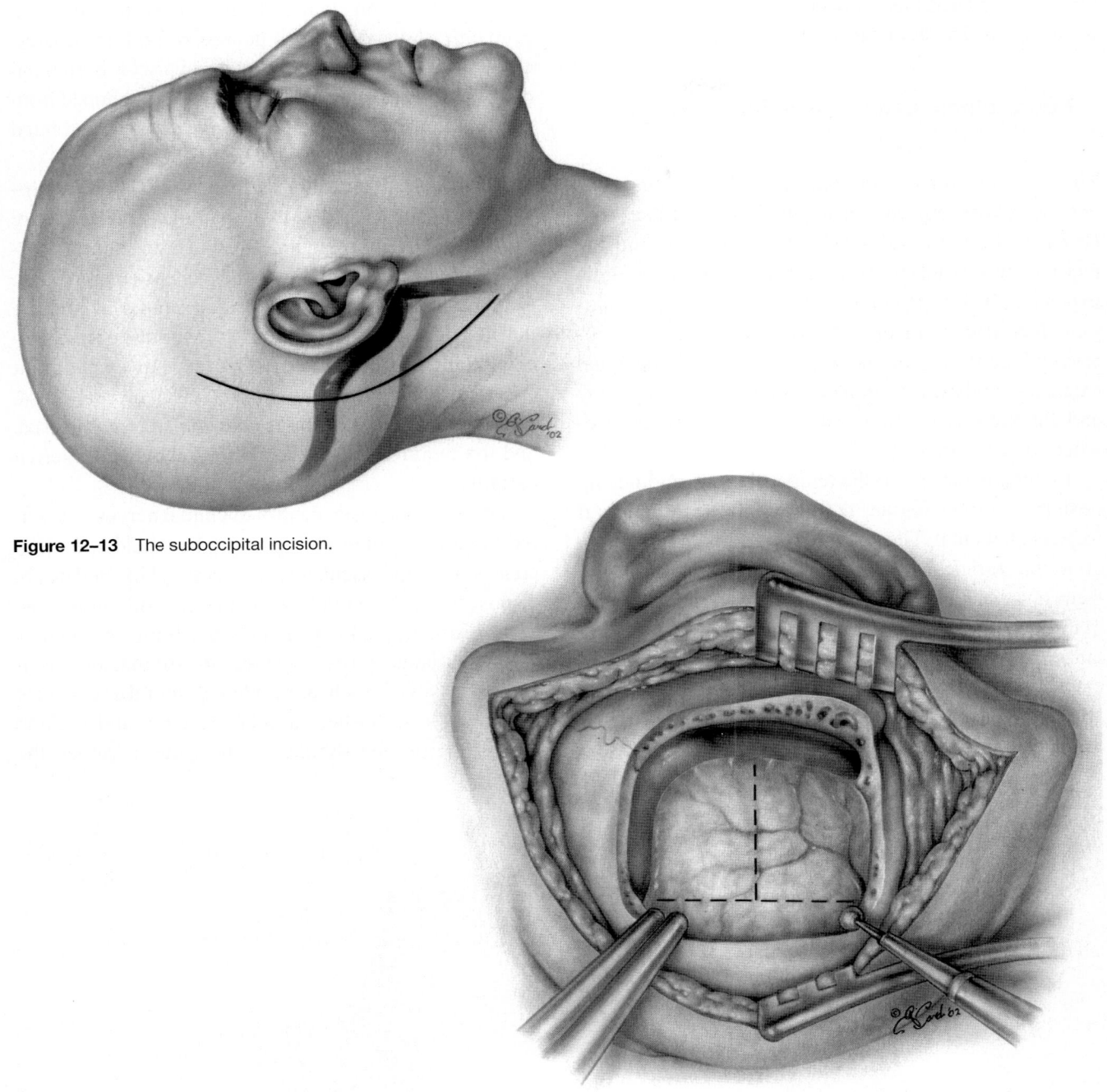

Figure 12–13 The suboccipital incision.

Figure 12–14 The suboccipital craniotomy.

its postauricular extent is approximately 7 cm. The skin is incised, and a 1.5-cm anteriorly based flap is created. The subsequent incision is carried down through the suboccipital soft tissue and upper cervical musculature to bone, again imbricated relative to the skin incision. Periosteum is elevated anteriorly and suboccipital pericranium posteriorly. Heavy retraction is required.

On completion of bony exposure, the suboccipital craniectomy is executed (Figure 12–14). Its anterior limit is the lateral venous sinus, whereas the superior limit is the transverse sinus. Posterior exposure is extended as needed. It is important to remove sufficient bone inferiorly and anterior-inferiorly. The resultant craniectomy is 4 × 4 cm. Emissary veins are isolated and electro-bipolar coagulated. Retrosigmoid air cells are assiduously bone waxed. The dura can then be incised.

Neurotologic Lateral Skull Base Exposure

The exposure for neurotologic lateral skull base surgery necessarily exceeds that required for procedures confined to the temporal bone. The approach, and the incision, must be adapted to each tumor and patient. Basic exposure objectives include exposure of all tumor margins, identification (for control) of vital regional neurovascular anatomy, access to all margins of intracranial extension, and preservation of as much normal anatomy and function as possible. Details are described elsewhere (see Chapter 36).

In general, access to the temporal bone, middle and posterior cranial fossae, the neck, and infratemporal fossa is elemental. The skin incision extends from 3 cm above the auricle, arches posteriorly behind it some 4 to 8 cm, and extends into the neck to approximately the level of the larynx. Should vascularized pericranium or cephalad middle cranial fossa access be required, a vertical extension can be added (Figure 12–15). An extensive, anteriorly based flap is elevated and retracted. If the external auditory canal is to be preserved, it marks the limit of dissection. If the canal is to be transected, a deep cuff of canal tissue is incised and reflected laterally. This cuff is everted and oversewn with horizontal mattress stitches. A subcutaneous flap is developed from tissue anterior and posterior to the canal and is rotated over the closure to further secure it as watertight.

An incision is created over the temporal bone to provide both adequate access to the pathology and to secure a watertight closure (Figure 12–16). Basic concepts parallel those of the less complicated postauricular incision for translabyrinthine acoustic neuroma removal but have the added element of preserving the tissue necessary to cover the temporal bone defect as well as excluding it and CSF from the neck and the infratemporal fossa. The extent of the incision is determined by tumor size and the requirements for control of the distal internal carotid artery.

Proximal and distal control of cranial nerves is essential to optimize their preservation. Proximal and distal control of major vasculature is a matter of life and death. Exposure here must define the element of control: the ability to manipulate structures yet limit unintended, collateral damage as we operate on, around, and occasionally in vessels such as the internal carotid artery. Such control is an established vascular principle, and addition of the microscope should not abrogate it; rather, the

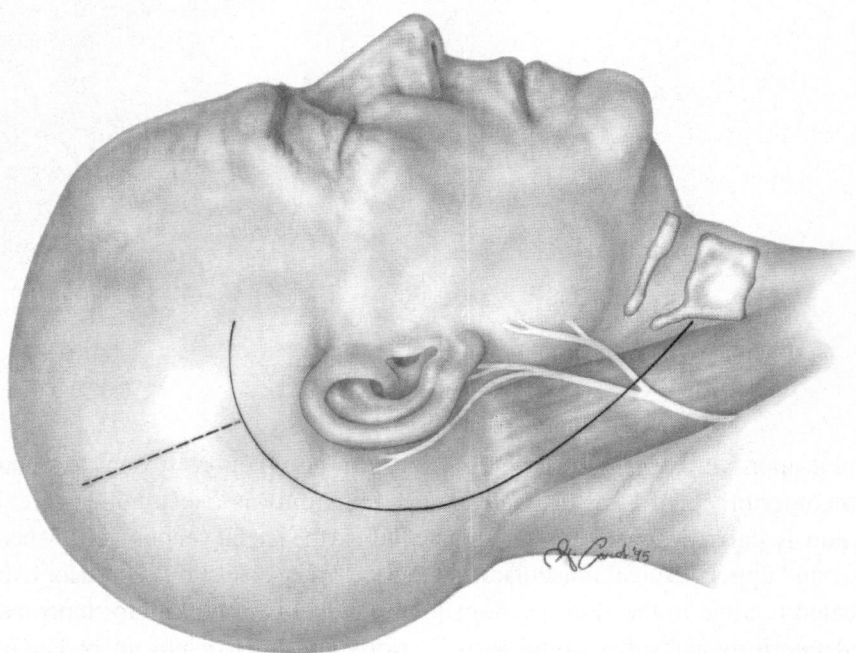

Figure 12–15 The incision used for neurotologic lateral skull base exposure.

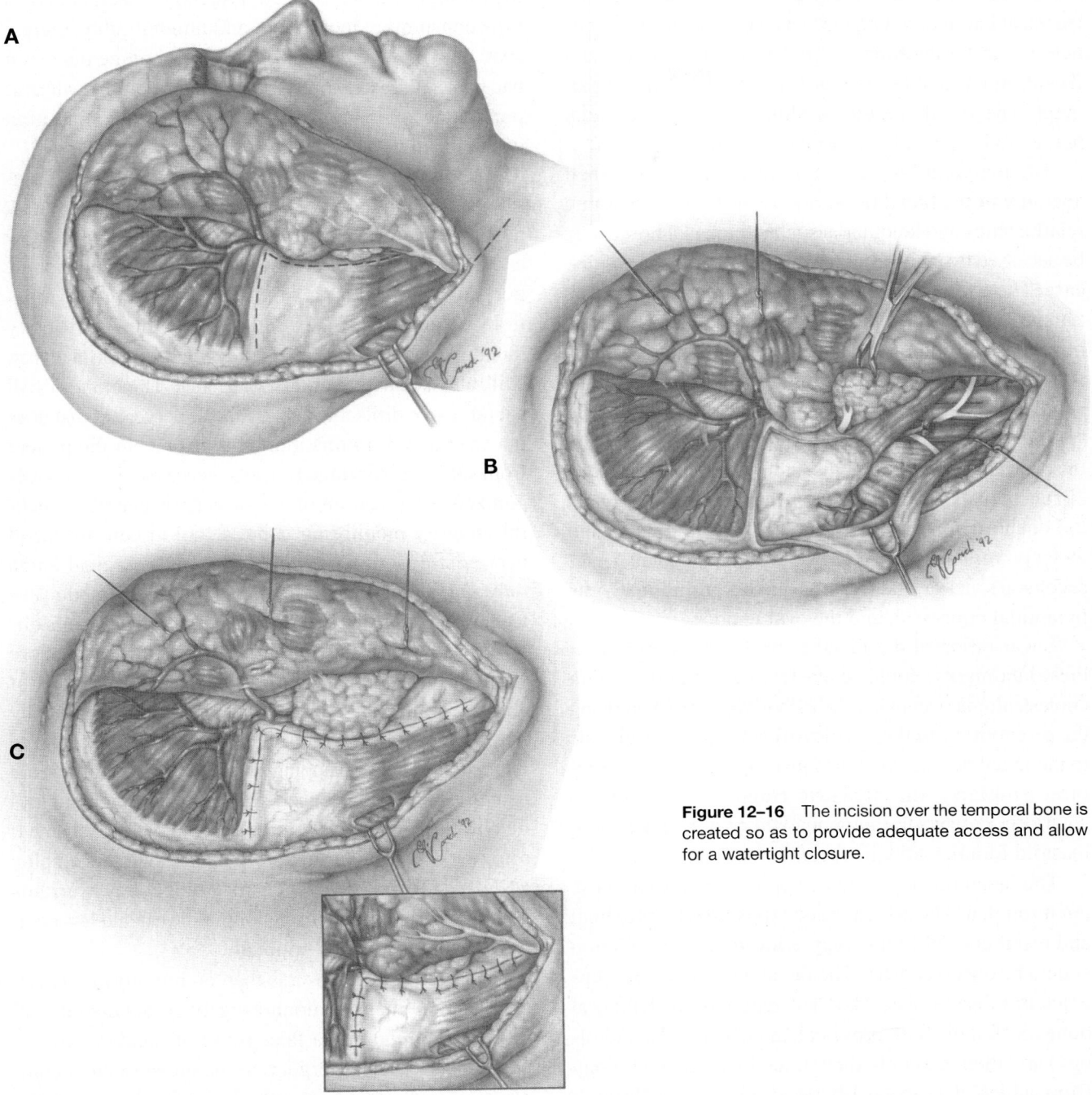

A

B

C

Figure 12–16 The incision over the temporal bone is created so as to provide adequate access and allow for a watertight closure.

exposure must ensure it. Seeing is not the same as being able to do something with "it," be "it" the facial nerve, the lateral venous sinus, or the internal carotid artery.

FACIAL NERVE

Otology is fortunate to be afforded the luxury of readily available anatomic material and systems by which the temporal bone can be studied and operations intensively practiced in the laboratory. There is no excuse for even the newest of ear surgeons feeling insecure with the anatomy of temporal bone structures, particularly the facial nerve—its location, its course, and its variations. Neurotology affords great confidence in the management of the facial nerve, its dissection, tolerance, and overall tactical familiarity, which translates very well to mastoid and middle ear operations. Successful surgery in and around the temporal bone requires both anatomic and technical familiarity with the facial nerve so that the facial nerve may be legitimately looked on as a procedural friend and valuable landmark rather than an impediment. The timid surgeon wishing to avoid the facial nerve "to keep it safe" is doomed to injure it.

The temporal bone surgeon must know the normal anatomy of the facial nerve and recognize its anatomic relationships and landmarks so that the facial nerve may be accessed by many alternative routes in the face of disease. The course of the facial nerve is most stable in its tympanic segment to the external genu, whereas variation is most common in the vertical segment. The facial nerve is most commonly exposed (dehiscent), bereft of any bony covering, in its tympanic segment. Anatomic "pointers" to the facial nerve include the digastric ridge, the chorda tympani nerve, the lateral and posterior semicircular canals, the facial recess, the incus/fossa incudis, the cochleariform process, the "cog," the greater and lesser petrosal nerves, Bill's bar, the eighth cranial nerve, Jacobson's nerve and vessels on the promontory, the pyramidal eminence, and the oval window.

Localization of the facial nerve by the use of all of these landmarks should be mastered. For example, with cholesteatoma occupying the mesotympanum, following the promontory to the cochleariform process leads one to the facial nerve, which lies just superior to this structure. Similarly, the digastric ridge, once dissected anteriorly, delivers the surgeon to the region of the stylomastoid foramen and the facial nerve.

The facial nerve should be approached into disease, not through it. The principles of exposure with proximal and distal control of anatomy prior to its manipulation should be observed here. The facial nerve must be identified in a disease-free, "known" region of the temporal bone (preferably both proximal and distal to the pathology) and then, and only then, traced into the pathology from which it is to be liberated. Operating through pathology to find the facial nerve courts disaster. Similarly, the facial nerve is identified distally at Bill's bar and proximally as well, at its root entry zone in the brainstem. Only then is dissection carried into the acoustic neuroma to separate it from the facial nerve. Cholesteatoma involving the facial nerve at the oval window is likewise challenging. Identifying the facial nerve distally as well as proximally at the cochleariform process facilitates efficient, yet safe, removal from the nerve. Work-ing through friable, infected tissue to the facial nerve is time consuming, inefficient, and unintelligibly aggressive. One may get away with such technique once, but bad habits ultimately breed poor outcomes. When all temporal bone landmarks fail, extratemporal identification of the facial nerve must be considered.

Facial nerve neural integrity monitoring has revolutionized temporal bone surgery as it relates to the facial nerve. Facial nerve neural integrity monitoring is now a recognized standard in most, if not all, neurotologic surgery and is becoming routinely employed in tympanomastoid surgery. Facial nerve neural integrity monitoring is no substitute for knowledge of the anatomy, skillful tissue handling, or experience. The monitor will sound as one drills through the facial nerve, but that does not save one from this indignity or prevent the patient from suffering this tragedy. Facial nerve paralysis is a recognized complication of ear surgery. Facial nerve neural integrity monitoring is but a tool to educate facial nerve dissection; it is to be viewed as a surgical guide only. Facial nerve neural integrity monitoring educates technique. Today the author places mastoid retractors differently because the monitor suggested facial nerve stress in a previously used technique. Dissection of cholesteatoma from the facial nerve is informed by FNNIM to define which maneuvers risk facial nerve injury. Facial nerve mapping and dissection from acoustic neuroma have made its sacrifice rare. The author employs FNNIM in all temporal bone cases, both otologic and neurotologic. All neurotologic procedures should employ FNNIM. Difficult, revision mastoidectomy warrants FNNIM, whereas monitoring for middle ear and less complicated cases remains optional.

Bad monitoring is worse than no monitoring. Facial nerve neural integrity monitoring that is not operational lulls the surgeon into a false sense of security. All OR personnel, from the surgeon to the nurse to the technicians, must be familiar with electrode placement, the monitor, its audio and video outputs, artifacts, and power supply.

As the facial nerve is dissected, technique must be appropriate to ensure integrity of the nerve and its intrinsic and extrinsic blood supplies. Guided by the FNNIM, there are some basic guidelines. Never drill bone off the facial nerve; rather, "eggshell" the bone covering the facial nerve and then flake this shell gently from the nerve. Violation of the nerve sheath increases the probability of injury. Hemostasis on the surface of the facial nerve is achieved with MBPE at a low setting. Removing the facial nerve from the fallopian canal for a short distance can be achieved without significant functional effect owing to the support of the intrinsic blood supply of the nerve. Mobilization of two consecutive segments usually adversely affects functional recovery. Proximal to the labyrinthine segment, the facial nerve has no sheath; small manipulations can have large consequences.

The facial nerve is the map and the highway that guides and illuminates our concourse through the temporal bone. Approaching it as an unwelcome intruder to be avoided breeds contempt, a spirit that underwrites outcomes downgraded from optimum, as well as injury.

MANAGING BONE

Bone is a tissue with inherent biologic and physical properties that requires techniques distinct from those applicable to soft tissue. In no other intraosseous human anatomy is there so much vital nonsupport function as exists within the temporal bone. Necessity has served as the mother of an evolution of strategies designed to meet this challenge. Magnification has served to induce *special* microsurgical techniques that serve as a collective fundamental for surgery of the ear. Modern otology and neurotology have far evolved from the elegantly deft artistry of our mallet-and-rongeur-tooled fore-fathers. Nowadays, the rapid removal of large expanses of bone as well as small patches of bone overlying incredibly delicate anatomy is required.

Otologic Drills

Unlike the belt-driven dental drills of the past, which struggled to produce a few thousand revolutions per minute (rpm), modern biotechnical industry has produced instrumentation of such scope and power that a concept of "bone dissection" has arisen. Pneumatic or electrical systems producing 50,000 to 70,000 rpm provide a technology in which bone literally melts away, allowing a surgical perception not unlike the touch of a scalpel on soft tissue (Figure 12–17). Tools of enormous elegance, they also are capable of enormous destruction.

Burs rotating at 50,000 to 70,000 rpm generate enormous heat capable of tissue destruction and thermal injury to immediately adjacent structures (eg, the facial nerve). The use of continuous irrigation in sufficient quantities is necessary to cool the field. The irrigation can be drill mounted, irrigated into the field by the nurse, or, as the author prefers, via a suction-irrigator. Copious irrigation also serves to prevent fouling of both cutting and diamond tools with bone dust. Fouled burs cannot remove bone efficiently and prompt the use of excessive pressure, which, in turn, risks thermal injury and surgeon error and defeats the technology.

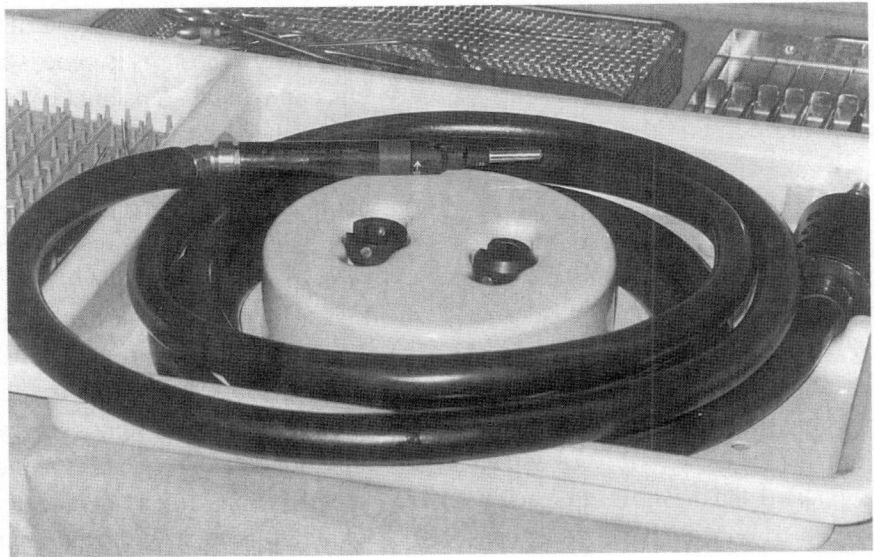

Figure 12–17 Currently available otologic drills, such as the one pictured here, have given rise to the concepts of bone dissection.

Drills of all size and shapes, equipped with a wide variety of bells and whistles, are available to the otologic surgeon. Although most current models are pneumatically powered, great interest is being afforded electrical power. Up until the last 10 years, a reliable electrically powered system did not exist. Now we are fortunate to have noteworthy alternatives that are multipurpose and of high quality. The device chosen should be capable of producing 50,000 to 70,000 rpm; be sized for microsurgical application; have a handpiece design that is ergonomic and appealing; have a bur-changing technology that is technically easy to understand and operate quickly; use low-cost, high-quality burs; be self-maintaining and self-oiling; be quiet and environmentally safe; be efficiently sterilizable; be totipotential to accommodate a wide variety of surgeon preferences (irrigating or not reversible, angled or straight handpieces, and neuro-attachments); be foot pedal controlled, with an ergonomic and safe design; and be reliable and supported by a sales force/service center of high quality and easy access. Products meeting these criteria are available from a number of companies (eg, Medtronix, Anspach, Inc., Smith + Nephew, Linvatec).

As in all surgery, control is an issue. The author prefers to concentrate on the surgical task at hand rather than search for and operate the drill foot pedal. The scrub nurse operates the pedal according to a precise communication protocol: "drill off" and "drill on" are the only variables. All other commands are disregarded. Drill speed is not a variable; the reverse function is not used. Working with a stable team in the OR is a distinct advantage. Alternatively, the surgeon may opt to control the drill foot pedal as a matter of preference.

Some drilling "do's and don'ts" have emerged as principles:

- The handpiece should be well balanced so as to allow the unit to be held like a pen. Unlike a pen, however, the cutting surface of the bur is its side, not its tip.
- Use the microscope for *all* drilling.
- The largest bur possible should be used. Small burs penetrate and injure.
- Hands should be supported and the drill held securely. When aggressively fluted burs approximate irregularities in bone, they have a tendency to skip or "flip." These terms imply loss of control and the potential for unintended consequences. Keeping the drilling landscape devoid of ledges/edges helps defeat this tendency.
- One purposeful, continuously pressured drill stroke is more efficient and safer than multiple inefficient, dangerous strokes.
- Keep the field clean. If necessary, stop frequently to irrigate away bone dust/bleeding. You will injure what you cannot see.
- The perforation of bone by a bur is to be avoided. Broad saucerization and wide-field exposure allow more light to reach the field and more room for instrumentation. Working under ledges or in holes is ill-conceived.
- Develop the existing anatomy; do not create it. Confident and broad exposure of the anatomy that exists transcends a timid dissection that creates confusing mounds, ledges, and edges that look like anatomy.
- The diamond bur is structurally and functionally different than a cutter. The cutter is designed to remove large expanses of bone rapidly, whereas the diamond bur is for less aggressive, finer tasks. The diamond bur removes bone, but slowly. It has less of a tendency to incise underlying soft tissue or sinuses as it pushes material ahead of it. Its smoother edge rejects the "flipping" noted above; hence, it is employed for delicate tasks such as exposing the facial nerve and the lateral venous sinus and blue-lining the semicircular canals. Because of its stability, it is preferred intracranially. The diamond bur generates great heat, and the field must be kept well irrigated. Hemostasis in bone is achieved by diamond bur application. As stated above, the diamond bur pushes bone dust ahead of it into open vessels and diploic canals in bone, obliterating them to achieve hemostasis. The incorrect assumption that the diamond bur cauterizes bone by heat is dangerous as it risks local thermal injury.
- Use all of your senses when drilling. Drilling through the aerated temporal bone generates a characteristic chatter. As the bur approaches the compact bone of the middle and posterior cranial fossae, the tegmen, the external auditory canal, or the bone overlying the lateral venous sinus, a characteristic, high-pitched whine is emitted. With experience and the elegance of 70,000 rpm, you will also develop a touch-sense for this auditory correlate.

- Like a sculptor, release the anatomy from the bone that holds it prisoner. Develop anatomy broadly, not at a focused point. For example, in approaching the vertical segment of the facial nerve, it is better to delicately develop the area both proximal and distal to the nerve rather than deepen a hole devoid of perspective.
- Beware of bone dust; it is osteogenic and can impair the vibratory function of the ossicular chain.

With the advent of laser technology, the popularity of microdrills has waned. Microdrills do exist, however, that are designed for maximum micropotential, as in drill-outs of obliterated footplates and in cochleostomies.

Curette

With both drill and laser technology at apparent zenith, the curette is rarely used. Nonetheless, the curette remains a popular tool for stapes exposure as the scutum must be removed for exposure of the oval window and related anatomy. Some principles regarding the use of the curette include the following:

- Like a bur, the cutting surface of the curette is its side. Use the largest curette possible.
- Curette bone parallel to, never across, the long axis of a vital structure, for example, the chorda tympani nerve.
- Sharp instruments require less force and lessen the likelihood of errors.
- Cutting strokes should be bold, long, and purposeful rather than whittling.
- Remove bone fragments and blood for better visualization.
- Never curette upwards from an undersurface. Work from visible exposure down.

Hemostasis in Bone

The special form and structure of bone dictate control of blood loss for exposure as unique. Summarized below:

- The diamond bur is efficient and usually employed.
- Bone wax is useful in controlling bleeding from bone surfaces such as the marrow in the mastoid tip. Bone wax is a foreign body; therefore, less is more. Caution must be used when obliterating large-caliber vessels, such as the lateral venous sinus or dural veins at the tegmen. Enormous amounts of bone wax can be forced into the vessel, beyond intended limits. Embolization is a risk in the lateral venous sinus, whereas at the tegmen, subdural collection is a hazard.
- Multiple, small areas of bleeding in diploic bone, or bleeding at the mastoid tip, are controlled well with Gelfoam soaked in epinephrine. Surgicel™ can be packed into sinuses in bone or used to compress bleeding sites while managing them.
- Monopolar electrocautery use risks injury to underlying soft tissue. It is not used in the temporal bone.
- The defocused laser beam offers excellent microsurgical-grade bone hemostasis.
- For vascular lesions of the temporal bone, embolization of the tumor and its bed affords considerable diminution of intraoperative bone bleeding.
- Copious cool irrigation evacuates bone dust, clot, and related debris. It also induces vasoconstriction of small diploic vessels, inducing an element of hemostasis.

POSTOPERATIVE CARE

The immediate postoperative care after general anesthesia or local anesthesia with heavy sedation is directed toward any respiratory depression. Until the patient is awake and responding, he/she should be under continuous observation, by a nurse if possible or by a relative if a nurse is not available.

Dehydration from persistent vomiting is seen occasionally after operations that open the labyrinth and requires appropriate intravenous fluid management.

Postoperative thrombophlebitis, although not at all as common as after abdominal operations, is nonetheless a potentially dangerous complication of ear surgery. If the patient cannot be out of bed within 24 hours, the wearing of elastic support stockings until he/she is ambulatory is a very simple and effective prophylactic measure that prevents stagnation of blood in the femoral veins.

Postoperative facial paralysis that is noted immediately after surgery and that does not disappear in 1 or 2 hours must be assumed to be caused by surgical trauma, with the possibility of a depressed fracture or severance of the nerve. Immediate (within 24 hours) exploration and decompression or repair of the facial nerve are indicated if the status of the nerve is not certain.

Facial paralysis that begins after an interval of several days may be assumed to be caused by edema of the nerve in the fallopian canal with the probability of spontaneous recovery without further surgery. Because the time of onset of facial paralysis is a determining factor in whether to explore surgically, facial nerve function must be determined after every temporal bone operation as soon as the patient can respond.

Intact canal wall types of procedures, such as routine stapedectomy, myringoplasty, tympanoplasty with and without mastoidectomy, and endolymphatic sac procedures, require only a mastoid-type dressing for approximately 24 hours. After application of the dressing, either a sterile cotton plug, a postauricular "Band-Aid" type of dressing, or both, is all that is required.

Postoperative dressing changes are at various intervals, depending on the procedure, but until the incision is healed should proceed as follows:

1. The surgeon scrubs the hands and arms with a soap containing pHisoHex™ or povidone-iodine and dries them with a towel.
2. The speculum is introduced and the cavity inspected. If there is no infection, nothing is introduced beyond the speculum, and the less done to the cavity, the better.
3. If there is beginning infection, there is an increase in the drainage, which begins to appear cloudy (instead of clear and serous) before it becomes frankly purulent. In this event, the cavity must be cleaned thoroughly using sterile microsuction. In addition, the patient should use antibiotic/steroid otic drops two to three times daily in the ear and should receive an appropriate oral antibiotic as determined by culture and sensitivity results. With such prompt and intensive treatment, the infection should subside quickly before it can penetrate deeply into pneumatic cells to become chronic.
4. In the absence of infection, intracavitary medications are not necessary and probably retard epidermization. An exception is the case in which the vertical portion of the endaural incision tends to close too rapidly. Aqueous gentian violet, 2%, applied to the incision every 4 to 7 days, retards adhesion of the cut surfaces and promotes epidermization of any unhealed areas.

Further details of postoperative care are considered with the individual surgical procedures that follow in subsequent chapters.

SUMMARY

Napoleon has been recorded to have said, "Manage the details and the war wins itself." Rigid adherence to the basic principles of temporal bone surgery ensures a concert of details, which, as a whole, generally portends a successful outcome. Surgery of the temporal bone, within which lies as complicated anatomy as the human knows, presents special challenges. Contained herein are time-tested fundamentals to help meet the challenges effectively.

SUGGESTED READING

Canalis RF, Lambert PR. The ear, a comprehensive textbook of otology. New York: Lippincott & Wilkins; 2001.

Doyle KJ, Brodersae BR. Anesthetic considerations. In: Jackler RK, Brackmann DE, editors. Neurotology. St. Louis: Mosby-Yearbook; 1994. p. 701–11.

Glasscock ME III, Hart MJ. Management of the patient undergoing neurotologic surgery. In: Jackler RK, Brackmann DE, editors. Neurotology. St. Louis: Mosby-Yearbook; 1994.

Jackson CG. Insuring success in tympanoplasty. Audio-Digest Otolaryngol Head Neck Surg 1996;29.

Jackson CG. The chronic draining ear. In: Gates GA, editor. Current therapy in otolaryngology—head and neck surgery. 6th ed. St. Louis: Mosby-Yearbook; 1998.

Jackson CG, Glasscock ME III. Neurotologic skull base surgery for glomus tumors. Diagnosis for treatment planning and treatment options. Laryngoscope 1993;103(11 Pt 2 Suppl 60):17–22.

Jackson CG, Glasscock ME III, Strasnick B. Tympanoplasty: the undersurface graft technique-postauricular approach. In: Brackmann DE, Shelton C, Arriga MA, editors. Otologic surgery. 2nd ed. Philadelphia: WB Saunders; 2001. p. 113–24.

Jackson CG, Netterville JL, Glasscock ME III, et al. Defect reconstruction and cerebrospinal fluid management in neurotologic skull base tumors with intracranial extension. Laryngoscope 1992;102:1205–14.

Jackson CG, Schall DG, Glasscock ME III, et al. A surgical solution for the difficult chronic ear. Am J Otol 1996;17:7–14.

Jackson CG, Storper IS. Antimicrobial prophylaxis in otology and neurotology. In: Johnson JT, Yu V, editors. Infectious diseases and antimicrobial therapy of the ears, nose and throat. 2nd ed. Philadelphia: WB Saunders; 1996.

Manolidis S, Pappas D Jr, Von Doersten P, et al. Temporal bone and lateral skull base malignancy: experience and results with 81 patients. Am J Otol 1998;19 Suppl 6:S1–15.

13

Lasers in Otology

S. GEORGE LESINSKI, MD

Over the past two decades, four lasers have been approved by the Food and Drug Administration for otologic surgery in the United States: two lasers in the visible light spectrum, argon (514 nm) and KTP (potassium titanyl phosphate) (532 nm), and two in the infrared, carbon dioxide, (10,600 nm) and erbium:YAG (yttrium-aluminum-garnet) (2,960 nm). These lasers have increased surgical precision while reducing mechanical trauma to the inner ear and facial nerve. Otologic lasers have now been widely accepted for otosclerosis surgery. Many studies have demonstrated improved clinical results for primary and, in particular, revision otosclerosis surgery compared to standard nonlaser techniques. Otologic lasers have been used successfully for vaporizing glomus tumors, acoustic neuromas, small arteriovenous malformations, and, in chronic ear surgery, granulation tissue and cholesteatomas, particularly on a mobile stapes. All four lasers have proven clinical efficacy and safety for these applications provided that the surgeon employs appropriate energy guidelines and microsurgical techniques. More recently, otologic lasers have been employed for myringotomies, coagulation of the membranous labyrinth for benign positional vertigo (BPV), tissue "welding," and stabilizing prostheses by drilling holes into the incus or malleus. These latter applications still lack convincing evidence that lasers offer a significant clinical advantage over alternative techniques.

Which laser is best for which otologic procedure? Is the laser's wavelength important? What potential future applications do lasers offer for otologic surgery? Understanding the biophysical effects resulting from the laser's electromagnetic (EM) energy being absorbed by the EM fields of the atoms in the target tissue provides the scientific foundation to answer these questions. This submicroscopic world is composed of powerful EM fields, a domain that is very different from the world we experience through our senses. It is governed by rules of physics (quantum mechanics) that are counterintuitive to our daily experience and often seem to contradict the laws of Newtonian physics, the physics that most of us studied in college.[1]

This chapter first focuses on essential principles of quantum mechanics that explain the interaction of light and matter. Then the results from relevant laboratory experiments that compare the effects of different lasers on water, bone, and collagen are cited. Medical lasers approved for otologic surgery and their safe energy parameters are detailed. Next, specific laser surgical procedures are discussed. Finally, with some reservation, the author speculates on potential future applications for otologic lasers.

INTERACTION OF LIGHT AND MATTER: QUANTUM THEORY

To understand how the EM energy fields of light interact with the EM fields of atoms and molecules, we must examine the submicroscopic structure of matter at dimensions unfamiliar to our senses (smaller than 10^{-10} meters). To journey into this submicroscopic realm, we will leave our familiar world of solid, stable matter and enter the violent world of charged particles vibrating, spinning, and orbiting at unimaginable speeds, creating powerful EM forces and containing kinetic energy beyond our imagination.[2] This is "where the action is" when light interacts with matter.[3]

Although matter appears solid and static to our senses, the atoms and molecules composing matter are neither solid nor static.[4] Molecules are 99.99% "empty space." Contemporary subparticle physics teaches us that all matter is composed of miniscule vibrating "strings" of energy.[5] The frequency and pattern of each string's vibration determine its charge, mass, and energy. The vibrating strings are thus divided into quarks, electrons, or force particles. Three strings combine to form either a positively charged proton (two "up" and one "down" quark) or a neutral neutron (two "down" and one "up" quark). Protons and neutrons vibrate and rotate at extremely high frequencies but are bound into a nucleus by strong nuclear force strings called "gluons." Almost unimaginable energy is released when a nucleus is split (nuclear fission in the first atomic bomb). Enormous nuclear energies are also generated when protons and neutrons fuse to make denser elements (nuclear fusion in the hydrogen bomb). The heat in the core of our sun is generated by the protons from four hydrogen atoms fusing to eventually form helium and radiating its lost energy.

The negatively charged, spinning, and vibrating electrons travel at close to the speed of light until they are trapped into an "orbit" by the positively charged protons of the nucleus. This EM force is thousands of times weaker than the strong nuclear force. Powerful EM force fields are created by the electrons spinning and orbiting at half the speed of light. The negatively charged electrons are captured by the positively charged protons within a nucleus. An "electron cloud" is produced because each electron "orbits" the nucleus at 1 billion trillion (10^{21}) times per second, essentially existing "everywhere" at the same instant; thus, the dimensions of our atom are now defined by this powerful EM field. The diameter of a carbon atom measures approximately 10^{-11}M, but, like all atoms and molecules, 99.9% of its volume is empty space. Visible lasers can be passed through optical fibers but are poorly absorbed by water, collagen, and bone.

Because negatively charged electrons repel each other, no two electrons can exist at the same energy level. Second, electrons possess wave properties and therefore can exist only at specific energy levels, mathematical integers of their wavelength. As electrons decay to a lower "allowable" orbit, they emit the exact quanta ("wavelength") of EM energy that is lost.[6] Conversely, because electrons are allowed to orbit only at very spe-cific energy levels, a molecule's electrons can absorb only that quanta ("wavelength") of EM energy that will move it precisely to an allowable higher level.

Nearly all atoms are bound into molecules by sharing their outer orbiting electrons. One or more outer shell electrons are either donated to another atom or are shared with another atom so that these outer electrons begin to orbit the second nucleus, thus binding the two atoms together with EM force fields. The covalent and ionic bonds pulling atoms together into a molecule are elastic. All of the atoms vibrate in relationship to the central core of the molecule. Similar to the "allowable" energy levels of electron orbits, atoms vibrate at specific resonating frequencies where the surrounding EM fields are balanced. As the frequency of the atoms' vibration increases or decreases, the exact amount (quanta) of energy gained or lost is emitted as an EM photon with a specific wavelength. Finally, the entire molecule rotates as a unit, and this molecular rotation absorbs or emits specific photons as the frequency of molecular rotation changes.

Table 13–1 indicates these four levels of kinetic energy stored within a molecule and the types of EM photons that each kinetic energy level will emit or absorb.[7]

The total amount of kinetic energy contained within a molecule imparts its translational energy, that is, the vibration of that entire molecule in relationship to its neighboring molecules. The average amount of translational energy of molecules within a system is termed "heat." The more three-dimensional motion each molecule has in relationship to its neighbors, the hotter it is. The amount of translational energy determines whether that group of molecules will exist as a solid (lowest), liquid, or gas (highest).

Light is a form of EM energy made up of units called photons. All EM waves travel at the speed of light (3×10^8M/s). The primary characteristic of an EM wave is its frequency or wavelength. One photon equals one complete wavelength of EM. The energy within a

Table 13–1 SITE OF EM PHOTON ABSORPTION	
Kinetic Energy	Electromagnetic Photon
Nucleus	Gamma
Electrons (orbital)	Ultraviolet, visible, and near infrared
Atoms (vibrational)	Infrared
Kinetic energy molecule (rotational)	Microwave

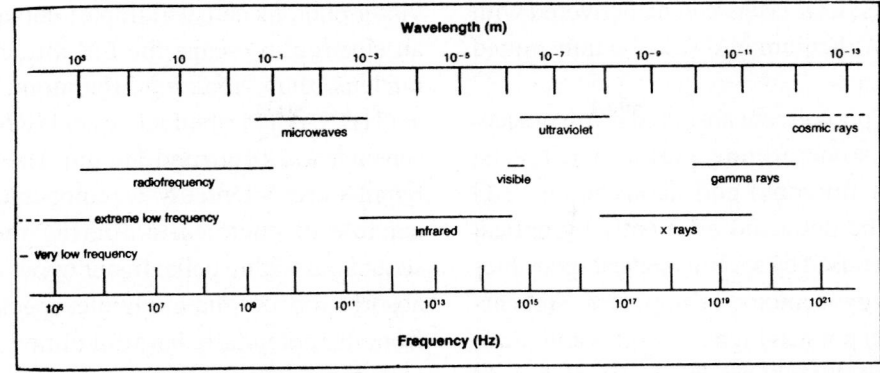

Figure 13–1 Electromagnetic spectrum showing wavelengths and meters and frequencies and Hertz. Photon energy is proportional to its frequency. Low-energy photons (low frequency, long wavelength) are on the left and high energy (high frequency, short wavelength) on the right.

photon increases proportional to its frequency and inversely proportional to its wavelength. The EM spectrum is represented in Figure 13–1, which shows its wavelengths in meters and its frequency in Hertz.[7] The lowest energy frequencies (longer wavelength radio waves) are on the left. As we move across the graph to the right, the amount of energy contained within each photon increases as its frequency increases and its wavelength shortens.

Electromagnetic radiation interacts with matter at all frequencies. Atoms and molecules can be viewed as radiators in which electrons and nuclei vibrate or oscillate at optical frequencies. Atoms and molecules exist in energy states of which only certain values or levels are possible. These values are governed by the laws of quantum mechanics. In emission, the transition is to a lower energy level, and the energy of the emitted photon is precisely equal to the energy given up by the atom or molecule. In absorption, this system is raised to a higher energy level, and then energy gained is equal to the energy of the absorbed photon. Emission or absorption occurs only at energies (wavelengths) corresponding to the transition between allowable energy levels.

Microwaves

The lower-energy photons of microwaves (10^{-1} to 10^{-3} M) are emitted and absorbed by the molecular rotation kinetic energy state. Although molecules can rotate at a large number of closely spaced frequencies, there are ideal "resonating" frequencies at which the molecule's EM fields are balanced. The ideal rotational kinetic energy state of water is 2,450 MHz—the frequency of an 11.8-cm microwave. Microwave ovens emit an 11.8-cm microwave because water selectively absorbs this EM wavelength; thus, more of the EM energy will heat the water of our coffee rather than its container.

Infrared

The infrared wavelengths include far infrared (1,000 to 50 microns), mid-infrared (50 ms to 2.5 microns), and near infrared (2.5 to 0.76 microns). Far infrared photons are emitted and absorbed by the translational motion and the molecular rotation of molecules. Every object warmer than its environment emits far infrared waves. "Night vision" optical instruments have photoelectric cells that detect this far infrared spectrum. There are no far infrared lasers.

Carbon dioxide (10.6 microns) and erbium:YAG (2.9 microns) are in the mid-infrared range. Atomic vibration kinetic energy states emit and absorb the mid-infrared spectrum. Atoms are allowed to vibrate at many closely spaced frequencies, but depending on its molecular bond, there are specific resonating frequencies whose quantum states are ideal. The hydrogen atoms of water ideally resonate at approximately 10^{14} Hz, the frequency of erbium:YAG (2.9 microns); thus, erbium:YAG is the EM photon best absorbed by water. Unfortunately, mid-infrared lasers are absorbed by most molecules. Every known material used for optical fibers absorbs carbon-dioxide laser energy. Therefore, handheld fiberoptic probes are not available for surgery with carbon-dioxide lasers; CO_2 lasers can be delivered with "hollow waveguides"; Erbium:YAG can be transmitted fiberoptically.

The near infrared photons are absorbed by outer electron orbits and by some atomic vibrational levels. Holmium:YAG (2.1 microns) and neodymium:YAG (1.06 microns) can be delivered efficiently by optical fibers. These lasers are used by several medical specialties including obstetrics/gynecology, orthopedics, and cardiology. Because they possess higher energies and fewer molecules can absorb them, these lasers can be passed through optical fibers but tend to penetrate tissue deeply and scatter more readily than mid-infrared lasers. These tissue characteristics make holmium:YAG and neodymium:YAG lasers undesirable for otologic surgery.

Visible Light

The visible spectrum (380 to 760 nm) is defined by those photons that are absorbed and activate photochemoreceptors in the human eye. Visible light photons are absorbed or emitted by the outer electron orbits of the atoms as these electron orbits rise and fall to very specific allowable energy levels. Enhanced studies of visible spectra are important means of spectroscopically analyzing the electron structure of atoms and molecules. The blue-green argon (488 and 514 nm) and KTP (532 nm) laser photons are not absorbed by water molecules and readily pass through most of the molecules of our atmosphere. Red hemoglobin selectively absorbs these blue-green wavelengths. An object appears "red" in visible light because it reflects the red portion of the spectrum while absorbing the remainder of visible light photons.

Ultraviolet

The ultraviolet spectrum (1 to 380 nm) results from large transitions between allowable outer electron orbits. Ultraviolet photons contain higher energy than visible light and thus are particularly useful for photodissociation of specific molecular bonds without heating molecules. The carbon-carbon double bond of collagen can specifically absorb 193-nm photons, the wavelength of one of the eximer lasers, argon fluoride. This laser has been enormously successful in dividing collagen and reshaping the cornea without heating tissue (LASIK [laser-assisted in-situ keratomileusis] procedure). Ultra-violet photons can also impart enough energy to cause an electron to escape the EM attraction of its original nucleus, thus "ionizing" the atom. Deoxyribonucleic acid (DNA) and ribonucleic acid (RNA) are particularly sensitive to 248 nm and 312 nm. These ultraviolet wavelengths are potentially carcinogenic because they are capable of chemically altering the DNA and RNA sequences within cells. In our upper atmosphere, ozone absorbs most of the ultraviolet spectrum, protecting us from the potentially harmful ultraviolet photons.

Laser Photon

Lasers are unique forms of EM energy in that they are monochromatic (one wavelength), coherent (phase locked), and collimated (parallel waves). Depending on the laser's wavelength, the photons will interact with the molecules of the target tissue to produce photothermal effects (eg, "heating" for coagulation or vaporization), photodissociation (eg, excimer laser for LASIK surgery), photoacoustic effects (eg, aluminum garnet laser for lithotripsy), and photochemical effects (eg, ultraviolet lasers for photodynamic therapy).[8]

Lasers have been employed in otology for their photothermal effects to vaporize bone (stapedotomy), collagen (stapedectomy revision), and tumors (acoustic neuroma, glomus tympanicum, cholesteatoma, granulation tissue) or to coagulate blood vessels. The EM laser energy is absorbed by the EM fields, thus raising the molecular translational energy of electron orbits, atom vibrations, or molecular rotations. As the molecule's translational motion (heat) increases, the physical state of those molecules will change from solid to liquid to gas. Coagulation of blood vessels occurs when the collagen translational energy is raised enough to liquify the collagen, and then, as it cools, it congeals into a solid mass, obliterating its lumen. Vaporization occurs when the molecules' translational energy is increased sufficiently to convert its physical state from solid to gas.

LASER–TISSUE INTERACTION: LABORATORY STUDIES

Early applications for otologic lasers focused on otosclerosis: laser stapedotomy and laser stapedectomy revision. Four requirements are essential to safely apply laser energy to the stapes footplate (stapedotomy) or to the collagen sealing the oval window (stapedectomy revision) without damaging the inner ear or facial nerve (Table 13–2): precise optics, efficient absorption by the bone and collagen, minimal heating of perilymph, and no damage to inner ear structures from photons transmitted through the perilymph.[7]

In the early 1980s, the use of argon and KTP lasers to perform stapedotomies became increasingly popular.[9–12] Until 1985, these were the only lasers that had satisfactory optical precision for microscopic ear surgery. Although little laboratory work had been done to establish their safety, clinical studies of visible laser stapedotomy demonstrated that they were safe and effective for vaporizing stapes bone. Could argon lasers be used for stapedectomy revision to improve our clinical results? If the oval window collagen neomembrane could gradually be vaporized without damage to the inner ear, the precise cause for the conductive hearing loss could be identified, the old prosthesis safely removed, and a new prosthesis stabilized in the center of the oval window. Argon lasers were being used by ophthalmologists to coagulate retinal blood vessels, specifically because they were not absorbed by the collagen of the cornea or the fluid inside the eye.

Thermocouple Experiments

By 1985, Sharplan had developed its first microscope delivery system that provided optical precision satis-

Table 13–2 LASERS FOR OTOSCLEROSIS SAFETY REQUIREMENTS
Optics
Bone and collagen absorption
No heating of perilymph
No damage to inner ear or facial nerve

factory for ear surgery. In the laboratories of the Midwest Ear Foundation (MEF), a series of thermocouple experiments were performed to evaluate the relative merits of argon, KTP, and carbon-dioxide surgical lasers and to establish safe energy parameters for both stapedotomy and stapedectomy revision (Figure 13–2).[13,14] Stapedotomies of 0.6 mm were vaporized in fresh human stapes footplates with appropriate energy settings using 0.2-mm "rosettes" for argon and KTP lasers and a 0.6-mm diameter pulsed carbon-dioxide beam. Thin allograft collagen was then placed in an open oval window and was vaporized to simulate stapedectomy revision. Finally, all of the lasers were focused on surface perilymph to evaluate the effects of heating and transmission into inner ears.

These thermocouple experiments were designed to test all four requirements for safely using a laser to perform stapedotomy and stapedectomy revision (see Table 13–2). Following data analysis, the author drew the following conclusions:

1. Provided that safe energy parameters were used, argon, KTP, and carbon-dioxide lasers could be used safely for laser stapedotomy.

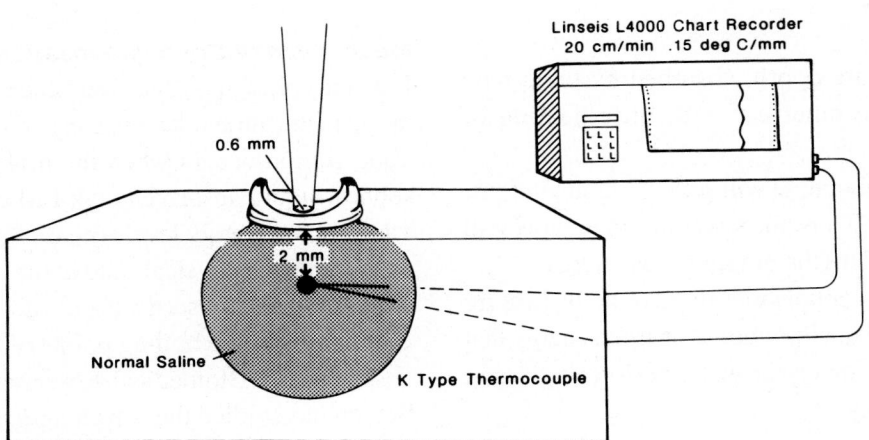

Figure 13–2 Laser stapedotomy performed with argon, KTP, and carbon-dioxide lasers. Ultrasensitive thermocouple in vestibule measures electromagnetic energy transmitted through the stapes footplate. (Midwest Ear Foundation—1984.)

2. The focused argon and KTP beam readily passes through the perilymph without absorption and potentially could damage the inner ear. Therefore, the author recommended using a pulsed carbon-dioxide beam for stapedectomy revision.

Many otologists who were successfully using argon and KTP lasers for stapedotomy challenged the experimental design of these thermocouple experiments, claiming that the black thermocouple did not measure perilymph temperature change.[15–17] This is true! However, the experiment was designed to measure all of the EM energy that passed through the stapes, both those photons that were absorbed by perilymph (heating it) and those that passed through the perilymph that could potentially damage the inner ear. A second criticism was that only a focused argon and KTP laser beam was used for stapedotomy. This also was true. The Gherini/Horn EndoOtoprobe® had not yet been invented for the argon laser.

Several years later, Gherini redesigned the thermocouple experiments and performed argon stapedotomy with the HGM EndoOtoprobe®.[17,18] He used a silver thermocouple positioned in the periphery of the vestibule, not aligned with the laser beam target area on the footplate. He stated that he found "no significant change in perilymph temperature," concluding that the argon EndoOtoprobe® is safe because of the rapid dilution of energy caused by the 14-degree tip diffusion angle of the EndoOtoprobe®. Gherini, indeed, was measuring only perilymph temperature change. He was not measuring the argon EM energy that was being transmitted into the inner ear for three reasons:

1. Argon photons are poorly absorbed by perilymph passing into the inner ear with little heating of perilymph.
2. The silver thermocouple will reflect argon photons, not absorb them. Thus, the silver thermocouple will not record wavelengths of argon EM energy.
3. The silver thermocouple measured only the heating of perilymph and not the amount of argon energy that traveled into the inner ear when performing argon laser stapedotomy.

There are many otologists who have reported the safe use of argon and KTP lasers for stapedotomy (both focused and fiberoptic).[9,10,12,19–22] The author, however, continues to warn the surgeon to avoid applying visible lasers directly into the open vestibule.[23,24]

Safe laser use is enhanced when the surgeon understands laser–tissue interaction. Isolated cases of laser-induced postoperative nerve deafness, facial paralysis, and dizziness have occurred, particularly following laser stapedectomy revision. After confidentially discussing specific cases of complications with the involved surgeon, it became evident that the inner ear or facial nerve damage was indeed caused by inappropriate use of the carbon-dioxide or visible laser. The most common error with the carbon-dioxide laser was using the wrong energy parameter setting ("average" power for pulsed lasers is very misleading; see below). The common error with argon or KTP lasers was employing these visible lasers for revision surgery but using techniques that were designed to be safe only with the carbon-dioxide laser. This chapter was written to help otologic laser surgeons avoid such complications in the future.

The controversy between visible and infrared otologic lasers continues to this day.[16,25–28] It can be resolved by understanding how EM energy interacts with tissue. The EM wavelength is the single most important factor that determines its absorption by water, collagen, or bone. The spectral characteristics of water have been known for over a century. Many spectroscopy and fluence threshold experiments have studied the absorption characteristics of bone and collagen from ultraviolet through the infrared spectrum.

Bone

Mechanism of Bone Vaporization

Izatt and colleagues vaporized bone with a dozen different lasers in the ultraviolet, visible, and infrared spectrums.[29] Vaporization occurs when the molecules composing a solid or liquid absorb enough EM energy to raise their translational energy levels (heat) to the boiling point, at which time the physical state of the molecule changes to a gas. Table 13–3 lists the chemical composition of bone and the respective boiling points of these components.

The Laser Biomedical Research Center at MIT in Boston has studied the wavelength dependency of bone vaporization. High-speed photography documented what occurred during laser vaporization of bone (Figure 13–3). Because the boiling point of hydroxyapatite is so high

Table 13–3 BONE VAPORIZATION BOILING TEMPERATURE	
Composition of Bone	BP
Hydroxyapatite 75%	~1,500°C
Collagen 20%	~300°C
Water 5%	100°C

BP = boiling point.

Table 13–4 BONE VAPORIZATION FLUENCE THRESHOLDS		
Laser	Wavelength (microns)	Bone Ablation Fluence Thresholds (mJ/mm²)
Xenon chloride	.308	12
ErbYAG (yttrium aluminum-garnet)	2.9	12
Carbon dioxide	10.6	15
Argon	.488 and .514	150
KTP (potassium titanyl phosphate)	.532	155

(1,500°C), both water (100°C) and collagen (300°C) are vaporized first, carrying the free hydroxyapatite crystals into the air. Therefore, to ablate bone, the ideal laser wavelength should be absorbed readily by water and collagen. This fact is particularly fortunate for choosing the ideal wavelength for otosclerosis surgery because the same wavelength would be ideal for laser stapedotomy (bone) and laser stapedectomy revision (collagen), while the surface perilymph will protect the inner ear.

Fluence Thresholds

Izatt and colleagues then performed fluence threshold experiments measuring the lowest energy levels (mJ/mm²) required for each laser to begin to vaporize bone molecules.[29] The lower the fluence threshold, the more efficiently the target bone absorbs that photon. Table 13–4 lists the mean fluence thresholds determined by their experiments for the wavelengths relevant to otologic surgery.

Histologic studies with both EM and light microscopy confirm that the more efficient wavelengths produce the "cleanest" ablation craters in bone, that is, less damage at the margins of the crater.

Transmission Spectroscopy: Stapes Bone

To evaluate which photons are best absorbed by the stapes bone, the Biomedical Laser Research Laborato-

ries performed transmission spectroscopy in the ultraviolet through far infrared range (research supported by the MEF).[30] Figures 13–4 to 13–7 graphically illustrate the results. Figure 13–4 graphs the percentage of ultraviolet and visible light that was transmitted through the center of three different fresh stapes footplates that varied in thickness from 130 to 160 microns. The energy that was not transmitted was absorbed by the footplate bone (reflection and scatter are negligible). The stapes footplate selectively absorbs nearly all of the energy in the 250- to 300-nm wavelengths (ultraviolet), and little is transmitted through even the thinnest footplate. The wavelengths of argon (488 nm and 512 nm) and KTP (532 nm) are highlighted with arrows. Absorption of these photons by the stapes footplate is only fair, and an average of 50% of argon and KTP EM energy is transmitted through the footplate.

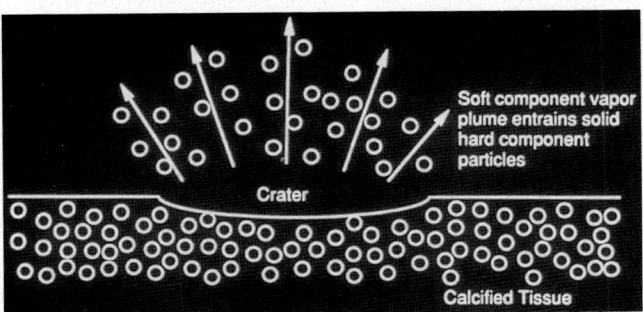

Figure 13–3 Bone vaporization with laser. With sufficient fluence, the photothermal effect of the laser boils water and collagen. Hydroxyapatite particles are entrained in the vapor flume.

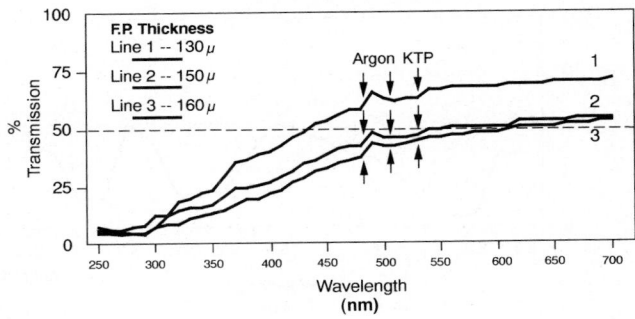

Figure 13–4 Wavelength dependency of stapes footplate absorption. Ultraviolet and visible wavelengths 250 to 300 nm (excimer lasers) are well absorbed. Visible photons around 500 nm (argon and KTP lasers—*arrows*) are not very well absorbed, with approximately 50% of this wavelength passing through a footplate of average thickness (150 microns).

Infrared Transmission Spectroscopy

Stapes Footplate

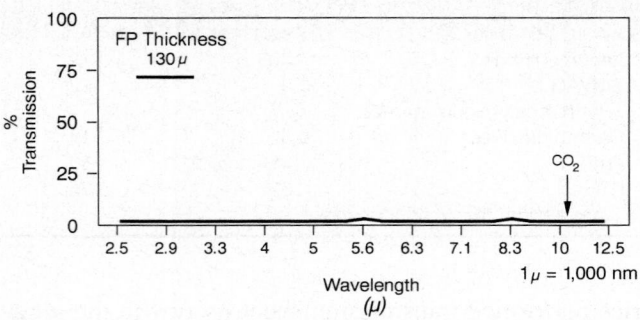

Figure 13–5 Wavelength dependency of stapes footplate (FP) absorption—infrared. The infrared spectrum from 2.5 to 12.5 microns is completely absorbed by even the thinnest stapes FP (130 microns).

Figure 13–5 illustrates the infrared transmission spectroscopy on the thinnest stapes footplate (130 microns). Essentially all of the infrared photons from 2.5 to 12.5 microns were completely absorbed. To evaluate which infrared wavelengths were best absorbed by the stapes, the 130-micron footplate was sectioned with the micrometer into 10-micron sections and transmission spectroscopy was repeated. Erbium:YAG photons (3 microns) are 100% absorbed and carbon dioxide (10.6 microns) are 75% absorbed by the stapes bone at a depth of 10 microns. Therefore, 100% of carbon-dioxide laser energy would be absorbed at a depth of 50 microns in

Infrared Transmission Spectroscopy

Stapes FP—Thin Section (10μ)

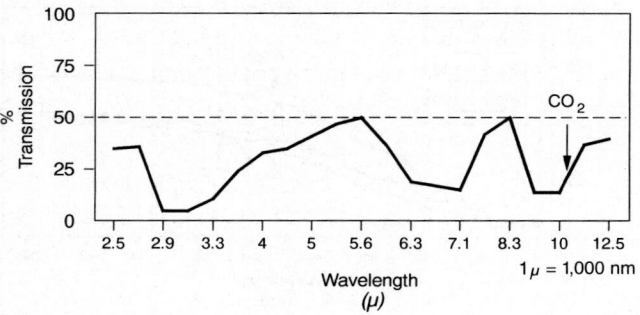

Figure 13–6 Selective infrared absorption by ultrathin (10 microns) stapes footplate (FP). Photons with wavelengths 2.9 to 3.1 microns (erbium:YAG 2.94 microns) are completely absorbed by the stapes FP within 10 microns. Seventy-five percent of carbon-dioxide laser photons (10.2 microns) are absorbed in the first 10 microns of stapes thickness.

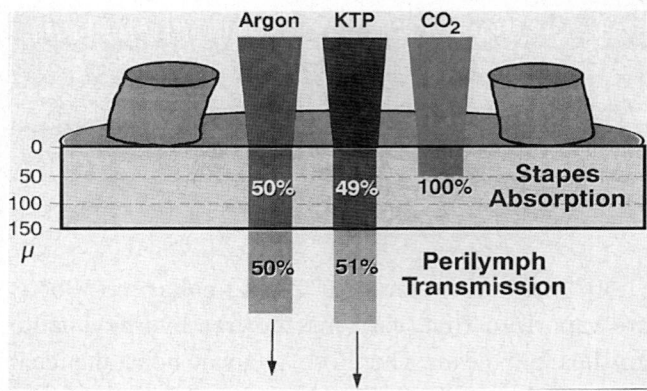

Figure 13–7 Summary of transmission spectroscopy of human stapes footplate for argon, KTP, and carbon-dioxide lasers.

the stapes bone. Figure 13–7 illustrates the amount of EM energy that is transmitted through an average stapes footplate (150 microns) during vaporization with argon, KTP, and carbon-dioxide lasers.

Water

Transmission Spectroscopy: Water

Most soft tissues in the human body contain 50 to 75% intracellular water. Laser ablation of soft tissue occurs when the intracellular water is heated to boiling, exploding the cell. The wavelength dependency of laser–tissue interaction becomes readily apparent because there is an enormous variability in water's ability to absorb photons from the ultraviolet through the infrared spectrum. Figure 13–8 illustrates the absorption coefficient of water based on wavelength.[31] This coefficient is used to calculate the distance that the photon will travel through water until 50% of irradiance is absorbed. The formulae to calculate these distances are beyond the scope of this chapter, but it is worth noting that the absorption coefficient for argon and KTP energy is 10^{-7}, smaller than that for carbon-dioxide energy and 10^{-8} smaller than erbium:YAG photons. In practical terms, an EM photon with a 0.5-micron wavelength must travel 229 feet in seawater before 50% of its energy is absorbed. Submerged submarines use KTP energy to communicate with orbiting navigational satellites because it is so poorly absorbed by water. Conversely, carbon dioxide is 50% attenuated after it travels a depth of 0.007 mm and erbium:YAG a depth of 0.0007 mm. Surface perilymph will rapidly absorb these two infrared beams, protecting the inner ear.

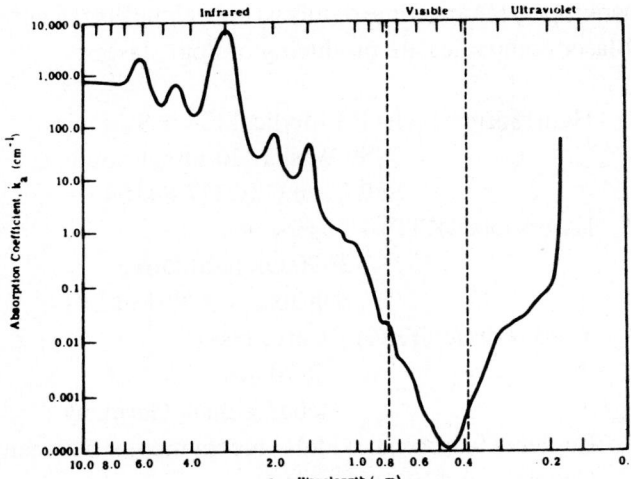

Figure 13–8 Attenuation of seawater as a function of wavelength. Electromagnetic wavelengths at 0.5 microns (Argon and KTP) will travel 229 feet before half of the energy is absorbed. Fifty percent attenuation of irradiance occurs within 0.0007 mm for erbium:YAG (2.94 microns) and 0.007 mm for carbon dioxide (10.6 microns). Reproduced with permission from The infrared handbook. Washington (DC): Office of Naval Research; 1978.

Table 13–5 TRANSMISSION SPECTROSCOPY: COLLAGEN (10 MICRONS)	
Laser	**Absorption (%)**
Argon fluoride (0.193 microns)	100
Erbium:YAG (2.9 microns)	93
Carbon dioxide (10.6 microns)	61
Argon (0.488 and 0.512 microns)	28
KTP (0.532 microns)	18

uate the relative merits of various lasers' wavelength for creating "a clean laser crater" with little damage to the surrounding tissue. In addition, the ideal energy parameters were determined.[38]

As one reviews the details of these histologic studies, a consistent theme resonates through all of them. The cleanest and safest stapedotomies were produced by those wavelengths that were best absorbed by the stapes bone. Because these wavelengths required less energy to vaporize the bone and because there was less photon scatter, laser energy was precisely converted to heating the tissue beneath the laser beam. Damage to the margins of the crater is further reduced by pulsing the laser in tiny microsecond bursts, limiting thermal spread by conduction through the tissue.

However, these infrared lasers must be pulsed in brief microsecond bursts to prevent thermal spread from the surface of the perilymph to deeper layers in the vestibule.

Collagen

Transmission Spectroscopy: Collagen

Yannas performed transmission spectroscopy in the ultraviolet through far infrared wavelengths on powdered bovine collagen and hot cast gelatin to determine which EM wavelengths collagen best absorbs.[32] Although various thicknesses of collagen were used for ultraviolet, visible, and infrared light, the author has extrapolated the data to compare the percentage of photon absorption by collagen at a depth of 10 microns (Table 13–5). Collagen absorbs argon fluoride (excimer laser) best and KTP worst.

Histologic Studies: Laser Stapedotomy

A wide range of surgical lasers as used to perform stapedotomy on both human and animal bones was then evaluated histologically with both light and electron microscopy.[33–38] These studies were performed to eval-

Summary

Quantum theory predicts that each molecule can absorb or emit only specific wavelength photons—those photons whose quanta of energy precisely equals the quanta of EM energy that has been gained or lost as the molecule moves among the various allowable energy levels in its four kinetic energy states. The laboratory studies confirm that laser–tissue interaction is dependent on the laser's wavelength. To produce photothermal effects (vaporize or coagulate), those wavelengths that are best absorbed by the target tissue are the safest to use because there is less energy transmission and scatter through the tissue and because lower power densities can be used. For the well-absorbed photon, thermal conductivity through the tissue should be limited by pulsing the laser beam. There was remarkable consistency between the data compiled with thermocouple studies; spectroscopy of the stapes bone, collagen, and water; and histologic studies. As applied to otosclerosis surgery, these laboratory tests, combined with the clinical experience of many surgeons, lead the author to the following conclusions:

1. Provided that safe energy parameters and surgical techniques are followed, argon, KTP, erbium:YAG, and carbon-dioxide lasers can be used safely for stapedotomy.
2. Because visible laser photons are poorly absorbed by both collagen and water, focused (microscope delivered) argon and KTP energy should not be aimed directly into the vestibule.
3. Infrared laser energy should be pulsed in microsecond bursts to minimize thermal spread to the inner ear.
4. The defocused argon EndoOtoprobe® beam is the safest visible laser to use for ear surgery.
5. The surgical techniques described for carbon-dioxide laser stapedectomy revision can also be performed with the erbium:YAG laser but should not be attempted with the argon or KTP laser.

OTOLOGIC SURGICAL LASERS

The medical laser industry is a rapidly changing, highly competitive business. New surgical applications for lasers are occurring in every specialty at a very rapid rate, often requiring unique laser delivery systems and energy parameters. Acceptance of these new procedures occurs at a more gradual pace, when clinical studies confirm the advantage of a new laser technique over nonlaser alternatives.

Laser companies are pressured to produce lasers with a great deal of versatility so that a particular surgical laser can be used by many surgical specialties. With dwindling resources, the laser committees of hospitals will usually approve the purchase of a new laser only if it has multispecialty applications. These laser committees usually require special certification training by the surgeon and the technical assistant because of perceived additional medicolegal risks. Finally, otologic lasers represent a tiny fraction (less than 0.1%) of the overall medical laser business. This limited "potential market" restricts the leverage that otologists have to influence both the manufacturer and hospitals' decisions.

Over the past two decades, nearly 20 laser companies producing otologic lasers have disappeared (merger or bankruptcy). At the time of this writing (June 2001), only 4 laser companies are producing otologic lasers:

1. HGM (argon)—HGM Medical Laser Systems
     3959 West 1820 Street South
     Salt Lake City, UT 84104
2. Laserscope (KTP)—Laserscope
     3070 Orchard Drive
     San Jose, CA 95134-2011
3. Zeiss (erbium:YAG)—Carl Zeiss
     D-73446
     Oberkochen, Germany
4. Lumenis (carbon dioxide)—recent merger between Coherent and ESC Sharplan
   2400 Condensa Street
   Santa Clara, CA 95051

Visible Lasers

In 1980, Perkins reported a small series of 11 successful laser stapedotomies performed with a microscope-mounted focused argon beam.[8] He concluded that the laser reduced mechanical trauma and increased surgical precision, should improve hearing results, and should reduce postoperative dysequilibrium compared with nonlaser stapedotomy. In 1983, McGee published a series of 100 consecutive argon laser stapedotomies.[9] Hearing results were similar between McGee's laser and nonlaser patients, but the laser patients were less dizzy postoperatively. These argon lasers had originally been designed for ophthalmology by Coherent. The continuous-mode argon energy was carried by a fiberoptic cable to a microscope-mounted "micromanipulator" that then delivered a focused argon beam to the operative field. At a 250-mm focal length, the spot size could be focused down to 0.05 mm.

The HGM argon EndoOtoprobe® developed under the guidance of Gherini and Horn was introduced to otologists in the late 1980s.[16] This handheld probe conveniently delivers an argon beam with a spot size of 200 microns. The 14-degree diffusion angle rapidly increases the spot size as the distance from the probe tip increases.

The KTP laser developed by Laserscope™ under the direction of Perkins is still the only 532-nm laser available for otologic surgery.[10] Its laser energy is delivered via a microscope-mounted micromanipulator. Laserscope has developed several fiberoptic handheld probes. They do not deliver sufficient power density to vaporize stapes bone.

These two visible lasers have ideal optical properties. The laser could be conveniently delivered to the microscope-mounted micromanipulator or a handheld probe through a fiberoptic cable. The micromanipulator can focus the visible beam down to a 0.05-mm spot size at a 250-mm focal length. Because argon and KTP are visible, the laser beam is used at a lower power for the "aiming" beam. Therefore, the laser will always hit the tissue exactly where it was aimed and with the same spot size (parfocal and coaxial). Until 1985, these two visible lasers were the only lasers that were optically precise enough to use for otologic surgery.

Infrared Carbon-Dioxide Lasers

Although carbon-dioxide lasers are the most widely used medical lasers for tissue coagulation and vaporization, the inherent optical properties of the infrared carbon-dioxide laser made the early models too imprecise for the rigid demands of microscopic surgery. Optical fibers will not transmit carbon-dioxide laser; therefore, the beam was delivered from the lasing counsel to a microscope-mounted micromanipulator by a series of 13 mirrors and lenses called the "flexible arm." A minimal amount of trauma (simply moving the laser from room to room) could misalign one or more of these mirrors. A second visible laser beam (helium-neon—632 nm) is required to aim the invisible carbon-dioxide laser beam. This introduces another optical problem: chromatic aberration. When light passes through a lens, it is refracted inversely proportional to its wavelength. As both beams pass through the same focusing lens the visible helium-neon beam is refracted (bent) to a much greater degree than the longer carbon-dioxide beam. It was nearly impossible to keep the helium-neon and carbon-dioxide beams parfocal and coaxial, and the separation worsened with optical misalignment of the mirrors and lenses. Finally, at a 250-mm focal length, the early carbon-dioxide beams could be focused only to a 2-mm spot size.

In the mid-1980s, researchers at Sharplan were experimenting with carbon-dioxide laser reanastomosis of small blood vessels. This application required much greater optical precision. Their engineers developed a microscope-mounted micromanipulator that could focus the carbon-dioxide beam down to 0.5 mm. This prototype model was used by the author for the stapes thermocouple experiments performed in the MEF laboratories and later was the first carbon-dioxide laser used in the operating room for stapedotomy and stapedectomy revision.[39,40]

The early carbon-dioxide lasers were less convenient to use in the operating room than the visible lasers. Each time the flexible arm was attached or detached from the micromanipulator, the operating microscope had to be rebalanced. To ensure proper alignment, the carbon-dioxide laser was test fired preoperatively. A technician routinely realigned the carbon-dioxide and helium-neon beams every few months. In the early models, the alignment of the helium-neon and carbon-dioxide beams could not be adjusted by the surgeon.

Since the mid-1980s, Sharplan continued to refine the optical precision and reliability of its flexible arm—stabilizing the reflecting mirrors and permitting quick readjustment should misalignment ever occur. Its micromanipulator also has been improved. The initial Microslad® allowed focusing the beam size down to 0.2 mm. In the mid-1990s, the Accuspot® could reliably focus the spot size to 0.05 mm at 275-mm focal length. Recently, Sharplan introduced Accublade®, a computer-driven vibrating mirror that distributes a 0.05-mm carbon-dioxide beam homogeneously throughout the area of a target whose shape and size are determined by the surgeon. Accublade vaporizes bone and collagen with remarkable precision and minimal thermal spread.

Finally, the convenience of carbon-dioxide lasers for otologic microsurgery has also been improved. The laser cabinet can be mounted on the base of an operating microscope. The flexible arm parallels the microscope arm, no longer limiting the freedom of motion of the microscope. The laser can now remain attached to the microscope at all times. Preoperative test firing and microscope counterbalancing are no longer required.

In 1989, IL Med introduced the Unilase®, a low-watt carbon-dioxide laser designed specifically for otologic surgery. The small lasing tube was mounted directly on the microscope, eliminating the need for a flexible arm delivery system. This removed 75% of the previous mirrors and lenses, simplifying the optic system and enhancing optical precision. This carbon-dioxide laser was much more convenient to use. The lasing tube remained on the operating microscope when not in use; thus, no additional counterbalancing was required. No pretest firing was necessary. Whenever the surgeon wished to use the laser, he/she merely turned it on. Energy was pulsed at the optimal safe parameters established by the thermocouple experiments. The Unilase proved to be a convenient, safe, reliable otologic laser and was being used by nearly 150 otologists. Unfortunately, this CO_2 otologic laser is no longer commercially available. Although many are still in use, maintenance and spare parts have become a serious problem.

Infrared Erbium:YAG

In the late 1990s, Zeiss perfected a microscope-mounted erbium:YAG laser designed specifically for ear surgery (OPMI®TwinER). As described earlier, spectroscopy studies on water, collagen, and bone and histologic experiments on both human and animal stapes suggested that this laser wavelength would be the most ideal for bone and collagen vaporization. After extensive animal experiments and clinical human trials, the OPMI®TwinER was approved for otosclerosis surgery in Europe in 1997 and in the United States in early 1999.[41–44] I have been using this laser for otologic surgery for 3½ years. As predicted, it vaporizes a precise stapedotomy with little lateral spread of energy (no charring and no significant heating of perilymph). However, this efficient photon absorption introduces two disadvantages:

1. Hemostasis is poor because the lack of lateral thermal spread prevents the coagulation of blood vessels at the periphery of the laser crater.
2. A photoacoustic wave is produced and, theoretically, if large enough, could damage hair cells.[35,38]

SAFE ENERGY PARAMETERS

Besides the laser's wavelength, two additional factors determine its effect on tissue: power density (watts/mm²) and fluence (mJ/mm²)—the time that the power density is applied to the tissue. Power density is determined by the watts of power delivered divided by its spot size. The power density will vary inversely to the area of the spot size. Therefore, reducing the diameter of the spot size in half increases the power density fourfold.

Fluence (mJ/mm²) is calculated by multiplying power density (watts/mm²) times the total time that power den-

sity is striking the tissue. Fluence calculations for visible lasers are straightforward because these beams are delivered in a continuous mode (KTP—quasicontinuous). Infrared lasers are pulsed. When the surgeon sets a Sharplan 1100 or a Coherent 500C laser on superpulse mode and then adjusts the power to 5 watts (average power) and a 0.1-second pulse duration, he/she is actually delivering a single micropulse with a peak power of 600 watts and a micropulse width of 0.075 milliseconds. This micropulse is too powerful for vaporizing the stapes!

Table 13–6 tabulates the safe energy parameters for stapedotomy that were established by thermocouple experiments in the MEF laboratories. The first four columns (average power, mode, pulse duration, spot size) are the variables that the surgeon adjusts. Only one column (peak power) is required for defining how the laser energy is being delivered for the continuous visible lasers. To determine energy characteristics of the pulsed infrared laser, the four characteristics of each micropulse must be known: peak power (W), pulse width (ms), work (mJ/micropulse), and number of micropulses. The final column compares the fluence levels (mJ/mm²) actually being delivered to the tissue.

Visible Lasers

Two watts of argon laser are delivered in a continuous mode by a 200-micron EndoOtoprobe® (Figure 13–9). Spot size at the probe tip is 0.2 mm and rapidly enlarges as the distance from the probe tip increases.

KTP lasers (Laserscope) are focused on the operative field by a microscope-mounted micromanipulator. Because KTP lasers are q-switched, an average power setting of 2 watts actually delivers 780 micropulses in 0.1 seconds (Figure 13–10). Each micropulse contains 6 watts of peak power. Q-switching behaves like a continuous beam (quasicontinuous) because there is not enough of a time interval between each micropulse to allow for tissue cooling. Therefore, average power (30% duty cycle × 6 watts peak power = 2 watts) can be used to define the laser/tissue effect.

Because these two wavelengths are particularly well absorbed by hemoglobin, argon and KTP can be used to efficiently vaporize small amounts of vascular tissue such as granulation tissue, small glomus, or small fragments of acoustic neuroma. Stapes bone vaporization can

Table 13–6 ENERGY PARAMETERS OF VISIBLE (NONPULSED) AND INFRARED (PULSED) LASERS

Visible (Nonpulsed) Laser	Settings				Energy Delivered	
	Average Power (watts)	Mode	Pulse Duration (seconds)	Spot Size (mm)	Peak Power (watts)	Total Fluence (mJ/mm²)
Argon (EndoOtoprobe)	2	Continuous	0.1	0.2	2	6,451
KTP (Laserscope)	2	Q-switched (quasicontinuous)	0.1	0.05	6 (30% duty cycle)	103,216
	2		0.1	0.2		6,450

Infrared (Pulsed) Laser	MD Settings				Micropulse Energy				
	Average Power (watts)	Mode	Pulse Duration (seconds)	Spot Size (mm)	Peak Power (watts)	Pulse Width (ms)	mJ/Pulse	Number of Pulses	Total Fluence (mJ/mm²)
Sharplan CO₂									
734	3.6	Superpulse	0.1	0.5	36	0.6	21.6	8	400
1040	2	Superpulse	0.1	0.5	280	0.09	25.2	2	117
1100A	Flexilase© #7	Chopped	0.1	0.5	130	0.075	9.75	20	450
Coherent CO₂									
5000C	Ultrapulse© #10	Chopped	0.1	0.5	120	0.08	10	20	465
IL Med CO₂									
Unilase	3	Superpulse	0.1	0.5	80	0.2	16	16	592
Erbium:YAG Zeiss									
OPMI®TwinER	(20 mJ)			0.2	200	0.1	20	1	639
	(70 mJ)			0.6	350	0.2	70	1	240

be enhanced by placing a small droplet of blood on the footplate (chromophore) or by overlapping rosettes (char). Because of poor absorption by water, visible lasers are inefficient for vaporizing most soft tissues and should not be aimed directly into the vestibule since the perilymph will not protect the inner ear.

Infrared Lasers

Focused carbon-dioxide laser energy is transmitted to the operative field by microscope-mounted micromanipulators. The energy can be delivered in one of three modes: continuous, chopped, or superpulsed.

When vaporizing tissue, efficiency is improved and thermal spread is reduced by pulsing the energy in a series of micropulses that are on for a fraction of a millisecond. Figure 13–11 illustrates the pulsing parameters of Sharplan 734, the first carbon-dioxide laser used by the author in 1985. Responding to demands by other specialties (obstetrics/gynecology, neurosurgery, general

surgery) for more efficient tissue vaporization, Sharplan began progressively increasing the peak power of each micropulse while reducing its pulse width. Within a decade, Sharplan had raised its superpulse from 36 watts (model #734) to 600 watts (model #1100). Average

ARGON
COHERENT 920

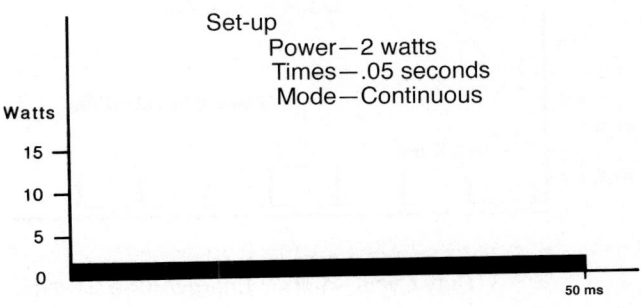

Set-up
Power—2 watts
Times—.05 seconds
Mode—Continuous

Watts

Energy/Pulse 100 mJ

Figure 13–9 Argon lasers are generated in continuous mode. With 2 watts of average power, 100 mJ of work are delivered to the operative field in 0.05 seconds.

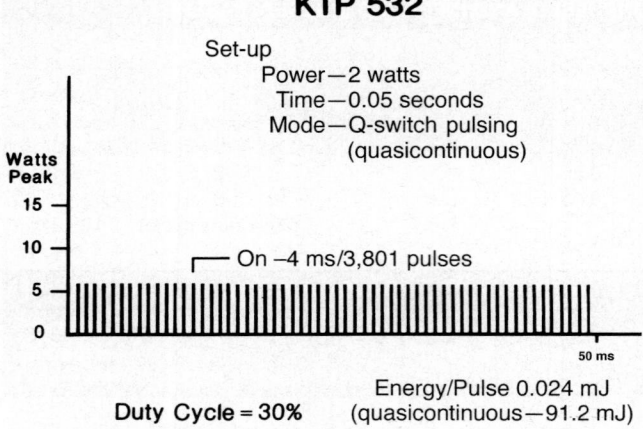

Figure 13–10 KTP lasers are q-switched in a rapid succession of microsecond pulses. Because the micropulse interval is extremely short (8 microseconds), there is little time for tissue cooling. Therefore, tissue response is similar to continuous beam (quasicontinuous). At 2 watts average power, the surgeon delivers 91.2 mJ of work in 0.05 seconds.

power setting do not change this peak power but merely change the number of 600-watt micropulses that were being delivered. At its lowest setting (5 watts average power), the model #110 delivers 600 watts of power, which is much too powerful for the delicate requirements for stapedotomy. Thus, despite a 5-watt "average" power setting, model #734 delivers 14 micropulses, each containing 36 watts of peak power, whereas the #1100 delivers one micropulse of 600 watts peak power. This progression in pulsing power is analogous to bombard-

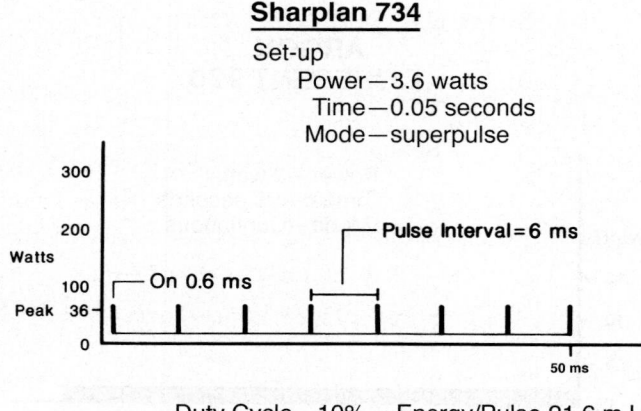

Figure 13–11 Carbon-dioxide laser for tissue vaporization is delivered in superpulse mode. This early Sharplan laser had ideal energy characteristics for laser stapedotomy. Each micropulse contained 21.6 mJ of energy, and a total of 173 mJ were delivered to operative field within 0.05 seconds at a setting of 3.6 watts average power.

ing the target with 14 B-B's (#734) versus one 70-mm caliber bullet (#1100).

The ideal energy parameters for laser stapes vaporization were established in the MEF laboratory. Each micropulse should contain between 10 and 20 mJ of energy (peak watts × micropulse width). Greater than 25 mJ/micropulse caused "flaring"—a literal microscopic "explosion" in which a microflame could be seen rising toward the facial nerve.

IL Med developed the Unilase, a microscope-mounted carbon-dioxide laser designed specifically for otologic surgery. On a superpulse setting, Unilase delivered a series of 16-mJ micropulses (80 watts × 0.2 milliseconds) (Figure 13–12).

By the mid-1990s, the two largest carbon-dioxide laser companies (Sharplan and Coherent) were producing pulsed carbon-dioxide lasers whose micropulses were delivering 500 to 600 watts of peak power. The problem was that average power was adjusted not by changing peak power but by changing the number of micropulses being delivered per second. New software programs were developed in the late 1990s to accommodate the needs of otologic microsurgery. Sharplan developed Flexilase© for its 1100A, 1041S, and 1055S—a chopped mode that delivers 130 watts of peak power and 9.75 mJ/micropip (Figure 13–13). Coherent 5000C followed suit with an ultrapulse setting. Ultrapulse© at a 10-mJ setting delivers 120 watts of peak power and 10 mJ/micropulse.

A word of caution. Several instances of thermal injury to the inner ear or facial nerve have been reported to the author by surgeons who performed laser stapedotomy with Coherent and Sharplan carbon-dioxide lasers in the superpulse mode. Guided by average power settings of 2 to 3 watts, they performed laser stapedotomy but were actually delivering 300 to 600 watts of peak power (one 70-mm machine gun bullets). When laser energy is pulsed, the average power setting is very misleading! Both laser companies have now stopped using the average power setting.

Because of its ideal tissue characteristics, vaporization of soft tissue and bone can be efficiently performed with the carbon-dioxide laser pulsed in brief microsecond pulses to minimize thermal spread. Slight thermal spread around the margins of the crater induces good hemostasis to coagulate blood vessels (or membranous labyrinth); the carbon-dioxide laser should be used on

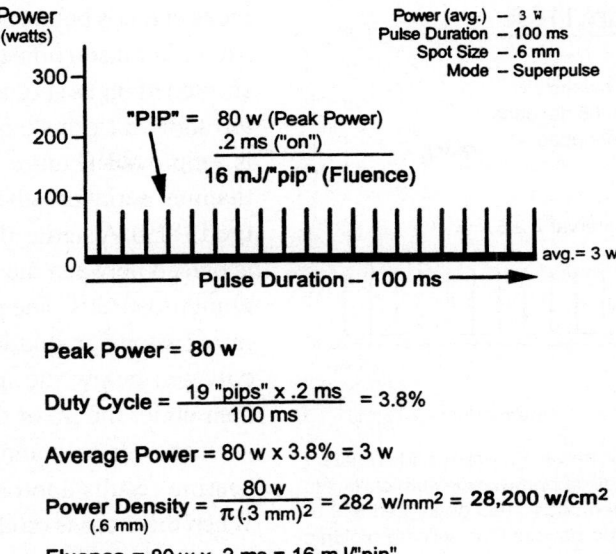

Peak Power = 80 w

Duty Cycle = $\dfrac{19 \text{ "pips" x .2 ms}}{100 \text{ ms}}$ = 3.8%

Average Power = 80 w x 3.8% = 3 w

Power Density = $\dfrac{80 \text{ w}}{\pi (.3 \text{ mm})^2}$ = 282 w/mm^2 = 28,200 w/cm^2
(.6 mm)

Fluence = 80 w x .2 ms = 16 mJ/"pip"

Total Work = 16 mJ x 19 "pips" = 304 mJ

Figure 13–12 IL Med's carbon-dioxide laser (Unilase®)—ideal safe energy parameters for tissue vaporization during stapedotomy and stapedectomy revision.

low power (2 to 3 watts) in a continuous mode for 0.1 to 0.2 seconds with a spot size of 0.5 to 1 mm.

Erbium:YAG

Zeiss's OPMI®TwinEr was designed specifically for otologic surgery. The surgeon can adjust only the milliJoules of the laser pulses (10 to 100 mJ) and the number that are delivered (frequency of 1 to 3 per second). The computer adapts the energy (mJ/pulse) by adjusting both the peak power (200 to 500 watts) and the pulse width (0.05 to 0.2 milliseconds). In Europe, stapedotomies are performed by vaporizing 0.2-mm rosettes at a 20-mJ setting. The author has been performing stapedotomies with a 0.6-mm spot size and a 70-mJ setting.

Erbium:YAG is an ideal laser for vaporizing bone. Soft tissue vaporization is too efficient. Because of lack of thermal spread to the periphery of the target spot, blood vessels are not coagulated; therefore, hemostasis is poor when vaporizing tumor cells. When aimed directly at a blood vessel, erbium:YAG will not coagulate the blood vessel because its pulse width is too short. Coagulation (raising collagen to 65 degrees) requires a continuous mode for hemostasis.

LASER OTOLOGIC PROCEDURES

Laser Stapedectomy Revision

Stapedectomy revision is presented first because in no other area of otology have lasers demonstrated such a profound advantage over nonlaser techniques. Nonlaser revision stapedectomies produce inconsistent hearing results and often damage the inner ear (3 to 20% surgical risk of significant postoperative nerve damage).[44–48] Lasers improve our ability to safely identify and repair the conductive hearing losses encountered and have reduced the risk of postoperative nerve damage to 0.5%.[26,49,50] Hundreds of patients who had undergone one to three unsuccessful nonlaser attempts at revision have had their hearing restored with laser techniques.

Figure 13–14 illustrates the revising surgeon's dilemma. After elevating the tympanotomy flap, the surgeon must identify the margins and depths of the oval window, any residual stapes footplate, and the relationship of the prosthesis to the vestibule. Palpations of the prosthesis and neomembrane can be misleading because the oval window collagen usually has contracted and lateralized above the level of the vestibule. The prosthesis is often eccen-

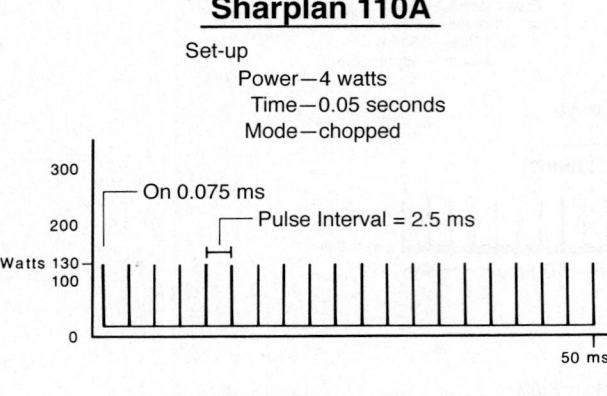

Sharplan 110A

Set-up
Power—4 watts
Time—0.05 seconds
Mode—chopped

Duty Cycle—3%   Energy/Pulse 9.75 mJ

Figure 13–13 Chopped mode for newer Sharplan and Coherent lasers. In superpulse mode, nearly all carbon-dioxide surgical lasers developed by Sharplan and Coherent after 1988 generated 500 to 600 watts of peak power—much too powerful for delicate otologic surgery. Sharplan adapted these lasers for ear surgery by adding Flexilase©, a chopped mode that delivers 130 watts of peak power and 9.75 mJ per micropip (model 1100A, 1041S, and 1055S).

tric, not reaching the vestibule or migrated against the fixed otic capsule bone. A fixed footplate may be present 2 to 3 mm below the lateralized neomembrane.

With appropriate energy settings, the carbon-dioxide laser progressively vaporizes (thins) the collagen neomembrane until the margins of the oval window can be precisely identified (Figure 13–15). The relationship of the prosthesis to the oval window can now be established. Next, tissue surrounding the prosthesis is vaporized, and the prosthesis is removed. Depending on the status of the incus, a 0.6- or 1-mm "stapedotomy" is vaporized through the center of the oval window neomembrane (Figure 13–16) to identify residual fixed stapes footplate, determine the exact length required for the new prosthesis, and stabilize the new prosthesis in the center of the oval window.

When the incus is intact, a 0.6-mm stapedotomy is used. A Teflon piston platinum ribbon stapedotomy prosthesis (0.25 mm longer than the distance between the entrance into the vestibule and undersurface of the incus) is inserted into the stapedotomy opening and crimped to the neck of the incus. Clotted blood is then used to seal the oval window.

If the incus is eroded, a 1-mm stapedotomy opening is vaporized into the center of the oval window. Thin tragal perichondrium (approximately 2 × 3 mm) is then layered over the oval window neomembrane and depressed into the enlarged stapedotomy opening. If 1 mm of the

incus extends below the level of the facial ridge, a Lippy Moon Robinson offset stapes prosthesis is attached to the shortened incus (Figure 13–17). If the incus is absent or too short, a Lesinski malleus to oval window prosthesis is employed (Figure 13–18). More recently, the new titanium aerial prosthesis from Kurz has been used (Figure 13–19). A sterile allograft collagen membrane (MEF) is placed between the tympanic membrane and the titanium prosthesis. The prosthesis is stabilized in the posterior superior quadrant by extending the allograft collagen below the malleus, over the prosthesis, and then under the lip of the bony canal.

If the malleus and incus are normal, postoperative hearing results approach that of primary stapedotomy. When the incus is eroded, 83% of the patients can expect to close the air–bone gap within 15 dB.[50] In a recent series of 300 consecutive carbon-dioxide laser stapedectomy revisions, two patients (0.7%) developed a mild (less than 25 dB) drop in the bone level (mean 500 Hz, 1 KHz, 2 KHz, 3 KHz).[51] No patient exhibited a greater loss.

A word of caution. The safe energy parameter used for carbon-dioxide laser revision techniques was established in the laboratory with human temporal bone thermocouple experiments prior to its use in the operating room. Understanding the absorption tissue characteristics of argon and KTP lasers for water, bone, and collagen, the focused visible lasers should not be employed in the manner described above. Focused argon and KTP laser energy (microscope mounted) readily penetrate perilymph, traveling into the inner ear with enough fluence to potentially damage inner ear structures. The argon EndoOtoprobe® offers a greater degree of safety by rapidly diluting the power density but still should be used with caution since collagen does not absorb this wavelength very well.

Laser Stapedotomy

The clinical advantages of stapedotomy versus stapedectomy include stabilization of the prosthesis in the center of the oval window, reduced trauma to the inner ear (less postoperative sensorineural loss and dizziness), and less mechanical trauma to the middle ear (reduced adhesions and less risk to facial nerve).[12,52–55] Mechanical stapedotomy techniques (trocar or low-frequency microdrill) do not consistently produce a round symmetric stapedotomy because the footplate frequently mobilizes or fractures.

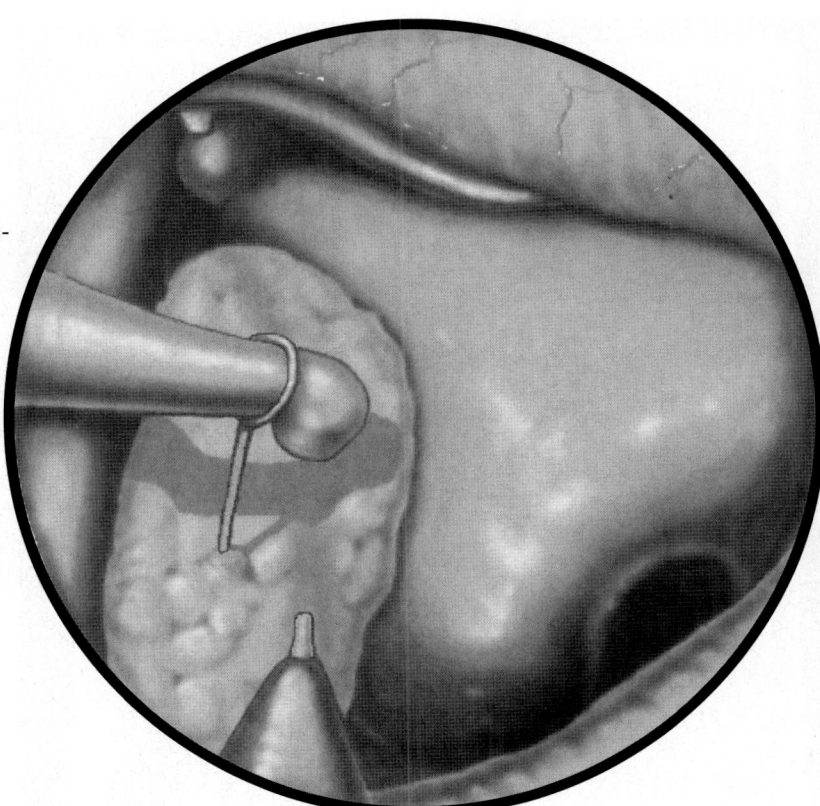

Figure 13–14 Stapedectomy revision: a surgical dilemma (right ear). The surgeon must identify the margins and depth of the oval window, any residual stapes footplate, and the relationship of the prosthesis to the vestibule. The dilemma, surgical manipulation of the obliterating soft tissue or the prosthesis, may produce significant dizziness and nerve deafness.

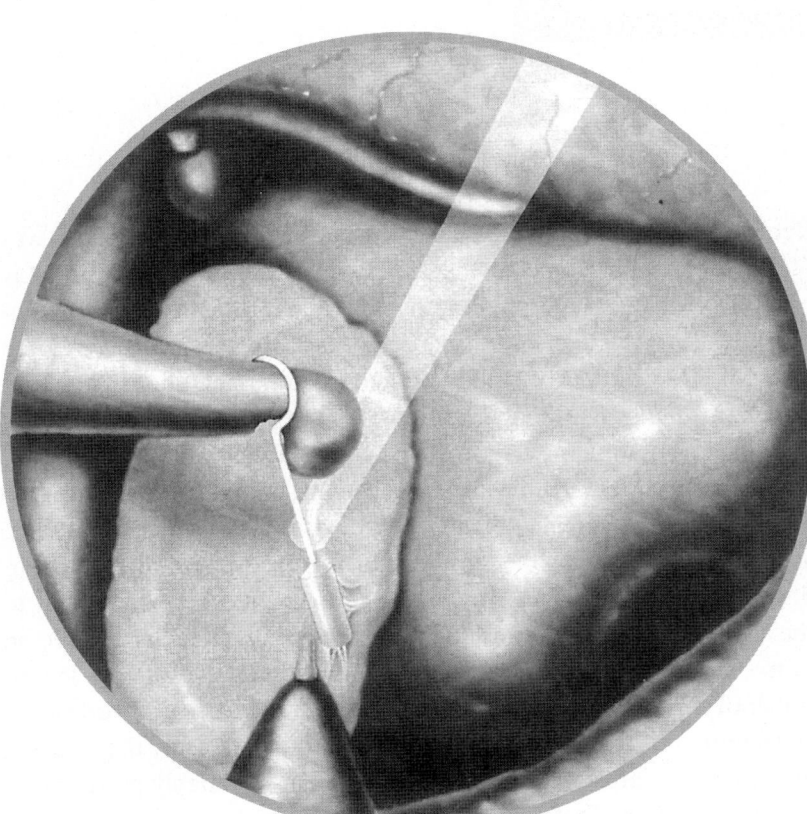

Figure 13–15 Laser stapedectomy revision—the solution. Carbon-dioxide laser vaporizes (thins) collagen until the margins and depth of the oval window can be identified. Laser vaporization of soft tissue attachments of the distal end of the prosthesis permits removal of the prosthesis without mechanical trauma to the inner ear.

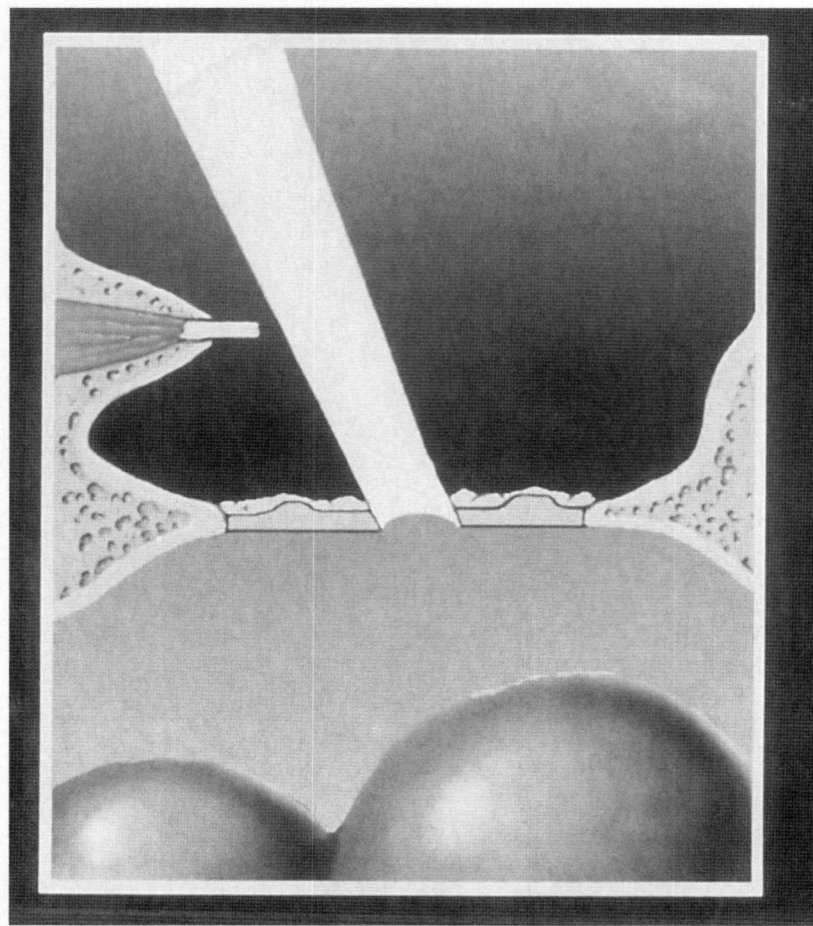

Figure 13–16 A stapedotomy is vaporized in the center of the oval window, through the sealing neomembrane, until perilymph of the vestibule is encountered. Note that fixed stapes footplate is found in 13%.

Laser vaporization of the stapes footplate offers a non-mechanical solution. Safe energy parameters for argon, KTP, carbon-dioxide, and, most recently, erbium:YAG lasers have been established by laboratory experiments and confirmed by scores of successful clinical studies.

Visible lasers require vaporizing a series of tiny "rosettes" (0.05 to 0.2 mm) in the center of the stapes footplate. The 200-micron EndoOtoprobe® is the most popular mode of delivery.

The result of this "rosette" technique is an irregular, scalloped stapedotomy, the precise diameter of which is difficult to control. Surgeons usually seal the visible laser stapedotomy with a vein or perichondrium.

For the past 16 years, the author has been identifying and tabulating the precise causes for stapedectomy failure that are found at the time of revision surgery. Analysis from the data on 279 consecutive patients with conductive hearing loss following stapedectomy was presented to the American Otologic Society in May 2001. Eighty-one percent of those patients had a conductive failure because their prosthesis had migrated out of the oval window fenestration. Collagen contracture lifted the prosthesis out of a stapedotomy opening, allowing the prosthesis to migrate onto the fixed footplate. Following stapedectomy, collagen contracture produced lateralization of the oval window neomembrane, allowing the prosthesis to migrate onto the fixed otic capsule bone (Figure 13–20). As the incus continued to vibrate against the fixed prosthesis, erosion occurred on the undersurface of the incus neck. Despite its inconvenience, the author prefers using a carbon-dioxide laser. A round symmetric stapedotomy precisely the size of a prosthesis piston (0.6 mm) can be reliably produced in the footplate. Because the stapedotomy is precisely the

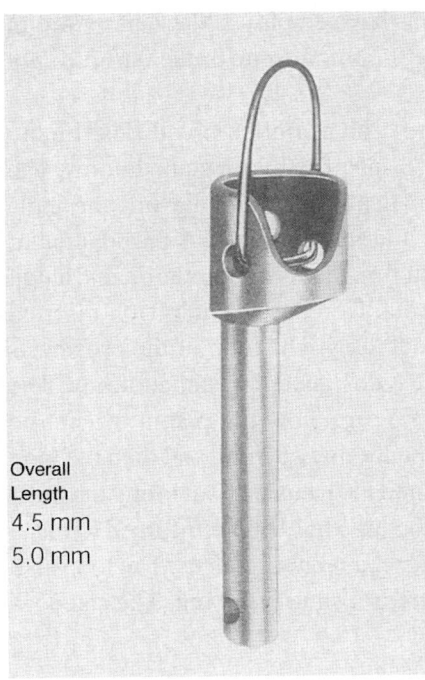

Overall
Length
4.5 mm
5.0 mm

Figure 13–17 Lippy Moon Robinson offset stapes prosthesis (Xomed/Medtronics #11-33009) for eroded incus when incus extends 1 mm or more below the facial ridge.

Figure 13–18 Conductive repair when incus is significantly eroded using Lesinski malleus to oval window prosthesis (Xomed/Medtronics #0320). Note perichondrial graft sealing 1 mm stapedotomy and supporting prosthesis.

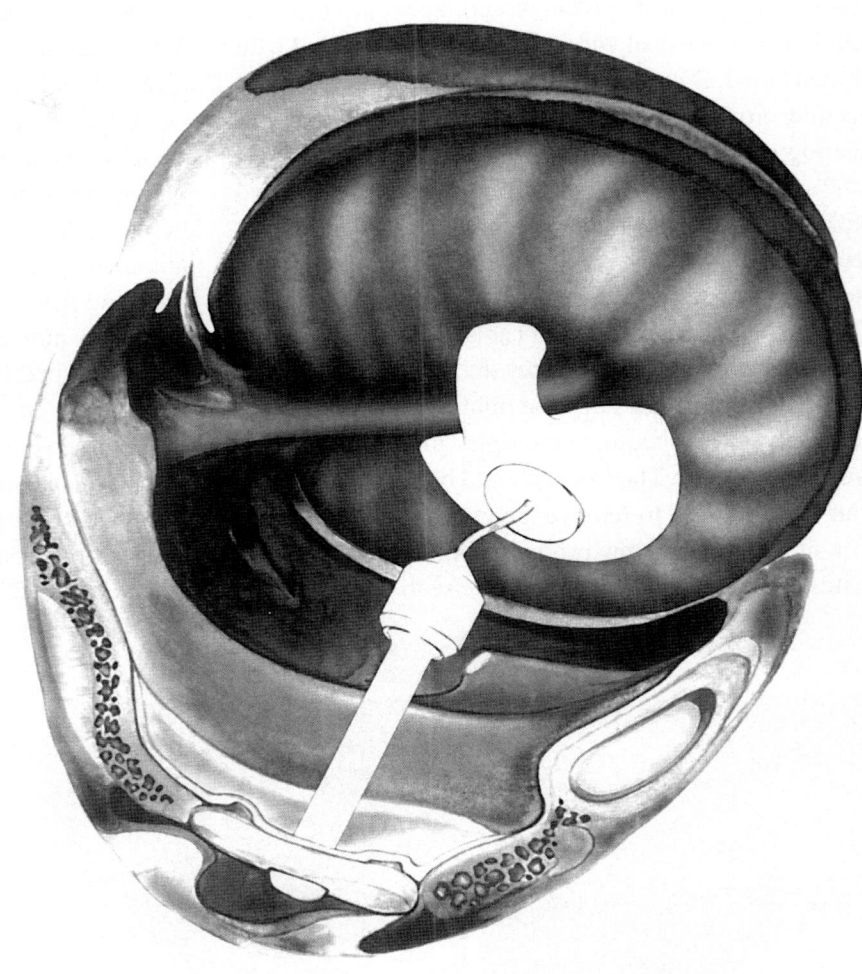

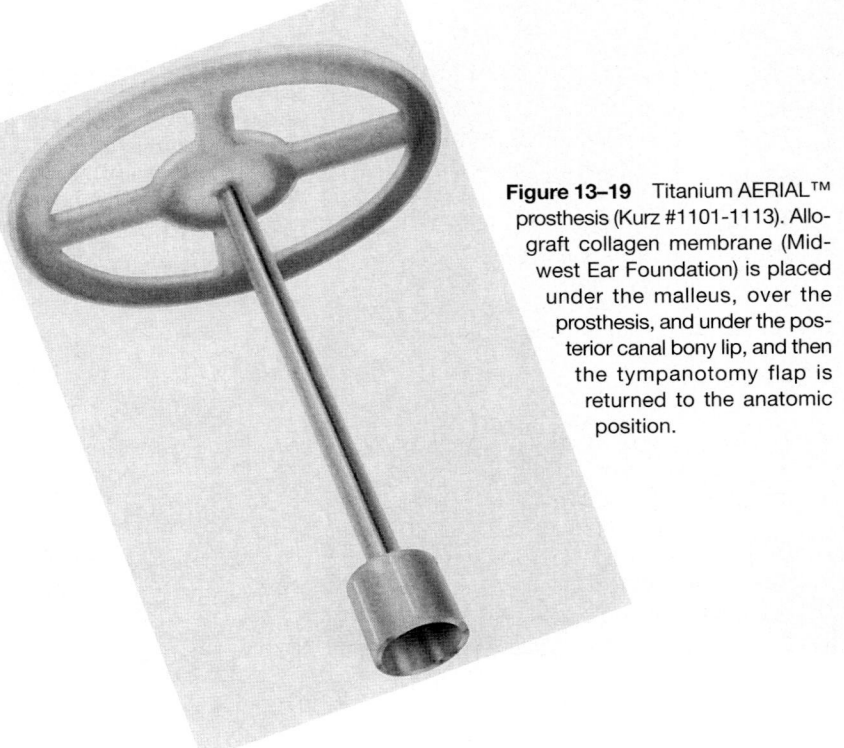

Figure 13–19 Titanium AERIAL™ prosthesis (Kurz #1101-1113). Allograft collagen membrane (Midwest Ear Foundation) is placed under the malleus, over the prosthesis, and under the posterior canal bony lip, and then the tympanotomy flap is returned to the anatomic position.

size of the prosthesis piston, no collagen tissue seal is required, and the oval window can be safely sealed with clotted blood. By avoiding a postoperative collagen contracture, prosthesis migration is minimized, and long-term hearing results are improved (Figure 13–21).[51]

Carbon-dioxide laser stapedotomies are produced with a few "hits" of a pulsed carbon-dioxide laser beam focused to a 0.6-mm spot size. The safe energy parameters for different carbon-dioxide models are listed in Table 13–7. A 0.6-mm Fisch trocar is then used to smooth the margins of the stapedotomy and ensure a symmetric 0.6-mm diameter. A thick or obliterated footplate can be fenestrated but requires multiple "hits" with the carbon-dioxide laser. The trocar should be used after every four or five "hits" to remove the crater char. The precision of the stapedotomy produced in this manner eliminates the need for a collagen tissue seal.

Otologic surgeons have employed the Zeiss erbium: YAG laser using the 0.2-mm rosette or the 0.6-mm spot size technique.

A Teflon piston/platinum ribbon prosthesis (Figure 13–22) was designed specifically for stapedotomy. The platinum ribbon is malleable to allow adjusting the angle between the piston and the footplate. A perpendicular alignment of the piston is necessary to minimize friction resulting from the snug fit of a 0.6-mm piston inserted into a 0.6-mm stapedotomy. The loop of the prosthesis also was specifically designed for stapedotomy. The loop opens on the side to allow the piston to first be inserted into the stapedotomy opening and then the loop can be slid laterally onto the incus without lifting the prosthesis. The base of the loop has been reinforced to resist downward pressure of the vibrating incus. The loop also should be offset to permit snug crimping. The stapedo-

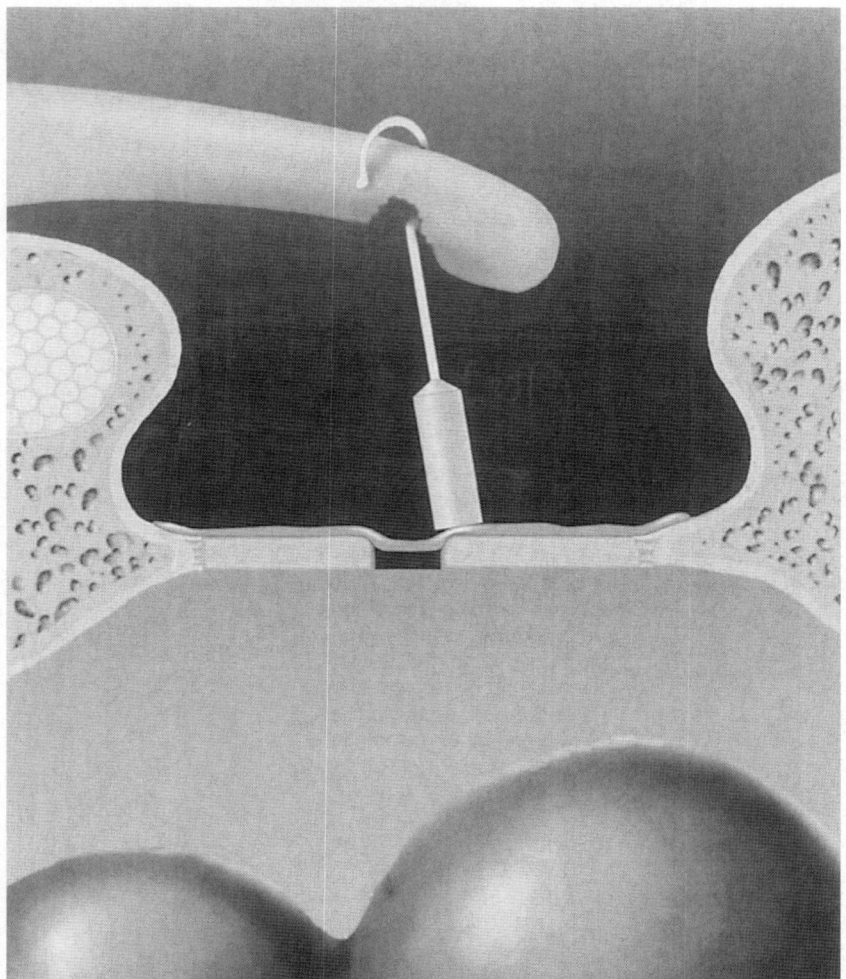

Figure 13–20 The most common cause for conductive hearing loss following stapedotomy is prosthesis migration out of stapedotomy and onto the solid fixed stapes footplate. Collagen contracture initiates the migration by lifting prosthesis out of the fenestration. Note that incus erosion occurs as the incus continues to vibrate against the fixed prosthesis.

tomy prosthesis should measure 0.25 mm longer than the distance between the undersurface of the incus and the footplate. Generally, a 4.5-mm and occasionally a 4.75-mm prosthesis is required. This longer prosthesis resists displacement out of the stapedotomy opening during Valsalva's maneuvers or head trauma.

No collagen tissue seal is used. The surgeon can now directly observe the position, length, and mobility of the prosthesis in relation to the stapedotomy. Postoperative contracture of the collagen neomembrane can lift the prosthesis out of the stapedotomy and is the most common cause for stapedotomy failures.[51] A drop of clotted blood reliably seals the oval window.

There are three instances when a thin tissue seal (vein or perichondrium) is recommended: "perilymph gusher," footplate fracture or mobilization, and stapedotomy that is too large for the prosthesis. If a collagen tissue seal is used, the author prefers a Lippy Robinson

bucket handle prosthesis because of its increased rigidity and stability. The platinum ribbon prosthesis is too malleable for the increased impedance of the collagen tissue seal.

Employing laser stapedotomy techniques, the surgeon can expect that 90% of his patients will close the air–bone gap to within 10 dB and 96% to within 15 dB.[30] Lasers reduce inner ear trauma as evidenced by less postoperative dizziness and sensorineural hearing loss. Finally, provided that the surgeon employs appropriate laser energy parameters and techniques, the risk to the facial nerve is nearly eliminated.

Lasers for Tympanoplasty/Mastoidectomy

Otologic lasers can assist the surgeon in several situations in which standard techniques are inadequate or

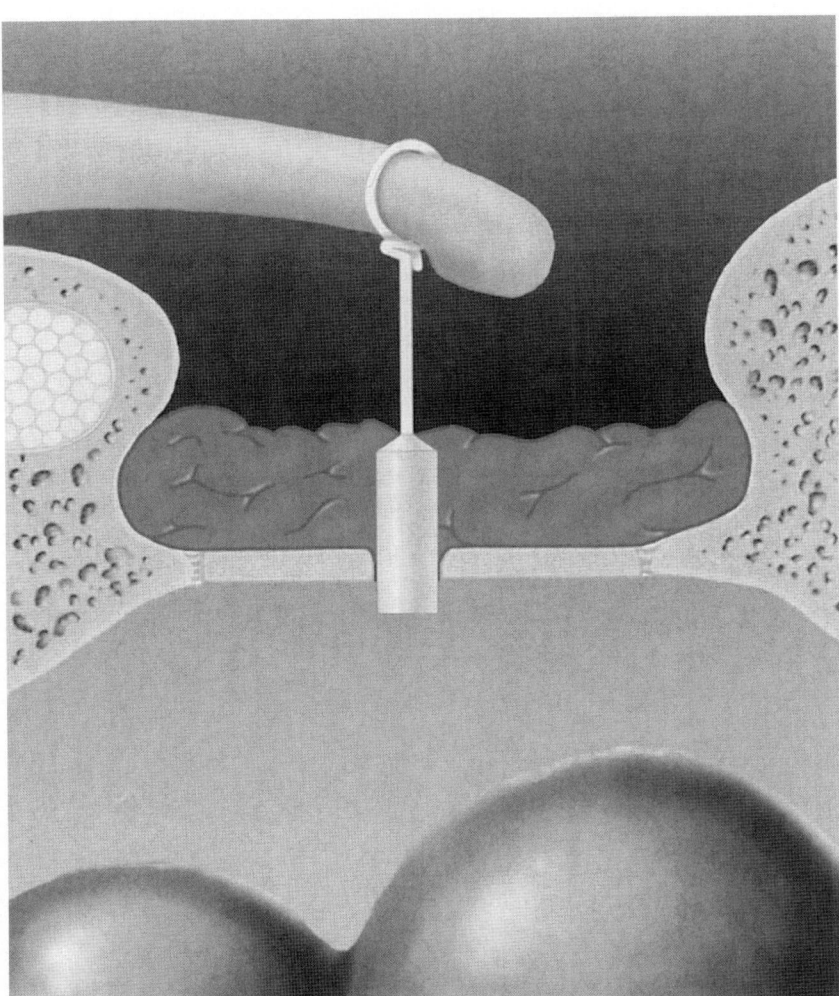

Figure 13–21 Carbon-dioxide laser produces round symmetric 0.6-mm stapedotomy opening. Clotted blood effectively seals the oval window. Collagen tissue seal is avoided, eliminating collagen contracture and reducing the risk of postoperative prosthesis migration.

potentially dangerous. Hemostasis can be obtained by coagulating blood vessels that are inaccessible to bipolar electrocautery. Frequently, the chronic ear surgeon encounters an oval window obliterated by cholesteatoma, granulation tissue, hyperplastic mucosa, and adhesions. In a chronically infected middle ear, dislocating the stapes bone potentially exposes the inner ear to bacterial contamination (bacterial labyrinthitis and meningitis). Visible or carbon-dioxide lasers are used to meticulously vaporize the abnormal soft tissue.[11,17,33,56] In addition, to facilitate complete tumor removal, the arch of a mobile stapes can be safely vaporized with a laser, providing free access to the footplate.

If the stapes head is eroded but the arch is intact, hearing reconstruction presents a challenge. Most prostheses designed for attachment to the stapes require an intact stapes head for stability. Optimal hearing results can be obtained by vaporizing the arch and centering a total ossicular replacement prosthesis (TORP) on the mobile stapes footplate. Mechanically crushing the arch (Wehr's or Fisch crura crusher) works well when the stapes footplate is fixed but will frequently dislocate a mobile footplate.

Vaporization and coagulation of granulation tissue and hyperplastic mucosa can also be safely done in delicate areas such as the round window niche or overlying a dehiscent facial nerve.

Tumor Ablation

In the late 1980s, there was considerable enthusiasm for employing both visible and carbon-dioxide lasers to vaporize acoustic neuroma, glomus tumors, and other base of skull tumors. The slow rate of laser tumor ablation coupled with the risk of adjacent tissue damage

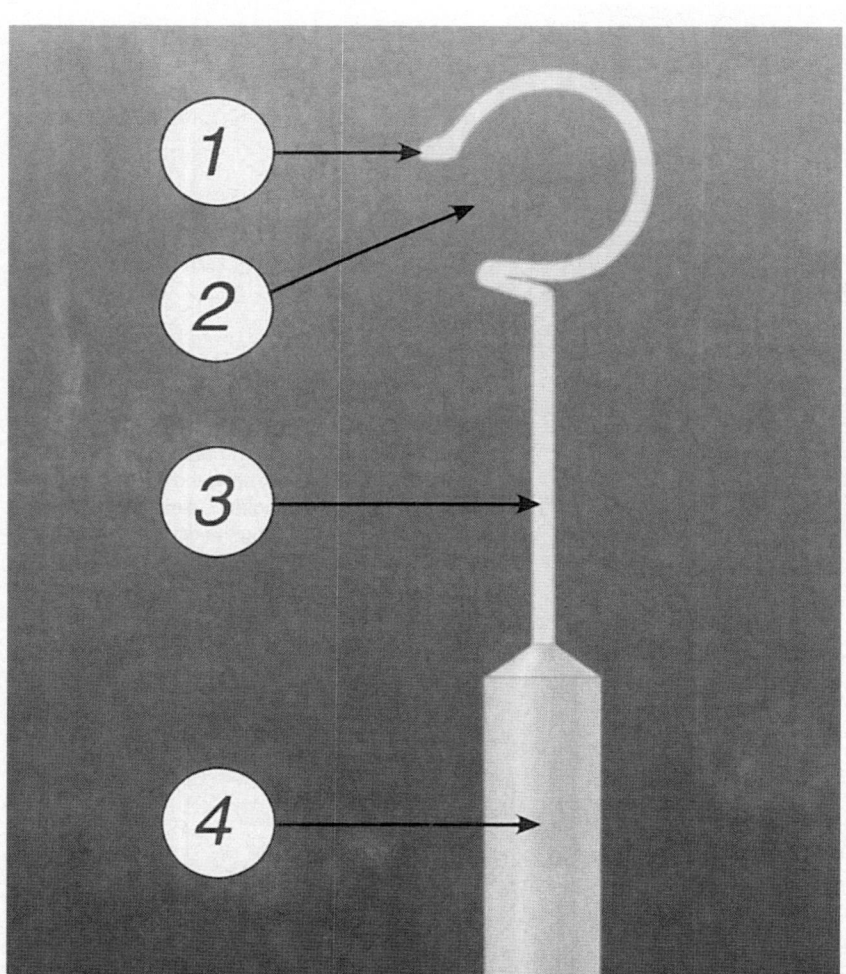

Figure 13–22 Improved stapedotomy prosthesis (Xomed/Medtronics #385): 1 = offset shepherd's crook, 2 = lateral opening, 3 = malleable platinum shaft is reinforced at the neck, and 4 = Teflon piston (0.6 mm diameter).

from thermal spread or a misdirected laser beam limited its advantages.[17] Just as for middle ear surgery, there are instances when the Argon EndoOtoprobe® or the carbon-dioxide lasers can be helpful (eg, vaporization and coagulation of small bits of acoustic neuroma still adherent to the facial nerve). The smaller feeding blood vessel can be coagulated.

With carefully controlled energy parameters, the author has used carbon-dioxide lasers to vaporize epidermoid carcinoma off the adventitia of the carotid artery and benign tumors off a dehiscent facial nerve. Stage I epidermoid carcinomas and papillomas of the external ear canal can be vaporized without extensive surgical dissection, although histologic evaluation of crater margins is required to ensure complete removal of the cancer cells. When the tumor is near the facial nerve, intraoperative electrical monitoring of the nerve is recommended.

Myringotomy

The OtoLam® carbon-dioxide laser was introduced by ESC Sharplan in 1997 as "a breakthrough in treatment of otitis media." It was marketed heavily by the company to both pediatricians and otolaryngologists as a possible alternative to tympanostomy tubes despite the absence of satisfactory scientific data to support its use. The Medical Devices and Drug Committee of the American Academy of Otolaryngology in Head and Neck Surgery investigated and subsequently published their opinion in the Academy bulletin in June 2001.[57] In their report, they summarized the findings of a multicentered clinical outcomes trial that used the OtoLam® for four indications: acute otitis media (AOM), persistent otitis media with effusion (OME), OME with adenoidectomy, and laser-assisted ventilation tube (PET) insertion in the office.

Laser myringotomy was compared with antibiotic treatment alone for AOM. At 3 months, residual middle ear effusion rates were equivalent—27% in the OtoLam® group and 21% in the group treated with antibiotics alone.

In this group, OtoLam® myringotomies were compared with standard myringotomy and PE tube insertion for the treatment of OME. At 3 months postoperatively, 36% of the OtoLam® group and 9% of the PET group had persistent fluid in the middle ear.

A third group of patients with OME underwent adenoidectomy along with either standard myringotomy or OtoLam myringotomy. Postoperative results were the same.

The fourth group represented the most attractive potential application for the OtoLam® laser: the ability to insert PE tubes in children in the office under local anesthesia. Eight percent tetracaine was used, but virtually all of the patients 4 years and younger required restraining with a papoose board. Despite the child's discomfort, 92% of the parents in this series preferred OtoLam® to tubes inserted under general anesthesia. Perhaps this statement best summarizes the opinion of the Medical Devices and Drug Committee: "Many questions still remain regarding the relative value of OtoLam® procedures compared with the traditional surgical intervention for otitis media."[57]

Laser Ablation of Membranous Labyrinth

Intractable benign positional vertigo symptoms have been successfully relieved by ablating the membranous labyrinth at the midpoint of the posterior semicircular canal.

Kartush and Sargent have accomplished this by removing the overlying bone and then using 1 to 2 watts of carbon-dioxide energy on a continuous mode for 1 to 2 seconds while observing the membranous canal shrink.[58] Parnes and McClure have had equal success by occluding this area of the posterior semicircular canal with bone paste.[59,60] This procedure carries less risk to the hearing nerve than singular neurectomy. The success of Epley maneuvers and the recent popularity of transtympanic chemical vestibular neurectomy for the intractable cases have limited the popularity of posterior semicircular canal membranous ablation.

THE FUTURE OF OTOLOGIC LASERS

Laser techniques are accepted by the otologic community only when the laser procedure offers significant clinical advantages over nonlaser techniques. When the first stapedotomy procedure was presented 20 years ago, many of the otologists in the audience were skeptical of the potential clinical advantages that lasers afforded. Ten years later, approximately half of the otologists were using lasers in the operating room; the other half maintained, "My results are just as good without the laser." Today, nearly every otologist employs a laser for specific otologic surgical circumstances when laser precision and lack of mechanical trauma offer a safer alternative.

Until now, lasers have been employed to vaporize or coagulate soft tissue or bone (photothermal effect). The photothermal effect of lasers is presently being tested for the following applications:

1. *Stabilizing middle ear prostheses.* Prostheses can be welded with lasers. Some polyethylene materials will shrink when heated. "Metals with memory" will reshape themselves when heated. Newer prostheses will incorporate these characteristics to stabilize their attachment to the malleus, incus, or stapes. In Europe, the erbium:YAG laser is used to vaporize a 0.1-mm hole into the incus to attach the microactuator arm of Implex's TICA®.[61]

2. *The ultrashort pulse lasers (USPLs).* This chapter has focused on the quantum mechanics principle that a molecule's ability to absorb (or emit) an EM photon is dependent on that photon's wavelength. If a laser's pulse is shortened to less than 10 picoseconds (10 trillionths of a second), the physics of laser–tissue interaction changes and is no longer wavelength dependent. The USPLs produce free electrons, which result in a plasma-mediated tissue ablation independent of the EM absorption characteristics of that tissue. The USPLs pulsed at 0.35 picoseconds (10^{-13} seconds) have produced precise stapedotomies in the laboratory at the University of California–Irvine Medical Center.[62]

3. *Interstitial laser photocoagulation (ILP) under direct imagery.* In Ontario, Drs. Wyman, Wilson, and Malone are performing this minimally invasive technique in animals.[63] Solid tumor tissue is destroyed thermally by directing near infrared laser energy into the center of the tumor through one or more optical fibers implanted interstitially. Ultrasonography and magnetic resonance imaging are simultaneously carried out, producing high-contrast images of the ILP lesions in real and near real time. These images provide feedback data that can be used to control the ILP lesion. This technique has potential applications for controlled destruction of inaccessible tumors deep in the brain or the skull base.

Besides its photothermal effects, EM energy could be used for many nonheating medical applications. Listed below are a few of the potential areas being explored in laser laboratories:

1. *Emission spectroscopy.* The electron orbits of molecules within tissue are excited with ultraviolet lasers. As their electron orbits decay, each molecule emits the exact photon (wavelength) of EM energy it loses. Molecules are identified by their spectral patterns. Cancer cells contain unique molecules (eg, primitive amino acids). Therefore, cancer cells could potentially be identified through emission spectroscopy with a great degree of accuracy.[64] Emission spectroscopy is presently being performed on many different types of tumors and being compared with histologic sections to determine its diagnostic potential.

What is even more intriguing about emission spectroscopy is its potential therapeutic benefits. If specific EM wavelengths can be identified that only cancer cells absorb, specific monochromatic x-rays or ultraviolet lasers could be used to ionize only those molecules in the cancer cells and not affect the molecules of normal cells. The potential medical implications are staggering. Quite simply, a woman with a breast mass could have a mammogram at 9:00 am. If suspicious, the tumor could be confirmed as malignant with laser emission spectroscopy at 10:00 am. At 11:00 am, the molecules of the cancer cells would then be ionized with a single high dose of radiation of monochromatic x-rays or ultraviolet lasers. The patient could return home in time for lunch, cured of her breast cancer!

In a similar manner, emission spectroscopy and then ionizing the tumor with selective monochromatic EM radiation offers major advantages for base of skull and intracranial tumors.

2. *LAS II®.* At MIT, Feld and colleagues have developed the LAS II: an integrated system for spectral diagnosis, guidance, and ablation in laser angiosurgery.[65] Researchers have developed a 1.5-mm diameter angiocatheter that contains 12 tiny silica optical fibers that are used for intraluminal spectroscopy and abla-

tion of atherosclerotic plaque-obstructing arteries. Using short pulses of ultraviolet light (480 nm), fluorescent spectroscopy is performed individually through each of the 12 optical fibers. A computer analyzes the returning spectrograph, and an image of the type, depth, and location of the obstructing atherosclerotic plaque is obtained. The computer then determines the dose for the ablating laser light (355 nm) for each of the 12 tiny optical fibers inside the catheter. The LAS II should significantly reduce the risk of laser damage to blood vessel walls and thus reduce the complications of perforation and restenosis seen with previous attempts at laser angiography.

3. *Inner ear endoscopy and spectroscopy.* Perhaps someday in the future surgeons will cannulate the inner ear with tiny optical fibers and perform emission spectroscopy at various sites in the vestibular and cochlear partitions. Cupulolithiasis could be identified and ablated with ultraviolet or photoacoustic laser effects. Do the dark cells have enough unique biochemistry that they could be partially ablated with appropriate ultraviolet lasers—reducing the production of endolymph in patients with Meniere's disease? Is peripheral tinnitus caused by excitable hair cells or neurons whose critical firing potentials have been biochemically altered? Could we biochemically re-engineer these aberrant molecules using the photodissection effect of EM energy?

Over the past 50 years, ear surgery has traveled from completely macroscopic techniques to exclusively microscopic. Perhaps in the next 50 years, otology will journey into the submicroscopic world. Surgeons will operate with EM energy on atoms and molecules, restructuring intracellular molecules to alter cell function. The road is well lit by the laws of quantum mechanics. Molecular physicists and biophysicists will guide us. Our ultimate destination is limited by our imagination.

REFERENCES

1. Ferris T. Quantum weirdness. In: Ferris T, editor. The whole shebang. Simon Schuster; 1997. p. 265–89.

2. Thuan TX. The unbearable strangeness of atoms. In: Thuan TX, editor. Chaos and harmony. Oxford University Press; 2001. p. 199–252.

3. Absten GT. Laser tissue interaction. In: Practical laser biophysics manual of American Society for Laser Medicine and Surgery. ASLMS April 2001. p. 1–70.

4. Lederman L, Teresi D. The naked atom. The God particle. Houghton Mifflin; 1993. p. 141–88.

5. Greene B. Tied up with string. In: The elegant universe. WW Notten & Co.; 1999. p. 3–22.

6. Bueche F. Electronic and electromagnetic waves. In: Principles of physics. 3rd ed. McGraw-Hill; 1977. p. 509–35.

7. Feld MD, Desari RR. Colliers encyclopedia. Vol 21. 1996. Spectroscopy; p. 414–24.

8. Perkins R. Laser stapedotomy for otosclerosis. Laryngoscope 1980;90:228–41.

9. McGee T. The argon laser in surgery for chronic ear disease and otosclerosis. Laryngoscope 1983;93:1177–82.

10. Perkins R. New instruments—the KTP/532 laser. Presented at the American Academy of Otolaryngology Head and Neck Surgery, Sept 1984.

11. DiBartolomeo JR. The argon laser in otology. Laryngoscope 1980;90:1786–96.

12. House J. The evolution of otosclerosis surgery. Otolaryngol Clin North Am 1993;26:323–33.

13. Lesinski SG. Lasers for otosclerosis: CO_2 vs. argon and KTP 532. Laryngoscope 1989;99:1–8.

14. Lesinski SG. CO_2 laser for otosclerosis: safe energy parameters. Laryngoscope 1989;99:9–12.

15. McGee TM, Kartush JM. Laser stapes surgery [letter]. Laryngoscope 1990;100:106–7.

16. Kartush JM, McGee TM. Controversies in laser stapedotomy. Insights Otolaryngol 1991;6:1–8.

17. Sargent EW, Kartush JM. Lasers in otology. Adv Otolaryngol Head Neck Surg 2000;8:187–201.

18. Gherini S, Horn KL, Causse JP, et al. Fiberoptic argon laser stapedotomy: is it safe? Am J Otol 1993;14:283–9.

19. Bartels L. KTP laser stapedotomy: is it safe? Otolaryngol Head Neck Surg 1990;103:685–92.

20. McGee TM, Diaz-Ordaz EA, Kartus J, et al. The role of KTP laser in revision stapedectomy. Otolaryngol Head Neck Surg 1993;109: 839–43.

21. Vernick DM. A comparison of the results of KTP and CO_2 laser stapedotomy. Am J Otol 1996;17:221–4.

22. Rauch SD, Bartley ML. Argon laser stapedectomy: comparison to traditional fenestration techniques. Am J Otol 1992;13: 556–60.

23. DiBartolomeo J. Argon and CO_2 lasers in otolaryngology: which one, when, and why? Laryngoscope 1981;91 Suppl 26:1–16.

24. Lesinski SG. Lasers in revision stapes surgery. Oper Tech Otolaryngol Head Neck Surg 1992;3:21–31.

25. Lesinski SG. Lasers for otosclerosis—which one and why? Lasers Surg Med 1990;10:448–57.

26. Horn KL, Gherini SG, Franz DC. Argon laser revision stapedectomy. Am J Otol 1994;15:383–8.

27. Rizer FM, Lippy W. Evolution of techniques of stapedectomy from the total stapedectomy to the small fenestra stapedotomy. Otolaryngol Clin North Am 1993;26:443–52.

28. House HP. The evolution of otologic surgery. Otolaryngol Clin North Am 1993;26:323–34.

29. Izatt JA, Albagli D, Britton M. Wavelength dependence of pulsed laser ablation of calcified tissue. Lasers Surg Med 1991;11: 238–49.

30. Lesinski SG, Newrock R. CO_2 lasers for otosclerosis. Otolaryngol Clin North Am 1993;26:417–42.

31. The infrared handbook. Washington (DC): Office of Naval Research. 1978.

32. Yannas I. Collagen and gelatin in the solid state. J Macromol Chem C7 1972;1:49–104.

33. Pfalz R, Hibst N. Suitability of different lasers for operations ranging from the tympanic membrane to the base of stapes. Adv Otorhinolaryngol 1995;49:87–94.

34. Nuss R, Fabian R, Sarkar R, et al. Infrared laser bone ablation. Lasers Surg Med 1998;8:381–391.

35. Hibst R. Mechanical effects of erbium YAG laser bone ablation. Lasers Surg Med 1992;12:125–30.

36. Stubig IM, Reder PA, et al. Holmium YAG laser stapedotomy: preliminary evaluation. Proc SPIE 1993;1876:10–9.

37. Scholz C, Grothues-Spork M. Comparison of experimental laser systems for in vitro osteotomy of human bone. Proceedings of the IX International Congress Laser '89. Berlin: Springer, 1990. p. 67–75.

38. Jovanovic S, Schonfeld U, Prapavat V, et al. Effects of pulsed laser systems on stapes footplate. Lasers Surg Med 1997;21: 341–50.

39. Lesinski SG. Stapedectomy revision with the CO_2 laser. Laryngoscope 1989;99:13–19.

40. Lesinski SG. CO_2 laser stapedotomy. Laryngoscope 1989;99: 20–4.

41. Nagel D. The ER:YAG laser in ear surgery: first clinical results. Lasers Surg Med 1997;21:79–87.

42. Lenarz T, Heermann R, Brandis A. Erbium YAG laser in middle ear surgery. In: Huttenbrink KB, editor. Middle ear mechanics in research and otosurgery. 1997. p. 233–7.

43. Pfalz R, Hibst, Bald N. Suitability of different lasers for operations ranging from the tympanic membrane to the base of the stapes. Adv Otorhinolaryngol 1995;49:87–94.

44. Glasscock ME. Revision stapedectomy surgery. Otolaryngol Head Neck Surg 1987;96:141–8.

45. Sheehy JL. Revision stapedectomy: a review of 258 cases. Laryngoscope 1981;91:43–51.

46. Lippy WH. Stapedectomy revision. Am J Otol 1980;2:15–21.

47. Crabtree JA. An evaluation of revision stapes surgery. Laryngoscope 1980;90:224–7.

48. Linthicum F. Histologic evidence of the cause of failure in stapes surgery. Ann Otol Rhinol Laryngol 1971;80:67–77.

49. Haberkamp TJ, Harvey SA. Revision stapedectomy with and without the CO_2 laser: an analysis of results. Am J Otol 1996; 17:225–9.

50. Lesinski SG. Revision surgery for otosclerosis—1998 perspective. Oper Tech Otolaryngol Head Neck Surg 1998;9:72–81.

51. Lesinski SG. Causes for conductive hearing loss following stapedectomy or stapedotomy. Presented at the American Otologic Society annual meeting, Palm Springs, CA, May 2001. [Accepted for publication Am J Otol]

52. Fisch U. Stapedotomy vs. stapedectomy. Am J Otol 1982;4: 112–7.

53. Smyth GDL. Eighteen years experience in stapedectomy. The case for small fenestra operation. Ann Otol Rhinol Laryngol 1978;87 Suppl 49.

54. Kursten R, Schneider B, Zrunek M, et al. Long term results after stapedectomy versus stapedotomy. Am J Otol 1994;15:804–6.

55. Marquet J. Stapedotomy technique and results. J Otol 1985;6: 63–7.

56. Vernick DM. Laser applications in ossicular surgery. Otolaryngol Clin North Am 1996;29:931–41.

57. Schroern S, Darrow D. Middle ear ventilation. Medical Devices and Drug Committee. Bull AAO-HNS 2001;20:45–7.

58. Kartush JM, Sargent EW. Posterior semi-circular canal occlusion for benign paroxysmal positional vertigo—CO_2 laser assisted technique: preliminary results. Laryngoscope 1995; 105(3 Pt 1):268–74.

59. Parnes LS, McClure JA. Posterior semi-circular canal occlusion for intractable benign paroxysmal positional vertigo. Ann Otol Rhinol Laryngol 1990;99(5 Pt 1):330–4.

60. Parnes LS. Update on posterior canal occlusion for benign paroxysmal positional vertigo. Otolaryngol Clin North Am 1996;29:333–42.

61. Zenner HP, Leysieffer H. Totally implantable hearing device for sensorineural hearing loss. Lancet 1998;352–9:#9142.

62. Armstrong WB, Neev, JA. Ultrashort pulse laser stapedotomy. Presented at the Western Section of American Laryngological, Pharmacological, and Otologic Society annual meeting, La Corte, CA, January 2001.

63. Wyman D. Medical imaging systems for feedback control of interstitial laser photocoagulation. Proc IEEE 1992;80:890–902.

64. Dept. of Biomedical Laser Research MIT. Richards-Kortum R. Fluorescence spectroscopy as a technique for diagnosis [PhD thesis]. Massachusetts Institute of Technology; 1990.

65. Feld M, Desari R. LAS II—an integrated system for spectral diagnosis, guidance and ablation in laser angiosurgery. In: Practice of interventional cardiology. 2nd rev ed. Mosby Yearbook; 1992.

14

Neurophysiologic Monitoring in Otologic/Neurotologic Surgery

ROBERTO A. CUEVA, MD, FACS
GAYLE E. HICKS, PhD, FASM

Whereas surgical experimentation with facial nerve electrical stimulation during cerebellopontine angle (CPA) surgery dates back to the late nineteenth century,[1] the modern era of neurophysiologic monitoring during otologic/neurotologic surgery begins in 1979, when Delgado and colleagues reported on their experience with intraoperative electromyographic (EMG) monitoring of the facial nerve during intracranial surgery.[2] Historically, various methods for detecting facial nerve irritation/trauma during surgery have been employed, varying from an observer watching the face during dissection[3,4] to the suturing of sterilized cat collar bells to specific locations on the face to signal facial movement by their ringing.[5] But it was Delgado and colleagues, along with the efforts of Møller and Jannetta,[6] Gantz,[7] Harner and colleagues,[8] Prass and Luders,[9] and others, using neurophysiologic equipment to monitor and record facial nerve activity, who ushered us into the modern era.

Soon after, in the early 1980s, Møller and Jannetta and others began to report their success in monitoring and recording cochlear nerve function during CPA surgery.[10,11] Facial nerve monitoring quickly became the standard of care during surgery for acoustic neuromas and other CPA pathology as studies indicated improved facial nerve function related to the use of monitoring.[12,13] Auditory monitoring, although initially reported using direct eighth nerve monitoring (DENM), came to be widely employed using auditory brainstem responses (ABRs).[14–16] Difficulties with maintaining electrode position and signal degradation in cerebrospinal fluid hampered successful DENM, but recent advances in electrode design have largely overcome these problems.[17] More recently, DENM is receiving increasing attention by surgeons and authors as it provides the most rapid feedback to the surgeon on the status of auditory function during CPA surgery.[18–20]

The techniques of EMG and direct nerve monitoring are being applied to monitor other cranial nerves in an effort to reduce patient morbidity following neurotologic surgery. Specifically, monitoring of the vagus, spinal accessory, and hypoglossal nerves is frequently done in skull base surgical cases.[21,22] Oculomotor and trigeminal nerve monitoring is also becoming more common.

As a whole, neurophysiologic monitoring during surgery continues to grow in routine use and advance in technological sophistication. The driving motivation for its application and ongoing development is the desire to keep morbidity related to complex neurotologic surgery to an absolute minimum. Clearly, monitoring the facial nerve during CPA surgery has had a positive effect on functional outcome.[23,24] The impact of facial nerve monitoring during routine otologic surgery remains less well defined. Auditory monitoring with DENM has been demonstrated as superior to ABR in facilitating hearing preservation during CPA surgery.[25,26] Future advances in application and technology hold the promise of better surgical outcomes.

FACIAL NERVE MONITORING

Neurophysiologic monitoring of the facial nerve most commonly involves EMG. Equipment for monitoring gross facial muscle contraction, via strain gauges, is commercially available, but the technique is not as sensitive as EMG at detecting facial nerve irritation. Like-

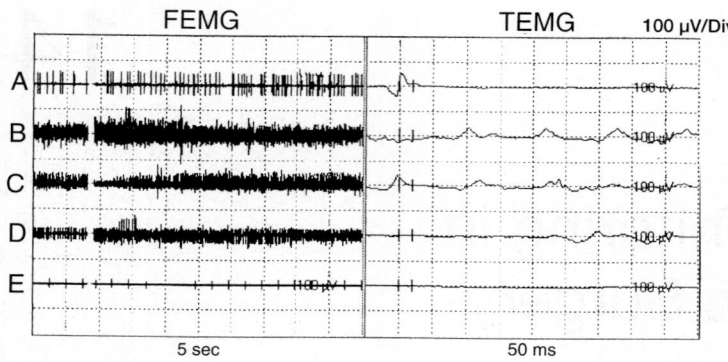

Figure 14–1 Simultaneous recordings of free-run electromyography (FEMG) and triggered EMG (TEMG) acquired during acoustic neuroma surgery are shown. Traces A through E reflect EMG from the orbicularis oculi (A), orbicularis oris (B), mentalis (C), masseter (D), and trapezius (E) muscles for both the FEMG and TEMG recordings. The five channels of FEMG to the left were recorded with a 5-second sweep window. All of the muscles, except the trapezius, exhibit spontaneous activity secondary to inadvertent stimulation of their respective nerves during tumor manipulation. The corresponding TEMG, to the right, is a 50-ms capture of the simultaneously recorded FEMG. In this recording, the trigger voltage was set at 50 μV. Any activity in the EMG exceeding 50 μV would trigger the capture.

wise, video monitoring of the face during surgery is likely to miss subclinical muscular contractions. Electromyographic voltages less than 100 μV are typically not visible as facial movement but are easily recorded using current technology. Hence, the sole advantage of strain gauge/video monitoring, relative to EMG, is the ability to continue monitoring during bipolar and monopolar electrocautery. Current artifact created during electrocautery effectively prevents EMG monitoring. Some authors employ both techniques simultaneously to avoid this latter problem associated with EMG monitoring.[27]

As a consequence of EMG's reliance on the neuromuscular junction, paralytic agents must not be used during surgery in which motor nerve monitoring is being performed. A short-acting neuromuscular blocker may be used during anesthetic induction, but motor nerve activity should be allowed to return to normal during the course of the surgical procedure. If significant facial nerve manipulation is anticipated, testing to ensure reversal of the anesthetic induction neuromuscular blockade should be done prior to beginning facial nerve dissection.

Electromyographic data may be recorded using three separate or simultaneous acquisition formats: continuous or free-run (FEMG), triggered EMG (TEMG), and stimulated EMG (SEMG). Free-run EMG is recorded in real time, typically employing sweep durations of 200 ms to 5 seconds. Triggered EMG allows the capture of spontaneous responses that exceed a preset voltage. Many commercial systems provide an audible warning when the EMG activity exceeds the preset voltage. Stimulated EMG records responses to a stimulus source such as a handheld probe designed specifically for cranial nerve stimulation. Figure 14–1 shows simultaneous recordings of FEMG and TEMG. Figure 14–2 demonstrates simultaneous recordings of FEMG and SEMG. Depending on the manufacturer, commercially available systems may employ one or a combination of the three acquisition formats.

Generally, two configurations may be employed for monitoring EMG from the face and other cranial nerves, monopolar and bipolar. In a monopolar and bipolar electrode configuration the amplifier records the difference in activity between two strategically placed electrodes. Monopolar recordings use active electrodes placed in the desired myotomes (eg, orbicularis oculi muscle for the facial [VII] nerve and the masseter muscle for the trigeminal [V] nerve) and a reference electrode neutrally placed (eg, lateral forehead on the opposite

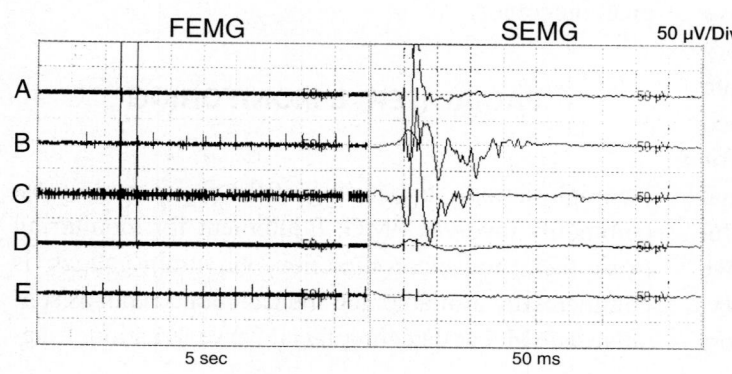

Figure 14–2 Simultaneous recordings of free-run electromyography (FEMG) and stimulated EMG (SEMG) acquired during acoustic neuroma surgery are shown. As in Figure 14–1, traces A through E reflect EMG from the orbicularis oculi (A), orbicularis oris (B), mentalis (C), masseter (D), and trapezius (E) muscles. The FEMG, to the left, is a second sweep of continuous EMG. Evident in traces B and E are regularly spaced artifacts from the probe stimulator. Two larger events are seen at the same intervals as the stimuli artifacts and reflect responses from the facial muscles to the probe stimuli. These responses are more clearly seen in a 50-ms sweep of SEMG to the right. In this recording, the probe stimuli triggered the capture.

side of the head from the active electrodes). Bipolar recordings are obtained by placing both the active and reference electrodes in the muscle. Both methods are acceptable and use a differential amplifier common to most current recording systems. True referential recorders may be used only with amplifiers specifically designed to provide this type of recording methodology. A referential amplifier subtracts the activity of the reference electrode from the activity of the active electrode or electrodes. This results in greater specificity, reduced noise, and the convenience of using fewer electrodes.

The most common EMG recording method employs paired subdermal needle electrodes in a bipolar configuration. Two subdermal needle electrodes are placed under the skin over the muscles or myotomes of the associated cranial nerve. Their distance is determined by the desired specificity. The closer the pair of electrodes are placed to each other, the fewer the muscle fibers represented in the EMG response. Electrode placement should take into consideration the size of the muscle group of interest as well as that of the surrounding muscles. For instance, the orbicularis oculi is in proximity to the frontalis and temporalis muscles. When placing electrodes to represent seventh nerve activity, the temporalis muscle should be avoided. Since the seventh nerve innervates the frontalis, activity from this muscle would be acceptable when the facial nerve is at risk. Thus, the recommended electrode placement for the orbicularis oculi muscle should be more centrally located over the orbit to avoid interference from temporalis electrodes reacting to inadvertent stimulation of the fifth nerve (Figure 14–3). In small tumors, overlap of activity from different cranial nerves is not usually a problem. However, for large tumors in which the anatomy may be significantly distorted, this overlap could be a critical issue. Figure 14–4 demonstrates a masseter response to fifth nerve stimulation and a "bleed-over" from the temporalis muscle to electrodes placed in the orbicularis oculi muscle. Note that these SEMG responses exhibit a simple biphasic waveform compared with typical multiphasic SEMG responses from the orbicularis oculi to stimulation of the seventh nerve, as demonstrated in Figure 14–5.

In most surgical conditions, two channels of facial nerve EMG are adequate. However, in large tumors in which the seventh nerve may be splayed over the tumor, three or four channels of EMG representing additional branches of the facial nerve provide greater sensitivity. Figure 14–6 shows EMG activity recorded continuously from four facial muscles. Electromyographic activity limited to the mentalis muscle in response to tumor manipulation is evident.

If the surgeon is very familiar with a particular, dedicated, motor nerve monitoring device and is able to differentiate true motor responses from artifact signals,

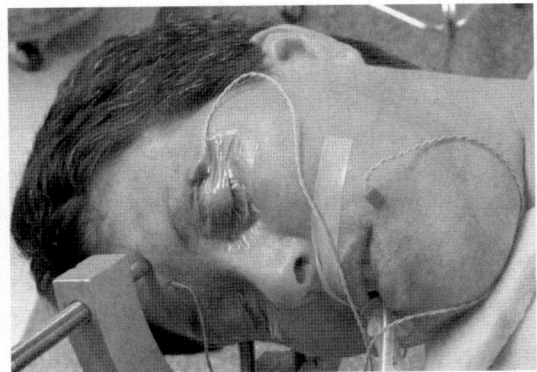

Figure 14–3 Subdermal bipolar needle electrodes are placed in the superior portion of the orbicularis oculi muscle away from the temporalis and masseter muscles to avoid bleed-over of electromyographic activity.

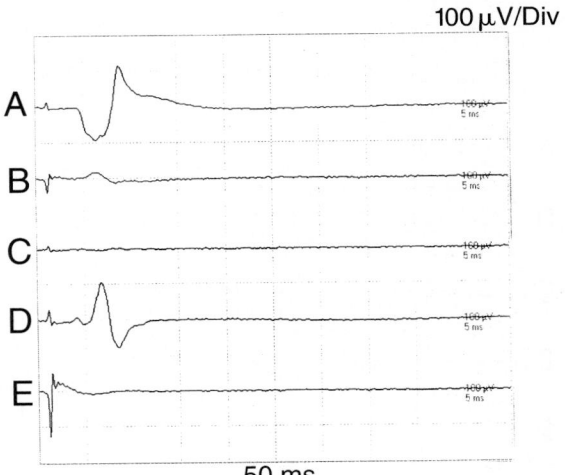

Figure 14–4 Recordings of stimulated electromyography (EMG) to probe stimulation of the motor branch (V3) of the fifth nerve are shown. Traces A through E reflect EMG from the orbicularis oculi (A), orbicularis oris (B), mentalis (C), masseter (D), and trapezius (E) muscles. Note the large biphasic responses from the orbicularis oculi and masseter muscles. The response exhibited in trace A reflects temporalis activity in the orbicularis oculi channel. These muscles are in such close proximity that electrode placement near the lateral orbital rim results in activity to stimulation of either nerve (V or VII).

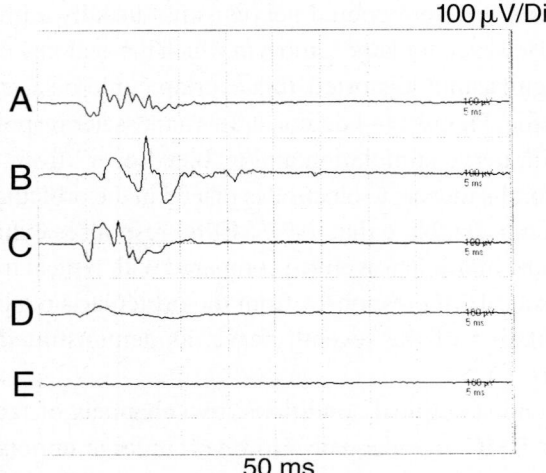

100 µV/Div

50 ms

Figure 14–5 Recordings of stimulated electromyography (EMG) to probe stimulation of the seventh nerve during the same surgery as those acquired in Figure 14–3 are shown. Traces A through E reflect EMG from the orbicularis oculi (A), orbicularis oris (B), mentalis (C), masseter (D), and trapezius (E) muscles. Note the complexity of the responses compared with those seen in Figure 14–3. The multiphasic and longer duration activity are typical of EMG responses to probe stimulation of the seventh nerve.

then he/she may be comfortable interpreting the output of the monitoring equipment himself/herself. Otherwise, the use of personnel trained and qualified to per-

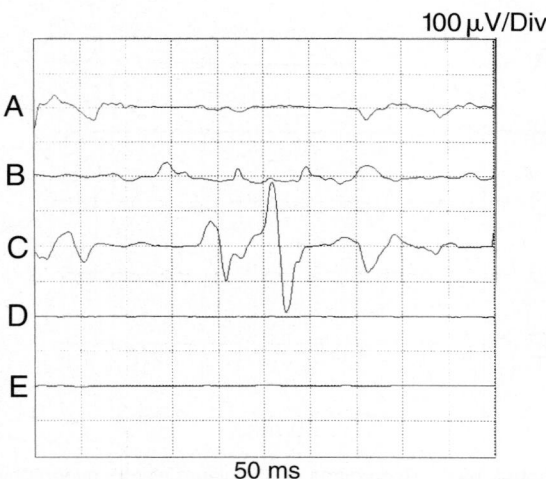

100 µV/Div

50 ms

Figure 14–6 Triggered electromyographic activity showing responses captured to a 100-µV trigger. Traces A through E reflect activity from the orbicularis oculi (A), orbicularis oris (B), mentalis (C), masseter (D), and trapezius (E) muscles. Note that the activity from the orbicularis oculi and oris muscles (traces A and B) did not reach an amplitude great enough to trigger a capture. Only the activity from the mentalis (trace C) reached adequate amplitude for a capture or an audible alert.

form neurophysiologic monitoring is strongly recommended. Using more sophisticated equipment and trained personnel has distinct advantages. As noted above, multichannel monitoring equipment allows monitoring of other motor nerves and helps differentiate true facial nerve stimulation from artifact or other cranial nerve stimulation. Additionally, a diffuse increase in EMG activity in multiple muscle groups may indicate reduced depth of anesthesia, which can be disastrous during posterior cranial fossa surgery. Furthermore, use of monitoring personnel allows the surgeon to concentrate on performing the surgery rather than having to divert attention to interpret the EMG feedback. Finally, for monitoring to be successful, the surgeon must respond appropriately to the feedback provided and alter activities to reduce or eliminate facial nerve irritation.

Stimulation of the nerve with electric current should be done at the lowest possible level. Pulse duration and the voltage or current determine the strength of the stimulus. Most commercial systems use a pulse width of 0.05 or 0.10 µs and provide intensity integrals of 0.05 or 0.10 mA. During initial stages of tumor resection, when the location of the seventh nerve may not be obvious, spontaneous EMG activity would suggest close proximity to the nerve. In this instance, a slightly higher pulse intensity (0.10 to 0.20 mA) is useful when searching for the nerve in a field in which anatomy is distorted. At the conclusion of surgery, the functional integrity of the facial nerve may be estimated by determining the lowest current level required for facial nerve stimulation. If robust amplitude motor responses are obtained from the facial nerve at its exit from the brainstem with stimulation at 0.05 to 0.10 mA, then good facial function is expected.

Facial nerve monitoring during otologic surgery may be helpful in reducing the risk of facial nerve injury during cases in which the facial nerve may be exposed by disease (cholesteatoma, granulation tissue) or congenital variation of anatomy. Because of the fibrous sheath surrounding the nerve in the temporal bone, higher current levels, in the 0.20 to 0.50-mA range, are required to stimulate EMG responses. If attempts to stimulate the nerve are being performed through a thin bony layer, higher current levels, 0.50 to 1.0 mA, are required.

There is no substitute for an intimate and thorough knowledge of facial nerve anatomy and its variations within the temporal bone. For the experienced surgeon, facial nerve monitoring may reduce the risk of facial nerve injury during dissection of cholesteatoma or granulation tissue from an exposed nerve. It should not serve as a crutch for finding the nerve during otherwise routine otologic surgery. Clearly, any patient who has had facial nerve symptoms related to cholesteatoma or ear infection or as a consequence of previous otologic surgery warrants facial nerve monitoring during surgery. These symptoms warn the surgeon of the high likelihood that the nerve is dehiscent and directly affected by the disease process, increasing surgical risk.

Routine facial nerve monitoring for otologic surgery remains somewhat controversial as there is disagreement regarding whether it provides significant, protective benefit to the nerve. Some authors express concern that routine use of facial nerve monitoring is no substitute for thorough knowledge of anatomy and may create a false sense of confidence for the inexperienced surgeon. For the experienced surgeon, medicolegal concerns may drive the decision regarding routine facial nerve monitoring during uncomplicated otologic cases. Although the senior author favors selective use of facial nerve monitoring for otologic surgery in his own practice, each surgeon must decide this issue for himself/herself.

AUDITORY MONITORING

Møller and Jannetta first reported recording compound action potentials from the auditory nerve in humans in 1981. This report focused on the correlation of anatomic locations and the different waveforms seen on ABR testing.[28] The year 1982 saw the first reports describing ABR, initially developed in the mid-1970s as a diagnostic tool, used for intraoperative monitoring during acoustic tumor surgery.[29,30] Although direct eighth nerve monitoring provides much larger amplitude responses and faster feedback than ABR, difficulties maintaining electrode position hampered its widespread use. As a result, ABR came to be the preferred method for monitoring auditory function during CPA surgery throughout the 1980s and 1990s.[31–34]

The mid-1990s saw a resurgence of interest in DENM.[35,36] With the traditional morbidities of CPA surgery greatly reduced owing to advances in surgical technique and motor nerve monitoring, increasing focus is being placed on improving rates of hearing preservation.

The best way to improve hearing preservation rates, apart from earlier diagnosis of smaller tumors, is to obtain the most rapid intraoperative feedback possible regarding the functional status of the cochlear nerve. Direct eighth nerve monitoring provides the nearest thing to real-time auditory function during CPA surgery and has been shown to be superior to ABR in facilitating hearing preservation.[25,26]

Scalp-recorded ABR is obtained by arranging surface or subdermal needle electrodes at opposing ends of the dipole or direction of the neuroelectric activity of the auditory neural pathway. Several hundred to several thousand click stimuli generated by a 100-µV square wave pulse are delivered to the ear via cushion or insert earphones. The small click-evoked responses (usually <1.0 µV) are computer averaged and appear within 10 ms of stimulus onset as a series of five to seven waves originally labeled with Roman numerals by Jewett and colleagues.[37] In the normal ABR (Figure 14–7, right ear) the post-stimulus latency of wave I evoked by a suprathreshold (60 to 80 dB nHL [normal hearing level]) click occurs at or before 2 ms. Subsequent waves exhibit latencies at approximately 1-ms intervals. Eighth nerve activity is reflected in waves I and II—the former near the cochlea and the latter near the brainstem.[38,39] The remaining waves are generated by brainstem structures rostral to the pontomedullary junction. Patients with eighth nerve or brainstem lesions rarely exhibit normal ABRs on the affected side and require interpretation by an experienced clinician or technologist. Figure 14–8 shows a series of

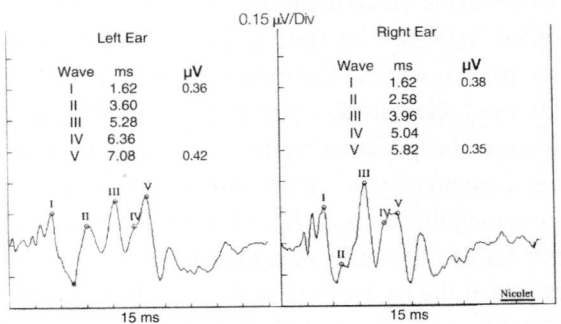

Figure 14–7 Scalp-recorded auditory brainstem response (ABR) traces for the left and right ears of a patient with a left-sided cerebellopontine angle lesion are shown. The left ear ABR exhibits relatively normal morphology. Wave I latency is normal, but the remaining peaks exhibit abnormal absolute and interpeak latencies. The right ear ABR exhibits normal morphology and normal absolute and interpeak latencies.

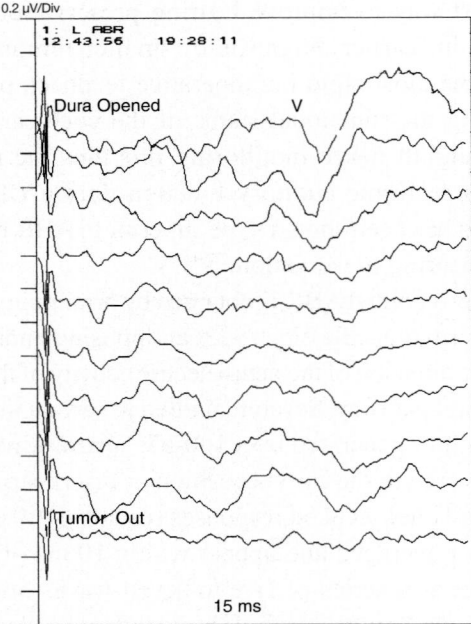

Figure 14–8 Serial recordings of scalp-recorded auditory brainstem responses acquired during resection of a 2.5-cm acoustic neuroma. The top trace was acquired just subsequent to opening the dura and was used as a baseline trace by which all subsequent traces were compared. Only wave V was clearly identified in the baseline trace. Subsequent traces exhibited even greater morphologic abnormality.

ABR tracings obtained during resection of an acoustic neuroma.

While recording the ABR during surgery, subdermal needle electrodes are preferred because of their impedance stability over long periods of time. An active electrode is placed at or near the vertex and a reference electrode on the mastoid, earlobe, or neck. Since the scalp-recorded ABR is a far-field response, slight variations in placing the vertex electrode are not critical. To optimize wave I, the reference electrode is placed on the mastoid or earlobe ipsilateral to the stimulated ear. However, this placement may be inconvenient for surgeries of the ear in which the surgical field lies close to the mastoid and/or earlobe. In such cases, placement of the reference electrode at the base of the skull or high cervical spine will yield a wave I comparable to the mastoid/earlobe placement.

Insert earphones with tube extensions deliver the acoustic click to the ear. The tube extension is secured in the ear with a flexible universal earmold (eg, Doc's Promold®) or a foam earmold. The universal mold is preferred to the foam earmold since it creates a more secure fit in the ear. However, the foam tip can be effective when secured in the ear with surgical bone wax. To avoid collection of preparatory or other fluids in the canal of the surgical ear, seal the earmold and tubing with a small adhesive drape (eg, Tegaderm®). A click of slow to moderate rate (7 to 27 per second) should be delivered with sufficient loudness to evoke the three most prominent waves (I, III, and V). Avoid click rates near or at multiples of 60 Hz that can result in cyclic interference from electrical lines and fields. Depending on the degree of hearing loss, 70 to 90 dB nHL is an adequate click intensity. Most patients who require monitoring of auditory function during surgery exhibit preoperative and intraoperative ABR abnormalities; a recording time window of 15 to 20 ms will account for any abnormally prolonged latencies. In an anesthetized patient, a reliable ABR can be identified within a few hundred averaged stimuli. Most difficulties in recording ABRs in the operating room are the result of technical conditions. A preoperative ABR study is recommended to determine the reliability of the ABR for the operative ear and will help avoid any questions regarding technical mishaps that can occur in the operating room. Additionally, occasional recording from the nonsurgical ear provides a control condition accounting for temperature and other nonpathologic events that can affect the ABR during surgery.

The operating room and surgical environment can create unpredictable events that can affect the reliability of the ABR. Continuous recording of the ABR during each stage of the surgery can help identify and troubleshoot these events. Although DENM recordings may be a more desirable method of monitoring during tumor resection, the scalp-recorded ABR is initially necessary to ensure technical reliability since the recording methodologies are similar, with the exception of the intracranial electrode. Additionally, brain retraction applied during initial exposure can alter eighth nerve function, and the scalp-recorded ABR can help identify this situation.

Technically, recording the cochlear nerve action potential (CNAP) is similar to recording the ABR, with some exceptions, including the placement of the reference electrode on or near the eighth nerve and the gain settings. The senior author has a long-standing interest in DENM and prefers an electrode of his own design (available through AD-Tech Medical Instrument Corporation, Racine, Wisconsin), which provides consistent

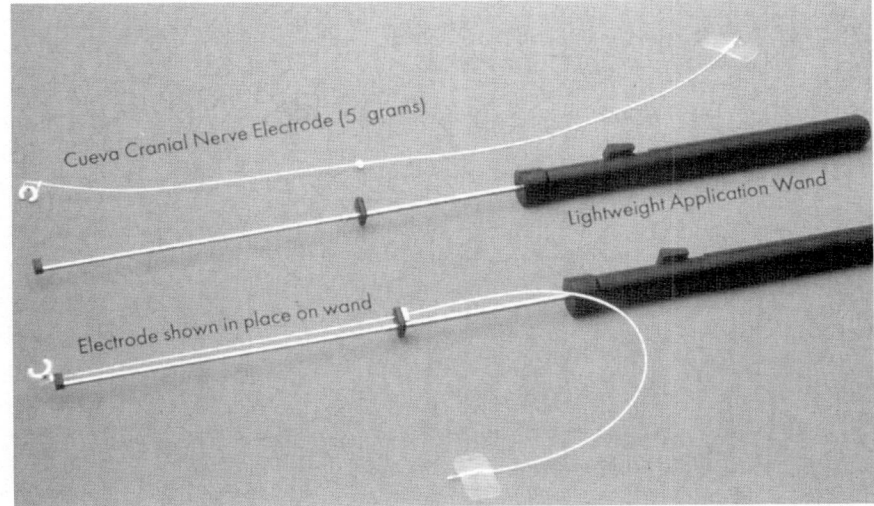

Figure 14–9 The Cueva cranial nerve electrode is shown with its application wand. When mounted on the wand, tension along the lead wire opens the C-shaped ring, allowing atraumatic placement on the cochlear nerve.

but gentle positioning on the cochlear nerve.[17,25] This electrode (Figure 14–9) partially encircles the cochlear nerve but allows atraumatic escape of the nerve should the electrode be accidentally displaced. When the electrode is mounted on the applicator, the opening in the C-shaped ring is opened widely, allowing for atraumatic insinuation of the electrode around the cochlear nerve. Simple digital pressure on the finger pad of the applicator allows closure of the ring, securing it gently on the nerve. The electrode wire is then disengaged from the proximal yoke of the applicator and the applicator is carefully withdrawn, leaving the electrode on the cochlear nerve as seen in Figure 14–10.

The amplitude of the CNAP is anywhere from 10 to 100 times larger than that of the scalp-recorded ABR since the impedance of the head significantly reduces the voltage of the ABR generators to an amplitude range of 0.50 to 1.0 µV. Because of the proximity of the intracranial electrode, the CNAP can be as large as 50 µV, depending on the extent of eighth nerve compromise and electrode location. Additionally, the voltage of the CNAP provides an improved signal-to-noise ratio, requiring fewer averaged responses to yield a reliable waveform. In the surgical environment, the scalp-recorded ABR may require 1 to 2 minutes to yield a reliable tracing, whereas the CNAP may be obtained in as little as six-tenths of a second. Figure 14–11 demonstrates a scalp-recorded ABR and a DENM from a patient undergoing surgery

for an acoustic neuroma. The DENM electrode was placed at the cochlear nerve root entry to the brainstem. The amplitude of the scalp-recorded ABR was less than 0.5 µV, whereas the DENM response exceeded 45.0 µV. Serially recorded DENM tracings acquired during removal of an acoustic neuroma are shown in Figure 14–12. The final tracing was recorded at the completion of tumor removal. Although the DENM response exhib-

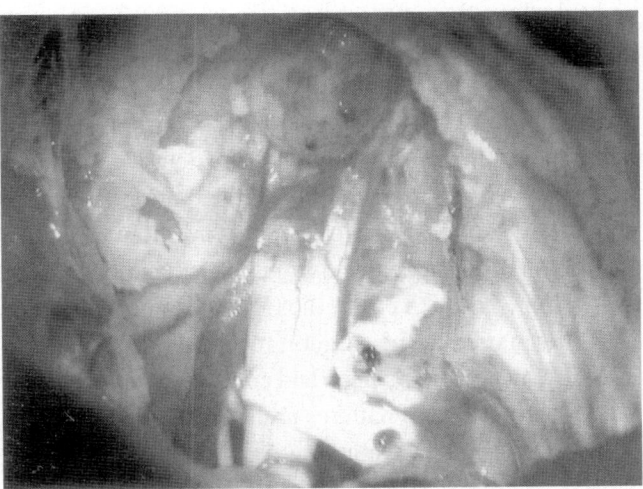

Figure 14–10 The electrode is in place on the cochlear nerve during retrosigmoid craniotomy for removal of a right, intracanalicular acoustic neuroma. The tumor arose from the superior vestibular nerve. Postoperative pure-tone levels were maintained within 5 dB of preoperative levels, and speech discrimination remained at 96%.

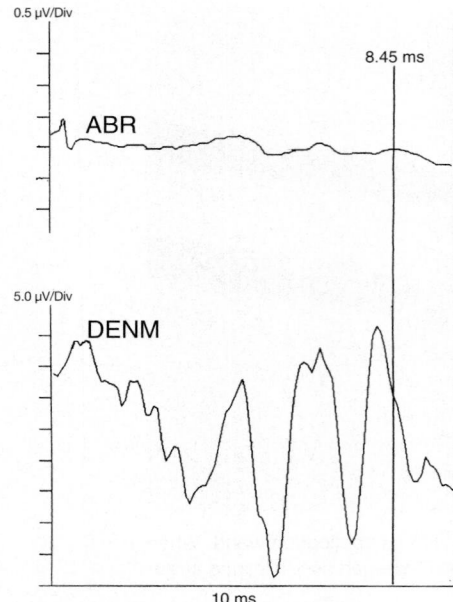

Figure 14–11 Scalp-recorded auditory brainstem response (ABR) and direct eighth nerve monitoring (DENM) traces recorded from the same patient undergoing craniotomy for acoustic neuroma removal are shown. The DENM electrode was placed at the eighth nerve entry zone at the brainstem. The ABR is the averaged response to 300 stimuli, and the DENM is the averaged response to 20 stimuli. Both were acquired with the same click rate (17.1/s) and click intensity (90 dB nHL), resulting in acquisition times of approximately 15 seconds and 1 second, respectively. Both traces are displayed with a 10-ms time window for comparison. A cursor is placed at wave V of the ABR (8.45 ms) and corresponds closely to the latest peak seen in the DENM. The amplitudes of the DENM waveforms exceed the ABR by nearly 100 times.

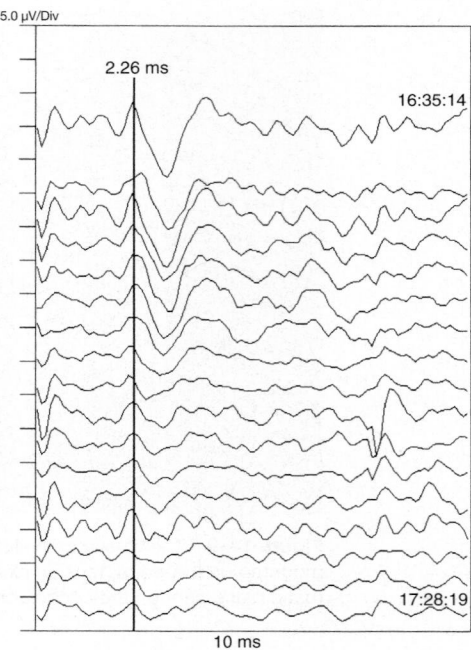

Figure 14–12 Serially recorded direct eighth nerve monitoring (DENM) traces acquired during tumor removal are shown. The first trace was recorded at 16:35:14 and the last trace at 17:28:19, just following removal of the remaining sections of the tumor. Although the last trace shows a decline in the DENM, evidence of activity consistent with neural continuity is evident.

ited a decline, there was still evidence of cochlear nerve continuity and function at the conclusion of surgery.

It is not unusual to observe a significant decline in the scalp-recorded ABR during tumor resection, and, in many cases, the ABR may be absent despite neural continuity. Authors have reported hearing preservation in a substantial percentage of surgical patients in whom the scalp-recorded ABR disappeared during surgical removal of the CPA tumor.[38] In such cases, the CNAP can provide valuable information to the surgeon regarding the condition of the eighth nerve. Roberson and colleagues reported their findings in a series of patients undergoing surgery for an acoustic neuroma in whom the ABR was absent, yet all had a detectable CNAP.[20] Figure 14–13 demonstrates the recordings from a patient in whom the ABR was absent, but a reliable CNAP was recorded using DENM.

Although the ABR will always be a part of auditory monitoring for CPA surgery, it has distinct disadvantages compared to DENM. The monitoring of cochlear nerve action potentials gives more rapid feedback with robust amplitudes. The CNAP can often identify neural integrity when ABR is no longer recordable. Hence, in their striving for optimal patient outcomes, an ever-increasing number of centers are using DENM as a routine part of CPA surgery.

OTHER CRANIAL NERVE MONITORING

Electromyography is widely used to monitor other motor cranial nerves during neurotologic surgery. The motor branch of the trigeminal nerve, the vagus nerve, the spinal accessory nerve, and the hypoglossal nerve are commonly monitored using EMG.[40,41] These nerves have been monitored primarily in patients undergoing surgery for tumors affecting the CPA, jugular foramen, and Meckel's cave.

Monitoring of the other motor cranial nerves involves placing either needle or surface electrodes in or near the muscles innervated by the nerve of interest. In the case

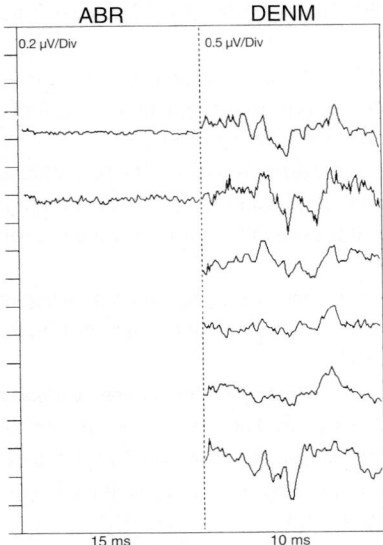

ABR   DENM

0.2 µV/Div   0.5 µV/Div

15 ms   10 ms

Figure 14–13 Simultaneous recordings of the auditory brainstem response (ABR) and direct eighth nerve monitoring (DENM) are shown. No response peaks were observed in the ABR recordings. Although the peaks seen in the DENM traces are abnormally reduced in amplitude (approximately 1.0 µV), they could be reliably recorded during tumor removal. The last DENM trace was acquired subsequent to tumor removal.

of the trigeminal nerve, the masseter or temporalis muscle may be used. Needle electrode placement into the trapezius and tongue muscles for monitoring the spinal accessory and hypoglossal nerves, respectively, is readily accomplished. Monitoring the vagus nerve is more challenging and requires either direct laryngoscopy for needle electrode placement into the vocalis muscles of the true vocal cords or use of a specially designed endotracheal tube that incorporates surface electrodes on its surface. As with facial nerve monitoring using EMG, neuromuscular paralysis must be avoided during the course of surgery.

Direct nerve monitoring of motor nerves has not been previously reported, but the senior author has used this technique with good results in surgery for tumors of the jugular foramen, low CPA, and foramen magnum. The same electrode used to monitor the cochlear nerve in the CPA is secured around the vagus, spinal accessory, and hypoglossal nerves in the neck. To ensure stable positioning, the open part of the C-shaped electrode is sutured with fine (4-0 or 5-0) silk to create a ring. The suture needle is passed through the soft silicone of the electrode at the edges of the opening.

Direct motor nerve monitoring does not rely on the neuromuscular junction and therefore allows ongoing

neuromuscular blockade, thereby simplifying the administration of anesthesia, which can be very helpful if use of the bipolar cautery is causing jerking muscular activity even from mild current spread. However, because the nerves of the jugular foramen are in direct contact with each other as they pass into the pars nervosa, electrical stimulation of one of the nerves intracranially often results in firing of all of the nerves. Mechanical stimulation of one of the nerves results in a compound action potential limited to that nerve; hence, the technique remains helpful during tumor dissection.

SUMMARY

Ever-growing numbers of surgeons are using neurophysiologic monitoring to help achieve optimal surgical outcomes for their patients undergoing neurotologic surgery. The last two decades have seen significant advances in technology facilitating routine use of these valuable monitoring methods. Future advances such as wireless connections between the monitoring head box/amplifiers and the averaging computer may reduce the impact of 60-cycle electrical interference in the operating room. The reader is encouraged to employ monitoring where judged appropriate in practice. In the final analysis, if the patient will likely have an improved result because neurophysiologic monitoring was used, then it should be used.

REFERENCES

1. Krause F. Surgery of the brain and spinal cord. Vol II. New York: Rebman Company; 1912.
2. Delgado TE, Buchheit WA, Rosenholtz HR, et al. Intraoperative monitoring of facial muscle evoked responses obtained by intracranial stimulation of the facial nerve: a more accurate technique for facial nerve dissection. Neurosurgery 1979;4:418–21.
3. Givre A, Olivecrona H. Surgical experiences with acoustic neuroma. J Neurosurg 1949;6:396–407.
4. Rand RW, Kurze TL. Facial nerve preservation by posterior fossa transmeatal microdissection in total removal of acoustic tumors. J Neurol Neurosurg Psychiatry 1965;28:311–6.
5. Williams JD, Lehman R. Bells against palsy. Am J Otol 1988;9: 81–2.
6. Møller AG, Jannetta PJ. Preservation of facial function during removal of acoustic neuromas. J Neurosurg 1984;61:757–60.
7. Gantz BJ. Intraoperative facial nerve monitoring. Am J Otol 1985;Nov. Suppl:58–61.

8.   Harner SG, Daube JR, Ebersold MJ. Electrophysiologic monitoring of facial nerve during temporal bone surgery. Laryngoscope 1986;96:65–9.

9.   Prass RL, Luders H. Evoked electromyographic activity during acoustic neuroma resection. Neurosurgery 1986;19:392–400.

10. Møller AG, Jannetta PJ. Compound action potentials recorded intracranially from the auditory nerve in man. Exp Neurol 1981;74:862–74.

11. Silverstein H, McDaniel AB, Norrell H. Hearing preservation after acoustic neuroma surgery using intraoperative direct eighth cranial nerve monitoring. Am J Otol 1985;6 Suppl: 99–106.

12. Harner SG, Daube JR, Ebersold MJ, et al. Improved preservation of facial nerve function with use of electrical monitoring during removal of acoustic neuromas. Mayo Clin Proc 1987;62:92–102.

13. Benecke JE, Calder HB, Chadwick G. Facial nerve monitoring during acoustic neuroma removal. Laryngoscope 1987;97: 697–700.

14. Ojemann RG, Levine RA, Montgomery WM. Use of intraoperative auditory evoked potentials to preserve hearing in unilateral acoustic neuroma removal. J Neurosurg 1984;61:938–48.

15. Abramson M, Stein BM, Pedley TA, et al. Intraoperative BAER monitoring and hearing preservation in the treatment of acoustic neuromas. Laryngoscope 1985;95:1318–22.

16. Schramm J, Mokrusch T, Fahlbusch R, et al. Detailed analysis of intraoperative changes monitoring brain stem acoustic evoked potentials. Neurosurgery 1988;22:694–702.

17. Cueva RA, Morris GF, Prioleau GR. Direct cochlear nerve monitoring: first report on a new atraumatic, self-retaining electrode. Am J Otol 1998;19:202–7.

18. Zappia JJ, Wiet RJ, O'Conner CA, et al. Intraoperative auditory monitoring in acoustic neuroma surgery. Otolaryngol Head Neck Surg 1996;115:98–106.

19. Colletti V, Fiorini FG. Advances in monitoring of seventh and eighth cranial nerve function during posterior fossa surgery. Am J Otol 1998;19:503–12.

20. Roberson JB, Jackson LE, McAuley JR. Acoustic neuroma surgery: absent auditory brainstem response does not contraindicate attempted hearing preservation. Laryngoscope 1999;109: 904–10.

21. Harper CM, Daube JR. Facial nerve electromyography and other cranial nerve monitoring. J Clin Neurophysiol 1998;15:206–16.

22. Romstock J, Strauss C, Fahlbusch R. Continuous electromyography monitoring of motor cranial nerves during cerebellopontine angle surgery. J Neurosurg 2000;93:586–93.

23. Hammerschlag PE, Cohen NL. Intra-operative monitoring of facial nerve function in cerebellopontine angle surgery. Otolaryngol Head Neck Surg 1990;103:681–4.

24. Kwartler J, Luxford W, Atkins J, et al. Facial nerve monitoring. Otolaryngol Head Neck Surg 1991;104:814–7.

25. Cueva RA, Mastrodimos B. An atraumatic, self-retaining electrode for direct cochlear nerve monitoring. In: Proceedings of the Third International Conference on Acoustic Neurinoma and Other CPA Tumors. Bologna: Monduzzi Editore; 1999. p. 505–8.

26. Jackson LE, Roberson JB. Acoustic neuroma surgery: use of cochlear nerve action potential monitoring for hearing preservation. Am J Otol 2000;21:249–59.

27. Bendet E, Rosenberg SI, Wilcox TO, et al. Intraoperative facial nerve monitoring: a comparison between electromyography and mechanical-pressure monitoring techniques. Am J Otol 1999; 20:793–9.

28. Møller AR, Jannetta PJ. Compound action potentials recorded intracranially from the auditory nerve in man. Exp Neurol 1981;74:862–74.

29. Rausdzens PA, Shetter AG. Intraoperative monitoring of brainstem auditory evoked potentials. J Neurosurg 1982;57:341–8.

30. Grundy BL, Jannetta PJ, Procoio PT, et al. Intraoperative monitoring of brain stem auditory evoked potentials. J Neurosurg 1982;57:674–81.

31. Abramson M, Stein BM, Pedley TA, et al. Intraoperative BAER monitoring and hearing preservation in the treatment of acoustic neuromas. Laryngoscope 1985;95:1318–22.

32. Ojemann RG, Levine RA, Montgomery WM, et al. Use of intraoperative auditory evoked potentials to preserve hearing in unilateral acoustic neuroma removal. J Neurosurg 1984;61: 938–48.

33. Schramm J, Mokrusch T, Fahlbusch R, et al. Detailed analysis of intraoperative changes monitoring brain stem acoustic evoked potentials. Neurosurgery 1988;22:694–702.

34. Møller AR. Use of brainstem auditory evoked potentials in intraoperative neurophysiologic monitoring. In: Kartush JM, Bouchard KR, editors. Neuromonitoring in otology and head and neck surgery. New York: Raven Press; 1992. p. 199–214.

35. Colletti V, Bricolo A, Fiorino FG, et al. Changes in directly recorded cochlear nerve compound action potentials during acoustic tumor surgery. Skull Base Surg 1994;4(1):1–9.

36. Nedzelski JM, Chiong CM, Cashman MZ, et al. Hearing preservation in acoustic neuroma surgery: value of monitoring cochlear nerve action potentials. Otolaryngol Head Neck Surg 1994;111:703–9.

37. Jewett DL, Romano MN, Williston JS. Human auditory evoked potentials: possible brain stem components detected on the scalp. Science 1970;167:1517–8.

38. Levine RA, Ronner SF, Ojemann RG. Auditory evoked potential and other neurophysiologic monitoring techniques during tumor surgery in the cerebellopontine angle. In: Intraoperative monitoring techniques in neurosurgery. McGraw-Hill; 1994. p. 175–91.

39. Martin WH, Pratt H, Schwegler JW. The origin of the human auditory brainstem response wave II. Electroencephalogr Clin Neurophysiol 1995;96:357–70.

40. Harper CM, Daube JR. Facial nerve electromyography and other cranial nerve monitoring. J Clin Neurophysiol 1998;15:206–16.

41. Romstock J, Strauss C, Fahlgusch R. Continuous electromyography monitoring of motor cranial nerves during cerebellopontine angle surgery. J Neurosurg 2000;93:586–93.

15

Endoscope-Assisted Middle Ear Surgery

Dennis S. Poe, MD, FACS

The introduction of endoscopy into the middle ear has opened up new opportunities for minimally invasive temporal bone surgery. The use of the surgical microscope brought revolutionary advances into the field of otologic surgery because its new technology expanded the ability of surgeons to see in limited confines of the temporal bone. Similarly, endoscopic imaging provides dramatic new vistas to the otologist, and we are just in the early exciting phases of developing the appropriate applications and supporting instrumentation. The endoscope lens brings the surgeon's view into the depths of the operative field and can provide a wide field of view with perspectives not possible through a surgical microscope.

The operating microscope provides magnified images in a straight line extending from the objective lens. Many deep recesses within the temporal bone cannot be visualized directly without the surgeon taking measures to expand the surgical exposure. Endoscopes have an immediate advantage with an inherently wide field of view that extends from the tip of the instrument's lens. Additional angulation of view is accomplished by placing prisms on the end. Endoscopes offer the surgeon the capability of wide field visualization with minimal exposure, looking behind the obstructions or overhangs and peering into recesses with much less requirement for surgical exposure than demanded by conventional techniques. Surgical morbidity and operating time can be substantially reduced. Endoscopy within the middle ear may be done through a myringotomy, offering spectacular in vivo examinations free of the artifacts of blood, tissue transudates, and injected local anesthetic agents. Accordingly, endoscopy may be useful for various diagnostic purposes, such as perilymphatic fistula explorations. Endoscopes also improve the ability to inspect the entire middle ear after cholesteatoma removal. Examination of the undersurfaces of the ossicles and tympanic membrane and the deep recesses of the mastoid cavity can reduce cholesteatoma residual rates.

BRIEF HISTORY

The first published description of visualization of the middle ear by endoscopy was by Mer and colleagues in 1967.[1] They passed a fiberoptic instrument through existing tympanic membrane perforations in two patients, but the image resolution of their instruments was quite limited. Eichner obtained much improved images using 2.7-mm-diameter rigid endoscopes; however, the much larger diameter significantly restricted the endoscope's utility within the small spaces of the temporal bone.[2] Nomura introduced the concept of middle ear exploration by passing a rigid endoscope through a myringotomy in an otherwise intact tympanic membrane.[3]

Rapid advances were subsequently made in fiberoptic resolution by reducing the size of individual fibers and packing more of them within the same outer diameter. Kimura and colleagues,[4] Chays and colleagues,[5] and Hopf and colleagues[6] passed high-resolution fibers through the nasal cavity to inspect the lumen of the eustachian tube, sometimes passing fibers all the way into the middle ear cavity for a limited view of its contents. Takahashi and colleagues inspected the bony eustachian tube orifices of children with 1.7-mm rigid endoscopes passed through an anterior myringotomy prior to the placement of ventilation tubes.[7] Poe and colleagues described the use of 1.9-mm rigid endoscopes through a myringotomy to aid in the diagnosis of perilymphatic fistulae.[8] Thomassin and colleagues developed successful rigid endoscopic techniques as an adjunct to conventional cholesteatoma surgery, dramatically reducing the residual rates of disease.[9] McKennan used minimally invasive endoscopic techniques to perform second-look operations to rule out residual cholesteatoma.[10] Magnan and colleagues[11] and O'Donoghue and O'Flynn[12] began to popularize the use of rigid endoscopes in cerebellopontine angle surgery.

EQUIPMENT

Rigid Hopkins rod endoscopes and fiberoptic endoscopes are both available for use in temporal bone surgery. Generally, the rigid endoscopes are preferred because of their superior resolution. Fiberoptic instruments are continually improving, allowing for ever-increasing numbers of individual light-carrying fibers to be packed into small (outer) diameter endoscopes. Each light fiber carries a portion of the image representing a single pixel, and increasing the number of pixels increases the resolution of the overall image. There is a finite amount of cladding and cement between fibers that creates a visible "chicken wire fence appearance" when images are sharply focused. Rod lens endoscopes avoid this problem, yielding images with superior clarity and resolution. Fiberoptic endoscopes can be constructed with smaller diameters than most rigid endoscopes, but the resulting image is generally considered to be impractical for surgical purposes owing to the consequent reduction in resolution. Newer generation rigid endoscopes, using gradient index of refraction lenses, are becoming ever smaller, and are closing the gap with fiber technology.[8] Charge-coupled device (CCD) camera microchips are now so small that they can be placed on the end of larger endoscopic instruments, eliminating the need for fiberoptic or long-lens systems entirely. As CCD chips become more miniaturized, they have the potential to further revolutionize the capabilities of endoscopes.

Endoscopic images have the disadvantage of spherical distortion ("fisheye views") and cannot provide the three-dimensional view afforded with the binocular operating microscope. Endoscopic magnification increases steeply as an object comes into close proximity to the lens and can approach the powers achieved with the operating microscope. Endoscopic surgeons learn to compensate for the variable magnification and two-dimensional views by watching how a structure and its surroundings change as the endoscope is moved in and out of proximity to it. The three-dimensionality of an image is re-created by these changes with endoscope motion.

Endoscopes intended for introduction through the tympanic membrane must be 1.9 mm in diameter or less. Operating room exposures permit the use of larger endoscopes, such as 2.7 to 4.0 mm, which are preferred since they yield larger images with improved brightness and clarity. Endoscopes typically have 0-, 30-, and 70-degree view angles.

Endoscopic illumination is provided by a halogen or xenon fiberoptic light source, generally using 150 to 300 watts. Images may be viewed directly through the endoscope lens, or, more commonly, a CCD camera is attached to the endoscope lens to deliver the images to a monitor. Computer interfaces, digital or video recording devices, and printing systems are optional.

ENDOSCOPY OF THE EXTERNAL AUDITORY CANAL AND TYMPANIC MEMBRANE

Endoscopes may be used in the office for inspecting areas of the ear that are inaccessible to the operating microscope and for photodocumentation. The panoramic view achieved with a 2.7- or 4-mm endoscope makes for excellent otologic photography. The endoscopes may be used to inspect the tympanic membrane or the medial external auditory canal when microscopic visualization is limited by canal stenosis or other obstruction. Bony canal defects or recesses and the depths of limited mastoid cavities may be easily visualized. Tympanic membrane retraction pockets may be inspected to determine their depth and the presence or absence of cholesteatoma. Surgeons may benefit from such information when considering whether a patient should undergo cholesteatoma surgery and determining the optimal approach.

TRANSTYMPANIC ENDOSCOPY

An endoscope may be passed through an existing perforation or myringotomy in the tympanic membrane to perform a limited middle ear exploration. The procedure may be performed in the office or operating room and is commonly done using Hopkins rod endoscopes with outside diameters of 1.7 or 1.9 mm. The 1.7-mm diameter endoscope is often preferred as it more readily passes through the tympanic membrane.

TECHNIQUE FOR OFFICE TRANSTYMPANIC ENDOSCOPY

The patient is reclined to the supine position in the office examination chair. The tympanic membrane is initially inspected with the operating microscope, and the location of the incision is planned to overlie the area of anticipated pathology. Working through an ear speculum, the tympanic membrane is anesthetized with topical phenol solution (USP) applied by dipping a 20-gauge suction tip into the solution and touching the adherent bead of solution to the tympanic membrane over the incision site only. Phenol is the preferred anesthetic because of its rapid onset of action and local cautery effect that provides a dry, bloodless field. A radial myringotomy is carried out from the umbo to the annulus, creating an opening sufficiently large to readily admit the endoscope without tearing the tympanic membrane. The incision for exploration of a possible perilymphatic fistula is made halfway between the shadow of the round window niche and the distal end of the long process of the incus seen through the tympanic membrane.

Defogger is applied to the endoscope lens at the tip. The drop of defogger is blotted with a cotton sponge, taking care to avoid contact with the lens, which would smear the solution and thus obscure the image.

Initial inspection of the middle ear is done with a 0-degree endoscope, which provides a good overall view of the middle ear. The 30-degree endoscope is usually required to obtain a definitive close-up view of areas with suspected pathology. The angled endoscope is more difficult to use, to a certain extent, because of its off-center view, and it requires some practice for atraumatic insertion through a myringotomy.

MIDDLE EAR ENDOSCOPIC SURGERY

Surgeons with little endoscopic experience would be well advised to introduce the endoscope through the tympanic membrane perforation while looking directly through the eyepiece. Although the image appears quite small to the eye, it allows for an adequate examination and it is easier to maintain control of the endoscope within the ear. Adding a CCD camera can cause disorientation by forcing the surgeon to look at a video monitor remote from the surgical field. Any rotation of the camera produces errors in hand-eye coordinated movements. The camera also adds additional weight to the endoscope system. With practice, most endoscopists eventually prefer video images, which are considerably enlarged and offer more detail of the surgical field.

Endoscopes are passed through a handheld ear speculum slightly smaller than would ordinarily be used with a microscope. The smaller speculum extends deeper into the external auditory canal and helps protect the sensitive canal skin from inadvertent contact with the endoscope shaft that could produce pain or bleeding. The speculum and endoscope shaft are supported by the surgeon's nondominant hand, and fine fingertip movements are used to guide the endoscope tip atraumatically through the myringotomy. The dominant hand is used to hold the eyepiece and camera, helping to guide the endoscope tip and allowing for some minimal rotation of the field of view as desired. With the endoscope fully passed through the tympanic membrane, a wide view of the middle ear can be appreciated (Figure 15–1). Close-up, angled views, especially beneath overhangs, are best achieved with a 30-degree endoscope, which is introduced by rotating the view angle to the appropriate direction prior to insertion into the middle ear (Figures 15–2 and 15–3). When viewing on the video monitor, it is especially important to ensure that the camera is properly oriented to avoid trauma to the ear from inadvertent movements. The endoscope is generally withdrawn and reinserted whenever a significant change in the direction of view angles is desired.

Patients may experience a heat-induced caloric effect with vertigo when using the 300-watt light source if the endoscope remains in situ more than 45 to 60 seconds. Withdrawal of the endoscope relieves the symptoms, and the examination may proceed, either with reduced brightness or by removing the endoscope periodically. The author has had no case of thermal injury, but elevations of temperature, up to 50°, have been produced in dry temporal bones exposed for 2 minutes or more.[13] Vertigo has not been seen with the 150-watt light source.

At the conclusion of the endoscopy, the myringotomy is inspected under the microscope to ascertain that the

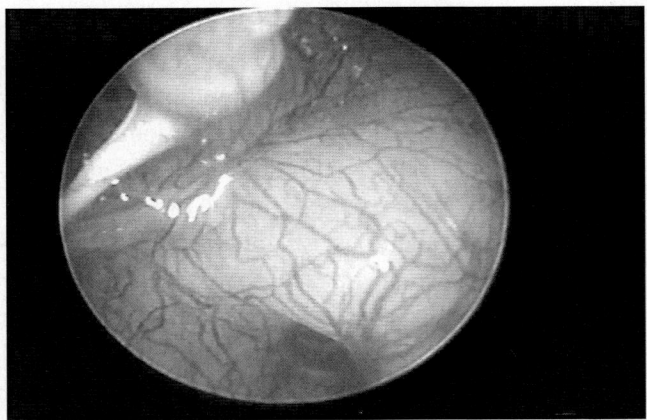

Figure 15–1 Transtympanic endoscopic view of the middle ear: 1.9-mm, 0-degree, angled Hopkins rod endoscope.

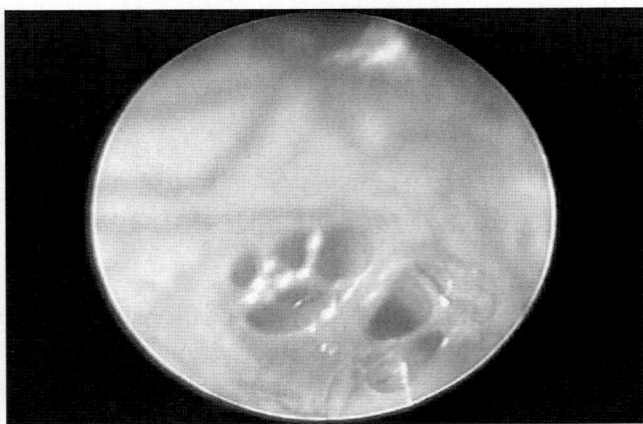

Figure 15–3 Transtympanic endoscopic view of the round window niche: 1.9-mm, 30-degree angled Hopkins rod endoscope.

margins were minimally traumatized and nearly in apposition. Wide gaps or inadvertent tears may be repaired with adhesive Steri-strip,™ cigarette paper, or Gelfilm™. This problem is usually avoided by making a sufficiently long myringotomy initially. The patient is advised to follow water precautions and avoid nose blowing for 2 weeks after the procedure.[14]

The author has performed 112 transtympanic endoscopic procedures in the office, and there have been no complications. There has been no instance of vertigo, persistent hearing loss, infection, or persistent perforation.

PERILYMPHATIC FISTULA EXPLORATION

Surgical exploration for perilymphatic fistula was once considered the gold standard for establishing the diagnosis. It has been learned that visualization of pooling

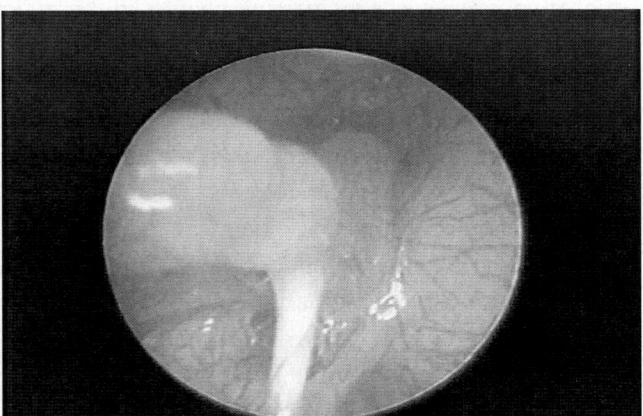

Figure 15–2 Transtympanic endoscopic view of the superior mesotympanum: 1.9-mm, 30-degree, angled Hopkins rod endoscope.

of fluid in the round and/or oval window niches, the previously accepted criterion for determining the presence or absence of a fistula, is inaccurate. Tissue transudates or residual injected anesthetic can also accumulate in these niches and appear identical to a presumed fistula.[15] Endoscopic exploration may help reduce some of the artifacts by using a topical cauterizing anesthetic such as phenol. The middle ear can be inspected in an undisturbed state. Transtympanic exploration for fistula may be done entirely in the office, or, if done in the operating room, there is also the capability to elevate a tympanomeatal flap for fistula repair, if a fistula is discovered.

Studies have been done to determine if endoscopy, in comparison to microscopic examination, has sufficient resolution to detect the presence of a leaking fistula.[16] Endoscopic and microscopic findings have been compared in temporal bone specimens and in the operating room.[17] Seventeen patients with a clinical history and findings suspicious for fistula underwent combined transtympanic endoscopy and microsurgical exploration. The middle ear endoscopy was performed first, with no local anesthetic, and findings were determined. One mL of lidocaine (1% solution with 1 to 100,000 epinephrine) was then infiltrated into the external auditory canal, and a standard tympanomeatal flap was elevated. In 8 of the 17 patients, thorough endoscopic examinations had showed no evidence of a fistula. However, microsurgical exploration, active pooling of clear fluid in the round or oval window, which would ordinarily have been regarded as a fistula, was seen. The preceding endoscopic exploration was done carefully and actually yielded more complete exposure of each window niche with superior magnification and resolution when compared to microscopic views. It was concluded that the pooling of fluids seen only on microscopic view must be artifactual.

There were four cases of probable true perilymphatic fistula identified with both endoscopic and microsurgical examinations. The site of each fistula was imaged better with the endoscope than by a microscope. Each case involved true trauma: barotraumatic injury in three cases and perforating trauma in one case. There were five patients, all of whom had undergone previous surgery and had inadequate endoscopic examination as a result of bleeding that occurred during the lysis of middle ear adhesions that resulted from the prior surgery (Figure 15–4).

The author has performed 75 transtympanic middle ear explorations for perilymphatic fistula in the office or in the operating room and has identified only 5 cases in which a fistula was seen. Other surgeons, using endoscopic techniques, have also reported a low incidence of fistulae, with Rosenberg and colleagues[18] seeing no cases in 13 endoscopic explorations and Pyykkö and colleagues[19] identifying only 2 fistulae in 350 endoscopies.

Middle ear endoscopic techniques probably improve the ability to identify true perilymphatic fistulas and reduce the number of false-positive examinations. Open surgical exploration cannot eliminate the artifactual pooling of infiltrated anesthetics and surgically induced transudates. Endoscopy is an excellent adjunct to microsurgical exploration (Figure 15–5).

Fistulae in adults most likely occur with significant trauma, such as barotrauma, head injury, and penetrating trauma and otologic surgery. Exploration is indicated in patients with sensorineural hearing loss or persistent vertigo or dysequilibrium associated with the trauma. A positive subjective or objective fistula test was present in each of the true fistula cases seen by the author. The diagnosis of perilymphatic fistula should be made only after exclusion of other possible etiologies. Consideration of additional evaluation, such as laboratory tests and imaging studies, should be individualized.

ENDOSCOPY IN CHRONIC EAR SURGERY

Endoscopes are best employed in chronic ear surgery as an adjunct to the removal of cholesteatoma.[20–24] Residual disease tends to occur in the sites hardest to visualize with the operating microscope, including the epitympanum, the sinus tympani, and the facial recess. Endoscopes may help detect residual disease in otherwise hidden recesses after microsurgical resection or may be used for a portion of the primary dissection of cholesteatoma. When cholesteatoma is limited to the attic, the aditus ad antrum, the facial recess, or the sinus tympani, endoscope-assisted surgery may eliminate the need for mastoidectomy in many cases. The enhanced ability to remove cholesteatoma reduces the incidence of residual disease and the frequency of planned second-stage procedures. In the event that a second-look oper-

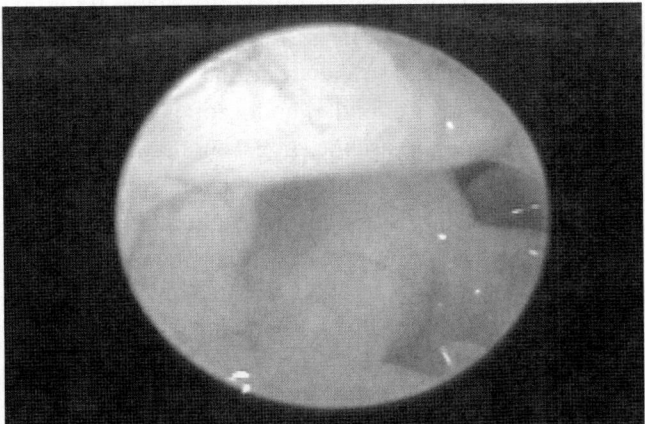

Figure 15–4 Transtympanic endoscopic view of the round window perilymphatic fistula: 1.9-mm, 30-degree, angled Hopkins rod endoscope.

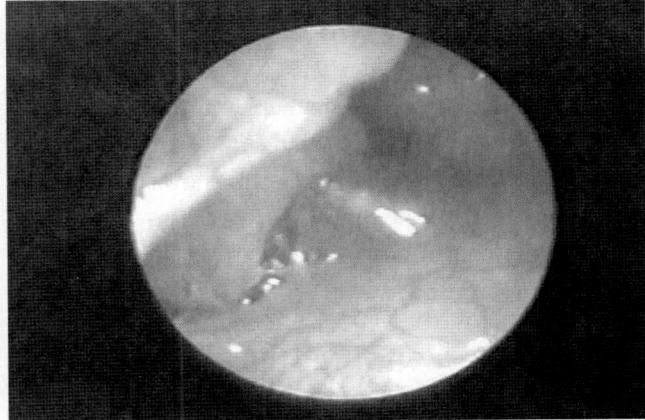

Figure 15–5 Transtympanic endoscopic view of the persistent stapedial artery: 1.9-mm, 30-degree, angled Hopkins rod endoscope.

ation is indicated, the procedure can most often be done as a transcanal approach with endoscopic assistance. Endoscopic visualization of the temporal bone recesses is far superior to the limited views obtained by microsurgical approaches.

The endoscope is not intended to replace microsurgical resection. It has several disadvantages. The endoscopes are held in the surgeon's nondominant hand, so that only one hand is free for surgery. The surgeon must often alternate between dissection and suction-aspiration of blood from the field, reducing operating efficiency compared to two-hand techniques. One should do as much dissection under the microscope as possible and reserve the endoscope for areas that are not easily visualized microscopically. Often an entire case is performed without endoscopes, and the endoscopes may be introduced only at the end of the procedure to inspect the recesses for residual disease. In other cases, microsurgical resection of cholesteatoma matrix may be hindered by firm adhesions in a recess such as in the sinus tympani, and continued "blind" elevation may risk tearing the matrix and leaving residual disease (Figure 15–6). The adhesion may be visualized endoscopically, allowing for expeditious lysis and resumption of microsurgical resection. It is often helpful to alternate between microscopic and endoscopic resections for this reason.

Cases of limited cholesteatoma or tympanic membrane atelectasis with deep retraction pockets are often approached by atticotomy or mastoidectomy. These are the standard microsurgical approaches to remove disease from the epitympanum, the mastoid antrum, and the medial surface of the scutum and within the facial recess itself. Removal of the cholesteatoma matrix is frequently piecemeal, and second-stage procedures are often recommended. These types of cholesteatoma cases are well-suited to endoscopic resection, which may often be performed as a transcanal procedure or through a postauricular exposure, working down the bony canal but without the need for an atticotomy or mastoidectomy. The matrix may be dissected under direct endoscopic visualization and can often be removed completely intact, obviating the need for second-look surgery.

TECHNIQUE

Use of the video monitor is preferred because the images are superior to those seen by viewing through the eye-

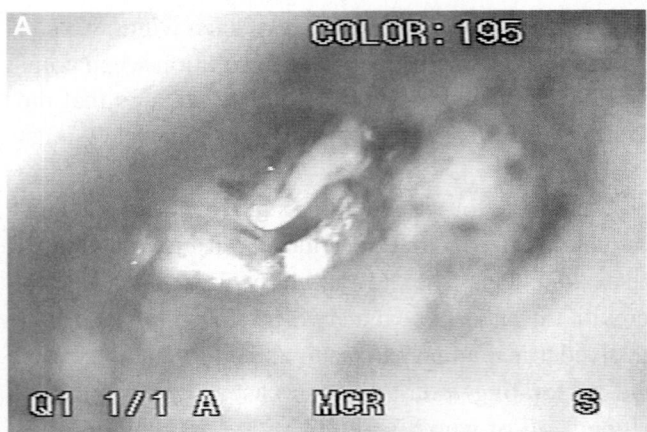

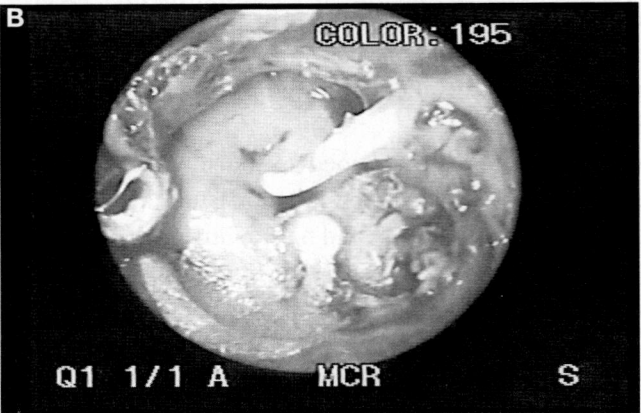

Figure 15–6 *A,* Microscopic view of the left ear with cholesteatoma in posterior-superior pars tensa retraction pocket. *B,* A 4-mm 0-degree Hopkins rod endoscopic view of the same ear.

piece. Prolonged endoscopic resection is optimized by using a monitor. If limited endoscopy is used for a brief section or just to inspect for residual disease, then viewing through the eyepiece is satisfactory and requires less setup time.

Endoscopy is used to view into the recesses so that the 30- and 70-degree angled endoscopes are the most often used. It is best to use the largest endoscope that will fit into the field while allowing sufficient room to pass instruments. The larger image and illumination afforded with the bigger endoscopes are preferred. Endoscopes of 30-degree angulation with a 2.7- or 4-mm outer diameter are often used. A 70-degree, 2.3-mm-diameter endoscope is most useful for viewing deep into the facial recess or aditus and yields excellent views far into the epitympanum and mastoid antrum. It requires considerable practice to use a 70-degree angled endoscope safely as there is no forward visualization. The endoscope is first inserted to nearly the full depth necessary while looking down the shaft of the endoscope with the naked eye and noting the location of the ossicles. The endoscope is then tilted to bring the ossicles into the monitor (or eyepiece) view, and the surgeon may then work through the endoscope or the monitor, carefully tilting the endoscope away from the ossicles into the appropriate recess, but always maintaining awareness of the location of the ossicles, which may now be out of view. The location of the ossicles should be periodically checked to confirm one's orientation and avoid inadvertent injury.

Retraction pockets and cholesteatoma that extend deep into the mastoid or epitympanum are beyond the reach of endoscopic resection and are best managed by open microsurgical techniques. Removal of shallow pockets and cholesteatoma may be assisted with endoscopic resection. The elevation of the atelectatic tympanic membrane or cholesteatoma matrix is begun with a conventional microsurgical technique, generally beginning with freeing up retractions into the attic. It is usually possible to elevate the adhesions off the neck of the malleus without difficulty. Elevation with two-hand techniques is continued until adhesions within the aditus, facial recess, or sinus tympani restrict further elevation. If the matrix cannot be mobilized without risking a tear, the endoscope may be inserted to visualize the adhesions limiting the dissection. The adhesions may then be lysed with long-angled scissors. The endoscope is held in the non-dominant hand, and one-handed dissection is performed using the dominant hand. It may be appropriate to obtain good hemostasis with Gelfoam™ soaked in 1 to 10,000 epinephrine solution placed in the middle ear for a few minutes prior to beginning endoscopic dissection. If bleeding occurs during the dissection, it will be necessary to alternate between suction and dissection. Frequent irrigation of the field aids with hemostasis. It may be beneficial to return to the microscope periodically to improve hemostasis, evacuate clots, and then continue with two-hand dissection until additional adhesions are encountered. Prototype-combined suction-dissectors are useful in improving endoscopic dissection efficiency but are not commercially available to date. Careful elevation of retraction pockets usually results in the intact removal of even very thin matrix in most cases, and, when successfully accomplished, a second-stage procedure is unnecessary (Figure 15–7).

Small cholesteatomas may be excised using techniques similar to those used to manage retraction pockets. The squamous debris are first removed, and in many cases the cholesteatoma matrix may be delivered intact. Large, bulky cholesteatomas are best excised with conventional microsurgical techniques, but endoscopes may be useful in inspecting the epitympanum, the supratubal recess, the facial recess, the sinus tympani, and other recesses. If residual matrix is identified, removal may be accomplished either with endoscopic or microscopic dissection.

It is helpful to use a diamond bur to drill on the medial surface of the scutum, the epitympanic tegmen, and into the supratubal recess to ensure maximal exposure and complete eradication of the disease. When the posterior bony canal wall obstructs the view into these areas, the drilling may be accomplished under endoscopic guidance (Figure 15–8).

Canal wall down mastoidectomy has a fundamental advantage over the intact canal wall technique in that visualization into the sinus tympani, facial recess, and epitympanum is less restricted and the risk of residual disease is appropriately reduced. Thomassin demonstrated that endoscopic visualization into recesses during canal wall up surgery may sufficiently improve residual disease removal as to become comparable with canal wall down surgery.[25] Initially, 44 of his patients underwent intact canal wall mastoidectomy and 47.7% were found to have residual disease at the time of planned second-stage surgery. Thirty-six patients underwent endoscopic inspection for cholesteatoma during the primary operation, and the rate of residual disease dropped

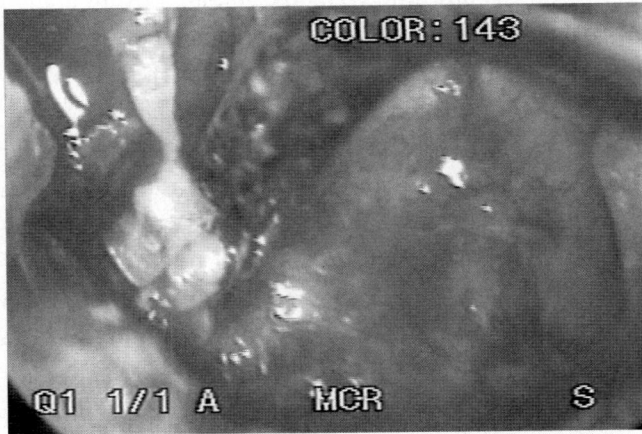

Figure 15–7 Endoscopic dissection of cholesteatoma using a suction dissector.

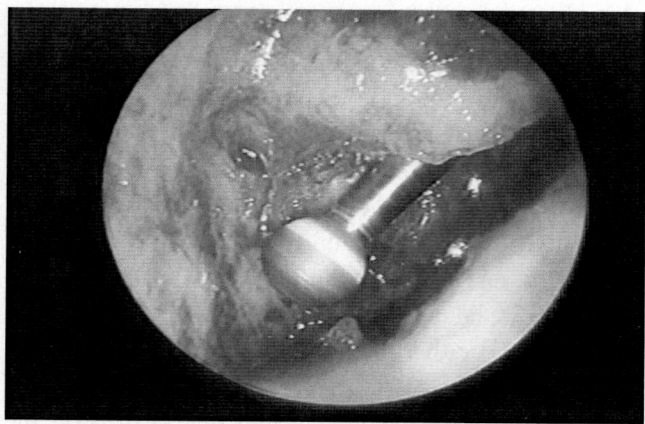

Figure 15–8 Endoscopic view of the right mastoid cavity after intact canal mastoidectomy. A diamond drill is passed down the bony canal to smooth the tegmen bone and ensure cholesteatoma removal.

to 5.5% at the time of the second-stage procedure, an incidence on par with published results from canal wall down operations.

SECOND-LOOK MASTOIDECTOMY

Endoscopic techniques reduce the necessity for second-look procedures and also facilitate them when they are required. Residual cholesteatoma is most commonly found in the epitympanum, sinus tympani, or facial recess rather than in the mastoid antrum or cavity. For this reason, the author prefers a transcanal approach for second-look procedures.[26] McKennan has advocated a small postauricular stab incision through which endoscopic inspection of the mastoid may be done,[10] but the view into the antrum is usually obtained using angled endoscopes introduced via the external auditory canal. Consequently, the author prefers elevation of a tympanomeatal flap through a transcanal approach. Middle ear adhesions are lysed, and hemostasis is obtained, all under microscopic visualization. Once exposure has been achieved, a 70-degree, 2.3-mm-diameter endoscope is introduced into the middle ear and rotated to give a panoramic view of the entire mesotympanum, the sinus tympani, the facial recess, the epitympanum, and the supratubal recess. Lysis of some adhesions is usually necessary to view through the attic and aditus far into the mastoid antrum and up to the tegmen. Satisfactory views are usually obtained. It is useful to alternate between

endoscopic and microsurgical techniques to lyse adhesions and obtain hemostasis (Figures 15–9 and 15–10).

It is especially important to inspect the supratubal recess and sinus tympani carefully as they are the most hidden from view when the posterior bony canal wall is intact. If residual cholesteatoma is identified, small lesions may be removed with endoscopic dissection, but large deposits may require further drilling for exposure and microsurgical removal. Patients are counseled preoperatively about the possibility of reopening the postauricular incision if necessary for cholesteatoma removal.

ENDOSCOPIC TYMPANOPLASTY

Anterior, marginal tympanic membrane perforations are frequently repaired using a postauricular approach to maximize exposure. The visualization of far anterior perforations may be especially difficult, and the anterior margin may be completely hidden from direct view behind a prominent anterior canal bony overhang. Anterior perforations may be managed through a transcanal approach, using the endoscope to visualize the anterior margin.[27,28] When the anterior margin is very narrow, lying quite close to the anterior canal and raising some question as to whether an underlay graft has sufficient contact to hold to the anterior drum remnant, an argon laser may be used to "spot weld" the graft in place. The fiber-delivered laser is convenient as the tip may be bent to accommodate the anterior bony overhang. A line-of-

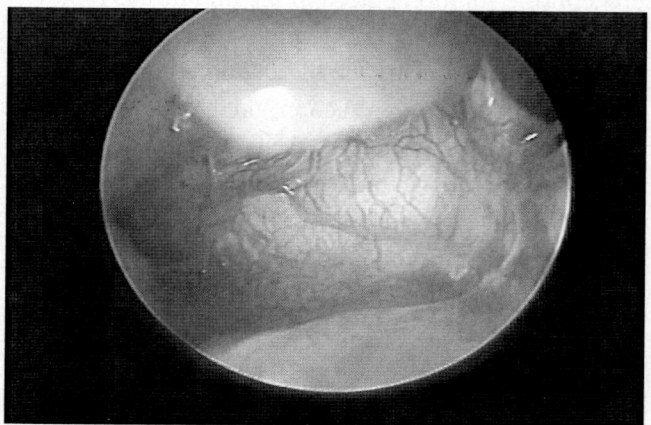

Figure 15–9 A 2.3-mm, 70-degree Hopkins rod endoscopic view of a "second-look" case after primary cholesteatoma removal from the cochleariform process and area medial to the malleus head.

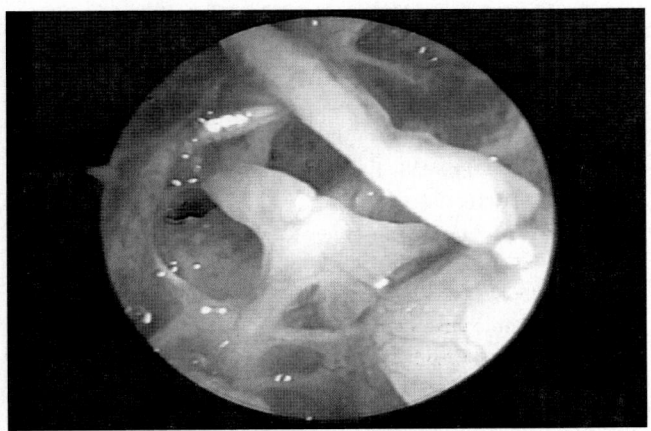

Figure 15–10 A 2.3-mm, 70-degree Hopkins rod endoscopic view of the superior mesotympanum and epitympanum at primary surgery after removal of anterior epitympanic cholesteatoma.

sight laser, such as a CO_2 laser, would not be useful in these circumstances.

ENDOSCOPIC ASSISTANCE IN STAPEDOTOMY

Laser stapedotomy minus prosthesis surgery is performed without prosthesis insertion.[29] An otosclerotic focus limited to the anterior one-third of the footplate may be managed by laser vaporization of the anterior crus and a laser cut made linearly and transversely to divide the stapes footplate between the anterior one-third and the posterior two-thirds. These cuts free the posterior footplate and posterior crus, restoring sound transmission without needing a prosthesis. The procedure differs from early mobilization techniques that fractured the otosclerotic focus but often necessitated postoperative refixation. Division of the footplate posterior to the otosclerotic focus provides lasting air–bone gap closure.[29–31]

Only rarely are the anterior crus and anterior footplate fully visualized with the surgical microscope, and the procedure may be facilitated with endoscopic assistance.

EUSTACHIAN TUBE ENDOSCOPIC SURGERY

Endoscopy of the eustachian tube may be performed from either the middle ear or nasopharynx and is giving new insights into tubal physiology and pathophysiology.[32,33]

The cartilaginous tube may be well studied by positioning an endoscope at the nasopharyngeal orifice, directing the angle of use superiorly into its lumen. Video capture of tubal function during swallows can be studied in slow motion to better understand the pathology cases of dysfunction. Endoluminal surgical procedures are now being performed on the basis of our growing understanding of many different mechanisms for failure of tubal ventilation.[33,34]

FUTURE PROGRESS

There is an ongoing need to develop specialized instruments to complement the minimally invasive endoscopic techniques that are rapidly being developed. Long, angled dissectors and suctions, laser probes, and forceps are being designed. Prototype-combined suction dissectors assist the one-hand techniques necessitated by hand-holding the endoscope.

An endoscope holder may prove useful in the future but should be used with caution to prevent catastrophic injury to the middle ear or ossicles in the event of unexpected patient movement. Fixation of any holder to the head of the patient will be necessary.

Charge-coupled device cameras are becoming smaller and ultimately may be sufficiently tiny to place directly into the middle ear without the need for optical endoscopes, improving the flexibility and versatility of visualizing instrumentation and allowing more working space for surgical dissecting tools.

Surgery of the temporal bone and middle ear will become increasingly minimally invasive with anticipated improved patient outcomes, reduced morbidity, and enhanced maintenance or restoration of function.

REFERENCES

1. Mer SB, Derbyshire AJ, Brushenko A, et al. Fiberoptic endoscopes for examining the middle ear. Arch Otolaryngol 1967;85:387–93.

2. Eichner H. Eline Mother-and Baby-Scope-Optic zur Trommelfell-und Mittelohr-Endoskopie. Laryngol Rhinol Otol (Stuttg) 1978;57:872–6.

3. Nomura Y. Effective photography in otolaryngology-head and neck surgery: endoscopic photography of the middle ear. Otolaryngol Head Neck Surg 1982;90:395–8.

4. Kimura H, Yamaguchi H, Cheng SS, et al. Direct observation of the tympanic cavity by the superfine fiberscope. Nippon Jibi-inkoka Gakkai Kaiho 1989;92:233–8.

5. Chays A, Cohen JM, Magnan J. La microfibroendoscopie tubo-tympanique. Presse Med 1995;24:773–4.

6. Hopf J, Linnarz M, Gundlach P, et al. Die Mikroendoskopie der Eustachischen Röhre und des Mittelohres. Indikationen und klinischer Einsatzpunkt. Laryngorhinootologie 1991;70:391–4.

7. Takahashi H, Honjo I, Fujita A, et al. Transtympanic endoscopic findings in patients with otitis media with effusion. Arch Otolaryngol Head Neck Surg 1990;116:1186–9.

8. Poe DS, Rebeiz EE, Pankratov MM, Shapshay SM. Transtympanic endoscopy of the middle ear. Laryngoscope 1992;102:993–6.

9. Thomassin JM, Korchia D, Duchon-Doris JM. Endoscopic-guided otosurgery in the prevention of residual cholesteatomas. Laryngoscope 1993;103:939–43.

10. McKennan KX. Endoscopic 'second look' mastoidoscopy to rule out residual epitympanic/mastoid cholesteatoma. Laryngoscope 1993;103:810–4.

11. Magnan J, Chays A, Lepetre C, et al. Surgical perspectives of endoscopy of the cerebellopontine angle. Am J Otol 1994;15:366–70.

12. O'Donoghue G, O'Flynn P. Endoscopic anatomy of the cerebellopontine angle. Am J Otol 1993;14:122–5.

13. Bottrill ID, Perrault DF Jr, Poe DS. In vitro and in vivo determination of the thermal effect of middle ear endoscopy. Laryngoscope 1996;106:213–6.

14. Poe DS. Transtympanic endoscopy of the middle ear. Oper Techn Otolaryngol Head Neck Surg 1992;3:993–6.

15. Friedland DR, Wackym PA. A critical appraisal of spontaneous perilymphatic fistulas of the inner ear. Am J Otol 1999;20:261–79.

16. Poe DS, Rebeiz EE, Pankratov MM. Evaluation of perilymphatic fistulas by middle ear endoscopy. Am J Otol 1992;13:529–33.

17. Poe DS, Bottrill ID. Comparison of endoscopic and surgical exploration for perilymphatic fistulas. Am J Otol 1994;15:735–8.

18. Rosenberg SI, Silverstein H, Wilcox TO, Gordon MA. Endoscopy in otology and neurotology. Am J Otol 1994;15:168–72.

19. Pyykkö I, Selmani Z, Ramsay H. Middle ear imaging in neurotological work-up. Acta Otolaryngol Suppl (Stockh) 1995;520:273–6.

20. Rosenberg SI. Endoscopic otologic surgery. Otolaryngol Clin North Am 1996;29:291–300.

21. Bottrill ID, Poe DS. Endoscope-assisted ear surgery. Am J Otol 1995;16:158–63.

22. Yung MM. The use of rigid endoscopes in cholesteatoma surgery. J Laryngol Otol 1994;108:307–9.

23. Bowdler DA, Walsh RM. Comparison of the otoendoscopic and microscopic anatomy of the middle ear cleft in canal wall-up and canal wall-down temporal bone dissections. Clin Otolaryngol 1995;20:418–22.

24. Karhuketo TS, et al. Endoscopy and otomicroscopy in the estimation of middle ear structures. Acta Otolaryngol (Stockh) 1997;117:585–9.

25. Thomassin JM, Korchia D, Doris JM. Endoscopic-guided otosurgery in the prevention of residual cholesteatomas. Laryngoscope 1993;103:939–43.

26. Youssef TF, Poe DS. Endoscopic-assisted second-stage tympanomastoidectomy. Laryngoscope 1997;107:1341–4.

27. el-Guindy A. Endoscopic transcanal myringoplasty. J Laryngol Otol 1992;106:493–5.

28. Pyykkö I, Poe DS, Ishizaki H. Laser-assisted myringoplasty: technical aspects. Acta Otolaryngol Suppl (Stockh) 2000;543:1–4.

29. Silverstein H. Laser stapedotomy minus prosthesis (laser STAMP): a minimally invasive procedure. Am J Otol 1998;19:277–82.

30. Poe DS. Endoscope-assisted laser stapedectomy: a prospective study. Laryngoscope Suppl 2000;110:1–36.

31. Silverstein H. Laser stapedotomy minus prosthesis (laser STAMP): absence of refixation. Presented at the American Otological Society, Palm Desert, CA, May 13, 2001.

32. Fabinyi B, Klug C. A minimally invasive technique for endoscopic middle ear surgery. Eur Arch Otorhinolaryngol Suppl 1997;1:S53–4.

33. Poe DS, Pyykkö I, Valtonen H, Silvolva J. Analysis of eustachian tube function by video endoscopy. Am J Otol 2000;21:602–7.

34. Poe DS, Abou-Halawa A, Abdel-Razek O. Analysis of the dysfunctional eustachian tube by video endoscopy. Am J Otol. [In press.]

THE LIBRARY
KENT & SUSSEX HOSPITAL
TUNBRIDGE WELLS
KENT TN4 8AT

16

Image-Guided Systems in Neurotology/Skull Base Surgery

M. MILES GOLDSMITH, MD, FACS

Traditional teaching of surgical technique emphasizes wide tissue exposure for progressive identification of surgical landmarks to safely navigate to the target. However, visualization beyond the exposed surface is often incomplete because the exposed surgical field lacks spatial clues orienting the surgeon to the underlying geometry of the target area.

In the past, integration of preoperative imaging information into the surgical field has been an intuitive process on the part of the operating surgeon. The surgeon relies on his/her ability to mentally reconstruct the image data in a three-dimensional fashion and transform this into the operative field. This ability may be adequate for simple routine cases with minimal distortion of normal anatomy. However, when routine anatomic landmarks are distorted by the pathologic lesion, the surgeon's ability to visualize damaged and functional anatomy is easily overcome.

The traditional open surgical approach has been dramatically impacted by the financial pressures of our managed care climate, as well as the rapid progression of technological advances within the health care system. So-called "minimally invasive" or "minimal access" surgical techniques have emerged that emphasize earlier functional recovery and cosmesis using a variety of technologies to minimize collateral tissue damage while achieving the surgical objective. Such minimally invasive surgical techniques often involve limited access and restricted visibility and thus mandate a precise knowledge of anatomy. Errors in localization of surgical position can result in damage to normally functioning tissue or failure to remove the pathologic lesion.

The emphasis on minimally invasive surgical techniques has increased the demand for sophisticated interactive radiographic guidance, which complements the eye that "sees the surface" with imaging to "see under the surface."[1] Real-time information from integrated multimodality image-based data can now be presented in an intuitive framework to facilitate precise preoperative visualization of pathologic anatomy as well as real-time interactive anatomic localization and targeting for surgical procedures.

The term *stereotactic surgery*, originally coined by Clarke in 1908,[2] refers to surgery incorporating devices that maintain spatial correspondence between the operating instrument and an image of the operative site. The term *virtual reality* has been described as the combination of human–computer interfaces, graphics, sensor technology, high-end computing, and networking to allow a user to become immersed in and interact with an artificial environment.[1] These terms are now very familiar to the modern-day surgeon as this technology is increasingly incorporated into preoperative planning, minimally invasive surgery, surgical education, and research.

In the field of otolaryngology, we have recently witnessed the rapid emergence of image-guided systems predominantly in surgeries of the anterior skull base (eg, functional endoscopic sinus surgery), and, to a lesser extent, these systems have found application in certain lateral skull base procedures. The purpose of this chapter is to present an overview of the history and technical aspects of current image-guided technology, its general and specific applications for the field of otology/neurotology, and its potential for the future.

HISTORY OF STEREOTAXY

Stereotaxy, before the age of computed tomography (CT), was based entirely on the use of equatorial head-frame systems.[2] Superimposition of frame-based Cartesian coordinate systems securely attached to the head, with calibration accomplished via orientation of the system to the anterior-posterior commissural line, provided an atlas for targeting cerebral lesions in animal models. Hoarsley and Clarke used these early stereotactic systems for placing electrodes in specific areas of animal brains and, although accurate for the purpose of their experiments, the system was not deemed sufficiently accurate or practical for human use.[2]

In 1947, Spiegel adapted the above stereotactic concepts to human use, employing pneumoencephalography and reference to internal tissues as opposed to external landmarks.[3] This technique was more precise than that of Hoarsley and Clarke,[2] but the methodology was tedious and laborious. With the increasing need to accurately localize deep intracranial structures, such as for the ablation of certain areas of the brain for the treatment of Parkinson's disease, there soon became a huge demand for more user-friendly stereotactic systems.

With the advent of CT, digital image databases, combined with more sophisticated surgical instrumentation, greatly enhanced the development of stereotactic surgery. Pioneered by Brown, Kelly, and other neurosurgeons, modern conventional stereotactic surgery employs a head frame to register image space to surgical space.[4–9] Preoperatively, digital image data via CT or magnetic resonance imaging (MRI) are obtained with a localization system (fiducials) attached to a head frame. The frame, which superimposes a Cartesian coordinate system on the head, provides attachment points for localization devices that are placed before imaging (Figure 16–1). Digital imaging allows the assignment of coordinates to any point in the image data. These image coordinates are then related to the coordinate system, which defines these points with respect to the head frame (stereotactic coordinates). Thus, stereotactic space is defined.

Although bulky and cumbersome, the head-frame systems have proven to be accurate in targeting intracranial lesions for stereotactic biopsy. The simplest form of preoperative planning with head-frame systems involves the selection of a point within the digital image of the head. This point will be transformed into a stereotactic coordinate for the purposes of surgically targeting a lesion, for example, to biopsy a brain tumor. More sophisticated preoperative planning may involve trajectory simulation to properly orient the surgeon and more safely guide the operative approach, minimizing collateral damage to normal tissues.

Since the accuracy of the head-frame systems is related to the rigid fixation of the frame to the skull, the frame must be securely bolted to the head, which causes considerable discomfort to the patient. This process often requires general anesthesia before the placement

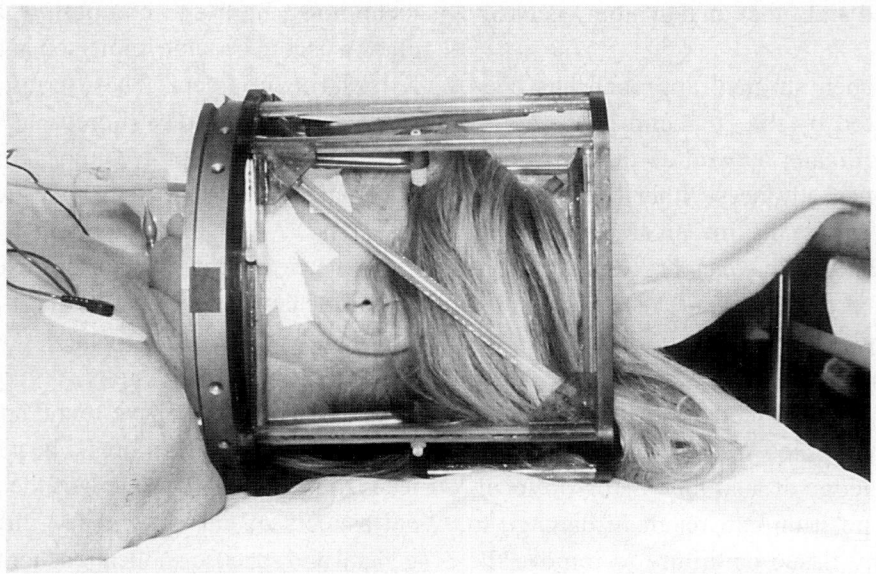

Figure 16–1 Conventional head-frame stereotactic system.

of the frame and the imaging; thus, the anesthesia time is lengthened and the potential for functional imaging is obviated. The frame is left on for the duration of surgery, committing both surgeon and anesthesiologist to a specific orientation with respect to the patient's accessible anatomy. The frame-based system presents a mechanical obstacle hindering a surgeon's ability to access particular areas such as the posterior fossa and skull base. Because of these drawbacks, frame-based stereotaxy has not been widely used in the operating theater, particularly not for neurotologic applications.

FRAMELESS STEREOTAXY

More recently, frameless stereotactic systems have been devised as a more sophisticated and yet user-friendly means of providing comparable stereotactic accuracy without the use of the aforementioned bolted head frame. Current systems consist of two basic components: the sensor, which relays positional information, and a computer, which translates the sensor's positional information to a visual aid for the corroboration of real-time anatomic information. In frameless stereotaxy, the transformation from image coordinates to stereotactic coordinates is defined by three or more noncolinear points (fiducials) in common between the two coordinate systems. Depending on the sensor technology employed, these fiducials may involve anatomic landmarks or reference markers attached to the head at consistent and immovable sites.

A variety of three-dimensional digitizers, or sensor technologies, have been employed to transform the coordinates in surgical space to the corresponding image space. These three-dimensional sensor technologies can be classified into two broad groups: those that require a mechanical link between the pointer and the sensor technology (mechanically linked systems) and those that do not (nonmechanically linked systems).

Mechanically Linked Systems

Mechanically linked systems are based on arms that are mounted to the operating table.[10–13] These mechanical arms are equipped with sensitive potentiometers, or angle detectors, located within their joints. By sampling the output of rotary optical encoders at each point,

a computer can determine the localization of the top of the arm and provide "arm coordinates" that are referenced to the base of the arm. Because the base of the arm is mechanically connected to the head, and the patient's head is registered to the image of the head by an appropriate method, a transformation can be calculated to map any common point in the two coordinate systems. For surgical purposes, real-time localization of the tip of the arm, or pointer, relative to preoperative images of the patient is possible. A variety of mechanically linked devices have been developed and are in the marketplace. These mechanically linked devices have proven to be accurate, although they are somewhat bulky and restrictive, depending on the size of the highly accurate joint detectors employed. Generally, these systems have more limited versatility of instrument use and are not as user friendly as the more current nonmechanically linked systems. To date, they have found limited application in the field of otology and neurotology.

Nonmechanically Linked Systems

More recently, nonmechanically linked sensor systems have been developed for the registration of image data to the surgical patient. These systems rely on the active or passive detection of signals generated by various emitters that are attached to surgical instruments (Figure 16–2). Using similar traditional triangulation concepts employed in the satellite industry, these frameless stereotactic systems are able to localize and track surgical instruments in three-dimensional space. There are essentially three types of nonmechanically linked digitizing systems: ultrasonic, electromagnetic, and optoelectric.

Ultrasonic digitizers determine position by measuring the time flight of sound from an emitter to at least three microphones.[14] The main advantage of ultrasonic digitizing systems is that a free line of sight between the receptor and the emitter arrays need not be maintained. The distinct drawback to ultrasonic digitizers is that the speed of sound varies with temperature and humidity gradients, which may result in positional error. Furthermore, ultrasonic digitizers may be compromised by echoes within the operating room or by interference from extraneous radiofrequency emissions. For these reasons, sonic referenced systems have fallen from favor.

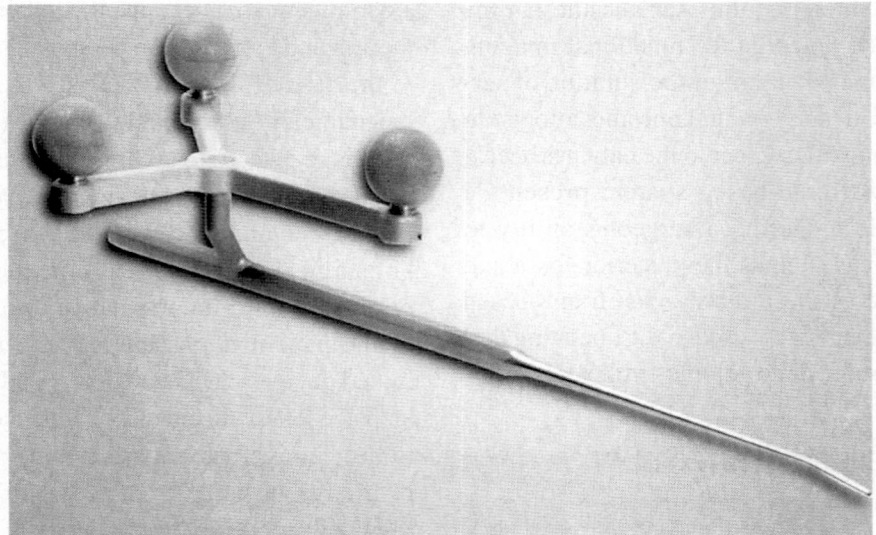

Figure 16–2 Passive surgical instrument employed by optoelectric system (LandMarx, Medtronic/Xomed, Inc).

Electromagnetic reference systems (eg, InstaTrak, VTI Inc) share similar advantages to the ultrasonic digitizers in terms of not needing to maintain a free line of sight between receptor and emitter arrays (Figure 16–3). These systems are referenced by a headset, which is worn by the patient during the CT scan and again later during the surgical procedure. Registration of this device is more rapid and user friendly than other commercially available frameless systems. However, electromagnetic referenced systems suffer the drawback of potential interference from other electromagnetic systems as well as certain ferromagnetic instrumentation in the operating arena. This interference, as well as minor inconsistencies in the repositioning of the headset for imaging and surgery, contributes to positional error and inaccuracy. These inaccuracies are relatively minor and inconsequential for most anterior skull base surgery (eg, endoscopic sinus surgery) where this system finds its primary application in otolaryngologic surgery. The automatic headset registration and referencing algorithm are currently not well suited for lateral skull base applications.

Optoelectric digitizers require an unobstructed path from the emitters to the overlying camera array.[15–17] Three cameras, containing a 1×4096 element linear-charged coupling device, are required to determine the three-dimensional position of infrared light-emitting

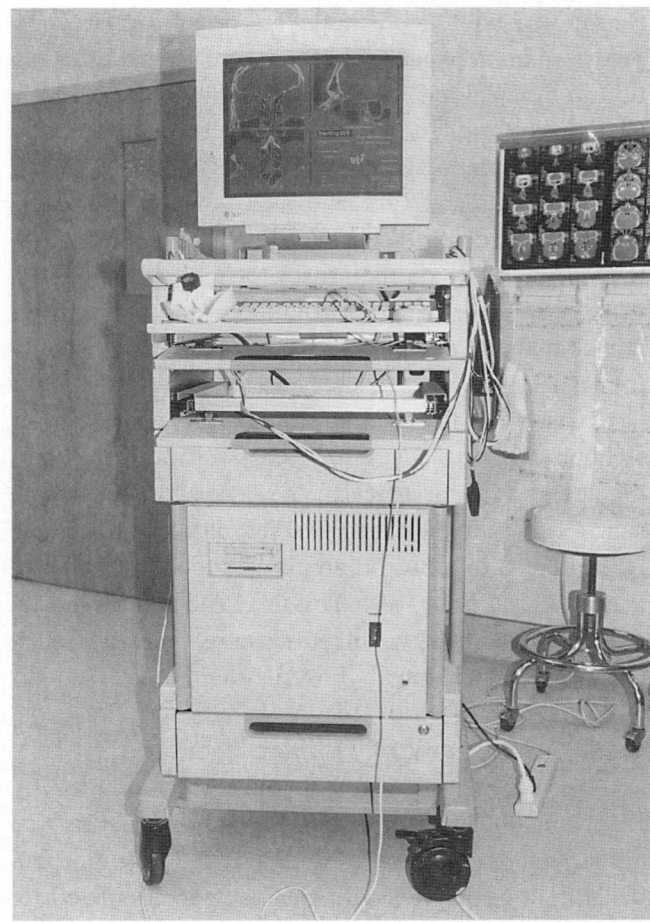

Figure 16–3 Electromagnetic referenced system (InstaTrak, VTI, Inc).

diodes (LEDs) attached to the surgical instruments (Figure 16–4). The overlying camera array is positioned 1.5 to 2 meters above the surgical field so that it can track the instrument-attached LEDs, and it thus detects and tracks the precise position of the surgical instrument in three-dimensional space. Multiple LEDs can be placed on different surgical instruments. Each instrument has a unique emitter spacing, and the computer software is able to recognize and differentiate between the various instruments based on the distance between the emitter pairs.

Optoelectric referenced systems are designated as active or passive, depending on whether the instrument reference points actively transmit or passively reflect the sensor medium (ie, infrared radiation). Active systems generally require wiring of the instruments, whereas passive systems do not.

The two commercially available optoelectric systems (Landmarx, Medtronic Xomed; Brainlab, Storz) are quite transparent and adaptable to different surgical instruments of various geometric configurations such as bipolar cautery, various suctions, and straight or curvilinear probes. A reference arc attached to the stabilized head allows adjustment in calibration with inadvertent movement of the operating room table or overlying camera array. Three-dimensional and three planar reconstructions of the data set are displayed on a video monitor,

permitting real-time interactive and positional information for the operating surgeon.

Soon to be available for optoelectric referenced systems is a new method of laser-contoured anatomic registration that does not use a contact probe. By attaching LEDs to a laser range finder and by moving the range finder over a part of the skull with anatomic diversity (such as the forehead), hundreds of points constituting a contour can be produced. This contour can then be matched to a corresponding contour of the scalp extracted from the image data set.[15] This method of registration will minimize set-up time while greatly minimizing registration error.

Generally, the author has found these optoelectric referenced systems to be the most accurate of the frameless stereotactic systems. The registration algorithms are currently better suited for lateral skull base orientations than the electromagnetic systems; however, anatomic landmark fiducial registration is typically a bit more lengthy and less user friendly. Maintaining line of sight with the overhead camera array of optoelectric systems can also be difficult in otologic/neurotologic procedures, depending on the size and orientation of the operating microscope to the surgical field. The latter concern is less apparent for the electromagnetic systems as they do not require a nonobstructed line of sight between sensor arrays and the detector.

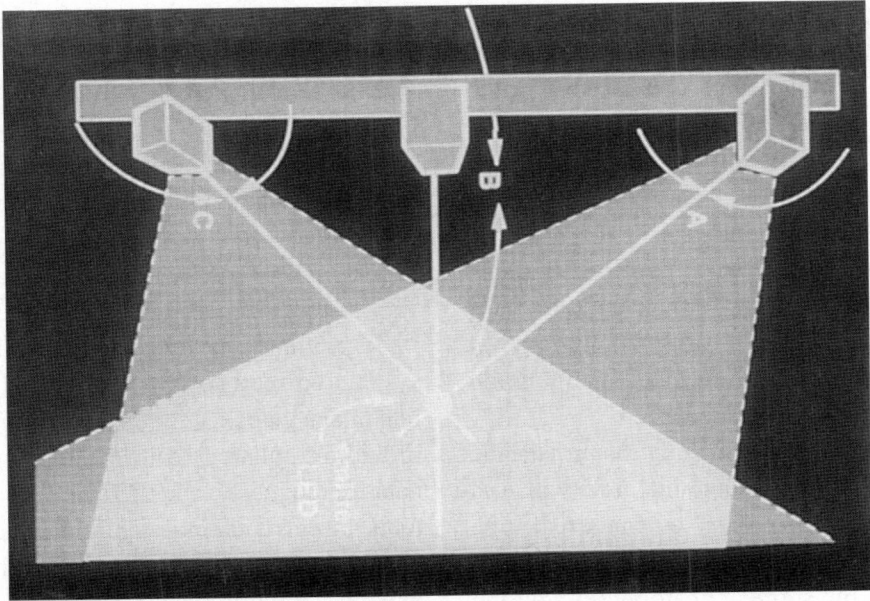

Figure 16–4 In optoelectric systems, three cameras triangulate position of surgical instruments based on the angle of light received from infrared light-emitting diodes attached to the surgical instruments.

VOLUMETRIC STEREOTAXY

Kelly and colleagues pioneered the next logical development in stereotactic surgery, interactive volumetric stereotaxy.[5–9] The name describes a process by which enhanced volumetric routines are reconstructed by the computer and stacked into a "volume" that can be displayed or manipulated in stereotactic space. Frameless stereotactic techniques have been adapted to operating microscopes by Kelly and Roberts so that image data can be displayed in the operating microscope in the correct scale, orientation, and position superimposed on the focal plane of the surgical field.[5–9,18] Kelly has recently adapted this system for interactive volumetric resection of intracranial tumors.[5,6] This system displays cross-sectional volumetric contours at progressive depths along the view line so that CT-defined margins of the tumor can be localized. The tissue volume can then be resected either passively or with laser ablation via the computer or actively by the surgeon. Although this system greatly enhances the integration of image data with the surgical field, it does not allow for soft tissue shifts caused by intraoperative manipulations because its information source is antecedent image data.

REAL-TIME INTRAOPERATIVE IMAGING

With all of the previously discussed frameless stereotactic systems, the computer algorithms and hence graphic image displays reflect antecedent imaging data. Intraoperative shifts and deformations of soft tissues can occur with surgical manipulations, swelling, or hemorrhage. These soft tissue shifts may thus distort accurate registration of image-based three-dimensional models with the patient's actual anatomy without full volumetric image update. This is particularly relevant for removal of intracranial tumors, for which surgical manipulation may produce edema and soft tissue shift.

Only real-time intraoperative imaging can provide the necessary updated positional data to integrate with and modify the volumetric image data set. Such real-time imaging provides updates about the position of instrumentation relative to the surgical anatomy without the fiducial registration process of frameless stereotactic systems.

X-ray fluoroscopy, ultrasonography, and CT have permitted sufficient interactive visualization for percutaneous biopsies and some intravascular interventions but are limited by the degree of spatial resolution of volumetric images as well as radiation exposure. Because of its improved soft tissue contrast, volumetric resolution, multiplanar and functional capabilities, and lack of ionizing radiation, MRI is ideally suited for real-time image-guided therapy. Mid-field open configurations with vertical magnets[1,19,20] are now available that permit full surgical access to patients. When combined with computer algorithms similar to those employed by the frameless stereotactic systems, these MRI systems permit the tracking and video display of nonferromagnetic MR-compatible instrumentation in real time for open surgeries.

A most exciting application for these intraoperative MR systems has been the removal of deep-seated brain tumors, particularly malignant intra-axial tumors.[21,22] Because surgical brain tumor margins are indistinct from normal tissues, real-time MRI may facilitate location of such tumor margins, thereby enhancing the likelihood of complete tumor resection while maximizing the integrity of surrounding normal brain.

Additionally, MRI can be used to control energy deposition of thermal ablative therapies because of the intrinsic sensitivity of MRI to both temperature and tissue integrity. Such thermal therapies have to date been applied to pathologies of the brain, spine, breast, and prostate.[21–23]

Multimodality preoperative image data sets from MRI, CT, positron emission tomography, and single-photon emission computed tomography scanning can now be integrated with intraoperative imaging data into a single data source. From this resource, enhanced visibility and virtual reality representation can be accomplished using various three-dimensional interactive display systems.[1]

In summary, the aforementioned interventional MRI systems currently offer the most sophisticated and accurate image guidance for the operating room of the future, providing updated real-time anatomic and functional data for diagnostic and therapeutic purposes. These systems are currently investigational and not commercially available, largely because of their complexity and expense. Finally, their ultimate role for otologic and neurotologic surgical procedures is less clear as MRI does not portray bony anatomy as well as CT.

APPLICATIONS OF IMAGE-GUIDED SYSTEMS IN OTOLOGY/NEUROTOLOGY

Traditional temporal bone surgery has involved a "funnel concept" (Figure 16–5) of methodical and progressive identification of key anatomic landmarks en route to the surgical target. For example, with routine mastoidectomy, the surgeon proceeds stepwise with initial identification of the mastoid antrum, the middle fossa dural plate, and lateral semicircular canal to achieve intuitive three-dimensional orientation within the surgical field. For the ordinary well-pneumatized mastoid, this funnel concept is routine and safely accomplished for the well-trained otologist without the need for real-time image guidance. However, for the nonroutine mastoid in which normal anatomic landmarks may be obscured by either pathologic disease, previous surgery, or anatomic variation, real-time image guidance may prove very helpful in safely navigating to the surgical target while minimizing collateral damage to vital anatomic structures. Such examples would include the sclerotic mastoid and congenital malformations such as cochlear dysplasia, enlarged vestibular aqueduct syndrome, and atretic ear malformations. In these situations, real-time image guidance may permit us to convert our traditional "funnel technique" to a "tunnel concept" of surgical navigation whereupon

we may virtually "see" these vital anatomic landmarks via interactive imaging rather than by direct surgical exposure (Figure 16–6).

Identification of the internal auditory canal via the middle fossa approach is another such example of this concept. The traditional "funnel" techniques of Fisch and House involve the sequential identification of certain neural and/or labyrinthine structures en route to the internal auditory canal. Using highly accurate frameless stereotactic guidance, the "tunnel" approach would permit direct localization of the internal canal with a pointer via interactive three planar and three-dimensional imaging, thus obviating the stepwise approach aforementioned. Theoretically, this should shorten surgical time and enhance safety, provided that the critical issue of clinically verifiable accuracy is achieved. For absent accuracy, the converse may be true.

Image-guided systems may greatly facilitate so-called "keyhole" surgical approaches to the posterior fossa and cerebellopontine angle. "Keyhole" is a term coined by neurosurgeons for the concept of operating through a minimal craniotomy using a variety of minimally invasive technologies to minimize collateral tissue damage— analogous to working through a keyhole. Interactive imaging is thus very useful in precisely orienting the minimal craniotomy necessary for achieving the desired surgical trajectory for accessing the surgical target (Fig-

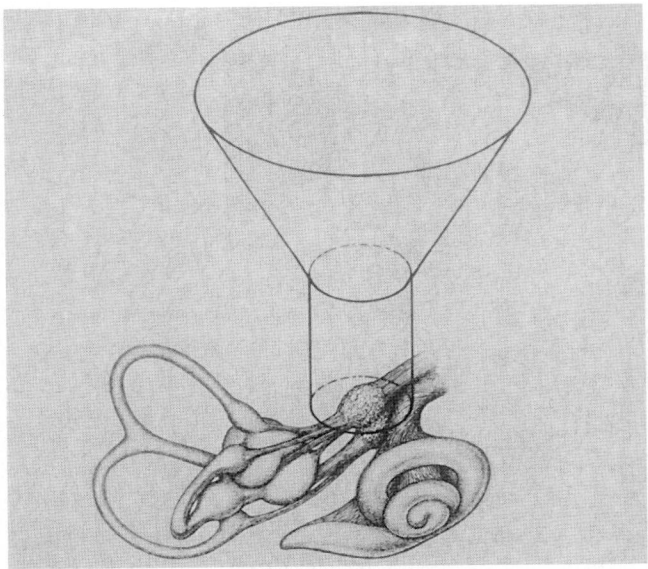

Figure 16–5 Traditional temporal bone surgery involves a "funneling" to the surgical target via exposure and progressive identification of key anatomic landmarks.

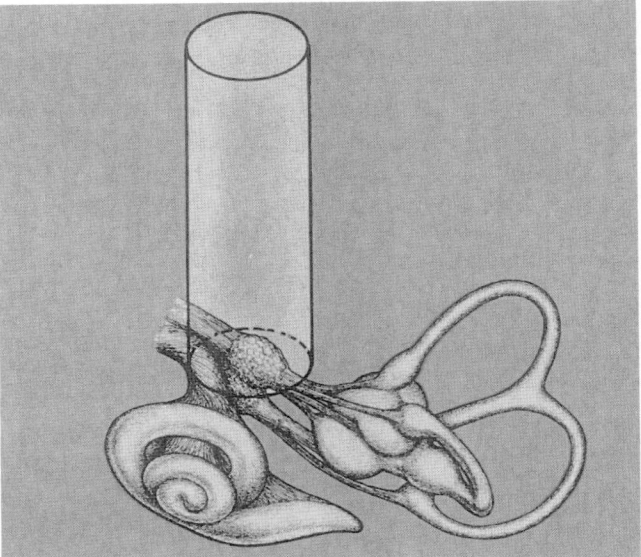

Figure 16–6 With image guidance systems, a "tunneling" to the surgical target may be achieved, whereupon vital anatomic landmarks are identified via interactive imaging rather than by direct surgical exposure.

ure 16–7). Postoperative healing is thus facilitated, and morbidity is decreased.

Another area of neurotologic application for these systems is the petrous apex. In this difficult to access, often poorly pneumatized anatomic area, we do not have a consistently defined series of anatomic landmarks for orientation as with conventional mastoidectomy or the middle fossa approach. Various pathologies of the petrous apex thus lie within very narrow confines bordered by vital structures such as the carotid artery and cranial nerves. In these situations, image guidance systems provide valuable preoperative planning, trajectory simulation, and target and entry formulation in addition to real-time intraoperative localization of these anatomic structures.

In certain other areas of neurotology/skull base surgery, frameless stereotactic systems may have less relevance. This largely relates to an accuracy issue related to soft tissue shifts during surgery. Because these devices are referenced to antecedent image data, without intraoperative updated information, inaccuracies develop as soft tissues are surgically manipulated. Thus, for procedures that are performed within an anatomic area confined to a "bony box" such as the mastoid, internal auditory canal, petrous apex, or sinus cavity, frameless stereotactic systems remain accurate without updated information. Outside of these bony confines, such as in the cerebellopontine angle and the soft tissue planes of

the infratemporal fossa, these systems are subject to positional error because of operative soft tissue shifts. The value of real-time image guidance in these anatomic areas is thus limited for the most part to localization and targeting within contiguous bony structures.

SUMMARY

Real-time image guidance employing computer interfaces and antecedent imaging can facilitate certain minimally invasive surgical approaches of the temporal bone. Current frameless stereotactic systems based on various referencing methodologies have individual advantages and disadvantages. In common between them all, the systems appear to be stable over time in the operating room and are generally transparent in use, permitting free movement of the surgeon and of the patient's head during the course of surgery. Optoelectric referenced systems, both active and passive, generally appear to be the more consistently accurate of the systems, whereas the electromagnetic referenced systems are generally the more user friendly in terms of the patient registration process and setup time. The latter systems are currently not as well suited for lateral skull base procedures with the automated headset algorithm.

There is a learning curve with these devices for everyone associated with their use, but software inter-

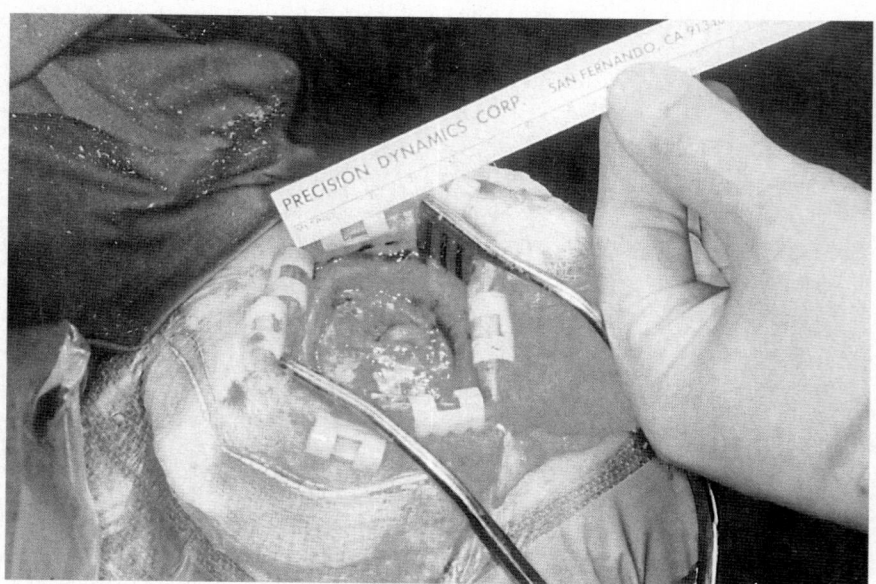

Figure 16–7 Keyhole craniotomy for removal of a posterior fossa meningioma.

actions are menu driven, user friendly, and simple enough to allow the surgeon to simply point and localize during the operative procedure. Clinical accuracy for all systems is generally 1 to 3 mm, which is sufficient for most neurotologic applications.

Interventional MRI represents the most sophisticated, exciting, and expensive of the image-guided systems available. Its chief advantage is the ability to provide real-time updated anatomic and functional information. Its chief disadvantages are its expense, complexity, and lack of commercial availability.

The operating room of the future is witnessing a paradigm shift from open surgical visualization to virtual visualization through integrated image data. The inherent complexity of image-guided therapies will require an increasing dynamic cooperation and interplay between the disciplines of surgery and radiology. Through the advancement of these technologies, we have the possibility of improving the safety, efficacy, and cost effectiveness of our diagnostic and therapeutic procedures.

Finally, it is important to remember that these adjunctive tools should never replace precise knowledge and visualization of anatomy when visualization is at all possible. That is, it is always preferable to visualize the runway before landing a plane rather than to rely solely on instrumentation.

REFERENCES

1. Jolesz FA. Image-guided procedures and the operating room of the future. Radiology 1997;204:601–12.

2. Hoarsley V, Clarke RH. The structure and function of the cerebellum examined by a new method. Brain 1908;31:45.

3. Zinreich J. Imaging of inflammatory sinus disease. Otolaryngol Clin North Am 1993;26:535–47.

4. Brown RA. A computerized tomography-computer graphics approach to stereotaxic localization. J Neurosurg 1979;50:715–20.

5. Kelly PJ. Volumetric stereotactic surgical resection of intraaxial brain mass lesions. Mayo Clin Proc 1988;63:1186–98.

6. Kelly PJ. Volumetric stereotaxis and computer-assisted stereotactic resection of subcortical lesions. In: Lunsford LD, editor. Modern stereotactic neurosurgery. Boston: Nijhoff; 1988.

7. Kelly PJ, Alker GJ. A stereotactic approach to deep-seated central nervous system neoplasms using the carbon dioxide laser. Surg Neurol 1981;15:331–4.

8. Kelly PJ, Farnest I 4th, Kall BA, et al. Surgical options for patients with deep-seated brain tumors: computer-assisted stereotactic biopsy. Mayo Clin Proc 1985;60:223–9.

9. Kelly PJ, Kall BA, Goerss SJ, et al. Computer-assisted stereotaxic laser resection of intra-axial brain neoplasms. J Neurosurg 1986;64:427–39.

10. Barnett GH, Barnett G II, Kormos DW, et al. Use of a frameless, armless stereotactic wand for brain tumor localization with two-dimensional and three-dimensional neuroimaging. Neurosurgery 1993;33:674–8.

11. Maciunas RJ, et al. Beyond stereotaxy: a computerized articulated localizing arm for all neurosurgical procedures [abstract]. Proc Am Assoc Neurol Surgeons 1990;254.

12. Watanabe E, Watanabe T, Manaka S, et al. Three-dimensional digitizer (Neuronavigator): new equipment for computed tomography-guided stereotaxic surgery. Surg Neurol 1987;27:543–7.

13. Watanabe E, Mayanagi Y, Kasugi Y, et al. Open surgery assisted by the Neuronavigator, a stereotactic, articulated, sensitive arm. Neurosurgery 1991;28:792.

14. Nitsche N, et al. Einsatz eines beruhrungsfreien computergestutzten Orientierungssystems bei Nasennebenhohlenoperationen. Otorhinolaryngol Nova 1993;3:57.

15. Bucholz RD, Ho HW, Rubin JP. Variables affecting the accuracy of stereotactic localization using computerized tomography. J Neurosurg 1993;79:667–73.

16. Bucholz RD, et al. Intraoperative localization using a three-dimensional optical digitizer. Proc Clin Appl Modern Imaging Technol 1894:1993.

17. Goldsmith MM, Bucholz RD, Smith KR, Nitsche N. Clinical applications of frameless stereotactic devices in neurotology: a preliminary report. Am J Otol 1995;16:475–9.

18. Roberts DW, Strohbehn JW, Hatch JF, et al. A frameless stereotaxic integration of computerized tomographic imaging and the operating microscope. J Neurosurg 1986;65:545–9.

19. Lufkin RB. Interventional MR imaging. Radiology 1995;197:16–8.

20. Gronemeyer DHW, Seibel RMM, Melzer A, et al. Future of advanced guidance techniques by interventional CT and MRI. Minimally Invasive Ther 1995;4:251–9.

21. Jolesz FA, Shtern F. The operating room of the future. Report of the National Cancer Institute Workshop, Imaging Guided Stereotactic Tumor Diagnosis and Treatment. Invest Radiol 1992;27:326–8.

22. Black PCL, Moriarity T, Alexander E, et al. Development and implementation of intraoperative magnetic resonance imaging and its neurosurgical applications. Neurosurgery 1997;41:831–43.

23. D'Amico AV, Cormack R, Tempany CM, et al. Real-time magnetic resonance image-guided interstitial brachytherapy in the treatment of select patients with clinically localized prostate cancer. Int J Radiat Oncol Biol Phys 1998;42:507–15.

IV

Surgery of the External Ear

17

Diseases of the Auricle, External Auditory Canal, and Tympanic Membrane

DAVID F. KROON, MD

BARRY STRASNICK, MD, FACS

The auricle and external auditory canal (EAC) serve to augment and transmit sound to the tympanic membrane. The shape of the EAC results in the optimization of sound conduction to the tympanic membrane in the frequencies of 2 to 4 kHz, those most important in human communication. Disorders of the pinna, EAC, and tympanic membrane are common entities in clinical otology. Successful diagnosis and management require a detailed knowledge of the embryology, anatomy, physiology, and bacteriology of these structures.

DEVELOPMENTAL CONSIDERATIONS

The auditory and vestibular systems develop as distinct anatomic units. During the sixth week of gestation, auricular development begins with the formation of the six hillocks of His, mesenchymal proliferations originating from the first and second pharyngeal arches. The first arch contributes three hillocks, which eventually form the tragus and the root and superior portion of the helix. The second arch also contributes three hillocks, destined to become the antihelix, antitragus, and lobule.[1] The definitive auricle develops from the fusion of the hillocks and is usually complete by the 12th week of gestation. The auricle will not reach its adult shape, however, until the 20th gestational week, and it continues to grow for the first 5 years of life. Given the complexity of this process, it is not surprising that developmental abnormalities of the auricle are common.

The ectoderm of the first branchial groove invaginates to form the primitive EAC. As the cells continue to grow inward, they eventually meet endodermal tissue of the developing tubotympanum, a derivative of the first pharyngeal pouch. Mesodermal anlages encroach on this area of apposition from ventral and dorsal sites. The resulting solid core of tissue is named the meatal plug or plate. By the 28th week of fetal development, the plate resorbs and the EAC recanalizes. Ectodermal elements from the meatal plate form the epithelial lining of the EAC and the lateral tympanic membrane, whereas mesodermal elements contribute to the development of the cartilaginous EAC, ossification centers of the tympanic ring, and the ossicular chain.[2] Failure of EAC recanalization results in congenital aural atresia.

THE AURICLE

Fibroelastic cartilage, perichondrium, and skin comprise the auricular framework. The cartilage of the auricle is continuous with that of the lateral EAC. The skin of the topographically complex lateral surface of the auricle is firmly attached to the perichondrium; however, the skin of the posterior auricle is less adherent, owing to a layer of loose areolar tissue between it and the perichondrium. The auricle is fixed to the temporal bone via its cartilaginous contribution to the external meatus and less so by the three auricular ligaments — anterior, superior, and posterior — as well as six poorly developed intrinsic muscles. Additionally, three distinctly better developed extrinsic muscles exist, also named anterior, superior, and posterior. Voluntary contraction of the extrinsic musculature is responsible for the ability possessed by some to "wiggle" the auricle. These muscles are innervated by the facial nerve.

Sensory innervation of the auricle is characterized by a great deal of overlap between multiple nerves.[3] The auriculotemporal branch of the mandibular division of the trigeminal nerve supplies sensation to the tragus and the helix and its crus; it also supplies sensation to the anterior and superior portions of the EAC and corresponding areas of the lateral surface of the tympanic membrane. Fibers from cervical sensory nerves, primarily contained in the great auricular nerve (C2, C3), innervate the posterior surface of the auricle, posterior region of the helix, antihelix, and lobule. Fibers from the ninth and tenth cranial nerves supply the majority of the conchal concavity and the posterior surface of the EAC.

The external carotid artery supplies blood to the auricle and external meatus via the postauricular and superficial temporal branches. Venous drainage parallels the arterial supply. The superficial temporal vein joins the retromandibular vein and ultimately the internal jugular system, whereas the postauricular vein joins the external jugular system. There also may be drainage to the sigmoid sinus via the mastoid emissary vein.

The lymphatics of the anterior auricle and meatus drain into the preauricular and periparotid nodes. Lymphatics of the posterior auricle, however, empty into the retroauricular (mastoid) and infra-auricular nodes.[3]

DISEASES OF THE AURICLE

Frostbite

Contemporary otolaryngologists rarely manage frostbite injuries of the auricle. The auricle, with its high ratio of surface area to mass, however, is at increased risk for this type of injury. Blood vessels supplying this region lie superficially within the subcutaneous tissues, increasing their exposure to colder temperatures. Prolonged exposure blocks afferent sensory nerve transmission, reducing the patient's awareness of ongoing injury. The initial physiologic response is vasoconstriction. Extracellular ice formation then results in cell lysis. As tissues warm, extravasated fluid causes edema and bullae formation, and pain is the rule.

Management consists of rapid tissue warming via circulating warm water or warmed moistened dressings. Use of radiant heat is contraindicated as it may worsen the injury. The pinna should be dressed aseptically with 1% silver sulfadiazine cream, similar to management of a burn injury. Secondary infection is treated with antimicrobial agents directed against *Pseudomonas aeruginosa* and *Staphylococcus aureus*. Frequently, tissue, initially appearing devitalized, will recover after a period of observation and conservative management. Therefore, débridement of necrotic tissue should be delayed until a reliable line of demarcation develops.

Hematoma

Blunt trauma to the auricle may result in hematoma. The trauma causes a shearing injury, resulting in separation of auricular cartilage from its associated perichondrium and bleeding into this newly created space. The cartilage is subsequently deprived of its perichondrium-dependent blood supply and may become ischemic.

Hematoma may present immediately following an injury or in delayed fashion as a painful swelling, which causes effacement of the normal topography of the auricle. Management consists of evacuation. This may be accomplished via aspiration if the hematoma is acute and small in size. For larger collections, an incision and drainage procedure is required. The incision is placed along the helical fold, thereby minimizing the conspicuousness of the resultant scar, and the blood clot is expelled. Occasionally, a curette must be used to completely remove all of the hematoma. Most important is the placement of a pressure dressing to prevent reaccumulation. Many prefer to use dental rolls secured with through-and-through sutures as bolsters on both the lateral and medial auricular surfaces.[4] Close follow-up is necessary to address recurrences in a timely fashion. Failure to evacuate a hematoma leads to fibrosis and new cartilage formation. The resulting deformity is permanent and ranges from mild cartilaginous thickening to the severe "cauliflower" ear seen most frequently in wrestlers and boxers.[5]

Perichondritis

Infection of the auricular perichondrium and underlying cartilage is a possible complication of surgery, trauma, or external otitis. Perichondritis presents with erythema, edema, and exquisite tenderness of the involved pinna. Progression of the infectious process can lead to abscess formation and loss of cartilage. The most common offending organism is *P. aeruginosa*. Diabetes and other causes of immunosuppression have been implicated as predisposing factors.[6]

If diagnosed early, perichondritis may be managed on an outpatient basis with oral antibiotics, aural toilet and débridement, and close observation. Because of its excellent cartilaginous penetration and high activity against *Pseudomonas* species, ciprofloxacin is the drug of choice.[7] The use of the fluoroquinolone class of antibiotics is contraindicated in the pediatric population, however, because of concerns regarding adverse effects on bone growth. In children with early perichondritis, outpatient management with antibiotics directed against gram-positive organisms can be initiated. If significant clinical improvement is not observed within the first 24 to 36 hours of oral therapy, or if the patient presents initially with severe infection, parenteral antibiotic therapy is warranted. An auricular abscess requires prompt incision and drainage. Additionally, all necrotic cartilage and tissue should be débrided and cultures obtained. Unfortunately, permanent auricular deformity is a likely consequence of abscess formation.

Cellulitis and Erysipelas

Cellulitis of the auricle refers to infection of the skin and subcutaneous tissue typically caused by streptococcal and staphylococcal species. Erysipelas is a similar entity resulting from a skin infection caused by beta-hemolytic streptococci. Both may result from minor trauma or surgical procedures and present with swelling, erythema, and tenderness of the auricle and surrounding tissue. In erysipelas, the region of inflammation tends to be well demarcated and shows more prominent induration, and even blistering, than what is observed with cellulitis. Constitutional symptoms of fever, chills, and malaise may be present with either process. Management consists of treatment with a penicillinase-resistant antibiotic, such as cephalexin or dicloxacillin, for cellulitis and penicillin G for erysipelas. If prompt response fails to occur, parenteral antibiotic therapy is warranted.

Herpes Zoster Oticus

Herpes zoster oticus represents a reactivation of infection caused by the varicella virus, which had lain dormant in the roots of cranial or dorsal nerves. The infection results in a painful vesicular eruption limited to the dermatome of the affected nerve. Pain usually precedes the appearance of dermatologic findings by hours to days. Constitutional symptoms of fever, chills, and malaise may also be present. The typical herpetic vesicle forms on an erythematous base and can be found on the skin of the pinna, conchal bowl, and EAC. As vesicles burst, amber fluid drains onto the skin and the lesions crust. Ramsay Hunt syndrome refers to herpes zoster oticus accompanied by facial palsy. Herpes zoster oticus commonly presents as a polyneuropathy with involvement of multiple cranial nerves, and patients must therefore be evaluated for associated hearing loss, vertigo, and dysphagia. Management consists of topical débridement of auricular lesions, pain control, and antiviral medications. Commonly used therapies include a 7-day course of either acyclovir (800 mg orally five times daily) or famciclovir (500 mg three times daily). Systemic corticosteroids (1 mg/kg/d × 7 days, then tapered) are added to this regimen when facial paralysis is present.

Sebaceous Cyst

Sebaceous cysts form as a result of sebaceous gland obstruction. The lobule and retroauricular area are common locations for these soft, mobile masses. Normally asymptomatic, sebaceous cysts do not require treatment unless cosmetic deformity exists. Occasionally, however, the cyst will become acutely infected and require antibiotic therapy. Formal excision should be delayed until the infection has resolved. When excision is performed, the entire cyst capsule must be removed, or recurrence is likely.

Preauricular Sinus

Preauricular pits and sinuses are commonly seen in the pediatric population. Resulting from abnormalities in the fusion of the hillocks of His during auricular development, these lesions present as pitlike depressions anterior to the root of the helix and superior to the level of the tragus. They may be unilateral or bilateral. Patients may present asymptomatically or report intermittent, scant drainage from the sinus. These lesions are prone to acute infection requiring antibiotic therapy. If significant fluctuance accompanies infection, incision and drainage may be necessary, but subsequent scarring and fibrosis will obliterate normal tissue planes and make future excision more difficult.

When symptomatic or associated with recurrent infection, surgical resection of a preauricular sinus is required. Placement of a lacrimal probe into the fistulous tract aids in determining its extent. Dissection is performed down to cartilage if necessary. To prevent recurrence, the sinus must be excised in its entirety.

Other related lesions include preauricular skin tags and first branchial cleft anomalies. Similar to preauricular sinuses, skin tags in this location represent duplication anomalies of the ectodermal hillocks of His. Although generally benign in their natural history, the skin tags may be excised for cosmetic purposes. First branchial cleft cysts, on the other hand, result from duplication anomalies of the membranous EAC. A fistulous tract exists between the external skin and an intact EAC. The Work classification divides first branchial cleft sinuses into two types.[8] Type I anomalies contain only ectodermal derivatives, whereas type II anomalies possess tissues of both ectodermal and mesodermal origin. Management of first branchial cleft lesions consists of surgical resection. Caution is required when dealing with type II anomalies as their mesodermal origin results in an intimate association with the parotid gland, placing the facial nerve at risk during attempts at excision.

Keloid

Keloids are benign, hypertrophic, fibrous lesions that generally develop following trauma or surgery. They are more common in darkly pigmented people and are frequently found on the lobule as a result of ear piercing. An excess of extracellular matrix, particularly glycoproteins, characterizes the histologic appearance of keloids.[9]

Treatment generally requires a combination of medical and surgical therapy. For small lesions or develop-

ing keloids, intralesional injections of triamcinolone acetonide may be used as first-line therapy. Because of their poor absorption through hypertrophic tissue, topical corticosteroids play a very limited role in the management of keloids. For larger and more mature lesions, excision is required. Intralesional corticosteroid injection is performed at the time of surgery and repeated every 4 to 6 weeks thereafter for a minimum of three postoperative injections. Patient compliance with this postoperative regimen is required to minimize the risk of recurrence. Some advocate additional pre-excisional injections to ensure that patients understand and accept the need for multiple treatments and are likely to adhere to the prescribed postoperative regimen.[10] Despite combined excision and intralesional corticosteroid therapy, recurrence rates approach 50%.[11] Low-dose radiation therapy can be considered for cases resistant to conventional therapy, but the risk of radiation-induced malignancy in these predominantly young patients tempers our enthusiasm for this aggressive approach.

Tophi

Gout is a severe monoarticular inflammatory arthritis triggered by the presence of urate crystals in synovial joint fluid. Tophaceous deposition of urate crystals in and around joints is one of the hallmark physical findings associated with hyperuricemia. Frequently, patients will present with deposits in the helix, appearing as moderately painful, salmon-pink nodules. When compressed, tophi exude a whitish, chalky substance consisting of sodium biurate. Crystals appear negatively birefringent when examined under polarized light. Treatment of acute attacks of gouty arthritis focuses on pain relief and correction of the underlying abnormality in uric acid metabolism.[12] No specific therapy directed at auricular tophi is necessary.

Prominent Ears

Abnormal protrusion of the auricle, also known as lop ear, is a common congenital deformity of the external ear. Patients may present with unilateral or bilateral deformities. Most frequently, the auricular cartilage is of appropriate size but lacks a well-defined antihelical fold. Occasionally, excess conchal cartilage and abnormal prominence of the lobule and antitragus also contribute to the deformity. The entity has no significant otologic ramifications; rather, its importance is determined by the psychological disturbance endured by the patient. By age 5, the auricle has essentially reached adult size, and children generally start school. Teasing from peers may become severe at this time, and surgical correction need not be delayed.

The goal of otoplasty is to correct abnormal prominence and create auricles that are symmetric in their appearance and position. Although differences in opinion regarding "normative values" for auricular position and protrusion exist, Tolleth provided some general guidelines on which surgical correction can be based.[13] With the head oriented vertically, the desired position of the auricle is approximately one ear length posterior to the lateral orbital rim. The level of the brow defines the preferred position of the top of the ear, whereas the base of the columella marks the appropriate inferior extent of the lobule. The axis of the auricle should not lie in the vertical plane; rather, it should be rotated 15 to 20 degrees in the posterior direction. A distance of 15 to 20 mm between the scalp and the anterior surface of the superior pole of the helix provides an esthetically pleasing degree of auricular protrusion.

Usually, the key element of otoplasty is the creation of a smooth antihelical fold. A wide variety of techniques can be used to reshape the auricular cartilage, including abrasion and scoring or suture fixation. We prefer a modification of the technique described by Mustarde, employing a combination of posterior auricular skin excision and mattress sutures.[14] The technique is relatively simple and provides predictable results. Posterior auricular skin and perichondrium are elevated to the helical rim, and nonabsorbable, buried horizontal mattress sutures are placed through cartilage and anterior perichondrium to shape the antihelical fold and its superior and inferior crura. Conchal excess is reduced by excising of a rim of cartilage from the distal bowl. Further retraction of the auricle can be achieved by tacking the proximal conchal soft tissue to the periosteum of the mastoid. Redundant posterior auricular skin is excised in elliptical fashion and the incision is then closed with a running 4-0 nylon suture.

EXTERNAL AUDITORY CANAL

The EAC is an S-shaped tube measuring approximately 2.5 cm in length that extends from the concha to the tympanic membrane. The most lateral one-third of the canal is cartilaginous, whereas the medial two-thirds are osseous. The narrowest segment of the EAC, the isthmus, corresponds to the junction of the cartilaginous and bony portions. The canal's anteroinferior wall is slightly longer than the posterosuperior wall, creating an acute angle between the anterior canal wall and the tympanic membrane. The EAC is also slightly concave anteriorly, which can prevent complete examination of the tympanic membrane. Improved tympanic membrane visualization is achieved by retracting the auricle in a posterosuperior direction during otoscopy.

The most critical pure-tone frequencies for understanding human speech fall between 500 and 4,000 Hz. The EAC entrance is of lesser diameter than its medial opening at the tympanic membrane, and, similar to an organ pipe, this shape helps to augment sound as it is transmitted through the canal. The average EAC length of 2.5 cm corresponds to an average resonant frequency of 3,500 Hz. The length added to the canal by the presence of the concha modifies its resonance characteristics somewhat, creating a resonance frequency of approximately 2,700 Hz.[15]

Skin and subcutaneous tissue surround the cartilage of the lateral EAC. Hair follicles and sebaceous and apocrine (ceruminous) glands exist within this subcutaneous tissue. These structures form an apopilosebaceous unit and produce a protective layer of cerumen. In contrast, the more medial, osseus EAC lacks glandular adnexae and consists only of the tympanic bone and a tightly adherent epidermis. The clinical significance of this difference lies in the fact that infected sebaceous cysts and furuncles occur only in the lateral EAC. The epidermis of the EAC is continuous with the squamous epithelial layer of the tympanic membrane. Infectious processes of the EAC may spread to the temporomandibular joint and periparotid soft tissue via inconstant dehiscences of the cartilaginous canal, the fissures of Santorini. An anterior gap of the tympanic bone, named Huschke's foramen, may permit similar spread of infection to the preauricular tissue. This dehiscence usually closes in late childhood but may persist into adulthood.[3]

The blood supply of the EAC is the same as that of the auricle, with additional contributions from the deep auricular artery. This vessel, a branch of the internal maxillary artery, passes through the substance of the parotid gland and travels posterior to the temporomandibular joint capsule before penetrating the EAC in the region of the isthmus. Venous drainage is via the superficial temporal and posterior auricular veins, which join the internal and external jugular systems, respectively. Lymphatics of the inferior EAC drain to the infra-auricular nodes, those of the posterior canal drain to the retroauricular nodes, and the periparotid, superficial, and deep cervical nodes receive drainage from the anterior region of the canal.

Sensory innervation of the EAC is variable, with suspected contributions from cranial nerves V, VII, IX, and X. Generally, the auriculotemporal branch of the mandibular division of the trigeminal nerve innervates the anterior and superior walls of the EAC. Fibers from the facial, glossopharyngeal, and vagus nerves, traveling with the auricular branch (Arnold's nerve) of the vagus nerve, enter the EAC through the tympanomastoid suture to supply the posterior and inferior aspects of the canal.[3]

DISEASES OF THE EXTERNAL AUDITORY CANAL

Exostoses and Osteoma

External auditory exostoses and osteomas are benign clinical entities characterized by hyperplastic growth of bone in the osseous EAC. Exostoses tend to be bilateral, broadly based protrusions originating from the anterior and posterior canal walls (Figure 17–1). In contrast, osteomas are more often unilateral, pedunculated growths located at suture lines and resulting in lesser degrees of EAC obstruction. Both types of lesions are most commonly noted incidentally in asymptomatic patients. However, as EAC obstruction worsens, symptoms of chronic debris trapping, recurrent otitis externa, and hearing loss develop.

External auditory exostoses occur most frequently in patients with interests in aquatic activities. A causal relationship between cold water exposure and the development of exostoses was first proposed by van Gilse.[16] His research revealed that irrigation of the EAC with water colder than 17°C results in prolonged meatal ery-

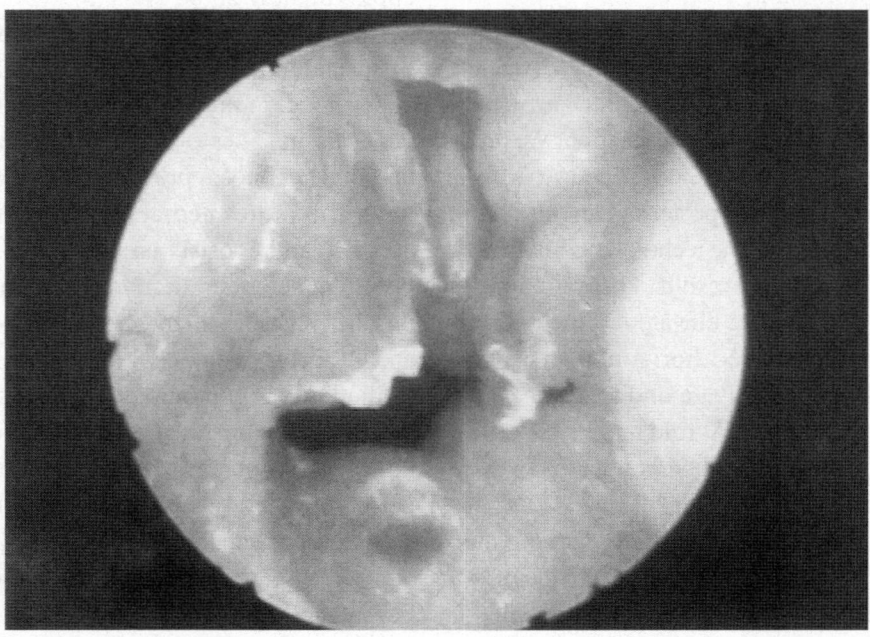

Figure 17–1 External auditory canal (EAC) exostoses. Right ear with near-complete EAC occlusion secondary to exostotic growth.

thema. Numerous prevalence studies demonstrate that surfers, especially those who surf in colder waters, are at increased risk for developing exostoses.[17,18] Continued cold water exposure generally results in progression of exostotic growth.

Management of exostoses and osteomas consists of periodic cerumen disimpaction and débridement and treatment of infection as necessary. Avoidance of further water exposure should be advised, but compliance with this recommendation is unlikely. Many surfers are, however, willing to wear earplugs or occlusive hoods to minimize water exposure. When conservative therapy fails, however, surgical excision of the bony obstruction is required.

Exostosis removal can be approached via a postauricular or endaural approach, depending on surgeon preference. Skin and periosteum overlying the mass are elevated, and an otologic drill is used to re-establish the normal bony contour of the canal. To avoid damage to the skin flap, drilling continues only until the exostosis has been "eggshelled." A curette can then be used to fracture remaining bone inward, allowing further dissection and separation of skin and periosteum away from adherent bone. A split-thickness skin graft or fascial graft may be necessary if significant areas of exposed bone remain following replacement of the skin flap. Placement of thin Silastic® or a piece of foil medial to the exostosis can protect the tympanic membrane from iatrogenic injury.[19] If a perforation results, however, it should be addressed at the time of surgery.

Keratosis Obturans

Keratosis obturans is characterized by the accumulation of large keratin plugs in the osseous EAC, resulting in acute, severe otalgia and hearing loss. Although its etiology is unknown, several authors link the process of chronic desquamation to protracted canal skin hyperemia.[19] Patients tend to be relatively young and have bilateral disease. Interestingly, upwards of 90% of patients suffering from keratosis obturans also have a past history of bronchiectasis or sinusitis.[20,21] Clinically, keratosis obturans presents as occlusion of the external meatus by tightly compacted plugs of desquamated keratin debris. The osseus external canal is often significantly widened, frequently to the point at which the tympanic membrane and annulus "stand out in relief." The tympanic membrane typically shows moderate degrees of thickening. Management consists of local débridement of the plug, occasionally requiring general anesthesia secondary to severe discomfort, and appropriate ototopical therapy to address residual tissue inflammation or secondary infection. Recurrent keratin accumulations are removed as needed. Infrequently, patients will suffer from repeated canal occlusion and pain despite vigilant office surveillance and débridement. In these difficult situations, we have found canalplasty to be an effective treatment option. The excessive desquamation characteristic of keratosis obturans is addressed by replacing chronically diseased epithelium with the healthy epidermis of a skin graft.

External Auditory Canal Cholesteatoma

Cholesteatoma of the EAC is similar to keratosis obturans in that each is characterized by the presence of keratin debris within the canal. They are, however, distinct clinical entities. Patients with EAC cholesteatoma are generally older and present with unilateral disease causing symptoms of otorrhea, dull pain, and hearing loss. This rare variety of cholesteatoma can be acquired secondary to trauma, surgery, stenosis, or chronic inflammation or arise spontaneously.[22] The precise etiology of spontaneous EAC cholesteatoma is unclear, but pathologic studies consistently cite a localized periosteitis and bone sequestra formation.[23]

Clinically, EAC cholesteatomas cause erosion of the bony canal wall, usually in an inferior and posterior location (Figure 17–2). The severity of the lesion can range from one causing limited, superficial erosion to one that invades deeply into the mastoid. Complete microscopic examination of the cholesteatoma is critical in determining its extent. For localized lesions, frequent office débridement of necrotic bone and debris may suffice. For those cholesteatomas eroding deeper pockets into the canal wall, a canalplasty may successfully exteriorize the defect. External auditory canal healing can be aided by placement of a skin or fascial graft. Disease involving the mastoid warrants tympanomastoidectomy.

Foreign Body

Children are frequently referred to otolaryngologists for the management of ear canal foreign bodies. Primary

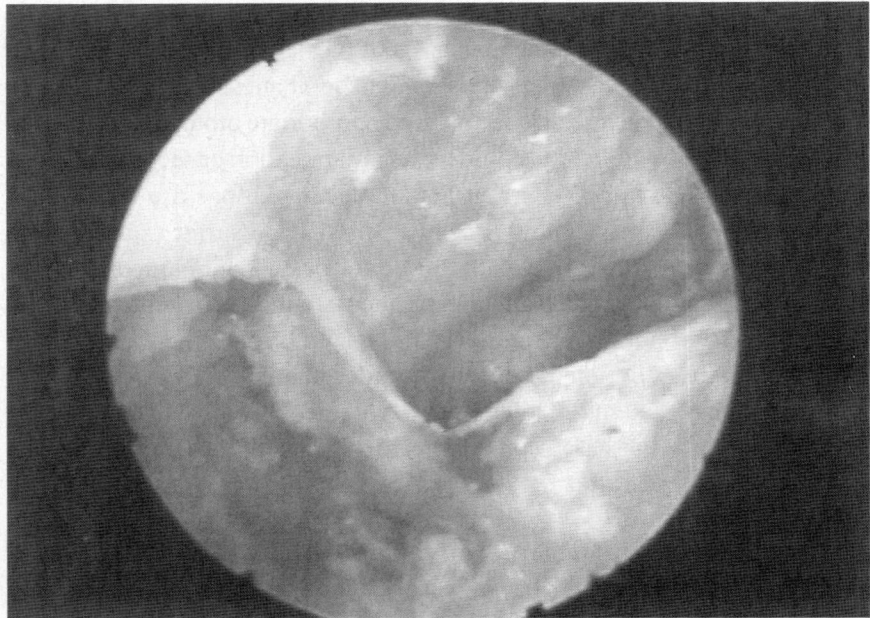

Figure 17–2 Right external auditory canal cholesteatoma resulting in erosion into the inferior canal wall. Note the intact tympanic membrane without evidence of chronic retraction.

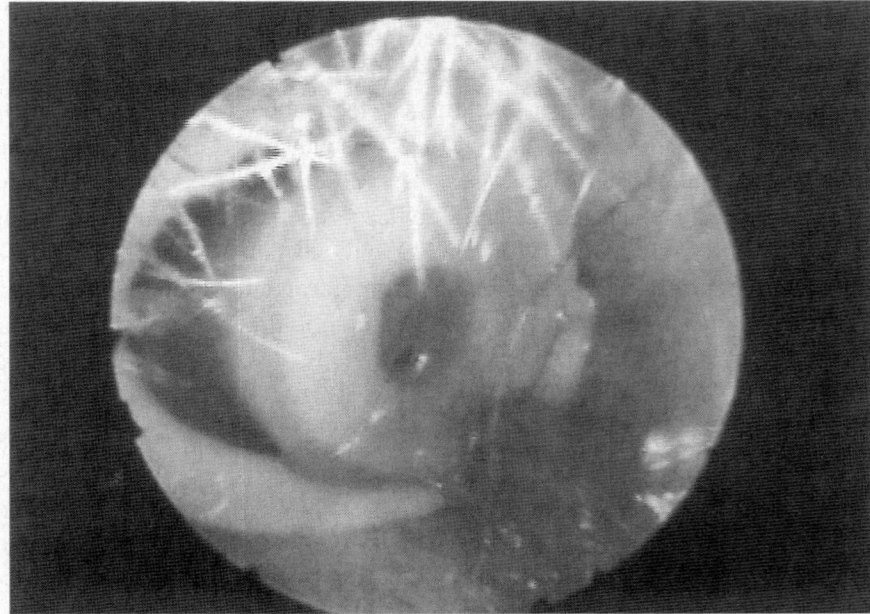

Figure 17–3 Left external auditory canal (EAC) foreign body. Tip of a hearing aid lodged in the lateral EAC.

care physicians often discover the foreign body when evaluating a child for possible otitis, or it may be found incidentally during a well-child visit. Inorganic objects are commonly present (Figure 17–3). A greater challenge to manage in the office, however, are organic objects, such as popcorn and peanut fragments, which tend to absorb moisture and swell to completely obstruct the meatus. Foreign bodies are removed under microscopic visualization with a cerumen loop, right-angle pick, or suction. For the uncooperative child, removal under general anesthesia is required, given the risk of tympanic membrane and ossicular chain injury that can result from the sudden movement of a distressed patient. Occasionally, an endaural incision is necessary to remove a severely impacted object. Postoperative antibiotic drops should be used when an incision is required or extensive trauma to the skin of the external canal is observed.

Furuncle

Also known as acute localized otitis externa, acute furunculosis is the result of obstruction of pilosebaceous glands present in the subcutaneous tissue of the cartilaginous EAC. Elevation of the tightly adherent skin of the external canal causes exquisite pain and discomfort. The pinna and preauricular soft tissue may display associated cellulitic changes. Treatment of acute furunculosis consists of antibiotics directed against *S. aureus* and warm compresses. If significant fluctuance develops, incision and drainage are required and generally provide welcome pain relief. If possible, a small wick of packing material should be placed into the abscess cavity following drainage to prevent recurrence.

Aural Polyp

Aural polyps are well-circumscribed, soft, fleshy masses frequently found in the EACs of patients presenting with otorrhea and hearing loss (Figure 17–4). They are usually inflammatory and suggest active middle ear disease. Polyps are frequently seen in pediatric patients, the result of a foreign body reaction to pressure equalization tubes. An association between aural polyps and cholesteatoma, especially in children, is well established and may be as high as 45%.[24,25] Most commonly, polyps originate from middle ear mucosa and protrude into the external meatus through a tympanic membrane perforation. Visualization of the tympanic membrane may be impossible as a result of EAC obstruction. The presence of a temporal bone malignancy must be considered, however, in any patient presenting with an aural polyp. Histopathologic analysis is therefore required when the etiology of a polyp is unknown.

The initial management of an aural polyp is focused on the identification of its etiology. Gentle aural cleansing and the application of antibiotic-corticosteroid–containing drops can effectively reduce a polyp's size to allow adequate examination of the medial EAC and tympanic membrane. Cauterization with silver nitrate can also be a helpful adjunctive measure in initial therapy. Aggressive débridement or avulsion of an aural polyp should be avoided as it may have attachments to a dehiscent facial nerve, the stapes footplate, or cholesteatoma overlying a labyrinthine fistula. Biopsy and histologic analysis should be performed on polyps of uncertain origin, both to rule out malignancy and possibly to help in diagnosing an underlying cholesteatoma. Unfortunately,

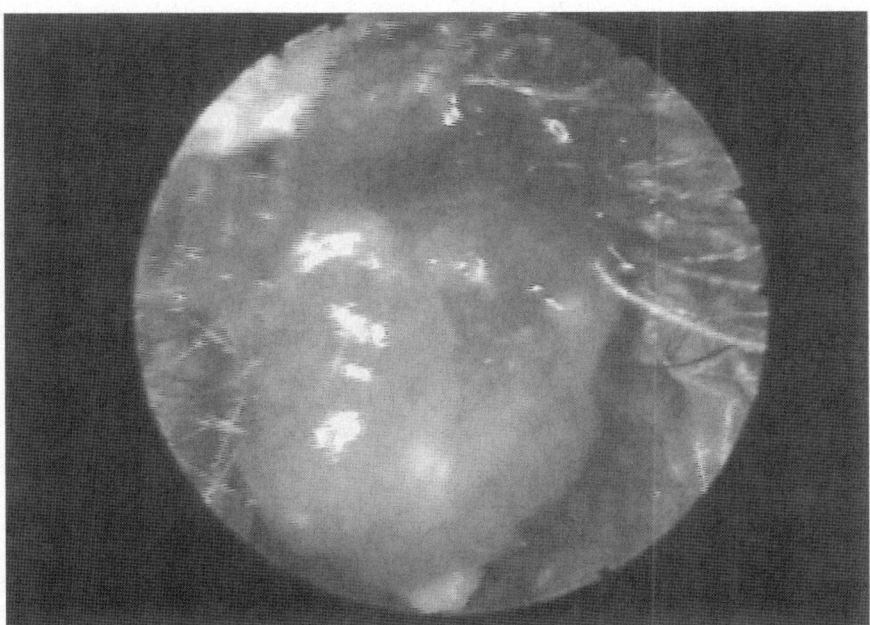

Figure 17–4 Left aural polyp. Mass of granulation tissue protruding into lateral external auditory canal.

reliable histopathologic features predicting cholesteatoma have not been established, and high false-positive rates have been reported.[24] Patients who fail to respond to medical management require surgery. Removal of aural polyps should be performed in conjunction with middle ear exploration. Noncholesteatomatous polyps of likely chronic mucosal otitis media origin may require mastoidectomy to adequately eradicate disease and provide ventilation to the mastoid antrum.[26]

Dermatologic Processes

The EAC is basically a blind pouch lined with skin. Its epidermis is susceptible to the same dermatologic processes encountered elsewhere in the body. Because it encompasses a small space and its skin is so thin, dermatitic processes of the external meatus produce troubling symptoms to afflicted patients.

Atopic dermatitis, also known as eczema, is a chronic pruritic skin condition commonly encountered in the external ear. Patients often report pruritus in other areas as well as associated medical histories of asthma and atopic rhinitis. Frequently, recurrent or chronic otitis externa generates the otolaryngologic referral. Clinically, the skin of the concha and lateral EAC appears hypertrophic and acanthotic (Figure 17–5). Evidence of excoriation reflects chronic pruritus and scratching. Most patients with atopic dermatitis are carriers of *S. aureus* on their skin, increasing their susceptibility to recurrent bouts of acute infection.[27] Treatment of the otologic component of eczematoid dermatitis requires control of acute flares of infection and suppression of pruritus. Acute episodes of otitis externa (discussed later in this chapter) are managed with local débridement and the application of antimicrobial drops. The underlying disease requires a regimen of topical corticosteroids. We have found that the combination of mometasone 0.1% (Elocon™) cream applied to the conchal region and 0.05% fluocinonide (Lidex™) drops in the EAC provides excellent results in the treatment of this disease.

Contact dermatitis is an inflammatory response triggered by contact with an irritant. The skin response is related to the potency of the irritant, such that a single exposure to a sufficiently strong stimulus may result in a significant reaction. Usually, however, the clinical picture of erythema, edema, and vesicular lesions does not develop until after repeated exposure to the offending agent. Contact dermatitis frequently occurs on the external ears and EACs. Allergy to grooming products such as hairsprays, shampoos, and fragrances may result in inflammation of the pinna and preauricular skin. Hypersensitivity to hearing aid molds has been reported, and,

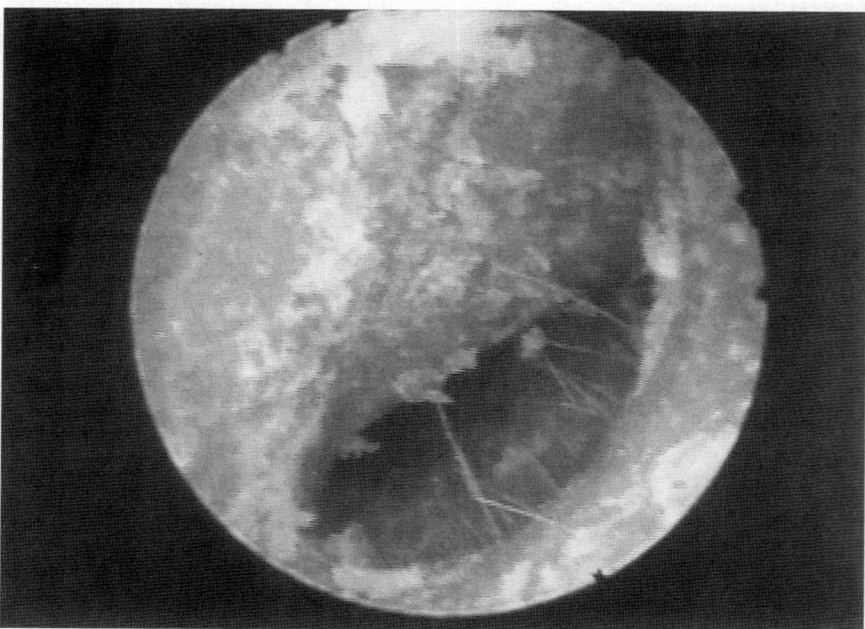

Figure 17–5 External auditory canal atopic (eczematoid) dermatitis.

if suspected, more hypoallergenic materials are available for substitution.

Neomycin hypersensitivity reactions deserve special mention. Many ototopical medications contain neomycin, including Cortisporin™, perhaps the most commonly used preparation. Objective evidence of neomycin allergy exists in approximately 1% of the population, but a hypersensitivity response develops in upwards of 15% of those who use the medication for otitis externa.[28] It presents as a worsening of the otitis for which it is being used along with a characteristic pattern of inflammation involving the skin of the concha and lobule. These dependent regions of the auricle endure the greatest exposure to the neomycin-containing preparation as it drains out of the external meatus following application. Effective treatment of all contact dermatoses requires identification and removal of the offending irritant. Topical corticosteroids provide symptomatic relief during acute flares. A short course of systemic corticosteroids can be useful in advanced cases to hasten resolution.

Acute Bacterial Otitis Externa

Acute diffuse otitis externa (swimmer's ear) refers to bacterial infection and inflammation of the skin and subcutaneous tissue of the cartilaginous EAC. Characteristic symptoms include itching, pain, and tenderness of the pinna with associated hearing loss and aural fullness. Examination typically reveals erythema and edema of the external canal skin, which may spread to involve the concha and lobule. Seropurulent otorrhea often results in crusting of the EAC and concha. Manipulation of the pinna and mastication generally elicit pain. In advanced cases, worsening edema significantly narrows the external canal lumen, preventing visualization of the tympanic membrane, and associated inflammatory changes may spread to involve preauricular soft tissue.

Cerumen plays an important protective role in EAC physiology. A relatively acidic pH and hydrophobic nature account for its bacteriostatic properties. A warm, moist environment favors bacterial growth, accounting for the increased incidence of acute otitis externa during summer months and in regions with tropical climates. Overzealous removal of cerumen not only compromises the natural defenses of the EAC, it may also cause sufficient trauma to allow for bacterial inoculation. Patients with pruritic dermatologic conditions often suffer from recurrent bouts of infection as a result of frequent scratching and excoriation of the canal skin.

Treatment of acute otitis externa requires the thorough removal of all purulent material and desquamated debris to allow penetration of antimicrobial therapy. The frequency of aural cleansing is dictated by the amount of debris present in the canal. When significant, débridement may be required several times per week. Ototopical preparations containing acidifying agents and antibiotics active against *P. aeruginosa*, *S. aureus*, and *Proteus mirabilis* address the infectious component of this process.[29] When edema is severe, inserting a wick into the canal aids in the delivery of medication to its deeper portions. Wicks should be replaced every 2 to 3 days until canal patency is restored. Many otic preparations contain a corticosteroid, helpful in reducing inflammation and edema of the canal as well as associated pain (see Table 17–1).[30] Oral antibiotics may be necessary when infection has extended to involve preauricular soft tissue. Pain control is another cornerstone in the treatment of otitis externa. Nonsteroidal anti-inflammatory medications or narcotic analgesics are required if over-the-counter analgesics fail to provide sufficient relief. The majority of treatment failures, particularly in those cases managed by primary care providers, are believed to result from inadequate skin penetration of the prescribed ototopical medication, further emphasizing the importance of adequate EAC débridement.[31]

Efforts to prevent recurrent episodes of otitis externa focus on minimizing the moisture content within the EAC. Water precautions should be recommended. Occlusive ear plugs are effective in preventing water entry into the canal. Directing a hair dryer at the EAC after water exposure followed by use of drying agents such as boric acid in ethyl alcohol can also be helpful.

The potential for ototoxicity must be considered when treating patients with tympanic membrane perforations or pressure equalization tubes. Instillation of ototopical drops into the middle ear of chinchillas was shown to result in cochlear toxicity.[32] Nevertheless, this appears to be an exceedingly rare complication in humans. In his review, Roland documented only four cases in the English literature of sensorineural hearing loss potentially related to topical antibiotic use.[33] A possible explanation is provided by the work of Schachern and colleagues, who demonstrated that the thickness of

Table 17–1   COMMONLY USED OTIC PREPARATIONS

Brand Name	Generic	Microbiology	Dosing*	Comment
CiproHC Otic	Ciprofloxacin Hydrocortisone	*Staphylococcus aureus* *Proteus mirabilis* *Pseudomonas aeruginosa*	3–5 drops bid × 7 days	No suspected ototoxicity
Floxin Otic	Ofloxacin	*Staphylococcus aureus* *Proteus mirabilis* *Pseudomonas aeruginosa*	5–7 drops bid × 10 days	FDA approved for middle ear use No steroid component
Cortisporin	Neomycin sulfate Polymyxin B Hydrocortisone	*Staphylococcus aureus* *Proteus mirabilis* *Pseudomonas aeruginosa*	3–7 drops tid	Neomycin sensitivity risk Potential ototoxicity
Gentamicin Ophthalmic	Gentamicin	*Staphylococcus aureus* *Proteus mirabilis* *Pseudomonas aeruginosa*	5–7 drops tid	Off-label use Potential ototoxicity No steroid component
Tobradex Ophthalmic	Tobramycin Dexamethasone	*Staphylococcus aureus* *Proteus mirabilis* *Pseudomonas aeruginosa*	5–7 drops tid	Off-label use Potential ototoxicity
Tobrex Ophthalmic	Tobramycin	*Staphylococcus aureus* *Proteus mirabilis* *Pseudomonas aeruginosa*	5–7 drops tid	Off-label use Potential ototoxicity No steroid component
Ciloxan Ophthalmic	Ciprofloxacin	*Staphylococcus aureus* *Proteus mirabilis* *Pseudomonas aeruginosa*	5–7 drops tid	Off-label use Potential ototoxicity No steroid component
Lotrimin	Clotrimazole	Broad-spectrum antifungal, especially *Candida*	5–7 drops tid	Off-label use Potential ototoxicity No steroid component
Cresylate	M-cresyl-acetate	Broad-spectrum antifungal	5–7 drops tid	Off-label use Potential ototoxicity No steroid component
Domboro	Acetic acid 2% in aqueous aluminum acetate solution	Antibacterial Antifungal	5–7 drops tid	Potential ototoxicity No steroid component

*Dosing information provided by Alcon Laboratories, Fort Worth, Tex.
FDA = US Food and Drug Administration.

the round window membrane increases while in the presence of inflammation or infection.[34] Use of potentially ototoxic medications in nondiseased middle ears should therefore be employed with caution as they lack this potentially protective characteristic.

Otomycosis

Otomycosis refers to an acute fungal infection of the EAC. Approximately 10% of cases of external otitis are related to fungal infection.[35] *Candida* and *Aspergillus* are the most common fungal species implicated in otomycosis.[36] The initial symptoms of fungal otitis externa mirror those of bacterial otitis externa, with the exception that associated pain is less severe. Intense pruritus is the most common complaint in otomycosis. Examination typically reveals canal skin erythema and the presence of abundant fungal debris, often embedded in a cheesy material thicker than that seen in bacterial otitis externa. Recognizing the white, gray, or black filamentous elements characteristic of fungal growth is critical to make the diagnosis of otomycosis. When unsure, a potassium hydroxide preparation can be helpful in demonstrating branching filaments or budding yeasts.

Treatment of otomycosis requires the removal of fungal debris and the application of appropriate topical antifungal medications. Many options are available and include M-cresyl-acetate (Cresylate™) or 1% clotrimazole (Lotrimin™) creams or solution, as well as vital dyes such as gentian violet. For recalcitrant cases, a topical preparation of 1% amphotericin B is available at compounding pharmacies and can be effective.

Malignant Otitis Externa (Skull Base Osteomyelitis)

Malignant otitis externa was first described by Meltzer and Keleman in 1959 and was later named by Chandler in 1958.[37,38] The term skull base osteomyelitis more accurately describes the pathophysiology of this life-threatening infection of the EAC and skull base. Usually seen in diabetic patients and those with other forms of immunocompromise, infection spreads from the skin and subcutaneous tissue of the cartilaginous canal to involve the tympanic bone. Skull base osteomyelitis spreads via the haversian system of compact bone, forming multiple abscesses and sequestra of necrotic bone. As infection progresses, periparotid and cervical soft tissues become involved. A facial nerve paralysis implies infection encasing the extratemporal portion of the nerve or involvement of the stylomastoid foramen. Palsies of cranial nerves IX, X, XI, and XII present as infection extends to involve the jugular foramen.[39]

The cerumen of patients with diabetes has been shown to be of higher pH than that of nondiabetics, perhaps responsible for the increased incidence of external otitis in this population.[40] Impaired polymorphonuclear leukocyte function characterizes the immunocompromise associated with diabetes. In addition, the microangiopathic disease typical of advanced diabetes inhibits delivery of systemic antibiotics to infected tissues. These factors contribute to the observation that progression of otitis externa to skull base osteomyelitis almost exclusively occurs in elderly diabetic patients.[41]

Patients with osteomyelitis of the skull base often report a previous history of otitis externa. Intense otalgia exceeding that expected for routine otitis is common and can be associated with otorrhea. Granulation tissue seen protruding into the EAC from the bony-cartilaginous junction is a cardinal sign of skull base osteomyelitis and should not be underestimated. Biopsy is required both to rule out malignancy and for culture purposes. Computed tomographic scans help to evaluate the extent of bony involvement. Magnetic resonance imaging provides more detail regarding soft tissue disease and, when combined with magnetic resonance angiography, can evaluate the patency of the dural sinuses. Technetium 99m

and gallium 67 bone scans help in confirming the diagnosis of skull base osteomyelitis. Only the gallium scan, however, can be used to monitor response to therapy. Gallium scans image the activity of white blood cells and proteins at sites of active infection. This study will normalize as infection resolves, whereas the technetium scan may remain positive for many months.[42]

Treatment of osteomyelitis of the skull base generally requires long-term administration of parental antibiotics in combination with daily aural débridement and vigilant management of diabetes and other compromising medical conditions. The vast majority of skull base osteomyelitis results from infection by *P. aeruginosa*.[28] Double coverage directed against *Pseudomonas* is empirically begun after cultures have been obtained. The emergence of fluoroquinolones, which offer potent activity against *Pseudomonas* via oral administration, permits the use of oral antibiotics after an appropriate response to several weeks of intravenous antibiotics has been observed. Some have reported success using oral ciprofloxacin alone, but further investigation is required before this mode of therapy can be endorsed.[7,43] Surgical therapy is rarely required and is usually mandated by progression of infection despite aggressive medical management. The role of surgery should be limited to the débridement of necrotic bone and granulation tissue and the drainage of abscesses. Decompression of the facial nerve for cases complicated by facial paralysis appears to have no role in the management of skull base osteomyelitis as it fails to address the extratemporal location of nerve involvement.[44]

Acquired Stenosis

Acquired stenosis of the medial EAC, also known as medial canal fibrosis, refers to a rare condition characterized by the cicatricial formation of fibrous tissue lateral to the tympanic membrane. A distinct clinical entity that must be differentiated from congenital aural atresia, acquired stenosis usually results from chronic infection and inflammation but may also represent a complication related to prior otologic surgery or EAC trauma.[45] As the developing stenosis progresses, affected patients suffer a worsening conductive hearing loss. Examination reveals edema and hypertrophy of the canal wall skin, and once fibrosis matures, the EAC becomes a blind, skin-lined pouch (Figure 17–6). The lateral aspect of the tympanic

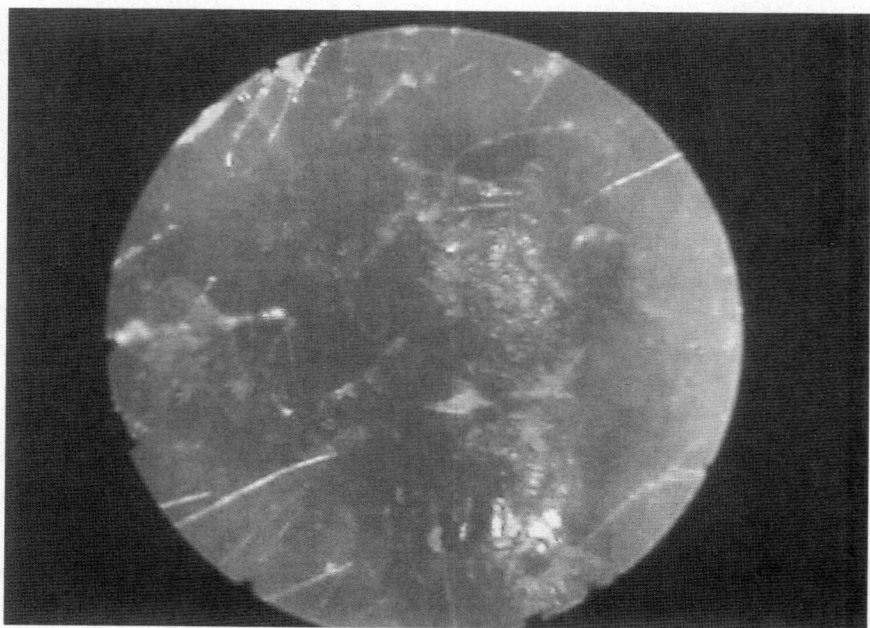

Figure 17–6 Right medial canal fibrosis.

membrane frequently becomes incorporated into the scar tissue, obliterating any potential intervening space.

The treatment of acquired stenoses of the EAC focuses on prevention. Chronic otitis externa refers to a diffuse inflammatory process of the external canal of long duration. Its etiology remains unclear, but it appears to be the most frequent cause of medial canal fibrosis.[46] Bilateral in 50% of cases and twice as common in women than men, this entity is probably related to a combination of infection, allergy, and dermatoses.[47] A paucity of literature analyzing treatment options for chronic otitis externa exists, but management is primarily medical until complete medial canal fibrosis develops. A regimen consisting of topical corticosteroid and antibiotic preparations in combination with periodic, atraumatic cleansing may prevent the need for surgical intervention.

Surgical therapy of acquired stenoses is indicated for correction of conductive hearing loss (hearing aids tend to exacerbate underlying inflammation) and to prevent cholesteatoma in those stenoses related to trauma or prior surgery. Generally, canalplasty with a wide meatoplasty is the procedure of choice. This may be performed endaurally if adequate exposure can be obtained but usually requires a postauricular approach (Figure 17–7). All involved skin must be removed and the bony canal enlarged to allow for some element of post-operative restenosis. The cicatrix can frequently be dissected free of the tympanic membrane, but, if not, a tympanoplasty is performed. Critical to the success of this procedure is resurfacing the osseous canal with epithelium. If bone is left exposed, and the formation of granulation tissue and healing by secondary intention are allowed, the risk of recurrent stenosis is unacceptably high.[42] Usually, a split-thickness skin graft is employed, but a variety of pedicled flaps, as well as full-thickness skin grafts, have been described.[48–50] A wide meatoplasty is a necessary addition to canalplasty to permit physiologic lateral migration of cerumen and squamous debris. A sterile gauze roll is typically placed into the canal as a stent for 10 to 14 days. The incidence of recurrence is difficult to determine since published series report results from small cohorts of patients without long-term follow-up.

MALIGNANCIES OF THE AURICLE AND EXTERNAL AUDITORY CANAL

The pinna and external auditory canal may be afflicted by cutaneous malignancies found elsewhere on the body. The most common form is squamous cell carcinoma, followed by basal cell carcinoma and melanoma. Adenoid

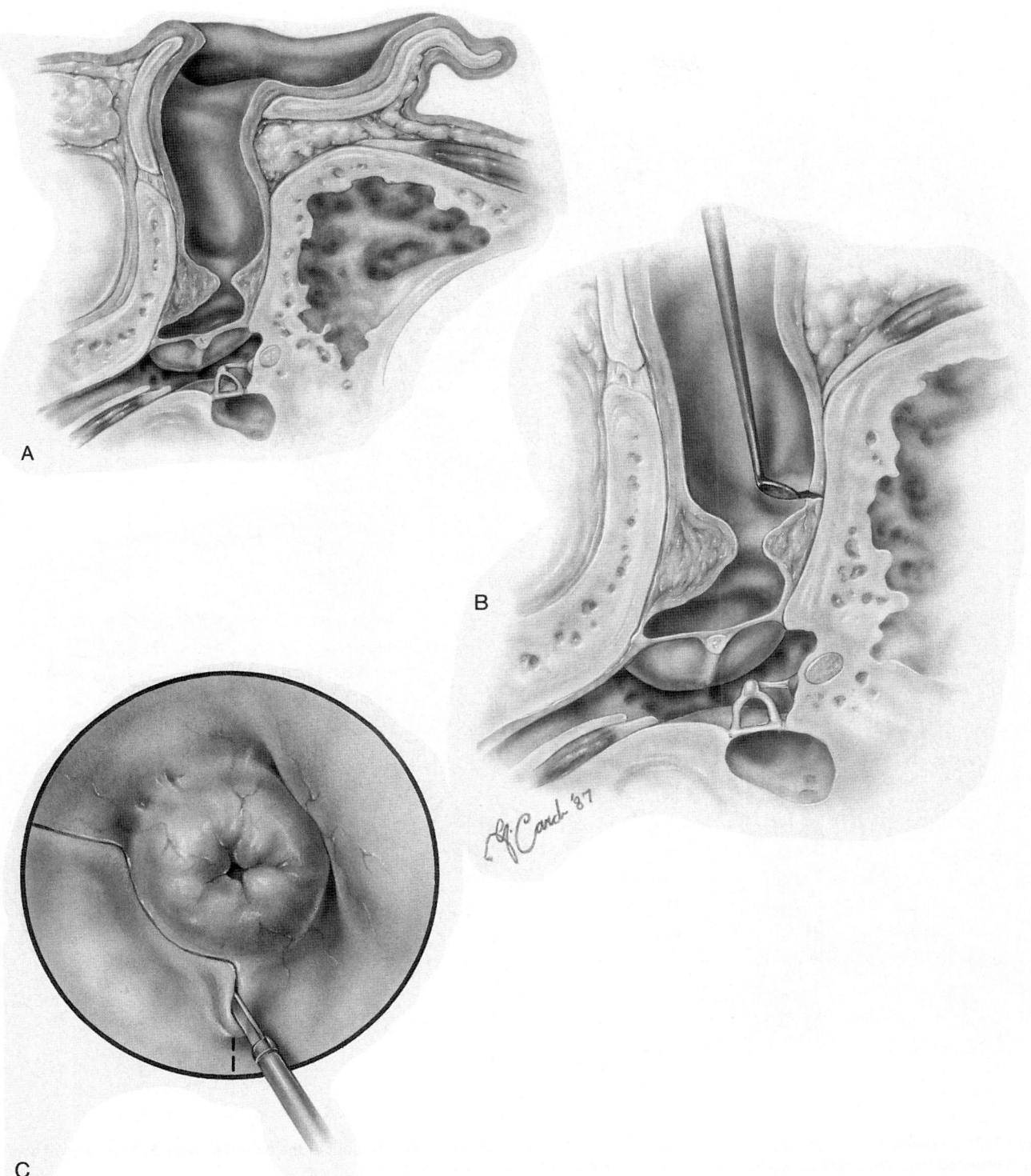

Figure 17-7 Surgical treatment of acquired external canal stenosis. *A,* Cicatricial fibrous stenosis at the level of the bony external auditory canal. *B* and *C,* Vascular strip incisions are made as far medial as is safe and practicable.

Illustration continued on following page

cystic carcinoma and ceruminal gland adenocarcinoma may also occur within the EAC. Malignancies of the auricle and EAC typically present as ulcerated or nodular skin lesions, which are associated with chronic bloody otorrhea when situated within the canal. Temporal bone invasion is classically heralded by complaints of a deep-

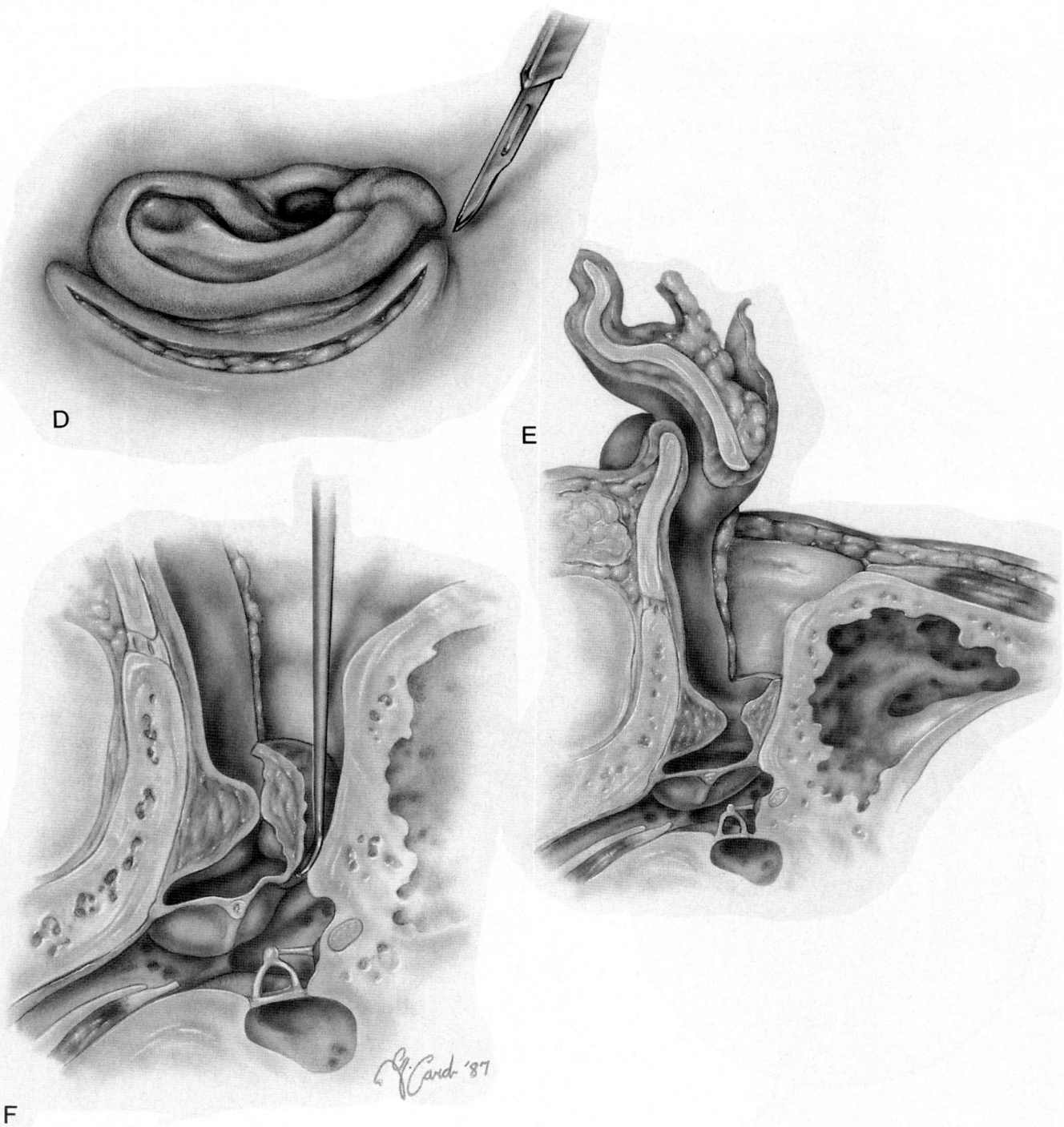

Figure 17–7 Continued *D*, A postauricular incision is made. *E*, The vascular strip is elevated out of the external canal. *F*, The mass of scar tissue is elevated from the posterior wall of the ear canal until the middle ear space is entered.

Illustration continued on following page

boring otalgia. Radiographic imaging helps define the extent of tumor invasion. Treatment usually requires wide excision but is frequently combined with postoperative radiation therapy. A thorough discussion of the management of this class of malignancy, however, is beyond the scope of this chapter (see Chapter 18).

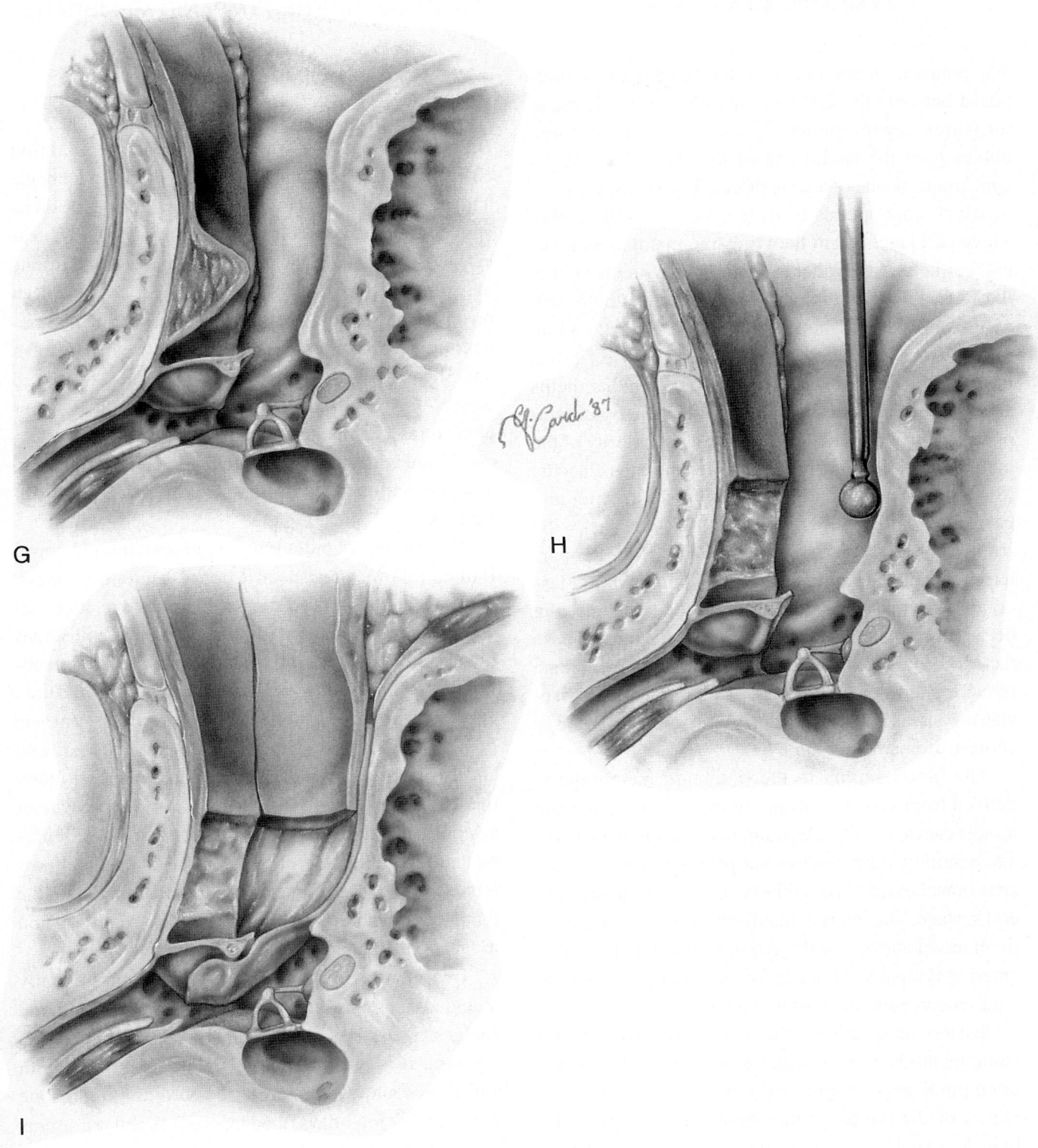

Figure 17–7   Continued *G*, Posterior fibrous stenosis excised. *H*, The stenotic scar tissue anteriorly is excised, leaving the anterior drum remnant if at all possible. The canal is enlarged with a drill until air cells can just be seen through bone. *I*, The drum and canal are grafted with fascia and the canal is filled with ointment.

TYMPANIC MEMBRANE

The tympanic membrane is a thin fibrous sheet interposed between the EAC and middle ear. Its diameter measures approximately 9 mm, and it is oriented obliquely at the lateral end of the external canal. Its appearance is one of a cone directed medially, the apex of which corresponds to its attachment to the umbo. Three cell layers form the tympanic membrane: a lateral epithelial lining that is continuous with the skin of the EAC, a middle fibrous layer composed of both radiating and circular fibers of connective tissue, and an internal mucosal layer. A coalescence of the fibrous layer at its rim, known as the fibrous annulus, helps anchor the tympanic membrane within the bony tympanic sulcus. The pars tensa refers to the majority of the membrane, which is separated from the pars flaccida (Shrapnell's membrane) superiorly by the anterior and posterior malleal folds. The pars flaccida lacks the strong fibrous layer of tissue present within the pars tensa; its collagen fibers are fewer in number and less organized. It also sits in a region of the tympanic ring deficient of bone, named the notch of Rivinus.[3] These factors account for the tendency for tympanic membrane retraction at the pars flaccida. Medial to the pars flaccida is Prussak's space, the most common site of primary cholesteatoma formation.

The blood supply to the tympanic membrane is derived from vessels that supply the external canal and middle ear cavity. The deep auricular branch of the internal maxillary artery forms a peripheral ring from which arise branches destined for the tympanic membrane's lateral surface. The internal maxillary artery also supplies the internal surface of the tympanic membrane via its anterior tympanic branch.[1] Venous drainage tends to parallel corresponding arterial anatomy.

Sensory innervation to the lateral surface of the tympanic membrane mirrors that of the EAC. The auriculotemporal nerve supplies the posterior and inferior region of the tympanic membrane, and the auricular branch (Arnold's nerve) of the vagus nerve innervates its anterior and superior aspects. The tympanic branch (Jacobson's nerve) of the glossopharyngeal nerve provides sensation to the medial surface of the tympanic membrane.

DISEASES OF THE TYMPANIC MEMBRANE

Bullous Myringitis

Bullous myringitis is a poorly understood condition characterized by inflammation of the tympanic membrane and the formation of serous or hemorrhagic bullae on its epithelial surface. Middle ear effusion may also be present. Most commonly, the disease is unilateral and results in severe otalgia, often disproportionate to findings seen on physical examination. Sensorineural hearing loss frequently accompanies bullous myringitis. In Hoffman and Shepsman's review of 15 patients with 21 affected ears, 67% showed evidence of sensorineural loss, either alone or as a component of a mixed loss.[51] Hearing loss associated with bullous myringitis is generally transient, and the majority of patients recover full auditory function.[52]

The etiology of bullous myringitis remains unknown. It often follows a nonspecific upper respiratory illness, and early studies indeed suggested a causal relationship with influenza infection.[53] Later, Rifkin and colleagues induced bullous myringitis in nearly half of healthy subjects inoculated with *Mycoplasma pneumoniae*.[54] However, when examining the acute and postconvalescent sera of patients diagnosed with bullous myringitis, Merifield and Miller found no consistent changes in antibody titers to suggest an etiologic role for *M. pneumoniae* or a variety of common upper respiratory viruses.[55] It may be that the bullous lesions characteristic of this illness represent a nonspecific response to inflammation of the tympanic membrane and that bullous myringitis is not, in fact, a distinct entity.

Treatment of bullous myringitis has traditionally included decompression of the painful vesicles and oral analgesics. In cases complicated by sensorineural hearing loss, it is our practice to treat aggressively with antibiotics and systemic corticosteroids (prednisone 1 mg/kg/day for 7 days, then tapered) as if it represents a complication of otitis media. Myringotomy is also performed if a middle ear effusion accompanies bullae formation. Randomized trials comparing management options for bullous myringitis with associated sensorineural hearing loss do not exist, however.

Granular Myringitis

Another poorly understood condition, granular myringitis is characterized by chronic inflammation of the tympanic membrane leading to the replacement of its epithelial surface and, occasionally, adjacent deep meatal skin with proliferating granulation tissue. The predominant presentation of granular myringitis is painless, unilateral otorrhea that is scant and malodorous. Symptoms of pruritus and aural fullness are also common. Otoscopy reveals a serous, mucopurulent, or frankly purulent discharge bathing the tympanic membrane. Careful aural cleansing is required to visualize characteristic granulation tissue, which may involve the tympanic membrane in focal patches, segmental distributions, or diffusely, where most of the pars tensa surface is replaced (Figure 17–8). Most agree that the tympanic membrane must be intact to diagnose granular myringitis and differentiate it from chronic suppurative otitis media.[56] Pneumatic otoscopy and tympanometry are helpful in confirming the absence of perforation and middle ear pathology when in doubt. A mild conductive hearing loss is frequently noted on audiometric evaluation.

The etiology of granular myringitis is unknown. Acute infection or mechanical trauma leading to loss of the squamous epithelial layer of the tympanic membrane appears to be a critical event in the development of granular myringitis, which disrupts normal epithelial migration responsible for the healing properties of the tympanic membrane.[57] In their review, Blevins and Karmody found that 60% of patients with granular myringitis had previously undergone an otologic procedure.[58] Once the epithelial layer has been exposed, infection by those organisms commonly responsible for otitis externa, especially *Pseudomonas* and *Staphyloccocus*, further inhibits healing of the tympanic membrane.

Management of granular myringitis often requires protracted therapy. Initially, external infection must be controlled. Topical antimicrobial drops or powders directed at gram-negative organisms and *Staphylococcus* species, as well as gentian violet, are effective. Once infection has been addressed, granulation tissue may be cauterized with silver nitrate, if abundant, and is controlled with daily use of topical corticosteroid drops (0.05% fluocinonide [Lidex™]) until resolution is observed. Unfortunately, recurrence is typical. The role of surgery in the management of granular myringitis remains controversial. It is generally reserved for those refractory cases that fail prolonged topical therapy. The involved area of the tympanic membrane is excised and repaired with an underlay or overlay graft. Some authors have reported excellent success rates for surgical therapy of granular myringi-

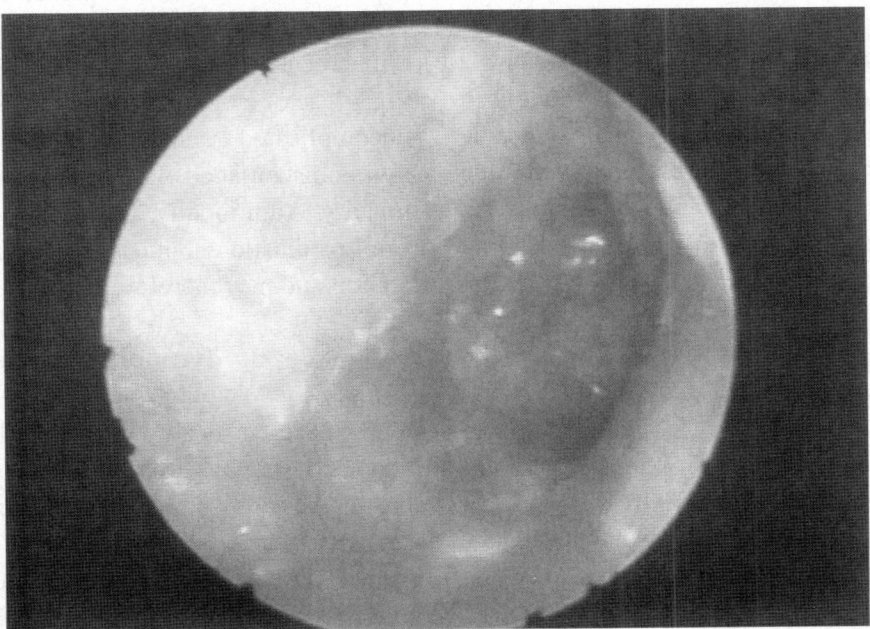

Figure 17–8 Right granular myringitis. Note granulation tissue present on the surface of the tympanic membrane with associated inflammatory changes to external auditory canal epithelium.

tis, but available data are sparse and limited by short follow-up periods.[59]

Traumatic Perforation

Acute perforations of the tympanic membrane generally result from episodes of acute otitis media or trauma. The majority of infectious perforations heal as the inciting condition resolves. Traumatic tympanic membrane perforation may result from blunt or penetrating injuries as well as rapid changes in barometric pressure (barotrauma). Slap injuries to the head, frequently encountered in cases related to assault or aquatic sports accidents, create a column of compressed air within the EAC of sufficient pressure to implode the tympanic membrane. Blast injuries inflict similar implosive forces on the tympanic membrane. Penetrating injuries are most frequently self-inflicted during overzealous cerumen removal. Barometric trauma commonly occurs following rapid airplane descent or deep-water diving or during hyperbaric oxygen therapy. Rather than causing a perforation, barotrauma generally results in hemorrhage of tympanic membrane vasculature. Thermal injuries to the tympanic membrane, commonly seen in welders and those struck by lightning, result in a small percentage of perforations. However, because of associated tissue necrosis, burn-related perforations have a high rate of nonhealing.

Most studies suggest that upwards of 90% of traumatic perforations heal spontaneously within 3 months of injury.[50,61] Epithelial migration patterns on the tympanic membrane and within the EAC responsible for the removal of desquamated cells and keratin debris form the basis for the tympanic membrane's impressive healing properties. Studies by Litton and Alberti used India ink to mark epithelial elements on the tympanic membrane and documented cell migration that originates from the region of the umbo and proceeds in a centripetal fashion.[62,63] Following an acute injury, platelets gather to cause vasoconstriction and form a thrombus. An inflammatory response ensues, attracting neutrophils, macrophages, and bioactive cytokines to the wound. A matrix of proteoglycans and glycosaminoglycans is formed and allows for proliferation of the tympanic membrane's squamous epithelial layer across the perforation, forming a scaffold on which the mucosal and, later, the fibrous layers of the tympanic membrane can grow. The squa-

mous elements responsible for bridging the perforation originate from "upstream" and must traverse the length of the defect. It is not surprising, therefore, that larger perforations are associated with delayed healing and higher rates of chronicity.[58]

Patients who have suffered a traumatic tympanic membrane perforation often complain of mild hearing loss and aural fullness. Vertigo is uncommon and should prompt concern for a perilymphatic fistula. Audiometric assessment often shows conductive hearing loss of varying severity. Some have proposed that ossicular injury may be predicted by more significant air–bone gaps, but studies have shown this not to be the case.[64] Management of traumatic perforations ranges from observation along with dry ear precautions to early myringoplasty. Either approach will result in perforation closure in approximately 90% of cases. Those who practice expectant management of traumatic tympanic membrane perforations cite the high likelihood of spontaneous healing, whereas supporters of early intervention report quicker resolution of hyperacusis and prompt return of patients to their preferred lifestyles. Myringoplasty can be performed as an office-based procedure under local anesthesia. After injecting the external canal with 1% lidocaine, the margins of the tympanic membrane are everted and aligned with a pick. A patch of moistened cigarette paper or Gelfilm™ is then placed over the perforation. Authors note that the patch helps prevent inversion of the tympanic membrane edges and promotes prompt healing.[16] Use of ototopical medications in the setting of an uncomplicated traumatic tympanic membrane perforation is discouraged. There is a theoretical risk of ototoxicity. Additionally, the wet environment resulting from medication application impairs fibroblast proliferation and may therefore hinder perforation healing.

Tympanosclerosis

Tympanosclerosis is characterized by hyaline degeneration of the fibrous layer of the tympanic membrane and the middle ear mucosa. Isolated involvement of the tympanic membrane is most common and is more appropriately named myringosclerosis, but tympanosclerotic plaques may also present within the middle ear cleft and mastoid. Tympanosclerosis is irreversible and results from infection or inflammation of the middle ear space. The incidence of tympanosclerosis in patients with a previous history of otitis media ranges from 14 to 43% in different clinical series.[65,66] In their review, Tos and Stangerup demonstrated an association between ventilation tube placement and tympanosclerosis.[67] Tympanosclerosis developed in 13% of ears with secretory otitis media treated with paracentesis compared with 59% treated with grommet tube insertion. Additionally, Kay and colleagues's recent meta-analysis of 134 studies regarding sequelae of tympanostomy tube insertion revealed a 32% incidence of postintubation tympanosclerosis compared with 10% of controls.[68]

Rarely does isolated tympanic membrane tympanosclerosis result in a clinically significant hearing loss requiring intervention. In one series, no difference in speech reception thresholds was found between ears with tympanosclerosis and those with healthy-appearing tympanic membranes.[69] In Tos and Poulsen's grommet tube study, the maximal conductive hearing loss associated with tympanosclerosis was 1 dB. Middle ear tympanosclerosis, on the other hand, can cause ossicular fixation and result in more severe degrees of conductive hearing loss.

MYRINGOTOMY FOR ACUTE SUPPURATIVE OTITIS MEDIA

Indications

Myringotomy by incision of the pars tensa of the tympanic membrane is indicated for acute suppurative otitis media with exudate under pressure in the tympanic cavity (see also Chapter 21). When otalgia and fever are mild, a 24-hour trial of antibiotic therapy is warranted, and in many cases, the infection clears without myringotomy. In severe infections (ie, those with a bulging drum, severe otalgia, high fever, and mastoid tenderness), as well as in persistent or recurrent infections that fail to resolve with antibiotic therapy, a myringotomy should be done.

Technique

For infants, no anesthesia need be used; the arms and legs are confined by being wrapped in a sheet "mummy fash-

ion" or a "papoose" board. An assistant holds the head. For children and adults, a brief general anesthetic is preferred. The topical application of phenol is not terribly effective for an acutely inflamed tympanic membrane but may be better than nothing.

Myringotomy should always be done under direct vision, not blindly, because of the risk of injuring the stapes or the facial nerve. The incision should be 2 to 3 mm in length in the postero inferior quadrant of the pars tensa and should be deep enough to go entirely through a thickened membrane. Culture of the tip of the blade provides an excellent opportunity for determining the causative organism(s) and appropriate antibiotic therapy.

MYRINGOTOMY AND VENTILATION TUBE INSERTION FOR SEROUS OTITIS MEDIA

Indications

Serous otitis media is an accumulation of clear (rarely opacified) straw-colored serous or tenacious mucoid fluid in the tympanomastoid compartment as a result of eustachian tube obstruction (see also Chapter 21). Myringotomy may be indicated for both diagnosis and treatment.

Diagnostic myringotomy for serous otitis media should be considered whenever there is a conductive hearing loss and a thickened tympanic membrane preventing otoscopic visualization of a fluid level or when otoscopy reveals the characteristic straw-colored fluid medial to the tympanic membrane.

Therapeutic myringotomy with insertion of a ventilating or pressure-equalizing (PE) tube is done whenever serous otitis media fails to resolve after adequate medical therapy.

Technique

Generally, myringotomy is performed in conjunction with the insertion of a PE tube. Infants and small children are best managed by performing this procedure under a general anesthetic. In older children and adults, local anesthetic can be used.

The incision in the tympanic membrane is usually made in the antero inferior quadrant. There are many commercially available PE tubes. Depending on the design of the tube, it stays in the drum for only a few months to several years. For example, a bobbin-type tube remains in place for 6 to 18 months; the tube is extruded as the tympanic membrane heals. On the other hand, T-type tubes remain in place for years, avoiding the need for repetitive insertion. Counterbalancing this advantage of the T tube are the heightened likelihood of permanent tympanic membrane perforation and cholesteatoma formation associated with the longer indwelling tube. In addition, like the short-term tubes, the long-term tubes can become obstructed with inspissated debris and require replacement. Consequently, long-term tubes are reserved for use in individuals with chronic eustachian tube difficulties.

REFERENCES

1. Storper IS, Canalis RF, Lambert PR. Diseases of the auricle and pericauricular region. In: Canalis RF, Lambert PR, editors. The ear: comprehensive otology. 1st ed. Philadelphia: Lippincott Williams and Wilkins; 2000. p. 325–39.
2. Sadler TW. Langman's medical embryology. 7th ed. Baltimore: Williams and Wilkins; 1995.
3. Hollinshead WH. Anatomy for surgeons: the head and neck. 3rd ed. Philadelphia: Lippincott-Raven; 1982.
4. Holt GR. Injuries of the external ear. Otolaryngol Clin North Am 1990;23:1003–18.
5. Schuller DE, Dankle SD, Strauss RH. Auricular injury and the use of headgear in wrestlers. Arch Otolaryngol Head Neck Surg 1989;115:714.
6. Bassiouny A. Perichondritis of the auricle. Laryngoscope 1981; 91:422–31.
7. Giamarella H. Malignant otitis externa: the therapeutic evolution of a lethal infection. J Antimicrob Chemother 1992;30:745–51.
8. Work WP. Newer concepts of first branchial cleft defects. Laryngoscope 1972;82:1581–93.
9. Kischer CW, Shetlar MR. Collagen and mucopolysaccharides in the hypertrophic scar. Connect Tissue Res 1974;2:205–13.
10. Sherris DA, Larrabee WF, Murakami CS. Management of scar contractures, hypertrophic scars, and keloids. Otolaryngol Clin North Am 1995;28:1057–67.
11. Farrior RT, Stambaugh KI. Keloids and hyperplastic scars. In: Thomas JF, Holt JR, editors. Facial scars, revisions, and camouflage. St. Louis: CV Mosby; 1989. p. 211–28.
12. Wortmann RL. Gout and other disorders of purine metabolism. In: Isselbacher, Kurt J, editors. Harrison's principles of internal medicine. 13th ed. New York: McGraw-Hill; 1994. p. 2079–88.
13. Tolleth H. A hierarchy of values in the design and construction of the ear. Clin Past Surg 1990;17:193.
14. Mustarde JC. The treatment of prominent ears by buried mattress suture—a ten years' survey. Plast Reconstr Surg 1967;39: 382.
15. Goode RL. Acoustical aspects of chronic ear surgery. Self-instructed package—American Academy of Otolaryngology Head and Neck Surgery 1987;16–24.
16. van Gilse PHG. Des observations ulterieures sur la genes des exostoses du conduit externe par l'irriations d'eau froide. Acta Otolaryngol (Stockh) 1938;26:343.
17. Wong BF, Cervantes W, Doyle KJ, et al. Prevalence of external auditory canal exostoses in surfers. Arch Otolaryngol Head Neck Surg 1999;125:969–72.
18. Kroon DF, Lawson ML, Derkay CS. Surfer's ear: external auditory exostoses are more prevalent in cold water surfers. Presented at the annual meeting of the American Academy of Otolaryngology-Head and Neck Surgery, Denver, 2001.
19. Fisher EW, McManus TC. Surgery for external auditory canal exostoses and osteomata. J Laryngol Otol 1994;108:106–10.
20. Corbridge RJ, Michaels L, Wright T. Epithelial migration in keratosis obturans. Am J Otolaryngol 1996;17:411–4.
21. Morrison AW. Keratosis obturans. J Laryngol Otolaryngol 1956;70:317–21.
22. Vrabec JT, Chaljub G. External canal cholesteatoma. Am J Otol 2000;21:608–14.
23. Piepergerdes JC, Kramer BM, Behnke EE. Keratosis obturans and external auditory canal cholesteatoma. Laryngoscope 1980;90:383–90.
24. Veitch D, Brockbank M, Whittet H. Aural polyp and cholesteatoma. Clin Otolaryngol 1988;13:395–7.
25. Gliklick RE, Cunningham MJ, Eavey RD. The cause of aural polyps in children. Arch Otolaryngol Head Neck Surg 1993;119: 669–71.
26. Tay HL, Hussain SSM. The management of aural polyps. J Laryngol Otol 1997;111:212–4.
27. Shea CR. Dermatologic diseases of the external auditory canal. Otolaryngol Clin North Am 1996;29:783–94.
28. Rietschel RL, Fowler JF Jr. Aquatic dermatoses. In: Rietschel RL, Fowler JF Jr, editors. Fisher's contact dermatitis. 4th ed. Baltimore: Williams & Wilkins; 1995. p. 958.
29. Linstrom JL, Lucente FE, Joseph EM. Infections of the external ear. In: Bailey BL, editor. Head and neck surgery—otolaryngology. 2nd ed. Philadelphia: Lippincott-Raven; 1998. p. 1965–81.
30. Bojrab DI, Bruderly T, Abdularazzak Y. Otitis externa. Otolaryngol Clin North Am 1996;29:761–82.
31. Hannley MT, Dennery JC, Holzer SS. Consensus panel report: use of ototopical antibiotics in treating 3 common ear diseases. Otolaryngol Head Neck Surg 2000;122:934–40.
32. Wright CG, Meyerhoff WL. Ototoxicity of otic drops applied to the middle ear in the chinchilla. Am J Otolaryngol 1984;5: 166–76.

33. Roland PS. Clinical ototoxicity of topical antibiotic drops. Otolaryngol Head Neck Surg 1994;110:598–602.

34. Schachern PA, Paparella MM, Goycoolea MV. Thickness of the human round window membrane in different forms of otitis media. Arch Otolaryngol Head Neck Surg 1987;110:630–4.

35. Mugliston T, O'Donoghue G. Otomycosis—a continuing problem. J Laryngol Otol 1985;99:327–33.

36. Lucente FE. Fungal infections of the external ear. Otolaryngol Clin North Am 1993;26:995–1006.

37. Meltzer P, Keleman G. Pyocyaneus osteomyelitis of the temporal bone, mandible and zygoma. Laryngoscope 1958;69:1300–16.

38. Chandler JR. Malignant external otitis. Laryngoscope 1968;78:1257–94.

39. Slattery WH, Brackman DE. Skull base osteomyelitis. Otolaryngol Clin North Am 1996;9:795–806.

40. Driscoll PV, Ramachandrula A, Drezner DA, et al. Characteristics of cerumen in diabetic patients: a key to understanding malignant external otitis? Otolaryngol Head Neck Surg 1993;109:676.

41. Smitherman KO, Peacock JE. Infectious emergencies in patients with diabetes mellitus. Med Clin North Am 1995;79:53–77.

42. Noyek AM, Kirsh JC, Greyson HD, et al. The clinical significance of radionucliotide bone and gallium scanning in osteomyelitis of the head and neck. Laryngoscope 1984;94 Suppl 34:1–21.

43. Hickey SA, Ford GR, O'Connor AF, et al. Treating malignant otitis externa with oral ciprofloxacin. BMJ 1989;299:550–1.

44. Neal GD, Gates GA. Invasive *Pseudomonas* osteitis of the temporal bone. Am J Otol 1983;4:332–7.

45. El-Sayed Y. Acquired medial canal fibrosis. J Laryngol Otol 1998;112:145–9.

46. Selesnick S, Nguyen TP, Eisenman DJ. Surgical treatment of acquired external auditory canal atresia. Am J Otol 1998;19:123–30.

47. Roland PS. Chronic external otitis. Ear Nose Throat J 2001;80 Suppl 6:12–6.

48. Adkins WY, Ogusthorpe JD. Management of canal stenosis with a transposition flap. Laryngoscope 1981;91:1267–9.

49. Heeneman H. Surgical correction of the stenosed ear canal. J Otolaryngol 1979;8:461–2.

50. McCary WS, Kryzer TC, Lambert PR. Application of split-thickness skin grafts for acquired diseases of the external auditory canal. Am J Otol 1995;16:801–5.

51. Hoffman RA, Shepsman MA. Bullous myringitis and sensorineural hearing loss. Laryngoscope 1983;93:1544–5.

52. Lashin N, Zaher S, Ragab A, et al. Hearing loss in bullous myringitis. Ear Nose Throat J 1988;67:206–10.

53. Milligan W. Hemorrhagic types of ear disease occurring during epidemics of influenza. J Laryngol Otol 1926;41:493–8.

54. Rifkin D, Chanock R, Kravetz H, et al. Ear involvement (myringitis) and primary atypical pneumonia following inoculation of volunteers with eaton agent. Am Rev Respir Dis 1962;85:479–89.

55. Merifield D, Miller G. The etiology and clinical course of bullous myringitis. Arch Otolaryngol 1966;84:41–3.

56. Stoney P, Kwok P, Hawke M. Granular myringitis: a review. J Otolaryngol 1992;21:129–35.

57. Makino K, Amatsu M, Kinishi M, et al. The clinical features and pathogenesis of granular myringitis. Arch Otorhinolaryngol 1988;245:224–9.

58. Blevins NJ, Karmody CS. Chronic myringitis: prevalence, presentation, and natural history. Otol Neurootol 2001;22:3–10.

59. El-Seifi A, Fouad B. Granular myringitis: is it a surgical problem? Am J Otol 2000;21:462–7.

60. Pulec JL, Kinney SE. Diseases of the tympanic membrane. In: Paparella MM, Shumrick DA, editors. Otolaryngology. 1st ed. Philadelphia: WB Saunders; 1973. p. 61–4.

61. Griffin WL. A retrospective study of traumatic tympanic membrane perforations in a clinical practice. Laryngoscope 1979:89;261–82.

62. Litton WB. Epithelial migration over the tympanic membrane and external auditory canal. Arch Otolaryngol Head Neck Surg 1963;77:254.

63. Alberti PWRM. Epithelial migration on the tympanic membrane. J Laryngol Otol 1964;78:808–30.

64. Camnitz PS, Bost WS. Traumatic perforations of the tympanic membrane: early closure with paper tape patching. Otolaryngol Head Neck Surg 1985;93:220–3.

65. Sheehy JL, House WF. Tympanosclerosis. Arch Otolaryngol 1962;76:151–7.

66. Bhaya MH, Paparella MM, Morizono T, et al. Pathogenesis of tympanosclerosis. Otolaryngol Head Neck Surg 1993;109:413–9.

67. Tos M, Stangerup SE. Hearing loss in tympanosclerosis caused by grommets. Arch Otolaryngol Head Neck Surg 1989;115:931–5.

68. Kay DJ, Nelson M, Rosenfeld RM. Meta-analysis of tympanostomy tube sequelae. Otolaryngol Head Neck Surg 2001;124:374–80.

69. Tos M, Poulsen G. Changes in pars tensa in secretory otitis. ORL J Otorhinolaryngol Relat Spec 1979;41:313–28.

18

Surgery for Cancer of the External Ear

Mark L. Gustafson, MD
Myles L. Pensak, MD, FACS

Cancer of the skin represents the most common form of diagnosed malignancy. In the last three decades, the lifetime risk of developing skin cancer has nearly tripled.[1] Over 600,000 new cases of cutaneous carcinoma are reported each year in the United States alone.[1] Otolaryngologists are frequently involved in the diagnosis, resection, and reconstruction of skin cancer of the head and neck. Over 80% of cutaneous carcinomas occur in the head and neck region, and 5 to 10% of these cases are localized to the ear.[2] Although eradication of the cancer is the goal of any treatment strategy, esthetics are an important factor in the management of tumors of the external ear. These competing concerns make auricular carcinoma a particularly challenging problem. This chapter reviews the diagnosis and management of auricular carcinoma. Tumors that originate or extend into the external auditory canal, middle ear, or temporal bone are covered separately in Chapter 37.

ANATOMY

Embryology

Development of the external ear begins at the fifth to sixth week of gestation. Six mesenchymal swellings, "hillocks," derived from the first and second branchial arches, form around the first branchial cleft. The first branchial arch hillocks go on to form the tragus, helix, and superior antihelix, whereas those from the second arch develop into the lateral helix, remainder of the antihelix, antitragus, and lobule. The fusion planes created between the first and second arch derivatives provide barriers to and define preferential paths of tumor spread.

The external auditory canal is formed from the first branchial groove. During the seventh week of gestation, a core of epithelium is canalized down to the tympanic ring and abuts the mucosa of the first pharyngeal pouch that forms the middle ear and eustachian tube. The lateral cartilaginous framework arises from mesenchymal tissue around the developing canal. The medial bony canal is formed from the tympanic portion of the temporal bone (anterior, inferior, and lower part of the posterior canal walls) and the squamous portion (posterior and superior walls).

Auricle

The appearance of the developed auricle comes from a folded framework of elastic fibrocartilage covered by perichondrium and skin. The skin on the lateral surface is firmly adherent, whereas that on the medial surface is looser secondary to the presence of a layer of areolar tissue. Hair follicles and sebaceous and sudoriferous glands are found on both surfaces.

The helix forms the external rim of the auricle, whereas the antihelix lies anterior to and parallels the helix. The concave surface between the two is the scaphoid fossa. Other concavities are the triangular fossa between the superior and inferior crura of the antihelix and the chonchal bowl inferiorly. The tragus represents an extension of the cartilaginous anterior canal wall and is mirrored by the antitragus posteriorly. The lobule, at the inferior extent of the auricle, contains no cartilage.

The ear is attached to the cranium through a series of ligaments, muscles, and skin. The muscles are innervated by the facial nerve but are normally only vestigial. The blood supply to the ear is from branches of the external carotid artery, which form arborizing anastomoses. The lymphatic drainage of the ear is to the parotid, preauricular, and retroauricular nodes, which then drain into the high cervical lymph nodes of the neck.

BASAL CELL AND SQUAMOUS CELL CARCINOMA

Epidemiology

As with all cutaneous malignancies, the reported incidence of basal cell carcinoma (BCC) and squamous cell carcinoma (SCC) has risen dramatically over the last half century.[3] This likely reflects both a greater awareness of the problem and an increased vigilance by physicians searching for suspicious lesions. Changing fashion and beauty ideals with an emphasis on skin exposure and tanned skin have also increased our exposure to damaging ultraviolet radiation.

Although skin cancer can occur in all age groups, the vast majority of patients presenting with cutaneous carcinoma are older. The mean age of patients with BCC or SCC is near 70 years.[4,5] The incidence of skin cancer is much lower in darker-skinned ethnic groups than in Caucasians, who represent 95% of patients.[4]

Basal cell carcinoma represents 65 to 85% of head and neck cutaneous malignancies and a similar proportion of auricular carcinomas.[6–11] Squamous cell carcinoma is the second most common, followed by melanoma. Some series have reported SCC to be the most common.[12] However, the different patient populations studied in these series likely arise from different patterns of referral or different treatment modalities offered.

Eighty-five to 95% of all BCCs and SCCs occur on the head and neck, and 12% of these are found on the auricle.[5,13] There are differences in the distribution of BCCs versus SCCs. Squamous cell carcinoma arises most frequently on the external ear and upper face, whereas BCC occurs most commonly in the midface, followed by the ear. When these lesions appear on the auricle, 72% of the BCCs and 61% of the SCCs are confined to a single subsite of the ear.[6] Basal cell carcinoma is found primarily on the posterior surface of the auricle, followed by the preauricular and then the retroauricular areas. Squamous cell carcinoma occurs in order of decreasing frequency on the helical rim, antihelix and triangular fossa, and posterior pinna and then the concha, lobule, or tragus.[4,5,14]

Pathophysiology/Risk Factors

Sun exposure is the number one risk factor for the development of cutaneous malignancies. The correlation between sun exposure and SCC is stronger than that with BCC.[9] Although sun exposure certainly increases the risk of developing BCC, the difference between the two types of cancer is reflected in the greater likelihood of BCC arising in areas that do not receive as much sun (posterior auricle, retroauricular, etc).

The sun is the primary source of human ultraviolet radiation. Ultraviolet radiation ranges in wavelength from 200 to 400 nm and has been divided into three groups.[15] Ultraviolet A rays (320 to 400 nm) make up the majority of the ultraviolet radiation reaching the earth and therefore produce most of the damage to our skin. They also represent the type of ultraviolet radiation used in tanning booths and for treatment of psoriasis. Ultraviolet B rays (290 to 320 nm) are the most efficient at enducing cutaneous changes but make up less than 10% of the solar ultraviolet radiation. Ultraviolet C rays (200 to 290 nm) are minimally involved in solar damage to the skin.[16] There are many factors that affect the amount and intensity of ultraviolet radiation to which we are exposed. Ultraviolet radiation increases with decreasing latitude, reduced cloud cover, and increasing altitude and during the summer months and the midday hours.[15,17]

Ultraviolet radiation affects the skin in multiple ways. In addition to inducing pigmentary changes and promoting photoaging of the skin, ultraviolet radiation also has a significant effect on local skin immunity. The disruption of local immune responses contributes as much to the development of cutaneous carcinomas as does direct molecular damage from the radiation.[5,15] Other mechanisms of cutaneous injury also increase the risk of skin cancer. Burn scars and skin damaged from gamma radiation treatments are more likely to develop

SCCs, which can be more aggressive and have a higher propensity to metastasize.[5]

Cutaneous carcinomas of the head and neck are almost exclusively confined to white and fair-skinned individuals. The natural pigmentation of black and darker-skinned people provides a natural protection from the damaging effects of solar radiation. Fitzpatrick developed a categorization of skin types to help him estimate dosing parameters for the treatment of psoriasis with ultraviolet radiation.[18] Now the Fitzpatrick scale (Table 18–1) can help identify patients who are at high risk of developing skin cancer. Those with type I and type II skins are at the most risk.

In addition to normal tanning, ultraviolet rays can induce other changes in the skin. Actinic keratoses are small, scaly, "stuck-on" lesions that occur in areas of sun-damaged skin. They are very common and are found in half of people with significant sun exposure.[15] Although benign, they should be considered precursor lesions for SCC. Sixty percent of cutaneous SCCs arise from actinic keratoses.[19] The transformation rate has been estimated to be 0.01 to 0.24% per year.[19,20] Other lesions that may be premalignant include keratoacanthomas and radiation keratoses.[21]

The damaging effects of ultraviolet rays on local immune systems are compounded in patients who have undergone transplants and are on immunosuppressive therapy. The rate of cutaneous carcinomas increases 5- to 16-fold in these patients.[22,23]

Several genetic syndromes have been shown to increase an individual's risk of developing skin malignancies. Nevoid basal cell syndrome (Gorlin's syndrome) is an autosomal dominant disease with complete penetrance and selective expressivity. Patients develop multiple pigmented BCC once they reach puberty. They often have characteristic facies (frontal bossing, hypertelorism, lengthened mandibles, and drooping lips) and

can develop other abnormalities including odontogenic keratocysts in the jaw, bifid ribs, and calcification of the falx cerebri.[24,25]

Xeroderma pigmentosum is an autosomal recessive disorder of the DNA repair system.[24] Patients develop numerous skin malignancies, primarily SCC and BCC, at a very young age. The mean age for the development of their first cancer is 8 years old. The cancers tend to be very aggressive because of the weak immune system. The syndrome is associated with photophobia, keratitis, and neurologic abnormalities, including deafness. Any patient diagnosed with either of these genetic syndromes should be monitored very carefully. Unfortunately, treatment of these patients is difficult because surgical excision of the multiple tumors results in significant deformities. Prevention with avoidance of the sun, sunscreen, and long clothing and hats is vital.

Pathology

The diagnosis of BCC or SCC can sometimes be difficult because of the variety of ways in which the tumors can appear. Pathologic analysis may be necessary to differentiate between the two. In addition, there are multiple pathologic subtypes of both tumors that can greatly influence the behavior of the lesion and prognosis.

Basal Cell Carcinoma

Basal cell carcinoma arises from the cells in the basal layer of the epidermis. The tumor cells will typically form lobules, cords, or nests extending from the basal layer of epidermis into more superficial or deep layers. The cells show little pleomorphism and have large oval hyperchromatic nuclei with minimal cytoplasm. There are several variants of BCC that differ both in their appearance histologically and grossly and in their behavior.[5,9] These include nodular, ulcerative, pigmented, superficial, morpheaform/sclerosing, and basaloid squamous.

Nodular BCC is the most common variant, accounting for 54% of all BCC.[5] It is also the least aggressive type. These tumors often appear as pearly gray nodules with a central telangiectasia. They typically bleed easily because of a lack of keratin on their surface. Ulcerative BCC (11% of BCCs) occurs when a nodular BCC outgrows its blood supply and the central portion

Table 18–1	FITZPATRICK CLASSIFICATION SYSTEM		
Skin Color	Skin Type	Sunburn	Tan
White	I	Always	Never
	II	Easily	Minimally
	III	Rarely	Yes
	IV	No	Yes
Brown	V	No	Yes
Black	VI	No	Yes

Adapted from Fitzpatrick.[18]

necroses. This forms the classic "rodent ulcer" in BCC. Superficial BCC (11%) looks like an indurated erythematous patch with pearly, scaly borders, and pigmented BCC (6%) resembles nodular BCC but has a tan color rather than the normal pearly gray. Two rare variants are particularly aggressive. Morpheaform BCC accounts for 2% of all BCCs but is the most aggressive and has the highest rate of recurrences.[9,26] It is almost always found on the head and neck and appears as a flat yellowish plaque with very poorly defined borders. Histologically, there are strands of tumor cells intermixed with the surrounding fibrous stroma, making the determination of the tumor margin difficult. Basaloid squamous carcinoma shows some squamous differentiation with keratin formation. It is generally considered more aggressive,[5,27,28] but not all studies support this finding.[29,30] Basal cell carcinoma can display other types of differentiation including adenoid, sebaceous, eccrine, and apocrine differentiation, but these variants are extremely rare.[9]

Squamous Cell Carcinoma

Like BCC, SCC may be confused with other types of lesions. Clinically, SCC can appear as anything from a plaque to a nodule or ulcerative lesion. Although there are variants of SCC, they are less common than those of BCC.

Squamous cell carcinoma is typically characterized by thickened, atypical keratinocytes with disruption of the normal maturation of cells from the basal layer to the upper layer of the epidermis. The cells form cords and islands that invade deep to the basement membrane. The tumor cells can have a great deal of pleomorphism and mitotic figures. The nuclei are hyperchromatic with large nucleoli. The tumors can show varying degrees of differentiation, with the more differentiated ones having large deposits of keratin labeled "keratin pearls." If the cells are poorly differentiated, they can be stained with cytokeratin to help with the diagnosis.[9]

Other variants of SCC include a pigmented variety that is often mistaken for melanoma. The spindle cell subtype is uncommon (1.5% of SCCs) and is seen more often arising from radiated skin. The cells have a fusiform pattern with poorly defined borders and infiltrate into the surrounding fibrous stroma.[13] Verrucous SCC is made up of bland epithelial cells that tend to heap up on the surface. Although not considered a risk for metastasis,

verrucous carcinoma can be locally destructive.[9] Other forms of squamous differentiation include basaloid squamous cell, discussed previously, and adenoid squamous cell.

Diagnosis and Imaging

The diagnosis of malignancies of the external ear relies on diligent clinical evaluation and a heightened sense of awareness. Often these lesions can be overlooked as benign, especially in elderly patients with extensively sun-damaged skin. Lesions that have changed in color, size, or shape or that are friable or ulcerated should be biopsied to ensure that they are not malignant. Early detection will result in better outcomes with less need for deforming aggressive surgery.

If a biopsy is performed, a punch biopsy is the preferred method. Complete excision of small simple lesions may be used if the resulting defect is minimal or easily closed. This is often difficult on the ear, however, given its complex structure. A punch biopsy preserves the architecture of the lesion, for histologic analysis, provides reliable information on the depth of the lesion, and, if needed, allows for definitive excision of the lesion with more precise margins. Shave biopsies often fail to demonstrate the full depth of the lesion.

Imaging studies (computed tomography [CT], magnetic resonance imaging [MRI]) are rarely needed for tumors of the external ear. If there is some question of parotid involvement or nodal metastases, a CT scan may offer some additional information. In addition, if the tumor extends near or involves the external auditory canal, CT scanning may provide information regarding bony invasion of the canal, mastoid cavity, or glenoid fossa.

Staging

There is no specific staging system for malignancies of the ear. The American Joint Committee on Cancer[10] (AJCC) includes auricular malignancies in their staging system for nonmelanomatous lesions of the skin (Table 18–2). This system, however, has many limitations when applied to the ear. The thin skin of the ear allows tumors to reach the deeper subcutaneous levels much sooner than

**Table 18–2 AJCC STAGING SYSTEM:
NONMELANOMA CANCER OF THE SKIN**

T Stage
  Tx   Cannot assess primary tumor
  T0   No evidence of primary tumor
  Tis Carcinoma in situ
  T1   Tumor ≤ 2 cm in greatest dimension
  T2   Tumor > 2 cm but not > 5 cm in greatest dimension
  T3   Tumor > 5 cm in greatest dimension
  T4   Tumor invades deep extradermal structures (bone,
       cartilage muscle)

N Stage
  Nx   Cannot assess regional nodes
  N0   No regional node metastasis
  N1   Regional lymph node metastasis

M Stage
  Mx   Distant metastasis cannot be assessed
  M0   No distant metastasis
  M1   Distant metastasis

Stage 0	Tis	N0	M0
Stage 1	T1	N0	M0
Stage 2	T2, T3	N0	M0
Stage 3	T4	N0	M0
Stage 3	Any T	N1	M0
Stage 4	Any T	Any N	M1

AJCC = American Joint Committee on Cancer.

they would at other sites. This results in many tumors being staged T4 that do not have similar prognoses or require as radical a treatment as T4 tumors in other locations. In addition, the unique anatomy of the ear makes a staging system based on size less practical. Even small tumors located in certain areas (eg, preauricular, choncha, tragus) can require more extensive surgery either because of the defect created or because of their proximity to other structures like the parotid gland. Finally, the AJCC system does not account for different histologies. Squamous cell carcinoma and BCC may act very differently from each other, and the histologic subtypes of BCC and SCC (eg, basosquamous, morpheaform) greatly influence a tumor's aggressiveness.

Prevention

Prevention is the mainstay of treatment for skin cancer. Decreasing one's exposure to ultraviolet radiation will have a significant impact on the risk of developing skin malignancies. Avoidance of midday sun (10 am to 3 pm), the use of broad-brimmed hats, and diligent application of sunscreen (at least SPF 15) on portions of the body that receive significant sun exposure will reduce the amount of ultraviolet radiation reaching the skin. Clouds do not block ultraviolet rays, so adequate protection is needed even on overcast days.[31]

Although the risks of skin cancer have been prominently reported and publicized, there remains a glorification in our society of tanned skin as both healthy and fashionable. Increased public awareness of skin cancer and continued diligence by health professionals in monitoring patients for signs of cutaneous malignancies are crucial components to a successful prevention policy. One-third of patients who have been diagnosed with one skin malignancy will develop others in the future and should be followed at least once a year, if not more often, to search for new lesions.[31,32]

Treatment of Primary Disease

There are many options available to the physician when deciding how to treat primary malignancies of the auricle. The choice of which modality to use will depend on the location and size of the lesion, the health of the patient, the expertise of the doctor in various techniques, and, ultimately, the desire of the patient once he/she is aware of the risks and benefits of each option.

Surgical Excision

Surgical extirpation of malignant lesions of the auricle is the most common form of treatment. Because of the complex anatomy of the ear, careful planning of the procedure must be done to ensure that a cosmetically acceptable repair can be performed if needed. Many small tumors can be excised, with little or no repair required.

Auricular neoplasms tend to follow consistent patterns of growth along embryologic fusion planes. Tumors in the pre- and postauricular areas grow onto the ear itself. Tumors that arise from the helix spread inferiorly and superiorly along the helix before extending onto the antihelix and the posterior auricle, whereas those that arise on the antihelix grow concentrically.[6] However, because of the thin skin of the auricle, tumors reach the dermis and subdermis quickly and tend to spread in those planes much sooner than expected. This rapid horizontal growth makes determining appropriate margins for resection difficult. Shockley and Stucker reported that 37% of auricular carcinomas excised using standard margins had tumor cells at the margin.[14] Bumsted and colleagues recommended 8-mm margins around BCC if the tumor is less than 3 cm and 1.5-cm margins if it is larger.[12] Others have advocated smaller 2- to 3-mm margins for solid well-circumscribed BCC less than 1 cm in size, 3- to 5-mm margins for those ≥ 1 cm but < 2 cm, and 7- to 10-mm margins for those with morpheaform histologies.[9] Surgical margins for SCC should be even larger (1 to 2 cm).[12]

By excising the tumor based on gross surgical margins, a larger amount of normal tissue is taken with the specimen. Bumsted and colleagues analyzed defects created with traditional wide local excisions and concluded that 1.8 to 3.5 cm more normal tissue was removed than needed.[12] The advantages of traditional surgery, however, are that it is easily performed, is relatively quick, and does not require advanced training.

The outcomes of patients with auricular carcinoma treated with standard surgical excision are good. Especially for smaller lesions, the cure rate approaches 100%. The overall cure rate is near 95% if one includes surgical salvage for recurrent tumors.[14] The recurrence rate for auricular carcinoma treated with conventional surgery ranges from 10 to 16%.[4,33,34] This must be taken into account when comparing conventional surgery to other methods of excision (Tables 18–3 and Table 18–4).

Mohs' Surgery

Mohs' surgical technique was developed in 1941 by a dermatologist, Dr. Frederick Mohs, at the University of Wisconsin.[35] The technique involves serial horizontal sectioning of the tumor and surrounding tissue with immediate microscopic analysis to confirm histologically that the margins are clear of tumor. Once the initial tissue is removed, the edges are color coded to ensure precise orientation of the specimen. Originally, the tumor and surrounding tissue were fixed in vivo with zinc chloride. Now the specimens are processed as frozen sections. The

Table 18–3 FIVE-YEAR RECURRENCE RATES FOR PRIMARY BASAL CELL CARCINOMA	
Treatment	Recurrence Rate (%)
Wide local excision	10.1
Radiation	8.7
Curettage and electrodessication	7.7
Mohs' surgery	1.0

Adapted from Rowe and colleagues.[34]

Table 18–4 FIVE-YEAR RECURRENCE RATES FOR PREVIOUSLY TREATED BASAL CELL CARCINOMA	
Treatment	Recurrence Rate (%)
Excision	17.4
Curettage and electrodessication	40.0
Radiation	9.8
Mohs' surgery	5.6

Adapted from Rowe and colleagues.[34]

tissue is cut horizontally, unlike the standard serial vertical sections, to ensure that all of the margins are analyzed. If any tumor cells are seen at the margins, the surgeon can immediately excise more tissue from that area.[36]

Mohs' surgery has several advantages over traditional wide local excision. The horizontal sectioning allows analysis of the entire margin to look for small islands or nests of tumor cells that may be missed with normal pathologic examination. It provides a means of ensuring that all of the tumor is removed without relying on unnecessary excision of normal tissue. This is especially important in areas such as the ear, nose, and eyelids, where preservation of as much tissue as possible is vital to maintaining good cosmesis.

The results with Mohs' surgery compare favorably with other modalities of treatment (see Tables 18–3 and 18–4). Overall cure rates for auricular carcinomas are near 98% for BCC and 92% for SCC.[7,11,12,37] Because of the ability to precisely follow the tumor margins with the Mohs' technique, the recurrence rates for auricular malignancies treated in this manner are lower than those treated with standard excision. The 5-year recurrence rate for BCC is barely 1% and that of SCC is under 3%, which is significantly lower than the 10 to 16% recurrence rate for tumors treated with wide local excision.[33,34,38]

Mohs' surgery is the recommended method of treatment for cancers arising in vital areas, for recurrent or previously treated tumors, for those tumors with aggressive histologies (morpheaform, basosquamous etc), for large carcinomas over 1 cm for which standard excision would require removal of significant amounts of normal tissue, and for tumors with poorly defined margins.[9,36]

Other Surgical Techniques

There are many methods of removing cutaneous malignancies, and for small nonaggressive tumors with clearly defined margins, curettage with electrodesiccation or cryosurgery is an effective technique. Curettage involves the use of a dermal curette to remove the tumor, and then the raw base is cauterized with an electrical bovie. The cure rates with curettage are greater than 90% with appropriately selected lesions.[39] Although easy to perform and cost effective, this technique is very skill dependent. It relies on the surgeon being able to feel the difference in texture between normal tissue and tumor. On the auricle, in particular, the thin skin and minimal subcutaneous tissue make curettage difficult to perform without damaging the underlying cartilage.

Cryosurgery, like curettage, is quick, is easily done, and can be used in settings outside of the office, making it a useful technique when seeing patients in nursing homes or other facilities. Thermocouples are placed at the deep margins of the tumor to ensure that appropriate temperatures are reached. The cryogen is then applied to the tumor to freeze it. Temperatures in the range of $-40°C$ are recommended. The cure rates for cryosurgery exceed 95% for nodular BCC and well-differentiated SCC.[39,40] Like curettage, however, cryosurgery is indicated only for small nonaggressive lesions with well-defined borders as neither technique provides marginal analysis to confirm that the cancer is completely removed.

Radiation Therapy

Radiation therapy offers several theoretical advantages over surgical excision of auricular malignancies. It avoids tissue defects in this anatomically complex area, allows treatment of patients who are medically unable or refuse to undergo surgery, and treats the tumor margins by radiating the surrounding tissue. However, multiple treatments may be needed, making radiation therapy less convenient and more costly than a simple excision. In addition, there is a risk of radiation-induced tumors, and scarring or notching can develop on the ear along with telangiectasias. For young patients, in particular, the likelihood that they will develop additional skin malignancies during their lifetime is high, and previous radiation can lead to more aggressive tumors, less clearly defined margins, and poorer surgical outcomes.[41]

Dosing regimens vary from center to center but common regimens are 20 Gy in one or two fractions for very small tumors, 30 to 40 Gy over 3 weeks for tumors with 2 to 4 cm³ volumes, and 60 to 65 Gy over 6 weeks for larger tumors.[42] The cure rates are comparable to surgery for small tumors less than 1.0 cm (97% for BCC and 91% for SCC).[43] Basal cell carcinomas larger than 1.0 cm treated with radiation therapy have recurrence rates of 10 to 13%.[43-45] The cure rate for SCC of similar size is much worse (76% for tumors 1 to 5 cm; 56% for tumors > 5.0 cm).[44]

Because of the excellent results achieved with surgery on the ear, radiation is rarely used for malignancies confined to the auricle. If tumor invades the parotid, temporomandibular joint, mandible, or temporal bone, adjunctive radiation is indicated because of the high risk of recurrence.

Other Nonsurgical Options

Topical 5-fluorouracil (5 to 20% concentrations) has been applied to premalignant lesions and select cutaneous carcinomas. The lesions are commonly treated for 4 weeks to 3 months. Only superficial BCC and Bowen's disease (SCC in situ) have responded with cure rates of over 80%.[39] Given the variable cure rates, this technique should only be used to treat patients in whom other methods of therapy are contraindicated.

Intralesional interferon-α has been shown to be effective for treatment of nodular and superficial BCC.[46,47] Patients receive low-dose (1.5×10^6 IU) injections three times a week for 3 weeks. Side effects are often minor (flulike symptoms, erythema, pain), although leukocytopenia and thrombocytopenia can develop. At this time, this treatment is still investigational.[39]

The use of photodynamic therapy for BCC and SCC has been studied. A photosensitizing drug is given that selectively localizes in the tumor and then, on exposure to light, causes tumor necrosis. The results have been inconclusive to date, and further study is needed before this technique is recommended.[48]

Treatment of Recurrent Disease

Although the recurrence rate for cutaneous malignancies is low, the ear has been shown to have a higher recurrence rate than any other region besides the midface.[26] The treatment of recurrent disease is more difficult because the tumors are often of an aggressive type, prior treatment has disrupted the normal anatomy, making reconstruction more difficult, and margins are much less precise. As with primary disease, treatment options depend on the size, location, and histology of the lesion, the skills of the physician, and the opinion of the patient.

Risk Factors

The overall recurrence rate for BCC of the ear is less than 5% and that of SCC is 10 to 15%. There are several factors, however, that increase the chance of tumor recurrence. The location of the tumor on the ear is the number one risk factor associated with recurrence of auricular carcinoma.[26] The postauricular area is the most likely site for recurrence in most studies,[6,7,12,26] although several studies have found preauricular lesions to recur at a much higher rate.[5,11] The cure rates for SCC and BCC are higher for lesions located on the helix, antihelix, and posterior surface of the ear. Tumors located on the concha, postauricular area, and canal had the worst prognosis (Table 18–5).[37]

Tumor size greatly affects the recurrence rate. Size greater than 3 cm increases the recurrence rate for BCC from 1 to 17% and for SCC from 2 to 31%.[38] Other authors have also shown that increasing tumor size correlates with poorer cure rates.[7,11,49]

The type of cancer and the histologic subtype can also increase the likelihood for recurrence. Squamous cell carcinomas generally have poorer results than BCCs.[5] Morpheaform BCCs are prone to recurrence because of their aggressive nature and poorly defined margins. They represent nearly one-third of the recurrent BCC of the head and neck.[26] Other aggressive histologic variants include basosquamous carcinoma, poorly differentiated SCC, and spindle cell variant of SCC.[26,50]

There is some debate as to whether positive microscopic margins affect outcomes. Some authors argue that positive margins do not affect recurrence of small tumors.

Menn and colleagues, however, found that the presence of tumor cells at the margin of resection greatly increased the risk of recurrence, especially for malignancies located in the skin of the ear, nose, or eyelid.[51] Other factors that have been shown to correlate with increased recurrence of skin malignancies include prior treatment,[7,37] the type of procedure used,[34] and cartilage invasion.[49]

The cure rates for recurrent BCC treated with various techniques are shown in Table 18–4. Similar results are found for SCC.[38] Mohs' surgery is the most effective technique for the treatment of recurrent carcinoma of the auricle. Because the margins of recurrent tumors are difficult to judge, Mohs' surgery offers an effective means of ensuring that all visible tumor is removed. If the recurrence is located in an area where additional surgery would be too morbid, radiation therapy is an alternative. Recurrent BCCs less than 1 cm are cured with radiation therapy approximately 95% of the time, and larger ones are cured in over 80% of cases.[52]

Treatment of Metastatic/Neck Disease

The rate of metastasis for cutaneous carcinoma is low. Auricular cancer, however, has an increased risk of metastasizing compared with other locations[5,11,38,53–55] Regional metastases occurs in approximately 5 to 18% of auricular SCCs and in 2 to 6% of BCCs.[1,53] Distant metastases are even rarer (0.3 to 3.7% for SCC and 0.003 to 0.1% for BCC).[4,10,55] When it does occur, nodal disease associated with auricular carcinoma is found most often in the parotid and preauricular nodes.[4,53] Neck disease is less common, and the upper jugulodigastric region is the primary site of involvement. Byers and colleagues found that only 3 of 486 patients with auricular SCC had nodal disease below the omohyoid, and none of these patients exhibited skip lesions.[4] They and others have noted that the suboccipital nodes are never involved in auricular skin carcinomas.[4,53]

Multiple studies have looked at the factors predisposing patients to regional and distant metastases. There are conflicting data as to which factors are important. Some authors have found that size and location on the ear (especially the preauricular area) correlate with increased risk of nodal disease.[5,10,49,53] Other studies, however, belie these findings.[4,53] Several histologic subtypes are more likely to metastasize, including basosquamous carcinoma and poorly differentiated carcinoma.[50,53]

Table 18–5 FIVE-YEAR CURE RATES (%) FOR AURICULAR CARCINOMAS BASED ON LOCATION		
Location of Tumor	Basal Cell Carcinoma	Squamous Cell Carcinoma
Helix	99.2	99.1
Antihelix and crus	99.0	94.6
Posterior surface	97.7	90.5
Lobe	97.4	90.0
Preauricular and tragus	97.0	80.9
Concha	94.0	78.4
Postauricular sulcus	92.0	81.3

Adapted from Mohs and colleagues.[37]

Other factors that have been implicated include perineural invasion,[56] cartilage invasion,[5] recurrent tumors,[5] and immunosuppresion.[10]

Patients who present with clinically node-positive necks should receive a modified radical neck dissection to remove the nodal disease. Sacrifice of the sternocleidomastoid muscle, cranial nerve XI, or jugular vein should be done only if the disease cannot be safely removed otherwise. The majority of patients present with single-node disease (N1).[4] If multiple nodes are positive or if there is evidence of extracapsular spread, postoperative radiation therapy should be considered.

The treatment of the N0 neck is more problematic. For patients with cutaneous carcinoma of the ear, elective lymph node dissection (ELND) has not been shown to increase survival over watchful waiting and treatment of the neck once disease appears. Given the overall low rate of metastatic disease in auricular carcinoma, ELND should be reserved for patients with multiple risk factors for nodal disease. Byers and colleagues recommended operating on people with poorly differentiated SCC greater than 3 cm in size.[4] They argued that a supraomohyoid neck dissection is sufficient given the very low rate of lower neck metastases (3 of 486 patients). Others have reported a greater percentage of mid and lower neck disease,[54] although in that study, there were no skip lesions (ie, all patients with lower neck disease also had disease in more proximal levels). It appears that a supraomohyoid neck dissection would be sufficient for the N0 neck. If disease is found intraoperatively, the procedure can be converted to a modified radical neck dissection, and if found by subsequent pathologic examination, postoperative radiation would be indicated to treat the remaining neck.

Prognosis/Outcome

The overall prognosis for cutaneous carcinoma of the external ear is good if caught early. Five-year survival is over 95%. Several factors can influence that outcome. Metastatic disease significantly reduces survival. Patients with multiple positive nodes have a 5-year survival rate of 25%.[4] Recurrent tumors, as discussed previously, are more difficult to treat and adversely affect outcomes.[7,37] Mohs and colleagues found that the cure rate for tumors ≥ 3 cm dropped to 83% for BCC and to 69% for SCC.[37] Freedlander and Chung found a correlation between

tumor size and outcome,[49] although other studies have not.[4,53] Tumor thickness has also been correlated with outcome, as have perichondrial invasion,[56] perineural invasion,[56] and immunosuppression.[23]

MALIGNANT MELANOMA

Malignant melanoma of the auricle is easily treated if diagnosed early but can be one of the most deadly cancers once it reaches an advanced stage. Like other cutaneous carcinomas, malignant melanoma is increasing in incidence, and a thorough knowledge of how to diagnose and treat this disease is needed by otolaryngologists as they are often the first physicians to identify lesions located on the head and neck.

Epidemiology

Malignant melanoma is now the sixth most common carcinoma in the United States.[57] The incidence of melanoma has tripled over the last 15 years and has reached 32,000 new cases per year, leading to 6,700 deaths per year.[58]

Twenty to 25% of melanomas occur on the head and neck. Melanoma is the third most common type of auricular carcinoma after SCC and BCC and accounts for 7 to 13% of all head and neck melanomas[59–62] and 1% of all melanomas.[61] The incidence of auricular melanoma is 0.1 to 0.6 in 100,000.[63] The most common site of origin on the ear is the helix (60%), followed by the lobule (25%).[59]

The average age of patients presenting with malignant melanoma is 65 to 79 years.[62] Like that of other cutaneous malignancies, the rate of melanoma is lower in blacks and dark-skinned people.[63] There is a lower incidence of auricular melanoma among women, likely owing to their longer hair lengths covering the skin of the ear.[62,63]

Pathophysiology

The primary risk factor for malignant melanoma is sun exposure. Interestingly, the type of sun exposure appears to make a difference in the risk of developing various subtypes of melanoma.[63–67] Superficial spreading melanoma (SSM), the most common type, seems to be more related to acute, severe sun exposure rather than cumulative ultraviolet damage to the skin. Patients with SSM are more likely to be younger and to develop lesions on their trunks and legs, areas of recreational sun exposure. Lentigo maligna melanoma (LMM), however, is just the opposite. It commonly develops from actinic precursors and is seen in older patients on average. It tends to develop on the ears and other areas of chronic sun exposure.[62,63] Why there are these differences in the reaction of the skin to ultraviolet radiation is unknown at this time.

The majority of malignant melanomas arise from preexisting nevi. Pigmented lesions that have changed in color, size, or shape should raise one's suspicion for melanoma. There are certain precursor lesions that are particularly high risk and should be looked for. Large congenital nevi present at birth carry a 5 to 20% lifetime risk of developing melanoma. Dysplastic nevi, which are often large (5 to 12 mm), with elevated irregular surfaces and variegated colors, almost always progress to malignant melanoma and should be excised. Lentigo maligna, so-called "Hutchinson's freckles," are superficial melanoma "in situ." Approximately 5% of these will develop into invasive, malignant tumors.[68]

As with other skin cancers, white and fair-skinned individuals are at increased risk for melanoma.[66] Patients who have undergone renal transplants and are on immunosuppressive agents have a greater chance of developing malignant melanoma.[69] A family history of malignant melanoma can double an individual's lifetime risk.[67,70] Finally, there are several inherited syndromes that predispose patients to developing melanoma. Xeroderma pigmentosa increases an individual's risk nearly 2,000 times above normal, and, although rare, these patients account for nearly 5% of all malignant melanoma cases.[24] Familial dysplastic nevus syndrome is an autosomal dominant disease with variable penetrance. Patients develop multiple dysplastic nevi all over their body and have a 400% increase in their risk for malignant melanoma. The large number of lesions makes surgical excision difficult, and these individuals represent a challenge for the treating specialist.[71]

Pathology

Melanoma can be exceedingly difficult to diagnose histologically. The individual malignant cells may be undif-ferentiated or, in some cases, even amelanotic. Melanocytes are normally located in the basal layer of the epidermis. Malignant cells may display nuclear/cellular atypia, mitotic figures, and vesicular nuclei with prominent nucleoli.[60]

Several different pathologic variants have been identified including SSM, LMM, and nodular melanoma (NM). Other variants include desmoplastic and neurotrophic malignant melanoma but account for less than 5% of the tumors.[61] Superficial spreading melanoma is the most common variant. Its incidence is 4.4 in 100,000,[63] and it represents nearly one-third of all melanomas[61,62] and 65 to 75% of head and neck melanomas.[60] Grossly, the lesions may be thin but are raised, palpable, and pigmented, with fairly regular borders. Histologically, there are melanocytes in all layers of the epidermis. These tumors tend to grow in a radial direction for 1 to 6 years before beginning their vertical growth phase into deeper tissue layers.[60]

Lentigo maligna melanoma occurs in 0.7 in 100,000 people[63] and accounts for 17 to 24%[62,63] of all melanomas and 5 to 15% of head and neck melanomas.[60] It is more common on the ear than SMM.[63] This reflects the differences in their etiologies. Lentigo maligna melanoma is flat and barely palpable, with irregular shapes and borders. There are nests of atypical melanocytes that are confined to the lower epidermis. This neoplasm has a very long radial growth phase, lasting up to 20 years.[60]

The incidence of NM is 1.1 in 100,000,[63] and it represents 28% of all melanomas[61,62] but 15 to 20% of head and neck melanomas.[60] Nodular melanoma is typically darkly pigmented, raised with a polypoid or nodular appearance. The malignant cells show a very early vertical growth phase, with very little involvement of the epidermis.[60] These tumors are particularly aggressive because of their deep invasion.

Diagnosis/Clinical Evaluation

The diagnosis of malignant melanoma requires a keen eye and a diligent physical examination to identify lesions when they are easily treated. The classic teaching is to remember ABCD: *A*symmetry in shape, *B*order irregularity, *C*olor variation, *D*iameter > 6 mm. Lesions that meet these criteria or lesions that have increased in

Table 18–6 CLARK AND BRESLOW STAGING SYSTEMS

Clark		Breslow	
Level I	Superficial epidermis	Stage I	< 0.75 mm
Level II	Basal cell layer of epidermis	Stage II	0.75–1.5 mm
Level III	Papillary dermis	Stage III	1.5–1.99 mm
Level IV	Reticular dermis	Stage IV	2.0–3.99 mm
Level V	Subcutaneous tissue	Stage V	> 4.0 mm

size or are ulcerated or bleeding are worrisome and should be biopsied.

If a biopsy is performed, the preferred method is an excisional biopsy. This allows the pathologist to examine the entire lesion and determine the greatest depth of invasion or tumor thickness. If a full excision cannot be performed, a punch biopsy into the subcutaneous tissue is warranted. This will still allow determination of tumor depth and thickness. Because they do not provide adequate information regarding tumor thickness, there is no place for shave biopsies in the treatment or diagnosis of malignant melanoma.

In addition to a biopsy, the patient should be examined from head to foot for other suspicious lesions. Any lymphadenopathy in the neck, occiput, or parotid should be palpated and a workup for metastatic disease, including a chest radiography and liver enzymes test, should be performed. Computed tomography or MRI of the neck is generally not required but may be considered if there is a question of cervical or parotid nodal metastasis.

The differential diagnosis includes a variety of other neoplasms: SCC, BCC, lymphoma, malignant fibrous histiocytoma, and fibrosarcoma, to name a few. If routine histologic examination is insufficient for diagnosis, immunohistochemical staining may help. Malignant melanoma stains positively with S-100 and HMB-45 stains. The latter is much more sensitive and specific.[61]

Staging

The staging of melanoma is based on tumor thickness and depth of invasion, as well as the presence of metastatic disease. The first prognostic staging system was devised by Clark in 1969 (Table 18–6) and analyzed the extent of tumor invasion into each histologic level of the epidermis and dermis.[72] Breslow published another system based on the absolute depth of tumor invasion (see Table 18–6).[73] The current AJCC staging system makes use of both systems (Table 18–7).[69]

Treatment of Primary Disease

Surgery
Surgical excision of the tumor with adequate margins is the primary treatment for malignant melanoma, especially if caught early. The excision should be full thickness, including the perichondrium and cartilage if necessary.[60] The amount of normal margin removed, however, is debated. A consensus panel sponsored by the National Institutes of Health (NIH) recommended a 1-cm margin of normal skin and subcutaneous tissue for melanomas less than 1 mm thick.[74] For tumors larger than that, a 2-cm margin is recommended.[60,75] Other studies have argued for larger margins,[76,77] but even the smaller margins are difficult to achieve on the ear and often entail wedge excisions or partial amputations of the pinna.

Mohs' surgery has been advocated for malignant melanoma and offers the theoretical advantage of reducing the amount of normal tissue needed to be excised.[78] There are several problems with Mohs' surgery for melanoma, however. Because of the difficulty in identifying malignant melanoma cells pathologically, precise identification of the tumor margins is more complicated

Table 18–7 AJCC STAGING SYSTEM FOR MALIGNANT MELANOMA

Stage	Pathologic Features*	Metastases
IA (T1N0M0)	Localized melanoma ≤ 0.75 mm or level II	None
IB (T2N0M0)	Localized melanoma 0.76–1.5 mm or level III	None
IIA (T3N0M0)	Localized melanoma 1.5–4.0 mm or level IV	None
IIB (T4N0M0)	Localized melanoma > 4.0 mm or level V	None
III (any T, N1, M0)	Limited nodal metastases involving only one regional lymph node basin or < 5 in transit metastases without any nodal metastases	
IV (any T, N2, M0)	Advanced regional metastases or distant metastases or (any T and N, M1)	

*If thickness and level of invasion do not coincide, then thickness takes precedence.
AJCC = American Joint Committee on Cancer.

than with other skin cancers. A consensus panel at the NIH has recommended against Mohs' surgery for this very reason.[74] The use of rapid immunohistochemical stains to help identify melanoma cells may increase the success of this technique in the future, but for now it should remain investigational.

The overall cure rates for surgical excision of malignant melanoma of the ear approach 68%. The success rate for early-stage disease is significantly higher.[74] Local recurrence rates are around 6.5% on the ear[79] and generally occur between 1 and 3 years after excision. The vast majority occur within the first 2 years; therefore, patients should be followed every 1 to 2 months during that period and then biannually for the next 2 to 3 years.[60]

Radiation

Melanoma has traditionally been considered to be radioresistant, but a few recent studies have shown that this may not be the case.[80,81] Radiation therapy has been shown to be effective for NM[43] and for local control of partially resected melanomas.[82] A study of patients with stage III melanoma showed a regional control rate of 75% at 5 years with adjuvant radiation therapy. Patients in whom all gross tumor had been removed had even better results (95% regional control).[83] There is some controversy over whether higher dose fractions will improve outcomes, but a prospective randomized study demonstrated no difference in results with larger dose fractions.[43,84,85]

Treatment of the Neck/Regional Metastases

Seventeen percent of patients with head and neck melanoma will have nodal disease at the time of presentation.[61] Auricular melanoma carries a risk of nodal metastases that approaches 42%.[60] The risk of nodal metastases correlates with tumor thickness, depth of invasion, presence of ulceration, and histologic subtype.[61,68,86–88] Tumor thickness is the most significant of these factors. The risk of developing nodal metastases from a tumor less than 0.75 mm is near zero. For thicker tumors, the risk increases significantly (Table 18–8). On the ear, melanomas under 3 mm thick have been shown to have a 21% chance of nodal disease. This risk increases to 61% for those over 3 mm thick.[59]

Table 18–8 RELATIONSHIP OF TUMOR THICKNESS TO OUTCOMES IN MALIGNANT MELANOMA			
Thickness (mm)	Recurrence Rate (%)	Metastases (%)	Survival (%)
< 0.75	2	0	85–99
0.75–1.49	5	20–25	65–88
1.50–3.99	15	51–57	58–71
> 4.0	20	62	25–57

Adapted from O'Brien and colleagues,[61] Ringborg and colleagues,[62] Medina,[68] Bauch and colleagues,[86] Fisher,[87] and Thorn and colleagues.[89]

The most common nodal areas involved with auricular melanoma are the parotid and upper jugulodigastric nodes. The retroauricular, preauricular, and submental nodes can also contain metastatic disease. If the tumor is located on the posterior portion of the pinna or in the retroauricular area, the suboccipital nodes are at risk.[60,68] Although there are patterns of nodal disease, there is no uniform sequential route of spread. Thirty-six to 43% of patients with auricular melanomas and neck metastases will have no disease in the parotid nodes.[90]

Patients with clinically positive necks should undergo a neck dissection. This is performed more for staging purposes than therapeutic ones. Although neck dissection in the patient with nodal metastases reduces regional recurrences, it has not been shown to improve survival, owing to the high rate of distant metastases (85%) in patients with neck disease.[91] Over 40% of necks identified as clinically positive, however, are ultimately found to be pathologically negative,[92] which has a significant impact on staging and therefore on prognosis and the need for adjuvant therapy. Radical neck dissections have been advocated, but there are no studies demonstrating a difference between radical and modified radical neck dissections for malignant melanoma. The use of a modified radical neck dissection should depend on the expertise and comfort of the surgeon with that procedure.

The risk of disease recurrence in the neck following neck dissection is 24 to 34%[61,62,87] and in the parotid it is 14%.[62] The use of radiation therapy following neck dissection has been shown to decrease recurrence in the neck but does not affect overall survival.[60]

The role of ELND in patients with melanoma is controversial. Overall, 7% of clinically negative necks will harbor disease.[61] Tumor thickness, however, greatly affects the risk of occult metastases.[68,86] Tumors less than 0.75 mm or LMM do not need ELND as the risk of nodal disease is negligible. For tumors > 4 mm, the risk of distant metastases is 75%; therefore, ELND would not alter prognosis.[93] For the intermediate tumors, there are arguments on both sides. Tumors 0.76 to 1.49 mm thick have a lower risk of nodal metastases, and ELND should be considered only in lesions with ulceration, nodular pathology, or Clark level IV or V invasion.[93] A few studies have shown that ELND for tumors 1.49 to 3.99 mm thick can improve survival.[94,95] Other studies do not support these findings and show that the survival advantage provided by ELND does not remain following multivariate analysis.[61,87,96,97] For auricular melanomas in particular, however, the high risk of nodal metastases may make ELND useful. No studies, unfortunately, have analyzed this subgroup specifically.

Lymphoscintigraphy and sentinel node biopsies have been advocated for head and neck melanoma to predict nodal metastases and to better define which nodal basins are involved. This technique involves identifying the primary nodal drainage basin for a specific tumor through the injection of methylene blue dye or a radioactive tracer that can be detected with a Geiger counter. The sentinel node is then dissected free and sent for frozen section. The presumption is that if the node is negative, the likelihood of more distant nodal disease is remote, and the patient is saved more aggressive surgery. If the node is positive, then further lymph node dissection can be undertaken. A few studies have shown promising results with head and neck melanoma, but the follow-up in these studies is short and the number of patients is small.[98,99] Intuitively, the use of sentinel node biopsies for auricular malignancies has several problems. There is no consistent pattern of nodal spread,[100] the actual biopsy of the lesion may alter lymphatic drainage patterns, and even if a sentinel node is identified, there is little evidence demonstrating a survival advantage with neck dissection in malignant melanoma. In addition, the technology is still in an early stage. The false-negative rate has been reported to be as high as 34%.[101] Sentinel node biopsies should continue to be considered investigational at this time.

Treatment of Advanced/Metastatic Disease

For patients in whom disease has spread distantly, the prognosis is dismal, with a 10% 10-year survival.[60] Surgery at the primary site is often performed but does not alter the prognosis owing to distant disease. In an attempt to improve survival, several other modalities of treatment have been investigated, including chemotherapy and immunotherapy.

The use of dimethyltrianzeno-imidazole-carboxamide (DTIC) or dacarbazine as a chemotherapeutic agent in patients with advanced melanoma has been studied. There was a 14 to 25% response rate to the drug, but no significant improvement in survival was shown.[60,68] An initial study with interferon-α2b showed a decrease in recurrence rates and distant metastases while patients remained on the treatment. Once off the therapy, however, the disease recurred, and there was no change seen in 5-year survival.[102] A later study by the Eastern Cooperative Oncology Group found that 1 year of treatment with interferon-α2b increased survival at the last follow-up period of 6.9 years from 37 to 46% in patients with melanomas > 4 mm and positive nodes.[103] Although statistically significant, the clinical improvement of a few percentage points is limited, and given the severe toxicity of interferon, it is unlikely that the drug will become widely used.

To avoid the toxicities associated with chemotherapy and interferon therapy, the use of melanoma vaccines has been investigated. Many studies are still ongoing, but one, using a polyvalent whole-cell melanoma vaccine, showed some survival benefit.[104] Further work is needed to determine if these or other investigational therapies will be truly effective for patients with advanced disease.

Outcomes/Prognosis

Melanoma accounts for the majority of deaths from skin malignancies,[57] but when treated at an early stage, the cure rates are excellent.[105] Despite the rising incidence in the disease, there has been a steady decrease in the death rate from melanoma. Five-year survivals have increased from 12.5% in the 1920s to nearly 80% today.[63] This drop in melanoma-related mortality rates is most likely attributable to increased awareness and prevention efforts.

For head and neck melanoma, the overall 5-year survival is 77%.[61] Melanomas of the auricle have been found to have a worse prognosis in some studies[62,89,97,106] but not in others.[59,79] The survival rate for auricular melanoma is 68 to 81% at 5 years[62,79] and 47% at 10 years.[79] The latter number likely reflects deaths from other causes as many patients with melanoma are older. The cure rate is higher in women than in men (96.2% versus 64.6%), perhaps because of more attention paid by women to their appearance and more regular physician visits for women.[62]

The risk factor that most strongly correlates with survival is tumor thickness.[61,62,79,89] Byers and colleagues have noted that on the ear in particular, thickness is a better predictor of outcome than Clark levels because of the thin skin of the auricle.[59] As tumor thickness increases, the chance for recurrence[61] and metastases[59] increases, resulting in decreased survival[61] (see Table 18–8). On the ear in particular, tumors > 3 mm thick have a much greater chance of metastases (61% versus 21%).[59]

The presence of metastatic disease carries a dismal prognosis. Some evidence suggests that for patients with nonpalpable nodal disease, the presence of less than three pathologically positive nodes does not alter survival.[107] However, patients with palpable nodes have a 20% 10-year survival.[108] Those with distant metastases have a 10% 10-year survival, and the mean time until death was 7 to 14 months.[60]

Other factors that have been shown to influence prognosis include ulceration,[87] tumor histology (NMs are worse than SSMs, which are worse than LMMs),[87,88] and sex.[62] Ultimately, however, early detection and diagnosis are the keys to improving the outcomes of our patients.

OTHER PATHOLOGY

The three most common types of malignancies of the auricle are SCC, BCC, and melanoma. Other rarer malignancies do occur and should be considered in the differential diagnosis of skin lesions.

Merkel cell carcinoma is one of the most aggressive skin malignancies. It is a neuroendocrine tumor that arises from pleuripotent basal cells in the epithelium.[109] They are typically rapidly growing firm nodular tumors with a bluish maroon hue. Histologically, the tumor cells are arranged in dense sheets and demonstrate aggressive growth into the deep dermal and subcutaneous tissue with sparing of the epidermis and superficial dermis.[109] The cells are small, with a high nuclear to cytoplasmic ratio and many mitotic figures. Electron microscopy, often helpful in making the diagnosis, will show perinuclear whorls of intermediate filaments.[110] The cells will stain positive for neuron-specific enolase, neurofilament, and cytokeratin.[109]

Merkel cell carcinoma is very aggressive, with a high propensity for recurrence and metastases. The recurrence rate after wide local excision can reach 90%,[111,112] and nearly two-thirds of patients will develop nodal metastases.[113,114] Wide local excision with large margins is recommended. Mohs' surgery may be helpful for tumors located on the ear to preserve normal tissue. These tumors are radiosensitive, and postoperative radiation can reduce the recurrence rate to 10 to 15%.[43,115] Neck dissection should be performed and postoperative radiation given to the neck if there is nodal disease.[109] Despite aggressive locoregional treatment, the 5-year survival rate is only 60%, mainly owing to distant metastases.[115]

Adnexal carcinomas are exceedingly rare, accounting for < 0.005% of all skin lesions.[116] Because of this, there are few data regarding outcome and therapy. They typically present in older patients and can appear as slowly growing nontender pink or yellow masses.[109] Despite their slow growth, they are locally very aggressive and insinuate themselves in the surrounding connective tissue. Recurrence rates are high despite wide local excision. Eighty percent of patients will develop at least one recurrence.[117] The role of radiation therapy has still not been defined.

Other malignancies that can occur on the auricle include malignant fibrous histiocytoma, dermatofibrosarcoma protuberans, angiosarcomas, and metastatic disease from other areas.

RECONSTRUCTION OF THE AURICLE

Because of the complex anatomy of the auricle, reconstruction of surgical defects requires great skill and planning. Efforts should be made during the resection to preserve as much normal tissue as possible. The approach to auricular repair can be divided into partial- (removal of skin and perichondrium) and full-thickness defects (removal includes cartilage). Next, the portion of the ear involved is assessed. For reconstructive purposes, the ear can be thought of in several parts: the external scaffolding including the helical rim and antihelix, the central cartilaginous portion made up primarily of the conchal bowl, the lobule, the preauricular area with the tragus, and the retroauricular region.

Partial-Thickness Defects

Most partial-thickness defects can be repaired with a split- or full-thickness skin graft or allowed to heal by secondary intention. If the cartilage exposure is > 1 cm, granulation tissue may not completely fill the defect from the edges. In these cases, perforations can be made in the cartilage every 5 mm to allow ingrowth of granulation tissue from behind.[5] Secondary intention is useful for patients in whom close surveillance of the site is desired or who have multiple cancers and little skin is left for grafting. Zitelli developed mnemonics for remembering areas appropriate for secondary intention.[118] Areas that lead to good cosmetic results after secondary intention include the concave surfaces of the nose, ear, eye, and temple ("NEET"). Convex surfaces of the nose, oral lips, cheeks, chin, and helix of the ear ("NOCCH") heal with unsightly depressed scars. Other areas on the forehead, antihelix, eyelids, and the remainder of the nose, lips, and cheeks ("FAIR") give variable results. If the defect is large, a skin graft will help to prevent the contraction that occurs as the wound granulates. It is impor-

tant to place skin grafts only in areas that have remaining perichondrium or subcutaneous tissue to provide nourishment to the graft. If bare cartilage is exposed, some of the cartilage can be resected to allow access to the perichondrium on the other side, or one can wait for some granulation tissue to form before applying the graft.

Defects of the Helical Rim and Antihelix

The majority of the full-thickness helical/antihelical defects can be closed primarily. Defects of the helix of up to 1 cm can be closed following a wedge excision (Figure 18–1).[119] As the wounds increase in size, closure of the space results in bowing of the ear as the more medial cartilage is compressed. To eliminate this and to close larger defects, there are several options. The most common is the use of a chondrocutaneous advancement flap (see Figure 18–1). Many variations of this flap have been devised.[120–122] The basic idea is the removal of a geometric portion of the more central cartilage to allow rotation of the outer rim. The space is then filled as cartilage is rotated up from below. Other alternatives include a composite cartilage graft[122,123] with local skin flap coverage, preauricular flaps if the defect is located along the

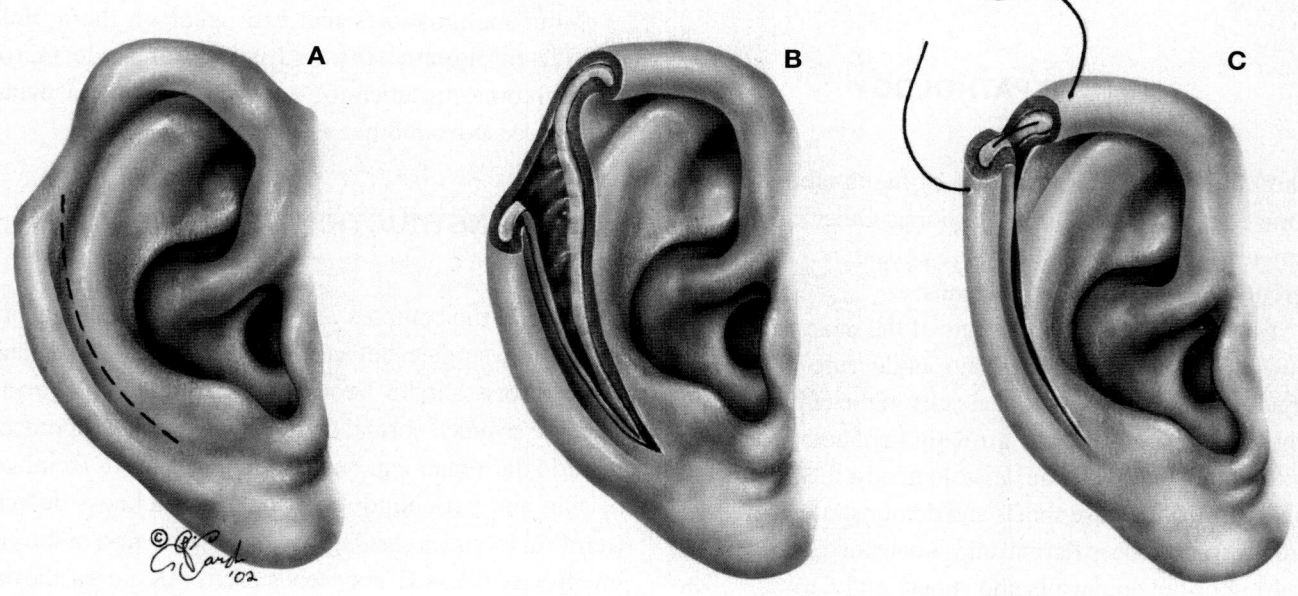

Figure 18–1   Chondrocutaneous helical advancement. A vertical releasing incision is made in the antihelical area extending into the lobule if needed (*A* and *B*). The helical rim can then be rotated and closed with minimal deformity (*C*).

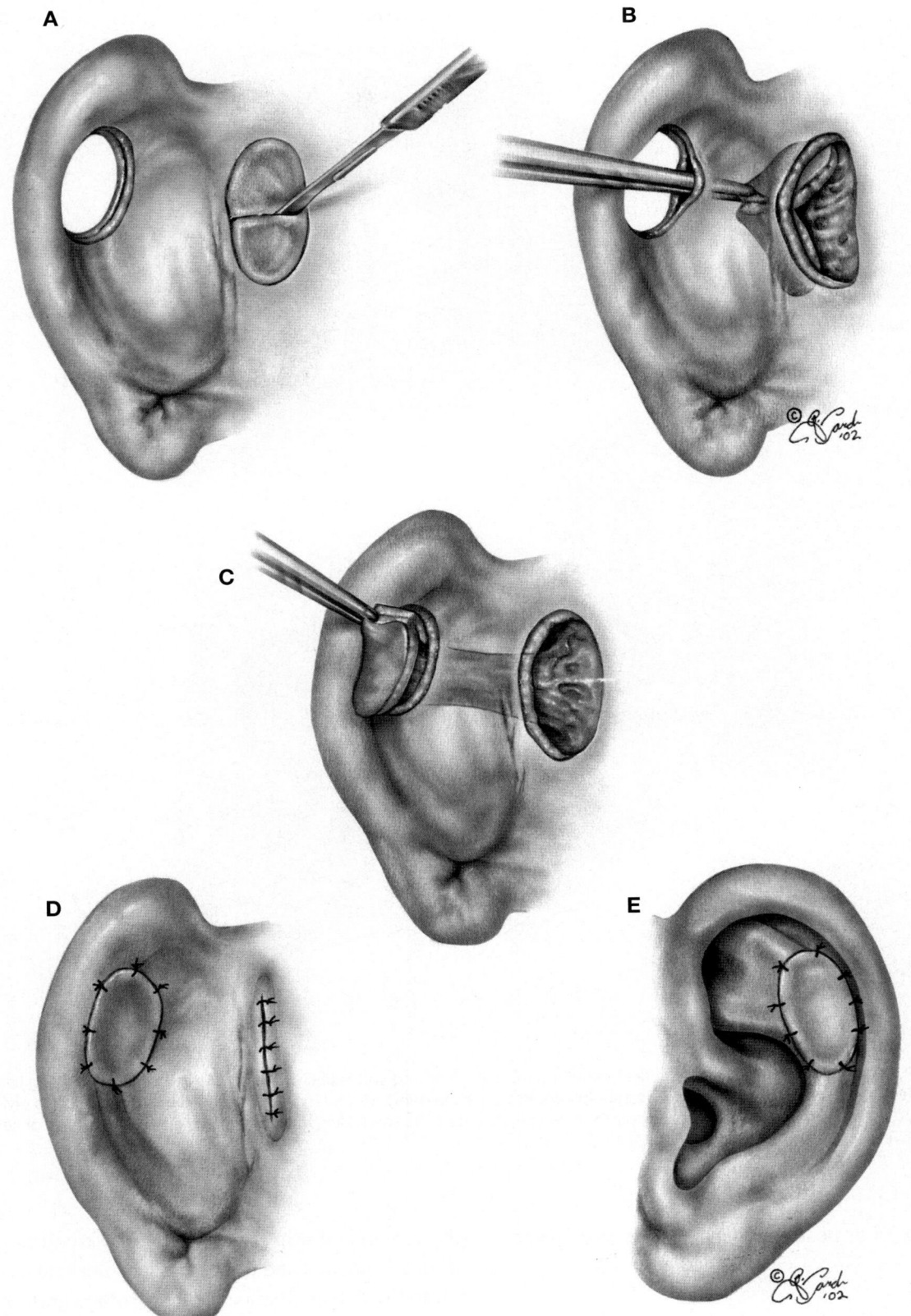

Figure 18–2   Posterior island flap. Defects of the conchal bowl can be repaired by lifting a flap of skin and subcutaneous tissue (*A*), which can be pedicled posteriorly and pulled through the defect (*B* and *C*). If skin is needed anteriorly and posteriorly, the flap can be folded on itself. The posterior defect is then closed primarily (*D* and *E*).

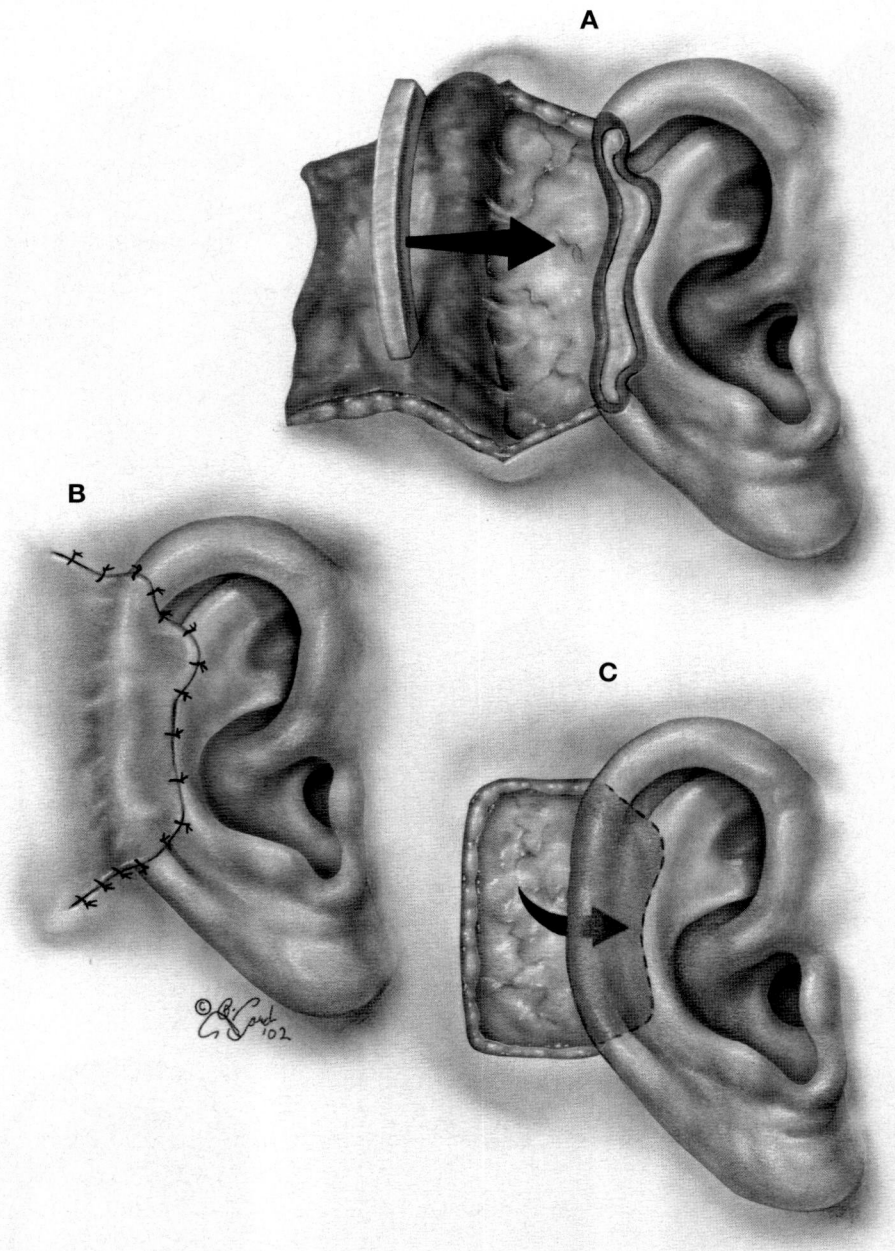

Figure 18–3 Postauricular graft. For defects of the posterior helical rim, skin and soft tissue coverage can be obtained by using tissue from the postauricular area. A posterior-based flap is raised and sutured over the defect (*A* and *B*). After 2 to 3 weeks, the pedicle is divided and closed primarily (*C*). If a cartilage defect is present, cartilage grafting can be performed using the contralateral auricular cartilage or septal cartilage prior to coverage with the flap.

anterior helix,[124] or postauricular flaps for more posterior defects.

Defects of the Concha

Because of the central location of the concha, rotational flaps are often difficult to devise. If the posterior peri-

chondrium and skin are intact, then a skin graft may be all that is needed and the cartilage is not replaced, similar to the defect after a conchal cartilage graft is taken. If there is a full-thickness defect including the posterior skin, then tissue must be brought in from another location. One effective means of doing this is with the subcutaneous island pedicle graft.[125] In this flap, an island of skin is taken from the postauricular area and then brought forward on a connective tissue pedicle and placed into the conchal defect. The posterior wound can easily be closed primarily (Figure 18–2).

Preauricular and Postauricular Defects, Reconstruction of the Lobule

Most defects anterior to the auditory canal can be closed primarily. If the tragus has been removed, reconstruction of the tragus may be performed with a cartilage graft, although the cosmetic results are often not as satisfactory as one would desire. Wide undermining in the postauricular area will provide considerable laxity in the tissue, and most wounds can be closed primarily. Otherwise, skin grafts work well in this area as it is often covered by hair and so is less noticeable. The lobule contains no cartilage and therefore is able to be recreated by the advancement of soft tissue either from the ear itself or from the surrounding skin, which is then folded over on itself and divided at a secondary procedure.

CONCLUSIONS

Auricular malignancies are becoming increasingly common as more and more people increase their exposure to solar radiation. Fortunately, there has also been an increased effort at educating the public of the dangers of skin cancer and a heightened sense of awareness of this problem by physicians. Early detection of skin cancer is the most effective form of treatment. When identified early, auricular malignancies are highly curable. More advanced disease, however, carries with it a poorer prognosis and requires surgical excision that can easily deform the complex anatomy of the ear. Mohs' surgery can provide a reliable means of preserving normal tissue during resection of SCC or BCC. Melanoma remains a difficult disease to treat if not identified at an early stage. Adjuvant therapies are being studied, but none have proven effective. If excision of a tumor on the ear is required, careful planning both during the surgery and for reconstruction of the resulting defect is needed (Figure 18–3).

REFERENCES

1. Glass AG, Hoover RN. The emerging epidemic of melanoma and squamous cell skin cancer. JAMA 1989;262:2097–100.

2. American Cancer Society. Cancer facts and figures—1992. New York: American Cancer Society; 1992.

3. Estrem SA, Remmer G. Special problems associated with cutaneous carcinoma of the ear. Otol Clin North Am 1993;26:231–45.

4. Byers R, Kesler K, Redmon B, et al. Squamous carcinoma of the external ear. Am J Surg 1983;146:447–50.

5. Balough BJ, O'Leary M, Martin P. Basal and squamous cell carcinoma of the auricle. In: Jackler RK, Driscoll CLW, editors. Tumors of the ear and temporal bone. Philadelphia: Lippincott Williams and Wilkins; 2000. p. 29–55.

6. Bailin PL, Levine HL, Wood BG, Tucker HM. Cutaneous carcinoma of the auricle and periauricular region. Arch Otolaryngol 1980;106:692–6.

7. Robins P, Nix M. Analysis of persistent disease on the ear following Mohs' surgery. Head Neck Surg 1984;6:998–1006.

8. Scotto J, Fears T, Fraumeni J. Incidence of non-melanoma skin cancer in the United States. Washington (DC): Dept. of Health & Human Services (US); 1983. NIH Publication No.: 83-2433.

9. Nguyen AV, Whitaker DC, Frodel J. Differentiation of basal cell carcinoma. Otolaryngol Clin North Am 1993;26:37–56.

10. Hayden RC III. Cutaneous squamous carcinoma and related lesions. Otolaryngol Clin North Am 1993;26:57–71.

11. Niparko JK, Swanson NA, Baker SR, et al. Local control of auricular, periauricular, and external canal cutaneous malignancies with Mohs' surgery. Laryngoscope 1990;100:1047–51.

12. Bumstead RM, Ceilley RI, Panje WR, Crumley RL. Auricular malignant neoplasms: when is chemotherapy (Mohs' technique) necessary? Arch Otolaryngol 1981;107:721–4.

13. Dinehart SM, Jansen GT. Cancer of the skin. In: Myers EN, Suen JY, editors. Cancer of the head and neck. Philadelphia: WB Saunders; 1996. p. 143–59.

14. Shockley WW, Stucker FJ. Squamous cell carcinoma of the external ear: a review of 75 cases. Otolaryngol Head Neck Surg 1987;97:308–12.

15. Buzzell RA. Effects of solar radiation on the skin. Otolaryngol Clin North Am 1993;26:1–11.

16. Urbach F. Potential effect of altered solar ultraviolet radiation on human skin cancer. Photochem Photobiol 1989;50:507–13.

17. Amron D, May R. Stratospheric ozone depletion and its relationship to skin cancer, J Dermatol Surg Oncol 1991;17:370–2.

18. Fitzpatrick T. The validity and practicality of sun reactive skin types I through VI. Arch Dermatol 1988;124:869–71.

19. Marks R, Rennie G, Selwood T. Malignant transformation of solar keratoses to squamous cell carcinoma. Lancet 1988;1:795–7.

20. Marks R, Foley P, Goodman G, et al. Spontaneous remission of solar keratoses: the case for conservative management. Br J Dermatol 1986;115:649–55.

21. Sanders GH, Miller TA. Are keratocanthomas really squamous cell carcinomas? Ann Plast Surg 1982;9:306–9.

22. Gupta A, Cardella C, Haberman H. Cutaneous malignant neoplasms in patients with renal transplants. Arch Dermatol 1986;122:1288–93.

23. Maize JC. Skin cancer in immunosuppressed patients. JAMA 1977;237:1857–8.

24. Shumrick KA, Coldiron B. Genetic syndromes associated with skin cancer. Otolaryngol Clin North Am 1993;26:117–37.

25. Gorlin RJ, Goetz RW. Multiple nevoid basal cell carcinomas, odontogenic keratocysts, and skeletal anomalies — a syndrome. N Engl J Med 1960;262:908–12.

26. Levine HL, Bailin PL. Basal cell carcinoma of the head and neck: identification of the high risk patient. Laryngoscope 1980;90:955–61.

27. Sloane JP. The value of typing basal cell carcinomas in predicting recurrence after surgical excision. Br J Dermatol 1977; 96:127–32.

28. Borel DM. Cutaneous basosquamous carcinoma: review of the literature and report of 35 cases. Arch Pathol 1973;95:293–7.

29. Jacobs GH, Rippey JJ, Altini M, et al. Predictions of aggressive behavior in basal cell carcinoma. Cancer 1982;49:533–7.

30. Von Domarus H, Steven PJ. Metastatic basal cell carcinoma: report of five cases and review of 170 cases in the literature. J Am Acad Dermatol. 1984;10:1043–60.

31. Buescher LS. Sunscreens and photoprotection. Otolaryngol Clin North Am 1993;26:13–22.

32. Robinson J. Risk of developing another basal cell carcinoma. A five year prospective study. Cancer 1987;60:118–20.

33. Blake GB, Wilson JSP. Malignant tumors of the ear and their treatment. Br J Plast Surg 1974;27:67–76.

34. Rowe DE, Carroll JR, Day CL Jr. Long term recurrence rates in previously untreated (primary) basal cell carcinoma: implications for patient follow up. J Dermatol Surg Oncol 1989;15: 315–28.

35. Mohs FE. Chemosurgery: a microscopically controlled method of cancer excision. Arch Surg 1941;42:279–95.

36. Clark D. Cutaneous micrographic surgery. Otolaryngol Clin North Am 1993;26:185–202.

37. Mohs F, Larson P, Iriondo M. Micrographic surgery for the microscopically controlled excision of carcinoma of the external ear. J Am Acad Dermatol 1988;9:729–37.

38. Rowe DE, Carroll RJ, Day CL. Prognostic factors for local recurrence metastasis and survival rates in squamous cell carcinoma of the skin, ear, and lip: implications for treatment modality selection. J Am Acad Dermatol 1992;26:976–90.

39. Limmer B, Clark D. Non-surgical management of primary skin malignancies. Otolaryngol Clin North Am 1993;26:167–83.

40. Kuflik EG. Cryosurgery for tumors of the ear. J Dermatol Surg Oncol 1985;11:1165–8.

41. Smith SP, Grande DJ. Basal cell carcinoma recurring after radiotherapy: a unique difficult treatment subclass of recurrent basal cell carcinoma. J Dermatol Surg Oncol 1991;17:26–30.

42. Westgate SJ. Radiation therapy for skin tumors. Otolaryngol Clin North Am 1993;26:295–309.

43. Lovett RD, Perez CA, Shapiro SJ, et al. External irradiation of epithelial skin cancer. Int J Radiat Oncol Biol Phys 1990;19: 235–42.

44. Fishbach A, Sause W, Plenk H. Radiation therapy for skin cancer. West J Med 1980;133:379–82.

45. Parker RG, Wildermuth O. Radiation therapy of lesions overlying cartilage: carcinoma of the pinna. Cancer 1962;15:57–65.

46. Klein E, Case RW, Burgess GH. Chemotherapy of skin cancer. Cancer 1973;23:228–31.

47. Sturm HM. Bowen's disease and 5-fluorouracil. J Am Acad Dermatol 1979;1:513–22.

48. Gluckman JL, Portugal LG. Photodynamic therapy for cutaneous malignancies of the head and neck. Otolaryngol Clin North Am 1993;26:311–8.

49. Freedlander E, Chung FF. Squamous cell carcinoma of the pinna. Br J Plast Surg 1983;36:171–5.

50. Borel DM. Cutaneous basosquamous carcinoma: review of the literature and report of 35 cases. Arch Pathol 1973;95:293–7.

51. Menn H, Robins P, Kopf AW. The recurrent basal cell epithelioma: a study of 100 cases of recurrent retreated basal cell epithelioma. Arch Dermatol 1971;103:628–31.

52. Wilder RB, Shimm DS, Kittelson JM, et al. Recurrent basal cell carcinoma treated with radiation therapy. Arch Dermatol 1991; 127:1668–72.

53. Lee D, Nash M, Har-El G. Regional spread of auricular and periauricular cutaneous malignancies. Laryngoscope 1996;106: 998–1001.

54. Lewis J. Cancer of the ear. Laryngoscope 1966;70:551–79.

55. Afzelius LE, Gunnarsson M, Nordgren H. Guidelines for prophylactic radical lymph node dissection in cases of carcinoma of the external ear. Head Neck Surg 1980;2:361–5.

56. Goepfert H, Dichtel WJ, Medina JE, et al. Perineural invasion of squamous cell skin carcinoma of the head and neck. Am J Surg 1984;148:542–7.

57. Landis SH, Manay T, Bolden S, Wingo PA. Cancer statistics 1999. CA Cancer J Clin 1999;49:8–31.

58. Boring C, Squires T, Tong T. Cancer statistics 1992. CA Cancer J Clin 1992;42:19–38.

59. Byers R, Smith J, Russel N, et al. Malignant melanoma of the external ear. Am J Surg 1980;140:518–21.

60. Beaver M, Chang CJ. Melanoma. In: Jackler RK, Driscoll CLW, editors. Tumors of the ear and temporal bone. Philadelphia: Lippincott Williams & Wilkins; 2000. p. 56–66.

61. O'Brien CJ, Coates AS, Petersen-Schaefer K, et al. Experience with 998 cutaneous melanomas of the head and neck over 30 years. Am J Surg 1991;162:310–4.

62. Ringborg U, Afzelius LE, Lagerlof B, et al. Cutaneous malignant melanoma of the head and neck. Analysis of treatment results and prognostic factors in 581 patients: a report from the Swedish Melanoma Study Group. Cancer 1993;71:751–8.

63. Elder DE. Skin cancer: melanoma and other specific non-melanoma skin cancers. Cancer 1995;75 Suppl 1:245–56.

64. Koh H, Kligler B, Lew R. Sunlight and cutaneous malignant melanoma: evidence for and against causation. Photochem Photobiol 1990;51:765–79.

65. Kopf A, Kripke M, Stern R. Sun and malignant melanoma. J Am Acad Dermatol 1984;11:674–84.

66. Osterlund A. Malignant melanoma in Denmark: occurrence and risk factors. Acta Oncol 1990;29:833–54.

67. Smith JF. Head and neck melanoma. Ear Nose Throat J 1991;70: 143–51.

68. Medina JE. Malignant melanoma of the head and neck. Otolaryngol Clin North Am 1993;26:73–86.

69. Greene MH, Young TI, Clark WH Jr. Malignant melanoma in renal transplant recipients. Lancet 1981;1:1196–9.

70. Holman CDJ, Armstrong BK. Pigmentary traits, ethnic origin, benign nevi, and familial history as risk factors for cutaneous malignant melanoma. J Natl Cancer Inst 1984;72:257–66.

71. Kraemer KH, Greene MA, Torone R, et al. Dysplastic nevi: cutaneous melanoma risk. Lancet 1983;2:1076–7.

72. Clark WH Jr, From L, Bernardino EA, Mihm MC. The histogenesis and biologic behavior of primary human malignant melanomas of the skin. Cancer Res 1969;29:705–26.

73. Bresslow A. Thickness, cross-sectional areas and depth of invasion in the prognosis of cutaneous melanoma. Ann Surg 1970;172:902–8.

74. National Institutes of Health Consensus Development Conference statement on diagnosis and treatment of early melanoma. Am J Dermatopathol 1993;15:34–43.

75. Balch CM, Urist MM, Karakousis CP, et al. Efficacy of 2-cm surgical margins for intermediate thickness melanomas (1–4 mm). Ann Surg 1993;218:262–9.

76. Veronesi U, Cascinelli N, Adamus J, et al. Thin stage I primary cutaneous malignant melanoma. Comparison of excision with margins of 1 or 3 cm. N Engl J Med 1988;318:1159–62.

77. Weiss RL Jr. Recent findings in melanoma research. In: Bailey BJ, Johnson JT, Kohout RI, Pillsbury HC III, editors. Head and neck surgery: otolaryngology. Philadelphia: JB Lippincott; 1993. p. 1087–90.

78. Coldiron BM. Current management of skin cancer. Curr Opin Otolaryngol Head Neck Surg 1997;5:214–22.

79. Cole DJ, Mackay GJ, Walker BF, et al. Melanoma of the external ear. J Surg Oncol 1992;50:110–4.

80. Trott KR, Vonliever H, Kummermehr J, et al. The radiosensitivity of malignant melanomas. part I: experimental studies. Int J Radiat Oncol Biol Phys 1981;7:9–13.

81. Trott KR, Vonliever H, Kummermehr J, et al. The radiosensitivity of malignant melanomas. part II: clinical studies. Int J Radiat Oncol Biol Phys 1981;7:15–20.

82. Harwood AR, Cummings BJ. Radiotherapy for malignant melanoma: a re-appraisal. Cancer Treat Rev 1981;8:271–82.

83. Harwood AR. The role of radiation therapy in the treatment of melanoma. In: Larson DL, Ballantyne J, Guillamondegui OM, editors. Cancer in the neck: evaluation and treatment. New York: Macmillan; 1986. p. 243.

84. Overgaard J. Radiation treatment of malignant melanoma. Int J Radiat Oncol Biol Phys 1980;6:41–4.

85. Sause WT, Cooper JS, Rush S, et al. Fraction size in external beam radiation therapy in the treatment of melanoma. Int J Radiat Oncol Biol Phys 1991;20:429–32.

86. Balch CM, Morad TM, Soong SJ, et al. A multifactorial analysis of melanoma: prognostic histopathologic features comparing Clark's and Breslow's staging methods. Ann Surg 1978; 188:732–42.

87. Fisher SR. Cutaneous malignant melanoma of the head and neck. Laryngoscope 1989;99:822–36.

88. Day C, Mihm M, Sober A, et al. Prognostic factors of melanoma patients with lesions 0.76–1.69 mm in thickness: an appraisal of thin level IV lesions. Ann Surg 1982;195:30–4.

89. Thorn M, Ponten F, Bergstrom R, et al. Clinical and histopathological predictors of survival in patients with malignant melanoma: a population based study in Sweden. J Natl Cancer Inst 1994;86:764–9.

90. Shah JP, Kraus DH, Dubner S, et al. Patterns of regional lymph node metastases from cutaneous melanomas of the head and neck. Am J Surg 1991;162:320–3.

91. Ballantyne AJ. Malignant melanoma of the head and neck: an analysis of 405 cases. Am J Surg 1970;120:425–31.

92. Byers RM. The role of modified neck dissection in the treatment of cutaneous melanomas of the head and neck. Arch Surg 1986;121:1338–41.

93. Medina JE, Canfield V. Malignant melanoma of the head and neck. In: Myers EN, Suen JY, editors. Cancer of the head and neck. Philadelphia: WB Saunders; 1996. p. 160–83.

94. Balch CM. Surgical management of regional lymph nodes in cutaneous melanoma. J Am Acad Dermatol 1980;3:511–24.

95. Milton GW, Shaw HM, McCarthy WH, et al. Prophylactic lymph node dissection in clinical stage I cutaneous malignant melanoma: results of surgical treatment in 1319 patients. Br J Surg 1982;69:108–11.

96. Sim FH, Taylor WF, Pritchard DJ, et al. Lymphadenectomy in the management of stage I malignant melanoma: a prospective randomized study. Mayo Clin Proc 1986;61:697–705.

97. Wanebo HJ, Cooper PH, Young DV, et al. Prognostic factors in head and neck melanoma. Cancer 1988;62:831–7.

98. Wagner JD, Hee-Myung P, Coleman JJ, et al. Cervical sentinal lymph node biopsy for melanomas of the head and neck and upper thorax. Arch Otolaryngol 2000;126:313–21.

99. Wanebo HJ, Chung M. Radionuclide lymphoscintigraphy to identify lymphatic drainage patterns of cutaneous head and neck melanoma. Diagn Oncol 1993;3:258–62.

100. Kapteijn BAE, Nieweg OE, Olmus RAV, et al. Reproducibility of lymphoscintigraphy for lymphatic mapping in cutaneous melanoma. J Nucl Med 1996;37:972–5.

101. Coldiron BM. Sentinel node biopsy: who needs it? Int J Dermatol 2000;39:807–11.

102. Kokoschka EM, Trautinger F, Knobler RM, et al. Long-term adjuvant therapy of high risk melanoma patients with interferon alpha-2b. J Invest Dermatol 1990;95 Suppl 6:193–7.

103. Kirkwood JM, Strawderman MS, Smith TJ, et al. Interferon alpha 2b adjuvant therapy of high risk resected cutaneous melanoma: an Eastern Cooperative Oncology trial EST 1984. J Clin Oncol 1996;14:7–17.

104. Morton DL, Nizze A, Hoon D, et al. Improved survival of advanced stage IV melanoma following active immunotherapy: correlation with immune response to melanoma vaccine. Proc Am Soc Clin Oncol 1993;12:391.

105. Balch CM, Karakousis C, Mettlin C, et al. Management of cutaneous melanoma in the United States. Surg Gynecol Obstet 1984;158:311–8.

106. Ames FC, Sugarbaker FV, Ballantyne AJ. Analysis of survival and disease control in stage I melanoma of the head and neck. Am J Surg 1976;132:484–91.

107. Olson R, Woods J, Soule E. Regional lymph node management and outcome in 100 patients with head and neck melanoma. Am J Surg 1981;142:470–3.

108. Singletary SE, Byers RM, Shallenberger R, et al. Prognostic factors in patients with cervical nodal metastases from cutaneous malignant melanoma. Am J Surg 1986;152:371–5.

109. Marenda SA, Otto RA. Adnexal carcinomas of the skin. Otolaryngol Clin North Am 1993;26:87–116.

110. Hitchcock CL, Bland KI, Laney RG, et al. Neuroendocrine (Merkel cell) carcinoma of the skin. Ann Surg 1988;207:201–7.

111. Marks ME, Kim RY, Salter MM. Radiotherapy as an adjunct in the management of Merkel cell carcinoma. Cancer 1990;65: 60–4.

112. Morrison WH, Peters LJ, Silva EG, et al. The essential role of radiation therapy in securing locoregional control of Merkel cell carcinoma. Int J Radiat Oncol Biol Phys 1990;19:583–91.

113. Goepfert H, Remmler D, Silva E, et al. Merkel cell carcinoma (endocrine carcinoma of the skin) of the head and neck. Arch Otolaryngol 1984;110:707–12.

114. Hanke CW, Conner AC, Temofrew RK, et al. Merkel cell carcinoma. Arch Dermatol 1989;125:1096–100.

115. Pacella J, Ashby M, Ainslie J, et al. The role of radiotherapy in the management of primary cutaneous neuroendocrine tumors (Merkel cell or trabecular carcinoma): experience at the Peter MacCallum Cancer Institute (Melbourne, Australia). Int J Radiat Oncol Biol Phys 1988;14:1077–84.

116. Smith CCK. Metastasizing carcinomas of the sweat glands. Br J Surg 1955;43:80–4.

117. Wick MR, Coffin CM. Sweat gland and pilar carcinomas. In: Wick MR, editor. Pathology of unusual malignant cutaneous tumors. New York: Marcel Dekker; 1985. p. 1–76.

118. Zitelli JA. Wound healing by secondary intention: a cosmetic appraisal. J Am Acad Dermatol 1983;9:407–15.

119. Menick FJ. Reconstruction of the ear after tumor excision. Clin Plast Surg 1990;17:405–15.

120. Chiu LD, Barber W, Chen A. J-shaped, conchal excision with rotation advancement for closure of large auricular wedge defects. Laryngoscope 1996;106:116–8.

121. Antia NH, Buch VI. Chondrocutaneous advancement flap for the marginal defect of the ear. Plast Reconstr Surg 1967;39: 472–7.

122. Millard DR Jr. Reconstruction of one third plus of the auricular circumference. Plast Reconstr Surg 1992;90:475–8.

123. Tanzer RC. Total reconstruction of the external ear. Plast Reconstr Surg 1959;23:1–6.

124. Lawson VG. Reconstruction of the pinna using preauricular flaps. J Otolaryngol 1984;13:191–3.

125. Fader DJ, Johnson TM. Ear reconstruction utilizing the subcutaneous island pedicle graft (flip-flop) flap. Dermatol Surg 1999;25:94–6.

19

Surgery for Congenital Aural Atresia

Robert A. Jahrsdoerfer, MD

Congenital aural atresia occurs once in every 10,000 births. Unilateral atresia is seven times more common than bilateral atresia. Aural atresia is associated with a recognizable syndrome in about 10% of cases. In about 5% of nonsyndromic cases, the birth defect is inherited.

Surgical correction of congenital atresia is a formidable operation and demands the best talent of the ear surgeon. This operation should not be performed by the novice. The patient is at risk of being harmed in the hands of an inexperienced operator. Facial nerve paralysis and sensorineural hearing loss are very real possibilities. However, in a patient with bilateral atresia, successful surgery that achieves normal hearing and allows the patient to discard his/her hearing device can be very gratifying for the otologist.

The opinions and recommendations presented here represent experience gained from over 1,300 operations on patients with congenital ear malformations.

SURGERY FOR UNILATERAL VERSUS BILATERAL ATRESIA

The older literature reiterates the theme that only bilateral cases of congenital aural atresia should be operated on. The reasoning behind this philosophy was that surgery would probably not produce serviceable hearing, and the risks of facial nerve injury and sensorineural hearing loss would outweigh any potential benefit. Moreover, postoperative meatal stenosis and the failure to maintain long-term hearing were cited as arguments against operating on unilateral atresia. If unilateral cases were to be operated on, it was stated, they should be operated on only when the child had reached adolescence or young adulthood and could share in the decision.

Times have changed. Unilateral atresia may be operated on routinely but under strict criteria. Unilateral atretic ears must be carefully selected for surgery. This selection involves sorting out the high-risk (poor result) patients in whom the preoperative evaluation has indicated a 50% chance or less of success. Success herein is defined as a postoperative speech reception threshold of 15 to 25 dB. This threshold is attainable in 75 to 80% of patients selected for surgery.

Criteria for surgical intervention may be more lenient in cases of bilateral atresia. In patients who are marginal surgical candidates, it is appropriate to operate on at least one ear in an attempt to render serviceable hearing. However, impossible cases should be avoided.

A grading system was developed in an effort to select those individuals who have the best chance of successful atresia surgery.[1] The system is based on a preoperative high-resolution computed tomographic (CT) scan of the temporal bones. In addition, the appearance of the external ear prior to microtia surgery is factored in. Previous studies have shown that the appearance of the external ear correlates well with the degree of development of the middle ear.[2]

To be a potential candidate, certain other criteria must be met. First, there must be audiometric or evoked response evidence of cochlear function, and second, there must be imaging evidence of normal inner ear architecture. A relative contraindication of surgery would be a nonaerated middle ear and mastoid. If the middle ear is not aerated, the best possible surgical result one can achieve is 35 dB. This would still require the use of amplification. The lack of aeration may be caused by fluid on a temporary or on a permanent basis by primitive mesenchymal tissue of a fibrous gelatinous nature. This is found in patients with absent or poor eustachian tube function in whom air has never reached the middle ear or mastoid.

There is no easy way to tell if the soft tissue density is fluid or tissue. To better define the condition, the author waits 1 year and then repeats the CT scan. If the soft tissue density persists for 2 years or more, it is probably primitive mesenchymal tissue, and surgery is not indicated. Otitis media with effusion will usually clear within 1 year, revealing a well-ventilated middle ear and mastoid on a subsequent CT scan.

The grading system currently in use is shown in Table 19–1. The stapes is assigned 2 points as this is the most important ossicle to be found in the middle ear and on which the success or failure of the operation hinges. In approximately 4% of patients, the stapes will be fixed. There is no way to diagnose this preoperatively. A fixed stapes requires that the operation be staged. The first stage includes the usual atresia repair with canalplasty, tympanoplasty, and meatoplasty, whereas the second stage requires that the stapes be mobilized or a stapedectomy/stapedotomy be done with ossicular chain reconstruction.

Most patients who are candidates for surgery will be graded 7 to 8 of 10. This translates to a 70 to 80% chance of achieving normal, or near normal, hearing through surgery.

Other Options

It is important for the ear surgeon and the family to realize that other options are available. A long-term bone-conducting hearing device may be used, and many patients with this device develop excellent speech. An implantable bone-conducting hearing device may be inserted in those patients in whom the middle ear architecture is so distorted as to preclude ossiculoplasty. The only implantable bone-conducting hearing aid currently on the market is the bone-anchored hearing aid. This is approved by the US Food and Drug Administration for use in adults and children. The Audiant® implant never lived up to its hype and is no longer commercially available. The surgeon may elect to make a new skin-lined ear canal in a patient with an otherwise uncorrectable middle ear to allow the use of an ear-level or in-the-ear hearing aid.

It is also important to consider congenital microtia and atresia as a single problem. The older and more traditional schools of thought tended to separate the problem into two parts, cosmetic and functional, and often corrective procedures were done without regard for one or the other. Under this philosophy, the patient was the ultimate loser because rarely was it possible to achieve both good hearing and good appearance.

WHO SHOULD OPERATE FIRST?

There continues to be controversy over who should operate first, the plastic or facial plastic surgeon or the ear surgeon. This is no longer a negotiable point. If the external ear requires reconstruction, the plastic or facial plastic surgeon should operate first. The reasons for this position are as valid today as they were years ago. It is imperative that the reconstructive surgeon have a virgin field in which to place the implant. It is far easier for the reconstructive surgeon to build an ear in the absence of scar tissue and a compromised vascular bed than it is to build an ear around a hole in the side of the head. However, the otologic surgeon is not constrained by an ear canal and has the latitude to position the reconstructed ear where it needs to be to align it with the newly created ear canal. In over 2,800 patients evaluated for atresia, the author has never seen a cosmetically acceptable external ear when the otologic surgeon has operated first (Figures 19–1 and 19–2).

One of the arguments used by those who favor atresia repair first is that "function is more important than appearance." This argument lacks merit. Function can be provided by a hearing device in the child's first few years of life. There is no "magic moment" when atresia surgery must be done for function. Close cooperation between the ear surgeon and the reconstructive surgeon

Table 1 GRADING SYSTEM OF CANDIDACY FOR SURGERY OF CONGENITAL AURAL ATRESIA	
Parameter	**Points**
Stapes present	2
Oval window open	1
Middle ear space	1
Facial nerve	1
Malleus/incus complex	1
Mastoid pneumatized	1
Incus-stapes connection	1
Round window	1
Appearance external ear	1
Total available points	10

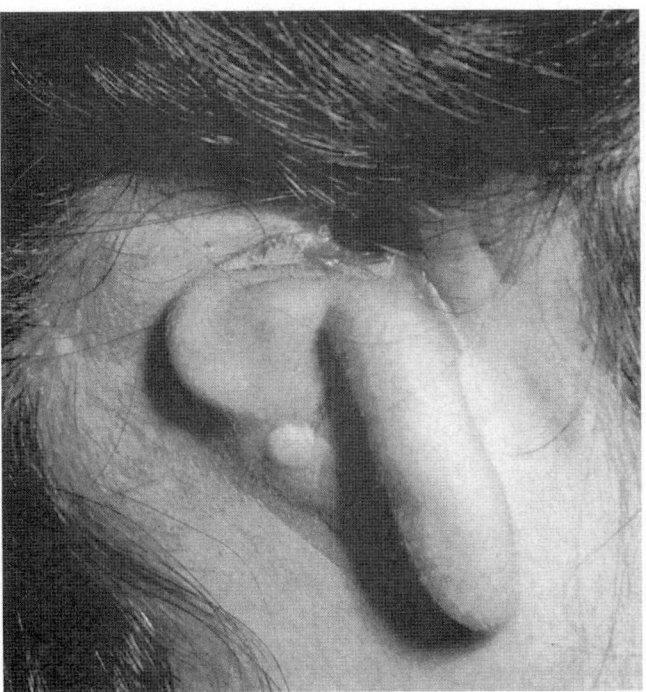

Figure 19–1 Failed attempt at atresia repair in a young boy. The ear had been operated on three times. Note the superiorly placed external ear canal, which is draining mucopurulent secretions. A large conductive hearing loss persists.

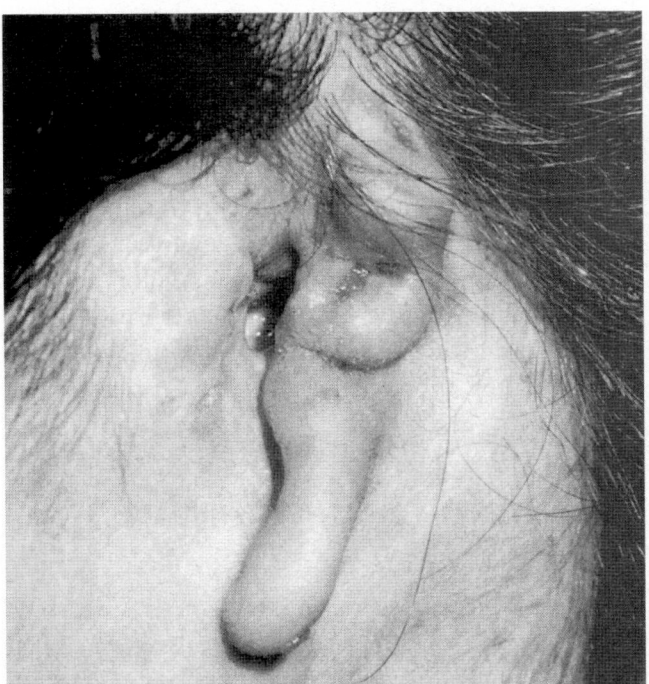

Figure 19–2 Failed attempt at atresia repair in the left ear (same patient as Figure 19–1). This ear had been operated on twice. The ear was draining, and there was a large conductive hearing loss. A skin pedicle had been placed in the ear canal, and hair was growing from the depths of the flap.

is what counts. The surgeons must combine their best efforts to create both good function and good appearance.

The surgical protocol that the author recommends depends on the grade of microtia. Grade III microtia, in which the external ear remnant is little more than a nubbin of skin on the lateral face, is routinely operated on first by the reconstructive surgeon (Figure 19–3). Grade I microtia, in which the external ear is slightly smaller but well formed, usually does not require the services of a reconstructive surgeon because this ear can rarely be improved on cosmetically (Figure 19–4). Grade II microtia, in which the external ear is about one half of normal size but has reasonably good shape, may be operated on by the otologic surgeon first if the atresia is bilateral (Figure 19–5). If the atresia is unilateral, it is a judgment call by the reconstructive surgeon, who must decide if his/her skills may improve the appearance of the external ear.

TIMING OF MICROTIA REPAIR

External ear reconstruction is usually delayed until the child is about 7 years of age. This delay allows for growth of the rib cage, enabling sufficient costal carti-

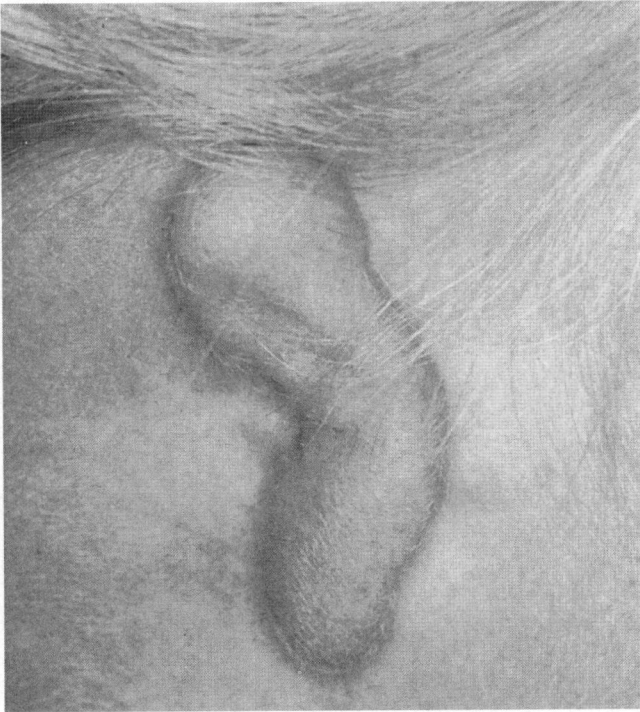

Figure 19–3 Grade III microtia. Note the poorly formed ear remnant on the lateral face.

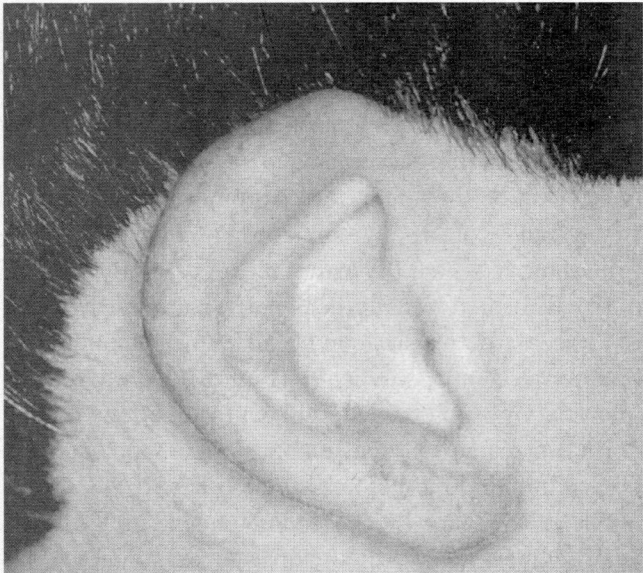

Figure 19–4 Grade I microtia. The appearance of the external ear is fairly well formed but smaller.

lage to be harvested for sculpturing of the implant. Younger children simply do not have enough cartilage to fashion an implant. A child who is large for his/her age may be operated on earlier. In my opinion, soft silicone (Silastic®) implants are contraindicated because the extrusion rate exceeds 50%.

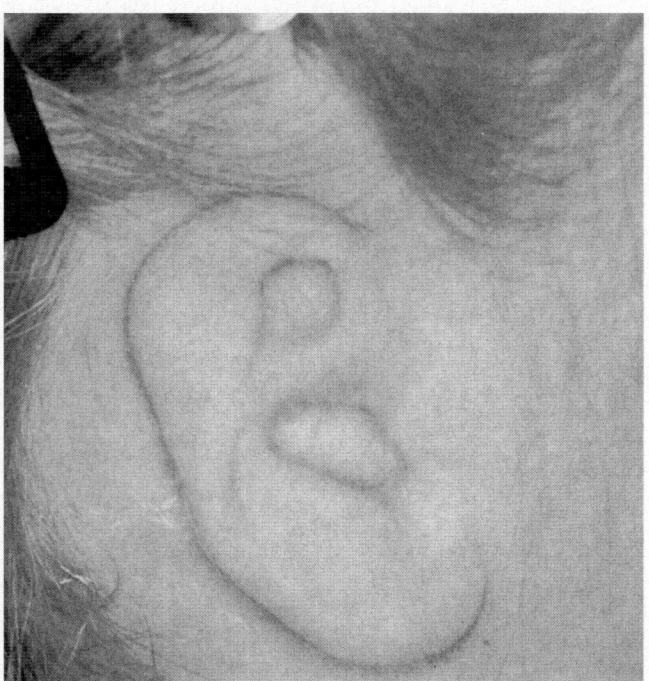

Figure 19–5 Grade II microtia. The external ear remnant is about one half of normal size and has some form.

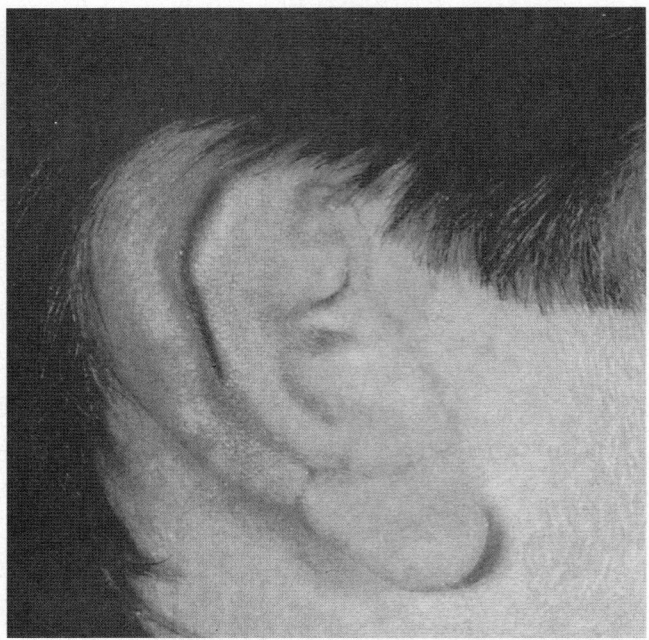

Figure 19–6 Appearance of the external ear after stages I and II of microtia repair. The ear is now ready for atresia repair.

The first stage of external ear reconstruction is harvesting, sculpturing, and implanting the contoured rib graft. A second-stage procedure is performed 3 to 6 months later in which the external ear remnant is repositioned as the lobule (Figure 19–6). After this stage, atresia repair, stage 3, may be performed. Stage 4 entails creating a tragus, and stage 5 involves lifting the ear off the head and skin grafting the postauricular sulcus. Many parents elect to terminate reconstructive surgery of their child's external ear once the atresia has been repaired. Indeed, some ears look better before they are elevated off the head. What really matters, however, is that the reconstructive surgeon and the otologist coordinate their best efforts for the good of the patient (Figure 19–7).

TIMING OF ATRESIA REPAIR

The age at which atresia repair is undertaken varies with the initial grade of microtia and whether the atresia is unilateral or bilateral. As mentioned previously, grade III microtia must always be first reconstructed by the plastic surgeon or facial plastic surgeon. Assuming that the earliest the reconstructive surgeon will operate is age 6 or 7 years, the otologist may then plan to open the ear for

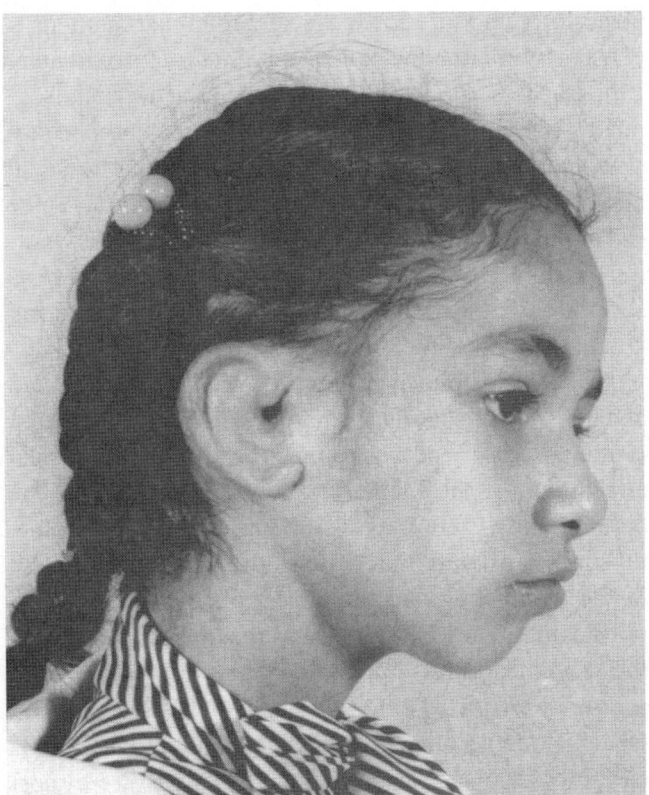

Figure 19–7 Final long-term appearance of repaired microtia/atresia.

hearing purposes when the patient is age 7 or 8 years. Although this dictum holds true for both unilateral and bilateral cases, in unilateral atresia, there is no urgency, and the repair can be delayed to suit the convenience of the patient, the parents, and the ear surgeon.

The earliest that atresia surgery should be performed in patients with grade I or II microtia is 5 years of age. The reason for this is that patient cooperation is of critical importance in the immediate postoperative period. A potentially poor result can be salvaged postoperatively in the office or clinic but requires the cooperation of the patient. One may argue that the child can always be returned to the operating room and given general anesthesia, but this is a poor alternative. Many of these children have mandibular hypoplasia that restricts easy access to the larynx. Endotracheal intubation is often difficult and sometimes dangerous. Most of these young children do quite well with their hearing device until surgery is electively performed. The only condition under which the author operates early is when the child refuses to wear a hearing device. In these rare cases, the author has operated as early as age 3 years.

SURGICAL TECHNIQUE

Preparation of the Patient

The lateral face and the skin graft donor site are prepared and draped. A $\frac{1}{2}$-inch swath of hair is shaved around the external ear. Infiltration anesthesia, using lidocaine (Xylocaine®) 1% with epinephrine 1:50,000, is routinely employed. The operation is usually planned for 5 hours, with a range of 3 to 6 hours. Urethral catheterization is avoided, and the anesthesiologist adjusts the intravenous fluid volume accordingly. In the past, all patients were routinely catheterized. However, urethral irritation evoked more patient complaints than any other aspect of the surgery, and catheterization was therefore discontinued. Nitrous oxide anesthesia is not routinely used. Even without nitrous oxide, a respirator using room air nitrogen may cause increased positive pressure in the middle ear and balloon the fascia graft.

Incision and Drilling

A postauricular incision is used routinely. In those patients with a well-formed auricle, the author has no objection to the otologist's using an endaural incision. Soft tissue is elevated off the mastoid process in a posterior to anterior direction. The temporal root of the zygomatic arch and the glenoid fossa are identified. A tympanic bone remnant is searched for because it points the way to the middle ear. If no remnant is found, the cribriform area of the mastoid process serves as a landmark for drilling.

Drilling is begun, staying superior and anterior (Figure 19–8). There is no rationale for doing a mastoidectomy. This procedure leaves a large, unsightly cavity that is difficult to graft and prone to postoperative infection. The superoanterior surgical approach should hug the tegmen and the glenoid fossa. This approach best avoids an aberrant facial nerve. The bone opening need not be large; about 1.5 cm in diameter is recommended. Dense atretic bone is followed medially. At a depth of about 1.5 cm, the fused incus-malleus complex is encountered. The first landmark the surgeon sees is the body of the incus. This landmark can be confirmed by gentle palpation, noting a slight displacement of the ossicle. The ossicular chain is fixed to the atretic plate medially at the level of the malleus neck (Figure 19–9). Therefore, there

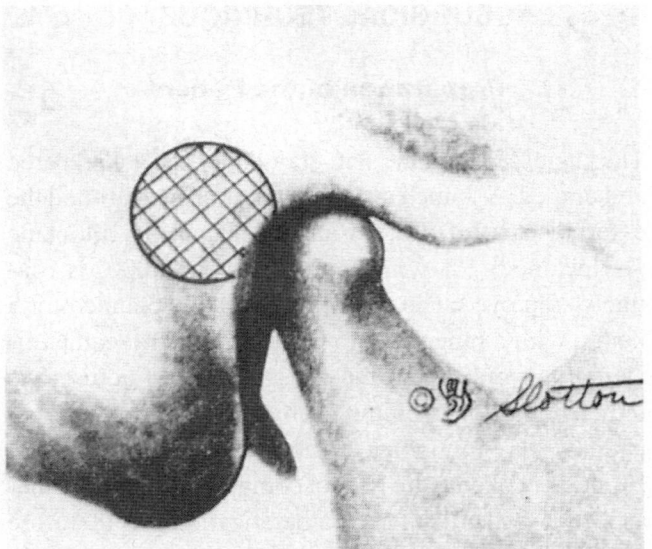

Figure 19–8 Lateral view of temporal bone showing the area where the ear surgeon should begin drilling for congenital atresia.

is almost always some motion of the fused malleus head and incus body on palpation.

Drilling is continued over the atretic plate, gradually thinning bone to eggshell thickness. A diamond bur is used in the final stages of drilling. As bone is drilled away

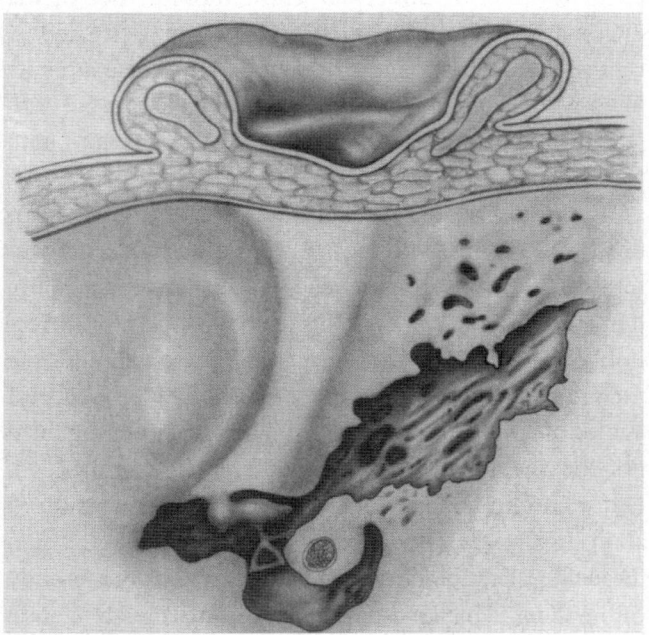

Figure 19–9 Sagittal view at the level of the epitympanum showing fused incus and malleus and bony attachment of the malleus neck to the atretic plate.

posteriorly and inferiorly, the surgeon must maintain a constant vigil for the facial nerve.[3] In approximately 25% of cases, the facial nerve has a short vertical segment (sometimes nonexistent). Instead, the nerve makes a sharp curve anteriorly at the second bend. The facial nerve is most vulnerable to injury in this location. A clue to the proximity of the facial nerve can be had by noting small blood vessels over the surface of the nerve as seen through the thinned bone. Facial nerve monitoring is used routinely.

The atretic bone overlying the middle ear is thinned and gently picked away in small pieces. Sharp dissection is often necessary because there is always firm periosteal attachment of the malleus to the undersurface of the atretic plate. There may also be a band of soft tissue, mostly periosteum, that courses through a bone defect in the wall separating the atretic plate from the temporomandibular joint. This band may be confused with the facial nerve. It is imperative that the facial nerve be positively identified before this band of soft tissue is cut. Once the atretic plate is removed, the ossicular chain is carefully assessed. The incus and malleus are almost always fused, although there may be some early demarcation of an incudomalleal joint. The handle of the malleus is often absent, having not yet developed (Figure 19–10), and the neck of the malleus is usually in firm bone union with the undersurface of the atretic plate. Care must be exercised in removing the overlying fragments of atretic bone so as not to subluxate the ossicles or impart vibratory trauma to the inner ear. The author finds that sharp dissection works best in this situation. The use of a small scalpel or alligator scissors is helpful in incising the periosteum and freeing the malleus from the remaining atretic plate. If necessary, a small fragment of atretic bone may be left attached to the malleus.

The shape and direction of the incus long arm are highly variable. What is important, however, is that the incus attaches to a stapes. The stapes superstructure may also be varied. In more extreme malformations, the superstructure may be monopedal with no connection to the incus. The mobility of the footplate must be determined. As mentioned earlier, congenital fixation of the stapes is found in 4% of cases. Conversely, congenital stapes fixation is common in minor ear malformations in which the problem is confined to the middle ear. This is not to say that the stapes is always of use to the

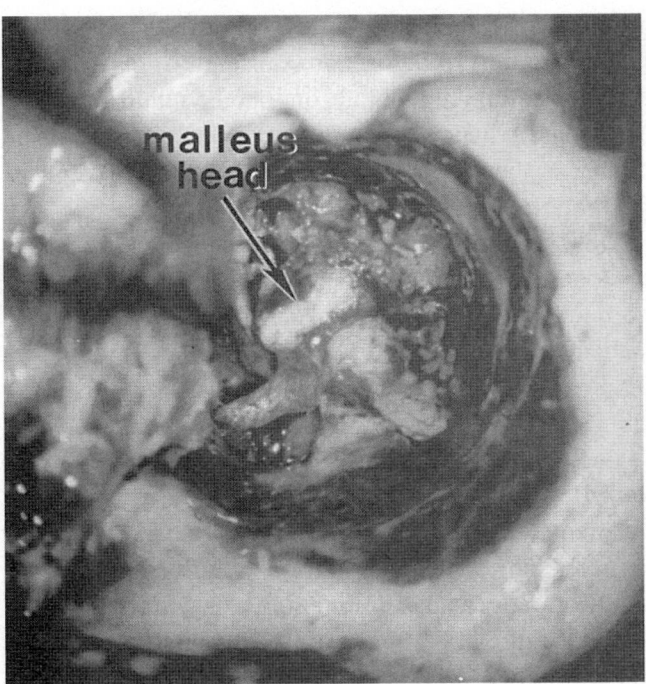

Figure 19–10 Atresia surgery of the left ear. Note the absent malleus handle, fused incus-malleus complex, and facial nerve.

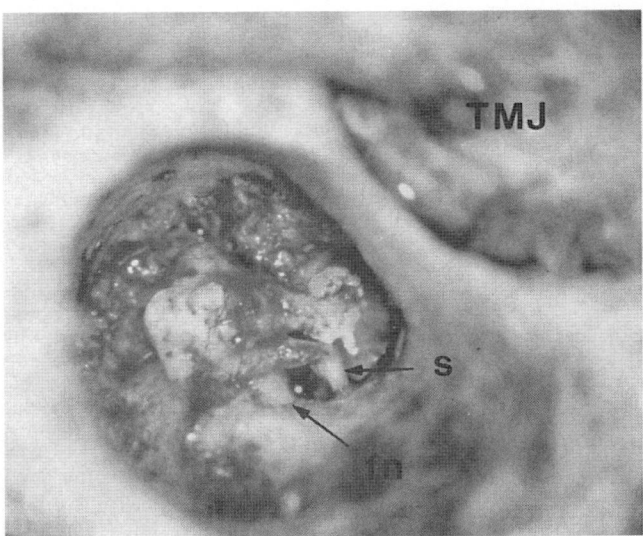

Figure 19–11 Atresia surgery of the right ear. Note the fairly well-formed ossicular chain, which was mobile. There is a fused incus and malleus. The periosteum has been left attached to the malleus handle. fn = facial nerve; s = stapes; TMJ = temporomandibular joint.

surgeon. The stapes may be markedly underdeveloped or even absent. However, this finding would have been noted on the preoperative CT scan, lowering the patient's score as a potential candidate for surgery.

It is common in congenital atresia to find a reasonably well-formed stapes with a mobile footplate. The oval window, in concert with the stapes footplate, may be smaller than normal, but this does not adversely affect either the reconstruction or the postoperative hearing result.

It may not be possible to visualize the round window. A sharp anterior bend to the facial nerve may prevent exposure of the round window. It is inadvisable to deliberately decompress and transpose the facial nerve simply to document the presence of a round window. Moreover, this information would have been gleaned from the preoperative CT scan.

The best possible circumstance in which to find the ossicles is for them to be intact (although malformed) and to move as a unit (Figure 19–11). In this condition, the fascia graft may be placed directly on the ossicular mass.

At this junction, an important step is undertaken that is critical to the success of the operation. This step entails drilling away bone peripherally to gain room for the placement of a new eardrum (fascia graft). The new tympanic membrane will be about 1 to 1½ times the diameter of a normal tympanic membrane. In drilling away bone peripherally, the surgeon is constrained in all directions: superiorly by the tegmen, anteriorly by the glenoid fossa, inferiorly by the facial nerve (if it takes a sharp bend), and posteriorly by the mastoid air cells. Failure to gain sufficient room compromises the hearing result.

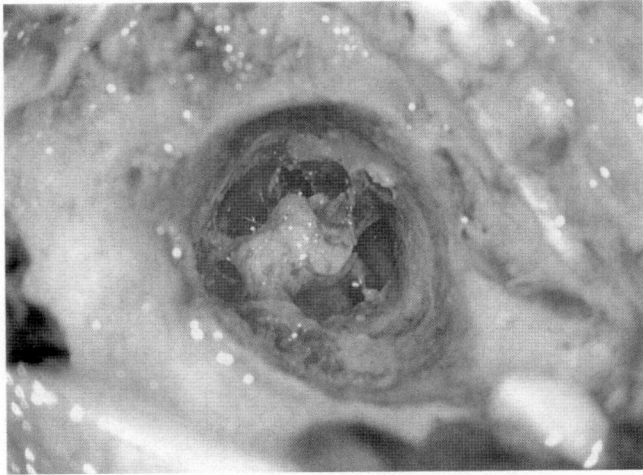

Figure 19–12 Atresia repair of the right ear. Note the fused incus/malleus and absent malleus handle.

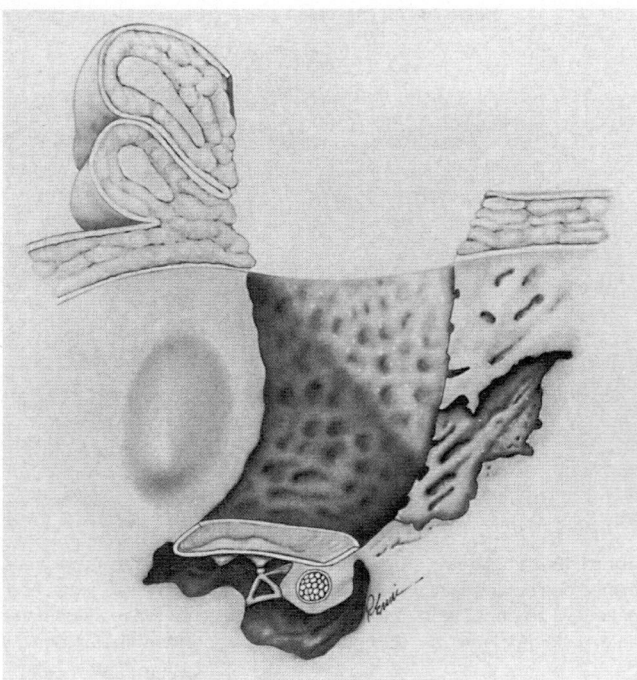

Figure 19–13 Illustration of atresia surgery showing placement of fascia graft for a new tympanic membrane.

tympanic membranes, it is my belief that the surgical technique described earlier consistently gives better hearing results. To reiterate, one should retain the ossicular mass whenever possible, and it should be positioned in the approximate center of the new tympanic membrane (Figure 19–12).

In preparation for placing the fascia graft for a new tympanic membrane, the anesthesiologist is instructed to decrease the expired oxygen to 25% or less. If a patient can be maintained on room air, that is preferable. Expired oxygen concentrations greater than 30% will almost routinely cause ballooning of the graft.

After harvesting the fascia graft, it is allowed to dry on a Petri dish. The fascia is cut to size—about 1.5 cm in diameter—and placed as an overlay graft on the ossicles. The edges of the fascia are reflected onto the new bony ear canal wall for a short distance only, about 2 mm (Figures 19–13 and 19–14). If the fascia is positioned higher, it serves as a barrier between the bare bone of the external ear canal and the skin graft. In this position, the fascia prevents blood vessels emanating from the bone from reaching the skin graft. This may delay or prevent vascularization of the skin graft and result in a devitalized area that will subsequently require débridement.

The ossicular mass should eventually be positioned in the approximate center of the new tympanic membrane. Although some surgeons advocate the use of homograft

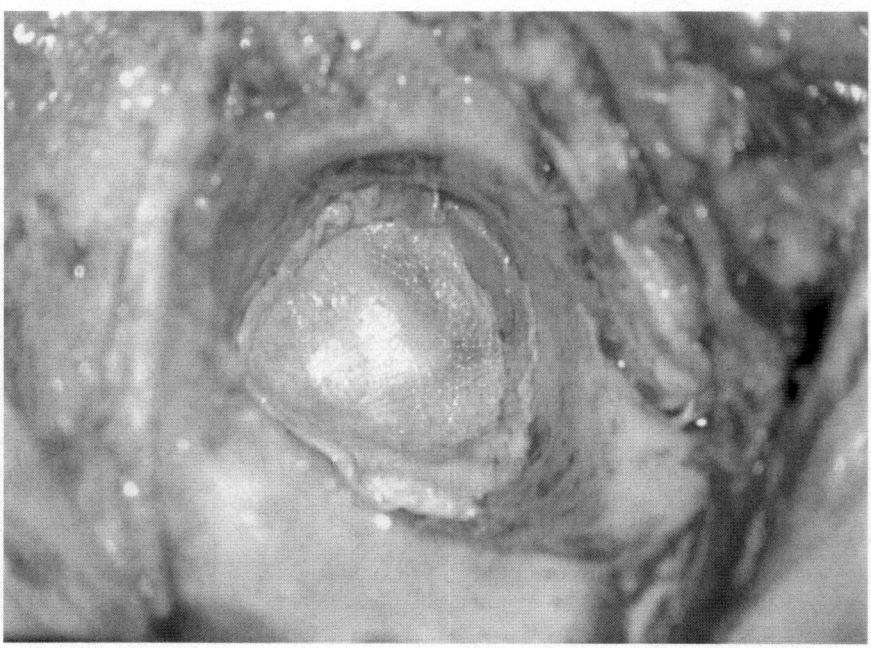

Figure 19–14 Same ear as in Figure 19–12. Note the malleus/incus complex beneath thin fascia graft.

Skin Graft

A split-thickness skin graft measuring 0.006 to 0.008 inches is harvested. The donor site depends on the surgeon's preference. The author prefers to use the medial aspect of the ipsilateral upper arm. The graft must be thin and should not contain hair follicles. A split-thickness skin graft that is thick has a tendency to curl at the edges. This tendency not only makes the graft more difficult to work with but creates a situation in which buried squamous epithelium may cause a cholesteatoma. If the skin graft is too thin, it withstands environmental abuse poorly. For example, although the author routinely allows patients to swim postoperatively, a graft that is too thin may slough after becoming wet.

When the skin graft is harvested, an uneven thickness to its parallel borders is frequently noted. In this case, the thinner border is used at the level of the eardrum, and the thicker border is sutured to the new meatus. The skin graft is cut to a size of 3 × 5 cm and notched (Figure 19–15). A final reduction in size is made if necessary by sharply trimming the edges of the skin graft once it has been positioned in the ear.

The skin graft is placed with the vertical slit facing anteriorly. This placement ensures that free edges will not grow into the mastoid air cells. The notched edges of the skin graft are reflected onto the fascia graft tympanic membrane (Figures 19–16 and 19–17).

The key to a successful hearing result is a thin tympanic membrane. A thick eardrum thwarts this goal. A Silastic button (1 mm thick) is cut to size and placed over the new tympanic membrane to hold the notched skin edges in place and prevent blunting. The Silastic button also gives the surgeon something to pack against and helps prevent displacement of the skin graft medially.

Packing is used in the ear canal to stabilize the skin graft. The author prefers to use Merocel® (Medtronic, Jacksonville, Fla.) wicks. The new ear canal is packed to the level of the bone opening. The skin graft is then folded over the packing, while the surgeon focuses attention on the meatus.

Meatoplasty

The meatoplasty is performed by first debulking the external ear posteriorly in the area where the new opening will be placed. This is unnecessary if the conchal bowl is deep. The external ear can be moved in any direction to align the ear canal with the new meatus. The ear will require relocation about half the time. Most often the direction in which the ear needs to be transposed is posterosuperior. The degree of transposition is a few mil-

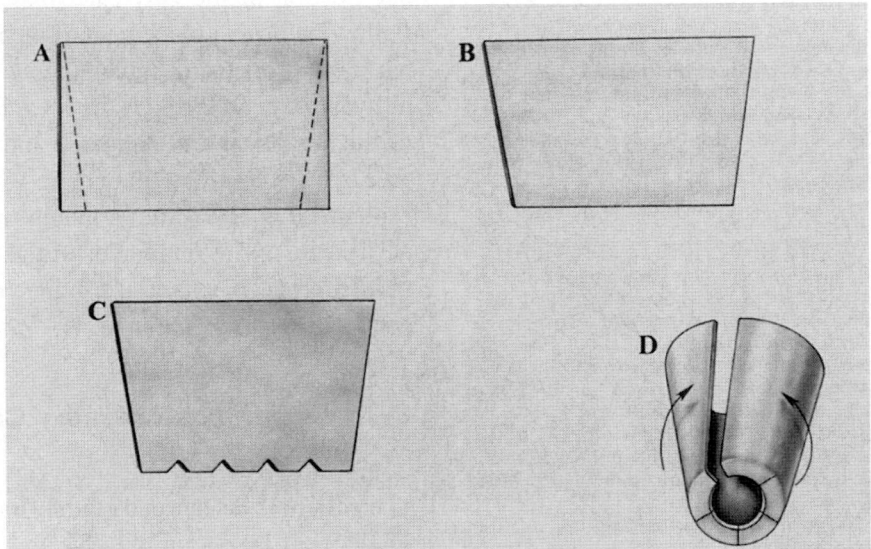

Figure 19–15 Preparation of split-thickness skin graft to line the new bony ear canal. Note that a center opening is no longer used, and the split-thickness skin graft covers the entire drum. The graft is placed on a derma carrier and shaped with a scapel as shown in steps A through D.

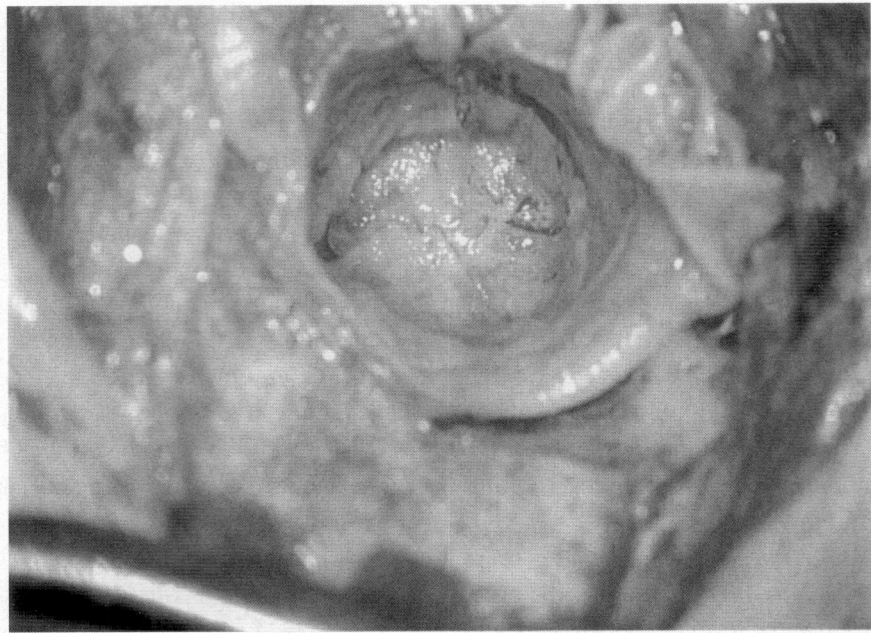

Figure 19–16 Same ear as in Figures 19–12 and 19–14. Note that skin tabs have been placed over fascia to provide a second epithelial layer to the tympanic membrane.

limeters to as much as 3 cm. As the ear is not yet tethered by an ear canal, this can be effected with relative ease.

The author now routinely develops a "U"-shaped pedicle flap hinged at the tragus. A marking pen is used to outline the flap, and an incision is made through the skin. A skin flap is raised from a posterior to anterior direction and left attached at the tragus. The underlying soft tissue is cored out using a #11 blade. This provides access to the new ear canal. The pedicle flap is then positioned into the new ear canal and sutured to a cuff of periosteum at the level of the glenoid fossa. The pedicle flap provides excellent skin coverage to the soft tissue portion of the new ear canal in its anterior part. Following proper placement of the meatus, the external ear is stabilized with subcutaneous sutures. Thereafter, all work is done through the meatus. The folded edges of the skin graft are identified and brought to the surface. Any excessive skin may be sharply excised. Interrupted 5.0 Vicryl sutures attach the skin graft to the new meatus. The remainder of the ear canal is packed with Merocel wicks and a bulky mastoid dressing is applied.

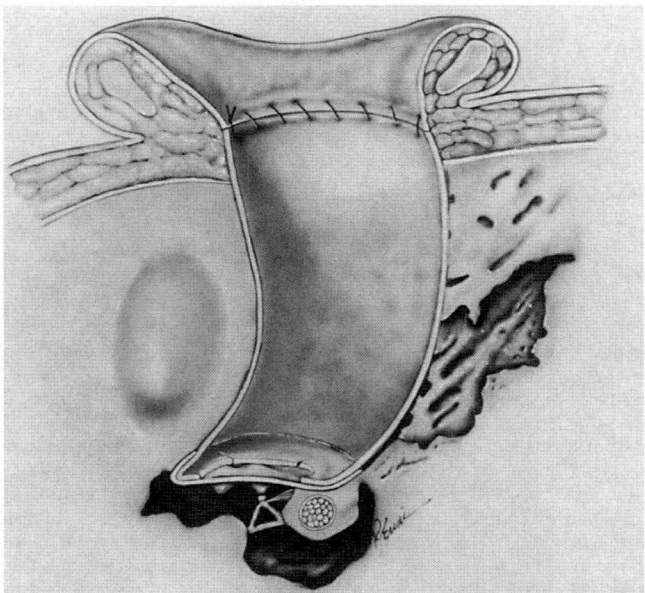

Figure 19–17 Skin graft in place. The center opening over the new tympanic membrane is no longer used.

Postoperative Care

The patient is discharged on the first postoperative day. The patient is seen in the office or clinic 1 week postoperatively, and all packing and sutures are removed. A corticosteroid antibiotic eardrop preparation is prescribed for 1 week. Thereafter, nothing is placed in the ear canal, and the canal is left open to the air. A second postoperative visit is made by the patient 3 weeks later. Extensive crusting will have occurred. However, beneath the crust there should be dry healthy skin. The skin graft is débrided and redundant skin folds are sharply excised if necessary. A postoperative audiogram may be obtained. Thereafter, the intervals between follow-up visits can be extended.

It is important that the patient be followed every 6 to 12 months indefinitely. Although the skin graft is healthy, it is not self-cleaning and must be carefully débrided of desquamated epithelium. Failure to adhere to this schedule may result in decreased hearing and chronic infec-tion. Postoperatively, the author places no restrictions on the patient. Swimming is permitted, but alcohol eardrops after each outing are advised.

REFERENCES

1. Jahrsdoerfer RA, Yeakley JW, Aguilar EA, et al. Grading sys-tem for the selection of patients with congenital aural atresia. Am J Otol 1992;13:6–12.

2. Kountakis SE, Helidonis E, Jahrsdoerfer RA. Microtia grade as an indication of middle ear development in aural atresia. Arch Otolaryngol Head Neck Surg 1995;121:885–6.

3. Jahrsdoerfer RA, Lambert PR. Facial nerve injury in congen-ital aural atresia surgery. Am J Otol 1998;19:283–7.

20

Closure of Tympanic Membrane Perforations

Spiros Manolidis, MD

HISTORICAL ASPECTS

From the seventeenth to the nineteenth centuries, several attempts at closing tympanic membrane perforations using prosthetic materials were made, culminating in the "paper patch" technique developed by Blake in 1887.[1-4] The use of cauterizing agents to promote healing of tympanic membrane perforations was introduced by Roosa in 1876, who used the application of silver nitrate to the rim of a perforation[5]; the use of trichloroacetic acid was first advocated in 1895. It was not until Joynt combined the cautery and paper patch techniques that closure results improved,[6] forming the basis of the modern-day use of the paper patch technique as popularized by Derlacki.[7]

The surgical repair of permanent tympanic membrane perforations was first attempted at the same time as the paper patch technique but did not produce adequate results until 1952, when Wullstein published a method of closing perforations with a split-thickness skin graft.[8] Only a year later, Zöllner described his experiences with a similar graft.[9] At the same time, Wullstein and Zöllner introduced the use of the operating microscope, significantly enhancing surgical results by improving the accuracy of the technique.

Problems with skin grafts as the closure material for tympanic membrane perforations soon became apparent, and in 1956, Zöllner first used fascia lata to close perforations.[10] In 1958, Heermann began to use temporalis fascia.[11] In 1960, Shea described the closure of tympanic membrane perforations using a vein graft.[12] The advantages of connective tissue over skin as a grafting material were confirmed by the higher percentage of successful closures; however, skin grafting of perforations was not completely abandoned. Meatal skin, which lacks glands and is elevated with the underlying periosteum, has distinct advantages over skin grafts, both full and split thickness, from other areas of the body. It has continued to be used in selective instances. In the 1960s and 1970s, homograft (cadaveric) materials, including tympanic membrane, dura, and pericardium, among others, were used with varying success.[13-18] None of these materials gained universal acceptance and today pose a problem because of the potential for transmitting disease (eg, Jakob-Creutzfeldt disease and HIV infection).

Temporalis fascia continues to be the material of choice for reconstruction of the tympanic membrane. Regardless of the technique employed, "take" rates of 93 to 97% are typically reported.[19,20] Certain refinements applicable in particular situations have diversified the types of tympanic membrane reconstructions that are part of our surgical armamentarium. Continuing improvement in surgical technology and a better understanding of wound healing will undoubtedly further improve our ability to reconstruct the tympanic membrane while reducing the magnitude of intervention required.

ETIOLOGY OF TYMPANIC MEMBRANE PERFORATIONS

Infectious

Bacterial

Bacterial infection of the middle ear causes acute otitis media, which often results in a small perforation through which purulent material discharges. These perforations heal spontaneously in a short time unless complicating factors coexist. Eustachian tube dysfunction is the major factor that results in a permanent perforation.[21,22] In such a middle ear, the mucous membrane is exposed to repeated infection, both through the external auditory canal and through the eustachian tube, with chronic continuous discharge or with recurring episodes of suppurative otitis media. Allergic sensitization of the exposed middle ear mucosa frequently occurs.[23,24] Such disease is termed active chronic otitis media without cholesteatoma. The incidence of this condition varies widely by geography, race, and genetic predisposition, as well as socioeconomic factors. Studies in the Caucasian population show the incidence to be approximately 2%.[25]

Beta-hemolytic streptococci are capable of inciting a necrotizing form of acute suppurative otitis media, especially in children suffering from measles or scarlet fever. The pathogenic characteristics of the infecting species of bacterium cause capillary infarction and subsequent ischemic necrosis of tissue. Thus, large portions of the tympanic membrane (where the blood supply is poorest) become necrotic and slough, usually leaving intact the better nourished annular rim, the area near the handle of the malleus, and the pars flaccida.[26] The resulting kidney-shaped perforation is called a central perforation because of the marginal rim that remains. After the acute episode of necrotizing otitis media has subsided, the perforation may heal spontaneously, leaving a thin atrophic scar, or may remain permanently open. The microcirculation of the middle ear also is disrupted, leading to tympanosclerosis, in which healing involves an ossification process with variable involvement of the middle ear structures.[27,28]

Mycobacterial

Mycobacterial infection of the tympanic membrane is primarily caused by *Mycobacterium tuberculosis* and, to a lesser degree, atypical mycobacteria. This condition manifests as a relentless, low-grade inflammation of the tympanic membrane that is refractory to conventional (oral or topical) antibiotic treatment. It eventually results in multiple small perforations that subsequently coalesce.[29]

TRAUMA

The incidence of traumatic perforations of the tympanic membrane has been estimated at 8.6 per 1,000 persons.[30] Three types of traumatic perforations can occur: penetrating, blunt, and iatrogenic. It is important to keep in mind that inner ear injury may accompany acute traumatic perforations, a possibility that should be evaluated by careful questioning for the presence of vertigo, hearing loss, tinnitus, or sound distortion. Physical examination should include a fistula test with pneumatic otoscopy. Audiometric evaluation is recommended to exclude the presence of sensorineural hearing loss and to document hearing status. The tympanic membrane has a great potential to heal such perforations without intervention; however, as a general rule, traumatic perforations that become infected will be permanent.

Penetrating Trauma

Penetrating trauma of the tympanic membrane occurs more commonly than expected, despite the protected location of the tympanic membrane. Most often it occurs as an inadvertent phenomenon from manipulation of the ear canal (eg, an accidental deep insertion of a probe such as a cotton swab). The vast majority of these perforations heal spontaneously or with minimal intervention; accordingly, the management of such perforations entails a period of observation, provided that injury to the labyrinth and ossicular chain has been ruled out.

An exception to this rule is the perforation caused by a hot slag seen in welders. These perforations do not heal spontaneously, possibly because of the devascularizing nature of the injury, and will require intervention subsequently.[31]

Blunt Trauma

Blunt trauma causing perforation of the tympanic membrane can result from sudden explosive or implosive alterations in air pressure in the vicinity of the patient such as blasts, firearm discharges, lightning strikes, or a direct slap to the auricle. In these situations, the vibratory force transmitted exceeds the mechanical capacity of the tympanic membrane with consequent rupture. The force required to rupture the tympanic membrane of cadavers has been estimated at 14 to 33 lb per square inch, which is equivalent to 195 dB.[32] Such perforations are stellate and are located in the central part of the tympanic membrane. Most such perforations heal spontaneously (generally within 1 month); thus, observation is recommended prior to any intervention. An exception to this general rule is any perforation that involves water entry, such as those seen in water sports (eg, water skiing). These perforations will become infected, resulting in a permanent perforation. Therefore, it is imperative to treat such perforations with antibiotics at presentation.[31]

Surgical Trauma

The most common surgical trauma resulting in tympanic membrane perforation is tympanostomy tube insertion.[33–35] The larger the diameter of the pressure-equalizing tube, the greater the incidence of perforation.[36] Similarly, the longer the ventilating tube remains in place, the higher the incidence of perforation.[37] In addition, underlying eustachian tube dysfunction increases the incidence of permanent perforation after ventilation tube removal.[38,39] Surgical trauma resulting in perforation may also occur with exploratory tympanotomy or transcanal stapedectomy, either as the result of improper identification of the sulcus with subsequent inadvertent dissection into the tympanic membrane or with poor technique in reflecting a tympanomeatal flap. Most of these perforations heal spontaneously but are best grafted (eg, with perichodrium or fascia) when identified during the initial operation.

PATHOLOGY OF TYMPANIC MEMBRANE PERFORATIONS

As documented in the experimental animal, proliferation of stratified squamous epithelium at the rim of a perforation begins within 12 hours, and granulation tissue growth begins at 36 hours.[40] Regeneration of the epithelium of the inner (mucosal) surface is more sluggish and begins only after several days. As long as there is a suitably flat surface, stratified squamous epithelium grows at the rate of 1 mm a day.[26]

Histopathologic examination of permanent perforations showed that stratified squamous epithelium grows medially over the edge of the perforation,[41–43] which appears to arrest the subsequent closure of the perforation. Removal of this medialized epithelium forms the basis of some of the treatments for tympanic membrane perforation. The cytokines implicated in this arrest of healing may be multiple, but transforming growth factor-β1 (TGF-β1) is found at the border of the chronic perforation and may mediate the arrest of healing.[41–43]

EFFECTS OF TYMPANIC MEMBRANE PERFORATIONS ON HEARING

A simple perforation of the tympanic membrane, with no additional lesion of the middle ear transformer mechanism, has two different effects on the hearing. First, there is the diminished surface area of tympanic membrane on which sound pressure is exerted, resulting in dampened ossicular chain excursion. For a small (1-mm) perforation, Békésy found that the effect on ossicular motion is confined to sounds below 400 Hz and is 12 dB at 100 Hz, 29 dB at 50 Hz, and 48 dB at 10 Hz.[44] The larger the perforation, the greater the loss of surface area on which sound pressure can act, with the additional factor that sound pressure entering the middle ear through the perforation can act on the posterior surface of the tympanic membrane against the sound pressure on the outer surface. In addition, the site of the perforation influences the degree of hearing loss; posterior perforations produce more severe hearing losses.[45]

A second effect of a simple perforation on hearing results from sound reaching the round window directly without the dampening and phase-changing effect of an intact tympanic membrane. Moreover, as the size of the tympanic membrane remnant decreases, the hydraulic advantage produced by a large tympanic membrane on a small oval window disappears, so that sound reaches both windows with more nearly equal force and at nearly the same time. The resultant cancellation of vibratory movement of the cochlear fluid column produces the maximum hearing loss observed in simple perforation, as much as 45 dB for the speech frequencies.[46,47]

Elimination of hearing loss by closure of a tympanic membrane perforation is not guaranteed. A persistent hearing loss may be caused by cochlear dysfunction and ossicular disruption, which contribute to the hearing loss caused by the perforation and are not addressed by the myringoplasty. A small perforation with a large audiometric air–bone gap likely reflects an ossicular chain problem and will most likely require correction by tympanoplasty. In general, the larger the perforation, the greater the hearing impairment, but this relationship is neither constant nor consistent in clinical practice; perforations seemingly identical in size and location produce different degrees of hearing loss.[47]

INDICATIONS FOR AND ADVANTAGES OF CLOSURE

Protection

Closing a tympanic membrane perforation isolates the middle ear from the external environment and prevents contamination by exposure to pathogens introduced via the external auditory canal. Repeated exposure to pathogens can lead to recurrent, acute otitis media with consequent permanent alteration of the middle ear and its sound-transmitting mechanism and/or active, chronic otitis media with otorrhea that is refractory to treatment.

Auditory

Closure of a tympanic membrane perforation restores the vibratory area of the membrane and affords round window protection, thus improving hearing and decreasing tinnitus; however, high-frequency audiometry demonstrates a persistent air–bone gap, despite successful closure of a perforation.[48] An approximate estimate of the improvement in hearing and tinnitus that may be expected from closure of a perforation is obtained by temporary patching with cigarette paper or cellophane. If a carefully applied airtight patch does not eliminate the conductive loss, one may assume that an additional ossicular lesion is present, either fixation or discontinuity. In such cases, simple myringoplasty will not suffice. Closure must be accompanied or followed by correction of the ossicular problem by tympanoplasty.

CONTRAINDICATIONS TO CLOSURE OF A PERFORATION

Not every perforation needs to, or should, be closed. Each patient must be managed in accordance with what is best for that patient. An elderly or debilitated patient with an asymptomatic perforation, or a patient with a perforation in an only hearing ear, is not a good surgical candidate. In a young child with a perforation from a ventilation tube inserted because of poor ear ventilation, it is unwise to repair the tympanic membrane until it is apparent that eustachian tube function has significantly improved lest the pathologic process repeat itself.

Absolute

The presence of cholesteatoma is an absolute contraindication for a myringoplasty. Active chronic otitis media with otorrhea refractory to medical management indicates the presence of an infectious focus, which needs to be surgically addressed prior to repair of the tympanic membrane. Medical contraindications to surgical intervention include advanced patient age. Last but not least, unrealistic patient expectations and/or the inability of the patient to understand the reasoning for the proposed intervention are contraindications for repairing a tympanic membrane through myringoplasty.

Relative

Eustachian tube dysfunction increases the chances of failure of myringoplasty. Myringoplasty in the only hearing ear should be evaluated carefully, and the potentially small risk of sensorineural hearing loss should be outweighed by the benefits of the operation. Such an example would be the presence of severe atelectasis, which has led to ossicular erosion, or atelectasis with changes indicating progression to cholesteatoma. Every attempt should be made to control allergies manifested by upper respiratory symptomatology that will increase the incidence of failure of myringoplasty.

MYRINGOPLASTY TECHNIQUES

Closure of Perforations by a Prosthesis

A paper disk, moistened on one side with a solution of 1% phenol in glycerin to make it adherent, is introduced with a small alligator-type forceps and teased into place with a tiny blunt ear hook or ring. After a week to 10 days, the patch migrates along with the exfoliated skin toward the external auditory meatus. Although patching is a temporary solution, it provides a measure of the improvement in hearing and tinnitus that the patient can expect with definitive repair and has been used in the past for this reason.

Splinting of Traumatic Perforations

A paper patch applied as a splint to a fresh traumatic perforation helps keep the edges approximated and prevents them from curling under. Since most traumatic perforations close spontaneously, no study has proven the utility of splinting; however, in large traumatic perforations and in perforations with inverted edges, splinting is helpful.[49] Splinting involves everting the margins of the perforation and supporting them by placing Gelfoam™ (Pharmacia-Upjohn, Kalamazoo, Michigan) into the middle ear through the perforation. A paper patch or additional Gelfoam can be used on the lateral surface of the tympanic membrane. Local anesthesia is required.

Technique of Closure by Promotion of Healing

Large perforations of the tympanic membrane heal by restoration of the epithelial layer only, producing a thin, atrophic tympanic membrane, termed a monomeric tympanic membrane, which is devoid of the middle fibrous elements that provide structural support. Although such a tympanic membrane is adequate for the purposes of sound conduction, it is vulnerable to repeated perforation by infection or eustachian tube dysfunction. The principle of closure by promotion of healing of the tympanic membrane involves inducing the fibrous layer to close the perforation prior to epithelial closure, restoring the normal anatomy of the tympanic membrane. An adequate trial of closure by acid cautery on several occasions, with or without marginal eversion, is an option for small and medium-sized central perforations before resorting to myringoplasty.[7]

Principles

- Based on the histopathology of perforations, the stratified squamous epithelium that has grown medially to cover the fibrous layer must be destroyed or removed, oftentimes repeatedly, to prevent it from obstructing healing by fibrous layer growth.
- The newly exposed fibroblasts at the rim of the perforation should be kept moist since desiccation kills the new fibroblasts but allows the stratified squamous epithelium to proliferate under the dry crust and bridge the defect to create a monomeric tympanic membrane.
- Mild irritation induces hyperemia and secondary fibroblast proliferation. Therefore, inducing hyperemia by mild irritation of the perforation is desirable.

Indications

Stable, small to medium-sized perforations in an ear with favorable external auditory canal dimensions and configuration are idea circumstances. The patient must be compliant and willing to participate in multiple treatments if necessary.

Contraindications

The presence of active infection or cholesteatoma is an absolute contraindication for this technique and, in general, for all techniques for myringoplasty. Ossicular chain abnormalities, if present, should be addressed through a tympanoplasty, with ossicular chain reconstruction. Patient noncompliance will guarantee the failure of this technique.

Technique

Anesthesia

Topical anesthesia of the perforation margins may be achieved by the application of 10% cocaine solution to the margins with a probe or with a cotton-tipped probe. Alternatively, topical application of phenol is expeditious because of the availability of prefabricated kits. Topical anesthesia by iontophoresis or the application of anesthetic creams that fill the ear canal is not recommended because of middle ear entry and alteration of the appearance of anatomic landmarks.

Cautery of Epithelium

Cautery of the perforation margin is accomplished with a saturated solution of trichloroacetic acid applied by a fine metal probe onto the end of which a "bead" of cotton is wound tightly. The trichloroacetic acid is then applied repeatedly until a white cauterized margin 0.5 mm in width is created. Care is taken not to cauterize the promontory. Derlacki,[7] who has the largest reported series, uses cautery alone to destroy the epidermis at the margin of the perforation.

Excision of the Epithelial Edge
Variations in this technique include the removal of the epithelial edge with the use of microhooks and micro-cupped forceps. This technique can be aided by the use of a very precise ophthalmology microblade (Beaver blade #5910).

Splinting and Aftercare
Repetition of the cautery at weekly intervals is required until a new, pink, and actively growing margin is seen around the entire perforation. The intervals may then be lengthened to 2 weeks as long as the margins continue to be active. Patching by a flat disk of cotton kept moist by eardrops twice daily is necessary to keep the cauterized edge from drying. Alternatively, Gelfoam and eardrops may be used.

Results
Closure is more likely when the perforation is small or medium in size and involves no more than 65% of the pars tensa. Eversion or cautery of the edges of the perforation produces similar success rates, approaching 90% after an average of 3.7 treatments per patient.[50,51] Derlacki[7] reported closure in 75% of 131 perforations, some as large as four-fifths of the pars tensa; 9 spontaneously reperforated and 8 of these were successfully closed again. The quickest closure in this series needed only two treatments, whereas the longest required 64 treatments.[7] All reports emphasized the need for persistence by both patient and physician if a high closure rate is to be realized.

MYRINGOPLASTY

The term myringoplasty is reserved for the simple repair of a tympanic membrane perforation in which no ossicular reconstruction is involved. Fascia is the graft material of choice, although perichondrium obtained from the tragus produces the same success rates; however, peri-

chondrium is not transparent and hinders future examination of the middle ear. Two basic grafting techniques have emerged, referred to as the overlay and undersurface (or medial onlay) techniques.

Patient Selection

Regardless of the grafting technique chosen, the preoperative evaluation and management of the patient with a tympanic membrane perforation remain the same. A proper history with sufficient detail as it relates to the tympanic membrane perforation is necessary as is a thorough examination of the ear in question under the examining microscope. A complete head and neck examination is essential in identifying risk factors for failure of the proposed myringoplasty. The record should document the findings, preferably diagramming the perforation in question; current technology enables the physician to obtain a high-quality photograph of the otoscopic findings. All patients should undergo pure-tone air and bone conduction audiometric testing along with speech discrimination evaluation. Tuning fork tests should be done on all patients to confirm the audiologic findings. If there is disagreement between the tuning fork examination and the audiogram, then the latter should be repeated. High-resolution computed tomographic (CT) scanning of the temporal bone is not indicated unless there is a suspicion of underlying pathology or separate indicators from the problem at hand such as revision surgery in association with chronic otorrhea.

The patient is counseled preoperatively as to the nature of the problem, the proposed treatment and alternative therapies, expected outcome, and potential complications. It is helpful to provide written explanations and instructions discussing pre- and postoperative care of the ear. Videotaped discussions of the proposed procedure are also useful.

The following factors must be considered and dealt with preoperatively.

Eustachian Tube Function
Assessing the function of the eustachian tube is difficult. Conflicting evidence exists in the literature as to the importance of eustachian tube function for the success of tympanic membrane repair,[52–56] reflecting the inac-

curacy of the methods available to assess the function of the eustachian tube.[57,58] From a practical point of view, one of the most useful indications of proper eustachian tube function is a normal contralateral ear.[59] Bilateral pathology is associated with decreased success of surgical intervention, especially in children.[59] Although a functioning eustachian tube is important to the success of the operation, a lack of eustachian tube function should not preclude surgical intervention. In fact, eustachian tube function may improve once the infection is removed and the middle ear space reconstructed through normalization of the mucosal inflammation seen in the presence of a perforation.[20,60]

Control of Infection

Eradication or control of active infection in the ear under question is crucial. Repeat visits for proper aural toilet and monitoring of improvement in otorrhea should be instituted prior to any consideration of surgery. The patient is instructed to irrigate the ear three times a day with a sterile 1.5% acetic acid solution using a small rubber bulb ear syringe. This procedure allows purulent material to be removed from the middle ear and external canal and restores a more physiologic pH. It is important that the solution be used at body temperature to avoid caloric stimulation of the labyrinth. Following acetic acid irrigation, three drops of an antibiotic otic solution are instilled into the ear. Depending on the severity of the infection, systemic oral antibiotics may also be prescribed. The fluid from draining ears is not routinely cultured because the majority will respond to local care. If the ear continues to drain despite aggressive medical treatment, culture and sensitivity testing is performed and the antibiotic regimen adjusted appropriately. The majority of patients will respond to this treatment. If treatment fails, consideration should be given to other factors such as patient compliance, mastoid involvement, severe allergies, and/or incomplete treatment of the offending organism(s).

Perioperative Antibiotics

In the absence of signs of active infection (purulent otorrhea), the perioperative administration of systemic antibiotics does not influence the results of myringoplasty.[61,62] Furthermore, perioperative antibiotics do not prevent the emergence of bacterial pathogens in the postoperative period.[63] Similarly, the presence of nonpurulent otorrhea preoperatively does not indicate the presence of pathogenic bacterial flora in the middle ear and external auditory canal.[63]

Control of Allergies and Rhinosinusitis

Every attempt is made to identify and treat coexistent inhalant allergies and sinus disease prior to surgery. The status of the upper respiratory tract directly influences eustachian tube function and therefore the eventual outcome of surgery. Therefore, a trial of antihistamines and/or nasal corticosteroid sprays may be indicated empirically based on the history and examination. If there is a strong history of allergies, skin testing with targeted desensitization should be considered.

Age of Patient

The success of tympanic membrane repair in the pediatric age group has been reported from as low as 35% to as high as 93%.[35,54,56,59,64–67] The consensus holds that myringoplasty in the pediatric age group has a lower success rate than in the adult age group.[56] The reasons for this discrepancy are not clear but may be related to the higher incidence of otitis media and its predisposing factors in children.

In children, it is best to avoid elective surgery for myringoplasty between the ages of 4 and 7 years because of the risk of otitis media and from a psychological point of view. At age 8 years and thereafter, the child should participate in the decision process for such elective surgery.

Status of Contralateral Ear

If the ear under question is the only hearing ear, no attempt should be made to repair a tympanic membrane perforation. A small but real risk of sensorineural hearing loss does exist with myringoplasty. The rate of such hearing loss has been reported to range from 0.1 to 2%.[68]

Often the contralateral ear may be involved by similar pathology. The choice of which ear to repair is then dependent on hearing status—the worse hearing ear should be operated first. An exception to this rule is a pathologic condition in a better hearing contralateral ear that threatens hearing or health such as cholesteatoma, active infection such as mastoiditis, or significant atelectasis with likely progression to cholesteatoma or ossicular chain erosion.

Hearing Status/Need for Hearing Aids

If there are bilateral perforations, with significant conductive hearing loss in the absence of otorrhea, hearing aid fitting may be preferable for children under the age of 8 years. If otorrhea is provoked by hearing aid use in this situation, the worse hearing ear should be repaired first.

A wet ear in and of itself is not a contraindication to myringoplasty, although purulent otorrhea is a contraindication. A wet ear should not be an absolute contraindication for myringoplasty, provided that factors such as allergies, eustachian tube function, and superinfection have been controlled. In selected patients, a mastoidectomy may be considered as an adjunct to the myringoplasty that can improve the success rate.[69,70]

Operative Technique

Patient Positioning

For the surgeon to accomplish the goal of grafting, the head must be positioned so that the ear canal can be viewed throughout its length while the surgeon is seated comfortably. Therefore, the angulation of the external auditory canal, location of the perforation, and local anatomy of the external auditory canal should be taken into consideration. Adjustments can then be made to achieve optimal position for myringoplasty.

Bringing the patient close to the edge of the bed prevents the surgeon from overextending his/her hands, thus increasing stability. It also assists in correct upright posture. The patient's arm on the operating side should be padded and tucked close to the body. This assists in visualizing the tympanic membrane when the canal has a superior angulation. Additionally, it provides an increased view of the anterior/superior tympanic membrane quadrant. The patient's head should be placed on a doughnut-shaped pillow approximately 3 to 4 inches thick. Care should be taken to ensure that the contralateral ear is not folded. This arrangement provides stability for the patient's head and allows the head to be rotated along the neck axis. Rotation toward the surgeon increases the view of the posterior quadrants, while rotation away from the surgeon increases the view of the anterior quadrants. Extending the patient's neck increases the visibility of the superior aspect of the tympanic membrane. Placing a folded blanked or a silicon gel roll under the patient's shoulders provides increased room for neck extension, which results in a more comfortable working position for the surgeon under the microscope by avoiding an extreme caudad placement of the microscope head in order to visualize the superior aspect of the tympanic membrane and ear canal.

A hydraulic chair without armrests greatly assists the surgeon by allowing better angles of approach with minimal repositioning. An operating table that can rotate about its long axis assists in obviating the need of the surgeon to change position and facilitates achieving the desired angle of exposure with less effort.

Finally, the patient's head needs to be placed at the foot of the bed so there is adequate room for the surgeon's legs beneath the table. The anesthesiologist should be at the foot of the bed. This positioning requires longer ventilation tubing and intravenous lines. The blood pressure cuff should be placed on the arm contralateral to the surgeon.

Skin Preparation and Sterility

If a postauricular approach is anticipated, or if fascia will be harvested, a small area of skin must be shaved so that approximately 2 to 3 cm of hairless skin are visible. The shaved hair is removed with adhesive tape. The skin is then cleaned and degreased using acetone and allowed to dry. Tincture of benzoin or adhesive spray is applied close to the hairline and around the auricle and allowed to dry thoroughly. Self-adhesive plastic drapes, cut in 10- to 15-cm strips, are applied precisely over the area of adhesive around the auricle, ensuring that 2 cm of skin remain exposed. The circulating nurse injects the postauricular region and tragus with a 2% lidocaine with 1:100,000 epinephrine solution. This procedure allows adequate time for the epinephrine to diffuse through the tissues, thereby reducing the amount of bleeding encountered at the time of incision. The auricle and external auditory canal are prepared with a sterilizing solution of the surgeon's preference or as per operating room routine. The external auditory canal is flushed with isopropyl alcohol (or povidone-iodine [Betadine] solution—surgeon's preference) and then sterile saline.

Sterile sponges are used to dry the auricle and adhesive drapes by gently dabbing and then discarding them from the field. The operative site is draped with a specialty drape prefabricated with a hole for the auricle and adhesive that approximates the underlying plastic drapes.

Final Preparation

Once the instruments, cautery, suction, and irrigation have been set up by the scrub nurse, the operating microscope is brought into position and the external auditory canal is inspected. The canal is then copiously irrigated with lactated Ringer's solution, and any debris and remaining fluid are removed. A small suction is used and is carefully held in a stable position distally in the canal close to the perforation so that a stream of continuous irrigation with distal to proximal flow is created. This positioning also avoids the danger of "bleb" formation on the external auditory canal skin, which will hinder exposure.

Anesthesia

The four quadrants of the cartilaginous external auditory canal and the "vascular strip" region of the bony canal are injected with a 2% lidocaine with 1:50,000 epinephrine solution. The local anesthetic reduces pain, decreasing the requirements for general anesthetic.

In the underlay technique, no limitation on the use of nitrous oxide during graft placement is necessary, whereas in the overlay technique, nitrous oxide should be discontinued during and after graft placement.

It is necessary to extubate the patient while still deeply anesthetized to avoid straining and potentially detrimental Valsalva's maneuver efforts.

Postoperative nausea and vomiting are avoided by the administration of antiemetics, tailored to the specific requirements of the patient based on the previous history of anesthetic reaction and the anesthesiologist's preference. Dopamine agonists such as ondansetron, butyrophenones such as droperidol, phenothiazines such as promethazine hydrochloride (Phenergan®), and/or a pulse dose of corticosteroids can avert this potentially damaging problem.

Overlay Technique of Myringoplasty

The following steps are the basic building blocks of the overlay myringoplasty surgical technique:

Surgical Technique

1. *A postauricular incision to harvest temporalis fascia.* Once the ear canal and postauricular area have been injected, an incision is made above and posterior to the auricle to obtain temporalis fascia.

2. *A series of transmeatal canal incisions that preserve but elevate the vascular strip.* A vascular strip is then created in the external auditory canal by making incisions at the tympanosquamous and tympanomastoid suture lines. These incisions converge near the annulus, and then a circumferential incision is made anteriorly at the level of the bony-cartilaginous junction.

3. *An optional full postauricular incision for exposure through a postauricular approach.*

4. *Removal of the anterior canal skin.* The skin of the anterior ear canal is dissected and removed as a free graft.

5. *Enlargement of the ear canal by removal of the anterior external auditory canal bulge.* This can be performed with the otologic drill or a curette, and care must be taken not to enter the temporomandibular joint or to injure the vascular strip.

6. *De-epithelialization of the tympanic membrane remnant.* The remnant of the tympanic membrane and malleus handle requires meticulous de-epithelialization.

7. *Placement and proper positioning of the fascia graft.* The fascia is prepared for insertion after a slit is placed into the graft so that it can accommodate the malleus handle lateral to the graft. The fascia may be left in its dehydrated state or slightly moistened. The fascia is then placed medial to the malleus handle, the skin of the vascular strip overlying its posterior edge.

8. *Replacement of the anterior external auditory canal skin as a free graft.* The canal skin is replaced into the ear, either totally over the fascia or back into its original position.

9. *Closure of the postauricular incision and replacement of the vascular strip transmeatally.* The vascular strip is replaced, and the ear canal is packed with Gelfoam pledgets soaked either in Tis-U-Sol® or in an antibiotic eardrop solution.

Postoperative Care

A mastoid dressing is applied for the first 24 hours postoperatively if a postauricular approach has been used. All patients are discharged on the day of surgery unless there are specific medical contraindications, or the patient is experiencing uncontrolled postoperative nausea and vomiting. Postoperatively, the patient is placed on topical antibiotics, which begin on the second week to soften the Gelfoam in the external auditory canal. The patient is then seen at the office in 4 to 6 weeks for follow-up examination. Complete epithelialization may not take place for 6 to 8 weeks.

Potential Pitfalls

There are several postoperative complications that may occur with the overlay procedure.

ANTERIOR ANGLE BLUNTING. Blunting of the anterior sulcus is the most frequent and bothersome complication with this technique. It can be so excessive as to fix the malleus handle and produce a significant conductive hearing loss, and is difficult to correct secondarily. Attention to detail with graft placement is important to avoid this problem. Compressed Gelfoam should be placed firmly against the annulus at the anterior sulcus, and the skin graft should reach its normal anatomic position at the annulus.

EPITHELIAL PEARLS. Another difficulty with the overlay technique is the inability of the surgeon to completely remove all of the squamous epithelium in denuding the drum remnant. Epithelial pearls can therefore arise anywhere in the new drumhead. Meticulous attention to removal of all epithelium from the remaining drumhead wholly avoids this problem.

GRAFT LATERALIZATION. Lateral migration of the tympanic membrane away from the malleus handle, resulting in a conductive hearing loss, may occur later and is most frequently seen when the graft is placed lateral to the malleus handle rather than medial to it. The graft should always be placed medial to the malleus handle when this technique is used.

PROLONGED HEALING. One other problem commonly associated with this technique is the relatively long duration of the healing process. Because the canal skin is completely removed and replaced as a free graft, there is a tendency for the ear to epithelialize slowly. The ear may easily take 6 weeks to heal completely.

If the blunting and lateralization are kept to a minimum, the hearing results of the overlay procedure can be quite good. The overlay technique is ideally suited for large central perforations in which minimal de-epithelialization is required. A prominent anterior bulge of the bony external auditory canal may also lend itself to this technique. Take rates are excellent and account for the popularity of this procedure early in the historical course of myringoplasty surgery.

Undersurface Technique of Myringoplasty

Connective tissue grafts (fascia, vein, and perichondrium) first began to be used in the late 1950s and early 1960s. With these tissues, it became possible to place the grafting material medial to the drum remnant rather than on top of it. In contrast, the overlay technique had its origin in the early days of myringoplasty when skin of various types was used to close the perforation. The concept of placing the graft medial to the drum remnant was first introduced by Shea and Tabb.[12,71,72] Their procedures were identical, employed vein as the grafting material, and were performed through an endomeatal (transcanal) approach.

The endomeatal approach starts with raising a tympanomeatal flap, with visualization through an aural speculum, just as one would for stapedectomy. The rim of the perforation must be excised and the undersurface of the drum remnant denuded of squamous epithelium. The middle ear is then packed with Gelfoam, and the graft is placed medial to the perforation. The Gelfoam holds the graft against the undersurface while epithelialization is taking place. The new drum is usually healed in 1 to 3 weeks.

There are several problems associated with the endomeatal undersurface (medial onlay) technique. First, unless the surgeon is experienced with the stapedectomy operation, he/she will not work well through a speculum. Second, if the external auditory canal is small and tortuous, it is extremely difficult to prepare the drum remnant or annulus, and graft placement is not as precise as it should be. For these reasons, the take rate for endomeatal undersurface grafting has never been as good as that obtained by the average surgeon using the overlay procedure.

By routinely approaching the ear through a postauricular incision, it is possible to work transmeatally without requiring a speculum, thus eliminating the technical difficulties of the endomeatal undersurface technique while combining the advantages of both undersurface and overlay techniques. Exposure is improved, graft placement is therefore more exact, and the resulting take rates are significantly better.

Surgical Technique

The procedure is performed in the following manner. The ear canal and postauricular area are injected with a 2% lidocaine with 1:100,000 epinephrine solution. Working endomeatally through a speculum, a vascular strip is outlined by making incisions at the tympanosquamous and tympanomastoid suture lines using a #67 Beaver knife blade. In addition, small inferiorly and superiorly based flaps are created by making right-angle incisions to the vascular strip incisions. The medial end of the vascular strip is formed by connecting the two primary incisions with a #72 Beaver blade approximately 2 mm lateral to the annulus (Figure 20–1, A).

A postauricular incision is made about 3 mm behind the postauricular crease using a #15 scalpel blade. The incision is made with the dominant surgeon's hand while the nondominant hand vigorously pulls the ear laterally. This manual retraction facilitates the rapid identification, without disruption, of the areolar tissue immediately lateral to the temporalis fascia (Figure 20–1, B).

Two Senn retractors placed in the superior aspect of the postauricular incision expose the areolar tissue, which is injected with anesthetic solution and incised along the linea temporalis. The areolar tissue is carefully harvested using nontoothed forceps and a fresh #15 scalpel blade to dissect the areolar tissue from the temporalis fascia. The angle of the blade is approximately 15 to 20 degrees with respect to the temporalis fascia. In this way, inadvertent perforation of the graft is prevented, and since the temporalis fascia is resilient, it guides the dissecting scalpel; a large piece of areolar tissue can be harvested without disturbing the temporalis fascia. The harvested graft is placed on a polytef (Teflon™) block, teased out to a thin uniform layer, and set on the back table under a heating lamp to dry to the consistency of parchment paper (Figure 20–1, C).

MIDDLE EAR EXPOSURE. Subsequently, a T-shaped incision is made through the subcutaneous tissue and periosteum to the bone overlying the mastoid and linea temporalis (see Figure 20–1, C). A Lempert elevator is used to mobilize the periosteum to the level of the ear canal. The vascular strip is then identified from posteriorly, elevated from the ear canal, and brought backward by grasping it with an Adson forceps. The postauricular incision, along with the vascular strip, is held open with a self-retaining retractor (Figure 20–1, D). A second self-retaining retractor can then be placed perpendicular to the first for additional exposure. The surgeon can now work with both hands, free of the constraints of the ear speculum. The ear canal is copiously irrigated with a physiologic saline solution to remove blood and debris.

With a 20-gauge needle suction in the left hand and a House #2 lancet knife in the right, the skin of the inferior ear canal is elevated down to the fibrous annulus, creating an inferiorly based flap. Next, a House #1 (sickle) knife is used to develop a superior flap just above the short process of the malleus. The fibrous annulus is mobilized out of its sulcus and displaced anterior to the malleus. The undersurface of the drum remnant is then denuded using a sickle knife and a cupped forceps (Figure 20–1, E and F). The manubrium of the malleus is denuded, preserving the fibrous annulus.

Working through the postauricular exposure, the surgeon can obtain an excellent view of the anterior annulus simply by rotating the patient away. Even with a prominent anterior canal wall bulge, it is seldom necessary to remove bone in this area to see the annulus. Hemostasis should be achieved prior to graft placement with Gelfoam saturated in 1:1,000 epinephrine packed into the middle ear space while the graft is being trimmed. The dried areolar tissue graft is removed from the polytef block and trimmed to size (approximately $2\frac{1}{2} \times 1\frac{1}{2}$ cm). A slit is made in the superior aspect of the graft to accommodate placement medial to the manubrium. The epinephrine-soaked gelatin sponge is removed and the middle ear space is filled with Gelfoam soaked in Tis-U-Sol (Figure 20–1, G). Particular care should be exercised in packing the middle ear with Gelfoam. Packing should start at the eustachian tube region and proceed posteriorly. Adequate Gelfoam should be used in the eustachian tube region to avoid medial collapse of the graft anteriorly, which results in failure. With a 22-gauge suction in one hand and

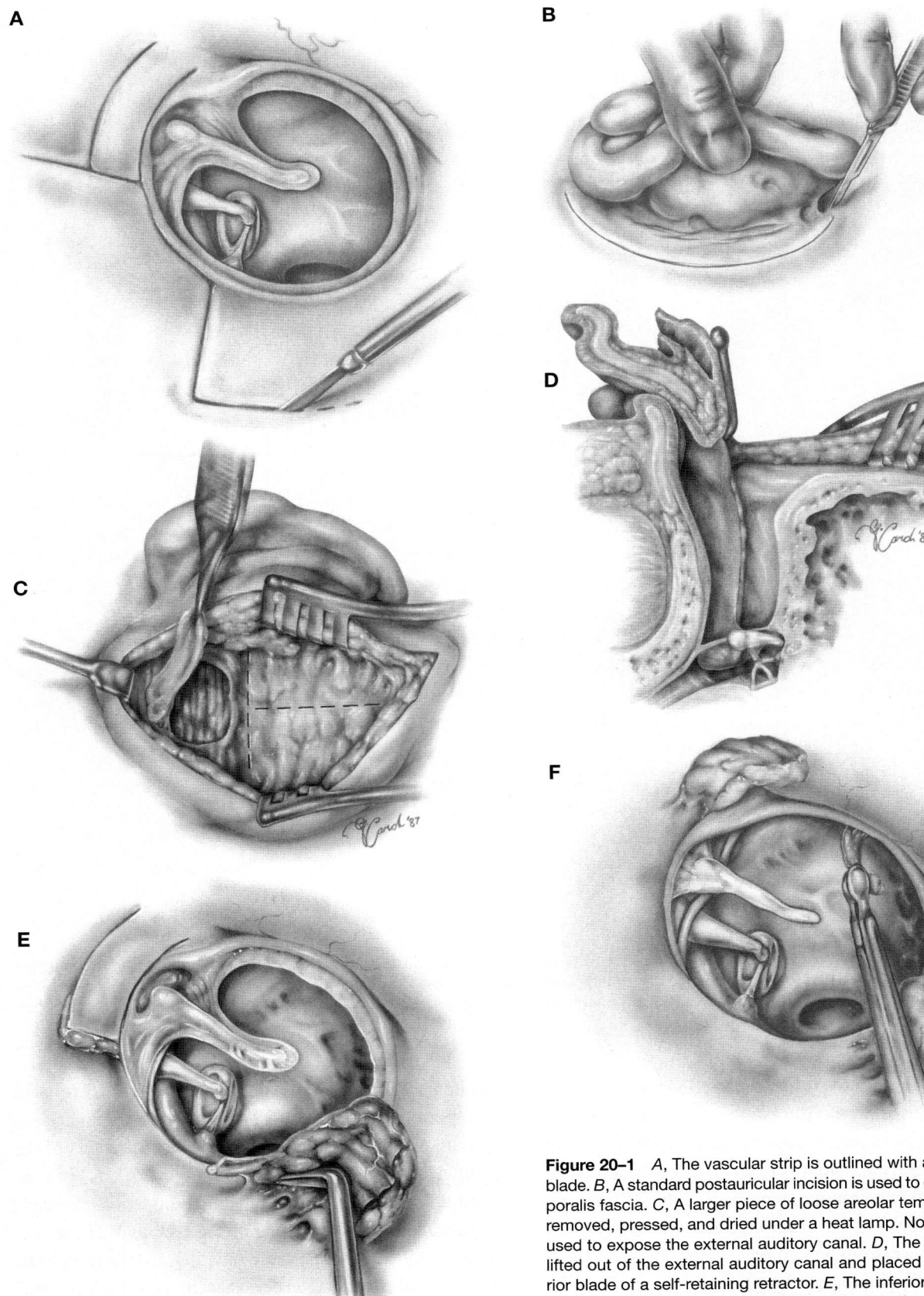

Figure 20–1 *A,* The vascular strip is outlined with a No. 67 Beaver blade. *B,* A standard postauricular incision is used to expose the temporalis fascia. *C,* A larger piece of loose areolar temporalis fascia is removed, pressed, and dried under a heat lamp. Note the T incision used to expose the external auditory canal. *D,* The vascular strip is lifted out of the external auditory canal and placed under the anterior blade of a self-retaining retractor. *E,* The inferior flap is elevated to the fibrous annulus with a House No. 2 knife. *F,* Cup forceps remove mucosa from under the fibrous annulus.

Illustration continued on following page.

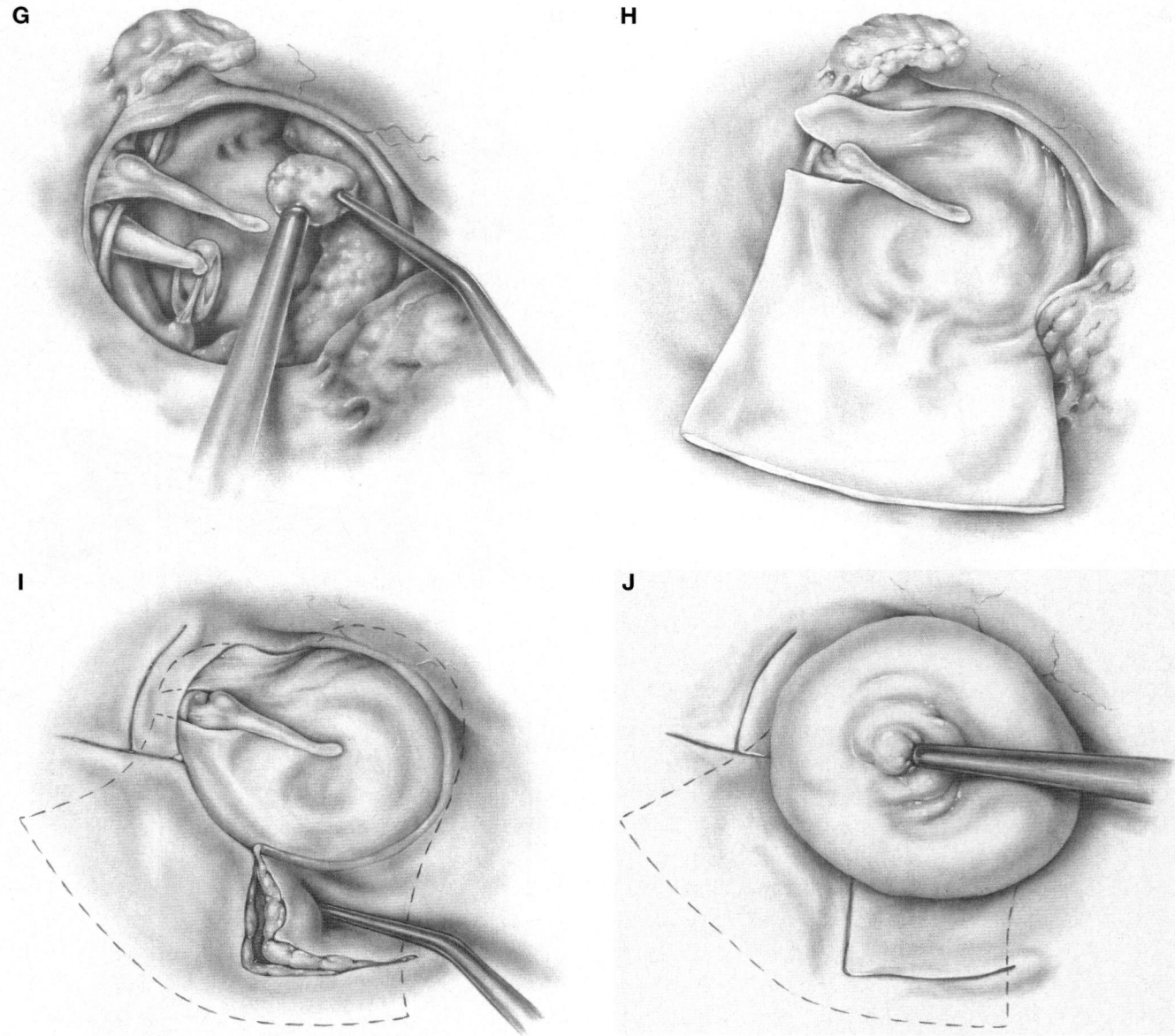

Figure 20–1   Continued. *G*, Moist absorbable gelatin sponge (Gelfoam) is packed into the entire middle ear space, starting in the eustachian tube orifice. *H*, The graft is placed into the middle ear so that it lies under the annulus anteriorly. *I*, When the inferior and superior flaps are replaced, the graft is held securely in position. *J*, The ear canal is filled with polymyxin B and bacitracin (Polysporin) ointment instead of packing at the end the procedure.

a right-angle hook in the other, the graft is slid medial to the manubrium and onto the lateral attic wall. A House annulus elevator is used to tuck the graft under the drum remnant anteriorly and inferiorly under direct vision. With the medial onlay technique, there is a point (at approximately 6 o'clock) in the inferior canal where the graft makes a transition from lying medial to the annulus to resting lateral to it. The remaining graft is draped along the posterior canal wall, and the inferior canal flap with

attached annulus is repositioned over the graft. Similarly, the superior flap is replaced, covering the graft anterior to the malleus. A gimmick is used to even all edges of the annulus and smooth out the graft (Figure 20–1, H to J).

Antibiotic ointment is placed into the anterior sulcus and the vascular strip is replaced into the ear canal. The retractors are removed, and the vascular strip is carefully replaced in its original position. The periosteal incision is closed with 3-0 absorbable suture in a purse-string fashion. The postau-

Author/Year	Patients	Technique	Result/Success, %	Comments
Sheehy, 1980	472	Overlay	97	88% > 10 dB No long-term follow-up
Tos, 1980	387	Mostly overlay	91.2	Long-term results >3-yr follow-up
Glasscock, and colleagues 1982	1556	Underlay	92	Long-term follow-up 663 tympanoplasties
Vartiainen, 1993	404	Underlay and overlay	88	Mean follow-up 5½ yr
Gersdorff, and colleagues 1995	320	Formaldehyde fascia	87.7	48% follow-up at 1 yr
Kotecha, and colleagues 1999	1,070	Underlay 92 Overlay 3.2	82	Audit of 405 surgeons

Table 20–1   RECENT SERIES OF MYRINGOPLASTY WITH NOTES ON THEIR AUTHORS' TECHNIQUE PREFERENCE AND RESULTS ACHIEVED

ricular incision is approximated with absorbable suture in an interrupted simple fashion using a subcuticular closure. Through an aural speculum, the position of the vascular strip can be checked and adjusted and the remainder of the ear canal filled with antibiotic ointment. A cotton ball is placed in the meatus and a mastoid dressing is applied.

Postoperative Care

On the first postoperative day, the mastoid dressing is removed. A fresh cotton ball is placed in the meatus of the ear canal to absorb the ointment as it liquefies. Patients are instructed to change the cotton ball at least three times per day and whenever it becomes soiled. Once the drainage stops, the cotton is discontinued, and the ear is allowed to ventilate. In the event that purulent discharge occurs, antibiotic otic drops are started and continued until the first postoperative visit. The patient is instructed regarding precautions to keep the ear dry and is advised to avoid nose blowing and the use of drinking straws. Follow-up is at 3 weeks. Each individual is counseled as to the warning signs of infection and instructed to contact the surgeon's office immediately should these occur. A prescription for a mild narcotic analgesic is given for a limited period of time. Antibiotics are not routinely prescribed unless there is an active infection at the time of surgery or other circumstances dictating their use.

By the first postoperative visit, the postauricular wound should be well healed, the ear canal free of ointment, and the tympanic membrane epithelialized. If the graft is intact but not completely epithelialized at the time of the first postoperative visit, antimicrobial drops or a vinegar-alcohol solution should be used for 1 to 3 weeks to promote healing. Although frank graft failure is a rarity, a small area of residual perforation will occasionally be found. If this occurs, the edges can be cauterized with trichloroacetic acid and then covered with a cigarette paper patch. If revision surgery is necessary, it should be delayed for at least 3 months to allow for resolution of postoperative inflammatory changes.

All simple myringoplasty patients undergo pure-tone audiometric testing at this or a subsequent visit. By 6 weeks, the grafted drum has thinned considerably and takes on the appearance of a normal tympanic membrane. Follow-up visits are arranged at 6 and 12 months; thereafter, the patient is seen at yearly intervals.

Results of Underlay Postauricular Myringoplasty

Early results for both the undersurface postauricular approach and the overlay techniques in the hands of expert surgeons show success rates of over 95%.[19,20] Others authors have repeatedly confirmed the high success rates in myringoplasty (summarized in Table 20–1).[20,22,68,73,74] Long-term results show a slight deterioration, but the overall success rates are maintained close to 90%.[13] More significantly, the undersurface postauricular approach to myringoplasty significantly reduces the problems of blunting, lateralization, pearl formation, and delayed healing associated with the overlay technique. It is particularly suited for surgeons who do not have extensive otologic experience or a high volume of otologic cases. Surgeon experience is known to be a significant factor in the success rate of myringoplasty.[75]

The initial report of this technique by Glasscock and colleagues[19] showed a success rate of 93%, although 34% of the 1556 cases were revision operations. Others, however, have found that revision and re-revision myringoplasty is fraught with poor results.[76] Furthermore, in the same report,[19] of the 110 failures, only 19 (17%)

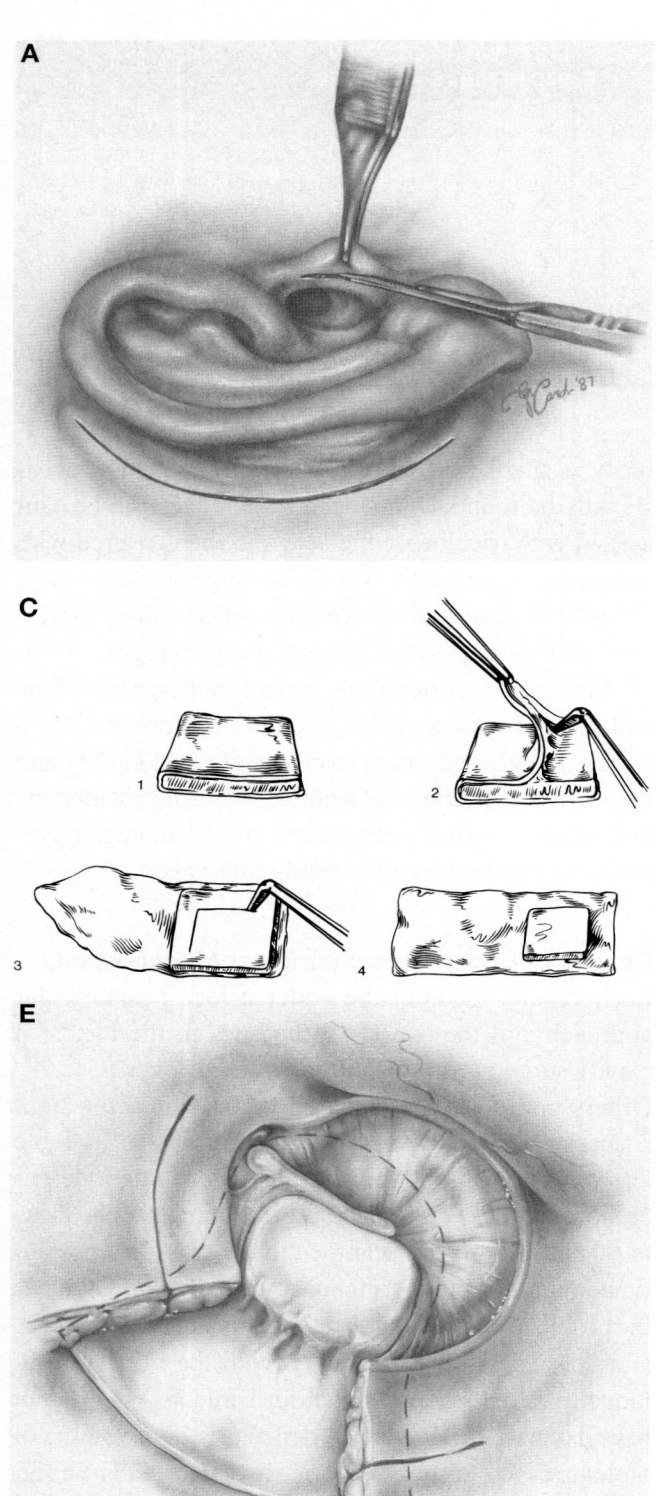

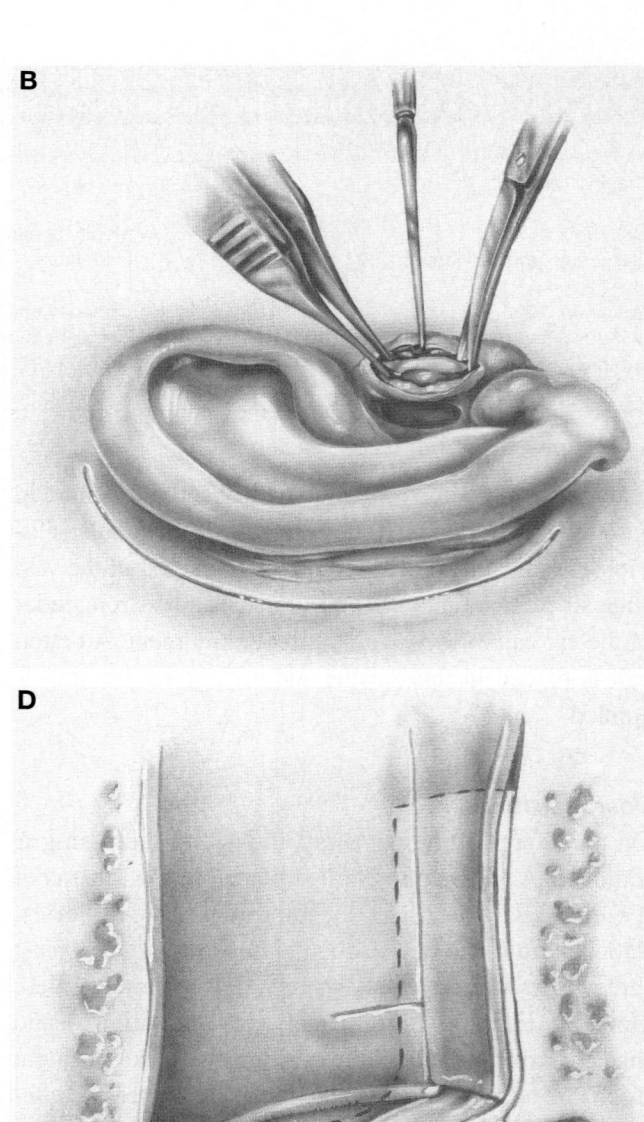

Figure 20–2   *A*, An incision is made in the posterior aspect of the tragus and carried through perichondrium and tragal cartilage. This leaves cartilage remaining at the tip of the tragus to maintain its shape. *B*, A piece of tragal cartilage with perichondrium is removed with the use of small-pointed scissors. *C*, The perichondrium is reflected from the surface of the cartilage similar to a book cover and the cartilage is trimmed to size. *D*, The perichondrium is placed under the malleus anteriorly and on to the posterior canal wall posteriorly. *E*, This view demonstrates how the cartilage becomes incorporated into the substance of the tympanic membrane to prevent recurrence of the disease process.

were early failures (within 3 weeks of surgery), whereas over a third of the failures (37%) were late surgical failures (more than 1 year after surgery).

Success rates in myringoplasty do not depend on the size of the perforation.[22,77] The site of the perforation also does not appear to influence the failure rate, and the site of failure is not consistent.[35,65,76] Similarly, the presence of tympanosclerotic plaques does not influence the take rate of the graft but may influence the degree of hearing improvement postoperatively.[78] When the graft is not anchored under the manubrium, but placed lateral to it and then under the tympanic membrane remnant edges, it appears to heal without problem, but, according to one study, in 31% of cases some degree of lateral graft migration was observed.[79]

Cartilage Grafting

Atelectasis is the collapse of the drum into the ossicular chain and on to the promontory. If the drum becomes adherent to these structures or retracts into the epitympanum, there is a tendency to form a cholesteatoma. Histologically, the atelectatic drum demonstrates an absent or diminished fibrous layer. Many patients have undergone fascia grafting in an attempt to recreate the fibrous layer and thereby strengthen the drum. However, long-term follow-up has shown that the newly formed drum has a tendency to retract and adhere again. This tendency has prompted the development of cartilage grafting of the drum.

Cartilage grafts can be harvested from a number of sites, but the most convenient sites are the tragus and the concha. A small incision is made on the posterior aspect of the tragus (Figure 20–2, A) and continued deep to incise through the tragal perichondrium and cartilage, leaving the dome of the tragal cartilage to maintain the normal shape of the tragus (Figure 20–2, B). An appropriate piece of tragal cartilage is removed, and the donor site is closed, using small (6-0) interrupted chromic sutures. The perichondrium is elevated from one side of the cartilage using the round House #2 knife (Figure 20–2, C). The cartilage is shaped to fit the posterior quadrant of the drum (Figure 20–2, D and E). After the middle ear is packed with Gelfoam, the cartilage graft is placed over the posterior quadrant with the perichondrial surface facing laterally. A second triangular wedge of cartilage can also be placed anteriorly to further reinforce this area.

The drum is grafted, with the fascia placed lateral to the cartilage graft(s).

Materials Used in Myringoplasty

Skin grafts were the first materials used in myringoplasty/tympanoplasty. However, they were quickly replaced because of problems with higher failure rates (reperforation in 11% of cases) and continuous desquamation with potential cholesteatoma formation (3%).[80] Fascia lata and subsequently temporalis fascia were established as the preferred materials for tympanic membrane reconstruction.[81] The advantages of the temporalis fascia include the ease of harvest from the same incision as the operation, availability of a large amount of graft, and very high take rates without subsequent problems.[82] Refinements in this technique have included the use of areolar tissue, which has similar success rates as temporalis fascia and has the additional advantages of resulting in a transparent tympanic membrane, and preserving the true temporalis fascia should revision surgery require additional grafting material.[13]

Xenograft (from a different species) materials, such as porcine dura and calf jugular vein, have been used to repair tympanic membrane perforations but were quickly abandoned because of their very high failure rates.[83–85]

Allograft and homograft materials (materials derived from genetically nonidentical humans) have been used extensively and include cadaveric dura, cadaveric tympanic membrane, pericardium, formaldehyde-preserved temporalis fascia, and sclera, among others.[13,86–89] These materials have the advantage of being readily available in any quantity without the need for additional surgery to harvest a graft. The results with such materials have been excellent, although in some instances, prolonged healing is seen. However, the main disadvantage of these materials that has led to their abandonment is the possibility of transmission of prion vector diseases such as Creutzfeldt-Jakob encephalopathy.[90,91] More recently, newer allograft materials, such as Alloderm,™ which is treated acellular human dermis that does not carry the risk of prion infection, have been successfully used in experiments with animals and in limited but successful repair of human tympanic membrane perforations.[92–94] Again, increased time of complete healing is required because of prolonged epidermization of the graft.

In an effort to increase the success rate of closure of tympanic membrane perforations while minimizing the surgery required, a variety of biomaterials have been used. Gelfilm™ has been used for small post–tympanostomy tube perforations, with good success rates.[95–98] Fibrin glue, which is derived from blood products and is nonototoxic, has been used in myringoplasty in combination with temporalis fascia.[99,100] It is unclear what, if any, advantage this technique affords. Fibrin glue, in combination with paper patches, appears to be very effective in repairing subtotal perforations in experimental animals, but this technique remains to be applied to humans.[101] Hyaluronic acid had been used for middle ear surgery and was found to be safe, without ototoxic potential.[102] Two double-blind, randomized studies have found this material to be superior to placebo and approximately equivalent to the paper patch technique in its ability to repair tympanic membrane perforations of limited extent.[103,104] More recently, epidermal growth factor has been used to repair tympanic membrane perforations in animal studies successfully, but there is yet no experience with this biologic modulator in humans.[105–107]

Technical Modifications in Myringoplasty

Several technical modifications have also been applied to myringoplasty. Attempts at endoscopic tympanic membrane repair have not found wide application, although endoscopic repair seems to offer the advantage of exposure without additional incisions.[108,109] Similarly, laser-assisted myringoplasty, in which a laser welds collagen from the graft to the tympanic membrane, appears to offer the advantages of a minimally invasive technique, rapidity in performing the procedure, and reduced healing periods.[110] However, to date, none of these methods have found wide application.

Fat graft myringoplasty is a technique that has been employed with consistently good results when patients are selected properly.[111–115] In this technique, a small amount of fat is removed from the ear lobe and applied through a perforation, the edges of which have been denuded of epithelium. It is ideally suited for small perforations and residual perforations after myringoplasty. The advantage of this technique is that it can be performed in the office setting under local anesthesia.

REFERENCES

1. Banzer M. Disputatio de auditione laesa. 1640.

2. Toynbee J. On the use of an artificial membrana tympani in cases of deafness dependent upon perforations or destruction of the natural organ. London: J. Churchill & Sons; 1853.

3. Yearsley J. Deafness, practically illustrated. London: Churchill & Sons; 1863.

4. Blake CJ. Transactions of the First Congress of the International Otological Society. New York: D. Appleton & Co; 1887.

5. Roosa DB. Diseases of the ear. New York: William Wood & Co.; 1876.

6. Joynt JA. Repair of drum. Iowa Med Soc 1919;9:51.

7. Derlacki EL. Repair of central perforations of tympanic membrane. Arch Otolaryngol 1953;58:405.

8. Wullstein H. Funktionelle Operationen im Mittelohr mit Hilfe des freien Spalt-lappen-Transplantates. Arch Ohren-Nasen-u Kehlkopfh 1952;161:422.

9. Zollner F. The principles of plastic surgery of the sound-conducting apparatus. J Laryngol Otol 1955;69:637.

10. Zollner F. Panel of myringoplasty. Second workshop on reconstructive middle ear surgery. Arch Otol 1963;78:301.

11. Heermann H. Tympanic membrane plastic with temporal fascia. Hals-Nasen-Ohrenh 1960;9:136.

12. Shea JJ. Vein graft closure of eardrum perforations. J Laryngol Otol 1960;74:358.

13. Glasscock ME, House WF, Graham M. Homograft transplants to the middle ear. A follow-up report. Laryngoscope 1972;82:868.

14. MacKinnon DM. Homograft tympanic membrane in myringoplasty. Ann Otol Rhinol Laryngol 1972;81:194–202.

15. Overbosch HC. Homograft myringoplasty with micro-sliced septal cartilage. Pract Otorhinolaryngol 1971;33:356–7.

16. Brandow EC Jr. Homograft tympanic membrane transplant in myringoplasty. Trans Am Acad Ophthalmol Otolaryngol 1969;73:825–35.

17. Packer P, Mackendrick A, Solar M. What's best in myringoplasty: underlay or overlay, dura or fascia? J Laryngol Otol 1982;96:25–41.

18. Zakzouk S, Attallah M. Transcanal tympanoplasty: dura versus temporalis fascia. Ear Nose Throat J 1992;71:590–2.

19. Glasscock ME III, Jackson CG, Nissen AJ, Schwaber MK. Postauricular undersurface tympanic membrane grafting: a follow-up report. Laryngoscope 1982;92:718–27.

20. Sheehy JL, Anderson RG. Myringoplasty. A review of 472 cases. Ann Otol Rhinol Laryngol 1980;89:331–4.

21. Holmquist J, Lindeman P. Eustachian tube function and healing after myringoplasty. Otolaryngol Head Neck Surg 1987;96:80–2.

22. Vartiainen E, Nuutinen J. Success and pitfalls in myringoplasty: follow-up study of 404 cases. Am J Otol 1993;14:301–5.

23. Torsney PJ. Allergic rhinitis and otologic allergy. Semin Drug Treat 1973;2:403–12.

24. Derlacki EL, Shambaugh GE Jr. Allergic management of some common ear conditions. Trans Am Acad Ophthalmol Otolaryngol 1953;57:304.

25. Browning GG, Gatehouse S. The prevalence of middle ear disease in the adult British population. Clin Otolaryngol 1992;17:317–21.

26. Gladstone HB, Jackler RK, Varav K. Tympanic membrane wound healing. An overview. Otolaryngol Clin North Am 1995;28:913–32.

27. Gibb AG. Tympanosclerosis. J Laryngol Otol Suppl 1983;8: 63–7.

28. Wielinga EW, Kerr AG. Tympanosclerosis. Clin Otolaryngol 1993;18:341–9.

29. Kirsch CM, Wehner JH, Jensen WA, et al. Tuberculous otitis media. South Med J 1995;88:363–6.

30. Griffin WL, Jr. A retrospective study of traumatic tympanic membrane perforations in a clinical practice. Laryngoscope 1979;89:261–82.

31. Kristensen S. Spontaneous healing of traumatic tympanic membrane perforations in man: a century of experience. J Laryngol Otol 1992;106:1037–50.

32. Keller AP Jr. A study of the relationship of air pressure to myringopuncture. Laryngoscope 1958;68:2015–29.

33. Hyden D. Ear drum perforations in children after ventilation tube treatment. Int J Pediatr Otorhinolaryngol 1994;29:93–100.

34. Pribitkin EA, Handler SD, Tom LW, et al. Ventilation tube removal. Indications for paper patch myringoplasty. Arch Otolaryngol Head Neck Surg 1992;118:495–7.

35. Te GO, Rizer FM, Schuring AG. Pediatric tympanoplasty of iatrogenic perforations from ventilation tube therapy. Am J Otol 1998;19:301–5.

36. Kay DJ, Nelson M, Rosenfeld RM. Meta-analysis of tympanostomy tube sequelae. Otolaryngol Head Neck Surg 2001;124: 374–80.

37. Nichols PT, Ramadan HH, Wax MK, Santrock RD. Relationship between tympanic membrane perforations and retained ventilation tubes. Arch Otolaryngol Head Neck Surg 1998;124: 417–9.

38. Holmquist J. Eustachian tube function and tympanoplasty. Acta Otorhinolaryngol Belg 1991;45:67–9.

39. Farrior JB. Eustachian tube function in tympanoplasty. Am J Otol 1989;10:234–6.

40. Taylor M. McMinn RM. Healing of experimental perforations of the tympanic membrane. J Laryngol Otol 1965;79:148.

41. Yamashita T. Histology of the tympanic perforation and the replacement membrane. Acta Otolaryngol (Stockh) 1985;100: 66–71.

42. Spandow O, Hellström S, Dahlstrom M. Structural characterization of persistent tympanic membrane perforations in man. Laryngoscope 1996;106:346–52.

43. Somers T, Goovaerts G, Schelfhout L, et al. Growth factors in tympanic membrane perforations. Am J Otol 1998;19:428–34.

44. Békésy G von. Uber die mechanisch-akustischen Vorganage beim Horen. Acta Otolaryngol (Stockh) 1939;27:281–388.

45. Yung MW. Myringoplasty: hearing gain in relation to perforation site. J Laryngol Otol 1983;97:11–7.

46. Derlacki EL. Residual perforations after tympanoplasty: office technique for closure. Otolaryngol Clin North Am 1982;15: 861–7.

47. Payne MC, Githler FJ. Effects of perforations of the tympanic membrane on cochlear potentials. Arch Otolaryngol 1951;54: 666.

48. Mair IW, Hallmo P. Myringoplasty. A conventional and extended high-frequency, air- and bone-conduction audiometric study. Scand Audiol 1994;23:205–8.

49. Oppenheimer P, Kaplan J, Harrison W, et al. Repair of traumatic myringorupture. Arch Otolaryngol 1961;73:328.

50. Juers AL. Perforation closure by marginal eversion. Arch Otolaryngol 1963;77:76.

51. Wright WK. Repair of chronic central perforations of tympanic membrane: by repeated acid cautery; by skin grafting. Laryngoscope 1956;66:1464.

52. Virtanen H, Palva T, Jauhiainen T. The prognostic value of eustachian tube function measurements in tympanoplastic surgery. Acta Otolaryngol (Stockh) 1980;90:317–23.

53. Andreasson L, Harris S. Tympanoplasty and eustachian tube function. Clin Otolaryngol 1978;3:421–30.

54. Gianoli GJ, Worley NK, Guarisco JL. Pediatric tympanoplasty: the role of adenoidectomy. Otolaryngol Head Neck Surg 1995; 113:380–6.

55. Virtanen H, Palva T, Jauhiainen T. Comparative preoperative evaluation of eustachian tube function in pathological ears. Ann Otol Rhinol Laryngol 1980;89:366–9.

56. Vrabec JT, Deskin RW, Grady JJ. Meta-analysis of pediatric tympanoplasty. Arch Otolaryngol Head Neck Surg 1999;125: 530–4.

57. Jonathan D. The predictive value of eustachian tube function (measured with sonotubometry) in the successful outcome of myringoplasty. Clin Otolaryngol 1990;15:431–4.

58. Sloth H, Lildholdt T. Tests of eustachian tube function and ear surgery. Clin Otolaryngol 1989;14:227–30.

59. Caylan R, Titiz A, Falcioni M, et al. Myringoplasty in children: factors influencing surgical outcome. Otolaryngol Head Neck Surg 1998;118:709–13.

60. Glasscock ME. Symposium: contraindications to tympanoplasty. II. An exercise in clinical judgment. Laryngoscope 1976;86: 70–6.

61. John DG, Carlin WV, Lesser TH, et al. Tympanoplasty surgery and prophylactic antibiotics: surgical results. Clin Otolaryngol 1988;13:205–7.

62. Jackson CG. Antimicrobial prophylaxis in ear surgery. Laryngoscope 1988;98:1116–23.

63. Carlin WV, Lesser TH, John DG, et al. Systemic antibiotic prophylaxis and reconstructive ear surgery. Clin Otolaryngol 1987;12:441–6.

64. Black JH, Hickey SA, Wormald PJ. An analysis of the results of myringoplasty in children. Int J Pediatr Otorhinolaryngol 1995;31:95–100.

65. Denoyelle F, Roger G, Chauvin P, Garabedian EN. Myringoplasty in children: predictive factors of outcome. Laryngoscope 1999;109:47–51.

66. Ophir D, Porat M, Marshak G. Myringoplasty in the pediatric population. Arch Otolaryngol Head Neck Surg 1987;113: 1288–90.

67. Vartiainen E, Vartiainen J. Tympanoplasty in young patients: the role of adenoidectomy. Otolaryngol Head Neck Surg 1997; 117:583–5.

68. Kotecha B, Fowler S, Topham J. Myringoplasty: a prospective audit study. Clin Otolaryngol 1999;24:126–9.

69. Jackler RK, Schindler RA. Myringoplasty with simple mastoidectomy: results in eighty-two consecutive patients. Otolaryngol Head Neck Surg 1983;91:14–7.

70. Jackler RK, Schindler RA. Role of the mastoid in tympanic membrane reconstruction. Laryngoscope 1984;94:495–500.

71. Tabb HG. Closure of perforations of the tympanic membrane by vein grafts. Laryngoscope 1960;73:699.

72. Tabb HG. Experience with transcanal and postauricular myringoplasty. Trans Pac Coast Otoophthalmol Soc Annu Meet 1968;52:121–5.

73. Vartiainen E, Karja J, Karjalainen S, Harma R. Failures in myringoplasty. Arch Otorhinolaryngol 1985;242:27–33.

74. Gersdorff M, Garin P, Decat M, Juantegui M. Myringoplasty: long-term results in adults and children. Am J Otol 1995;16: 532–5.

75. Palva T, Virtanen H. Pitfalls in myringoplasty. Acta Otolaryngol (Stockh) 1982;93:441–6.

76. Berger G, Ophir D, Berco E, Sade J. Revision myringoplasty. J Laryngol Otol 1997;111:517–20.

77. Yung MW. Myringoplasty for subtotal perforation. Clin Otolaryngol 1995;20:241–5.

78. Wielinga EW, Derks AM, Cremers CW. Tympanosclerosis in the tympanic membrane: influence on outcome of myringoplasty. Am J Otol 1995;16:811–4.

79. Stage J, Bak-Pedersen K. Underlay tympanoplasty with the graft lateral to the malleus handle. Clin Otolaryngol 1992;17:6–9.

80. Wright WK. Tissues for tympanic grafting. Arch Otolaryngol 1963;78:291.

81. Cable HR. Surface tension and temporalis fascia grafts. J Laryngol Otol 1981;95:667–73.

82. Wormald PJ, Alun-Jones T. Anatomy of the temporalis fascia. J Laryngol Otol 1991;105:522–4.

83. Puls T. Myringoplasty: is molded collagen xenograft a valid alternative for fresh temporalis fascia? Acta Otorhinolaryngol Belg 1996;50:111–4.

84. Callanan VP, Curran AJ, Gormley PK. Xenograft versus autograft in tympanoplasty. J Laryngol Otol 1993;107:892–4.

85. Zini C, Sanna M, Bacciu S, et al. Molded tympanic heterograft. An eight-year experience. Am J Otol 1985;6:253–6.

86. Pfaltz CR, Griesemer C. Pericard: a new biomaterial for tympanoplasty. Preliminary report. Am J Otol 1985;6:266–8.

87. Thawley SE, Smith PG, Faw KD. The use of sclera in tympanic membrane reconstruction. Laryngoscope 1982;92:1360–2.

88. Perkins R, Bui HT. Tympanic membrane reconstruction using formaldehyde-formed autogenous temporalis fascia: twenty years' experience. Otolaryngol Head Neck Surg 1996;114: 366–79.

89. Yetiser S, Tosun F, Satar B. Revision myringoplasty with solvent-dehydrated human dura mater (Tutoplast). Otolaryngol Head Neck Surg 2001;124:518–21.

90. Tange RA, Troost D, Limburg M. Progressive fatal dementia (Creutzfeldt-Jakob disease) in a patient who received homograft tissue for tympanic membrane closure. Eur Arch Otorhinolaryngol 1990;247:199–201.

91. Glasscock ME III, Jackson CG, Knox GW. Can acquired immunodeficiency syndrome and Creutzfeldt-Jakob disease be transmitted via otologic homografts? Arch Otolaryngol Head Neck Surg 1988;114:1252–5.

92. Laidlaw DW, Costantino PD, Govindaraj S, et al. Tympanic membrane repair with a dermal allograft. Laryngoscope 2001; 111:702–7.

93. McFeely WJ Jr, Bojrab DI, Kartush JM. Tympanic membrane perforation repair using AlloDerm. Otolaryngol Head Neck Surg 2000;123:17–21.

94. Saadat D, Ng M, Vadapalli S, Sinha UK. Office myringoplasty with alloderm. Laryngoscope 2001;111:181–4.

95. Hekkenberg RJ, Smitheringale AJ. Gelfoam/Gelfilm patching following the removal of ventilation tubes. J Otolaryngol 1995; 24:362–3.

96. Handler SD. Gelfilm myringoplasty. Laryngoscope 1992;102: 1198–9.

97. Lehrer JF. Gelfilm myringoplasty. Laryngoscope 1992;102: 1198; discussion 1199–200.

98. Baldwin RL, Loftin L. Gelfilm myringoplasty: a technique for residual perforations. Laryngoscope 1992;102:340–2.

99. Sataloff RT, Feldman MD. Fibrin glue in myringoplasty. Laryngoscope 1987;97:1111–2.

100. Wood AP, Harner SG. The effect of fibrin tissue adhesive on the middle and inner ears of chinchillas. Otolaryngol Head Neck Surg 1988;98:104–10.

101. DiLeo MD, Amedee RG. Fibrin-glue-reinforced paper patch myringoplasty of large persistent tympanic membrane perforations in the guinea pig. ORL J Otorhinolaryngol Relat Spec 1996;58:27–31.

102. Bagger-Sjöback D, Holmquist J, Mendel L, Mercke U. Hyaluronic acid in middle ear surgery. Am J Otol 1993;14: 501–6.

103. Stenfors LE. Repair of tympanic membrane perforations using hyaluronic acid: an alternative to myringoplasty. J Laryngol Otol 1989;103:39–40.

104. Rivas Lacarte MP, Casasin T, Pumarola F, Alonso A. An alternative treatment for the reduction of tympanic membrane perforations: sodium hyaluronate. A double blind study. Acta Otolaryngol (Stockh) 1990;110:110–4.

105. Lee AJ, Jackler RK, Kato BM, Scott NM. Repair of chronic tympanic membrane perforations using epidermal growth factor: progress toward clinical application. Am J Otol 1994;15: 10–8.

106. Somers T, Goovaerts G, Schelfhout L, et al. Growth factors in tympanic membrane perforations. Am J Otol 1998;19:428–34.

107. Amoils CP, Jackler RK, Lustig LR. Repair of chronic tympanic membrane perforations using epidermal growth factor. Otolaryngol Head Neck Surg 1992;107:669–83.

108. el-Guindy A. Endoscopic transcanal myringoplasty. J Laryngol Otol 1992;106:493–5.

109. Usami S, Iijima N, Fujita S, Takumi Y. Endoscopic-assisted myringoplasty. ORL J Otorhinolaryngol Relat Spec 2001;63:287–90.

110. Pyykko I, Poe D, Ishizaki H. Laser-assisted myringoplasty—technical aspects. Acta Otolaryngol Suppl (Stockh) 2000;543:135–8.

111. Gross CW, Bassila M, Lazar RH, et al. Adipose plug myringoplasty: an alternative to formal myringoplasty techniques in children. Otolaryngol Head Neck Surg 1989;101:617–20.

112. Mitchell RB, Pereira KD, Younis RT, Lazar RH. Bilateral fat graft myringoplasty in children. Ear Nose Throat J 1996;75:652, 655–6.

113. Mitchell RB, Pereira KD, Lazar RH. Fat graft myringoplasty in children—a safe and successful day-stay procedure. J Laryngol Otol 1997;111:106–8.

114. Ringenberg JC. Closure of tympanic membrane perforations by the use of fat. Laryngoscope 1978;88:982–93.

115. Terry RM, Bellini MJ, Clayton MI, Gandhi AG. Fat graft myringoplasty—a prospective trial. Clin Otolaryngol 1988;13:227–9.

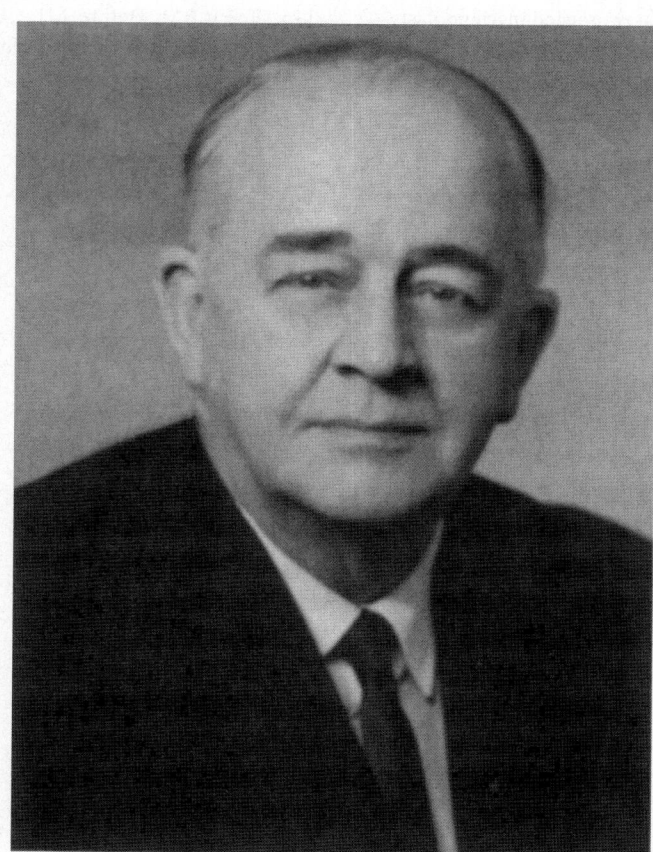

Sir Terence Cawthorne (1902–1970). Eminent London aural surgeon who helped to bridge the transition from surgery for the evacuation of pus to surgery in a clean field under the operating microscope.

V

Surgery of the Tympanomastoid Compartment

21

Pathology and Clinical Course of Inflammatory Diseases of the Middle Ear

WILLIAM H. SLATTERY III, MD

Otitis media is defined as "an inflammation of the middle ear without reference to etiology or pathogenesis."[1] Otitis media also implies concomitant inflammation, to a greater or lesser extent, of the mastoid air cell system, owing to its anatomic linkage to the middle ear cleft (ie, the tympanic cavity). Accordingly, otitis media is more correctly conceived of as an inflammatory disorder of the entire tympanomastoid compartment.

Otitis media is one of the most common diseases of children, and it is estimated that there are over 3 million patient visits annually in the United States for this condition. Placement of tympanostomy tubes is the most common procedure performed in the United States; more than 1 million tubes are inserted every year.[2] The cost of treating otitis media has been estimated as at least $3.8 billion in 1995.[3]

Because of the strategic location of the tympanomastoid compartment, separated from the middle and posterior cranial fossae by the thinnest of bony partitions, otitis media has the potential for intracranial extension. As cited in Cawthorne, Hippocrates stated that "Acute pain of the ear, with continued strong fever, is to be dreaded, for there is danger that the man may become delirious and die."[4] Fortunately, with progress in medical diagnosis and antibiotic therapy, it is unusual for otitis media to manifest its lethal potential. Nonetheless, a clear understanding of the pathology of otitis media is important for the clinician to be able to distinguish between infections that can be controlled by antibiotics and those that require surgical intervention.

STRUCTURE AND DEFENSE MECHANISMS OF THE MIDDLE EAR

The Eustachian Tube

The tympanomastoid compartment and the eustachian tube are derived from the tubotympanic recess, an extension of the first pharyngeal pouch. The medial part of the tubotympanic recess becomes elongated to form the pharyngotympanic (eustachian) tube. Posterior expansion of the tympanic cavity gives rise to the mastoid antrum and air cell system. Pneumatization progresses as mesenchyme is resorbed.

The eustachian tube has at least three physiologic functions: (1) protecting the middle ear from nasopharyngeal pressure changes and secretions, (2) draining middle ear secretions into the nasopharynx, and (3) ventilating the middle ear to equilibrate pressure with ambient atmospheric pressure and to replenish absorbed oxygen. The normal eustachian tube is closed at rest. Intermittent active dilation (opening) of the tube maintains near-ambient pressures in the middle ear. Therefore, middle ear pressure is largely regulated by the exchange of gas between the middle ear and nasopharynx that accompanies eustachian tube opening. A gradient-driven, transmucosal exchange of gases between the middle ear and blood also participates in the regulation of middle ear pressure.

Individuals with impaired eustachian tube function are prone to middle ear inflammation. The eustachian tubes of children are both smaller in diameter and more horizontally oriented than those of adults. As flow through a tube is inversely proportional to the fourth power of the radius, ventilatory function is considerably reduced in the child. Consequently, the prevalence of negative middle ear pressure is greater in children, which, in turn, contributes to the greater prevalence of middle ear disease. For example, in a study conducted by Bylander and colleagues, 35.8% of children without otologic disease, as compared with only 5% of adults, could not equilibrate an applied negative intratympanic pressure by swallowing.[5] Understandably, ventilation of the middle ear of the child is exquisitely sensitive to inflammatory edema of the lining epithelium of the eustachian tube. The tendency toward negative middle ear pressure in children improves with maturation, paralleling the decreased incidence of otitis media in adolescence as compared with infancy.

The horizontal angulation and shorter length of the eustachian tube of the child favors reflux of nasopharyngeal contents into the middle ear with consequent inflammation and infection. With maturation, the eustachian tube assumes a more vertical position, which also serves to diminish proclivity for inflammation.

The Epithelium

The lining of the tympanomastoid compartment comprises a modified respiratory epithelium, similar to that lining the nasal cavity and sinuses. The mucosa of the eustachian tube and much of the middle ear is a ciliated, columnar epithelium with a subepithelial layer of connective tissue. Goblet cells, as well as mucous glands, can be found throughout the middle ear but are concentrated near the eustachian tube orifice. The thin layer of the mucus they produce, consisting mainly of glycoproteins and containing lysozyme, blankets the mucosa (the "mucociliary blanket"). Continuous action of the cilia propels the mucus film, and its contents, from the tympanic cavity to the nasopharynx, serving to cleanse the middle ear space.

The lining epithelium becomes more cuboidal and loses its cilia as it reaches the floor of the tympanum and then changes to a flat pavement epithelium in the epitympanum, antrum, and mastoid air cells. The subepithelial connective tissue becomes progressively thinner as one progresses from the cartilaginous to bony portion of the eustachian tube and from the tympanic cavity to the mastoid antrum and air cells.

CLASSIFICATION OF INFLAMMATORY MIDDLE EAR DISEASE

The following six distinct clinical types of inflammatory reaction occur in the mucoperiosteum of the middle ear space:

1. Acute viral otitis media
2. Acute suppurative otitis media
3. Acute necrotizing otitis media
4. Serous otitis media
5. Chronic otitis media
6. Tuberculous otitis media

The microorganisms of prime importance in acute middle ear infection are *Streptococcus pneumoniae*, *Haemophilus inffluenzae*, and *Moraxella catarrhalis*.[6] Although gram-negative coliforms and *Staphylococcus aureus* have been reported to predominate as etiologic agents in neonatal otitis media,[7] more recent studies report that the usual pathogens are the same as those encountered in older children and adults.[8]

Several researchers have emphasized the contribution of viruses, particularly the respiratory syncytial virus, influenza A and B viruses, and the rhinovirus, to the pathogenesis of otitis media.[9,10]

The bacteriology of chronic otitis media is more diverse, including both aerobes and anaerobes. The predominant organisms recovered are *Pseudomonas aeruginosa*, *S. aureus*, *Klebsiella pneumoniae*, and *Bacteroides* species.[11,12]

Tuberculosis, considered rare in the 1950s, has reemerged as an important consideration in the differential diagnosis of chronic otitis media, its prevalence fueled by homelessness and the acquired immune deficiency syndrome (AIDS) epidemic of the 1990s and perpetuated by immigration from endemic areas.[13]

ACUTE VIRAL OTITIS MEDIA

Viral upper respiratory infections (URIs) can involve the middle ear. As in viral infection of the nasal passages, the pathologic change is in the ciliated columnar cells, which degenerate and slough, leaving a basal, germinal layer of nonciliated cuboidal cells. From these cells, the ciliated columnar epithelium regenerates after approximately 10 to 14 days, and the nasal mucosa returns to normal.[14]

Similar sloughing of the ciliated epithelium may occur with viral infection of the eustachian tube. The loss of ciliary activity, inflammatory edema, and increased mucus production result in a temporary obstruction of the eustachian tube with negative middle ear pressure and a tendency for the accumulation of transudate. In addition, respiratory viruses induce the release of cytokines and other inflammatory mediators (eg, histamine, bradykinin, and a number of the interleukins), which have been shown to provoke eustachian tube dysfunction.[10] Accordingly, serious otitis media is a common complication of a viral URI.

Upper respiratory tract viral infection of the nonciliated epithelium of the middle ear and mastoid appears to have a less drastic effect than seen with infection of the ciliated epithelium and may be lacking the clinical signs of otitis media. Clinical involvement of the mucoperiosteum is suggested by the observations made by George E. Shambaugh Jr during fenestration operations carried out on patients with acute "head colds."[15] He noted hyperemia and excessive bleeding from the mucosa and bone of the epitympanum and antrum despite the absence of signs of otologic infection and attributed these finding to viral injection. He also theorized that this subclinical, mucoperiosteal hyperemia accounted for the temporary worsening of hearing during head colds so often mentioned by patients.

Secondary bacterial infection can complicate a viral URI. A viral URI seems to alter both bacterial colonization of the nasopharynx and bacterial adherence to epithelial cells. For example, experimental influenza A viral infection in adults was associated with enhanced colonization of the oropharynx with *S. pneumoniae*.[10] The ciliated epithelium is the first line of defense against bacterial infection, and the loss of this layer as a result of viral infection as described above permits bacterial invasion and delayed clearance from the middle ear.[9] In addition, some respiratory viruses (eg, the influenza viruses) have an immunosuppressive effect on polymorphonuclear leukocytes, further impairing host defenses to infection.[10]

Acute bacterial otitis media complicating a viral URI or influenza can be differentiated from an uncomplicated viral otitis by the fever, hearing impairment, and positive culture results of middle ear fluid in the former.

ACUTE SUPPURATIVE OTITIS MEDIA

Acute suppurative otitis media refers to a bacterial infection of the middle ear.

Epidemiology

Acute suppurative otitis media is an extremely common illness; 70% of all children have at least one episode. In the United States, the peak age-specific incidence of acute suppurative otitis media is in the first 2 years of life, perhaps linked to daycare entry; there is a second peak of incidence at age 5 years, coincident with school attendance.[3] Infantile proclivity for otitis media relates to their immature immune systems and the easy access bacteria have to the middle ear through a short, horizontally oriented eustachian tube. Additional factors implicated in the tendency for otitis media in the child include child care attendance, parental smoking, and respiratory virus exposure (eg, siblings).[3]

Etiology

With rare exception, such as following traumatic tympanic membrane rupture or imperfect otologic surgery sterile technique, the infecting organisms of acute suppurative otitis media gain entry into the middle ear via the eustachian tube. Forcible blowing of secretions, or water entry, carries the organisms through the eustachian tube lumen to the middle ear; alternatively, middle ear extension of infecting agents occurs through the subepithelial connective tissue of the tube.

The bacteria most commonly implicated in acute suppurative otitis media are *S. pneumoniae*, *H. influenzae*, and *M. catarrhalis*.[6]

Clinical Course

Acute suppurative otitis media runs a typical clinical and pathologic course with successive stages that can be distinguished by symptomatology and otoscopic findings. Depending on the virulence of the infecting organism, host immune resistance, and antibiotic therapy, the infection may pass through all of the stages or resolve after any stage. Typically, acute suppurative otitis media is a self-limiting disease, with resolution and return of infected tissues to normal, barring the development of a complication. Nevertheless, owing to absent or inadequate antibiotic therapy, or to the antibiotic resistance of the infecting organism, cases of acute suppurative otitis media that progress to the stage of bone erosion and mastoid coalescence and that require surgical intervention are still encountered. Accordingly, the treating physician must have a firm grasp of the stages through which the disease may advance.

Acute suppurative otitis media typically progresses in four stages: hyperemia, exudation, suppuration, and resolution. Depending on the virulence of the infecting organism, the resistance of the host, and the adequacy of antibiotic therapy, the otitis may progress to the stage of coalescence and surgical mastoiditis and the stage of complication.

The initial infection by bacteria results in simple *hyperemia*, causing otalgia, ear fullness, and fever. The hearing may be normal, or slightly impaired, depending on the rapidity of the development of the hyperemia and intratympanic air pressure. The pathologic change of this stage comprises edema of the mucoperiosteum owing to vascular engorgement; beginning in the eustachian tube and tympanic cavity, the hyperemic edema usually involves the mucoperiosteum of the mastoid antrum and air cells. The otologic examination demonstrates injection of the vessels of the tympanic membrane in the vessels along the manubrium, the periphery of the pars tensa, and the pars flaccida. The drum is edematous, although landmarks can still be distinguished. Antibiotic therapy should be initiated; usually, amoxicillin in appropriate dosages will suffice.[6] Symptom relief should occur within the first 12 to 24 hours.[16]

Absent therapy, the stage of hyperemia is soon followed by the stage of *exudation*, an outpouring of fluid (serum containing fibrin, red blood cells, and polymorphonuclear leukocytes) from the dilated, permeable capillaries of the mucoperiosteum (Figure 21–1). Very quickly in virulent infections, and after 12 to 24 hours in milder infections, the tympanomastoid compartment

becomes filled with exudate under pressure. Manifestations of this stage are increased otalgia and fever, accompanied by a considerable, conductive hearing loss. In infants, a very high fever may be accompanied by vomiting, convulsions, and meningismus. On otoscopy, the tympanic membrane is red, thickened, and bulging, with loss of landmarks. Occasionally, the drum may appear pale instead of red, owing to thickening and desquamation of the outer, stratified squamous epithelium. There may be mastoid tenderness, a consequence of the exudate under pressure in the mastoid air cells. In infants, there may be edema and hyperemia over the cribriform area of the antrum. Although imaging studies reveal opacification of the tympanomastoid compartment, mastoid surgery is not indicated. Rather, simple myringotomy to release the exudate under pressure, along with appropriate antibiotic therapy, suffices at this stage.

The otorrhea following myringotomy (or spontaneous perforation) is initially hemorrhagic or serosanguinous but then becomes mucopurulent—the stage of *suppuration*. The mucoperiosteum of the tympanomastoid compartment is progressively thickened with the formation of new capillaries and fibrous tissue, infiltrated with lymphocytes, plasma cells, and polymorphonuclear leukocytes to form a very thick mucosal lining resembling granulation tissue. The bony trabeculae of the mastoid air cells remain intact. The otalgia and fever abate with the release of the exudate under pressure; hearing impairment worsens somewhat as increased stiffness of the ossicular chain owing to the thickened mucoperiosteum accompanies the mass of the purulent exudate. On otoscopy, a small perforation in the pars tensa discharging mucopus distinguishes acute suppurative otitis media from acute necrotizing otitis media, with its large, pars tensa perforation. Therapy can be tailored to the etiologic organism(s) by culture and sensitivity testing of the discharge. Toilet of the external auditory canal comprises frequently replaced cotton wicks and 1.5% acetic acid irrigation with an ear/ulcer syringe. Antibiotic eardrop therapy may not be efficacious as it cannot penetrate to the seat of the infection.

When the infection is severe and persists beyond 2 weeks, progressive thickening of the mucoperiosteum—especially in the epitympanum and in the smaller periantral cells—obstructs drainage of the mucopurulent secretions. Reaccumulation of pus under pressure, combined with marked hyperemia, results in venous stasis,

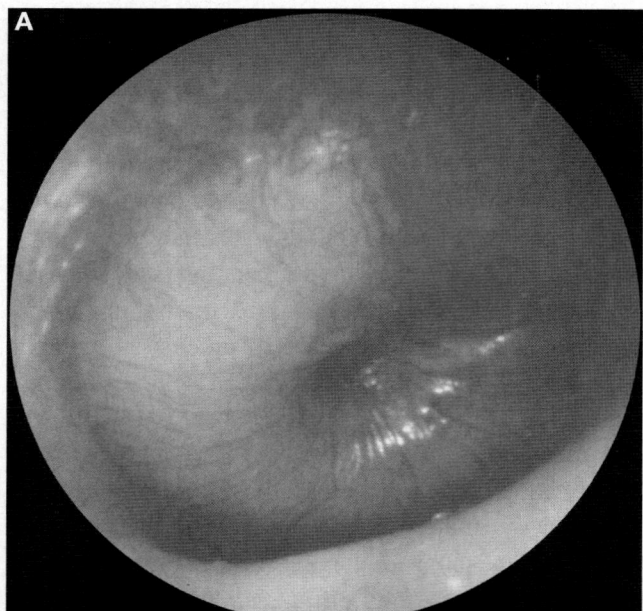

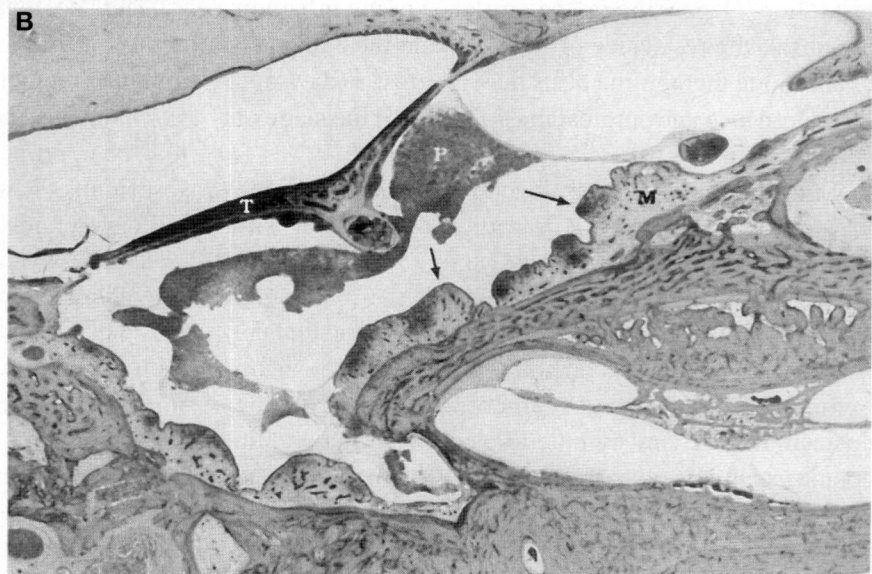

Figure 21-1. *A*, Right ear, otoscopic view. Acute suppurative otitis media, 12 hours after onset; the erythematous tympanic membrane is bulging and the tympanic cavity is filled with purulent exudate. Reproduced with permission from Chole RA, Forsen JW. Color atlas of ear disease. 2nd Ed. Hamilton (ON): BC Decker Inc; 2002. *B*, Left temporal bone (×8.5 original magnification). Acute otitis media (*H. influenzae*) in a 7-month-old girl. The tympanic membrane (T) and middle ear mucosa (M) are thickened due to vascular engorgement, polymorphonuclear leukocytic and lymphocytic infiltration, and edema; polyps (arrows) are forming on the medial wall of the tympanic cavity. There is pus (P) in the middle ear. Reproduced with permission from Schuknecht HF, Kerr AG. Pathology of the eustachian tube. Arch Otolaryngol Head Neck Surg 1967;86:497–502.

local acidosis, and the dissolution of calcium from the adjacent bony walls. Continued new blood vessel formation in bone, along with the activity of numerous osteoclasts, acts to soften and destroy the decalcifying septa, resulting in the stage of *coalescence* of the mastoid air cells and *surgical mastoiditis*. Bony erosion can also occur in the lateral mastoid cortex and in the bone overlying the lateral venous sinus and the dura. Symptomatology, in comparison to the stage of exudation, is deceptively mild. It is the *timing* of the symptomatology rather than its *severity* that is critical to the correct diagnosis of surgical mastoiditis. Reaccumulation of pus under pressure manifests with recurrence of otalgia and

low-grade fever. Otorrhea continues, varying with the extent of obstruction and degree of infection. On examination, the mastoid is tender to palpation and its periosteum is thickened as the abscess begins to surface; with perforation of the outer cortex, the fluctuant subperiosteal abscess displaces the auricle outward and downward. There is sagging of the posterosuperior wall of the external auditory canal owing to periosteal thickening adjacent to the antrum, and the thickening of the tympanic mucosa results in a nipple-like protrusion through the tympanic membrane perforation. Imaging studies reveal opacification of the tympanomastoid compartment with loss of the bony septa. In most cases, uncomplicated acute mastoiditis resolves with myringotomy and intravenous antibiotic therapy directed at the organism(s) detected by Gram stain and culture. Complicated acute otitis media (eg, the development of a subperiosteal abscess) necessitates surgical drainage, either an incision and drainage procedure or a formal tympanomastoidectomy. The advantage of the former approach is that the acutely infected ear can "cool down," and tympanomastoidectomy can be performed at a later date with less blood loss and better assessment of the status of the ear.

As intimated above, extension of infection beyond the confines of the tympanomastoid compartment to adjacent structure(s) heralds the onset of the stage of *complication*. The aural complications of otitis media are detailed in Chapter 22 and the intracranial complications are reviewed in Chapter 23. Fortunately, as for surgical mastoiditis, acute otitis media rarely progresses to the stage of complication.

The end result of acute suppurative otitis media is the stage of *resolution*, beginning with lessening and finally cessation of otorrhea. Closure of the tympanic membrane perforation follows, and any exudate remaining within the tympanomastoid compartment is absorbed rapidly. The reversal of mucoperiosteal thickening progresses more slowly. Osteoblastic activity repairs any partially decalcified septa. The healing of a large coalescent cavity involves initial filling with vascular connective tissue, which later becomes pale (referred to as "chicken fat" granulations) and is eventually replaced with osteoid. It is rare for acute suppurative otitis media to leave any permanent residua, and the hearing usually returns to normal.

ACUTE NECROTIZING OTITIS MEDIA

Acute necrotizing otitis media is a special form of acute suppurative otitis media that occurs predominantly in infants and young children who are acutely ill from scarlet fever, measles, pneumonia, influenza, or some other systemic febrile infection. This form of otitis media, which is accompanied by true necrosis and sloughing of considerable areas of tissue of the tympanomastoid compartment, was a frequent source of chronic suppurative otitis media and, fortunately, is now rarely encountered. The infecting organism is nearly uniformly

β-hemolytic Streptococcus. Distinguishing acute necrotizing otitis media from the usual otitis are early spontaneous tympanic membrane perforation, malodorous purulent discharge, and profound sensorineural hearing loss (although, in most cases, there is a moderate conductive hearing loss). The key finding on otoscopy is that of a large, tympanic membrane perforation; occasionally, necrotic ossicle can be seen. Intravenous antibiotics comprise initial therapy, with surgery according to the same indications as for acute suppurative otitis media.

SEROUS OTITIS MEDIA

Serous otitis media (Figure 21–2) follows acute suppurative otitis media or arises from eustachian tube dysfunction associated with allergies. The fluid found in the middle ear space is considered sterile ("noninfected"), although the thought that bacteria are present in the fluid remains controversial. Allergic otitis media tends to be more mucoid or secretory, reflecting its origin from antigenically sensitized middle ear mucosa. Symptoms include conductive hearing loss and aural fullness; in the young child, there may be no symptoms. On otoscopy, the tympanic membrane appears retracted, with diminished mobility to pneumatic massage. On occasion, the drum appears full or bulging, and, in addition to fluid, an air-fluid level and/or air bubbles can be seen medial to the drum. The manubrium of the malleus may appear unusually white as it contrasts with the fluid. Therapy spans the gamut of myringotomy to tympanostomy tube insertion, as well as medical management of any underlying etiology.

TUBERCULOUS OTITIS MEDIA

Tuberculous otitis media usually develops in a patient with tuberculosis who infects the middle ear via the eustachian tube by coughing up sputum laden with tubercle bacilli. Less commonly, it may be acquired by contact with infected sputum or, in children without pulmonary tuberculosis, by drinking unpasteurized milk from infected cows. Tuberculosis, thought to be virtually eliminated in the 1960s, has re-emerged as a diagnostic consideration, fueled in the 1990s by homelessness and the AIDS epi-

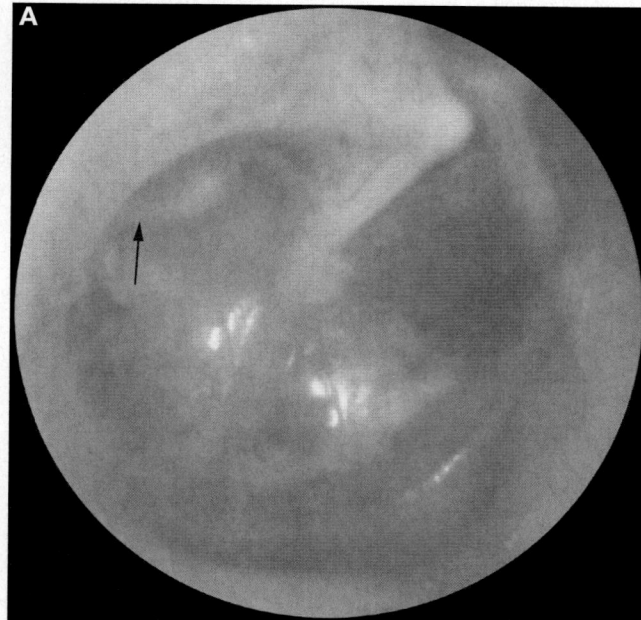

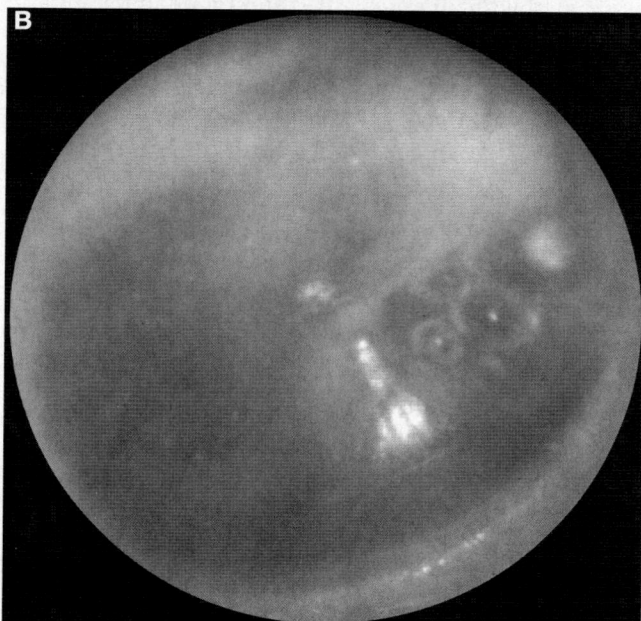

Figure 21-2. *A*, Right ear, otoscopic view. Serous otitis media. The tympanic membrane is slightly retracted and the tympanic cavity is filled with thin, watery fluid. The stapedius tendon is indicated by the arrow. *B*, Right ear, otoscopic view. Serous otitis media. Air bubbles can be seen in the anterior-superior quadrant. Reproduced with permission from Chole RA, Forsen JW. Color atlas of ear disease. 2nd Ed. Hamilton (ON): BC Decker Inc; 2002.

demic and perpetuated in the twenty-first century by immigration from areas of endemic infection.[13] Tuberculous otitis media is insidious in onset, with involve-ment of the tympanic membrane resulting in thickening, spontaneous perforation, and an aural discharge that is thin, scanty, and odorless. In particular, the finding of multiple perforations and extensive granulation tissue in the middle ear, especially if associated with facial paralysis, should suggest to the clinician the possibility of tuberculous otitis media.[17] Infection begins with extensive edema and infiltration of the mucosa and tympanic membrane by round and giant cells. As the infection progresses, numerous tubercles are formed, consisting of epithelioid, round, and multinucleated Langerhans' cells. Invasion of soft tissue and bone lead to caseation necrosis, sequestration and facial paralysis. *Mycobacterium tuberculosis* is detected by stain, by culture, or on examination of biopsied middle ear granulation tissue. Pulmonary screening should be performed in individuals diagnosed with tuberculous otitis media. Medical therapy precedes any surgical treatment as surgical therapy may fail absent systemic medical therapy.

CHRONIC SUPPURATIVE OTITIS MEDIA

Chronic suppurative otitis media is characterized by intermittent or persistent, chronic purulent drainage through a perforated tympanic membrane (Figure 21–3) and can be associated with cholesteatoma. On occasion, a permanent, central perforation of the tympanic membrane can remain dry, with only rare intermittent drainage, that is, inactive chronic otitis media. More typically, chronic or recurrent mucoid otorrhea, that is, active chronic otitis media, is provoked by exposure of the tympanic mucosa to bacteria of the external auditory canal as well as of the eustachian tube.

The most common bacterial isolate of chronic otitis media is *P. aeruginosa*.[12,16] Other isolates include aerobic organisms, such as enteric gram-negative bacilli, *S. aureus, streptococci, K. pneumoniae,* and *H. influenzae.* Anaerobic isolates, associated with a malodorous otorrhea, include *Peptostreptococcus* and *Bacteroides* species.[11,12]

Otoscopy, or preferably examination with an operating microscope, reveals a tympanic membrane perforation and, in active disease, mucoid or mucopurulent discharge. The presence of an aural polyp or malodorous otorrhea should raise the clinician's suspicion regarding the presence of cholesteatoma. After careful aspiration of any debris, the status of the middle ear mucosa can be assessed through the perforation and can appear only slightly thickened, with ciliary activity visualized, or can be markedly thickened, with polypoid degeneration. The ossicular chain can be intact, or disrupted, with the long process of the incus most prone to resorption. The mobility of the stapes can be assessed by microscopic examination combined with Bárány noise box stimulation of the contralateral ear, taking advantage of the crossed stapes reflex.

On histopathologic examination, the middle ear mucosa is edematous, with submucosal fibrosis and infiltration by chronic inflammatory cells. The mucosal edema can lead to the formation of aural polyps, which can even project into the external auditory canal.[17] Bone erosion, including ossicular resorption, mucosal ulceration, and the formation of granulation tissue, is the correlate of persistent otorrhea.[17] Mucosal thickening can impair ossicular and tympanic membrane mobility, aggravated by the deposition of hyalinized cartilage (ie, tympanosclerosis).[17]

The treatment of chronic otitis media focuses on the mucosal infection in the tympanomastoid compartment. After aspiration of retained debris, aural toilet comprising 1.5% acetic acid (one part white vinegar to two parts water) irrigation (at body temperature, three times daily with an ear/ulcer syringe) followed by the instillation of topical antibiotic drops (eg, ciprofloxacin, sulfacetamide) suffices to bring most infections under control. The acetic acid irrigation removes accumulated debris and acidifies the external auditory to canal, discouraging growth of *Pseudomonas* and other bacteria. Any underlying allergies and/or nasopharyngeal disorder should be managed and closure of the tympanic membrane perforation undertaken as soon as the ear becomes dry.

CHOLESTEATOMA

Cholesteatoma (more correctly keratoma) represents squamous epithelium and its exfoliated keratin debris trapped within the tympanomastoid compartment. Cholesteatomas are classified, according to pathophysiology, into congenital and acquired types; the acquired type is further subdivided into primary and secondary types.

The congenital cholesteatoma is believed to arise from a squamous epithelial rest in the temporal bone. There are four basic theories for the development of acquired cholesteatomas: invagination of the pars flaccida,[18] perforation of the tympanic membrane with epitthelial ingrowth,[19] basal cell hyperplastia,[20–22] and mucosal metaplasia.[23] Invagination of the pars flaccida (retraction of Shrapnell's membrane)—or of the posterosuperior pars tensa—occurs as a consequence of persistent negative middle ear pressure (Figure 21–4). As the retraction pocket deepens, keratin debris is trapped, resulting in a *primary acquired cholesteatoma*. The basal cell hyperplasia theory is a modification of the invagination theory and proposes that cone-like extensions of the basal layer of the epidermis can become invasive as a result of infection; microcholesteatomas arise as prickle cells invade the subepithelial layer through breaks in the basal lamina. Perforation of the tympanic membrane, particularly a marginal (extending to the tympanic annulus) perforation, allows squamous epithelial invasion of the tympanomastoid compartment; entrapment of the epithelium and its exfoliated keratin results in a cholesteatoma—a *secondary acquired cholesteatoma*. The mucous metaplasia theory proposes that the transformation of middle ear mucosa into keratinizing squamous epithelium underlies cholesteatoma development; no evidence supports this theory.

Regardless of origin, cholesteatomas inexorably expand as desquamated keratin debris accumulates; moisture and infection serve to accelerate the process. With growth, the cholesteatoma sac invades regions of the tympanomastoid compartment adjacent to its region of origin and envelops the ossicles. Cholesteatomas erode adjacent bone, both through the pressure effect of the expanding keratin mass and osteoclast-mediated enzyme activity, for example, collagenase, abundant in the epidermis of cholesteatoma.[17] Bone resorption results in destruction of mastoid trabeculae, ossicular erosion, labyrinthine fistulization, and exposure of the dura, facial nerve, and lateral venous sinus. Infection by the bacteria populating the sac results in labyrinthitis, facial paralysis, brain abscess, meningitis, and lateral venous sinus thrombophlebitis (see Chapters 22 and 23).

There is no medical therapy for cholesteatoma. In the majority of cases, surgical intervention is required, either extirpation or exteriorization. The goal of the

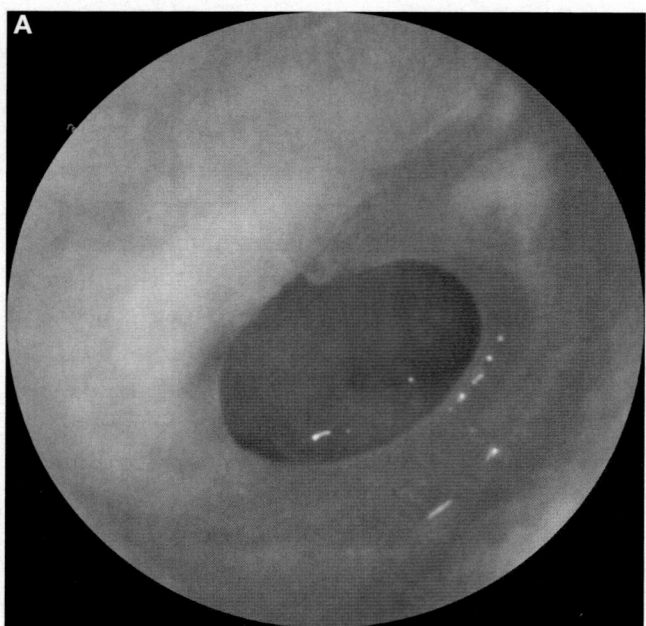

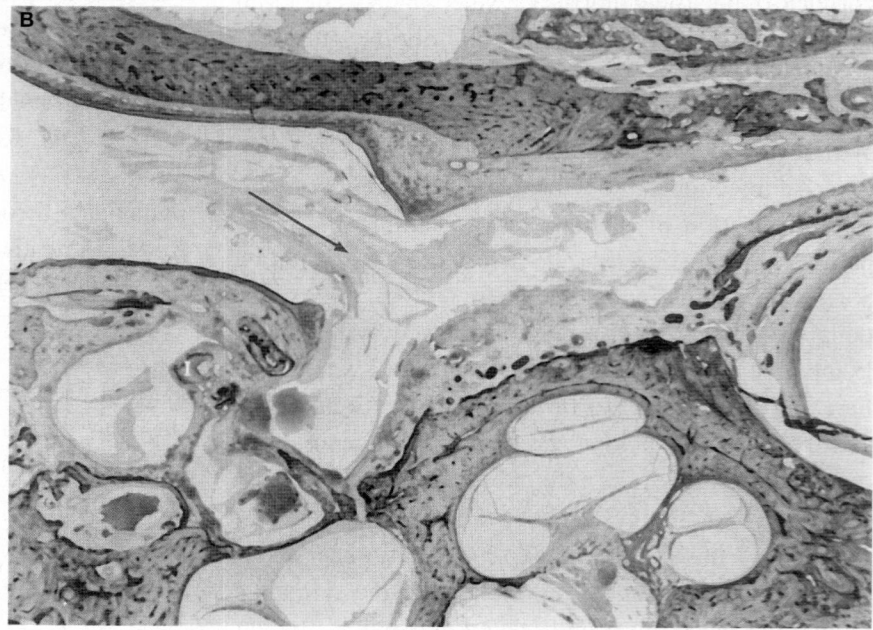

Figure 21-3. *A*, Right ear, otoscopic view. There is a moist, chronic perforation in the anterior-inferior quadrant, fringed by patches of tympanosclerosis. The mucosa of the tympanic cavity is thickened. Reproduced with permission from Chole RA, Forsen JW. Color atlas of ear disease. 2nd Ed. Hamilton (ON): BC Decker Inc; 2002. *B*, Left temporal bone (×14 original magnification). Chronic otitis media in a 76-year-old man. There is an anterior tympanic perforation (*arrow*), and the tympanic membrane remnant and the middle ear mucosa are thickened. There is pus in the middle ear and the long process of the incus (I) has been partially eroded. Reproduced with permission from Schuknecht HF. Pathology of the ear. 2nd Ed. Philadelphia (PA): Lippincott, Williams and Wilkins; 1993.

surgery is to render the affected ear clean, dry, and "safe." The surgical options are further detailed in Chapters 24, 25, and 26.

CONGENITAL CHOLESTEATOMA

Congenital cholesteatomas arise from epithelial remnants of embryonic development. The progression and histopathology of the congenital cholesteatoma is similar to secondary cholesteatoma, excepting the lack of concomitant infection as it is isolated from the environment (Figure 21–5). A congenital cholesteatoma arising in the cerebellopontine angle causes slowly progressive sensorineural hearing loss, loss of caloric respose, and facial nerve paralysis, mimicking a vestibular schwannoma. The congenital cholesteatoma of the middle ear presents as a white mass visible through an intact tympanic membrane in an individual with no prior history of otitis media. Similar to acquired cholesteatomas, surgical intervention is the management of choice.

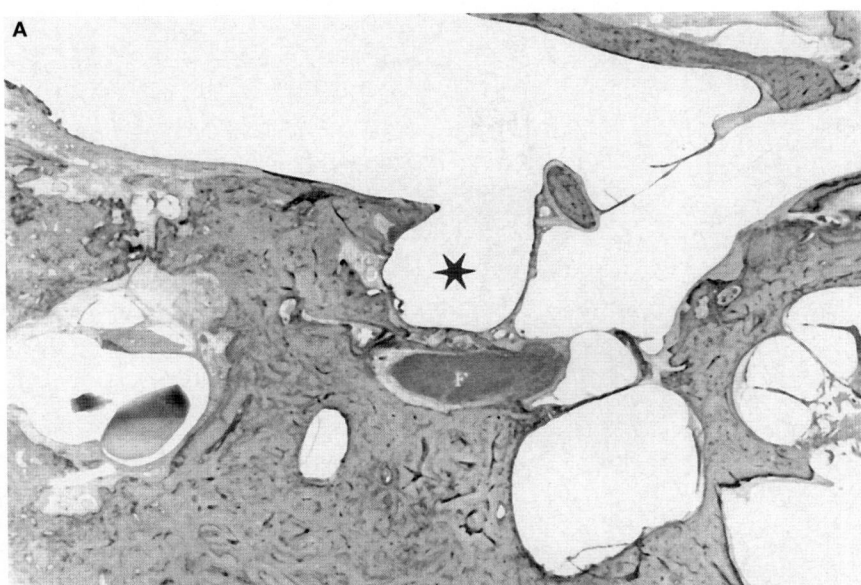

Figure 21-4. A, Left temporal bone (×6.75 original magnification). Posterior retraction pocket (at star) in a 47-year-old woman. The retraction pocket, which extended to the level of the body of the incus, is adherent to the fallopian canal (F indicates facial nerve). The long process of the incus has been eroded. Reproduced with permission from Schuknecht HF. Pathology of the ear. 2nd Ed. Philadelphia (PA): Lippincott, Williams and Wilkins; 1993. *B*, Right ear, otoscopic view. Primary acquired cholesteatoma. Keratin debris are evident superior to the lateral process of the malleus and the superior canal wall has been eroded. Reproduced with permission from Chole RA, Forsen JW. Color atlas of ear disease. 2nd Ed. Hamilton (ON): BC Decker Inc; 2002.

Illustration continued on next page

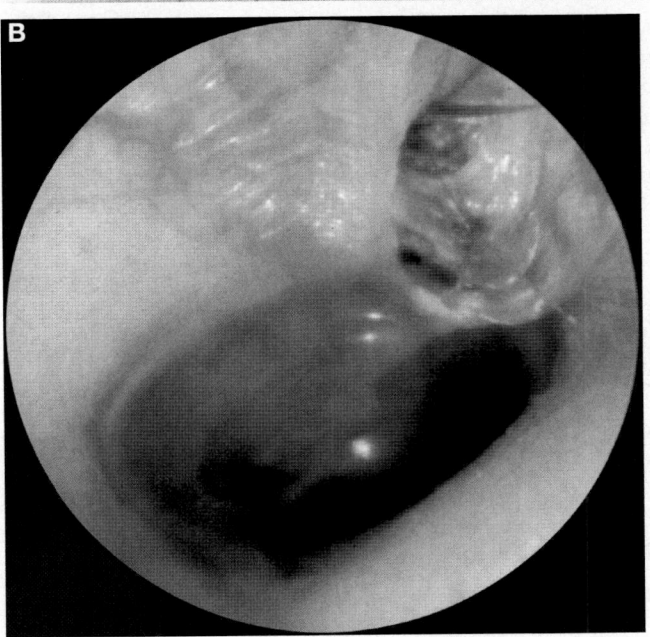

CHRONIC OSTEITIS OR OSTEOMYELITIS

Unusually severe acute necrotizing otitis media, involving bone around the antrum or the petrous pyramid, can result in the development of a bony sequestrum that is surrounded by infected granulation tissue and that serves as a source of chronic otorrhea. Occasionally, acute suppurative otitis media can be complicated by the development of chronic osteomyelitis of nonpneumatized areas of the petrous portion of the temporal bone. Osteomyelitis is less likely to develop in a well-pneumatized bone because of its much lesser amount of

residual, marrow-containing diploic bone. The offending organism is usually *Staphylococccus* spp or anaerobic *Streptococcus*. The primary clinical manifestation in either case is persistent, purulent nonmucoid discharge unresponsive to medical therapy. On otoscopy, there is a tympanic membrane perforation but no sign of cholesteatoma. Pain or headache, low-grade fever, and malaise are associated with cessation of discharge and improve when the ear drains. If there is a bony sequestrum, like any foreign body, it requires removal. Chronic osteitis or osteomyelitis also requires surgery; when the focus is in the petrous pyramid, it is difficult

Figure 21-4. (Continued.) *C*, Right temporal bone (×13 original magnification). Cholesteatoma (at star) in a 64-year-old man. The long process of the incus and the stapes have been destroyed. Reproduced with permission from Schuknecht HF. Pathology of the ear. 2nd Ed. Philadelphia (PA): Lippincott, Williams and Wilkins; 1993. *D*, Histopathologic detail of acquired cholesteatoma. Keratin debris are evident.

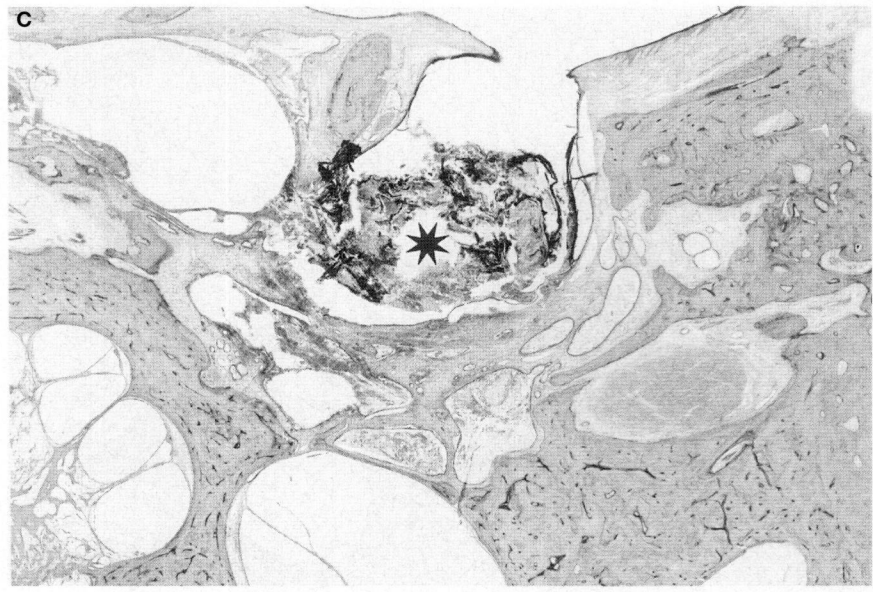

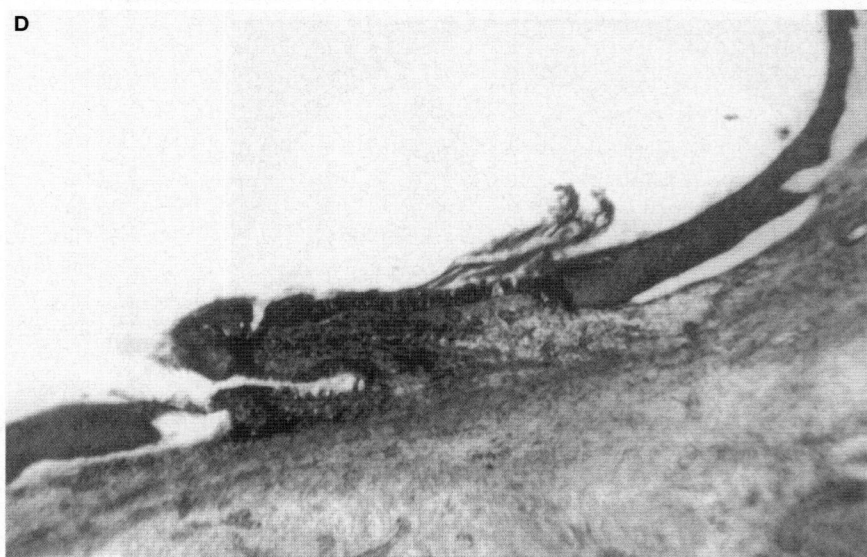

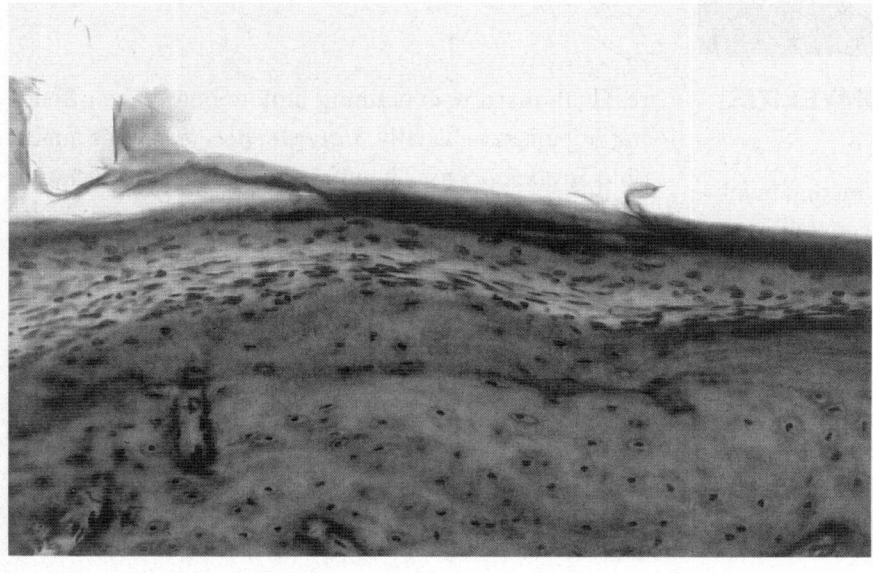

Figure 21-5. Histopathologic detail of congenital cholesteatoma matrix. Note similarity to Figure 21-4, D.

to eradicate and may recur or persist despite multiple surgeries and repeated courses of antibiotics.

REFERENCES

1. Bluestone CD, Gates GA, Klein JO, et al. Panel reports: 1. Definitions, terminology, and classification of otitis media. Ann Otol Rhinol Laryngol 2002;111 Suppl 188:8–18.

2. Isaacson G, Rosenfeld RM. Care of the child with tympanostomy tubes. Pediatr Clin North Am 1996;43:1183–93.

3. Daly KA, Giebink GS. Clinical epidemiology of otitis media. Pediatr Infect Dis J 2000;19:S31–6.

4. Cawthorne T. Surgery of the temporal bone. J Laryngol Otol 1953;67:377.

5. Bylander A, Tjernstrom O, Ivarsson A. Pressure opening and closing functions of the eustachian tube by inflation and deflation in children and adults with normal ears. Acta Otolaryngol (Stockh) 1983;96:255–68.

6. Celin SE, Bluestone CD, Stephenson J, et al. Bacteriology of acute otitis media. JAMA 1991;266:2249–52.

7. Bland RD. Otitis media in the first six weeks of life: diagnosis, bacteriology, and management. Pediatrics 1972;49:187–97.

8. Burton DM, Seid AB, Kearns DB, et al. Neonatal otitis media: an update. Arch Otolaryngol Head Neck Surg 1993;119:672–5.

9. Chonmaitree T. Viral and bacterial interaction in acute otitis media. Pediatr Infect Dis J 2000;19:S24–30.

10. Heikkinen T. The role of respiratory viruses in otitis media. Vaccine 2001;19:S51–5.

11. Erkan M, Aslan T, Sevük E, et al. Bacteriology of chronic suppurative otitis media. Ann Otol Rhinol Laryngol 1994;103:771–4.

12. Fliss DM, Dagan D, Meidan N, et al. Aerobic bacteriology of chronic suppurative otitis media without cholesteatoma in children. Ann Otol Rhinol Laryngol 1992;101:866–9.

13. Linthicum FH Jr. Temporal bone histology case of the month: tuberculous otitis media. Otol Neurotol 2002;23:235–6.

14. Hilding AC. Summary of known facts concerning the common cold. Ann Otol Rhinol Laryngol 1944;53:444.

15. Shambaugh GE Jr. Pathology and clinical course of inflammatory diseases of the middle ear. In: Glasscock ME III, Shambaugh GE Jr, editors. Surgery of the ear. 4th ed. Philadelphia: WB Saunders; 1990. p. 167–93.

16. Bluestone CD. Clinical course, complications and sequelae of acute otitis media. Pediatr Infect Dis J 2000;19:S37–46.

17. Schuknecht HF. Pathology of the ear. 2nd ed. Philadelphia: Lea & Febiger; 1993. p. 191–253.

18. Witmaack K. Wie entsteht ein genuines Cholesteatom? Arch Ohren Nasen Kehlkopfh 1933;137:306.

19. Habermann J. Zur Entstechung des Cholesteatoms des Mittelhors. Arch Ohrenh 1888;27:42.

20. Lange W. Tief eingezogene Membrana flaccida und Cholesteatom. Hals Nasen Ohrenh 1932;30:575.

21. Nager F. The cholesteatoma of the middle ear. Ann Otol Rhinol Laryngol 1925;34:1249.

22. Ruedi L. Pathogenesis and treatment of cholesteatoma in chronic suppuration of the temporal bone. Ann Otol Rhinol Laryngol 1957;66:283.

23. Sadé J. Cellular differentiation of the middle ear lining. Ann Otol Rhinol Laryngol 1971;80:376.6

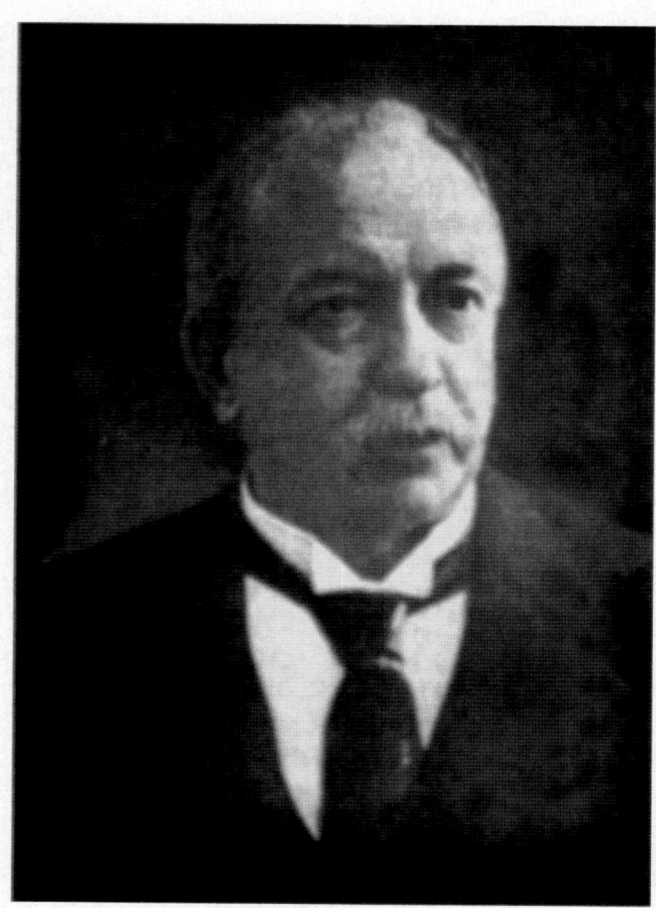

Giuseppe Gradenigo (1859–1926). Described the syndrome of suppuration of the apical portion of the petrous pyramid.

22

Aural Complications of Otitis Media

NEIL D. GROSS, MD
SEAN O. MCMENOMEY, MD

Otitis media is one of the most commonly treated infections in clinical practice today. The majority of patients with otitis media do well with or without antimicrobial therapy. However, there is a subset of patients who develop serious complications from this otherwise self-limiting disease. In the preantibiotic era, acute otitis media (AOM) frequently led to intratemporal and intracranial complications. The mortality rate of patients with such complications was high.

Complications can occur in the acute phase of an infection (ie, AOM) or as result of bony destruction from chronic bioenzymatic activity (ie, cholesteatoma). The most common intratemporal complications include tympanic membrane (TM) perforation, acute mastoiditis, facial nerve paralysis, acute labyrinthitis, and petrositis. If left unchecked, infection can spread beyond the temporal bone as a subperiosteal abscess or intracranially. Potential intracranial complications include acute meningitis, epidural abscess, subdural empyema, brain abscess, lateral venous sinus thrombosis, and otitic hydrocephalus.

With the introduction of modern antibiotic therapy, the incidence of such complications has declined dramatically. Nevertheless, the mortality rates of patients with intracranial otogenic complications remain substantial, ranging from 10 to 31%.[1] Therefore, it is incumbent upon the otolaryngologist to be familiar with the evaluation and management of the aural complications of otitis media and to stand vigilant against extratemporal or intracranial spread of disease. When an intracranial complication is identified, it is especially important to seek out an occult second complication.

INTRATEMPORAL COMPLICATIONS

Tympanic Membrane Perforation

Tympanic membrane perforation is a well-known complication of untreated otitis media. It can develop in the setting of either acute or chronic ear disease. The common pathogenic pathway is excessive pressure on the TM, either from pressurized purulent matter in the middle ear or from long-standing eustachian tube dysfunction and its associated atelectasis. The resulting defect usually occurs in the pars tensa and can vary considerably in size, depending on the virulence of the organism.

Although most TM perforations heal spontaneously, some patients are left with a persistent hole in the eardrum. A patient with a chronic perforation classically presents with a mild conductive hearing loss with or without otorrhea. Hearing loss associated with a TM perforation can range from 0 to 40 dB, varying also with the status of the ossicular chain. Direct visualization of the defect is best performed with the otomicroscope. Careful binocular examination is important for ruling out occult cholesteatoma or potential ossicular pathology.

The results of tympanoplasty for chronic TM perforations are excellent in experienced hands. Successful closure of the perforation and improvement in hearing are typically seen in greater than 90% of patients, even in the face of nonsuppurative otorrhea.

Acute Mastoiditis

Fluid in the mastoid cavity is a universal finding in patients with AOM because of the direct connection between the middle ear and mastoid. Acute mastoiditis, on the other hand, is relatively rare. Acute mastoiditis may manifest in one of two ways: acute periostitis (spread of infection via venous channels resulting in inflammation of the periosteum) or acute osteitis (bony destruction of mastoid air cell trabeculae). The latter is often referred to as "coalescent" mastoiditis. Acute mastoiditis can develop from AOM despite prior antibiotic treatment.

The hallmark triad of symptoms of acute mastoiditis comprises (1) otalgia, (2) postauricular pain, and (3) fever. Otorrhea and hearing loss are less frequently reported. The most common presenting sign, postauricular tenderness, is seen in over 80% of cases.[2] In addition, protrusion of the pinna and postauricular erythema and swelling are classic findings. Induration over the mastoid is thought to be a harbinger of impending subperiosteal abscess. Temporal bone computed tomographic (CT) scanning is the diagnostic study of choice to detect coalescent mastoiditis, which is characterized by a loss of bony trabeculae (Figure 22–1). Computed tomographic scanning may also identify an occult second complication, such as an intracranial or neck (Bezold's) abscess.

The majority of cases of acute mastoiditis can be treated conservatively with intravenous antibiotics and myringotomy, with or without tympanostomy tube placement. Culture-directed antimicrobial therapy is paramount to the successful treatment of acute mastoiditis. Therefore, a culture should always be obtained. Mastoidectomy is required whenever there is significant bony destruction or a poor response to up to 2 weeks of conservative management. The goal of surgery is to débride necrotic bone and to prevent intracranial extension of infection.

Facial Nerve Paralysis

Prior to the advent of antibiotics, the prevalence of facial nerve paralysis in chronic otitis media (COM) was greater than 2%.[3] More recent reports indicate that this complication is now exquisitely rare.[4] Facial nerve paralysis may be a complication of either AOM or COM.

Facial nerve paralysis within the first 10 days of AOM is believed to be caused by edema of the nerve within the fallopian canal, similar to Bell's palsy. In these cases, complete recovery from facial paralysis

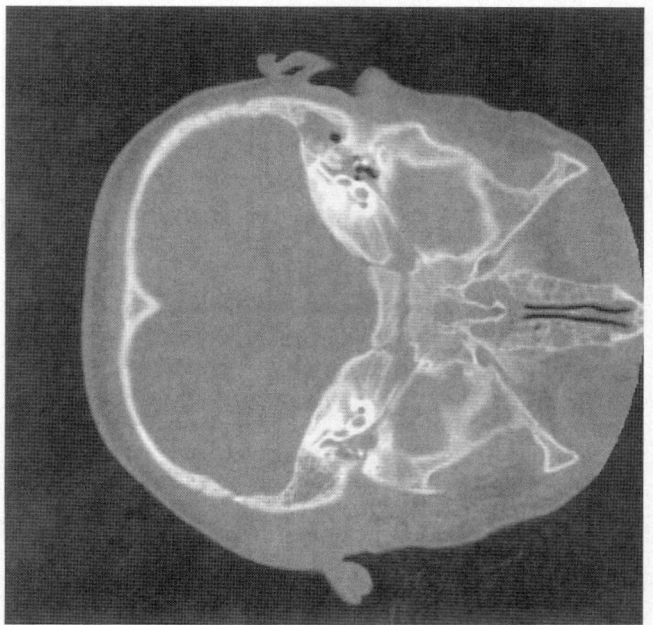

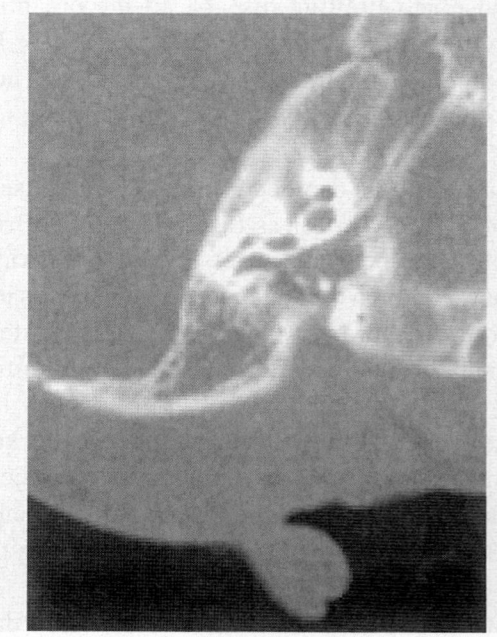

Figure 22-1   Acute coalescent mastoiditis. A characteristic loss of bony trabeculae is noted as well as adjacent soft tissue thickening.

may be expected with conservative treatment. On the other hand, facial paralysis seen beyond 2 weeks of infection should be assumed to be the result of erosion of the osseous facial canal with exposure of the nerve to advancing suppuration.

When facial nerve paralysis is noted in a patient with COM, cholesteatoma should be suspected. In these cases, osteitis and subsequent bone erosion likely expose the nerve to infection. The result is inflammation and ultimately facial nerve compression. Ironically, the epidermal lining of the cholesteatoma may act as a protective covering for the nerve as the bone is being destroyed. It is not surprising, then, that exposure of the facial nerve by cholesteatoma without paralysis is more common than exposure with paralysis.

High-resolution temporal bone CT scanning is essential in the evaluation of facial nerve palsy associated with otitis media. Computed tomography can best delineate the extent of disease and identify contributing pathology, such as cholesteatoma or neoplasm. Electrical testing of nerve function is rarely required.

Treatment of facial nerve paralysis as a complication of otitis media requires the use of intravenous antibiotics and prompt surgical intervention. Surgery is indicated to arrest the coalescent process and to protect the nerve from partial destruction. The tympanic segment is the most common area of involvement, suggesting that the surgical procedure should, at a minimum, eradicate infection from the middle ear. For an incomplete paralysis associated with protracted AOM, intravenous antibiotics and wide-field myringotomy or tympanostomy tube placement may be adequate. Some authors also advocate the use of concomitant corticosteroids.[5] A simple mastoidectomy is recommended for recalcitrant cases.

Facial nerve decompression is infrequently indicated. However, for complete facial paralysis with loss of electrical excitability, facial nerve exploration from the first genu to the stylomastoid foramen should be accomplished. Decompression of the nerve above and below the area of disease should be carried out until healthy nerve is visualized. If a dehiscence of the nerve trunk is identified, repair should be performed using a nerve graft or nerve rerouting and end-to-end anastomosis.

Labyrinthitis

Labyrinthitis is the most frequent intratemporal complication of otitis media, owing to extension of infection within the temporal bone. Similar to meningitis, labyrinthitis has two clinically distinguishable subtypes: (1) localized, circumscribed, or *serous labyrinthitis* without total and permanent loss of function and (2) diffuse, purulent or *suppurative labyrinthitis* with permanent total destruction of the sensory elements within the labyrinth.

Serous Labyrinthitis

Inflammation of the labyrinthine contents is rarely hematogenous.[6] It is nearly always the result of osteitis of the labyrinthine capsule or of extension by preformed or acquired pathways. Potential pathways include the annular ligament of the oval window, the round window membrane, and the cholesteatomatous fistula.

The symptoms of serous labyrinthitis are the result of disturbed vestibular and cochlear function, nearly always with a depression of sensory response. The vestibular symptoms precede the cochlear symptoms by hours to days when the site of invasion is a semicircular canal. These symptoms typically consist of profound vertigo, nausea, and vomiting. Patients usually demonstrate spontaneous nystagmus toward the unaffected ear and some degree of ataxia with past-pointing. The cochlear symptoms of serous labyrinthitis consist of primarily high-frequency sensorineural hearing loss with distortion of hearing and diplacusis.[7]

Prior to treatment, it is imperative to rule out suppurative labyrinthitis, which can be accomplished by identifying definite retention of labyrinthine function (eg, by means of a caloric test). Treatment of the serous labyrinthine inflammation is directed toward the etiologic factor. If the cause is an early acute suppurative otitis media, myringotomy and antibacterial therapy will suffice. If the cause is perilabyrinthine osteitis or cholesteatoma, mastoidectomy with removal of diseased bone should be combined with parenteral antibiotics.

Suppurative Labyrinthitis

The same etiologic factors and pathways of invasion pertain to diffuse suppurative labyrinthitis as to serous labyrinthitis, that is, a stage of localized serous inflammation generally preceding the stage of diffuse purulent involvement. An exception to this rule is involvement of the labyrinth secondary to generalized meningitis, in which case, purulent labyrinthitis usually occurs without a prodrome of serous labyrinthitis.

The symptoms of suppurative labyrinthitis are similar to those of serous labyrinthitis, including the lack of fever. However, there are some key differences. The symptoms of suppurative labyrinthitis are more rapid and intense, with gradual improvement over the ensuing days. Also, the onset of severe vestibular symptoms is accompanied by a complete loss of cochleovestibular response. Notably, the caloric response is conspicuously absent from the diseased ear.

The most important treatment of suppurative labyrinthitis is close and continuous monitoring for symptoms of intracranial extension. Antibiotics should be administered, albeit more to aid in preventing the spread of infection than in the expectation that the drug will enter the infected labyrinth in therapeutic concentrations. If meningeal signs are noted, then a lumbar puncture should be performed immediately. Any evidence of intracranial spread warrants surgical labyrinthectomy.

Labyrinthine Fistula

A fistula of the labyrinth may be surgically produced or may occur as a consequence of suppurative or neoplastic ear disease. The vast majority of cases of fistula, however, occur as a result of bone erosion by cholesteatoma. In fact, the development of a labyrinthine fistula is so characteristic of cholesteatoma that a thorough evaluation should be initiated even in the absence of typical findings such as granulation tissue and drainage.

Patients with labyrinthine fistulae most often present with episodic vertigo. However, differentiating between a labyrinthine fistula and other benign vestibular and nonvestibular disorders based on history alone can be difficult. Thus, the "fistula test" can be helpful in making this clinical distinction. It is easily performed using either pneumatic insufflation or manual tragal pressure to apply positive or negative pressure to the ear. Pressure perturbations of the soft tissue covering a fistula result in nystagmus (produced by the movement of endolymph toward or away from the ampulla) and vertigo. A positive test consists of a quick component of nystagmus toward the affected ear with the application of positive pressure. As the vast majority of fistulae occur in the lateral semicircular canal, the nystagmus is most frequently horizontal.[8] Conversely, the nystagmus is vertical with a fistula of either vertical canal. With a large (> 2 mm), far-anterior fistula, which exposes simultaneously the ampullae of the horizontal and superior canals, the nystagmus is rotary.

It is important to remember that the fistula test can be elicited only when vestibular function is retained. Thus, a negative fistula test does not rule out fistula. In fact, the fistula test is positive in less than half of all patients with confirmed fistulae.[9] A false-negative fistula test occurs when the fistula is accompanied by a localized loss of function of the ampulla of the involved canal or by a generalized loss of labyrinthine response. A false-positive fistula test can be seen in the rare condition of a hypermobile stapes without other ear disease. Occasionally, patients with a labyrinthine fistula will experience momentary vertigo when exposed to loud noise, that is, the Tullio phenomenon.

Computed tomographic scanning of the temporal bone is the diagnostic test of choice to rule out cholesteatoma and to evaluate the status of the otic capsule. Labyrinthine fistulae can be readily identified on CT scan, which can help direct surgical management (Figure 22–2). A fistula of the labyrinth owing to cholesteatoma is an indication for surgery to remove the cholesteatoma and to prevent the retention of infected debris.

Fistulae should be managed according to their location, size, and the status of hearing.[10,11] Even in experienced hands, there is considerable risk to the inner ear in patients with labyrinthine fistula, with rates of total hearing loss between 8 and 56%.[8] The conservative management of a labyrinthine fistula consists of a canal

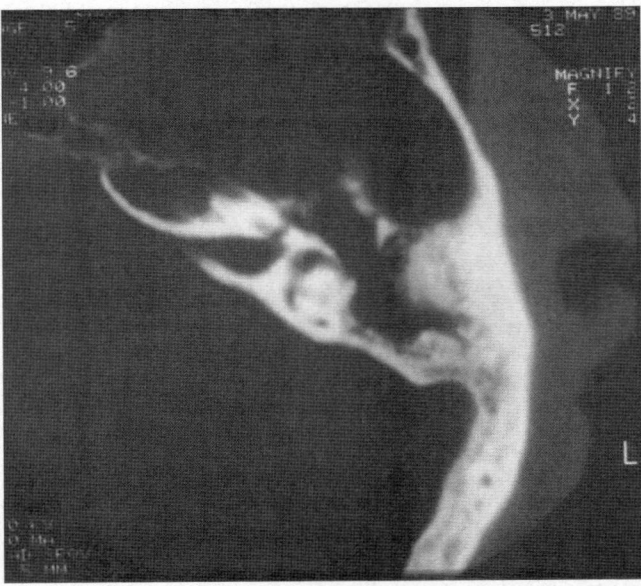

Figure 22-2 Labyrinthine fistula. The vast majority of fistulae involve the lateral semicircle canal.

wall down mastoidectomy with exteriorization of the cholesteatoma matrix overlying the fistula. This approach is best suited for fistulae that involve more than one semicircular canal, the cochlea, the vestibule, or the internal auditory canal. Even attempted removal of the matrix overlying a large fistula involving a single semicircular canal can result in deafness and therefore should be avoided if possible. On the other hand, the matrix can generally be removed from fistulae measuring less than 2 mm in size (ie, "small" fistulae).[11] Small fistulae involving the semicircular canals can be managed more aggressively by removing cholesteatoma matrix from the fistula at the end of a canal wall up procedure. The fistula is then "repaired" with a soft tissue graft (eg, fascia, perichondrium), bone paté, or a similar covering. When infection is present, the management of the fistula should be staged.[9]

Acute Petrositis

Petrositis (also known as petrous apicitis) is an inflammation of the petrous portion of the temporal bone. Except for the rather rare acute, fulminating osteomyelitis of the petrosa seen in infants, petrositis occurs only in temporal bones with pneumatic cells in the petrous pyramid.[12] Because less than one-third of petrous bones are pneumatized into the apex,[13] petrositis is an uncommon complication of otitis media. When it does occur, however, petrositis can be a devastating complication. The absence of natural drainage pathways, with a "bottleneck" to drainage posed by the bony labyrinth that nearly fills the base of the petrous pyramid, and the close proximity to the central nervous system make the petrosa a particularly dangerous site of infection when occupied by virulent organisms.

Inflammation of the petrous air cells behaves similarly to that of the mastoid system. Any middle ear infection will result in fluid in pneumatized cells. As in the mastoid process, this inflammation recedes in the great majority of cases as the otitis media subsides without producing symptoms referable to petrous involvement and without producing bone changes in the cell walls. Such cases are not clinically diagnosed as petrositis. The diagnosis of petrositis is reserved for infected petrous cells with inadequate drainage causing bone changes of coalescence in the cell walls and resulting in symptoms referable to the petrosa.

Although the symptoms of acute petrositis can be subtle, the two most constant complaints are deep-boring pain and aural drainage. The nature of the pain associated with petrositis depends on the area of the petrous pyramid affected. Air cells extend into the petrous pyramid in two main groups: a posterior group of air cells from the epitympanum and antrum that finds its way around the semicircular canals into the base of the pyramid, frequently extending to the apex, and an anterior group of cells from the tympanum, hypotympanum, and eustachian tube that finds its way around the cochlea into the apex of the pyramid. The posterior group of cells is more common and is present in about 30% of temporal bones. In the case of posterior petrositis, the pain is occipital, parietal, or temporal, and the discharge is from the mastoid. In the case of anterior petrositis, the pain is frontal or behind the eye, and the discharge is from the tympanum.

Diplopia caused by sixth cranial nerve paralysis may occur when the apex is involved, the nerve being compressed by edema where it passes through Dorello's canal beneath the petroclinoid (Gruber's) ligament at the tip of the petrous apex. The three cardinal symptoms of diplopia (from ipsilateral abducens nerve palsy), retrobulbar pain, and persistent otorrhea constitute Gradenigo's syndrome. Yet petrositis often occurs without the full triad. Less common symptoms of petrositis include transient facial nerve paresis, mild recurrent vertigo, and fever that is usually low grade and intermittent.

The diagnosis of petrositis should be suspected whenever there is persistent, purulent discharge and pain, despite a well-done mastoidectomy. The diagnosis is made on clinical suspicion and can usually be confirmed with a high-resolution temporal bone CT scan. Gallium 67 and technetium 99m bone scans are also occasionally helpful, showing increased radioactive uptake on the affected side.

Management of acute petrositis includes parenteral antibiotics and surgical drainage. The object of surgery is to provide adequate drainage from the suppurative focus in the petrosa without damage to either the facial nerve or labyrinth. Although symptoms and imaging studies may point toward one particular group of cells as the site of disease, a systematic surgical routine should be employed. There are several viable surgical approaches to the petrous apex, all of which include a preliminary complete simple mastoidectomy with skeletonization of the semicircular canals.

The primary factors that determine the surgical drainage routes for petrous apicitis are (1) the location of the infection, (2) the pneumatization of the temporal bone, and (3) the status of the hearing. In the absence of hearing, the translabyrinthine approach affords excellent exposure of the entire posterior portion of the petrous apex. If more anterior exposure is required, then the transcochlear approach should be considered. This approach can usually be accomplished without rerouting the facial nerve. If anterior drainage is necessary in a patient with hearing, either a subtemporal or an infracochlear approach can be considered. The infracochlear approach provides a very narrow window of access as compared with the subtemporal but does provide a route for sustained, gravity-dependent drainage. Posterior apicitis can be approached and drained via a retrolabyrinthine or subarcuate route. Both approaches provide adequate access in a well-pneumatized bone, as well as allowing both hearing preservation and drainage.

EXTRATEMPORAL COMPLICATIONS

Subperiosteal Abscess

As many as 50% of patients with mastoiditis seen today develop a subperiosteal abscess.[14] Such an abscess forms as a result of either direct destruction of cortical bone or hematogenous spread through small vascular channels. Well-pneumatized mastoids are believed to be more susceptible to forming subperiosteal abscesses than sclerotic mastoids because of increased capacity for the accumulation of pus and decreased capability of resorption.

The most common site of cortex breakdown is through the thin trabecular bone of Macewen's triangle. As a result, the auricle is displaced forward and outward, and a fluctuant mass can be palpated behind the ear. When pus breaks through the tip of the mastoid process and into the digastric groove (incisura mastoidea), infection can extend into the neck. This abscess typically forms deep to the sternocleidomastoid muscle and is referred to as a Bezold's abscess. Patients uniformly present with a fluctuant neck mass and otitis media. This infectious process can rapidly prove fatal if left unchecked as the carotid

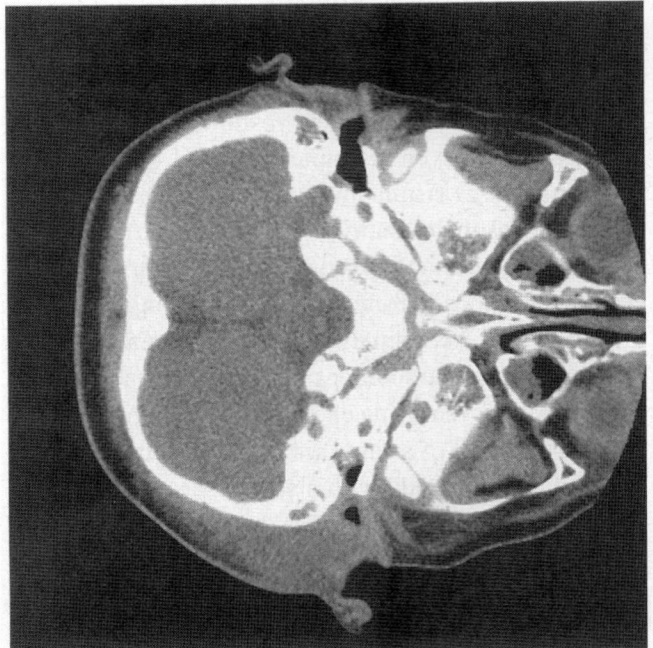

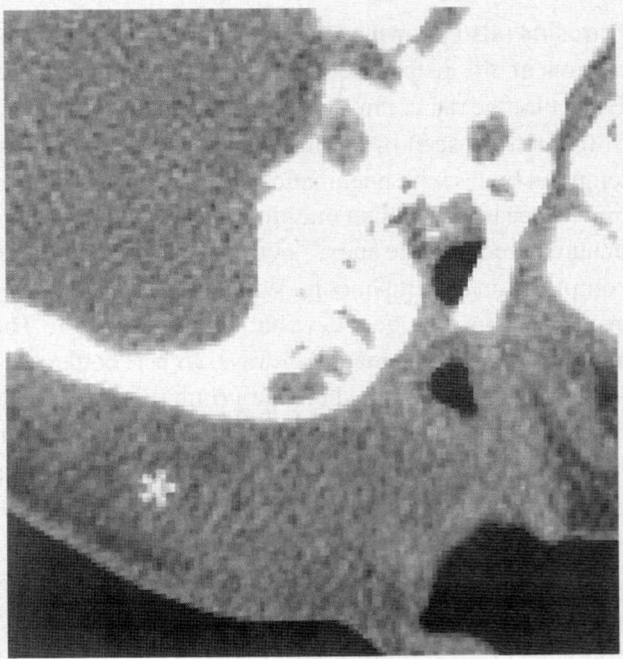

Figure 22-3 Subperiosteal abscess. Early abscess formation noted on high resolution computed tomography (CT) scan of the temporal bone (abscess is seen anteromedial to asterisk).

sheath, parapharyngeal space, and mediastinum can all be involved.

Infrequently, purulent secretions can perforate the periosteum and collect deep to the temporalis muscle. When this process occurs from infection tracking along the external auditory canal, it is called a Luc's abscess. An alternative and even more uncommon pathway for pus to spread to the temporalis fossa is via a pneumatized zygomatic arch. In either case, patients present with induration and tenderness over the temporalis muscle with projection of the upper half of the pinna away from the calvarium.

Imaging is critical to the diagnosis and management of subperiosteal abscesses, which occur with relatively low frequency and can present with variable symptoms and signs. Computed tomographic scanning is essential to the detection of a subperiosteal abscess and to the delineation of the full extent of disease (Figure 22–3).

Although some subperiosteal abscesses in young children can be managed with intravenous antibiotics and myringotomy alone, treatment generally requires more aggressive surgical intervention. A simple mastoidectomy is first performed to allow drainage and ventilation of the mastoid space. The postauricular incision can then provide access to other areas that require drainage. Penrose drains are frequently employed, and culture-directed oral antibiotics should be given for 2 weeks postoperatively.

REFERENCES

1. Kangsanarak J, Navacharoen N, Fooanant S, Ruckphaopunt K. Intracranial complications of suppurative otitis media: 13 years' experience. Am J Otol 1995;16:104–9.

2. Goldstein NA, Casselbrant ML, Bluestone CD, Kurs-Lasky M. Intratemporal complications of acute otitis media in infants and children. Otolaryngol Head Neck Surg 1998;119:444–54.

3. Nissen AJ, Bui H. Complications of chronic otitis media. Ear Nose Throat J 1996;75:284–92.

4. Wetmore RF. Complications of otitis media. Pediatr Ann 2000;29:637–46.

5. Joseph EM, Sperling NM. Facial nerve paralysis in acute otitis media: cause and management revisited. Otolaryngol Head Neck Surg 1998;118:694–6.

6. Torok N. Tympanogenic labyrinthitis. Otolaryngol Clin North Am 1972;5:45–57.

7. Shambaugh GE. Diplacusis: a localizing symptom of disease of the organ of Corti. Arch Otol 1940;31:160–84.

8. Sheehy JL, Brackmann DE. Cholesteatoma surgery. Management of the labyrinthine fistula — a report of 97 cases. Laryngoscope 1979;89:78–87.

9. Mandolis S. Complications associated with labyrinthine fistula in surgery for chronic otitis media. Otolaryngol Head Neck Surg 2000;123:733–7.

10. Vartianinen E. What is the best method of treatment for labyrinthine fistula caused by cholesteatoma? Clin Otolaryngol 1992;17:258–60.

11. Gacek RR. The surgical management of labyrinthine fistulae in chronic otitis media with cholesteatoma. Ann Otol Rhinol Laryngol 1974;84 Suppl 10:1–19.

12. Lindsay JR. Suppuration in the petrous pyramid. Ann Otol Rhinol Laryngol 1938;47:3.

13. Rainer A. Development and construction of pyramidal cells. Arch Ohren Nasen Kehlkopfh 1938;145:3.

14. Spiegel JH, Lustig LR, Lee KC, et al. Contemporary presentation and management of a spectrum of mastoid abscesses. Laryngoscope 1998;108:822–8.

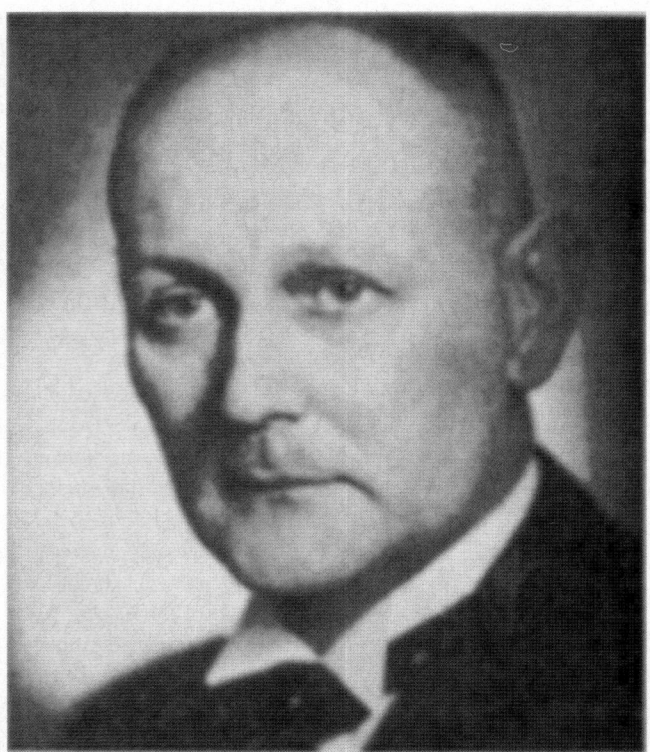

Gerhard Domagk (1895–1964). In 1932 demonstrated the curative effects of Prontosil, a red dye containing sulanilamide, in streptococcal infection in mice, for which he received the Nobel Prize for Medicine.

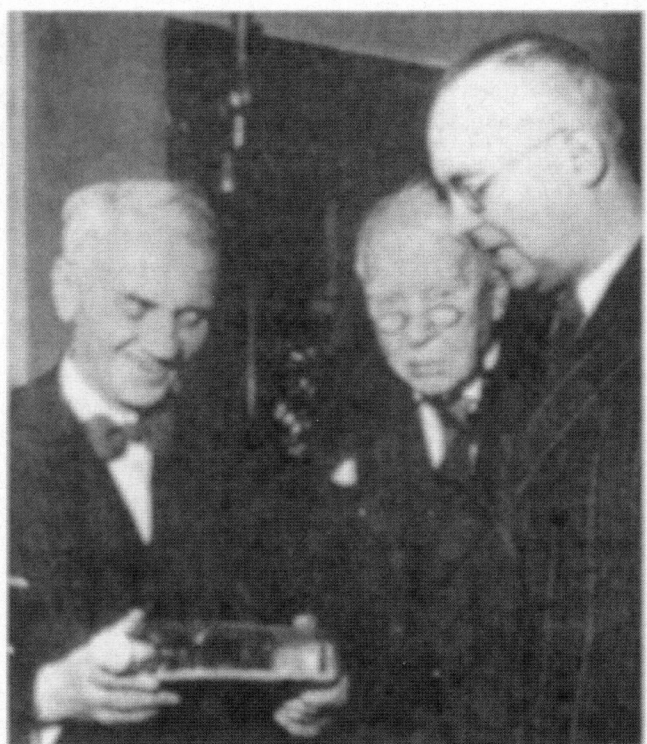

Alexander Fleming left, holding a vial containing Penicillium notatum mold) (1881–1955). Observed and recorded, in 1928, the lysis of Staphylococcus colonies by Penicillium mold. The 1945 Nobel Prize was awarded to Fleming, Florey, and Chain "for the discovery of penicillin and its therapeutic effect for the cure of different infectious maladies."

23

Intracranial Complications of Otitis Media

SAMUEL C. LEVINE, MD, FACS

CHRIS DE SOUZA, MD, FACS

HISTORICAL PERSPECTIVE

Hippocrates noted in 460 BC that "acute pain in the ear with continued high fever is to be dreaded for the patient may become delirious and die."[1] In the preantibiotic era, complications from otitis media occurred abundantly, accompanied by a high morbidity. This was recognized by the Roman physician Celsius (25 AD) and the Arabian physician Avicenna (980 to 1037 AD).[2] It was Morgagni (1682 to 1771 AD) who recognized that the ear infection came first and the brain abscess was secondary.[2]

Brain abscess was the first complication of otitis media to be recognized and the first one successfully treated by operation. It was in 1768 that Morand reported a successful operation for brain abscess.[3] In 1856, Lebert accurately described the pathology of brain abscess, confirming the fact that it follows infection of the ear, not the reverse.[4] It was in 1881 that MacEwen reported a successful series of brain abscesses that were operated on by him.[5] Körner, in 1908, was able to find 268 reported operations with 137 recoveries.[6]

The surgery of brain abscess had reached its peak of otologic interest by the time of Eagleton's text in 1922.[7] The management of this relatively common complication of otitis media remained chiefly in the hands of the otologic surgeon until sulfonamides began to be used for acute otitis media in 1935 and penicillin was introduced in 1942. Thereafter, the incidence of brain abscess, which may already have begun to decline, decreased abruptly. The relative success of surgery for brain abscess remained in sharp contrast for many years to the almost invariably fatal outcome of purulent meningitis, the most dreaded complication of otitis media and the most frequent cause of death. Because therapy of generalized otitic meningitis was rarely successful, the efforts of the otologic surgeon were directed toward prevention. Whenever possible, bone-invading types of acute and chronic otitis media were operated on before a complication had occurred. Careful clinical observation of patients with middle ear infections would not infrequently permit the detection of the earliest stages of beginning meningeal involvement. With prompt and thorough surgical drainage of the suppurative focus in the temporal bone, considerable success was achieved in arresting the meningeal invasion, in many cases while it was still localized, preventing the development of otherwise fatal generalized meningitis.[8] Despite these advances, meningitis remained the most frequent cause of death in otitis media, and otitis media was by far the most frequent cause of meningitis not due to *Neisseria meningitidis*.

The last of the three major intracranial complications of otitis media to be related to ear disease was infective thrombosis of the lateral sinus, first described in 1826. Thirty years later, Lebert accurately described the pathology of otitic sinus thrombosis.[9] In 1880, Zaufal proposed an operation for this complication and first attempted it in 1884, but the patient died.[10]

The surgical treatment of sinus thrombosis was finally established by the publications of Lane[11] in 1889 and Ballance in 1890.[12] However, a controversy over whether, as part of the surgical management, to ligate the jugular vein in all cases, in some cases, or in no case continued for many years, only to be resolved by the introduction of effective antibacterial and anticoagulant medication in favor of nonligation for most cases.

The two complications of otitis media caused by expansion within the temporal bone that often lead to a fatal intracranial extension, namely, purulent labyrinthitis and petrositis, were the last serious complications to be defined and effectively treated. A technique for draining the infected labyrinth was first described in 1895 by Jansen.[13] In 1904, Gradenigo described the syndrome of continuing aural discharge, severe fifth cranial nerve pain, and sixth nerve paralysis caused by infection of pneumatic cells in the petrous portion of the temporal bone with adjacent meningitis.[14] Kopetsky and Almour[15] in 1930 and Eagleton[16] in 1931 described the first systematic attempts to drain an abscess of the petrous apex. Other methods for reaching this relatively inaccessible area were soon described. For a few years, the literature contained numerous reports of successful operations for petrositis, many of them in patients with early meningitis. Just at the time that this frequent cause of otitic meningitis began to yield surgical therapy, it virtually disappeared from the scene of otologic experience as a result of effective antibacterial medication for acute otitis media.

The frequency of complications of otitis changed dramatically with the introduction of effective antibiotics. In the 5-year period immediately preceding the introduction of these agents, from 1928 to 1933, approximately 1 in every 40 deaths in a large general hospital was caused by an intracranial complication of otitis media, with meningitis heading the list, sinus thrombosis second, and brain abscess last.[17] In a subsequent 5-year period (from 1949 to 1954), only 1 in every 400 deaths was the result of ear disease—an amazing 10-fold reduction in less than 20 years. The decrease in fatalities following acute otitis media was greatest because this disease previously accounted for the majority of serious complications.

Of the three major intracranial complications of otitis media, the reduction in mortality has been greatest for thrombophlebitis of the lateral sinus, which has nearly disappeared as a cause of death.[17] This fact is easily understood because infection of the bloodstream was the usual mechanism of death from sinus thrombosis, and antibiotics act best in the bloodstream. The incidence of brain abscess has been greatly reduced by antibiotics. Purulent meningitis, though reduced, persists today as by far the most frequent intracranial complication of otitis media. However, it has changed from a nearly 100%

fatal disease to one in which recovery can be expected in the majority of instances if diagnosed early and treated adequately.

The family physician has come to rely more on drugs to take care of ear disease than on careful clinical study and early otologic consultation. The diagnostic acumen of the otologist has been blunted by diminished experience and lessened familiarity with the symptoms of otitic complications. The situation has been made more difficult by the masking effect of antibiotics on the symptoms of continued infection. These factors may be resulting in an increase in serious complications of otitis media, particularly in proportion to the number of cases of surgical mastoiditis.[18] In a report of 50 intracranial complications of otitis media from 1961 to 1977, more than half were caused by brain abscess, with involvement of the temporal lobes five times more frequent than that of the cerebellum.[19] Meningitis was second in frequency. Lateral sinus thrombosis and cortical thrombophlebitis each caused two cases. There was one case of a cerebral hernia and three of otitic hydrocephalus. All but 3 of the 50 complications were in cases of chronic otorrhea with cholesteatoma, granulations, or both. Three cases were unresolved acute otitis, two of which were caused by *Streptococcus pneumoniae*.

Today the neurosurgeon is often the first to be called in consultation for intracranial complications. Most otologists work in combination as a team with a neurosurgeon. Treatment involves both specialties. Although the neurosurgeon should direct therapy of the complication, he/she must recognize the frequent otitic (sometimes nasal accessory sinus) origin and always request otologic consultation and help in the management, with surgical removal of the suppurative focus, which is usually in the ear.

The patient with chronic suppurative otitis media who is not doing well may indicate trouble. Earache with chronic otitis means that something has gone wrong, and if pus is under pressure in the middle ear cleft, an intracranial complication may be impending. Certainly, headache and drowsiness are signs of danger. One of the earliest signs of brain abscess is a visual field defect, which is almost invariably present if the patient is carefully examined. A fever suggests meningitis or sinus thrombosis. Awareness of the significance of the symptoms and signs results in earlier diagnosis, prompt treatment, and further reduction in mortality.

Although the incidence of the complications of otitis media has declined and a whole new range of antibiotics has been introduced, complications have not been eradicated completely. Complicating early identification and timely intervention when complications occur is the fact that most patients have been treated with one or more courses of antibiotic therapy.

FACTORS THAT INFLUENCE THE DEVELOPMENT OF COMPLICATIONS

Intracranial complications occur as the result of many factors, often acting simultaneously, causing the infection to spread from the ear and into the intracranial cavity. In general, intracranial complications occur when ear infections are either uncontrolled or inadequately controlled.

The tendency of middle ear infection to spread beyond the confines of the middle ear and its adjacent spaces is influenced by a number of factors, including the virulence of the infecting organism and its sensitivity to antibiotics, host resistance, the adequacy of antibiotic therapy, the anatomic pathways and barriers to spread, and the drainage of the pneumatic spaces, both natural and surgical.

The microbiology of middle ear infections remains relatively constant over time. *Streptococcus pneumoniae*, *Haemophilus influenzae*, and *Moraxella catarrhalis* cause most acute infections.[20] As new antibiotics are introduced, however, the patterns of antibiotic resistance seem to change and may vary from one location to another.

The microbiology of chronic infection is different from the acute process. Organisms such as *Pseudomonas aeruginosa* are much more common.[21] The treatment of a *Pseudomonas* infection requires a higher dosage of less routinely used antibiotics. The benign type of chronic otorrhea with mucoid discharge coming from a central perforation does not by itself invade bone and cause complications. There is, however, nothing to prevent a fresh virulent organism from entering such an ear and causing an acute exacerbation and a complication by the same mechanism as in any case of acute otitis media. Unfortunately, the new organism is likely to display some greater resistance to antibiotics since the patient is likely to have received treatment for the otorrhea.

Immunocompromised individuals are at risk of developing not only otitis media but also complications of otitis media. The organisms causing the infection are more likely to be atypical pathogens. Individuals may be taking immunosuppressive medications, rendering them immunocompromised and susceptible to infection, or may have acquired immune deficiency syndrome (AIDS).

Intracranial extension of acute otitis media occurs somewhat more often from poorly pneumatized than well-pneumatized temporal bones and even ears with a history of previous attacks of otitis media. The likelihood of a complication arising from chronic middle ear infections depends on the pathologic lesion causing the chronic otorrhea. The middle ear cleft has bony barriers that prevent the middle ear infection from extending intracranially. However, these barriers may be eroded by antecedent infections, granulation tissue, or cholesteatoma, thus allowing infection to spread into the cranial cavity from the middle ear. Trauma with fracture can create passages that allow infections to bypass these natural defenses.

The natural drainage of the mastoid cavity (approximately 5 cc in volume) is into a relatively smaller space, the middle ear cavity (capacity approximately 0.9 cc), which then drains through the eustachian tube. Drainage may be inadequate, allowing infected secretions to accumulate and then erode through the middle ear cleft to extend intracranially.[22]

PATHWAY OF SPREAD IN THE PRODUCTION OF A COMPLICATION

As stated above, the infection spreads beyond the confines of the ear because it may be uncontrolled or poorly controlled. The infection from the middle ear cleft may enter the intracranial cavity through any of three routes.

Bone Erosion

Extension by bone erosion is the most frequent manner of spread, leading to a complication in cases of acute otitis media in well-pneumatized temporal bones, and it is nearly always the manner of spread in cases of chronic suppurative otitis media. In acute otitis media, bone erosion is the result of coalescent mastoiditis. In chronic otitis media, the bone erosion is usually caused by a cholesteatoma; less often, it is caused by chronic osteomyelitis.

The bone-eroding process first exposes the soft tissue of a neighboring structure. Protective granulations form on the structure as a last line of defense. Then, after a period of time that varies with the virulence of the organism, the pus under pressure finally penetrates the wall of protective granulations by pressure necrosis. Bone erosion as the pathway of spread may be recognized by the following characteristics:

- The complication occurs several weeks or more after the onset of acute otitis media or in chronic otitis of long duration.
- A prodromal period of partial or intermittent involvement of the structure frequently precedes the diffuse involvement. Thus, a milder, intermittent facial weakness may precede complete facial paralysis; recurrent mild vertigo may precede diffuse purulent labyrinthitis, and localized meningismus may precede diffuse purulent meningitis.
- At operation, a dehiscence of the bone barrier is found between the suppurative focus and the neighboring structure. A layer of granulations covers the exposed soft tissue of the neighboring structure.
- The treatment of a complication by bone erosion is directed toward the complication and always includes surgical removal of the suppurative, bone-eroding focus in the temporal bone. If such removal is neglected, the complication is likely to recover or respond poorly to treatment.

Direct Extension along Preformed Pathways

Extension by preformed pathways (Figure 23–1, A) may occur in either acute exacerbations of chronic otitis media or acute otitis media. The preformed pathway may be a normal anatomic opening in the bony wall, such as the oval or round window, internal auditory canal, cochlear aqueduct, or endolymphatic duct and sac. The pathway may be a developmental dehiscence such as a patent suture or a dehiscent floor of the hypotympanum over the jugular bulb. The preformed pathway may be the result of a skull fracture or previous surgery. A perilymph fistula, either congenital or acquired, can also serve as a pathway. Occasionally, previous otitis media with coa-

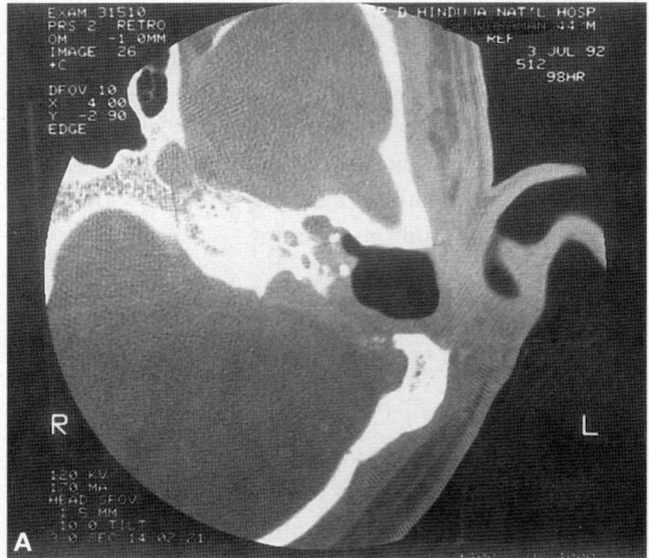

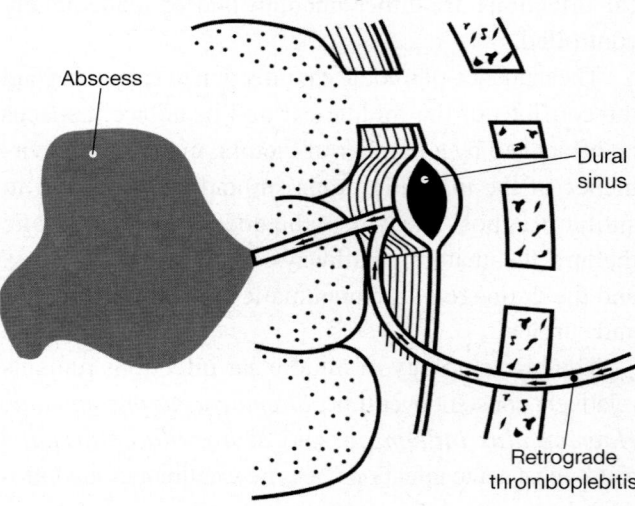

Figure 23–1 *A,* Temporal bone computed tomographic scan, axial section. There is considerable erosion of the temporal bone and a high likelihood of an intracranial complication developing. *B,* Schematic representation of the development of a brain abscess from otitis media. Spread of infection can occur by direct extension or by retrograde thrombophlebitis.

lescent mastoiditis heals but leaves a scar tissue tract to a neighboring structure. This tract acts as a preformed pathway for succeeding infections. Extension by a preformed pathway is not always easily diagnosed preoperatively. The diagnosis is suggested by the following characteristics:

- There is a history of repeated attacks of meningitis, skull fracture, operation on the temporal bone, or previously healed otitis media.

- The complication occurs early in the acute infection, thus resembling extension by thrombophlebitis.
- At operation, a dehiscence of the bone barrier not caused by bone erosion is found.
- The patient has an intracranial complication following suppurative labyrinthitis.

The treatment of a complication by a preformed pathway is directed toward the complication along with closure of the fistula and surgical evacuation of any collection of pus within the temporal bone. An example is beginning meningitis via the internal auditory canal from suppurative labyrinthitis; the labyrinth should be drained at the same time that the meningitis is treated by antibacterial medication.

Thrombophlebitis

In 1902, Körner demonstrated by histopathologic studies that it is possible for infection to pass from the lining mucosa of the middle ear and mastoid through intact bone by means of a progressive thrombophlebitis of small venules (Figure 23–1, B).[6] This manner of spread may occur in acute middle ear infections or in acute exacerbations of a chronic infection. Progressive retrograde thrombophlebitis is the usual route for the formation of a brain abscess. Infection spreads through veins contiguous with either the infected pneumatized spaces of the temporal bone or the previously thrombosed dural venous sinus. There is a rich network of veins within the temporal bone that is in direct communication within the temporal bone and that, in turn, is in direct communication with the extracranial, intracranial, and cranial diploic veins. The extracranial veins are closely associated with the arterial supply of the temporal bone. The extracranial and intracranial venous systems anastomose through the mastoid emissary veins that enter the sigmoid sinus, which drains the superior and inferior petrosal sinuses. All of the dural venous sinuses are interconnected. Thus, sigmoid sinus thrombosis can lead to thrombophlebitis of other sinuses as well.

A complication caused by thrombophlebitis may be recognized by the following characteristics:

- The complication occurs early in the acute infection, sometimes within a day or two of the onset, usually within the first 10 days.

- In certain complications, such as purulent meningitis, the prodromal period of beginning invasion with localized meningitis, commonly called menigismus, such as is usually seen in extension by bone erosion, is lacking.
- At operation, the bony walls of the middle ear and mastoid cells are intact. The bone and mucoperiosteum lining of the mastoid cells may be inflamed and bleed easily, but there is no coalescent abscess, and the bone is not dehiscent.
- Hematogenous spread of infection usually results in meningitis. Whereas venous thrombophlebitis usually leads to cerebellar abscesses, arterial spread leads to temporal lobe abscesses and diffuse septicemia.

SPECIFIC COMPLICATIONS

It is uncommon for an intracranial complication to occur without a temporal bone complication occurring first. Common symptoms of an impending intracranial complication are as follows:

- Persistence of otorrhea. The otorrhea is particularly foul smelling, and the pus becomes more viscous. The pus is thicker and creamier and may be blood stained. When intracranial complication is imminent, the discharge becomes scanty, indicative of poor drainage.
- Pain is an ominous sign that an intracranial complication is imminent. The pain is typically of a deep boring nature and is accompanied by a change in the quality of the pus emanating from the ear. Patients may also complain of a generalized headache that is "the worst headache" they have ever had.
- High-grade fever, altered sensorium, toxemia, photophobia, and irritability are other signs of impending intracranial complication.
- Neck stiffness and generalized malaise are signs that the organism has reached the cerebrospinal fluid (CSF) space.

The principles of ear surgery remain unchanged in these complications:

- Eradication of disease

• Establishment of adequate drainage for accumulated material

Eradication of disease requires a thorough and complete mastoidectomy. All of the diseased air cells are exenterated. Pus, wherever it is encountered, is drained. All diseased or dead tissue is removed. There are some general remarks that can be made concerning all complications of mastoid disease. Specific recommendations are made in the following sections concerning each complication. Creating adequate drainage usually requires a canal wall down approach, with exceptions in certain situations. In the presence of acute otitis media that has caused meningitis, usually antibiotics and a myringotomy with tube insertion suffice to provide adequate drainage. In the presence of overwhelming disease and cholesteatoma, most reports advocate canal wall down techniques. To make the ear disease free, the canal wall down technique should be performed so that the ear is made disease free. Equally important is creating a wide meatoplasty. A wide meatoplasty permits adequate drainage and allows easy inspection and cleansing of the mastoid cavity.

Each diagnosis of intracranial disease is defined and discussed individually. The diagnoses are presented in order of decreasing frequency. Meningitis is the most common complication in this group of diagnoses in most traditional articles, but CSF otorrhea is used in the broad sense here and is reviewed first. Brain abscess and lateral sinus thrombosis are the next most common. Finally, other diagnoses, including otitic hydrocephalus, and subdural and epidural processes are reviewed. Pathophysiology, including microbiology, unique symptoms, specific evaluation methods, and treatment, is outlined.

CEREBROSPINAL FLUID OTORRHEA

Drainage of CSF from the ear may be a complication of chronic ear disease or the result of surgery. A frequent cause is a fracture of the temporal bone. Drainage may also develop following irradiation of tumors involving the temporal bone. In rare cases, drainage begins spontaneously without previous ear disease, usually a consequence of a congenital malformation. Regardless of origin, the symptoms, diagnosis, and treatment of CSF otorrhea are the same.

Special mention should be made of the profuse flow of clear fluid from the oval window that can occur in stapes surgery, sometimes referred to as a "gusher." On penetrating the footplate, a gush of clear, colorless fluid that rapidly fills the field and overflows the ear identifies a gusher; an oozer comprises a slower, less profuse flow of fluid. Schuknecht and Reisser[23] described the pathology associated with the gusher and the oozer. The oozer reflects an enlarged cochlear aqueduct, which may be seen on computed tomographic (CT) scan.[24] Gushers are associated with a modiolar defect. Prevention is thought to be the primary means of treatment. Patients who are identified with a large cochlear aqueduct and abnormally dilated vestibule, or a modiolar defect, should be considered candidates at risk for a vigorous flow of fluid (initially perilymph and then CSF). Because gushers result in sensorineural hearing loss, it is important to avoid stapes surgery in such ears.[25] If encountered inadvertently, elevation of the patient's head during and after surgery can reduce the rate of flow. It is important to seal the oval window with a tissue graft and a prosthesis. In some cases, particularly in anacusic ears, it may be necessary to obliterate the vestibule with a tissue graft.

More difficult, insidious, and controversial is a perilymph fistula (PLF), which may occur following stapes surgery or other trauma. Rupture of the oval or round window can occur with barotrauma, as seen in divers and aviators, or a lifting/straining effort. Perilymph fistulae of spontaneous origin are controversial.[26]

Clinical Presentation

Clear, colorless, watery fluid draining from the mastoid cavity or the external auditory canal that reaccumulates immediately after removal by suction or cotton applicator should be assumed to be CSF; however, aspirating clear, watery fluid from the middle ear does not suffice to confirm the diagnosis. The β_2 transferrin test is conclusive. Initial screening may be accomplished by testing for glucose. Glucose levels in the 60 to 80 mg/100 mL range suggest CSF. Occasionally, there is no external drainage from the ear, but the patient complains of aural fullness caused by fluid accumulation behind an intact tympanic membrane. There may also be CSF escape down the eustachian tube, and, if the patient leans forward, rhinorrhea may be seen. The most conservative form of treatment is bed rest, with the head elevated at 30 degrees. If leakage or symptoms persist, surgical repair is indicated.

Surgical Repair

The technique used to repair a CSF leak varies with the source, the size of the defect, and the status of the hearing. In general, the goal is to isolate the CSF from the middle ear space, or at least from the eustachian tube orifice, thus preventing retrograde infection and troublesome headaches from decreased CSF pressure.

When a CSF leak occurs through a minute dural tear, the dura should be exposed on all sides of the tear. A small graft of temporalis muscle, fascia, or even Gelfoam® can usually tamponade the leak. Larger or more extensive tears may require suturing or larger grafts. Acute tears are easier to repair than chronic ones. Defects that are larger than 1 to 2 cm may require an alternate route of repair. Usually, a defect in the middle fossa will require a craniotomy and defect repair from above. Repairs may be completed using muscle, fascia, or bone. A middle fossa defect occurring near the ossicular chain may be small, but repair from above may be necessary to prevent ossicular chain injury. Use of a lumbar drain can reduce pressure on the repair and improve the chances of success.

In the anacusic ear, eustachian tube obliteration, using muscle, bone, or foreign materials, may be indicated.

Repair of a PLF generally involves "patching" of the oval and/or round window areas with perichondrium. Recovery of hearing is possible but unlikely in some cases of traumatic PLF.[27]

MENINGITIS

Generalized bacterial meningitis is defined as an inflammatory response to bacterial infection of the pia-arachnoid and the CSF of the subarachnoid space. Since the subarachnoid space is continuous around the brain, spinal cord, and optic nerves, infections of this space usually involve the entire cerebrospinal axis.

Localized meningitis may be defined as a localized inflammation of the dura and pia-arachnoid confined to the region adjacent to a suppurative focus or dural irritation, without viable organisms in the CSF.

Meningitis was the most frequent intracranial complication of otitis media in the preantibiotic era. With the introduction of antimicrobial drugs, recovery from meningitis improved from 10 to 86%,[28] whereas recovery from otogenic meningitis was 59%.[29] Other clinicians[30–32] have confirmed that meningitis is the most common intracranial complication of otitis media. Some workers find that acute otitis media is more likely to cause meningitis than chronic otitis media.[30]

Pathophysiology

The major meningeal pathogens are *H. influenzae* and *S. pneumoniae*.[33] *Streptococcus pneumoniae* infections of the meninges are often associated with acute otitis media.[34] Recovery of anaerobic organisms from the CSF suggests intraventricular rupture of a brain abscess. Polymicrobial infection of CSF resulting from otogenic complications is uncommon and accounts for less than 1% of cases.

Meningitis may result from infection spreading from the ear via retrograde thrombophlebitis, bone erosion, and preformed pathways. An important route through which infection can gain access to the CSF is via the labyrinth through the round and oval windows. Nager[35] and Kaplan[36] stressed that this mode of extension is via the perineural spaces to the internal auditory canal and less frequently via the endolymphatic ducts. Proctor[37] postulated that otitic meningitis occurs as the result of infection spreading via the labyrinth and petrous apex. Meningitis can develop following trauma to the ear with fracture, dural tear, and CSF leak. Meningitis can also occur following any middle ear and mastoid surgery.

Clinical Presentation

Otogenic meningitis often goes unrecognized. It is imperative for the physician who is treating a patient with meningitis to rule out a possible otologic cause. Most physicians will suspect an otologic cause in the presence of otorrhea or obvious long-standing ear disease. It is imperative to rule out otitis media in the patient who does not have otorrhea or long-standing otologic complaints.

Cawthorne[38] noted that the symptoms tend to be more rapid when associated with acute otitis media. The earliest symptoms are headache, fever, vomiting, photophobia, irritability, and restlessness. Infants may have seizures. As the infection progresses, the headache increases, and vomiting becomes more pronounced. Neck stiffness, with resistance to flexing the neck so that the chin does not touch the chest, may start with minimal discomfort and progress. Brudzinski's sign, the inability to flex the leg without moving the opposite leg (or flexion of the neck resulting in flexion of the hip and knee), is a sign of meningitis. Similarly, Kernig's sign, an inability to extend the leg when lying supine with the thigh flexed toward the abdomen, is suggestive of meningitis.

Management

Computed tomographic scanning of the temporal bones demonstrates the status of the temporal bone and that of surrounding structures (Figure 23–2). High-resolution CT scanning is very useful and is the imaging modality of choice. Rapid CT scanning is now available that reduces the time to take a high-resolution scan of the temporal

bones, which is particularly important in children in whom a congenital malformation of the ear needs to be ruled out. Computed tomographic scanning helps rule out the presence of congenital ear malformations that permit leakage of CSF through an associated inner ear fistula. Bony details are best visualized with CT scanning.

Magnetic resonance imaging (MRI) provides better resolution of the brain substance and shows middle ear fluid and inflammatory changes in the brain and meninges. No bone detail is possible. The relationship of middle ear disease to the surrounding bone is not well visualized.

Either CT scanning or MRI can identify a mass effect that could lead to herniation. Thus, imaging usually precedes lumbar puncture. Although fundoscopic examination may show indistinct disk margins or even choking of vessels, it is sometimes difficult to perform in an uncooperative patient.

It is imperative to identify the causative organism and the source of infection. Accordingly, a lumbar puncture is performed to obtain CSF for bacteriologic analysis. In meningitis, the CSF is cloudy or yellow (xanthochromic); an elevated white blood cell count, low glucose, and high protein are expected. The pathogen is identified by microscopic examination of Gram-stained fluid with confirmation by culture; sensitivity testing aids in the

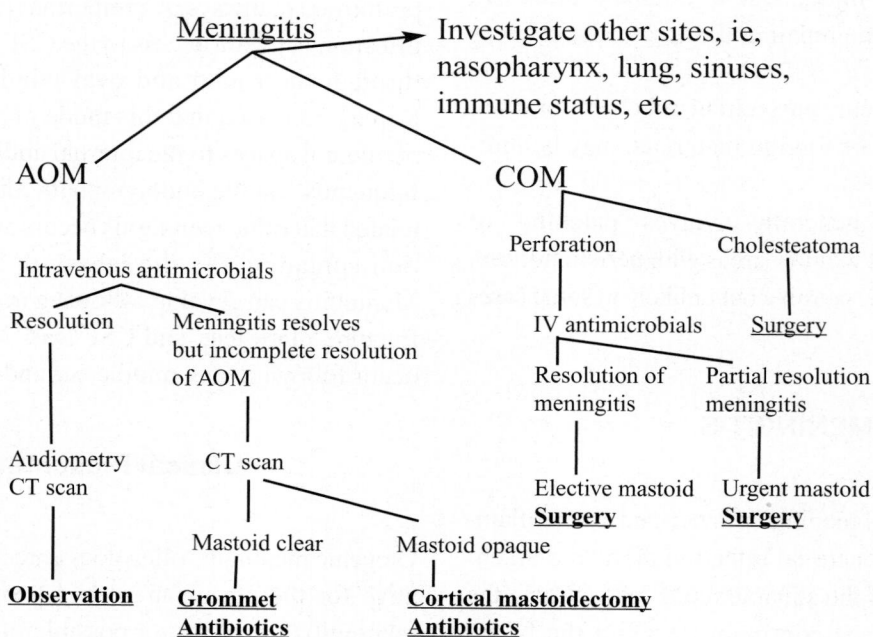

Figure 23–2 Management of otogenic meningitis. AOM = acute otitis media; COM = chronic otitis media; IV = intravenous; CT = computed tomography.

selection of a suitable antimicrobial drug. A sample should be taken from the ear as well, especially if pus is present.

Treatment

Antimicrobial drugs are essential in the treatment of meningitis. Treatment for meningitis resulting from acute otitis media should be directed at *H. influenzae* type B with second- or third-generation cephalosporins.[39]

The advantages of third-generation cephalosporins are their bactericidal activity, ability to penetrate the blood-brain barrier and enter the CSF, their expanded activity against β-lactamase-producing organisms and gram-negative organisms, and low toxicity.[40] Bactericidal drugs are preferred over bacteriostatic drugs.[41,42]

Rapid bacteriolysis releases large amounts of inflammatory fragments that have severe neurologic and auditory sequelae (sensorineural hearing loss—glucocorticoids, such as dexamethasone, have been shown to decrease these sequelae).[43,44] However, corticosteroids have been found to be useful only for meningitis caused by acute otitis media and only if there are no other intracranial complications. To be effective, dexamethasone should be administered shortly before or concurrently with the first dose of antimicrobial medication to decrease the CSF inflammatory response.

Role of Surgery

In acute otitis media with an intact tympanic membrane, surgery consists of myringotomy with evacuation of the fluid from the middle ear, which is sent for examination and culture.

For the patient with coalescent mastoiditis or with a history of ear trauma and precipitous meningitis, a complete mastoidectomy with middle ear exploration should be performed. In the latter circumstance, the surgeon should look for and repair the route of CSF leakage. Computed tomographic scanning usually reveals the fracture line, allowing the surgeon to identify the site of the leak.

If cholesteatoma is present, a radical mastoidectomy is usually performed; the goal of surgery is to rid the ear of disease and provide adequate drainage.

BRAIN ABSCESS

A brain abscess is a focal suppurative process within the brain parenchyma surrounded by a region of encephalitis.[34]

Brain abscess secondary to otitis media displays a bimodal age distribution, with peaks in the pediatric age group and in the fourth decade.[45] In most series, the male-to-female ratio has been approximately 3 to 1.[46] Otitis media was an important cause of brain abscess in the past but has been much less significant more recently. Chronic otitis media is much more likely to cause brain abscess than acute otitis media,[47] and cholesteatoma now accounts for most cases.[48] Most authors report that otogenic brain abscesses are more likely to be located in the cerebrum (temporal lobe) than in the cerebellum[32,49]; however, the majority of cerebellar abscesses are associated with middle ear infections.[34] On the other hand, Murthy and coworkers[50] found that otogenic abscesses occurred more frequently in the cerebellum. The mortality associated with brain abscess of otogenic origin in the antibiotic era is about 25%.[51] Cerebellar abscesses have a greater likelihood of fatal outcome.[52]

Pathophysiology

Multiple organisms are usually present in brain abscesses.[53] Polymicrobial cultures with a high incidence of anaerobes are reported in various studies.[54] Streptococcus and staphylococcus are common gram-positive organisms that are isolated from brain abscesses. *Escherichia coli* and *Proteus*, *Klebsiella*, and *Pseudomonas* species are typical gram-negative isolates. The microbiology of a brain abscess is influenced by the immune status of the host. It is interesting to note that *H. influenzae* is rarely found in otogenic brain abscesses.[38]

Brain abscess can result from any of three processes: (1) a contiguous focus of infection, such as otitis media (Figures 23–3, A and B); (2) hematogenous spread from a distant focus of infection, such as chronic pyogenic lung disease; and (3) head injury or cranial surgery.

Otogenic brain abscesses are often the result of venous thrombophlebitis rather than direct dural extension.[55] Five percent of brain abscesses occur soon after mastoidectomy,[46] for example, when an open mastoid cavity has been created but residual disease persists.[56]

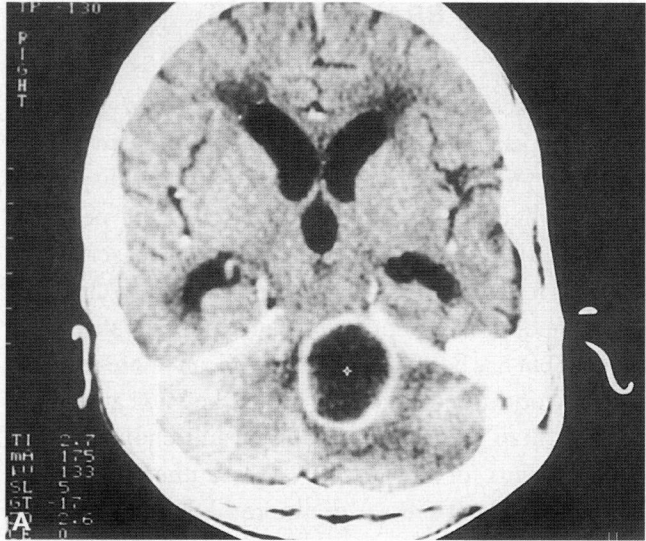

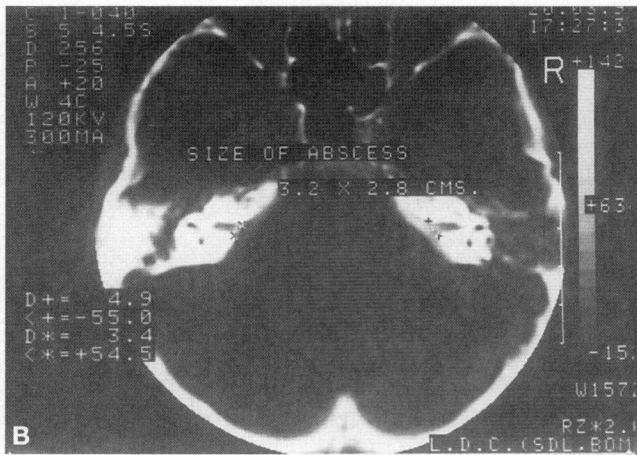

Figure 23–3 *A*, A well-encapsulated brain abscess complicating otitis media. *B*, Temporal bone computed tomographic scan, bone algorithm, axial section (same case as in *A*). The temporal bone has been largely destroyed. The contralateral temporal bone is normal.

Thrombophlebitis usually accompanies the formation of a brain abscess and must be managed appropriately. Osteitis or granulation tissue causes retrograde thrombophlebitis of dural vessels that terminate in the white matter of the brain,[57] producing encephalitis. This localized encephalitis progresses to necrosis and liquefaction of brain tissue (focal suppuration) with surrounding edema.[51] Within approximately 2 weeks, an abscess capsule surrounded by granulation tissue forms. Brain

abscess formation is a continuum from cerebritis to a well-encapsulated necrotic focus; nonetheless, many authors[37,58] have described stages of the formation of a brain abscess (Figure 23–4). Encapsulation is more well defined on the cortical side as compared with the ventricular side, perhaps explaining the propensity of abscesses to rupture medially into the ventricular system rather than into the subarachnoid space (Figure 23–5).

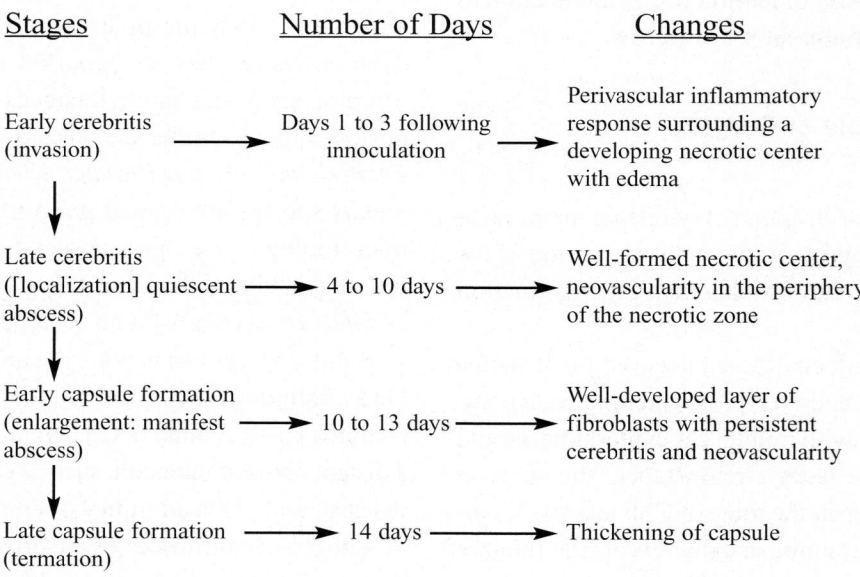

Figure 23–4 Stages of formation of brain abscess and changes that occur.

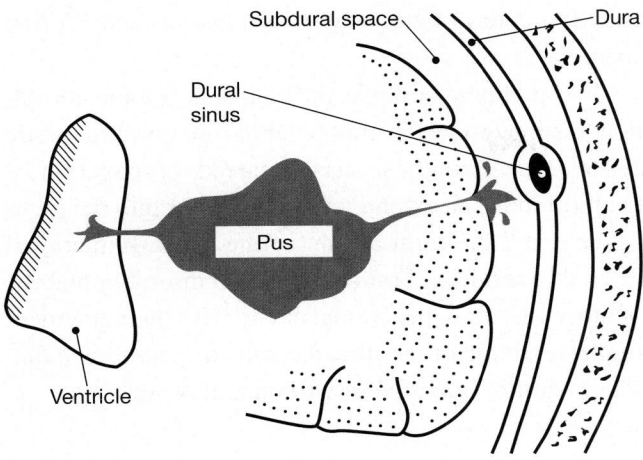

Figure 23–5 Schematic illustration demonstrating brain abscess rupture into the ventricle and into the subdural space.

The maturity of the brain abscess depends on the local oxygen concentration, the offending organism, and the host immune response.

Clinical Presentation

The patient appears very "toxic" and drowsy and often complains of deep bony pain. Occasionally, indolent mastoiditis can cause a brain abscess. Foul-smelling, creamy otorrhea indicates a fulminant, destructive process. Brain abscess formation is indicated by the presence of the triad of (a) headache, (b) high-grade fever, and (c) focal neurologic deficits. In more recent times, the complete triad is not frequently encountered. Symptoms may be present for 2 weeks before the brain abscess is fully formed.[34] Focal deficits depend on the location of the abscess. Cerebellar abscesses provoke dizziness, ataxia, nystagmus, and vomiting. Temporal lobe lesions may result in seizures. Associated signs of meningitis are usually present.[55] Papilledema is frequently seen in stage 3 of abscess formation.[59]

Imaging

Computed tomographic scanning is very useful in the evaluation of the patient suspected of having an otogenic brain abscess. Scanning may allow for earlier detection of abscesses and improved outcomes.[60] The brain abscess appears as a hypodense area surrounded by an area of edema, a configuration known as the "ring" sign. Serial CT scanning can be used to follow the effects of treatment, determine if the abscess is resolving, and assist in the timing of surgical intervention.

Magnetic resonance imaging has also proven to be useful and is superior to CT scanning in detecting subtle changes in the brain parenchyma and in detecting the spread of the abscess into the subarachnoid space or into the ventricle.[61]

One limitation of MRI is that it cannot provide detailed information about the temporal bone; thus, a separate CT scan is required to assess the temporal bone.

Management

The patient must be hospitalized and treated with appropriate, high-dose antimicrobial medication immediately. The management of the brain abscess takes precedence over that of the primary infective source because the patient is seriously ill and the neurosurgical procedure may be the life-saving procedure. The patient should be first stabilized neurologically; only then should the ear causing the infection be operated on.

Currently, the management of brain abscesses is a controversial issue owing to improved imaging and more effective antibiotics. The decision to excise or drain a brain abscess is one such controversy. Williams[62] recommends aspiration with high doses of appropriate antibiotics because he finds that this regimen is associated with fewer permanent neurologic sequelae. Le Beau and colleagues[63] recommend total excision because they find that this leads to lower mortality. Another controversy exists as to whether neurosurgical intervention is required at all because the intravenous administration of newer and more effective antibiotics can result in the complete resolution of small brain abscesses,[64] obviating neurosurgical intervention.

OTOGENIC SUPPURATIVE THROMBOPHLEBITIS

Otogenic suppurative thrombophlebitis is defined as the simultaneous presence of venous thrombosis and suppuration in the intracranial cavity.

Formation of a thrombus occurs after the infection has spread to the intima. The mural thrombus becomes infected and may propagate; as it increases in size, it occludes the lumen. Embolization of septic thrombi or extension into tributary vessels may produce further disease.

Infectious thrombophlebitis of the sigmoid sinus is a well-known intracranial complication of otitis media. The advent of antibiotics has brought about a decline in this condition,[65] yet the mortality associated with this condition remains high.[32] Suppurative thrombophlebitis of the sigmoid sinus can be seen with acute and chronic otitis media.

Pathophysiology

The β-hemolytic streptococcus was the most common organism associated with this condition; however, more recently, cultures have revealed mixed flora, including *Bacteroides* and *Streptococcus* species as well as gram-negative rods. Seid and Sellars[66] have reported the rel-ative frequency of culturing *Pseudomonas* and *Proteus* species.

Two pathophysiologic mechanisms for the formation of suppurative thrombophlebitis are given in Figure 23–6. Once thrombosis has occurred, propagation of the thrombus can extend intracranially or into the jugular vein and the right atrium of the heart. Intracranial extension results in brain abscess and thrombophlebitis of other vessels in the cranial cavity with their attendant sequelae. Intracardiac spread results in widespread dissemination of infection and fulminant septicemia.

Clinical Presentation

High-grade fever is a sign of suppurative thrombophlebitis. The fever may have a "picket fence" appearance or may be high grade without returning to baseline.[67] The patient will typically be toxic and restless and will complain of otalgia. The otalgia, described as a deep, boring pain, usually heralds a worsening neurologic status. Otorrhea will be foul smelling and usually blood stained.

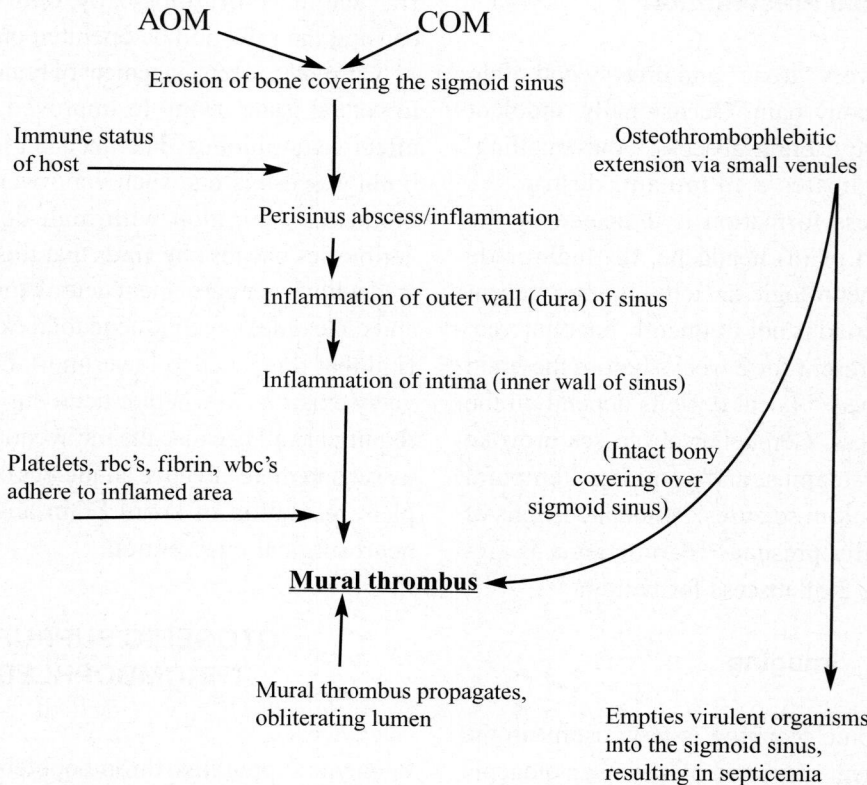

Figure 23–6 Pathogenesis of thrombophlebitis in the sigmoid sinus. AOM = acute otitis media; COM = chronic otitis media.

Neck stiffness and papilledema are usual findings. If beta-hemolytic streptococci are responsible for the infection, the patient may present with anemia, manifesting in pallor and low hemoglobin levels. Proptosis, ptosis, chemosis, and ophthalmoplegia indicate that the thrombus has spread to the cavernous sinus. Tenderness and edema over the mastoid (Griesinger's sign) are pathognomonic for suppurative thrombophlebitis of the sigmoid sinus and reflect thrombosis of the mastoid emissary veins. Propagation of the thrombus into the internal jugular vein causes it to become hard, cordlike, and very tender to palpation, and results in a stiff neck. The lymph nodes along the internal jugular vein are enlarged and tender. Involvement of the torcular and sagittal sinuses can result in otitic hydrocephalus.

Imaging

Computed tomographic scanning and MRI are the current imaging tools of choice in making the diagnosis. Before the advent of these imaging tools, cerebral angiography with observation of the venous phase was used to determine if thrombosis was present; however, cerebral angiography is no longer routinely performed because of its potential to dislodge the clot.[65]

Computed tomographic scanning usually demonstrates the "delta sign"—an empty triangle at the level of the sigmoid sinus, consisting of the clot surrounded by a high-intensity rim of contrast-enhanced dura (Figure 23–7)—when thrombosis is present.[68] However, this sign is not always detectable, and not all thrombi can be documented by CT scanning.[69]

Magnetic resonance imaging is more sensitive than CT scanning in detecting thrombosis. Magnetic resonance imaging shows blood flow, sinus obstruction, and subsequent reversal of flow.[70] Magnetic resonance imaging also provides higher resolution in detailing nerve tissue. Thus, MRI allows for earlier and more precise diagnosis of sinus thrombosis and better delineates both its extent and the involvement of surrounding structures. On gadolinium-enhanced MRI, the thrombus appears as a soft tissue signal associated with a vascular and bright appearance of the dural walls—the "delta" sign as seen with gadolinium-enhanced MRI.[71,72]

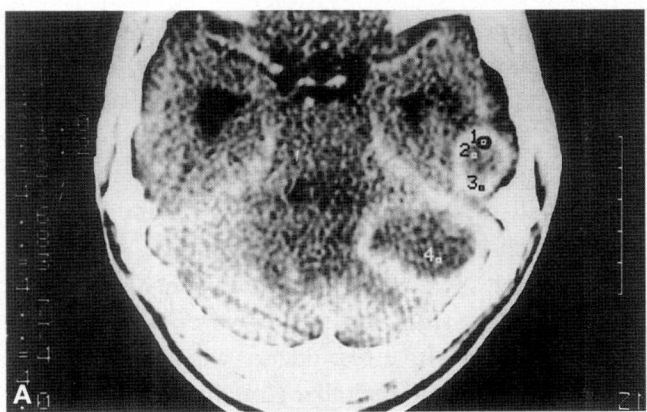

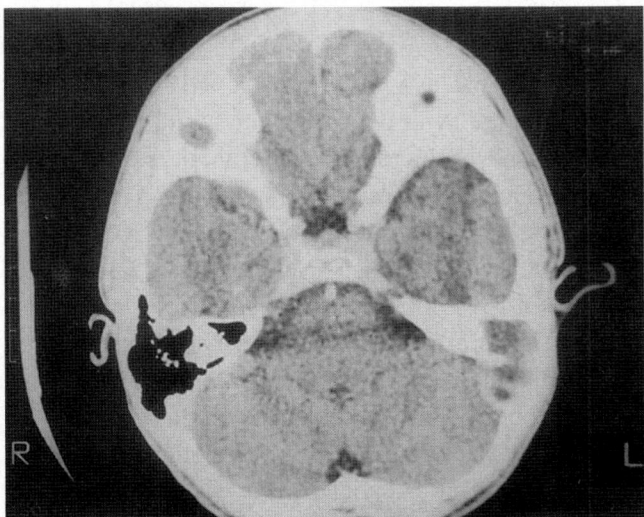

Figure 23–7 A computed tomographic scan of sigmoid sinus thrombophlebitis. The mastoid is eroded, particularly at the sigmoid sinus. The pathognomonic "delta" sign is seen. The contralateral temporal bone is normal.

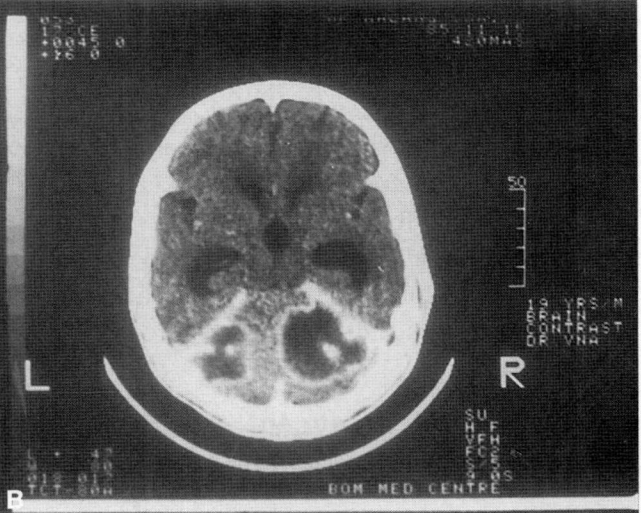

Figure 23–8 *A*, Multiple, ipsilateral otogenic brain abscesses. The anterior abscess is located in the temporal lobe, whereas the posterior abscess is located in the cerebellum. *B*, Bilateral cerebellar brain abscesses of otogenic origin.

Early thrombus, as it is rich in deoxyhemoglobin, has an intermediate density on T_1-weighted images and a low intensity on T_2-weighted images. As the clot matures, methemoglobin forms and the MRI appearance changes so that the clot is hyperintense on both T_1- and T_2-weighted images.

Management

Sigmoid sinus thrombophlebitis manifesting the classic signs and symptoms outlined above is unmistakable. However sigmoid sinus thrombophlebitis can present in an atypical manner, and additional evaluation may be necessary. Queckenstedt's (or the Tobey-Ayer) test is used to detect lateral venous sinus thrombosis and is performed as follows: a spinal needle is inserted into the subarachnoid space, a manometer is attached, and the resting CSF pressure is recorded. The change in pressure produced by digital compression of first one internal jugular vein and then the other, and then both at once, is noted. When the pressure fails to rise after compression of the internal jugular vein on the side of the diseased ear and fails to fall when the vein is released, with a prompt contralateral response, the test is positive. A positive Queckenstedt's test is very strong evidence in favor of occlusion of the sigmoid sinus; however, it is not infallible. A false-positive test occurs when one sigmoid sinus is smaller than the other (usually the left one). A false negative test occurs when there is unusually good collateral circulation around the obstructed sigmoid sinus via the mastoid emissary vein, the inferior petrosal sinus, and the sinus of Englitsch.

Any contraindication to performing a lumbar puncture (eg, elevated intracranial pressure) is also a contraindication to performing Queckenstedt's test.

A positive blood culture provides good evidence of sigmoid sinus thrombosis, especially when accompanied by the clinical signs and symptoms of thrombosis.

Treatment

Before the development of antibiotics, the treatment of lateral sinus thrombosis comprised surgery. A complete mastoidectomy was performed, and the entire sigmoid sinus was unroofed. Often a perisinus abscess was encountered and drained. Once the entire sinus was exposed, it was inspected and palpated; if it was soft and pliable, and the patient's symptoms were not serious, the sinus was left alone. However, if a rubbery clot was felt, then the sinus was carefully aspirated with a small-gauge needle and syringe. Lack of blood flow indicated a clot. The sinus was then opened in such a way that the medial dural wall was not traumatized. The clot was evacuated as completely as possible. Prior ligation of the internal jugular vein was carried out to prevent propagation of the thrombus into the heart.

Currently, complete mastoidectomy with evacuation of all middle ear and mastoid disease, drainage of the perisinus abscess, and clot removal, along with high-dose, appropriate antimicrobial medications administered intravenously, is considered to be adequate to control suppurative thrombophlebitis.

Ligation of the internal jugular vein is reserved for those cases in which sepsis continues despite an adequate surgical procedure and appropriate intravenous antibiotic therapy. In addition, there should be evidence that the sigmoid sinus thrombophlebitis is propagating into the heart before resorting to ligation.[73]

Anticoagulants arrest the spread of thrombosis but may increase the risk of venous infarction and therefore are no longer recommended.

OTITIC HYDROCEPHALUS

Otitic hydrocephalus is the term suggested by Symonds[74,75] to describe the syndrome associated with otitis media characterized by increased intracranial pressure, normal CSF findings, spontaneous recovery, and no abscess. Although the term otitic hydrocephalus was coined by Symonds, the condition itself was first described by Quincke in 1897.[76] As there is no associated ventricular dilation, it is more appropriately termed "benign raised intracranial tension"[76]; however, the term "otitic hydrocephalus" has persisted and is used in this chapter.

Otitic hydrocephalus is a rare complication of otitis media and stems from either acute or chronic otitis media. Otitic hydrocephalus has a favorable prognosis and is very commonly associated with sigmoid sinus thrombophlebitis; however, not all patients with sigmoid sinus thrombophlebitis develop otitic hydrocephalus.

Pathophysiology

The precise mechanism underlying the development of otitic hydrocephalus is unknown. Symonds[74,75] provided the explanation seen in Figure 23–9. An alternative theory postulates an increase in CSF volume.[77] Sahs and Joynt[78] theorized that the hydrocephalus is secondary to brain edema as brain biopsies reveal interstitial edema, yet electroencephalograms and neurologic function are normal. Weed and Flexner[79] postulated disruption in venous circulation as a cause since changes in CSF pressure are directly related to intracranial venous pressure.

Clinical Presentation

Headache, drowsiness, vomiting, blurring of vision, and diplopia are typical symptoms. Acute or chronic otitis media is also seen.

Papilledema and sixth cranial nerve palsy are usually evident. Optic atrophy can eventually develop.

Elevated CSF pressures with normal CSF biochemistry comprise the classic findings of otitic hydrocephalus. A lumbar puncture should be done with caution lest herniation of the cerebellar tonsils occur.

Magnetic resonance imaging is the imaging modality of choice as it allows for superior evaluation of the venous sinuses.

Retrograde extension of thrombophlebitis from sigmoid sinus to superior sagittal sinus

↓

Blockage of arachnoid villi

↓

CSF decreased absorption/increased secretion

↓

Raised CSF pressure

Figure 23–9 Pathophysiology of otitic hydrocephalus. CSF = cerebrospinal fluid.

Management

The goals of therapy are eradication of ear disease and lowering of the elevated intracranial pressure. O'Connor and Moffat[80] recommend decompression of the sigmoid sinus. Cerebrospinal fluid drainage procedures, such as shunts, have been recommended. Optic sheath decompression has been recommended to prevent optic atrophy.[81] Medical therapy includes corticosteroids, mannitol, diuretics, and acetazolamide.

SUBDURAL EMPYEMA

A subdural empyema is a collection of pus in the space between the dura mater and the arachnoid membrane. This condition was almost always fatal prior to the advent of antibiotic therapy. Today, subdural empyema is the rarest of the complications of otitis media.

Pathophysiology

The subdural space, normally a potential space rather than an actual one, is divided into several large compartments by the foramen magnum, tentorium cerebelli, base of the brain, and the falx cerebri (Figure 23–10). Since these spaces are anatomically confined, a developing empyema can quickly evolve into a fatal mass lesion (Figure 23–11).

Clinical Presentation

Headache of abrupt onset and unusually severe nature is typical of subdural empyema. Fever and vomiting are other symptoms that accompany this disease. The rapidity with which the patient deteriorates points to a subdural empyema.

Magnetic resonance imaging is the imaging modality of choice.[82] It has been found to be superior at detecting the presence and extensions of the infection and can also distinguish between epidural and subdural infection. Multiple, discrete, loculated subdural collections may occasionally be seen. Magnetic resonance imaging is particularly useful because of the absence of bone artifact, heightened contrast between bone, CSF, and brain parenchyma, as well as because of its multiplanar imaging capability.[83] Magnetic resonance imaging can also

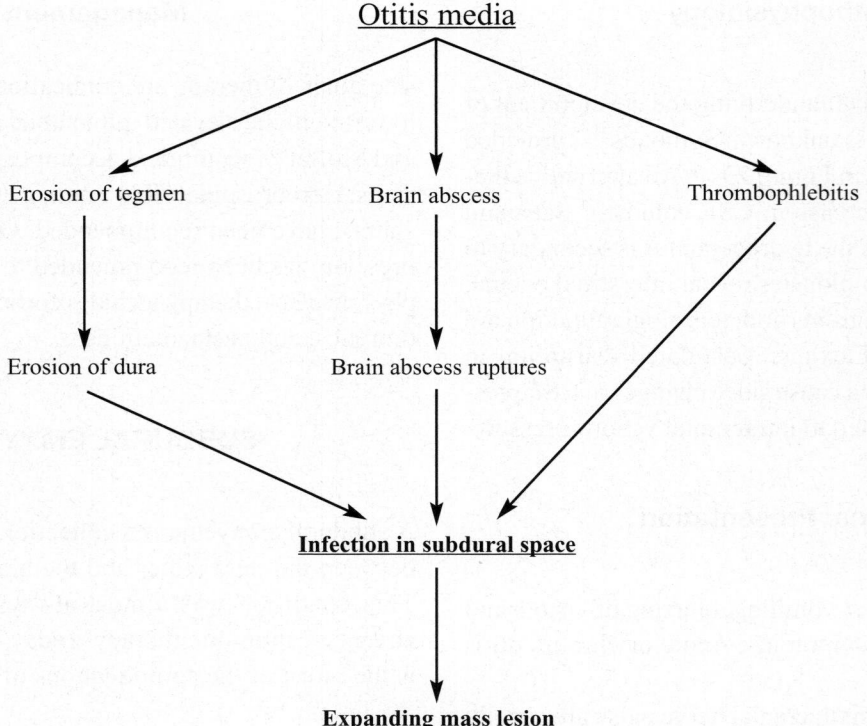

Figure 23–10   Pathology of subdural empyema.

characterize subdural collections, allowing differentiation of sterile, bloody, and infected collections. Computed tomography is unable to perform these functions.

Treatment

Subdural empyema is a surgical emergency, and prognosis is related to the promptness of diagnosis and drainage. Lumbar puncture is contraindicated as it could precipitate herniation of the cerebellar tonsils. Emergency drainage with high-dose, intravenous antimicrobial medication is the treatment of choice. Once the patient has been stabilized neurologically, the underlying ear disease can be managed.

EPIDURAL (EXTRADURAL) ABSCESS

The epidural (extradural) space is a potential space between the dura mater and the bone of the intracranial cavity. Infection here usually manifests with granulation tissue that is in direct continuity with the suppurative process. Large accumulations of pus are rare. Granulation along the dura mater is seen more commonly than an actual abscess (Figure 23–12, A and B). An epidural abscess usually precedes other intracranial complications, especially sinus thrombophlebitis and brain abscess. Sinus thrombophlebitis is the complication that most frequently coexists with an epidural abscess.

Pathogenesis

Coalescent mastoiditis entails bone reabsorption, especially in the areas adjacent to the sigmoid sinus; these areas of bone give way, resulting in a pocket of granulation tissue/pus that expands along the sigmoid sinus. Ultimately, the granulation tissue also infects the sigmoid sinus. Chronic suppurative otitis media without cholesteatoma is usually associated with granulation tissue that invades the perisinus air cells. A single acute exacerbation of infection may cause silent extradural granulation tissue to progress into more serious complications.

Epidural abscesses are rarely symptomatic unless they are very large. Usually, they are noted as incidental findings during surgery performed for another complication;

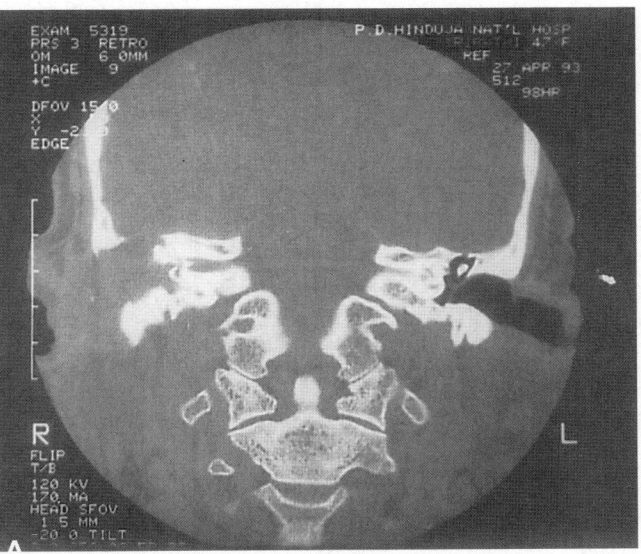

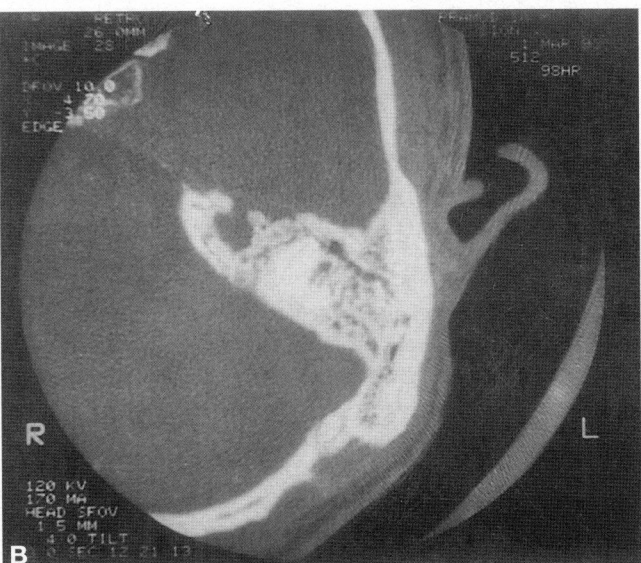

Figure 23–12   *A,* Temporal bone computed tomographic (CT) scan, coronal section. There is mastoiditis and dural elevation, indicative of an epidural abscess. The contralateral temporal bone is normal. *B,* Temporal bone CT scan, axial section. Petrous apicitis is associated with a small epidural abscess.

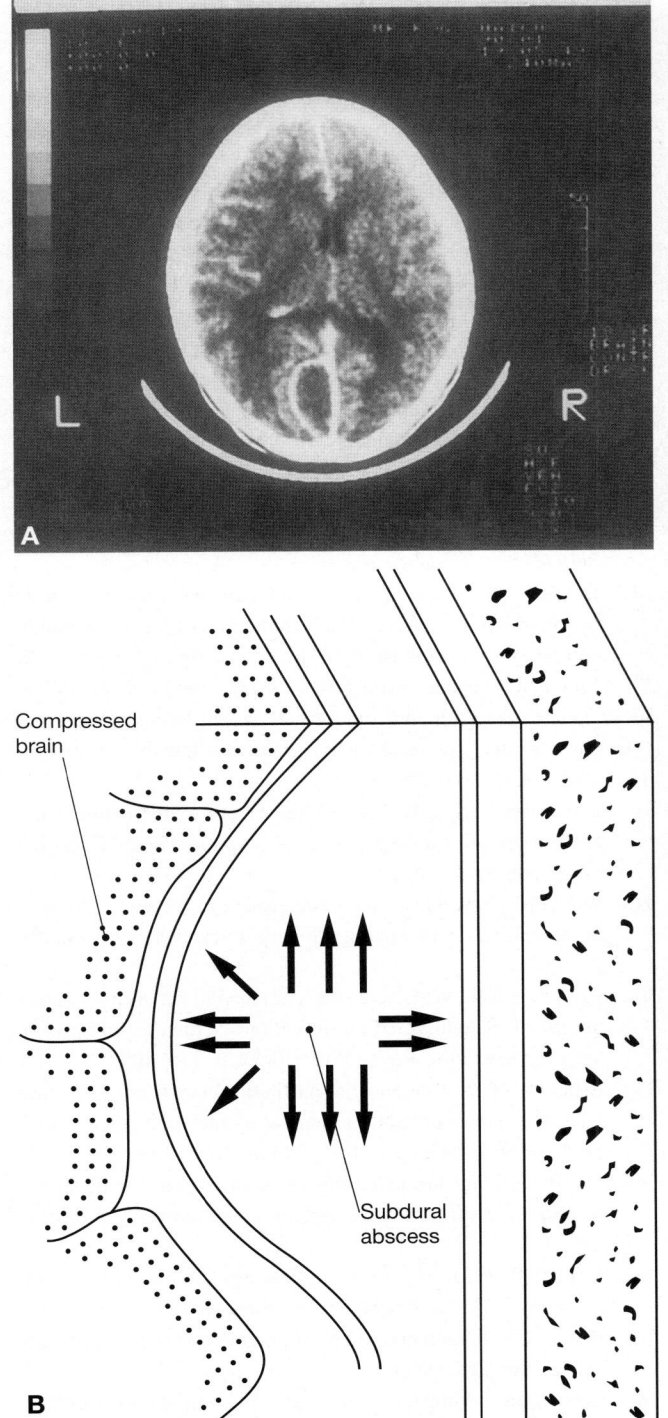

Figure 23–11   *A,* A computed tomographic scan of a loculated subdural abscess in the falx. *B,* Schematic illustration of the mass effect related to an expanding abscess in the subdural space.

however, with the radiologic imaging modalities of today, epidural abscesses can be visualized prior to surgery.

Management

The discovery of granulation tissue penetrating bone or granulation tissue along the sigmoid sinus should prompt further exploration. The surrounding bone should be gently removed and the abscess drained. Care should be taken not to perforate the dura, which could result in a CSF leak and allow the infection to spread directly into the brain. Excessive granulation tissue should be gently trimmed.

REFERENCES

1. Quoted in Cawthorne T. The surgery of the temporal bone. Laryngol Otol 1953;67:377.

2. Quoted in Heine B, Beck J. Handbuch der Hals-Nassen-Ohr-enheilkunde. In: Denker A, Kahler O, editors. Berlin: 1927.

3. Morand SF. Opuscules de chirurgie. Paris: 1768.

4. Lebert. Ueber Entzundung der Hirn-Sinus. Virchows Arch 1856;9:381.

5. MacEwen W. Pyogenic infective diseases of the brain and spinal cord. Glasgow: 1893.

6. Korner O. Die Otitischen Erkrankungen des Hirns, der Hirnhaute und der Blutleiter. Wiesbaden: 1908.

7. Eagleton WP. Brain abscess: its surgical pathology and operative technic. New York: Macmillan; 1922.

8. Shambaugh GE Jr. The surgical treatment of meningitis of otitic and nasal origin. JAMA 1937;108:696.

9. Lebert. Ueber Gehirnabscesse. Virchows Arch 1856;10:78.

10. Zaufal E. Operation der Sinusthrombose und Versuche mit Cocain am Gehororgane. Prag Med Wochenschr 1884;9:474.

11. Lane WA. Middle ear suppurations and their complications. BMJ 1889;1:998.

12. Ballance CA. Pyemic thrombosis of the lateral sinus. Lancet 1890;1:1057.

13. Jansen A. Referat die Operations methoden bei den verschiedenen otitischen Gehirnkomplikationen. Verhandl Deutsch Otol Gesellsch 1895;4:96.

14. Gradenigo G. Sulla leptomeningite circoscritta e sulla paralisi dell' adducente di origine otitica. Gior Accad Med Torino 1904;10:59.

15. Kopetsky SJ, Almour R. Suppuration of the petrous pyramid. Ann Otol Rhinol Laryngol 1931;39:996.

16. Eagleton WP. Unlocking the petrous pyramid for localized bulbar meningitis secondary to suppuration of the petrous apex. Arch Otol 1931;13:386.

17. Courville CB. Intracranial complications of otitis media and mastoiditis in the antibiotic era. Laryngoscope 1955;63:31.

18. Rosenwasser H, Adelman N. Otitic complications. Arch Otol 1957;65:225.

19. Lund WS. A review of 50 cases of intracranial complications from otogenic infection between 1961 and 1977. Clin Otolaryngol 1978;3:495–501.

20. Bluestone CD, Stephenson JS, Martin LM. Ten-year review of otitis media pathogens. Pediatr Infect Dis J 1992;11 Suppl 8:S7–11.

21. Feinmesser R, Wiesel YM, Argaman M, Gay I. Otitis externa—bacteriological survey. ORL J Otorhinolaryngol Relat Spec 1982;44:121–5.

22. Neely G. Complications of suppurative otitis media, Parts 1 and 2. Washington (DC): American Academy of Otolaryngology Head and Neck Surgery; 1978.

23. Schuknecht HF, Reisser C. The morphologic basis for perilymphatic gushers and oozers. Adv Otorhinolaryngol 1988;39: 1–12.

24. Jackler RK, Hwang PH. Enlargement of the cochlear aqueduct: fact or fiction? Otolaryngol Head Neck Surg 1993;109:14–25.

25. Glasscock ME 3rd. The stapes gusher. Arch Otolaryngol 1973; 98:82–91.

26. Hughes GB, Sismanis A, House JW. Is there consensus in perilymph fistula management? Otolaryngol Head Neck Surg 1990;102:111–7.

27. Glasscock ME 3rd, McKennan KX, Levine SC. Persistent traumatic perilymph fistulas. Laryngoscope 1987;97(7 Pt 1): 860–4.

28. House H. Acute otitis media. A comparative study of the results obtained before and after the introduction of the sulfonamide compounds. Arch Otolaryngol Head Neck Surg 1946;43:371–5.

29. McLay K. Otogenic meningitis. J Laryngol Otol 1954;68:140–6.

30. Gower D, McGuirt WF. Intracranial complications of acute and chronic infectious ear disease: a problem still with us. Laryngoscope 1983;93:1028–33.

31. Habib RG, Girgis NI, Abu el Ella AH, et al. The treatment and outcome of intracranial infections of otogenic origin. J Trop Med Hyg 1988;91:83–6.

32. Samuel J, Fernandes CM, Steinberg JL. Intracranial otogenic complications: a persisting problem. Laryngoscope 1986;96: 272–8.

33. Roos K, Scheld WM. Acute bacterial meningitis in children and adults. In: Scheld W, editor. Infections of the central nervous system. New York: Raven Press; 1991. p. 335–409.

34. Scheld W. Bacterial meningitis and brain abscess. In: Isselbacher K, et al, editors. Harrison's principles of internal medicine. 13th ed. New York: McGraw-Hill; 1994. p. 2296–309.

35. Nager GT. Mastoid and paranasal sinus infections and their relation to the central nervous system. Clin Neurosurg 1966;14: 288–313.

36. Kaplan R. Neurological complications of infections of the head and neck. Otolaryngol Clin North Am 1976;9:729–49.

37. Proctor CA. Intracranial complications of otitic origin. Laryngoscope 1966;76:288–308.

38. Cawthorne T. Otogenic meningitis. J Laryngol Otol 1939;54: 444–70.

39. Neely G. Intratemporal and intracranial complications of otitis media. In: Bailey B, editor. Otolaryngology-head and neck surgery. Philadelphia: Lippincott; 1993.

40. Jacobs R. A prospective randomised comparison of cefotaxime vs ampicillin and chloramphenicol for bacterial meningitis in children. J Pediatr 1985;107:129–35.

41. Quagliarello V, Scheld W. Bacterial meningitis: pathogenesis, pathophysiology and progress. N Engl J Med 1992;327:864–72.

42. Weiner GM, Williams B. Prevention of intracranial problems in ear and sinus surgery: a possible role for cefotaxime. J Laryngol Otol 1993;107:1005–7.

43. Lebell M. Dexamethasone therapy for bacterial meningitis: results of 2 double blind placebo controlled trials. N Engl J Med 1988;319:964–6.

44. Odio CM. The beneficial effects of early dexamethasone administration in infants and children with bacterial meningitis. N Engl J Med 1991;324:1525–31.

45. de Souza CE GM. Complications of otitis media in children. In: de Souza CE SJ, Pellitteri PK, editors. Pediatric otorhinolaryngology head and neck surgery. San Diego, London: Singular; p. 115–35.

46. Yen P, Chan S, Huang T. Brain abscess with special reference to otolaryngologic sources of infection. Otolaryngol Head Neck Surg 1995;113:5–22.

47. Meyers E, Ballantine H. The management of otogenic brain abscess. Laryngoscope 1965;75:273–88.

48. Sennaroglu L, Sozeri B. Otogenic brain abscess: review of 41 cases. Otolaryngol Head Neck Surg 2000;123:751–5.

49. Stuart E, O'Brien F, McNally W. Some observations on brain abscesses. Arch Otolaryngol Head Neck Surg 1955;104:542–3.

50. Murthy PS, Sukumar R, Hazarika P, et al. Otogenic brain abscess in childhood. Int J Pediatr Otorhinolaryngol 1991; 22(1):9–17.

51. Kornblut AD. Cerebral abscess—a recurrent otologic problem. Laryngoscope 1972;82:1541–56.

52. Quijano M, Schuknecht HF, Otte J. Temporal bone pathology associated with intracranial abscess. ORL J Otorhinolaryngol Relat Spec 1988;50:2–31.

53. Ingham H, Selkon J, Roxy C. Bacteriological study of brain abscesses: chemotherapeutic roles of metronidazole. BMJ 1977;2:991–3.

54. Brook I. Bacteriology of intracranial abscesses in children. J Neurosurg 1981;54:484–8.

55. Nissen A. Intracranial complications of otogenic disease. Am J Otol 1980;2:164–7.

56. Keet PC. Cranial intradural abscess management of 641 patients during the 35 years from 1952 to 1986. Br J Neurosurg 1990;4: 273–8.

57. Maniglia AJ, VanBuren JM, Bruce WB, et al. Intracranial abscesses secondary to ear and paranasal sinuses infections. Otolaryngol Head Neck Surg 1980;88:670–80.

58. Ward PH, Setliff RC, Long W. Otogenic brain abscess. Trans Am Acad Ophthalmol Otolaryngol 1969;73:107–14.

59. Buchheit WA, Ronis ML, Liebman E. Brain abscesses complicating head and neck infections. Trans Am Acad Ophthalmol Otolaryngol 1970;74:548–54.

60. Nalbone VP, Kuruvilla A, Gacek RR. Otogenic brain abscess: the Syracuse experience. Ear Nose Throat J 1992;71:238–42.

61. Maniglia A, Goodwin J, Arnold J, Ganz E. Intracranial abscesses secondary to nasal, sinus and orbital infections in adults and children. Arch Otolaryngol Head Neck Surg 1989;115:1424–9.

62. Williams MR. Open evacuation of pus: a satisfying surgical approach to the problem of brain abscess? J Neurol Neurosurg Psychiatry 1983;45:697–700.

63. LeBeau J, King S. Surgical treatment of brain abscess and subdural empyema. J Neurosurg 1973;38:198–203.

64. Brand B, Caparosa RJ, Lubic LG. Otorhinological brain abscess therapy—past and present. Laryngoscope 1984;94:483–7.

65. Teichgraeber J, Perlee H, Turner J. Lateral sinus thrombosis: a modern perspective. Laryngoscope 1982;92:744–51.

66. Seid A, Sellars S. The management of otogenic lateral sinus disease at the Groote Schuur Hospital. Laryngoscope 1973;83: 397–403.

67. Wolfowitz BL. Otogenic intracranial complications. Arch Otolaryngol 1972;96:220–2.

68. Buonanno F, Moody D, Ball M, Laster D. Computed cranial tomographic findings in cerebral sinovenous occlusion. J Comput Assist Tomogr 1978;2:281–90.

69. Harris T, Smith R, Koch K. Gadolinium DTPA enhanced MR imaging of septic dural thrombosis. J Comput Assist Tomogr 1989;13:682–4.

70. Doyle WJ, Webster DB. Neonatal conductive hearing loss does not compromise brainstem auditory function and structure in rhesus monkeys. Hear Res 1991;54:145–51.

71. Fritsch M, Miyamoto R, Wood T. Sigmoid sinus thrombosis diagnosis by contrasted MRI scanning. Otolaryngol Head Neck Surg 1990;103:451–6.

72. Davison SP, Facer GW, McGough PF, et al. Use of magnetic resonance imaging and magnetic resonance angiography in diagnosis of sigmoid sinus thrombosis. Ear Nose Throat J 1997;76: 436–41.

72. Rizer FM, Amiri CA, Schroeder WW, Brackmann DE. Lateral sinus thrombosis: diagnosis and treatment—a case report. J Otolaryngol 1987;16:77–9.

74. Symonds C. Otitic hydrocephalus. Brain 1931;54:55–71.

75. Symonds C. Hydrocephalic and focal cerebral symptoms in relation to thrombophlebitis of the dural sinuses and cerebral veins. Brain 1937;60:531–50.

76. Foley J. Benign forms of intracranial hypertension "toxic" and "otitic" hydrocephalus. Brain 1955;78:1–41.

77. Calabresse V, Selhorst J, Harbison J. Cerebrospinal fluid infusion test in pseudotumor cerebri. Ann Neurol 1978;4:173.

78. Sahs A, Joynt R. Brain swelling of unknown cause. Neurology 1956;6:791–802.

79. Weed L, Flexner L. The relations of the inracranial pressure. Am J Physiol 1933;105:266–72.

80. O'Connor A, Moffat D. Otogenic hypertension. J Laryngol Otol 1978;92:767–75.

81. Horton J. Decompression of the optic nerve sheath for vision threatening papilledema caused by dural sinus occlusion. Neurosurgery 1992;31:203–12.

82. Weingarten K. Subdural and epidural empyema. MR imaging. Am J Radiol 1989;152:615–21.

83. Baum PA, Dillon WP. Utility of magnetic resonance imaging in the detection of subdural empyema. Ann Otol Rhinol Laryngol 1992;101:876–8.

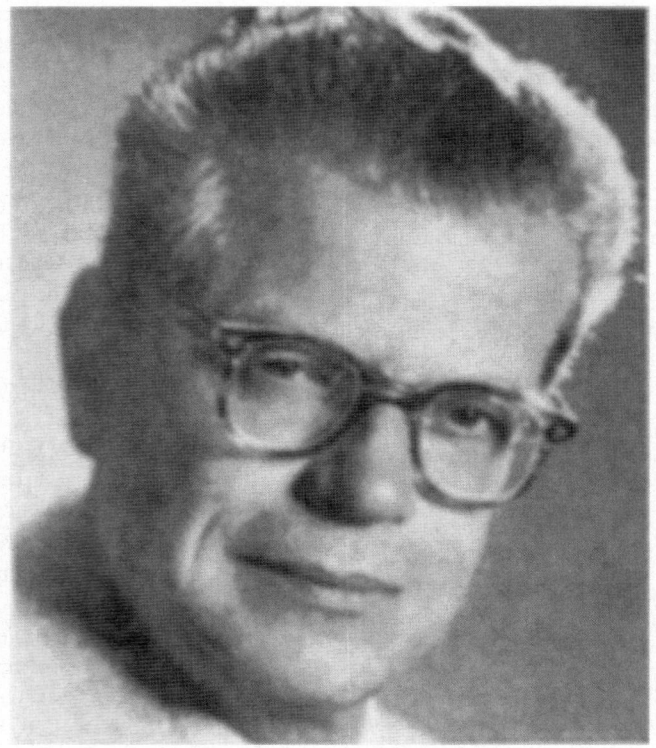

Fritz Zöllner (born 1901).

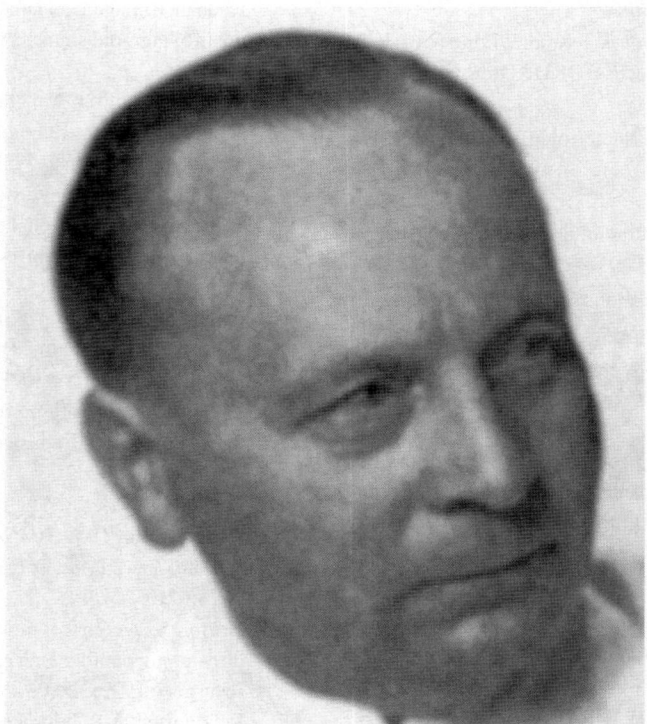

Horst Wullstein (born 1906).

Eminent otologic surgeons who developed the concepts and techniques of tympanoplasty.

24

Tympanoplasty

ARISTIDES SISMANIS, MD

HISTORICAL ASPECTS

The term tympanoplasty was first used in 1953 by Wullstein[1] to describe surgical techniques for reconstruction of the middle ear hearing mechanism that had been impaired or destroyed by chronic ear disease.

Tympanoplasty is the final step in the surgical conquest of conductive hearing losses and is the culmination of over 100 years of development of surgical procedures on the middle ear to improve hearing. The first of these procedures was the stapes mobilization of Kessel[2] in 1878, soon followed by Berthold's[3] plastic repair of a perforated tympanic membrane in the same year and Kiesselbach's[4] attempt in 1883 to correct a congenital meatal atresia. These 7 eventful years might well have been the beginning of a fruitful development of operations for conductive hearing losses because the mechanics of the middle ear had been defined clearly by Helmholtz[5] shortly before, in 1868. However, despite the successes with stapes mobilization reported by Boucheron[6] in 1888 and Miot[7] in 1890, the new surgery for deafness declined and almost died out for reasons that are not entirely clear. By the end of the nineteenth century, a determined opposition by the leaders in otology had arisen toward all attempts to improve hearing by operations on the middle ear.

The strong opposition against surgery for deafness was reflected in the standard texts of otology and otologic surgery, which scarcely mentioned or mentioned only to condemn such operations. For example, Kerrison's[8] 627-page *Diseases of the Ear*, published in 1930, devoted less than a single page to surgical measures for relief of deafness, concluding that "These operations, mentioned for their place in otological history, are quite obsolete today." It is even more surprising that Sir Charles Ballance,[9] in his two-volume text, failed to mention any sort of operation to improve hearing.

Reasons for the opposition toward reconstructive surgery of the middle ear were no doubt the lack of surgical microscopes, imperfect sterilization techniques, and the absence of protective antibiotics, possibly resulting in iatrogenic injuries and infections. There were few reports of serious infections following the early operations, but one can surmise that some unfortunate unreported results contributed to the opposition. An additional reason for the skepticism toward operations to improve hearing may have been the lack of audiometers for quantitative measurements of hearing before and after surgery.

Probably the greatest reason for the lack of interest in reconstructive operations on the ear was the intense preoccupation of the otologists of those days with infections of the ear and their complications. It is interesting that Schwartze and Eysell[10] described the simple mastoid operation just 3 years before Kessel[2] mobilized the stapes, and Küster,[11] Zaufal,[12] and Stacke[13] described the radical mastoidectomy at exactly the time that Boucheron[6] and Miot[7] were reporting successes with stapes mobilization. It is evident that the climate of otologic thought was favorable toward procedures to control infection and quite unfavorable toward operations on the ear to improve hearing.

The revival of interest in the surgery of deafness began when Holmgren,[14] with considerable courage in the face of the concerted opposition, began his long series of operations on the labyrinth for otosclerosis, demonstrating that with modern methods of aseptic technique, the noninfected mastoid process and labyrinth could, after all, be opened safely. The development of the operating microscope, first by Nylén[15] in 1921, who used a monocular instrument, and then by Holmgren, who introduced the binocular operating microscope in 1922, was an important advance destined to play an increasing role in the perfection of fenestration, stapes operations, and tympanoplastic surgery. Sourdille's[16] ingenious and successful tympanolabyrinthopexy for otosclerosis added to the reviving interest in surgery for deafness.

The real turning point in the reorientation of otologic surgery away from operations for infection toward reconstruction of the hearing mechanism occurred when Lempert[17] combined Sourdille's several-stage operation into a more practical one-stage fenestration operation. At this time, sulfonamide therapy of acute otitis media and otitic complications had begun to lessen the urgency and frequency of operations for acute mastoiditis. Lempert emphasized careful aseptic technique in the postoperative period as well as during the fenestration operation. With the later addition to sulfonamides of prophylactic penicillin, postoperative infections lost much of their threat. Most important of all, Lempert taught his operation to otologists from all parts of the world. It was inevitable, as the number of patients successfully treated by Lempert and his pupils increased to hundreds and then thousands, that the traditional and often bitter opposition started to decline. Thanks to Lempert, the climate of otologic thought finally became favorable toward surgery for deafness. This led first to the successful operations for congenital meatal atresia in 1947 by Pattee[18] and Ombrédanne[19] and finally to the revival of stapes mobilization by Rosen in 1953.[20]

It is a remarkable fact that during all these years, clinicians and surgeons failed to see clearly the applications to surgical techniques of the principles of the middle ear sound-pressure transformer, as described by Helmholtz.[5] Holmgren, Sourdille, and Lempert had no clear idea of how the fenestrated ear functions and why the fenestration operation cannot restore hearing to normal. Likewise, Pattee and Ombrédanne failed to appreciate the need to restore sound-pressure transformation by placing the substitute tympanic membrane in contact with the mobile stapes.

The mechanics of the fenestrated ear remained obscure until Békésy and Juers began to study the problem. In 1948, Juers[21] noted that the tympanic membrane of the fenestrated ear must be intact "to protect the round window somewhat from sound pressure." Two years later, Davis and Walsh[22] defined the residue of unrestored conductive loss after successful fenestration as being "due to loss of the impedance-matching mechanism of the drum membrane, ossicular chain and oval window." The two basic principles of tympanoplasty had now been defined, namely, sound protection for the round window and sound-pressure transformation for the oval window.

It is interesting that tympanoplasty techniques for chronic otitis media began in Germany rather than in the United States, where fenestration surgery had reached a high degree of maturity and perfection.

In 1950, Moritz[23] first described the use of pedicled flaps to construct a closed middle ear cavity in cases of chronic suppuration, to provide sound shielding or protection for the round window in preparation for a later fenestration of the horizontal semicircular canal.

The principles of Moritz's procedure were immediately apparent. Zöllner,[24] in 1951, and Wullstein,[25] in 1952, reported similar operations to provide sound protection for the round window and to reconstruct sound-pressure transformation for the oval window. Early on, Wullstein advocated free skin transplants rather than pedicle grafts used by Moritz, and Zöllner soon after changed from pedicle to free grafts as well.[24,25]

Tympanoplastic techniques have subsequently undergone major changes. Zöllner replaced distant free skin grafts with meatal skin removed as a free full-thickness graft. Shea and Tabb[26,27] reported the use of vein as a grafting material independently. Temporalis fascia was described by Heermann and was introduced in the United States by Storrs.[28]

Plastic prostheses for reconstruction of the ossicular chain were tried early on and abandoned by Zöllner and Wullstein; however, they continued to be used in the United States both for tympanoplasty and stapedectomy. Soon after, the tendency toward rejection and extrusion of the plastic prostheses used in tympanoplasties and stapedectomies became evident. Following these initial failures, it was soon realized that wire prostheses made of stainless steel, platinum, or tantalum were better tolerated in the middle ear.

Ossicular repositioning was described by Hall and Rytzner[29] and first used at about the same time by Wullstein and Zöllner.[30]

Homograft ossicles for reconstructing the ossicular chain in tympanoplasty became popular in the early 1960s.[31] Glasscock and House reported the first large series of homograft tympanic membrane procedures in 1968.[32]

The risk of disease transmission, imaginary or real, as well as the need for an easily available prosthesis, led to the development of alloplastic ossicular prostheses. The longest clinical experience exists with Plastipore®, an alloplast made from a high-density polyethylene sponge (HDPS) that has nonreactive properties and sufficient porosity to encourage tissue ingrowth. In 1976, a Plastipore stapes to tympanic membrane partial ossicular replacement prosthesis (PORP) for use in cases with an intact stapes superstructure and a stapes footplate to eardrum total ossicular replacement prosthesis (TORP) for use when the stapes superstructure is absent were developed.[33] A thermal-fused HDPS was also developed, known as Polycel®.[34] Histologic examination of HDPS alloplasts that have been implanted from 1 to 4 years has shown extensive invasion of the porous spaces with fibrocytes, small round cells, and foreign-body giant cells. An envelope often forms around the implant composed of fibrous tissue with a lining membrane of mucosal epithelium.[35] Clinical experience has shown the necessity of covering these alloplasts with cartilage to minimize the incidence of extrusion.[34] Extrusion rates have been reported between 3 and 5% in large series with 5 to 10 years of follow-up.[36,37] Most of the extrusions occur within the first year postoperatively; however, some extrusions have occurred up to 5 years postoperatively.[37] Brackmann was able to attribute 70% of the extrusions in his series to middle ear pathology, such as atelectasis, middle ear fibrosis, and otitis media.[36] Satisfactory long-term results have been reported with the Plastipore prosthesis by various authors.[38,39]

Ceramic implants were introduced in 1979 with the anticipation that this new material would have a lower incidence of extrusion than the porous polyethylene implants.[40] Ceramic prostheses have been developed as either bioinert or bioactive materials. Bioactivity refers to the property of the ceramic to react with surrounding soft tissue and to coalesce with adjacent bone, allowing a coupling to occur between the implant and the ossicle in contact.[40] An extrusion rate of 8% over 5 years has been reported with this type of prosthesis.[41] The author abandoned using ceramic prostheses soon after their introduction because of poor hearing results.

Another biocompatible implant material with chemical composition similar to living bone that has been used successfully since the early 1970s in reconstructive procedures is hydroxylapatite.[42] Satisfactory long-term results have been reported with this type of ossicular prosthesis.[43,44]

Development of new ossicular prosthesis materials may be challenging in the future because of strict regulatory rules by the US Food and Drug Administration for medical implants and high cost. It has been estimated that testing such implants in animals may cost between $500,000 and $5 million, and this may make support of such studies by sponsoring companies less attractive.[45]

PHYSIOLOGIC PRINCIPLES OF TYMPANOPLASTY

When animals emerged from the sea onto dry land, a mechanical device was needed to overcome the air-water sound barrier. The middle ear mechanism, developed from the discarded bronchial apparatus no longer needed for breathing, was the answer. By means of a rather large hydraulic ratio of large tympanic membrane acting on the small stapes footplate, combined with a rather small lever ratio of the longer handle of the malleus acting on the slightly shorter long process of the incus, airborne sound vibrations of large amplitude but small force are transformed to fluidborne sound vibrations of small amplitude but large force. Békésy's calculations of effective vibrating surface of tympanic membrane area compared with the stapes footplate area of 17 to 1 and lever effect of ossicular chain of 1.3 to 1 are generally accepted rather than the somewhat larger ratios calculated by Helmholtz.[5] The 17 to 1 hydraulic ratio times the 1.3 to 1 lever ratio yields a total increase of pressure at the oval window of 22 times. This is termed the sound-pressure transformer ratio of the normal human ear. The 22 times increase of pressure equals 26.8 dB.[46]

The round window in the normal ear acts as a relief opening at the opposite end of the cochlear duct from the stapes footplate to permit maximum to-and-fro vibratory movements of the relatively noncompressible cochlear fluid column in the rigid bony cochlea. In the intact ear, the round window membrane movements are largely passive in response to the stapes footplate movements. This is partly because the 22 times pressure increase at the oval window far exceeds any competitive pressure exerted on the round window from the tympanic cavity side. Furthermore, round window membrane movements are largely passive in response to the stapes footplate movements because the intact tympanic membrane "protects" the round window from competitive sounds, partly by damping and partly by a phase lag, so the modest intensity of sound that reaches the round window may actually strengthen rather than cancel the movements of the cochlear fluid column. The relative importance of damping and phase shifting in the sound protection afforded to the round window by the intact tympanic membrane remains to be determined.

In the diseased ear impaired by chronic ear disease, the round window begins to play a more active and disturbing role in the mechanics of hearing. A perforation of the tympanic membrane removes sound protection from the round window, with a tendency for sound to reach both windows at nearly the same moment, thus canceling the resultant movements of the cochlear fluid column. As long as the transformer ratio of the middle ear is larger, as in the case of a small tympanic membrane perforation with an intact ossicular chain, the canceling effect of sound reaching the round window is small. As the perforation enlarges and the transformer ratio diminishes, the canceling effect of sound on the unprotected round window rises rapidly until with a total perforation there is a loss of 40 to 45 dB or a loss of sound energy transmission of 10,000 times or more. An interruption of the ossicular chain does not add much to the loss of a large perforation, but behind an intact tympanic membrane, an interrupted ossicular chain produces an enormous and maximum loss of hearing of the conductive type because now both windows lie behind sound protection and there is no sound-pressure transformation for the oval window. This is one situation in which the 60- to 65-dB loss, representing a loss of sound energy transmission of a million times or more, may be improved to a 40-dB loss simply by removal of the tympanic membrane.

The ideal tympanoplasty restores sound protection for the round window by constructing a closed and air-containing middle ear and rebuilds the sound-pressure transformation mechanism for the oval window by con-necting a large tympanic membrane with the stapes footplate via either an intact or a reconstructed ossicular chain.

To accomplish the two physiologic principles of tympanoplasty, sound protection for the round window must first be provided by means of a tissue graft to repair the tympanic membrane defect, and the middle ear must be lined with mucosa and must contain air to the protected window. Then sound-pressure transformation for the oval window must be provided by mobile ossicular continuity between the large tympanic membrane and small oval window.

DEFINITION OF TYMPANOPLASTY

In 1965, the American Academy of Ophthalmology and Otolaryngology Subcommittee on Conservation of Hearing set forth a standard classification for surgery of chronic ear infection and defined tympanoplasty as "a procedure to eradicate disease in the middle ear and to reconstruct the hearing mechanism, with or without tympanic membrane grafting."[47] This operation can be combined with either an intact canal wall (ICW) or a canal wall down (CWD) mastoidectomy to eradicate disease from the mastoid area. Tympanoplasty with or without mastoidectomy is indicated for chronic ear disease processes such as tympanic membrane perforations resulting from previous middle ear infections, atelectatic tympanic membranes, retraction pockets, cholesteatomas, tympanosclerosis, and chronic otitis media with effusion or mastoid cholesterol granuloma. In the same report, myringoplasty is defined as "an operation in which the reconstructive procedure is limited to repair of a tympanic membrane perforation."

In this classification, types of tympanoplasty are distinguished according to the method of ossicular reconstruction. In other words, the surgeon is expected to describe what was done. The original classification system of Wullstein is illustrated in Figure 24–1. This classification system is still used in the vernacular of otology (eg, a "type III mechanism" or a "type I tympanoplasty") but is not used in reporting results.

The Subcommittee's classification also enumerates a set of rules for describing the gross pathology present at the time of surgery for chronic suppurative otitis media. These rules have to do with the type and location of a perforation of the tympanic membrane, status of the

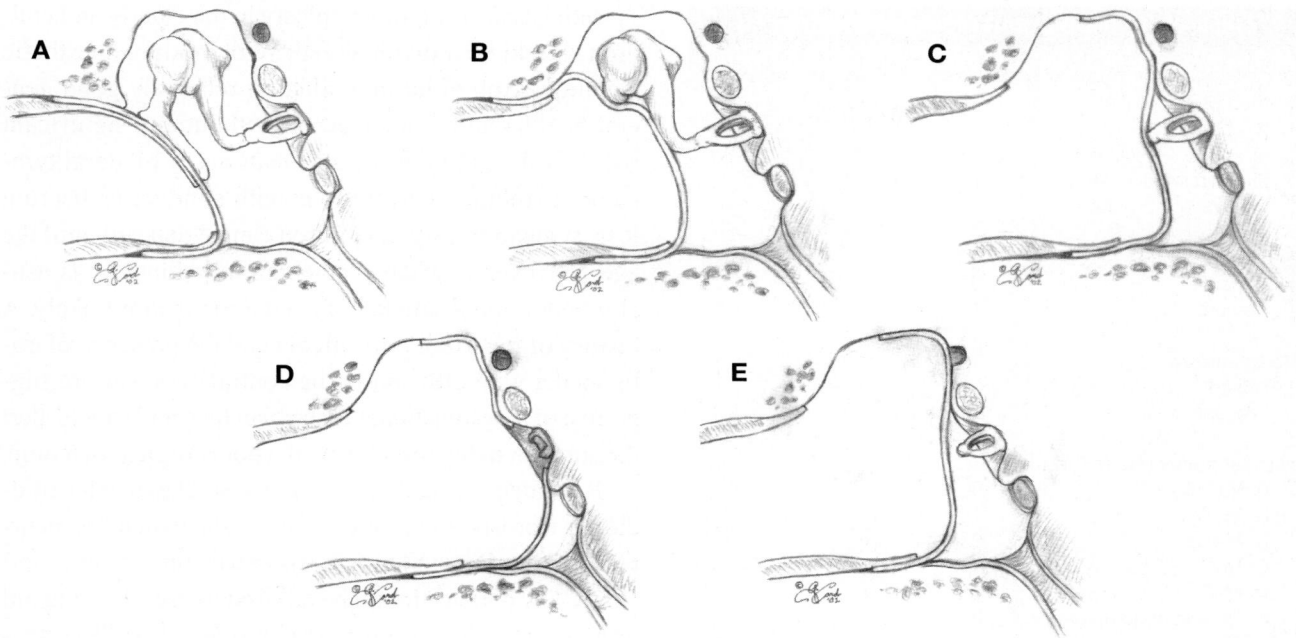

Figure 24–1 Types of tympanoplasty according to Wolfstein . *A*, Type I with restoration of the normal middle ear. *B*, Type II. Ossicular chain partially destroyed but preserved and continuity restored. Skin graft laid against the ossicles after removal of the bridge. *C*, Type III. Myringostapediopexy producing a shallow middle ear and a columella effect. *D*, Type IV. Round window protection with a small middle ear mobile footplate left exposed. *E*, Type V. Closed middle ear with round window protection; fenestra in the horizontal semicircular canal covered by a skin graft.

ossicular chain, presence of otorrhea, and status of the mucosa and eustachian tube. In addition, guidelines have been set forth for reporting results. In the past, most workers described success in terms of hearing improvement only when, in fact, elimination of infection and preservation or restoration of anatomy are of equal importance. Therefore, results today are reported in relation to control of pathology, anatomic status, hearing improvement, and postoperative complications.

A more practical tympanoplasty reporting protocol, developed by Kartush, generates a numeric indicator of the severity of the middle ear disease (Table 24–1).[44] In this protocol, a Middle Ear Risk Index (MERI) is used to stratify patient groups and allow for meaningful study comparisons.* Suggested risk categories can be derived from the MERI as follows: MERI 0, normal; MERI 1 to 3, mild disease; MERI 4 to 6, moderate disease; and MERI 7 to 12, severe disease.

Regarding reporting hearing results, the following guidelines for air–bone closure have been recommended

by the same author: 0 to 10 dB, excellent; 10 to 20 dB, good; 20 to 30 dB, fair; and more than 30 dB, poor.[44] It is recommended that the postoperative bone line be used.[44]

INDICATIONS AND CONTRAINDICATIONS FOR TYMPANOPLASTY

Reconstruction of the conductive hearing mechanism is clearly useless in an ear without useful residual cochlear function unless the patient wishes to participate in water activities. Tympanoplasty is contraindicated in malignant neoplasms of the outer or middle ear in which eradication of the tumor must take precedence; in invasive, life-threatening *Pseudomonas* infection of the outer or middle ear in diabetics; and in intracranial complications of ear disease.

Relative contraindications to tympanoplasty include an acute exacerbation of chronic otitis media, which must first be brought under control by appropriate antibiotic therapy, and chronic mucoid discharge associated with allergic rhinosinusitis. Chronic external otitis caused

---

*A free database is avalable in both Mac and Windows versions for use of MERI 2001 at <222.michiganear.com>.

Table 24–1 MIDDLE EAR RISK INDEX (MERI)*		
Risk Factor	**Risk Value**	**Assigned Risk**
Otorrhea (Bellucci)		
☐ I: Dry	0	
☐ II: Occasionally wet	1	
☐ III: Persistently wet	2	
☐ IV: Wet, cleft palate	3	___
Perforation		
☐ Absent	0	
☐ Present	1	___
Cholesteatoma		
☐ Absent	0	
☐ Present	1	___
Ossicular status (Austin/Kartush)		
☐ 0: M+I+S+	0	
☐ A: M+S+	1	
☐ B: M+S–	2	
☐ C: M–S+	3	
☐ D: M–S–	4	
☐ E: Ossicle head fixation	2	
☐ F: Stapes fixation	3	___
Middle ear: granulations or effusion		
☐ No	0	
☐ Yes	1	___
Previous surgery	0	
☐ None	1	
☐ Staged	2	
☐ Revision		
	Total	___ MERI

*A value is assigned for each risk factor, and then the values are added to determine the MERI.

by *Pseudomonas aeruginosa, Aspergillus niger*, or *Staphylococcus aureus* should be controlled by appropriate local cleaning and antibiotics. A nonfunctioning eustachian tube is a relative contraindication to tympanoplasty; however, functional status is not always easily determined preoperatively.

Tympanoplasty is contraindicated in the only or significantly better hearing ear to avoid the risk of irreversible sensorineural hearing loss. Tympanoplasty can be considered on the better hearing ear only in patients who can use a hearing aid in the opposite ear with satisfactory results. Finally, patients with chronic cough such as smokers and those with chronic obstructive pulmonary disease are not good candidates for tympanoplasty.

Indications for tympanoplasty in the elderly and children should be individualized. With modern anesthetic techniques, an older individual in relatively good general health can be operated on without any significant risk.[48] Unless there is a cholesteatoma or bilateral tympanic membrane perforations with conductive hearing loss, tympanoplasty in children can be delayed until the age of 10 years, when eustachian tube function is usually better and a satisfactory outcome is more likely. A history of recurrent otitis media and the presence of otitis media with effusion in the contralateral ear are suggestive of a dysfunctional eustachian tube and should alert the surgeon to the possibility of a poor surgical outcome.

Repeated surgical failures because of extensive middle ear fibrosis, a nonfunctioning eustachian tube, recurrent perforation, and prosthesis extrusion are better left alone. The patient should be advised to use a hearing aid provided that there is no recurrent or residual cholesteatoma. Recently, bone-anchored hearing aids have provided very promising results for patients who cannot tolerate conventional hearing aids because of recurrent otitis externa, draining mastoid cavities, and active chronic otitis media.[49]

PREOPERATIVE EVALUATION AND MANAGEMENT

A complete history and head and neck examination should be performed on all patients with chronic ear disease. The otoscopic examination is best accomplished with the operating microscope.

An audiogram is essential and should consist of puretone air and bone conduction thresholds as well as speech discrimination scores. All hearing test results should be confirmed with tuning forks.

Computed tomography (CT) of the temporal bones may be helpful, particularly in cases with cholesteatoma, in determining the degree of mastoid pneumatization, possible intracranial involvement, the presence of labyrinthine fistulae, tegmental defects, and fallopian canal anatomy. If tegmental defects are identified, diagnosis of brain herniation is best established with a magnetic resonance imaging (MRI) study.[50] In the author's experience, CT of the temporal bones is not entirely accurate in predicting extension of disease or the presence of recurrent/residual cholesteatoma.

For an actively draining ear, the external auditory canal and tympanic cavity should be cleaned of any purulent material with a small otologic suction (Baron #3 or #5) under the surgical microscope. The patient should be instructed to observe water precautions. For refractory cases, irrigation of the ear with a solution of 1.5% acetic acid using a bulb syringe two to three times a day can be helpful. The patient is asked to obtain a 1-oz rubber-bulb syringe and, with the involved ear down, to squeeze the bulb so that its contents are forced into the ear canal to wash out the purulent material. Following irrigation, the ear should be allowed to drain and antibiotic drops covering *P. aeruginosa* should be instilled while the affected ear is turned up. Digital pressure should then be applied several times over the tragus to drive the antibiotic solution deeper into the ear canal and middle ear cavity. Oral antibiotics with activity against *P. aeruginosa* should be considered for patients not responding to local treatment. Culture and sensitivity should be obtained for refractory cases, in immunosuppressed patients, and when an unusual infectious process, such as tuberculosis, is suspected. Although most surgeons would prefer to operate on a "dry" ear, there is no contraindication to tympanoplasty in an actively draining one. Cholesteatoma may render the ear refractory, and often it may have to be treated surgically to achieve a "dry ear."

In addition to the aforementioned measures, an effort should be made to control any contributing factors, such as allergic rhinitis, sinusitis, and nasal obstruction secondary to a deviated septum. The status of the upper respiratory tract directly influences eustachian tube function and therefore the outcome of any surgery in the tympanic cavity.

Poor eustachian tube function prior to surgery may improve following removal of disease processes such as polyps, granulation tissue, infection, and purulent debris.

Closure of the perforation, in combination with insertion of a sheet of absorbable gelatin film (Gelfilm®) from the eustachian tube orifice to the round window niche, may result in an improvement in eustachian tube function.

Prior to surgery, patients should properly be informed regarding the nature of the disease process, the proposed surgical procedure including expected outcomes, potential complications, the possibility of a second-stage procedure, and alternative treatments. Written instructions regarding the proposed surgical procedure and postoperative care are very useful.

ANESTHESIA FOR TYMPANOPLASTY

General anesthesia is preferred for all chronic ear surgery procedures and is particularly helpful for children and excessively apprehensive patients. General anesthesia can be used as well in an outpatient setting.

TYMPANOPLASTY (OSSICULAR RECONSTRUCTION) IN CASES WITH AN INTACT TYMPANIC MEMBRANE

Conductive hearing loss in association with an intact tympanic membrane is usually caused by fixation of one or several ossicles or interruption of the ossicular chain, most often the incudostapedial articulation. The majority of these cases can be operated by elevating a tympanomeatal flap through a transcanal approach. The Shea speculum holder is very helpful for this type of procedure. In cases with a narrow ear canal or bulging of the anterior wall obstructing visualization of the anterior sulcus area (Figure 24–2, A), a canalplasty is necessary prior to exploration of the middle ear.

The canalplasty is performed as follows: with a Beaver blade (#74), a "horizontal" incision is made medial to the area of the anterior wall bulge and lateral to the annulus. Two incisions are then extended "vertically" from the horizontal incision to the lateral aspect of the meatus (Figure 24–2, B). The resulting skin flap is elevated laterally to the level of the bony-cartilaginous junction and the bony protuberance is exposed (see Figure 24–2, C). Using continuous suction-irrigation and a high-speed drill, the obstructing bony area is removed until adequate exposure of the anterior sulcus area is achieved. Meticulous dissection is needed to avoid injury to the glenoid fossa capsule (Figure 24–2, C and D).

The Austin/Kartush classification of ossicular defects has been found practical and includes the following types: 0, ossicular chain intact (M+I+S+); A, malleus present, stapes present (M+S+); B, malleus present, stapes absent (M+S–); C, malleus absent, stapes present (M–S+); D, malleus absent, stapes absent (M–S–); E, ossicular head fixation; and F, stapes fixation.[44,51] The most commonly encountered ossicular defect is

A

B

C

D

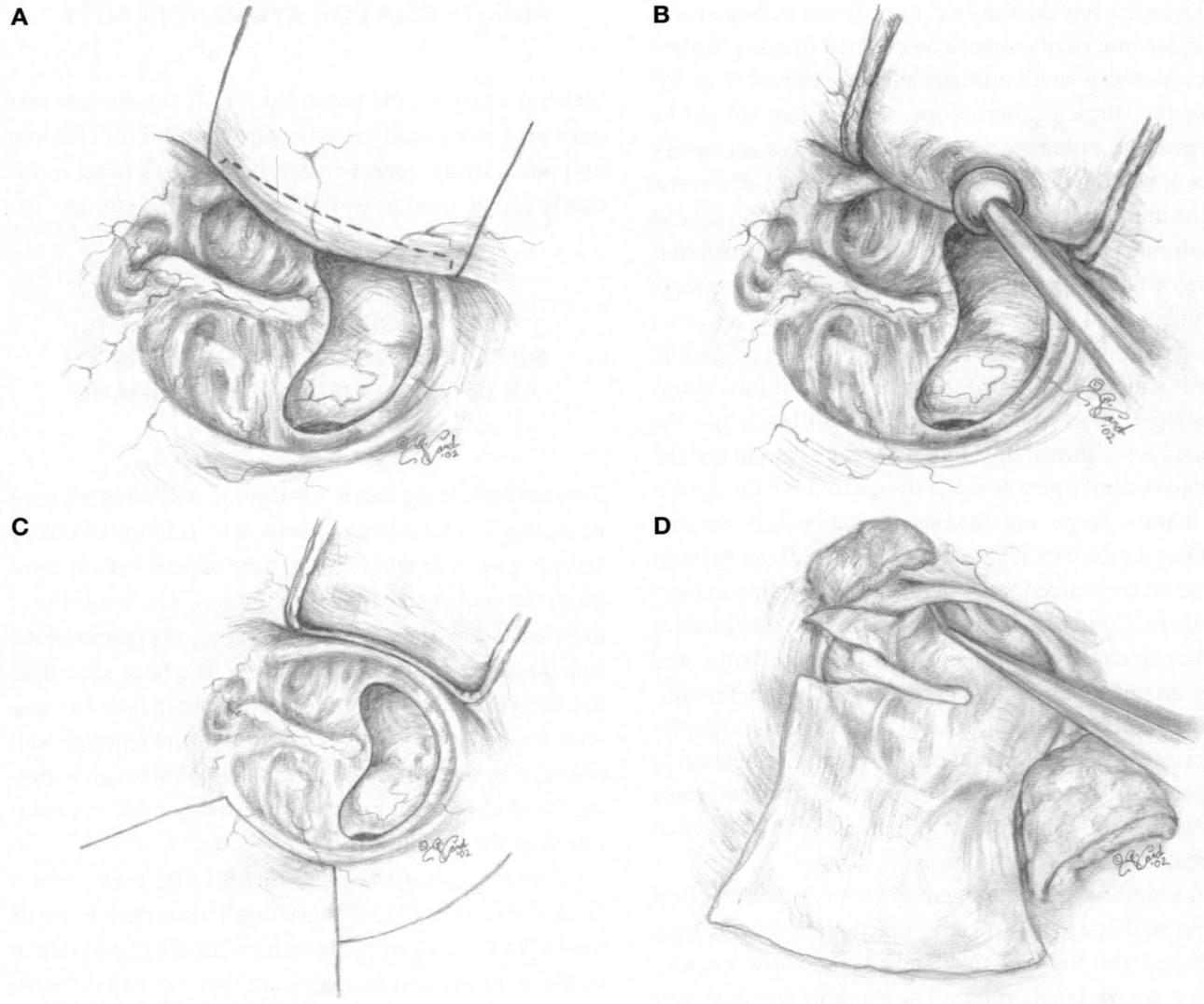

Figure 24–2 The canalplasty.

that of erosion of the long process of the incus with an intact malleus handle and stapes superstructure (type A).

OSSICULAR PROSTHESES

The ideal prosthesis should be made of a durable, biocompatible, and easy to manipulate material. As mentioned previously in this chapter, during the past 25 years, otologists have used numerous types of ossicular prostheses made of various alloplastic materials such as Plastipore®, Proplast®, polyethylenes, polytetrafluoroethylene, ceramics, Teflon®, and hydroxylapatite.

In a recent study, hydroxylapatite and Plastipore PORPs and TORPs were reported to be the preferred ossicular prostheses by 48 and 16%, respectively, of otologists in the United States.[42] Both materials have withstood the test of time and are suitable for ossicular reconstruction prostheses. The advantage of hydroxylapatite is that it can come into direct contact with the tympanic membrane, obviating the need for cartilage interposition. In one report, however, extrusion of hydroxylapatite prostheses occurred in 16% of patients when placed in direct contact with the tympanic membrane.[52] In cases with thin tympanic membranes, insertion of a tissue graft such as fascia or perichondrium between the prosthesis platform and the tympanic membrane may decrease the likelihood of extrusion. Placing the head of the prosthesis medial to the manubrium, if present, is another way to decrease extrusion.

Hybrid prostheses, composed of hydroxylapatite heads and shafts made of Teflon, Plastipore, fluoroplastic, platinum, or stainless steel, are easier to trim to the appropriate length.[53–56]

Recently, prostheses made of glass ionomer cement, titanium, and gold have been reported to have promising results.[57–61] The use of homograft ossicular grafts has been abandoned by many in this country because of the risk of transmission of viral and other diseases.[62]

TECHNIQUES AND RESULTS

For type A defects (M+S+), two ossicular reconstruction techniques are available:

1. In cases with an eroded lenticular process of the incus in which the manubrium is in close proximity to the stapes superstructure, a sculpted, incus autograft is an excellent choice. This technique has been described by Pennington[63] and Austin[64] and is performed as follows: the incus is held with the Sheehy ossicle holder and sculpted with an otologic high-speed drill to make a groove in its articular surface with the malleus and an acetabulum in the short process (Figure 24–3). When properly fitted (Figures 24–4 and 24–5), there should be just enough tension to hold the incus firmly in place between the manubrium and the stapes capitulum with no need to pack the middle ear with Gelfoam. The sculpted incus must be neither too long nor too short to prevent fixation and displacement, respectively. The sculpted incus affords excellent hearing results; the air–bone gap closure has been reported within 20 dB or less in 68% of patients.[65]

2. In cases with an eroded lenticular process of the incus and an anteriorly positioned manubrium, placement of a sculpted incus prosthesis is not recommended because of the instability of the graft. Air–bone gap closure within 20 dB using a PORP in this situation has been reported in 49% of such cases.[65]

For type B (M+S–) and D (M–S–) defects, a TORP can be used. In an effort to decrease extrusions, it is preferable to place the platform of the prosthesis medial to the malleus handle when this structure is present. In cases

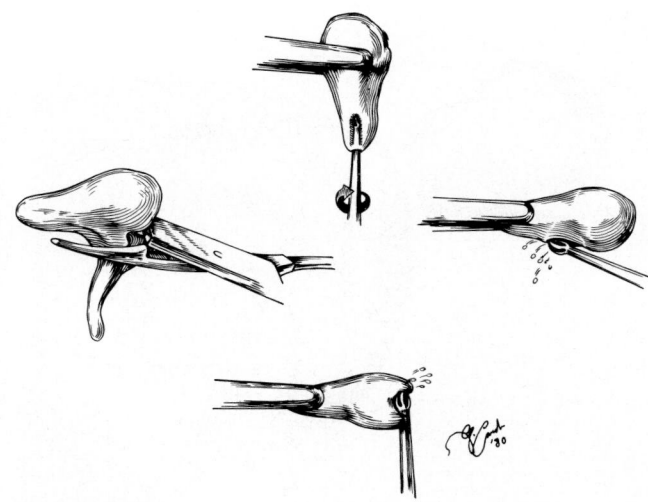

Figure 24–3 Sheehy clamp being used to hold incus while it is sculptured with a small cutting bur.

with a medially displaced manubrium, often encountered in chronic otitis media because of unopposed medial traction by the tensor tympani muscle, stretching or sectioning the tendon just lateral to the cochleariform process allows for lateralization of the manubrium. For type C defects (M–S+), a PORP can be used.

Long-term results in 233 patients undergoing ossicular reconstruction with the Goldenberg hydroxylapatite prostheses (incus replacement, incus-stapes replacement, PORP and TORP) revealed an air–bone gap of 21.1 dB in 56.8% of patients with a 5.29% extrusion rate.[53] With the criterion of a postoperative air–bone gap of 20 dB or less, there was an overall success rate of 64.8% for all prostheses. The results were best for the incus replacement prosthesis (76.0%) and the incus-stapes prosthesis (85.7%), with considerably lower success rates for the PORP (44.4%) and the TORP (61.9%). Overall, 50.6% of patients met the criteria for a successful hearing result, with a dry ear and without extrusion.[53] Better hearing before surgery, presence of the malleus handle, tympanoplasty alone, and canal wall up tympanomastoidectomy were factors associated with a successful hearing result.[53] Similar results with this type of prosthesis have been reported by others.[66,67]

In one report, a comparison of hearing results obtained with 247 Plastipore versus 265 hydroxylapatite prostheses revealed no statistically significant difference. However, five features—surgical, prosthetic, infection, tissue, and eustachian tube—were found to be predictive of

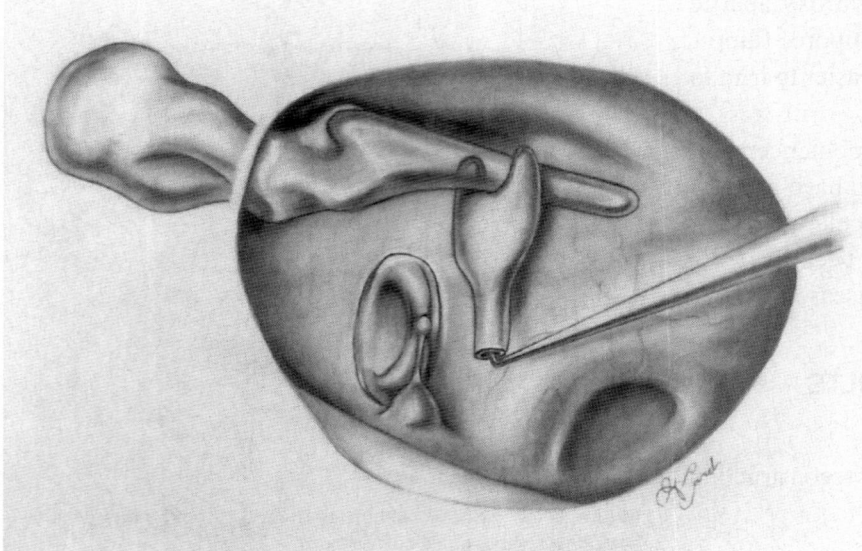

Figure 24–4 Fitted incus prosthesis being put into position with a right-angle hook.

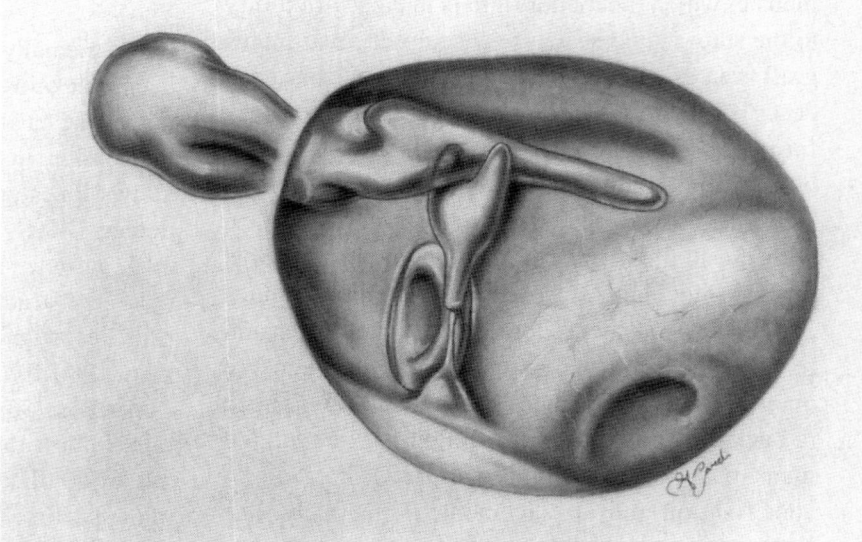

Figure 24–5 Fitted incus prosthesis in position between the malleus and the capitulum of the stapes.

ossicular reconstruction success. These factors allow for an accurate preoperative individual assessment when counseling patients regarding the likelihood of success or failure of a proposed ossicular reconstruction.[68] Extrusion and displacement of ossicular prostheses have been reported in association with eustachian tube dysfunction, chronic infection, mucosal adhesions, and atelectasis.[69–71] At the author's institution, the incidence of prosthesis displacement has been found to be higher in cases undergoing synchronous total tympanic membrane replacement and ossicular reconstruction. For this reason, such cases are staged.

The type of ossicular reconstruction performed in conjunction with CWD mastoidectomy depends on the presence and relationship of the stapes superstructure to the level of the facial nerve. When the stapes superstructure is located below the level of the facial nerve, a PORP or a sculpted middle ear bone such as the malleus head should be considered. In cases with absent stapes superstructure, a TORP is a good option.

In cases with a stapes footplate fixed by otosclerosis or tympanosclerosis, a stapedectomy can be performed (see Chapter 27) if there is no tympanic membrane perforation or infection; otherwise, this procedure should be performed at a second stage to avoid sensorineural hearing loss.

Fixation of the incus and/or malleus is uncommon and difficult to diagnose preoperatively. Conductive hearing loss in these cases can often be mistaken for otosclerosis, and diagnosis is made only after palpation of the ossicular chain during surgery. Tympanosclerosis, ligament ossification, and otosclerosis have been reported as etiologic.[72,73] An effective procedure to correct this problem is to reconstruct the ossicular chain with a sculpted incus prosthesis after removing the incus and amputating the head of the malleus with the House malleus nipper. To prevent noise-induced hearing loss, it is essential that the otologic drill does not come in contact with the ossicular chain until the incudostapedial joint is disarticulated. In cases with associated stapes fixation, stapedectomy and insertion of a TORP can be performed.[72] Mobilization of the fixed ossicles in the attic without disruption of the ossicular chain has also been reported.[74]

TYMPANOPLASTY FOR CHRONIC OTITIS MEDIA

Disease processes such as tympanosclerosis, tympanic membrane perforation/retraction, and cholesteatoma limited to the middle ear cavity can be managed effectively with tympanoplasty alone. In these cases, the transcanal approach is preferable since it avoids the inconvenience of a mastoid dressing, overnight hospitalization, and the slightly higher morbidity (pain, hematoma, infection) associated with the postauricular approach. The transcanal approach requires an adequately sized ear canal and good visualization of the anterior annulus. For cases with a small ear canal, either a canalplasty or a postauricular approach should be considered.

TECHNIQUE

In the transcanal approach, the edges of the tympanic membrane perforation are "freshened," denuded of any squamous epithelium, and tympanosclerotic plaques are completely removed prior to elevation of the tympanomeatal flap. Complete removal of tympanosclerosis from the remnants of the tympanic membrane is necessary to optimize graft "take."

The middle ear is then explored by elevating the tympanomeatal flap, diseased tissue is removed, and the ossicular chain is repaired as described above. Should polypoid mucosa and/or adhesions have been removed, Gelfilm is placed over the medial wall of the middle ear to prevent adhesion formation. The middle ear is packed with Gelfoam and the tympanic membrane graft is placed medial to the tympanic membrane remnant or tympanic annulus and medial to the manubrium.

If a postauricular approach is selected, vascular strip incisions are performed and access to the middle ear is gained through the postauricular incision, as described in Chapter 20. The remainder of the procedure is carried out in a similar fashion as in the transcanal approach.

RESULTS

The two goals of tympanoplasty are to eliminate disease and improve hearing. The results of tympanoplasty are measured in terms of success ("take") or failure of the graft and hearing improvement. To obtain a fair assessment of the long-term success of tympanoplasty, it is important to separate cases with benign central perforation from those with cholesteatoma and/or atelectasis. Benign perforations and simple ossicular chain deficits (M+S+) have a very good to excellent chance of resulting in a dry ear with normal hearing. Graft "take" in such cases should be in the 93 to 97% range, and there is an 85 to 90% chance of air–bone closure within 20 dB.

However, ears with cholesteatoma, severe mucosal disease, poor eustachian tube function, and total loss of the ossicular chain (M–S–) do not fare as well. Some patients do satisfactorily and others do not, depending on the extent of disease present at the time of surgery and the manner in which the disease is managed. It must be remembered that a tympanoplasty may be considered partially successful if a dry, intact ear is obtained regardless of whether there is any hearing improvement.

Ears with atelectasis and poor eustachian tube function do not do well unless middle ear aeration is achieved. Tympanoplasty followed by placement of a long-indwelling ventilating tube is sometimes the solution to this problem.

TYMPANOPLASTY WITH INTACT CANAL WALL MASTOIDECTOMY

Involvement of the attic, antrum, and mastoid cavity with cholesteatoma necessitates either a CWD mastoidectomy (described in Chapter 26) or an ICW mastoidectomy. The ICW technique can be used in the majority of cholesteatoma cases and is the author's preferred method since it avoids the creation of an open mastoid cavity with the associated need for long-term cleaning, restriction of water activities, and the possibility of recurrent infections. The postoperative result with this technique is a more anatomically and functionally normal ear. This technique, however, is associated with a higher incidence of residual[†] and recurrent[‡] cholesteatoma, and for this reason, a second-stage procedure, usually 1 year later, is required.

The ICW technique is technically more challenging, especially in a poorly pneumatized temporal bone, and requires special training. However, when properly performed, the ICW technique can produce a very satisfactory functional result.

Contraindications to ICW mastoidectomy include cholesteatoma in the only hearing ear, the presence of intracranial complications such as epidural abscess, and large (> 2 mm) fistulae of the semicircular canals.

TECHNIQUE

After the induction of general anesthesia and prior to draping, the postauricular area is injected with 2% lidocaine (Xylocaine) with 1:100,000 epinephrine to allow adequate time for the onset of hemostatic effect. Since facial nerve function must be assessable throughout the procedure, short-acting paralytic agents can be used only at the induction of anesthesia. Administration of nitrous oxide should be avoided because it diffuses into the middle ear and can displace the graft.

After the surgical field has been prepared and draped, the cartilaginous and bony canals are injected with the

---

[†]Residual cholesteatoma is defined as persistent cholesteatoma in the middle ear or mastoid cavity following incomplete removal.

[‡]Recurrent cholesteatoma is classified as cholesteatoma developing following complete removal as a result of retraction of the tympanic membrane.

local anesthetic solution described above and vascular strip incisions are made (Figure 24–6). Subsequently, a postauricular incision is made approximately 5 mm behind the postauricular sulcus (Figure 24–7). Hemostasis is obtained with electrocautery, and a self-retaining retractor is placed to expose the surgical field. Areolar tissue overlying the temporalis fascia is harvested for grafting (Figure 24–8). This tissue is considered a superior grafting material because it is located in an avascular plane, it is easy to handle during grafting, and the temporalis fascia is preserved for future use. Identification of the avascular areolar tissue layer is greatly facilitated by lateral (outward) traction of the auricle while making the postauricular incision. Injection of local anesthetic solution elevates (balloons) the areolar tissue from the underlying temporalis fascia. An incision is made over the linea temporalis and is carried down to the level of the temporalis fascia; the areolar tissue is dissected using Metzenbaum scissors. The areolar tissue thus obtained is squeezed out on a Teflon block and placed under a gooseneck lamp for dehydration (Figure 24–5).

A T-shaped incision is then made in the musculoperiosteal tissue overlying the mastoid cortex. The horizontal component of this incision is made in the (avascular) plane of the linea temporalis, and the vertical component connects the mastoid tip to the mid portion of the horizontal incision. Using a Lempert elevator, musculoperiosteal flaps are elevated posteriorly, superiorly, and anteriorly. The vascular strip is elevated out of the ear canal and is kept in place by repositioning the previously placed self-retaining retractor. A second self-retaining retractor is placed perpendicular to the first, allowing for excellent exposure of the bony canal, tympanic membrane, middle ear, and mastoid and eliminating the need for an ear speculum (Figure 24–9).

Following elevation and anterior reflection of the tympanic membrane, the middle ear is explored and the status of the ossicular chain, as well as any extension of disease within the middle ear, is assessed.

Using continuous suction-irrigation and a high-speed otologic drill, a simple mastoidectomy is performed (Figure 24–10). In "chronic ear" cases, the mastoid is usually poorly pneumatized. It is important to identify the middle fossa dura and the sigmoid sinus immediately after removing the mastoid cortex to avoid injuring these structures and to aid in identifying the facial nerve and

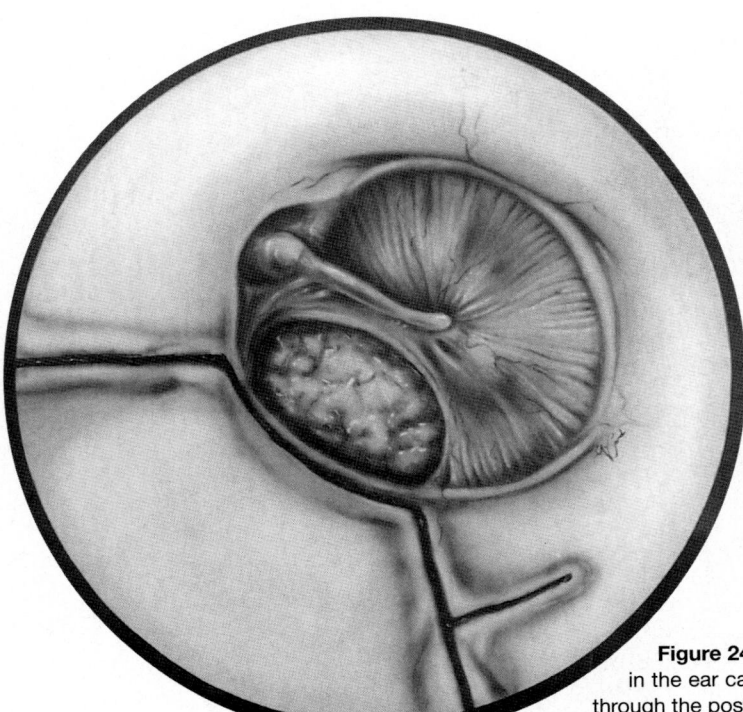

Figure 24–6 This illustration demonstrates the vascular strip incisions in the ear canal. Note the cholesteatoma debris in the middle ear as seen through the posterior-superior perforations.

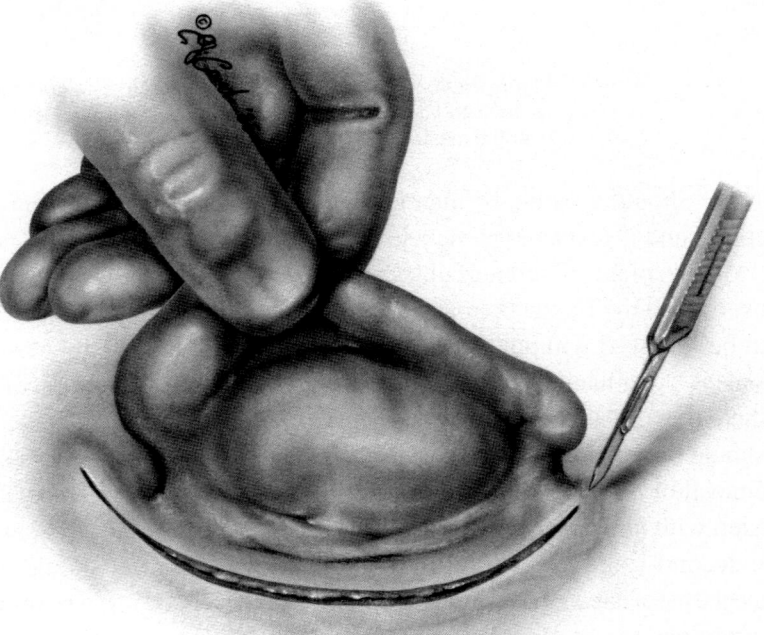

Figure 24–7 A routine postauricular incision is made about 5 mm behind the postauricular fold.

horizontal semicircular canal. Adequate identification of these structures can be accomplished while leaving intact a thin, bony covering.

Cholesteatoma is usually encountered on entering the antrum. In sequence, the sac is opened, its contents are evacuated, and the matrix is dissected with extreme caution to avoid exposing possible fistulae of the semicircular canals. With microscopic visualization and gentle palpation of the cholesteatoma matrix, fistulae and facial nerve exposure can be identified prior to removal of the

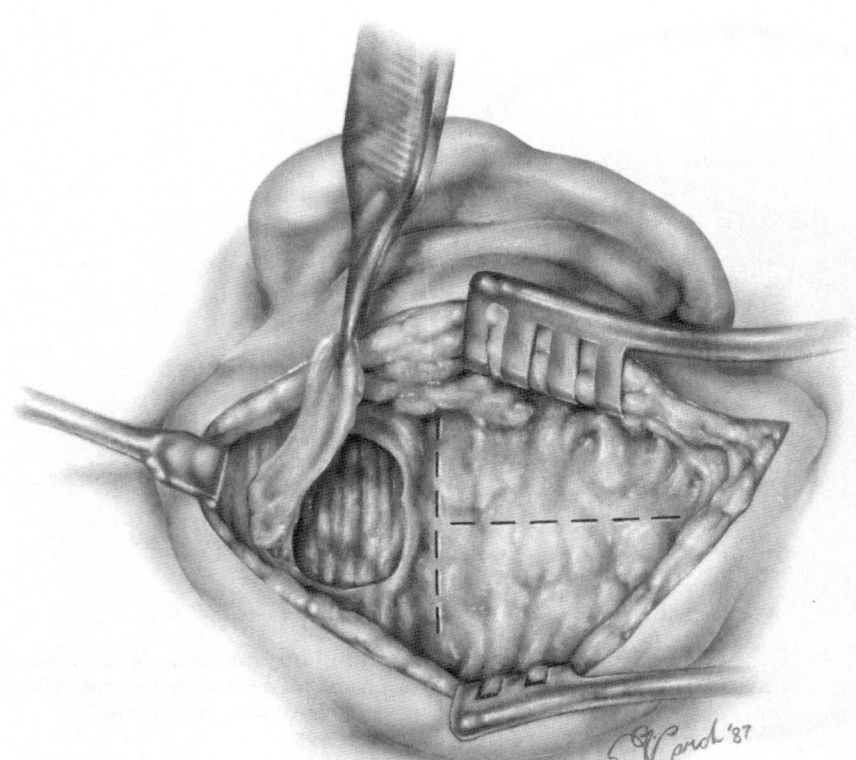

Figure 24–8   Superficial areolar tissue is removed from the temporalis fascia and put aside to be used later as a grafting material. A T-shaped incision is then made in the soft tissue over the mastoid.

matrix. Should a fistula be identified, the matrix is left in place and is managed at the end of the procedure.

Management of semicircular canal fistulae is controversial. If the fistula is smaller than 2 mm, the matrix can be removed without injuring the inner ear.[75] If the fistula is larger than 2 mm (especially if the matrix is very adherent) or located over the promontory of the cochlea, it should be left alone to avoid sensorineural hearing loss. Removal of remaining cholesteatoma matrix is usually easier, with less possibility of inner ear damage, during the second-stage procedure. Some fistulae will heal once the associated infection is controlled.[75,76] Others have recommended exteriorization of the matrix with the CWD technique,[77] which may be the most appropriate management of semicircular canal fistulae in the only hearing ear, large fistulae (> 2 mm), or fistulae of the promontory of the cochlea. In another report,[78] eradication of the cholesteatoma matrix with interruption and obliteration of the semicircular canals with autologous materials such as fascia, perichondrium, bone chips, and cartilage resulted in preservation, or improvement, of

hearing in seven of eight patients; in one patient only, hearing deteriorated 12 dB.

The incus and malleus are frequently engulfed by cholesteatoma; extension of cholesteatoma medial to these ossicles mandates removal of the incus and amputation of the malleus head to ensure complete removal of disease. The latter maneuver also allows exposure of, and cholesteatoma removal from, the anterior epitympanic recess (Figures 24–11 and 24–12). Prior to removing the incus, and under direct vision, the incudostapedial joint should be disarticulated if intact. Removing the incus exposes the fossa incudis and allows the surgeon to open the facial recess by dissecting lateral to the facial nerve (Figure 24–13). Another method of exposing the facial recess, especially appropriate if the incus has been left in place because of limited cholesteatoma extension, involves first identifying the facial nerve in its vertical segment and then dissecting the area between the facial and the chorda tympani nerves (Figure 24–14). This latter approach is very challenging or even impossible in a poorly pneumatized mastoid owing to the extreme restric-

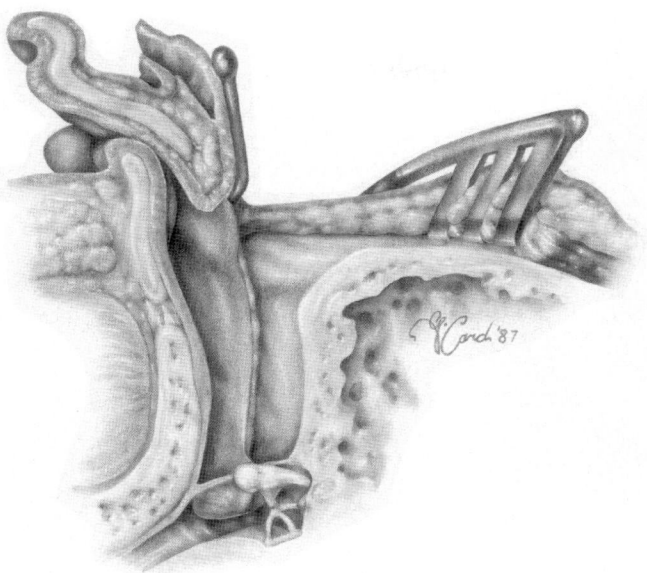

Figure 24–9 The vascular strip is elevated out of the ear canal and held in place with Weitlaner's retractor.

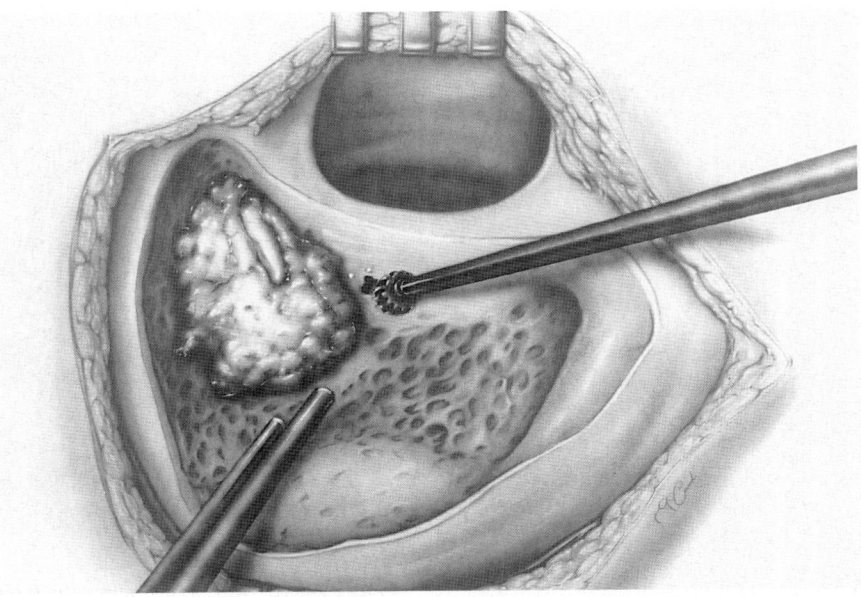

Figure 24–10 A simple mastoidectomy is performed with the aid of a pneumatic drill and irrigation suction. Note the cholesteatoma lying in the antrum.

tion of the surgical field. Useful landmarks for identifying the vertical segment of the facial nerve are the fossa incudis, short process of incus, horizontal semicircular canal, and digastric ridge inferiorly. Adequate thinning of the superior-posterior bony canal wall and delineation of the sinodural angle are very helpful in identifying the facial nerve. Landmarks for the tympanic segment of the facial nerve include the cochleariform process, Jacobson's nerve, and the stapes in the oval window.

In the majority of cases, a combined approach through the facial recess and the external auditory canal permits sufficient access to the middle ear for adequate removal of disease. After squamous debris has been evacuated from the cholesteatoma sac, the matrix is completely removed from the antrum, attic, mastoid, and middle ear.

Meticulous technique is required when separating the matrix from the tympanic segment of the facial nerve and the stapes. Dissection of the matrix from the facial

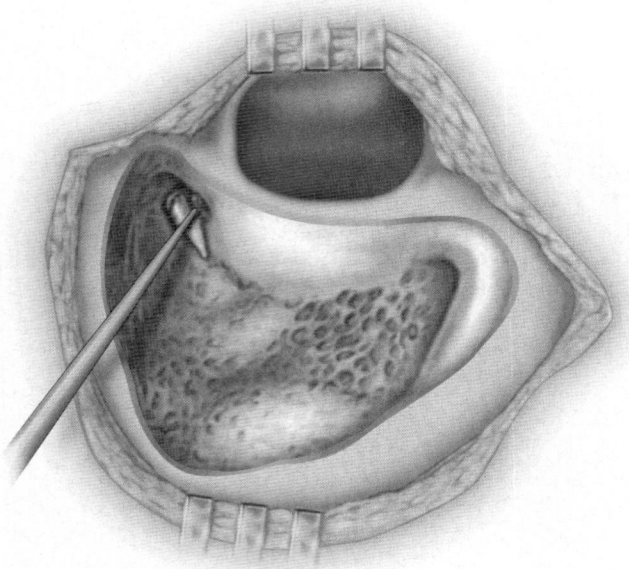

Figure 24–11   Once the incudostapedial joint has been disarticulated, a right-angle hook is used to remove the incus.

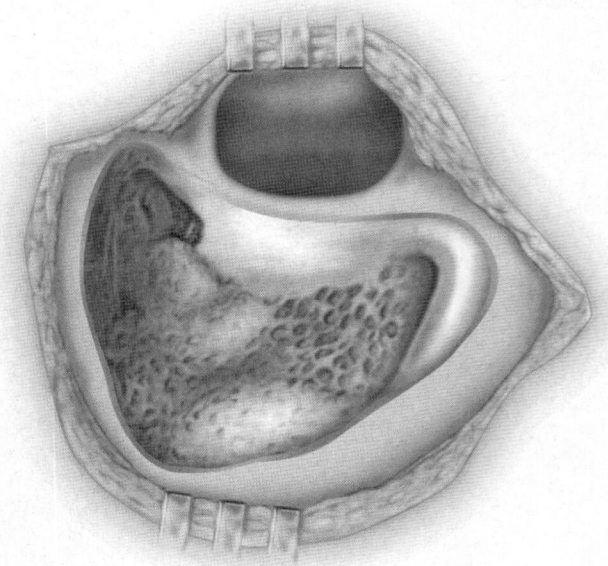

Figure 24–12   In this illustration, the facial recess has been made continuous with the oval window area.

nerve should be done with a blunt instrument, such as the back of a sickle knife or a House annulus elevator ("gimmick"). Dissection of the matrix from the stapes should proceed in a posterior to anterior direction to take advantage of the stabilization provided by the stapedius tendon. If the matrix is very adherent to the stapes superstructure, it can be left in place to avoid injury and the resulting hearing loss. Usually, during the second-stage procedure 1 year later, the cholesteatoma has formed a "pearl," which can be removed with ease. Caution is sim-

ilarly required in cases with cholesteatoma matrix overlying or adherent to an exposed facial nerve. Again, the matrix can be left in place for removal at the second stage.

The sinus tympani cannot be accessed directly by any approach to the middle ear; marginally adequate visualization can be accomplished either indirectly using a small mirror (Buckingham) or directly with an endoscope.

Markedly thickened polypoid mucosa and granulation tissue should be removed completely from the middle ear, along with scrupulous removal of every vestige

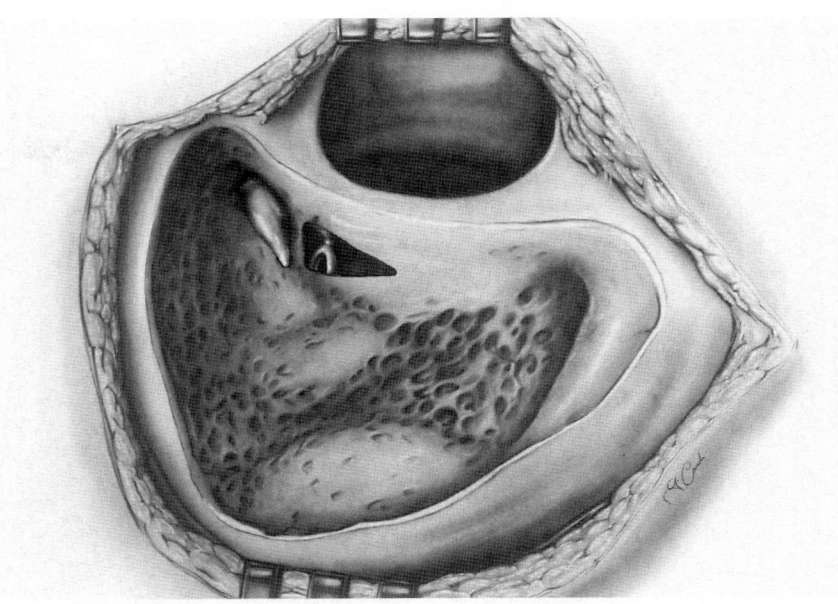

Figure 24–13 In this illustration, the cholesteatoma debris and matrix have been removed from the antrum, and the facial recess has been opened by identifying the facial nerve first and preserving the fossa incudis bone intact.

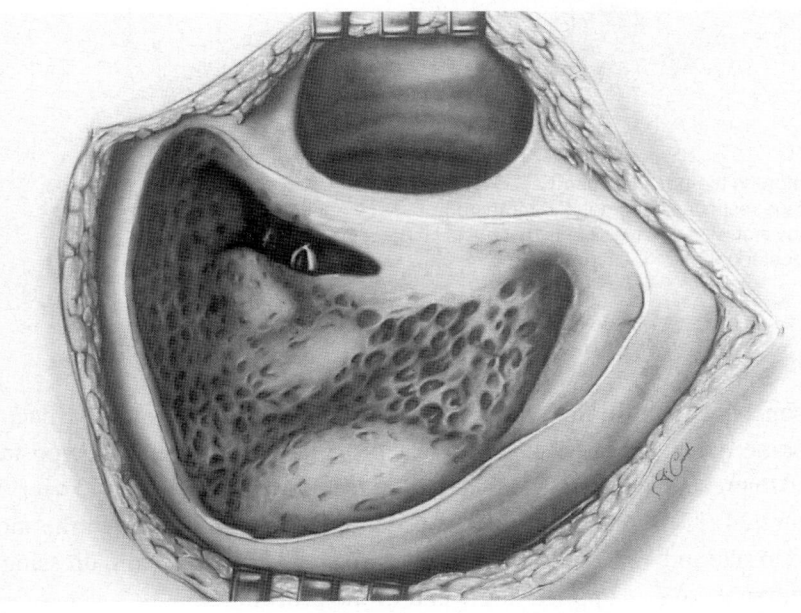

Figure 24–14 In this illustration, the facial recess has been made continuous with the attic by extending the fossa incudis lateral to the facial nerve.

of stratified squamous epithelium. Mildly diseased mucosa generally reverts to normal once the perforation is closed and all cholesteatoma has been removed.

After complete removal of all diseased tissue, preparations are made for grafting. The undersurface of the tympanic membrane remnant (or tympanic annulus) and manubrium of the malleus are denuded of squamous epithelium and mucosa. In the majority of cases, ossicular reconstruction is performed during the second-stage procedure.

Bony canal flaps are created, as described in Chapter 20. Gelfilm is placed over the medial wall of the middle ear to prevent adhesion formation and the middle ear is packed with absorbable Gelfoam. Tragal cartilage

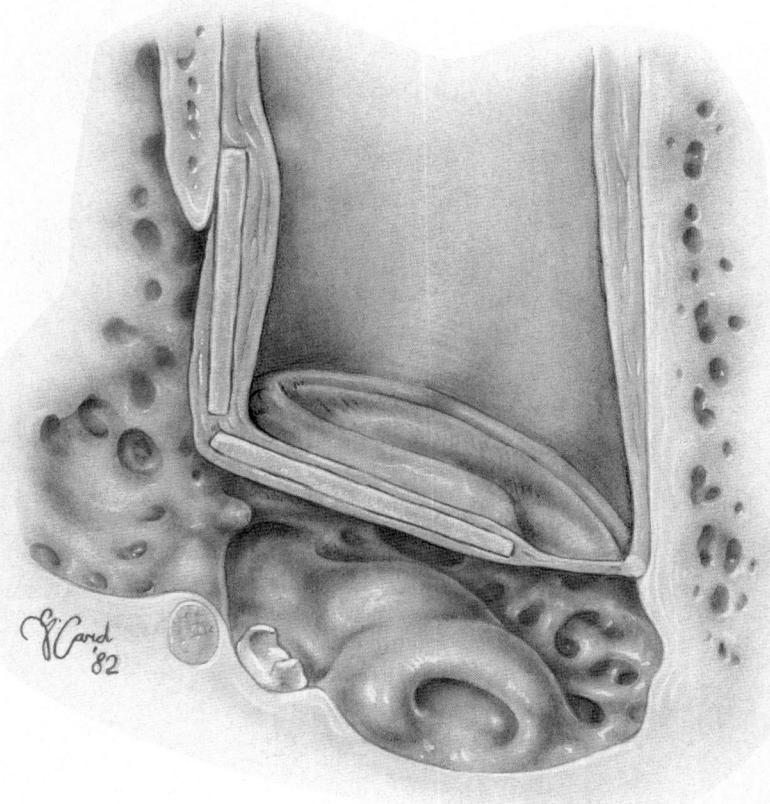

Figure 24–15   Cartilage reinforces the posterior quadrant. The absorbable gelatin sponge (Gelfoam) on which the cartilage rests has been deleted for the purposes of illustration. The attic defect is reconstructed by a curved cartilage piece that nests on the superior aspect of the cartilage occupying the posterior half of the tympanic membrane.

(harvested as described in Chapter 20) or conchal cartilage is used to repair the tympanic membrane defect in the posterior-superior quadrant and/or attic to prevent retraction and recurrent cholesteatoma (Figure 24–15). The dehydrated areolar tissue graft is trimmed to size and placed medial to the tympanic membrane remnant, lateral to the cartilage graft and extending posteriorly over the posterior canal wall (Figure 24–16). For total tympanic membrane perforations, a notch is made in the superior aspect of the graft to accommodate insertion medial to the manubrium. Small pledgets of Gelfoam are placed over the graft for stabilization and the canal skin flaps are replaced into anatomic position (Figure 24–17). A layer of antibiotic ointment is placed over the Gelfoam. Using an ear speculum, the ear canal is inspected and proper position of the canal skin flaps is ensured. One or two Pop's® (Merocel®) ear wicks impregnated in

antibiotic ointment are inserted in the lateral aspect of the ear canal to keep the flaps in position. The postauricular incision is closed in two layers with 4-0 Vicryl®, and a rubber band drain is extended through the most dependent portion of the incision. A mastoid dressing is applied at the end of the procedure.

CARTILAGE "SHIELD" TYMPANOPLASTY TECHNIQUE

Total tympanic membrane replacement with cartilage (cartilage "shield" tympanoplasty) has proved very useful in atelectatic ears, previous tympanoplasty failures, and cases with suspected eustachian tube dysfunction.[79] The canal incisions, flap elevation, and preparation of the middle ear and tympanic membrane remnant are as

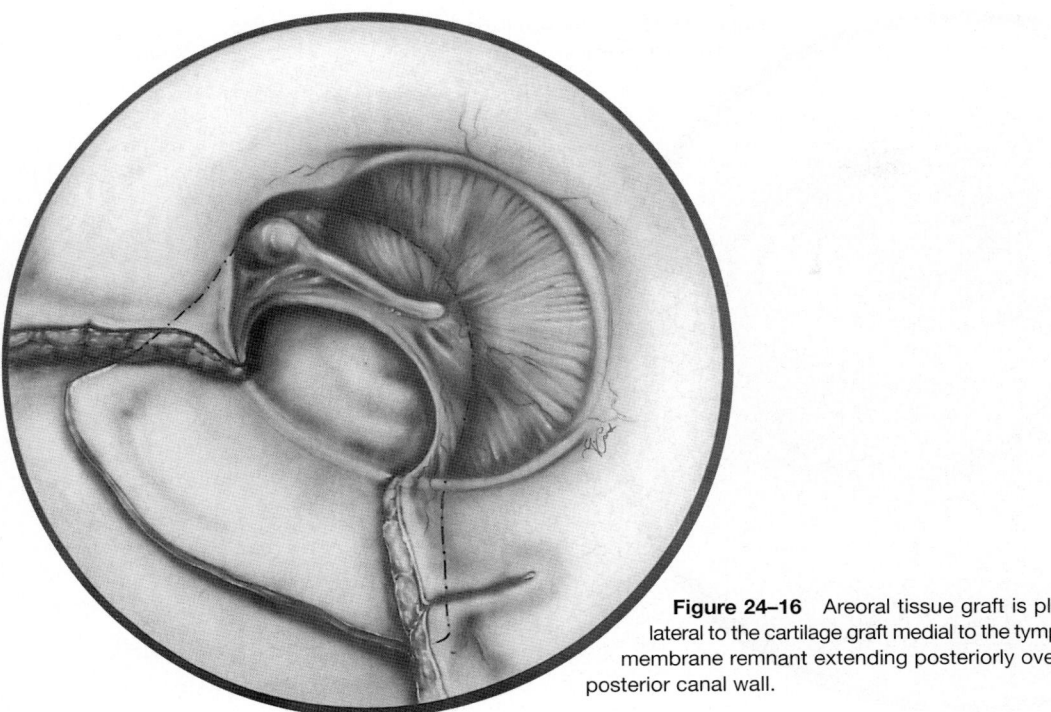

Figure 24–16 Areoral tissue graft is placed lateral to the cartilage graft medial to the tympanic membrane remnant extending posteriorly over the posterior canal wall.

described above. Cartilage is removed either from the posterior aspect of the concha or from the tragus using sharp and blunt dissection. The cartilage graft is stripped of its perichondrium, sized to the dimensions of the tympanic membrane defect, and thinned. A wedge is removed at the upper portion of the graft to accommodate the malleus handle. After the middle ear is packed with Gelfoam, the cartilage graft is placed medial to the manubrium and the tympanic sulcus. An areolar tissue graft is placed lateral to the cartilage and medial to the edges of the perforation and extended posteriorly onto the canal wall. The procedure is completed as previously described.

POSTOPERATIVE CARE

The mastoid dressing and drain are removed the next morning and the patient is instructed to instill antibiotic drops in the ear canal at bedtime. Showering is allowed provided that the patient places a cotton ball impregnated with petroleum ointment at the meatus. Oral antibiotics are prescribed for patients with ears found to be infected at the time of surgery. At the first postoperative visit

(1 week following surgery), the Merocel ear wick is removed. The Gelfoam over the graft is removed, if still present, at the second visit 3 to 4 weeks later. An audiogram is obtained 3 to 4 months after surgery.

SECOND-STAGE PROCEDURE

A second-stage procedure is recommended for all cholesteatoma cases requiring an ICW mastoidectomy to detect recurrent or residual disease and to perform ossicular reconstruction. This procedure is usually done 1 year following the initial operation. In selected cases, such as small cholesteatomas limited in the middle ear and retraction pockets, staging can be avoided and ossicular reconstruction can be performed during the original operation.

During the second-stage procedure, vascular strip incisions can be avoided and the middle ear approached directly from the postauricular area. Avoiding the vascular strip incisions provides a more stable tympanic membrane since its continuity with the posterior canal skin has not been disrupted. Ossicular reconstruction techniques are the same as previously described.

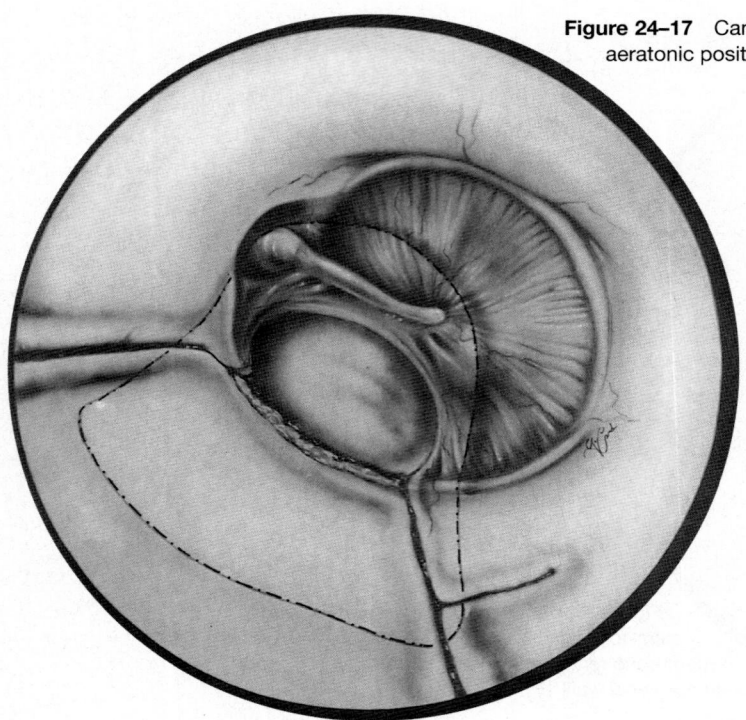

Figure 24–17   Canal skin flaps have been replaced into aeratonic position.

RESULTS

Long-term follow-up of cholesteatoma cases is imperative for the detection of recurrent and residual disease. Recurrent and residual cholesteatoma have been reported in 14 and 12%, respectively, of staged ICW mastoidectomies.[80] The incidence of recurrent and residual cholesteatoma with the ICW technique has been variably reported to be greater than, or less than, that associated with the CWD technique.[81,82]

Cholesteatomas in children behave more aggressively, and the 3- and 5-year recurrence rates have been reported to be as high as 48 and 57%, respectively.[83] In another report,[84] the cumulated total recurrence rate was 24% using standard incidence rate calculation and 33% applying Kaplan-Meier survival analysis. Recurrent disease occurred significantly more frequently in children less than 8 years of age.[84] In a study of 199 children (215 procedures) with cholesteatoma, the residual cholesteatoma rate with the ICW technique was 20.5%, and recurrent cholesteatoma occurred in 8.9%. With the CWD technique, the residual and recurrent cholesteatoma rates were 23.8% and 19%, respectively. Eighty-eight per-

cent of the procedures were performed with the ICW technique. It was concluded that the ICW technique should be used in most cases of pediatric cholesteatoma.[85]

COMPLICATIONS

Complications associated with chronic ear surgery are either secondary to damage caused by the disease process itself or are iatrogenic. Most of the iatrogenic complications can be prevented by using meticulous surgical technique and by having a comprehensive knowledge of temporal bone anatomy. Preoperative patient education includes a discussion of potential complications and is documented in the medical record.

The most common early complications are facial nerve injury; sensorineural hearing loss; dysequilibrium; chorda tympani nerve injury; wound infection and perichondritis; injury of the sigmoid sinus, jugular bulb, and dura; and cerebrospinal fluid leakage.

Facial nerve injury is perhaps the most devastating complication of otologic surgery and is preventable in the majority of cases. The facial nerve is at greatest risk during mastoidectomy, although it can be injured in tympanoplasty and in canalplasty, as for removal of exostoses. In one study, it was determined that the most commonly injured segments are the tympanic and the mastoid[86]; in addition, the injury was not identified intraoperatively in 79% of the patients.[86] If facial nerve injury is recognized intraoperatively, the bone overlying the involved segment of the nerve should be gently removed and the nerve sheath slit open. Immediate administration of corticosteroids such as dexamethasone may be helpful. If 35% or more of the nerve circumference has been destroyed, the involved segment should be removed and grafted.[87] In the majority of cases, the greater auricular nerve can be used as a graft (see harvesting technique in Chapter 31) since it is located in close proximity to the surgical area and has the same diameter as the facial nerve. Facial paralysis manifest immediately postoperatively should be managed according to whether the nerve was positively identified during surgery. Early facial paralysis may be secondary to local anesthetic, and a few hours should suffice to allow the anesthetic effect to subside. In those cases in which the nerve has been positively identified and is known not to have been injured, the paralysis should be managed expectantly. Corticosteroids may be helpful. In the majority of such cases, the paralysis will resolve with no need for surgical intervention.[86] If the surgeon is uncertain as to the integrity of the facial nerve, exploration should be performed as soon as possible. Delayed facial paralysis has a good prognosis and should be monitored with serial electrophysiologic testing.

Sensorineural hearing loss may result from direct injury to the stapes, as in manipulation during dissection of disease. Should the stapes be avulsed, it should be repositioned in its original position and stabilized with a tissue graft. Other causes of sensorineural hearing loss include labyrinthine fistulae and acoustic trauma resulting from contact of the drill with the ossicular chain. Iatrogenic semicircular canal fistulae should be covered immediately with a tissue graft such as areolar tissue, fascia, or perichondrium.

Dysequilibrium can result either from iatrogenic vestibular injury or a labyrinthine fistula caused by the disease process. Management of fistulae has been discussed above.

Injury to the chorda tympani nerve, by stretching, drying, or direct instrumentation, can result in taste disturbance. In the majority of cases, the taste disturbance is self-limiting, and recovery occurs within several months.

Wound infection and perichondritis are rare complications, the manifestations of which are pain, erythema, and swelling of the surgical wound or auricle. Perichondritis is usually a consequence of procedures violating the integrity of the cartilaginous auricle or external auditory canal. Intravenous antibiotics effective against *P. aeruginosa* and gram-positive organisms are indicated. Incision and drainage should be performed in cases with abscess formation. Meticulous aseptic surgical technique with minimal tissue damage and frequent irrigation of the surgical field are key to avoiding this complication.

Bleeding from a small area of the bone overlying the sigmoid sinus can be controlled with an otologic drill using a diamond bur. Tears in the wall of the sinus can be controlled with bipolar cauterization or by applying a piece of saline-soaked Gelfoam over the bleeding point while exerting pressure with a moist cottonoid. Profuse bleeding from the jugular bulb can be managed by packing with Surgicel® (oxidized cellulose). Overpacking and occlusion of the jugular bulb should be avoided.

Dural injury with cerebrospinal fluid leakage can be controlled with a piece of fascia or temporalis muscle graft placed over the dural tear. The edges of the graft should be tucked beneath the edges of the bone. The graft is reinforced with Gelfoam or Surgicel.

Late complications include recurrent cholesteatoma, graft failure, blunting of the anterior tympanomeatal angle, stenosis of the external auditory canal, and prosthesis displacement/extrusion. The most effective way to avoid blunting of the anterior tympanomeatal angle is meticulous graft placement medial to the edges of the tympanic membrane remnant or tympanic annulus and packing with pledgets of Gelfoam.

REFERENCES

1. Wullstein H. Die Tympanoplastik als gehorverbessernde Operation bei Otitis Media chronica und ihr Resultate. In: Proceedings of the Fifth International Congress on Otorhinolaryngology. 1953.
2. Kessel J. Uber das Mobilisieren des Steigbulgels durch Ausschneiden des Trommelfelles, Hammers und Amboss bei undurchgangigkeit der Tuba. Arch Ohrenh 1878;13:69.
3. Berthold E. Ueber Myringoplastik. Wien Med Bl 1878;1:1627.

4. Kiesselbach W. Versuch zur Anlegung eines ausseren Gehorganges bei angeborener Missbildung beider Ohrmuscheln mit Fehlen der ausseren Gehorgange. Arch Ohrenh 1882;19:127.

5. Helmholtz HLF. Die Mechanik der Gehorknochelchen und des Trommelfelles. Pflugers Arch 1868;1:1.

6. Boucheron E. La mobilisation de l'etrier et son procede operatoire. Union Med Paris 1888;46:412.

7. Miot C. De la mobilisation de l'etrier. Rev Laryngol 1890;10:49.

8. Kerrison PD. Diseases of the ear. 4th ed. Philadelphia: JB Lippincott; 1930.

9. Ballance CA. Surgery of the temporal bone. New York: Macmillan; 1919.

10. Schwartze HH, Eysell CG. Ueber die kunstliche Eroffnung des Warzenfortsatzes. Arch Ohrenh 1873;7:157.

11. Küster E. Ueber die Grundsatze der Behandlung von Eiterungen in starrwandigen Hohlen, mit besonderer Berucksichtigung des Empyems der Pleura. Dtsch Med Wochenschr 1889;15:254.

12. Zaufal E. Technik des Trepanation des Proc. mastoid nach Kusterschen Grundsatzen. Arch Ohrenh 1890;30:291.

13. Stacke L. Stacke's Operationsmethode. Arch Ohrenh 1893;35:145.

14. Holmgren G. Some experiences in surgery for otosclerosis. Acta Otolaryngol (Stockh) 1923;5:460.

15. Nylén CO. The microscope in aural surgery, its first use and later development. Acta Otolaryngo Suppl (Stockh) 1954;116:226–40.

16. Sourdille M. New technique in the surgical treatment of severe and progressive deafness from otosclerosis. Bull N Y Acad Med 1937;13:673.

17. Lempert J. Improvement of hearing in cases of otosclerosis: new one-stage surgical technique. Arch Otolaryngol 1938;28:42.

18. Pattee GL. An operation to improve hearing in cases of congenital atresia of the external auditory meatus. Arch Otolaryngol 1947;45:568.

19. Ombrédanne M. Surgery of deafness: fenestration in cases of congenital atresia of the external auditory canal. Otorhinolaryngol Int 1947;13:229.

20. Rosen S. Mobilization of the stapes to restore hearing in otosclerosis. N Y J Med 1953;53:2650.

21. Juers AL. Observations on bone conduction in fenestrated cases. Ann Otol Rhinol Laryngol 1948;57:28.

22. Davis H, Walsh TE. The limits of improvement of hearing following the fenestration operation. Laryngoscope 1950;60:273.

23. Moritz W. Horverbessernde Operationen bei chronischentzundlichen Prozessen beider Mittelohren. Ztschr Laryngol Rhinol Otol 1950;29:578.

24. Zöllner F. Die Radikal-Operation mit besonderem Bezug auf die Horfunktion. Ztschr Laryngol Rhinol Otol 1951;30:104.

25. Wullstein H. Funktionelle Operationen im Mittelohr mit Hilfe des freien Spaltlappen-Transplantates. Arch Ohren-Nasen-u Kehlkopfh 1952;161:422.

26. Shea JJ. Vein graft closure of eardrum perforations. J Otolaryngol 1960;74:358.

27. Tabb HG. Closure of perforations of the tympanic membrane by vein grafts: a preliminary report of 20 cases. Laryngoscope 1960;70:271.

28. Storrs LA. Myringoplasty with the use of fascia grafts. Arch Otolaryngol 1961;74:65.

29. Hall A, Rytzner C. Stapedectomy and autotransplantation of ossicles. Acta Otolaryngol (Stockh) 1957;47:318.

30. Kley W, Dra FW. Histologic studies of autotransplanted ossicles and bone in the human middle ear. Acta Otolaryngol (Stockh) 1965;59:593.

31. House WF, Patterson ME, Linthicum FH. Incus homografts in chronic ear surgery. Arch Otol 1966;84:148.

32. Glasscock ME, House WF. Homograft reconstruction of the middle ear. Laryngoscope 1968;78:1219.

33. Shea JJ, Homsy CA. The use of proplast in otologic surgery. Laryngoscope 1974;84:1835.

34. Emmett JR, Shea JJ, Moretz WH. Long-term experience with biocompatible ossicular implants. Otolaryngol Head Neck Surg 1986;94:611.

35. Schuknecht HF, Shi SR. Surgical pathology of middle ear implants. Laryngoscope 1985;95:249–58.

36. Brackmann DE. Porous polyethylene prosthesis: continuing experience. Ann Otol Rhinol Laryngol 1986;95:76.

37. Sheehy JL. TORPs and PORPs: causes of failure—a report on 446 operations. Otolaryngol Head Neck Surg 1984;92:583.

38. Hicks GW, Wright JW Jr, Wright JW 3rd. Use of plastipore for ossicular chain reconstruction: an evaluation. Laryngoscope 1978;88:1024–33.

39. Brackmann DE, Sheehy JL. Tympanoplasty: TORPs and PORPs. Laryngoscope 1979;89:108–14.

40. Niparko JK, Kemink JL, Graham MD, Kartush JM. Bioactive glass ceramic in ossicular reconstruction: a preliminary report. Laryngoscope 1985;95:249–58.

41. Babighian G. Bioactive glass ceramic in ossicular reconstruction: a preliminary report. Am J Otol 1985;6:285–90.

42. Goldenberg R, Emmet JR. Current use of implants in middle ear surgery. Otol Neurotol 2001;22:145–52.

43. Wehrs RE. Hydroxylapatite implants for otologic surgery. Otolaryngol Clin North Am 1995;28:273–86.

44. Kartush JM. Ossicular chain reconstruction. Capitulum to malleus. Otolaryngol Clin North Am 1994;27:689–715.

45. DeMane CQ. The development of implants and implantable materials. Otolaryngol Clin North Am 1995;28:225–34.

46. Schmitt H. Uber die Bedeutung der Schalldrucktransformation und der Schallprotektion fur Horschwelle. Acta Otolaryngol (Stockh) 1957;49:71.

47. Committee on Conservation of Hearing, American Academy of Ophthalmology and Otolaryngology: standard classification for surgery of chronic ear disease. Arch Otol 1965;81:204.

48. Saito T, Tanaka T, Tokuriki M. Recent outcome of tympanoplasty in the elderly. Otol Neurotol 2001;22:153–7.

49. Wazen JJ, Caruso M, Tjellstron A. Long-term results with the titanium bone-anchored hearing aid: the U.S. experience. Am J Otol 1998;19:737–41.

50. Mosnier I, Fiky LE, Shahidi A, Sterkers O. Brain herniation and chronic otitis media: diagnosis and surgical management. Clin Otolaryngol 2000;25:385–91.

51. Austin DF. Ossicular reconstruction. Arch Otol 1971;94:525.

52. Shinohara T, Gyo K, Saiki T, et al. Ossiculoplasty using hydroxy-apatite prostheses: long-term results. Clin Otolaryngol 2000; 25:287–92.

53. Goldenberg RA, Driver M. Long-term results with hydroxyl-apatite middle ear implants. Otolaryngol Head Neck Surg 2000;122:635–42.

54. Goldenberg RA. Hydroxylapatite ossicular replacement prostheses: results in 157 consecutive cases. Laryngoscope 1992; 102:1091–6.

55. Black B. A universal ossicular replacement prosthesis: clinical trials of 152 cases. Otolaryngol Head Neck Surg 1991;104: 210–8.

56. van Blitterswijk CA, Hesseling SC, Grote JJ, et al. The bio-compatibility of hydroxyapatite ceramic: a study of retrieved human middle ear implants. J Biomed Mater Res 1990;24: 433–53.

57. Maassen MM, Zenner HP. Tympanoplasty type II with ionomeric cement and titanium-gold-angle prostheses. Am J Otol 1998;19:693–9.

58. Milewski C, Giannakopoulos N, Muller J, et al. Tragus peri-chondrium-cartilage island transplant in middle ear surgery. Method and results after 5 years. HNO 1996;44:235–41.

59. Muller J, Geyer G, Helms J. Restoration of sound transmission in the middle ear by reconstruction of the ossicular chain in its physiologic position. Results of incus reconstruction with ionomer cement. Laryngorhinootologie 1994;73:160–3.

60. Schwager K. Titanium as an ossicular replacement material: results after 336 days of implantation in the rabbit. Am J Otol 1998;19:569–73.

61. Wang X, Song J, Wang H. Results of tympanoplasty with tita-nium prostheses. Otolaryngol Head Neck Surg 1999;121:606–9.

62. Glasscock ME, Jackson CJ, Knox GW. Can acquired immun-odeficiency syndrome and Creutzfeldt-Jakob disease be trans-mitted via otologic homografts? Arch Otolaryngol Head Neck Surg 1988;114:1252.

63. Pennington CL. Incus interposition techniques. Ann Otol Rhi-nol Laryngol 1973;82:518–31.

64. Austin DF. Ossicular reconstruction. Arch Otolaryngol 1971;94: 525–35.

65. Jackson CG, Glasscock ME, Schwaber MK, et al. Ossicular chain reconstruction: the TORP and PORP in chronic ear dis-ease. Laryngoscope 1983;93:981.

66. Grote JJ. Reconstruction of the middle ear with hydroxylap-atite implants: long-term results. Ann Otol Rhinol Laryngol Suppl 1990;144:12–6.

67. Wehrs RE. Incus replacement prostheses of hydroxylapatite in middle ear reconstruction. Am J Otol 1989;10:181–2.

68. Black B. Ossiculoplasty prognosis: the spite method of assess-ment. Am J Otol 1992;13:544–51.

69. Jackson CG, Glasscock ME, Schwaber MK, et al. Ossicular chain reconstruction: the TORP and PORP in chronic ear dis-ease. Laryngoscope 1983;93:981–8.

70. Brackmann DE, Sheehy JL, Luxford WM. TORPs and PORPs in tympanoplasty: a review of 1042 operations. Otolaryngol Head Neck Surg 1984;92:32–7.

71. Brackmann DE. Porous polyethylene prosthesis: continuing experience. Ann Otol Rhinol Laryngol 1986;95:76.

72. Vincent R, Lopez A, Sperling NM. Malleus ankylosis: a clin-ical, audiometric, histologic, and surgical study of 123 cases. Am J Otol 1999;20:717–25.

73. Moon CN, Hahn MJ. Primary malleus fixation: diagnosis and treatment. Laryngoscope 1981;91:1298–307.

74. Armstrong BW. Epitympanic malleus fixation: correction without disrupting the ossicular chain. Laryngoscope 1976;86: 1203–8.

75. Gacek RR. Surgical management of labyrinthine fistulae in chronic otitis media with cholesteatoma. Ann Otol Rhinol Laryngol 1974;83:19.

76. Dawes JD, Watson RT. Labyrinthine fistulae. J Laryngol Otol 1978;92:83–98.

77. Namyslowski G, Orecka B, Misiolek M. The management in chronic otitis media complicated by labyrinthine fistula. Oto-laryngol Pol 1997;51:371–6.

78. Kobayashi T, Sato T, Toshima M, et al. Treatment of labyrinthine fistula with interruption of the semicircular canals. Arch Oto-laryngol Head Neck Surg 1995;121:469–75.

79. Duckert LG, Muller J, Makielski KH, et al. Composite auto-graft "shield" reconstruction of remnant tympanic membranes. Am J Otol 1995;16:21–6.

80. Glasscock ME, Miller GW. Intact canal wall tympanoplasty in the management of cholesteatoma. Laryngoscope 1976;86: 1639–57.

81. Jansen CL. The combined approach for tympanoplasty. J Laryngol Otol 1968;82:776.

82. Sheehy JL, Patterson ME. Intact canal wall tympanoplasty with mastoidectomy. Laryngoscope 1967;77:1502.

83. Rosenfeld RM, Moura RL, Bluestone CD. Predictors of resid-ual-recurrent cholesteatoma in children. Arch Otolaryngol Head Neck Surg 1992;118:384–91.

84. Stangerup SE, Drozdziewicz D, Tos M. Cholesteatoma in chil-dren, predictors and calculation of recurrence rates. Int J Pedi-atr Otorhinolaryngol 1999;49 Suppl 1:S69–73.

85. Darrouzet V, Duclos JY, Portmann D, et al. Preference for the closed technique in the management of cholesteatoma of the middle ear in children: a retrospective study of 215 consecu-tive patients treated over 10 years. Am J Otol 2000;21:474–81.

86. Green JD Jr, Shelton C, Brackmann DE. Iatrogenic facial nerve injury during otologic surgery. Laryngoscope 1994;104(8 Pt 1):922–6.

87. Adkins WY, Osguthorpe JD. Management of trauma of the facial nerve. Otolaryngol Clin North Am 1991;24:587–611.

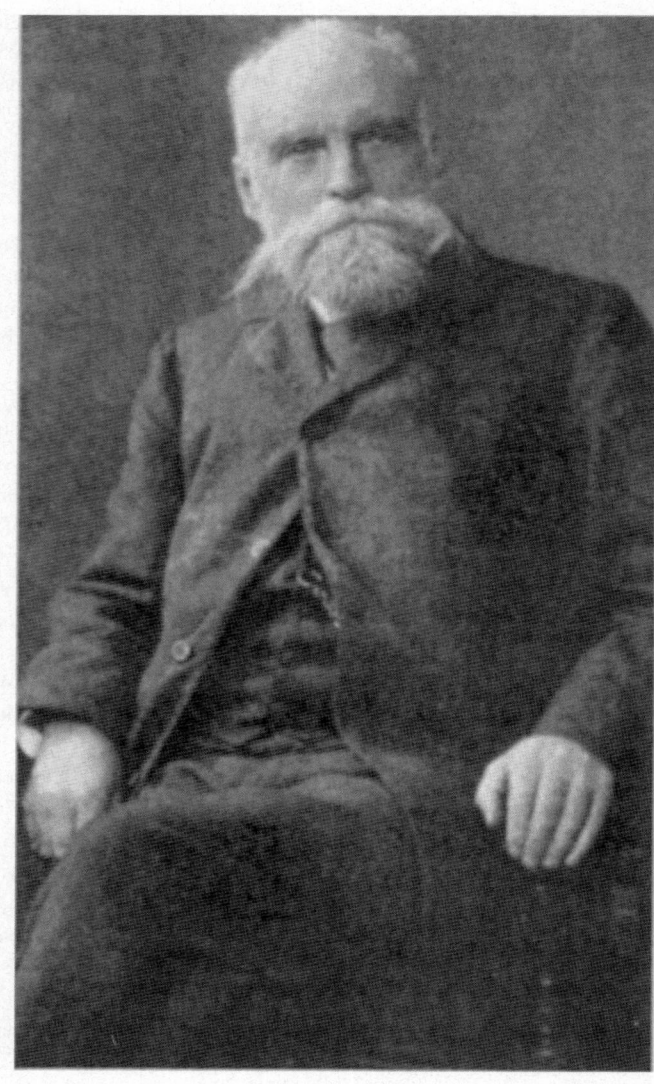

Hermann Schwartze (1837–1910). Established the indications and technique of the simple mastoid operation.

25

Simple Mastoid Operation

GLENN D. JOHNSON, MD, FACS

The simple mastoid operation to evacuate a coalescent abscess from within the mastoid process is seldom required today. This operation was formerly the one most frequently performed on the temporal bone, and the story of its rise and decline for this indication is an interesting one.

Although rarely done today for coalescent mastoiditis, the simple mastoid operation remains an important tool of the otologic surgeon. Although antibiotics have dramatically reduced the morbidity of otitis media, complications of acute otitis media still occur. Mastoidectomy continues to play a role in the management of these, as discussed in Chapter 23. The management of chronic otitis media, with or without cholesteatoma, is probably the most common reason why the simple mastoid operation is performed today. The surgical approach of the simple mastoid operation for removal of cholesteatoma combined with tympanoplasty was covered in Chapter 24.

The simple mastoid operation is also performed not to remove disease but to provide access to the deeper structures of the temporal bone. Cochlear implantation, insertion of implantable and semi-implantable hearing aids, translabyrinthine approaches to the inner ear and posterior fossa, endolymphatic sac procedures, perilabyrinthine approaches to the petrous apex, and extended facial recess approaches to tumors of the middle ear all depend on a well-performed simple mastoidectomy as the first step. It is therefore critical for the modern otologic surgeon to become competent through an understanding of the technique and practice in the performance of this operation.

HISTORICAL NOTES

The potential seriousness of ear suppuration was appreciated by Hippocrates, but the idea of operating to relieve the condition seems to have occurred for the first time about four centuries ago to the great medieval surgeon Ambrose Paré. Called to the sickbed of the young King Charles II of France and finding him delirious, in a high fever, and with a discharging ear, barber-surgeon Paré proposed an operation of the skull to drain away the pus. The boy-king's bride, Mary, Queen of Scots and of France, assented, but the king's mother, Catherine de'Medici, forbade an operation, so Mary lost her first husband and her first throne when she was only 18 years old.[1]

The first recorded successful mastoid operation for the relief of aural suppuration was by Jean Petit[2] of Paris. Independently, a short time afterward in 1776, Jasser, a Prussian military surgeon, successfully operated on a soldier's mastoid process. But the new operation was doomed to a long period of eclipse when Baron Bergen, personal physician to the King of Denmark, hearing of Petit's successful operation, persuaded a surgical colleague to operate on his mastoid to relieve deafness and tinnitus. It is not surprising that this operation, undertaken before any knowledge of surgical asepsis, ended in infection. When Bergen died 12 days later in great pain from the mastoid operation for mistaken indications, the procedure fell into a disrepute that lasted nearly 100 years.[3]

In 1853, Sir William Wilde[4] of Dublin introduced his famous postaural incision for suppuration of the ear with postaural abscess. Still, Wilde advised against opening the bone unless there were symptoms threatening to life, and apparently he never carried out a mastoidectomy. It remained for Schwartze and Eysell,[5] in 1873, to describe the indications and technique of the mastoid operation thoroughly enough to overcome the century of prejudice against it. So well did they succeed that by the end of the nineteenth century, the operation had attained general acceptance and such importance that Whiting[6] wrote, "As a life saving measure few surgical procedures equal and none surpass in efficiency the modern mastoid operation."

The dread with which a mastoid operation was often regarded by the laity came not from the timely interventions by qualified surgeons but from their efforts to save patients whose infections had already extended beyond the mastoid process and who died despite and not because of their mastoid operations.

It is true indeed that a skillfully performed and properly indicated mastoidectomy for a well-localized coalescent infection proved remarkably effective not only in removing the risk of serious complication from the abscess within the mastoid but also in very quickly bringing to an end the continued aural suppuration. The mastoidectomy needed only the addition of criteria and techniques for dealing with a similar process in the less accessible apex of the petrous pyramid[7-10] to bring this triumph of otologic surgery to final fruition. Almost at that precise moment appeared the revolutionary antibacterial therapy destined to do more for acute coalescent mastoiditis and other complications of acute otitis media than all of the most elaborate and highly developed surgery.

Sulfanilamide was first employed in 1935, in the form of Prontosil, for the serious complications of acute ear infection, especially for almost invariably fatal otitic meningitis. The favorable results that began to follow the use of sulfanilamide in some of these cases encouraged its application to earlier stages of severe ear infection. At first, otologic surgeons were loathe to abandon the tried and proven surgical procedures, fearing and predicting that sulfonamides would mask the clinical picture and lead to late dire results. But very soon it became clear that the earlier the sulfonamide and the even more effective penicillin could be given before localized collections of pus had begun to form, the fewer the complications and the indications for surgery.

The credit for the rapid decline of the need for the simple mastoid operation of Schwartze goes to Domagk and Fleming, the discoverers of sulfanilamide and penicillin. But credit should also go to the multitude of family doctors and pediatricians who put these antibacterial agents to such early and effective use that today few acutely infected ears ever drain and even fewer reach the operating table. To put the influence of antibiotics on the development of mastoiditis in perspective, at the start of the twentieth century, 50% of patients who had otitis media developed mastoiditis, compared with 0.24% of contemporary patients with otitis media.[11] But, perhaps because of the decreased familiarity with the presentation of coalescent mastoiditis and delay in surgical treatment, nearly 50% of modern patients with mastoiditis develop subperiosteal abscess compared with 20% at the turn of the twentieth century.[12]

COALESCENT MASTOIDITIS

The simple mastoid operation is indicated for cases of acute suppurative otitis media that fail to respond to antibiotic therapy and that proceed to a coalescent mastoiditis. In the presulfonamide era, the simple mastoid operation was sometimes required for certain early cases of acute suppurative otitis media with a beginning complication by osteothrombophlebitic extension. Today antibacterial medication may be relied on for cases complicated by osteothrombophlebitic extension, confining the simple mastoidectomy to cases of coalescent mastoiditis.

In Chapter 21, the pathology of acute suppurative otitis media in its various stages was described, including the stage of coalescent mastoiditis. At this point, certain fundamental characteristics of mastoiditis in acute otitis media bear repeating.

The physician should remember that the pneumatic cells of the mastoid process are lined by a continuation of the tympanic mucoperiosteum, which is simultaneously involved to some degree in every acute bacterial invasion of the middle ear, with purulent exudate in the mastoid cells and the tympanum. This involvement was never by itself an indication for surgery because the normal process of localization of the infection led to spontaneous resolution of the infection of the mucoperiosteum without bone involvement in the great majority of cases. In the presulfonamide era, not more than 1 to 5% of patients with acute suppurative otitis media required a mastoidectomy, the percentage depending on the virulence of the organism in different epidemics.

The involvement of bone with development of areas of coalescent bone erosion requires at least 10 days to 2 weeks or more of a severe untreated middle ear infection; the average duration of the otitis media before mastoidectomy becomes necessary is 3 to 5 weeks.

Areas of coalescent bone erosion are always associated with adjacent areas of beginning healing, and only evacuation of trapped pus from involved mastoid cells is required to replace the coalescent process of bone removal with active osteoblastic bone repair. Mastoidectomy is performed in acute otitis media with coalescent mastoiditis to accomplish just this evacuation of pus. Mastoidectomy is not done to remove "necrotic bone" because there is none in usual acute coalescent mastoiditis. Nor is mastoidectomy done to prevent chronic suppurative otitis media because this disorder rarely results from neglected acute suppurative otitis media of the usual non-necrotizing variety.

Symptoms and Signs of Surgical Coalescent Mastoiditis

It should be re-emphasized that many of the symptoms and signs of coalescent mastoiditis that require a simple mastoidectomy are exactly the same as those of early severe acute suppurative otitis media but with one essential difference. When the symptoms occur early in the first few days or week of an acute middle ear infection, they do not call for surgical opening of the mastoid, but, when they persist or recur after several weeks of acute otitis media, they point toward a developing coalescent process in the mastoid air cells that may require a mastoidectomy. Failure to appreciate this difference in the significance of symptoms in the first few days of acute otitis media, compared with the same symptoms after the ear had drained for several weeks, led to errors of both commission and omission in mastoid surgery. On the one hand, some surgeons would open a mastoid process in early "red hot" otitis media caused by hemolytic *Streptococcus* before any sort of localization of the infection had occurred. The result of such untimely surgery was an extraordinarily high incidence of intracranial and distant complications caused by dissemination of the infection. On the other hand, complacency toward persistent pain and low-grade fever from an ear that had drained for a month or more sometimes allowed a coalescent abscess to erode the inner plate, producing fatal meningitis. The time at which symptoms and signs

appear is more important than their severity in evaluating the need for a mastoidectomy in acute suppurative otitis media.

Persistence of aural discharge for more than 3 weeks in acute suppurative otitis media is the most constant symptom pointing toward a coalescent process, especially when the discharge is profuse or creamy (rather than thin and mucoid) or varies in amount with periods of copious drainage alternating with periods of scant or absent drainage. With an understanding of the normal tendency toward localization and resolution of an acute infection of the middle ear, the physician appreciates that the persistence of a purulent discharge beyond 3 or 4 weeks indicates that the normal tendency toward healing is being prevented by inadequate drainage from coalescing pneumatic cells. As the mastoid abscess develops, the discharge not only persists but usually becomes more purulent and creamy and may begin to vary in amount as the pus forces its way out of the abscess cavity from time to time. In rare cases, the discharge may actually cease, yet a walled-off abscess may remain to cause symptoms and radiographic changes. This situation occurs especially when a coalescent abscess develops in the petrous apex, in otitis media caused by pneumococci, or in acute otitis media partially arrested but not eradicated by inadequate or ineffective antibacterial medication.

Pain localized deep in or behind the ear is the next most common symptom of coalescent mastoiditis. The pain is caused by the pressure of the trapped pus on the inflamed tissues and diminishes when drainage increases. Severe pain suggests an extradural abscess. The pain is typically worse at night, perhaps because of increased venous congestion in the recumbent position that increases the pressure. If the pain is felt deep behind the eye, a coalescent process in the petrous apex is suggested.

The physician should remember that the time of appearance of pain after the onset of otitis media is the factor that determines its surgical significance. The extreme, even excruciating pain of an unruptured drum membrane in the first day or two of otitis should not alarm the physician, whereas comparatively mild pain that recurs after several weeks of painless discharge should cause deep concern.

Persistence of pain for longer than 2 weeks after the onset of otitis media has the same significance as recurrence of pain after several weeks of acute otitis media. Pain is not an invariable symptom of surgical mastoiditis and may be absent in the presence of a well-localized coalescent abscess.

Tenderness over the mastoid process is the most consistent physical sign of coalescent mastoiditis. Tenderness in the first few days of acute otitis media may be considerable, yet it does not indicate a surgical process, whereas after several weeks of draining of the ear, even a slight detectable difference of sensitivity to deep pressure between the affected and normal mastoid process points toward a coalescing process.

The tenderness is greatest where the trapped pus is nearest to the periosteum: in adults, over the tip of the mastoid process and in children with incomplete pneumatization, more often over the fossa mastoidea near the antrum. Periosteal thickening is caused by edema where the abscess is approaching the lateral surface of the mastoid process by bone erosion. To demonstrate slight but significant degrees of periosteal thickening, the examiner should stand behind the patient and palpate both mastoids at the same time. The irregularities of the bone surface seem to be obscured or "ironed out" by a thickened periosteum on the involved side.

Subperiosteal abscess occurs when the eroding pus perforates the outer cortex. The usual perforation on the lateral surface of the mastoid process is above the insertion of the sternocleidomastoid muscle and produces the typical displacement of the auricle downward, outward, and forward (Figure 25–1). Owing to the thickness of the overlying tissues, fluctuation may not be easy to detect at first, but, as the subperiosteal abscess enlarges, deep fluctuation can be demonstrated.

Less often the perforation occurs over the posterior root of the zygoma, producing a zygomatic abscess. The periosteum under the lower edge of the temporal muscle is elevated, and the upper half of the auricle is displaced away from the skull by the abscess.

Perforation on the medial aspect of the mastoid tip into the digastric groove (incisura mastoidea) produces

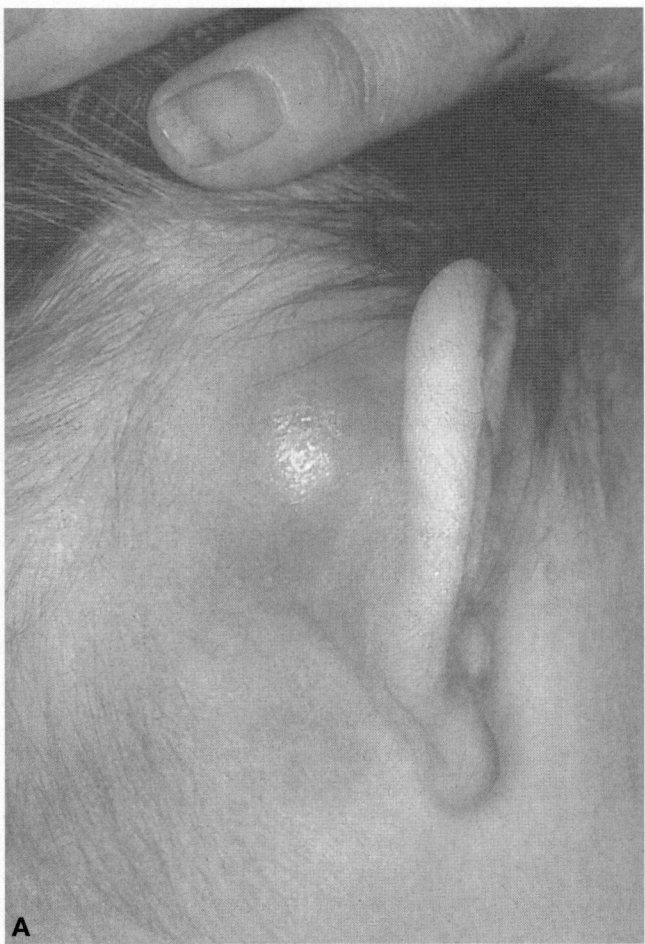

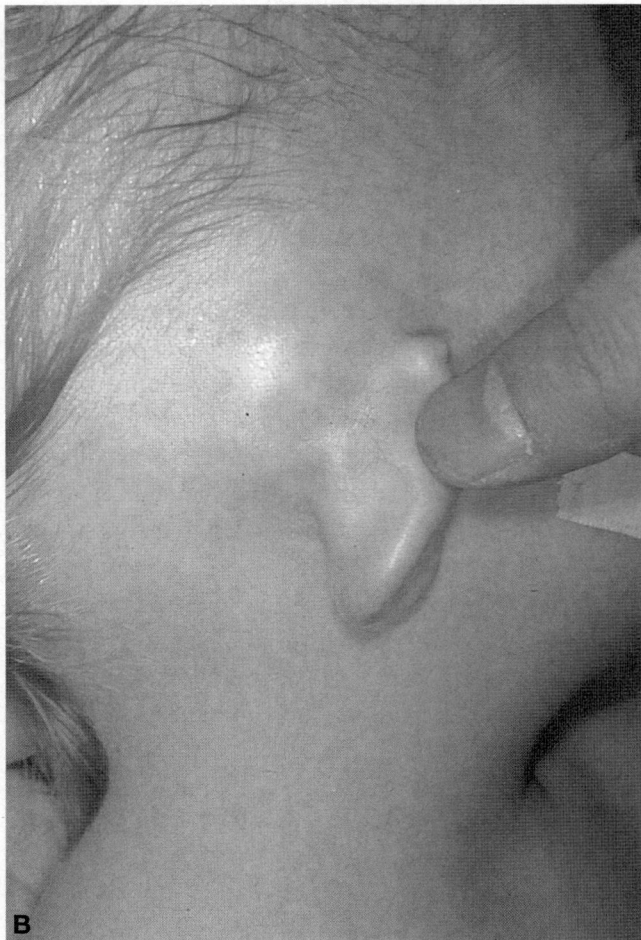

Figure 25–1 *A* and *B*. Mastoid subperiosteal abscess. Courtesy of Eiji Yanagisawa, MD, FACS.

a deep abscess of the neck, known as Bezold's abscess. To quote from Bezold:

> Exceptionally large cells are often found in the adult…on the inner surface of the mastoid process, sometimes extending from the incisura mastiodea as far as the bulb of the jugular vein. Perforations at these places produce a very distinct clinical picture…The pus cannot reach the surface…No fluctuation can be felt. A moderately sensitive swelling develops rather suddenly in the lower surroundings of the mastoid process concealing its contours…The suppuration spreads gradually in all directions…below the fascia of the neck. The pus may descend along the sheaths of the large vessels and may reach the larynx and even the mediastinum. The pus may descend…along the muscles of the vertebral column. A burrowing of pus leading to the formation of a retropharyngeal abscess was observed…
>
> A perforation of the tympanic membrane…did not precede the descensions of pus in the neck in 29 percent of the cases I observed. Pneumococci were found most frequently to be the cause of the suppuration.[13]

To this explanation we may add that an empyema of the apex of the petrous pyramid can produce a similar deep abscess of the neck.

A very rare type of perforation of the outer cortex is from the cells of the root of the zygoma downward and forward into the mandibular fossa.[14] A tender fluctuant abscess appears just in front of the tragus, with a displacement of the mandible toward the normal side so that the teeth no longer meet in occlusion.

Sagging of the posterosuperior meatal wall is a very frequent and dependable sign of coalescent mastoiditis. The sagging is caused by thickening of the periosteum of the osseous meatus adjacent to the antrum. Should the bone perforate at this point with the formation of a subperiosteal abscess, the sagging becomes so great as to nearly obliterate the lumen of the meatus. Today this is much less likely to happen in acute otitis media than in chronic otitis with cholesteatoma formation.

The tympanic membrane continues to be markedly thickened and red with loss of landmarks. A nipplelike protrusion through the small central tympanic membrane perforation, caused by the marked thickening of the tympanic mucoperiosteum, often accompanies a coalescent process within the mastoid. The purulent discharge may be seen coming from the tip of the conical

elevation. In recent reports of coalescent mastoiditis, tympanic membrane perforation is often absent, probably the result of aggressive antibiotic use.[15]

Fever, usually low grade and intermittent, is caused by toxic absorption from the trapped pus under pressure. Because by the third or fourth week of the middle ear infection the process of localization and production of specific antibodies is well advanced, any fever, leukocytosis, and malaise caused by toxic absorption are very much less than during the first week, yet they are now far more ominous as evidence of a dangerous bone-eroding process.

Fever may be absent or so occasional as to escape detection unless the temperature is taken regularly every 4 hours. Leukocytosis and increased sedimentation rate in an acutely diseased ear that has discharged for more than 3 weeks are indicative of retained pus and may be present without fever.

Secondary anemia may develop in hemolytic streptococcal infections that persist, especially when they are complicated by sigmoid sinus thrombophlebitis and septicemia. Anemia may also develop as a toxic reaction to sulfonamides and less often to an antibiotic. In these cases, anemia is associated with leukopenia.

The conductive hearing impairment of acute suppurative otitis media continues as long as the ear drains and the mucoperiosteal lining in the epitympanum and tympanum remains thickened. The presence of normal hearing speaks against mastoiditis secondary to otitis media and in favor of a large furuncle of the meatus, which may cause signs and symptoms that simulate coalescent mastoiditis.

Radiographic changes of coalescent mastoiditis are very characteristic and diagnostic. To the opacification of the pneumatic cells, which always occurs in acute suppurative otitis media as their content of air is replaced by exudate, are added a fading out and beginning fuzziness and indistinctness of the discrete bone cell partitions as decalcification and osteoclastic bone removal proceed. Serial radiographs made of the mastoid once a week during the course of acute otitis media help to demonstrate the progressive bone changes of coalescence. Computed tomography (CT) findings in coalescent mastoiditis include erosion of the mastoid septa and lateral cortical wall. Antonelli and colleagues found erosion of the cortical plate over the sigmoid sinus to be the most sensitive and specific CT finding distinguishing surgical acute coalescent mastoiditis from medically treatable mastoiditis.[16]

Differential Diagnosis of Coalescent Mastoiditis

Suppuration of the mastoid lymph node and furuncle of the meatus are two conditions that may be confusing and must be differentiated from surgical mastoiditis. The mastoid lymph node, lying on the lateral surface of the mastoid process, drains the scalp and becomes inflamed in hair follicle infections or pediculosis capitis. The normal hearing and absence of history and symptoms of otitis media should make the differentiation easy. Furuncle of the meatus secondary to external otitis is easily differentiated from surgical mastoiditis by the normal hearing, provided that the meatus is patent. When a furuncle complicates otitis media, the diagnostic problem is more difficult. Extreme sensitiveness of the cartilaginous meatus to pressure suggests a furuncle, but absence of great discomfort when the cartilaginous meatus is manipulated speaks for mastoiditis.

Atypical Mastoiditis

The terms atypical, latent, silent, and masked mastoiditis have been applied to cases of coalescent mastoiditis without a draining ear or the other usual symptoms and signs of this condition. Cases of this sort were encountered in the preantibiotic era, especially in pneumococcus infections. The patient's symptoms might consist of slight stuffiness in the ear or tinnitus. The tympanic membrane was intact with only minimal thickening or inflammatory change. Mastoid tenderness was slight or absent. Because of persistent fever or meningitis or other complication, a radiograph of the mastoid would be taken and would reveal extensive changes of decalcification and coalescence.

The early use of antibacterial medication in acute otitis media modifies the clinical course in some cases, causing otitis media to resemble pneumococcus infection. When the antibacterial agent is given in insufficient quantity or for too brief a period, when the antibiotic of choice for a particular organism has not been selected, or when the organism is one that has developed a resistance to the administered antibiotics, the infection in the middle ear is slowed down but not checked.

The acute symptoms subside, and the patient appears well for a time, but after a period of weeks, fever of unknown origin, recurring attacks of acute otitis media or meningitis, facial paralysis, or labyrinthitis calls attention to possible atypical mastoiditis. The only evidence of widespread suppurative disease within the temporal bone may be slight, persistent, inflammatory thickening of the drum membrane; persistent impaired hearing; or slight deep bone tenderness over the mastoid. Plain mastoid radiographs may show definite changes or may be reported as normal. The diagnosis of coalescent mastoiditis is strongly enhanced if those changes described in the previous section are seen on temporal bone CT images.

Whereas cases of typical acute coalescent mastoiditis have become rare indeed, otitic complications from atypical mastoiditis continue and may even be on the increase.[17,18] The diagnosis of atypical mastoiditis requires not only a careful history of an earache following a respiratory infection but also a complete otologic examination, including hearing tests and radiographic studies of the temporal bone. When the clinical picture is suggestive but not clear, the findings on CT scanning of erosion of the mastoid septa, lateral cortical wall, and/or cortical plate over the sigmoid sinus are strong indicators of coalescent mastoiditis. As stated by Antonelli and colleagues,[16] temporal bone demineralization that is imaged on CT scanning occurs on a continuum, so there can never be an absolute radiographic threshold for surgical treatment. The decision to treat a patient with mastoiditis by a simple mastoidectomy must take into account many factors, including the history of the infection, response to parenteral antibiotics, clinical findings, and radiologic evidence of bony erosion.

In every case of acute suppurative otitis media, including atypical cases without rupture of the tympanic membrane, when evidence of active infection persists beyond 3 to 4 weeks, the physician must weigh any symptoms and signs of a coalescent process against whatever evidence there is of spontaneous resolution. In case of doubt, a period of watchful waiting is indicated, with the patient in the hospital, where he/she may be given a trial of a more appropriate antibiotic as determined by culture and sensitivity tests and where the signs and symptoms, temperature, and radiographic and blood changes may be watched closely.

A simple mastoidectomy is not an emergency operation that must be performed immediately unless there are signs and symptoms of a threatened complication.[19,20] These signs and symptoms are considered in detail in Chapters 22 and 23.

TECHNIQUE

The early operations on the mastoid process for an acute coalescent abscess consisted of removing the cortex from the lateral surface of the mastoid process, locating the antrum, opening the abscess cavity widely, and scooping out adjacent softened cell remnants and granulations. Intact pneumatic cells were not disturbed. The wound was packed with a long strip of iodoform gauze and left open. The packing was replaced every few days for 3 to 5 weeks until the purulent drainage had ceased and the mastoid cavity filled with healthy granulations.

As the technique of the operation improved, it was found that the more complete the exenteration of all accessible pneumatic cells from the mastoid process, squama, and posterior perilabyrinthine petrous area medial to the antrum, the quicker the cessation of purulent discharge and the less often it became necessary to revise the operation to remove remaining coalescent foci of persistent suppuration. As the simple mastoidectomy changed to a complete anatomic dissection of all accessible pneumatic cells, the name complete mastoidectomy was proposed as being more appropriate. However, just as the name otosclerosis has persisted, the term simple mastoidectomy remains the most commonly used term for the operation.

Anesthesia

General anesthesia is usually selected. If for any reason a general anesthetic is contraindicated, a very satisfactory and excellent local anesthesia may be secured, as described in Chapter 12.

Incision

The endaural incision may be used for the simple mastoid operation on a mastoid process with restricted pneumatization, as advocated by Lempert,[10] but, for the usual well-pneumatized bone, the postaural Wilde incision gives far better exposure (Figure 25–2). There is one word of caution: if there is a subperiosteal abscess or if the mastoid was previously operated on, a bold incision through skin, subcutaneous tissue, and periosteum in a single stroke is contraindicated, and the tissues should be incised cautiously in layers to avoid possible injury to an exposed middle fossa dura or wall of the sigmoid sinus.

Remember that in the infant there is not yet a mastoid process, so that the usual postaural incision sections the facial nerve. Until the age of 2 years, a modified incision should be used, as described in Chapter 12.

Removal of the Cortex

The key to successful mastoid surgery is good exposure and early identification of the relevant anatomy. Using a large cutting bur (6 to 7 mm) and continuous suction irrigation, the cortex should be removed from the entire lateral surface, from the temporal line above to the mastoid tip below and from the posterior osseous meatal wall in front to the probable extent of pneumatization behind, as seen on the radiograph. The initial bur stroke is usually along the temporal line, continuing superiorly until the middle fossa dura is identified. The cortical opening is then made as wide as the surgeon thinks the pneumatization extends to give the best exposure. The ability to identify relevant anatomy, as well as the removal of disease within the mastoid, is greatly aided by the best exposure possible.

Exenteration of Mastoid Cells

If a coalescent abscess is opened into when the cortex is removed, it should be examined carefully for exposed wall of the sigmoid sinus or middle fossa dura before pneumatic cells are removed.

An orderly systematic removal of cell tracts saves a great deal of time and ensures complete exenteration of all accessible cells. After the cortex is opened, the air cells just below the cortex are thoroughly exenterated, using the middle fossa dura medially and the posterior bony canal wall as anatomic landmarks. The surgical depth is not increased until the more superficial layer is opened as widely as possible for the given extent of

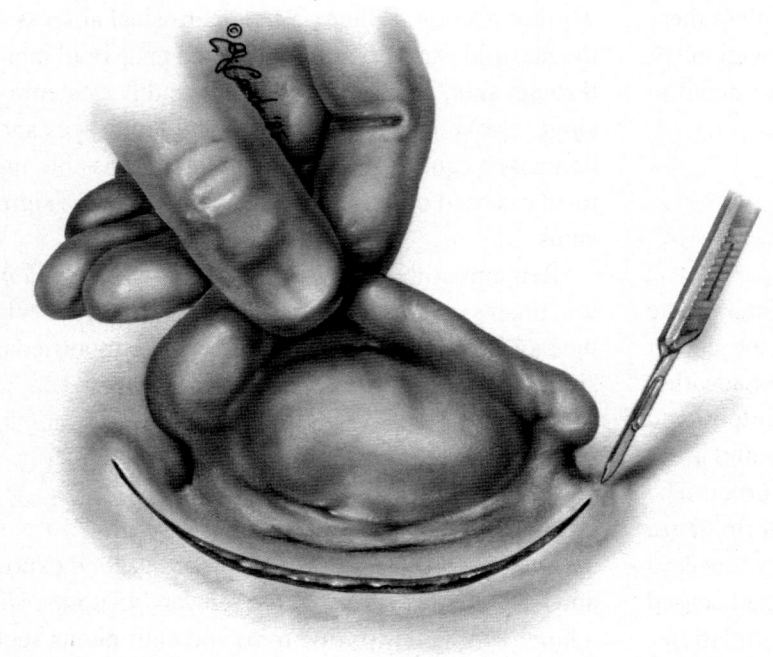

A

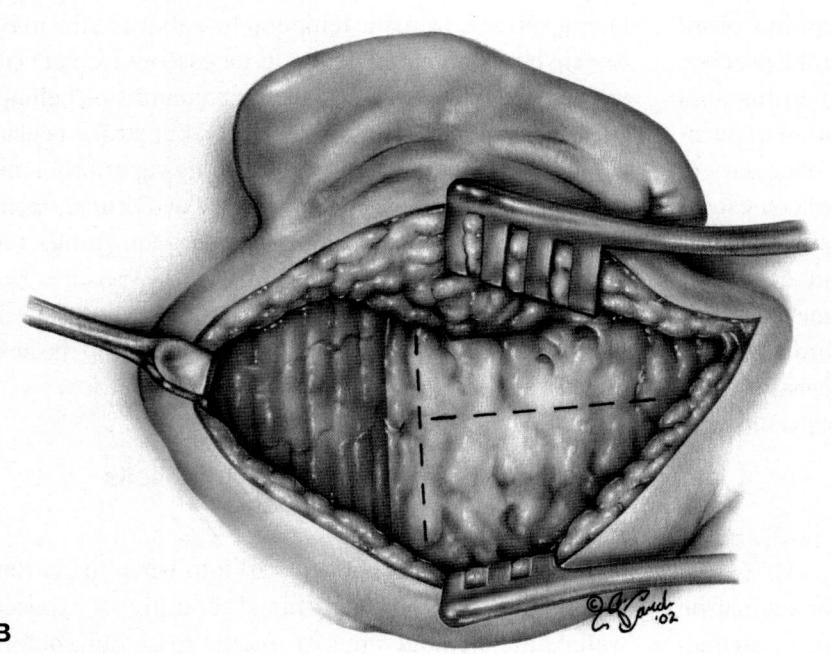

B

Figure 25–2   Incision and exposure for simple mastoidectomy. *A*, Line of postaural incision. *B*, Exposure of the mastoid cortex.

pneumatization. As the depth is increased, additional landmarks are identified. Posteriorly, the sigmoid sinus is identified. The sigmoid can then be followed inferiorly into the mastoid tip. The tip of the mastoid process contains one or several large cells. These cells are cleaned out; the lateral wall of the tip is removed, and, within the mastoid, the digastric ridge, which corresponds to the digastric groove (or incisura mastoidea), is defined.

Remember that the stylomastoid foramen containing the facial nerve lies at the anterior end of this ridge, and by staying close to the sigmoid inferiorly, the bur is kept posterior to the location of the vertical portion of the facial nerve.

The air cells in the sinodural angle are opened until the tegmen plate meets the sigmoid sinus plate at a sharp angle. The antrum is typically visualized at this time. The most common error in locating the antrum is to seek it too far below the temporal line. Opening the mastoid as far anteriorly above the bony external auditory canal into the zygomatic root will help avoid this error.

Very carefully clean out all small pneumatic cells medial to the antrum down to the hard bony posterior and superior semicircular canals. Define the posterior end of the bony horizontal semicircular canal very carefully, avoiding injury to or dislocation of the incus. The landmarks for the vertical portion of the facial nerve may now be located; the posterior end of the bony horizontal semicircular canal, the posterior semicircular canal, and the anterior extent of the digastric ridge. The anterior bony wall between the posterior end of the lateral semicircular canal and anterior digastric ridge is now gently drilled with a diamond bur, stroking the bur horizontally in the direction of the facial nerve. This movement may be likened to making light brush strokes with a paint brush. Ideally, the facial nerve is identified in the mid section of its vertical course rather than at the second genu. Since the nerve may course more posteriorly at the second genu, it is more prone to injury here than at the mid section of its vertical course through the mastoid.

In the completed simple mastoid cavity, the osseous superior and posterior meatal wall has been left standing; the tegmen and sinus plates are defined but intact; and the cell tracts have been followed to their termination from the antrum inferiorly to the tip, posteriorly to the junction of sinus plate and cortex, superiorly to the junction of tegmen plate and cortex, anteriorly to the limit of pneumatization in the posterior root of the zygoma, and medially to the superior and posterior osseous semicircular canals (Figure 25–3).

Should the sinus plate or tegmen plate be softened by disease, it should be carefully elevated from the underlying sigmoid sinus or dura and removed in small bites with a small rongeur until firm, healthy bone and healthy sinus or dura without granulations are encountered. Unnecessary exposure of sinus or dura under healthy bone should be avoided because it only lays open fresh tissue to the infecting organism.

Coalescent mastoiditis occurs most often in a well-pneumatized temporal bone. However, coalescent mastoiditis may occur in a partially pneumatized bone with peripheral areas of diploic marrow-containing bone in the mastoid process and petrous pyramid. A coalescent

osteitis in such a bone may extend to adjacent diploic bone to produce a localized osteomyelitis. With the bur, it is not difficult to determine when diploic bone is softened by disease. When this bone is softened, it should be burred away down to firm healthy bone exactly as is done with coalescent pneumatized bone.

Suture of the Wound

A complete mastoidectomy on a well-localized coalescent mastoiditis no longer needs to be packed and left open but may be sutured, with a small drain, leading to the antrum, left protruding from the lower end of the incision. With antibiotic coverage, the wound may be sutured without any drainage in selected cases, but, as a rule, the surgeon prefers to leave a small, soft rubber tube drain from the antrum for 3 or 4 days. To keep the drain in position, it may be sutured to the skin.

After the cavity is débrided of any loose fragments of bone, it is irrigated with warm sterile saline solution for hemostasis and removal of any remaining smaller particles of bone. The skin and periosteum are approximated by interrupted sutures. The meatus is packed firmly with a strip of petroleum jelly gauze, compressed absorbable gelatin sponge (Gelfoam®) moistened with saline or antibiotic solution, or antibiotic ointment to prevent stenosis. A mastoid dressing is applied.

POSTOPERATIVE CARE

The patient should be encouraged to ambulate as soon as the patient recovers from anesthesia. The mastoid dressing is changed daily with sterile technique (see Chapter 12). If there is no purulent discharge from the drain, it may be removed; otherwise, the drain should be left until the purulent drainage ceases. The appropriate antibiotic, as determined by sensitivity tests for the organism cultured from the mastoid at the time of surgery, should be administered until all aural or postaural discharge has ceased and then for 5 more days.

The patient usually leaves the hospital as soon as the drain is removed. The mastoid dressing may be dispensed with as soon as the wound is dry. Persistence of discharge from the ear or mastoid process may be attributable to one of the following:

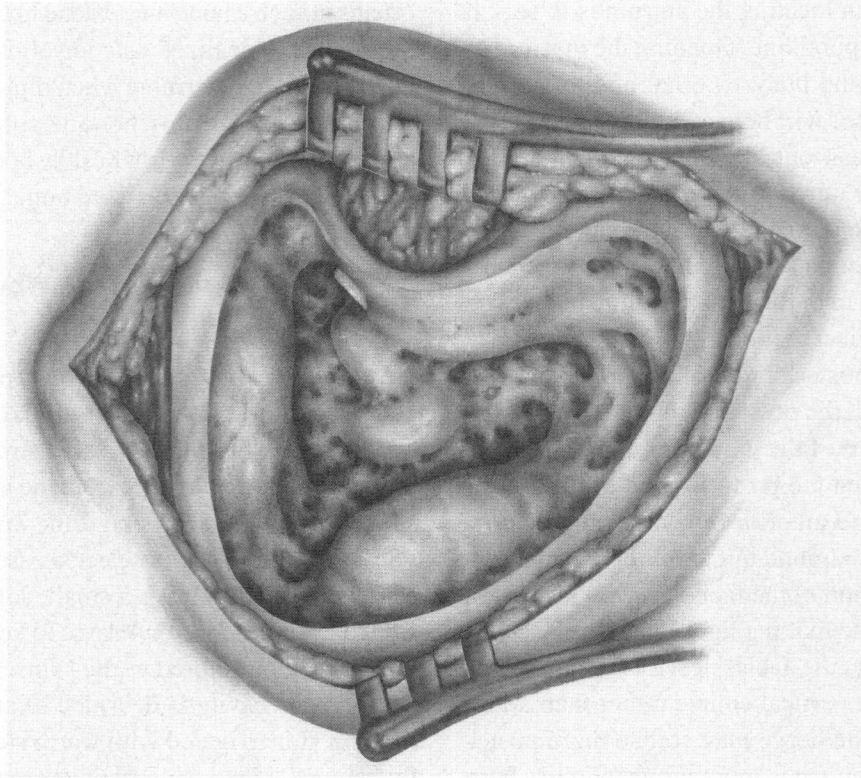

Figure 25–3 Completed mastoidectomy.

1. The operation was performed too soon, before localization of the infection had occurred.
2. There was incomplete removal of mastoid cells.
3. There is a coalescent process in the petrous pyramid (petrositis).
4. A simple mastoidectomy was erroneously performed for allergic otitis media or for cholesteatoma.

COMPLICATIONS DURING SIMPLE MASTOIDECTOMY

The most common serious surgical accident during the simple mastoid operation is injury to the facial nerve. This injury occurs most often in operations by poorly trained or occasional operators, but it can happen to the most skilled and experienced temporal bone surgeon when the nerve has an anomalous course.

Facial paralysis occurring during the operation or noticed immediately afterward means a probable injury or severance of the facial nerve. An exception is transitory facial paralysis caused by a local infiltrating anesthetic agent, in which case complete recovery occurs within a few hours. Prompt exploration with decompression and repair of the injured nerve is indicated within 24 hours of the operation, before granulations and degeneration of the severed ends of the nerve make it difficult to identify.

If the paralysis does not begin until several days after operation, an edema of the nerve is likely, with the probability of spontaneous recovery without surgical intervention. Thus, the time after operation that the paralysis is first noted is of decisive importance in determining the therapy. Therefore, as soon after the operation as the patient can respond, the patient should be asked to "show his/her teeth" so that the facial muscles can be observed for weakness or paralysis.

Injury to the sigmoid sinus, superior petrosal sinus, jugular bulb, or mastoid emissary vein results in an alarming profuse venous bleeding, which, however, is easily controlled by compressed absorbable gelatin sponge (Gelfoam) moistened with saline held against the vessel by cottonoid for at least 2 minutes by the clock. As soon as the field is dry, the cottonoid may be removed with the Gelfoam left in place, and the operative procedure may be resumed. Be sure that a spicule of bone is not left projecting into the sinus. Bone wax to control bleeding may act later as a foreign body and should be avoided.

Injury to the dura with the escape of spinal fluid is less common than injury to the aforementioned structures and is more dangerous. Carefully remove sufficient bone around the tear to expose a margin of intact dura all around, and be sure there is not a fragment of bone holding the tear open. Place a piece of temporal fascia over the tear; the muscle should be tucked under the margin of bone to hold it in place. Gelfoam is then used to reinforce the muscle.

As a rule, a tear of the middle fossa dura closes rapidly as fibroblastic proliferation of the adjacent arachnoid mesh walls off the area. Tears of the posterior fossa dura near the sinodural angle heal more slowly because of the arachnoid-free lateral prolongation of the basal cistern. Provided that the surgeon observes the strict technique described in Chapter 12, supplemented by prophylactic antibiotic therapy, accidental tears of the dura should heal without producing meningitis or brain abscess.

Dislocation or removal of the incus results in a particularly severe permanent conductive hearing loss. Later on, hearing may be improved by a tympanoplasty operation.

REFERENCES

1. Kemble J. Hero-Durst. London: Methuen; 1936.
2. Petit JL. Traité des maladies chirurgicales. Paris: 1774.
3. Balance CA. Essays on the surgery of the temporal bone. London: Macmillan; 1919.
4. Wilde W. Practical observations on aural surgery and the nature of the ear. Dublin: Maclachlan & Co.; 1853.
5. Schwartze HH, Eysell CG. Ueber die künstliche Eröffnung des Warzenfortsatzes. Arch Ohrenheilkunde 1873;7:157–87.
6. Whiting T. The modern mastoid operation. Philadelphia: P. Blakiston's Son & Co.; 1905.
7. Eagleton WP. Unlocking of petrous pyramid for localized bulbar meningitis secondary to suppuration of petrous apex. Arch Otol 1931;13:386.
8. Kopetsky WP, Almour R. Suppuration of petrous pyramid: pathology, symptomatology and surgical treatment. Ann Otol Rhinol Laryngol 1930;39:999. 1931;40:157.
9. Ramadier J. Les ostéites pétreuses profondes (pétrosites). Otorhinolaryngol Int 1933;17:816–21.
10. Lempert J. Complete apicectomy (mastoidotympanoapicectomy), new technique for complete apical exenteration of apical carotid portion of petrous pyramid. Arch Otol 1937;15:144.
11. Kangsanarak K, Fooanant S, Ruckphaopunt K, et al. Extracranial and intracranial complications of suppurative otitis media. Report of 102 cases. J Laryngol Otol 1993;107:999–1004.
12. Spiegel JH, Lustig LR, Lee KC, et al. Contemporary presentation and management of a spectrum of mastoid abscesses. Laryngoscope 1998;109:822–8.
13. Bezold F, Siebenmann F. Textbook of otology. Chicago: EH Cosgrove and Co.; 1908.
14. Shambaugh GE Jr. Involvement of the jaw joint in acute suppurative otitis media. Arch Otol 1941;33:975.
15. Holt R, Young WC. Acute coalescent mastoiditis. Otolaryngol Head Neck Surg 1981;89:317–21.
16. Antonelli PJ, Farside JA, Mancuso AA, et al. Computed tomography and the diagnosis of coalescent mastoiditis. Otolaryngol Head Neck Surg 1999;120:350–4.
17. Rosenwasser H, Adelman N. Otitic complications. Arch Otol 1957;65:225–34.
18. Courville CB. Intracranial complications of otitis media and mastoiditis in the antibiotic era. Laryngoscope 1955;65:31.
19. Shambaugh GE Jr. The surgical treatment of meningitis of otitic and nasal origin. JAMA 1937;108:696.
20. Kopeteky SJ. Otologic surgery. New York: Paul B Hoeber; 1929.

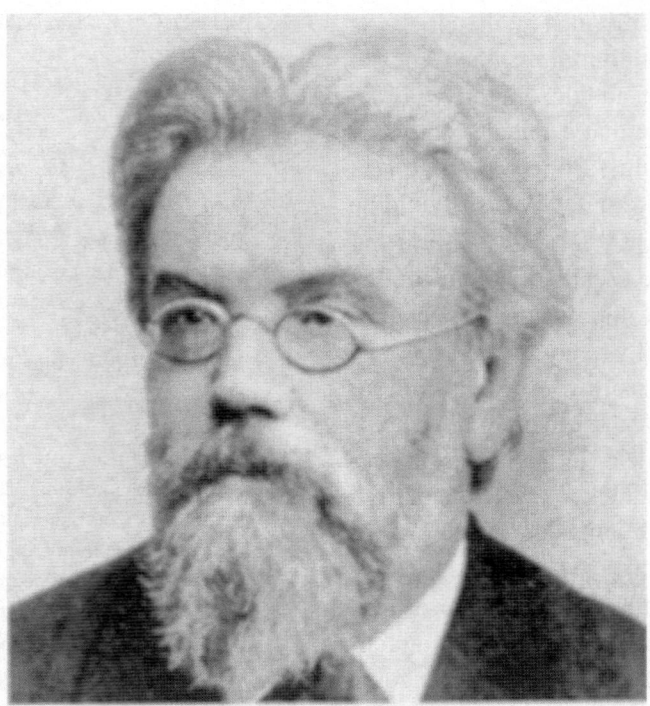

Emanuel Zaufal (1837–1910). With Küster and Stacke, developed the indications and technique of the radical mastoid operation.

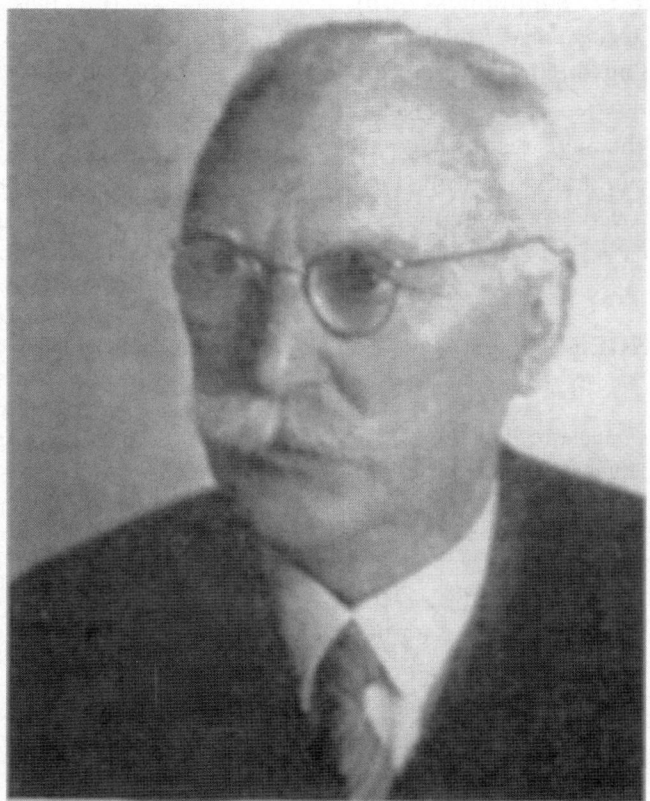

Fritz Thies (1873–1957). Rediscovered and used extensively the endaural approach for the radical mastoid operation.

26

Open Cavity Mastoid Operations

JOHN F. KVETON, MD

Open cavity procedures can be broadly defined as those requiring the removal of the posterior wall of the external auditory canal. These procedures are identified by many names—canal wall down mastoidectomy, modified radical mastoidectomy, radical mastoidectomy, and the Bondy mastoidectomy—depending on how the middle ear and the disease are managed. The purpose of open cavity procedures is to exteriorize the mastoid cavity for future monitoring of recurrent cholesteatoma, provide drainage for unresectable temporal bone infection, and, occasionally, provide exposure for difficult-to-access areas of the temporal bone.

HISTORICAL NOTES

In 1873, Von Tröltsch[1] was the first surgeon to suggest that Schwartze's[2] simple mastoidectomy technique needed to be modified to reduce persistent otorrhea after initial surgery. He had observed that remnants of cholesteatoma in the attic, antrum, or mastoid process would invariably result in chronic drainage. Von Bergmann[3] applied the term "radical" to any case in which the posterior and superior bony canal walls were removed to develop an open cavity. In 1890, Zaufal[4] described in detail the technique of the radical mastoidectomy to eradicate disease in the middle ear and mastoid. This operation converted the attic, antrum, mastoid process, tympanum, and external auditory canal into a common "radical cavity" that could be inspected and cleaned for the rest of the patient's life. Access to these areas involved in cholesteatoma would therefore prevent recurrence of bone-invading, life-threatening cholesteatoma. One year later, Stacke[5] described the addition of a plastic meatal skin flap, and the radical operation was referred to as the Zaufal or Stacke operation.

The effect of the radical operation on hearing was minimal in most cases in which it was employed. Initial severe necrotic otitis acquired in childhood had already destroyed much of the tympanic membrane, ossicles, and middle ear mucosa, allowing stratified squamous epithelium to extend from the external meatus into the tympanum, attic, antrum, and mastoid process as healing had occurred. Hearing was poor in these cases and so was not made worse by removal of the remnants of the tympanic membrane and ossicles or scraping of the middle ear mucosa in an attempt to close the eustachian tube.

Hearing, however, was at times quite good in patients who presented with cholesteatoma confined to the attic in which the pars tensa of the tympanic membrane was intact. Körner[6] recognized this situation in 1899 and suggested that the tympanic membrane and ossicles could be left in place during radical operations in certain cases of chronic otitis. In 1910, Bondy[7] described the indications and technique for a modification of the radical operation in cases involving a pars flaccida perforation with an intact pars tensa. In this technique, the superior osseous meatal wall and a portion of the posterior osseous meatal wall were removed without disturbing the intact tympanic membrane (except for the attic perforation), ossicles, or tympanic cavity. This technique thus exteriorized the attic and antral cholesteatoma into a permanently open "modified radical" cavity that could be cleaned through the external meatus without further destroying hearing.

Despite the clear indications that Bondy set forth, this modification of the radical mastoid operation was slow to become accepted into practice. In fact, as late as 1929, the Bondy modification was not even mentioned in a standard text of otologic surgery.[8] The overriding concern of otologic surgeons continued to focus on the prevention of intracranial complications of chronic otorrhea, regardless of the effect on hearing. The purpose of surgery was to produce a safe and hopefully dry ear, with little regard for a functioning ear.

Concern for preservation or improvement of hearing in addition to the prevention of complications from chronic otorrhea began to evolve after the introduction of Lempert's one-stage fenestration operation in 1938.[9] The early advocates of the Bondy modified operation soon were joined by otologic surgeons in the United States and abroad. The Bondy procedure rapidly evolved as the preferred method for the management of chronic otorrhea with cholesteatoma rather than the classic radical operation, as noted by Baron in 1944.[10] The introduction of tympanoplastic techniques by Zöllner[11] and Wullstein[12] in the early 1950s directed attention to reconstruction of the sound-conducting apparatus of the middle ear, further altering the philosophy regarding radical destructive procedures. Successful tympanoplasty required features such as an open, functioning eustachian tube, normal middle ear mucosa, and portions of normal tympanic membrane and ossicles, present in many ears undergoing radical procedures. In contrast, the radical operation attempted to close the eustachian tube and remove all remnants of the tympanic membrane, middle ear mucosa, and ossicles, eliminating any possibility of reconstruction. The introduction of tympanoplastic techniques, therefore, was responsible for the emergence of the modified radical mastoidectomy procedure.

Refinements in the modified radical mastoidectomy technique developed because of the drawbacks in the Bondy procedure. Recurrent or persistent aural discharge often occurred because of incomplete removal of infected mastoid air cells. Allowing the cholesteatoma matrix to remain in the attic frequently led to continued bone erosion and granulation tissue formation by the osteolytic enzymes produced by the matrix. Squamous debris accumulation, often resulting in recurrent infection, occurred because of incomplete tip cell removal and high facial ridge. These problems resulted in the Bondy procedure losing favor as the preferred open cavity technique.

The description of the intact canal wall tympanomastoidectomy for removal of cholesteatoma by

Jansen[13] in 1958 placed further emphasis on the status of the middle ear in the surgical management of cholesteatoma. Using a postauricular incision, the mastoid air cells are exenterated and the facial recess is opened to access the middle ear. This approach provides improved exposure of the anterior epitympanum and the whole mesotympanum while allowing tympanic membrane reconstruction. Theoretically, maintenance of an aerated middle ear with a normal external auditory canal and tympanic membrane should result in improved postoperative hearing. Hearing restoration has not been consistent using this technique, underscoring the importance of a functional eustachian tube and the dilemma associated with diagnosing a functional middle ear. The emphasis on eustachian tube function prompted by the intact canal wall mastoidectomy aided in the evolution of the modified radical mastoidectomy from the Bondy procedure to the complete mastoidectomy with tympanoplasty. Through a postauricular approach, all mastoid air cells are exenterated, the facial nerve is identified, and the facial ridge is taken down to the level of the fallopian canal. Tympanoplasty is performed and a large meatoplasty is created. The details of this technique will be described in greater detail in this chapter.

INDICATIONS FOR THE CLASSIC RADICAL MASTOID OPERATION

Antibiotic therapy, ventilating tube placement, and early identification of ear disease have reduced the incidence of secondary acquired cholesteatomas extensive enough to require treatment by a radical mastoidectomy. Even in the few remaining cases with a large tympanic membrane perforation associated with ossicular destruction and cholesteatoma, the eustachian tube should not be obliterated, the middle ear mucosa should not be stripped, and the ossicular and tympanic membrane remnants should not be removed, as in the case of the classic radical mastoidectomy, because these structures can be used in future tympanoplasty. The middle ear space should therefore be sealed except when access to the mesotympanum is needed. Thus, indications for the classic radical mastoidectomy are limited to the following unusual situations:

1. Unresectable cholesteatoma extending down the eustachian tube or into the petrous apex

2. Promontory cochlear fistula caused by cholesteatoma
3. Chronic perilabyrinthine osteitis or cholesteatoma that cannot be removed and must be cleaned or inspected periodically
4. Resection of temporal bone neoplasms with periodic monitoring

INDICATIONS FOR MODIFIED RADICAL MASTOIDECTOMY

Modified radical mastoidectomy is an effective method to manage cholesteatoma in a single-stage approach. Because there are potential disadvantages to the procedure, the author prefers to manage cholesteatoma with the staged intact canal wall technique whenever possible. If successful, this technique eliminates the need for periodic cleaning, avoids the caloric vertigo effect with water exposure, and provides the possibility of improved hearing. As described in Chapter 24, the intact canal wall technique is performed in two stages. The first operation is performed to remove all cholesteatoma and repair the tympanic membrane. Six months later, the second operation is performed to inspect the mastoid and middle ear for residual or recurrent cholesteatoma and to improve hearing by ossicular reconstruction. Since the canal wall up technique is technically more demanding, the modified radical mastoidectomy is recommended for the occasional otologic surgeon when confronted with a cholesteatoma extending into the attic, antrum, or mastoid process. The modified radical mastoidectomy should also be selected for patients who are unwilling to submit to the two-stage approach or are in circumstances for which the second procedure would be impractical.

The diagnosis of cholesteatoma in cases of chronic otorrhea deserves brief mention. Most cholesteatomas are associated with a pars flaccida or a marginal tympanic membrane perforation or retraction, in which stratified squamous epithelium extends into the attic. Rarely, a central perforation with mucoid discharge is associated with cholesteatoma in the middle ear and attic. An attic or pars flaccida perforation (actually an invagination) always means a cholesteatoma. Noninfected cholesteatoma debris may be present behind a dry attic perforation. Granulation tissue or a polyp protruding from an attic perforation indicates an infected cholesteatoma in the attic region.

The size of the attic defect bears little relation to the extent of the cholesteatoma in the attic, antrum, or mastoid. Preoperatively, the extent of the cholesteatoma can best be estimated by imaging studies. Noncontrast computed tomography (CT) of the temporal bone provides excellent definition of erosion of vital structures including the semicircular canals, cochlea, fallopian canal, dural plates, and sigmoid sinus. The diagnosis of attic cholesteatoma is made by noting erosion of the scutum with soft tissue accumulation in the attic on CT scan. Surgical planning is enhanced by identifying the degree of mastoid sclerosis and involvement of vital structures. Gadolinium-enhanced magnetic resonance imaging (MRI) may be used as an adjunct to CT to better define pathologic situations. In cases of extensive tegmen plate erosion on CT, MRI will demonstrate the presence of meningoencephalocele, dural inflammation, or intracranial infection. Sigmoid sinus thrombosis, suspected in cases of erosion of the posterior fossa dural plate and sigmoid sinus, may be confirmed by magnetic resonance angiography.

Conservative management of cholesteatoma can be attempted when the attic defect is large and the cholesteatoma sac shallow, allowing the accumulated desquamated debris to be removed by microdébridement and suction. Conservative management is contraindicated when

1. Radiographic evidence of an enlarged, smooth-walled antrum indicates a large cholesteatoma cavity.
2. Otorrhea persists after several cleanings.
3. A very small attic perforation makes cleaning painful, difficult, and unsatisfactory.
4. Cholesteatoma is observed behind the pars tensa.
5. There are symptoms or signs of erosion of vital structures such as the fallopian canal, semicircular canals, cochlea, or dura.
6. Hearing loss, either conductive or sensorineural, indicating progression of cholesteatoma.
7. The patient is uncooperative or is geographically unable to return for necessary management.

In actual clinical situations, the management of cholesteatoma is surgical. It is rare that an otologist will treat cholesteatoma medically. Modified radical mastoidectomy should be considered in cases of cholesteatoma in which there is a high risk of residual disease or risk of recurrence. The indications for modified radical mastoidectomy can be divided into absolute and relative indications. Absolute indications include unresectable disease, an unreconstructable posterior canal wall, failure of a first-stage canal wall up procedure because of poor eustachian tube function, and inadequate patient follow-up. The relative indications for an open cavity procedure include disease in an only hearing ear or in a dead ear, medical illness, severe otologic or central nervous system complications, and neoplasms. An additional relative indication is poor eustachian tube function.

CONTRAINDICATIONS FOR THE OPEN CAVITY MASTOID OPERATION

Removal of the posterior canal wall is contraindicated in cases of chronic otitis media without cholesteatoma. Unless the surgeon is certain of the diagnosis of cholesteatoma, the procedure should begin as a simple mastoidectomy, preserving the posterior canal wall until cholesteatoma is identified. Extensive débridement of mastoid or atticoantral infection can be accomplished with preservation of the posterior canal wall. Open cavity procedures are contraindicated in cases of acute otitis media with coalescent mastoiditis, persistent secretory otitis media, or chronic allergic otitis media. Tuberculous otitis media should be treated primarily with chemotherapy, with surgical intervention reserved for persistent drainage. Relative contraindications for open cavity procedures include wide exposure of the sigmoid sinus, dura, and the facial nerve caused by aggressive disease.

TECHNIQUE OF RADICAL MASTOIDECTOMY AND BONDY MODIFIED RADICAL MASTOIDECTOMY

The techniques of the radical mastoidectomy and the Bondy radical mastoidectomy are presented for historical interest and perspective. The objective of these procedures was to remove safely all bone-invading disease; create an accessible, exteriorized cavity for lifelong cleaning and care; and promote epithelialization of the cavity with healthy skin. Hearing improvement was of secondary importance.

The radical and Bondy operations began with exposure of the attic and antrum, followed by removal of the superior and posterior canal walls. By performing the "inside-out" mastoidectomy, the resultant cavity was smaller than if a complete mastoidectomy with tympanoplasty were performed. However, as a result of this approach, peripheral air cells were isolated from the eustachian tube. If the mucosa continued to produce mucus, it discharged into the mastoid cavity.

Atticotomy Bone Removal

The incision and atticotomy bone removal are the same for the classic radical mastoidectomy and for the Bondy modification. The endaural incision is made in two steps, with either a Lempert triangular knife or a Bard-Parker scalpel with a #15 blade, as follows:

1. Beginning at "12 o'clock" on the superior canal wall and about 1 cm from the outer edge of the canal, the first incision extends at about the same depth down the posterior canal wall in the incisura terminalis nearly to "6 o'clock," then at right angles outward about 2 or 3 mm to the edge of, but not into, the conchal cartilage.
2. Beginning again at "12 o'clock" on the superior canal wall where the first incision began, the second incision extends directly upward, still in the incisura terminalis, to a point about halfway between the meatus and the upper edge of the auricle. For greater exposure, this vertical incision can be extended as far upward as desired without encountering any important structure except for the temporalis muscle and branches of the superficial temporal artery and vein.

The two incisions, now continuous and at first through the skin only, are deepened to include periosteum, with the knife held at an angle so that it will not plunge into the bony canal. A broad periosteal elevator is inserted into the incision, directed posteriorly, and the periosteum over the entire mastoid process is elevated posteriorly and anteriorly only over the posterior root of the zygoma. Failure to elevate the periosteum sufficiently widely is a common cause of failure to obtain adequate exposure by this approach.

The self-retaining (Shambaugh) endaural retractor is inserted with retraction of periosteum, exposing the bone above and behind the osseous meatus, from the posterior root of the zygomatic process to 2 or 3 cm posterior to the suprameatal spine of Henle and from the temporal line above to the lower portion of the mastoid process below. Wide retraction of periosteum is essential to "mobilize the incision," as emphasized by Lempert.[9]

Atticotomy by means of a surgical cutting bur removes outer cortex just above and behind the meatus over a semi-lunar area. As the surgeon deepens the initial groove, he/she watches for the pink color shining through the bone and then for a little bleeding as the middle fossa dura is approached. An effort is made to avoid unnecessary dural exposure as the groove between the dura and the superior meatal wall is deepened. The notch of Rivinus is located by passing a narrow periosteal elevator inward along the superior osseous meatal wall. The epitympanum is encountered shortly before the groove reaches the depth of the notch of Rivinus, and if the preoperative diagnosis was correct, the white smooth wall of the cholesteatoma sac is identified. The middle fossa dura might resemble the wall of the cholesteatoma, requiring careful removal of bone anteriorly, inferiorly, and posteriorly before the surgeon is sure.

The sac is opened cautiously (in case dura is mistaken for the sac wall), the cholesteatoma contents are removed by suction and instrumentation, and the sac's furthest extensions anteriorly, superiorly, and posteriorly are explored with a blunt mastoid searcher. Bone cortex and overhang removal proceeds with a cutting bur, curet, or rongeur until the entire cholesteatoma sac lies exposed. In some cases, the cholesteatoma lining or matrix is smooth, with a thin layer of connective tissue between it and eburnated surrounding bone. More often, the cholesteatoma matrix is closely applied to bone with fingerlike extensions into small cells and haversian canals. All cholesteatoma extensions must be followed to their end with the aid of the operating microscope. All matrix is removed, with the following exceptions:

1. Matrix firmly adherent to exposed dura or sigmoid sinus may be left rather than risk injury to these structures.
2. Matrix over a fistula of a semicircular canal may be left to avoid postoperative serous labyrinthitis. Some surgeons prefer to dissect matrix from the fistula and immediately apply a thin fascia graft.
3. Matrix firmly attached to exposed facial nerve may be left.
4. Matrix extending into the mesotympanum and covering the stapes footplate may be left at the initial operation rather than opening the vestibule, with the risk of serous or suppurative labyrinthitis. At a second operation, after the ear is dry and healed, cholesteatoma matrix can be dissected from the oval window, and tympanoplasty can proceed, as described in Chapter 24.

Bone Removal beyond Cholesteatoma

Remembering that chronic otorrhea is the result of infected epidermal debris in the cholesteatoma sac, in most cases, evacuation of the sac, removal of matrix (epithelial lining), and curettage of softened osteitic bone adjacent to the matrix suffice to control the disease. The surgeon needs to exercise prudent judgment with regard to mastoid cells outside the cholesteatoma sac. These cells may be infected and osteitic (softened), with granulations requiring removal, but in many cases, mastoid cells are intact and need not be removed.

Taking Down the Bridge and the Facial Ridge

The remaining superior osseous meatal wall bridging the notch of Rivinus is removed in small bites with a narrow rongeur after first elevating the meatal skin from bone. With a small (000) curet, always working outward away from the fallopian canal and facial nerve, the anterior and posterior spines of the notch of Rivinus, composing the anterior and posterior buttresses of the bridge, are taken down. The tympanic segment of the facial canal is identified and kept in view while ossicles or remnants of ossicles are inspected. Wherever cholesteatoma envelops or extends onto the medial surface of the malleus head or incus, these ossicles must be removed. When cholesteatoma matrix lies against and lateral to these ossicles, the matrix may be left or carefully removed and the ossicles left undisturbed. When the long process of the incus is absent and matrix lies against the mobile stapes head, with excellent hearing producing nature's myringostapediopexy, this portion of the matrix is left undisturbed.

The step in the radical or Bondy operations most often accomplished poorly is taking down the posterior osseous meatal wall, which, deeper in, houses the posterior bend and vertical facial nerve and thus is called the facial ridge. The approximate position of the facial nerve is located by three usually dependable landmarks: the bony horizontal semicircular canal above, the tympanomastoid suture in the posterior meatal wall, and the digastric ridge in the mastoid tip. Because the tip cells rarely require removal in radical and Bondy mastoidectomies, the surgeon needs to dispense with the digastric ridge in the mastoid tip as a dependable landmark.

The bony facial ridge is taken down slowly and carefully with a drill or curet, working under the operating microscope, always parallel to and never across the direction of the facial nerve, until the bowl of the surgical cavity after removal of disease is flush with intact (or perforated) tympanic membrane. A pinkish color and bleeding are encountered when the facial nerve is approached. It is better not to expose the nerve unnecessarily because a Bell's palsy–type paresis occurs more often when this nerve is exposed than when not. Whereas this paresis, beginning 1 to 6 or 7 days postoperatively, generally recovers completely in a matter of weeks, residual weakness with synkinesis and spasm can ensue, just as occurs after recovery of some cases of Bell's palsy.

Preparation of the Meatal Plastic Skin Flap

The plastic pedicled skin flap that is turned back to cover the facial ridge and the floor of the completed operative cavity consists of the skin and periosteum of the entire superior osseous meatal wall and most of the posterior meatal wall. As the atticotomy proceeds and the bridge is being taken down, a narrow periosteal elevator separates the skin and periosteum from the superior and posterior meatal walls. With a curved meatal knife and iris scissors, an incision along the anterosuperior angle of the meatus frees the plastic flap anteriorly. The connective tissue band that enters the tympanosquamous suture needs to be cut, and posteriorly similar but less pronounced connective tissue in the tympanomastoid suture needs to be separated, beginning at the annulus and working outward. The outer edge of the meatal flap may need to be thinned to make it lie smoothly over the facial ridge.

Toilet of the Tympanum

In the classic radical mastoidectomy, the tympanic cavity is inspected minutely under the operating microscope. Healthy skin and remnants of tympanic membrane closing off the eustachian tube are not disturbed, but any polyps, granulations, or remaining mucosa are removed. Instrumentation in the oval window and round window niches should be avoided because of the possibility of opening the labyrinth. If the eustachian tube orifice is open and lined with mucosa, an attempt is made to close it in the classic radical operation after curetting its mucosa. In curetting the mouth of the eustachian tube, remember that the internal carotid artery is separated from it only by a thin plate of bone. Should curettage produce brisk bleeding, the bleeding is usually from the venous plexus that surrounds the carotid artery in its journey through the temporal bone and not from the artery.

In removing a mass of granulations from the stapes and the oval window, start at the pyramidal eminence and strip the granulations in a forward direction parallel to the stapedius tendon to keep from dislodging the stapes. Once the bone-invading infected cholesteatoma in the attic, antrum, and sometimes the mastoid process has been removed, any small granulations in the middle ear caused by the purulent drainage soon dry up with local conservative treatment.

Final Inspection of the Cavity

The completed open radical or Bondy cavity is irrigated with warm saline (Tis-U-Sol® or Ringer's) solution for hemostasis and for removal of any bone particles or other debris. Under the operating microscope, the cavity is inspected minutely for any remaining osteitis or cholesteatoma remnants. There must be no cortical overhang and no part of the cavity not perfectly accessible and exteriorized from the external meatus.

Atticotomy from within the Meatus

For a small cholesteatoma sac lateral to the incus and malleus head and with a large external meatus, it may be possible to perform an endomeatal atticotomy as follows:

1. A stapes type of meatal flap extended forward superiorly and outwardly is followed by removal of the meatal rim to exteriorize the small attic cholesteatoma sac.
2. The surgeon may then dissect the sac and remove it intact, or he/she may leave the matrix and exteriorize the sac as a small Bondy radical cavity.
3. Should the surgeon find that the cholesteatoma pocket is larger than anticipated, he/she should proceed with an endaural incision and atticotomy, as described previously.

Placement of the Meatal Flap and Packing of the Cavity

The plastic flap of meatal skin is turned back to cover the facial ridge, taking care not to cover areas of remaining matrix or even area that had been covered by matrix. A closed sleeve of surgical rayon or wide strips of surgical rayon are inserted to line the cavity, with cotton balls soaked in sulfisoxazole otic (or ophthalmic) solution placed firmly, but not tightly, to fill the cavity. At no point should cotton touch raw surface. One or two sutures partially close the endaural incision, but the final meatal opening must be packed wide open to three or four times the original size so that when healing is complete, the final meatus is twice the former size, and the healed exteriorized cavity can easily be inspected and kept clean.

Skin Grafting the Radical or Bondy Cavity

Siebenmann[14] was the first to recommend skin grafting by the method of Thiersch to promote rapid healing of the radical cavity. Experience in nearly 100 fenestration operations treated in this manner convinced Shambaugh[15] that primary split-thickness skin grafting of the operative cavity is not desirable. When such a graft took by first intention, the epidermal lining of the healed cavity was closely applied to the bone without an intervening layer of connective tissue. Not only was the surface of the stratified squamous epithelium rough and uneven, but it continued to desquamate excessively, was very subject to localized areas of breakdown and granulations with discharge, and demonstrated a distinct tendency to invasion of crevices and cells requiring a later revision. With a thoroughly performed radical or Bondy operation with removal of matrix, the cavity nearly always heals without troublesome granulations or suppuration provided that careful sterile technique is observed in the operations and postoperative dressings.

Should the surgeon wish to shorten the time of final healing, a skin graft may be applied to the cavity 2 or 3 weeks postoperatively after it has become lined by a thin layer of healthy granulations that then provide the desired subepithelial connective tissue layer.[16]

TECHNIQUE OF MODIFIED RADICAL MASTOIDECTOMY

Modified radical mastoidectomy, also known as complete mastoidectomy and tympanoplasty, is an evolutionary surgical development that attempts to incorporate the major goal of cholesteatoma surgery (ie, exteriorization of disease) with sealing of the middle ear space to avoid chronic drainage from exposed mucous membrane. A primary feature of the modified radical procedure is complete removal of the posterior canal wall, the major reason for failure of the Bondy procedure. The Bondy procedure was predicated on the philosophy of limited dissection of the canal wall and mastoid region, and this technique, although often sparing hearing in the short term, resulted in recurrent cholesteatoma or at least persistent aural discharge because of subsequent infection of the remaining mastoid air cells. The radical mastoidectomy, although effectively dealing with the shortcoming of the Bondy procedure by more extensive bone dissection, results in chronic aural drainage because of the impossibility of removal of all remaining mucosa in the exposed middle ear. The modification of the radical procedure (ie, adding the technique of tympanoplasty) potentially eliminates the expected intermittent discharge from the middle ear mucosa. Hearing, it should be noted, is a secondary consideration of the modified radical procedure.

Preoperative Assessment

The decision to perform a modified radical mastoidectomy rather than a staged intact canal wall approach depends on the extent and location of the disease, previous surgery, eustachian tube function and patient age, medical condition, and aftercare preference. Careful microscopic inspection and cleaning of the ear aid in the decision. Pus, mucus, and cholesteatomatous debris should be removed under microscopic suction. Polyps can be removed with gentle traction with the suction or microcup forceps. Significant retraction should be avoided since the polyp may be attached to the facial nerve, matrix of a labyrinthine fistula, or stapes superstructure or footplate. Extensive destruction of the posterior canal wall with obvious cholesteatoma invading the mastoid indicates the need for modified radical mastoidectomy. Active suppuration should be controlled prior to surgery whenever possible. Acetic acid (1.5% solution) irrigations followed by antibiotic otic drops should be instituted for several weeks prior to surgery. Acetic acid solution is made by mixing one part of white vinegar to two parts of boiling water. After cooling, the solution is instilled into the ear several times using an infant nasal-bulb syringe to mechanically débride the area. Antibiotic eardrops are instilled after the irrigations, which should be performed two to four times daily. The author prefers to use neomycin or aminoglycoside-based corticosteroid otic preparations rather than the newer flouroquinolone preparations in these cases. In cases of extensive mucosal infection and cellulitis, a 10- to 14-day course of oral fluoroquinolones with gram-positive coverage is indicated prior to surgery.

Surgical Procedure

After induction of general anesthesia, the ear is prepared by pouring povidone-iodine solution into the ear canal and scrubbing the auricle and postauricular area with povidone-iodine. One percent lidocaine with 1:100,000 epinephrine is injected into the postauricular region and the ear canal for hemostasis. Incisions are made in the ear canal for the vascular strip (Figure 26–1, A).[17] A postauricular incision is made about 1 cm behind the postauricular crease and a plane is developed between the subcutaneous tissue and the temporalis muscle and periosteum of the mastoid. Several large pieces of areolar tissue and temporalis fascia are harvested and set aside to dry. A horizontal incision is made superior to the temporal line through the temporalis muscle and a

vertical incision is carried down to the mastoid tip, perpendicular to and bisecting the horizontal incision (Figure 26–1, B). The mastoid bone is exposed using a Lempert elevator, and as the periosteum is raised into the ear canal, the vascular strip is elevated and reflected out of the ear canal anteriorly using a self-retaining retractor (Figure 26–1, C). In revision cases, elevation of the scarred musculoperiosteum must be done carefully to avoid injury to exposed dura or sigmoid sinus. Canal wall flaps are elevated and rotated anteriorly (Figure 26–1, D) prior to entering the middle ear. Disease in the mesotympanum is first removed, using the malleus handle and incus as landmarks. Cholesteatoma, polyps, and granulation tissue are removed from all areas except the posterosuperior quadrant; any atrophic tympanic membrane is removed and the middle ear is prepared for grafting. Once all available landmarks have been identified, the posterosuperior quadrant is inspected. If disease extends into the attic, dissection of disease ceases and Gelfoam with epinephrine is packed into the middle ear.

Bone Work

A simple mastoidectomy is now begun using a large cutting bur. The canal wall should be left up in all but the most contracted mastoid cavities. All mastoid air cells should be removed with exposure of the middle fossa and posterior fossa dural plates, the sigmoid sinus, digastric ridge, and bony canal wall (Figure 26–1, E). Cholesteatoma and granulations filling the central mastoid tract can be removed at this time. As the labyrinth is approached, the lateral capsule of the cholesteatoma should be opened and the cholesteatoma removed, leaving the medial matrix of the cholesteatoma on the bony labyrinth. Under higher-power magnification, the matrix can be inspected for the telltale blue line or palpated for the presence of a labyrinthine fistula. The vertical segment of the facial nerve should now be identified, followed by opening of the facial recess (Figure 26–1, F). This is best accomplished by using the digastric ridge and the lateral semicircular canal as landmarks. If the incus is involved with cholesteatoma, the incudostapedial joint is identified through the facial recess and cut and the incus removed. The posterior canal wall can now be safely taken down with a rongeur and the facial ridge lowered until a thin layer of bone remains over the vertical segment

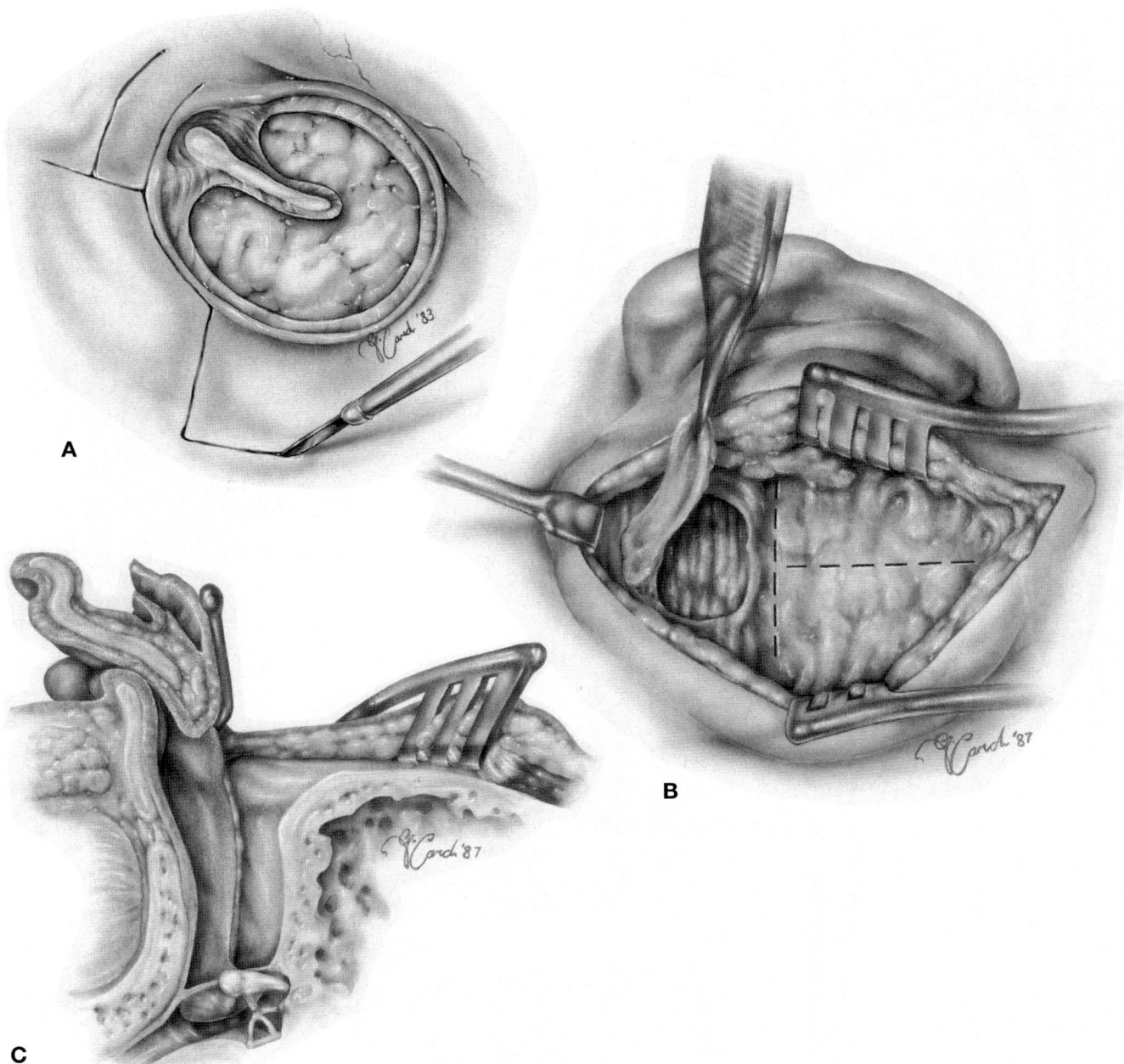

Figure 26–1   *A,* Standard tympanoplastic canal incisions outline the vascular strip as well as the superior and inferior canal wall flaps. *B,* Loose areolar fascia is harvested from temporal muscle, and a T-shaped incision is made in soft tissue over mastoid. *C,* Exposure of mastoid in cross-section showing vascular strip held forward under anterior blade of retractor.

Continued on next page.

of the facial nerve (Figure 26–1, G). The chorda tympani nerve must be sacrificed. Disease can now be removed from the oval window region and horizontal segment of the facial nerve. The malleus, or any remnant of the malleus, is removed by cutting the tensor tympani tendon at the cochleariform process, which provides access to the anterior epitympanum. The anterior epitympa-

num should be drilled down to become continuous with the anterior canal wall. The inferior canal wall must be drilled away until the inferior external canal wall and mastoid tip are confluent, with no bony overhang to obscure the mastoid tip. This dissection more widely exposes the middle ear, which can now be reinspected for residual disease. The sinus tympani is the most difficult region

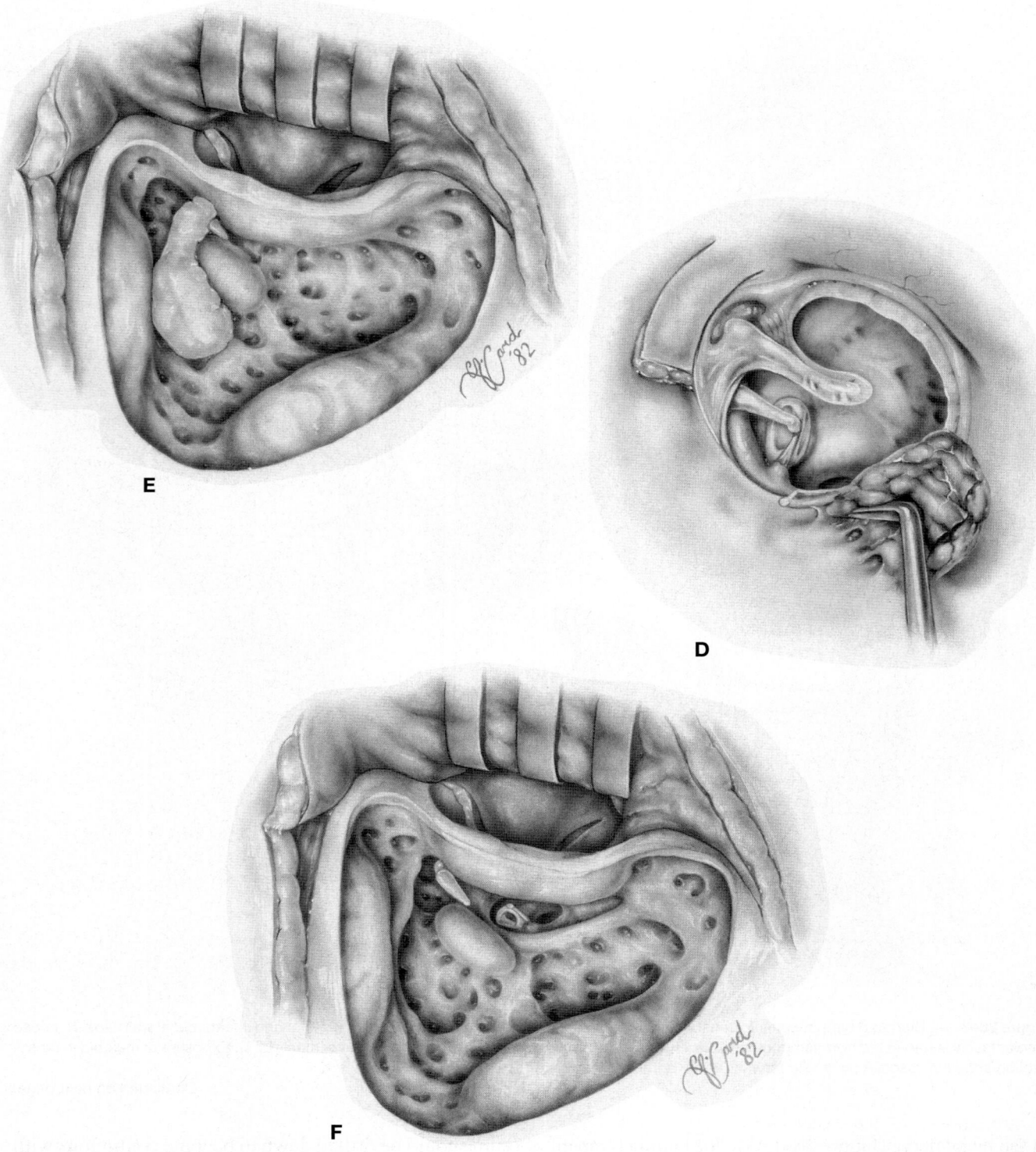

Figure 26–1   Continued. *D*, The inferior flap is elevated to the fibrous annulus with a House #2 knife. *E*, With the posterior external auditory canal (EAC) wall preserved, a complete, simple mastoidectomy demonstrates the anatomy and the pathology. *F*, Through the facial recess, disease can be well managed in an intact canal wall (ICW) context. The malleus head and incus are shown for orientation only. They are customarily removed. Incudostapedial disarticulation is demonstrated.

Continued on next page.

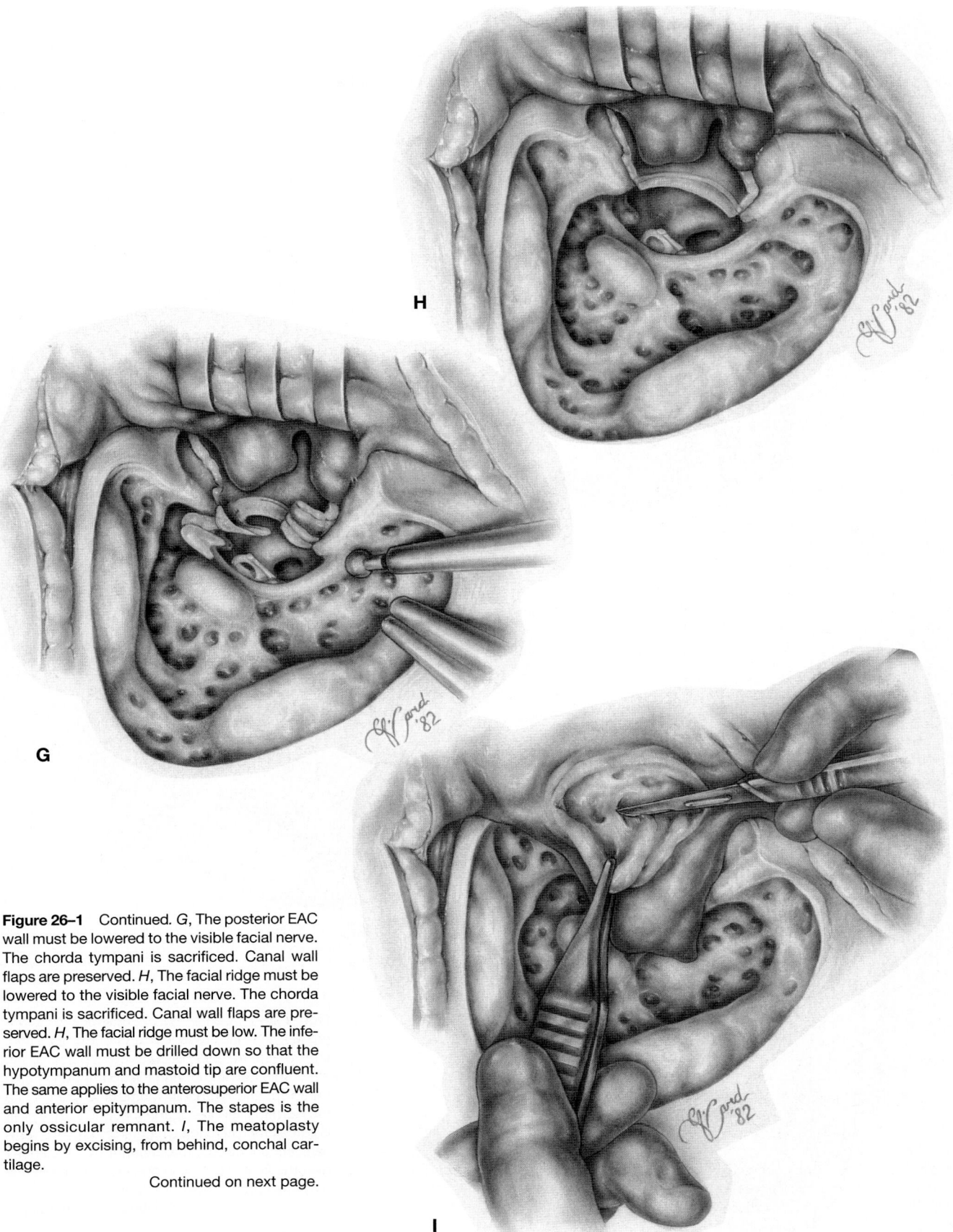

Figure 26–1 Continued. *G*, The posterior EAC wall must be lowered to the visible facial nerve. The chorda tympani is sacrificed. Canal wall flaps are preserved. *H*, The facial ridge must be lowered to the visible facial nerve. The chorda tympani is sacrificed. Canal wall flaps are preserved. *H*, The facial ridge must be low. The inferior EAC wall must be drilled down so that the hypotympanum and mastoid tip are confluent. The same applies to the anterosuperior EAC wall and anterior epitympanum. The stapes is the only ossicular remnant. *I*, The meatoplasty begins by excising, from behind, conchal cartilage.

Continued on next page.

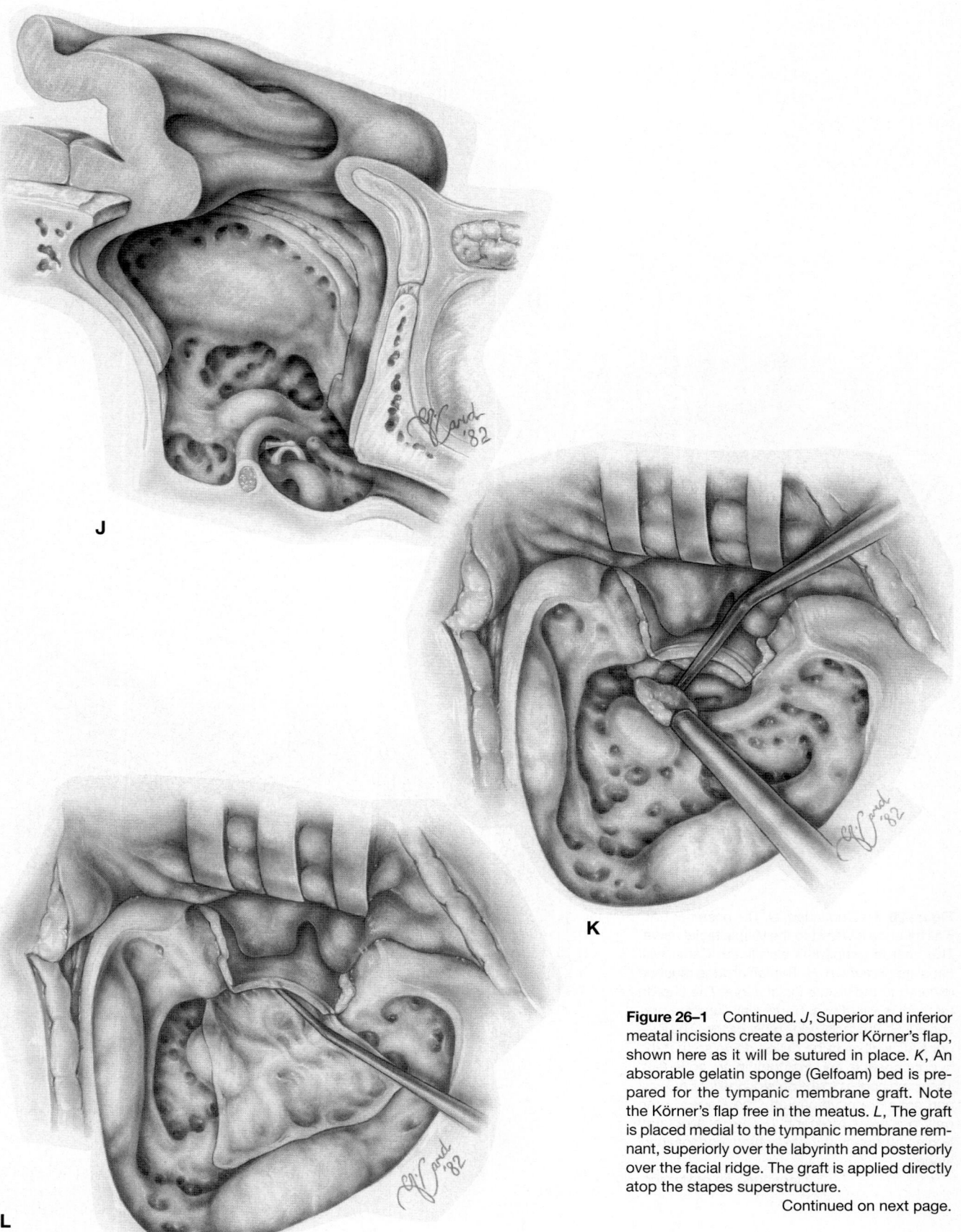

Figure 26–1 Continued. *J,* Superior and inferior meatal incisions create a posterior Körner's flap, shown here as it will be sutured in place. *K,* An absorbable gelatin sponge (Gelfoam) bed is prepared for the tympanic membrane graft. Note the Körner's flap free in the meatus. *L,* The graft is placed medial to the tympanic membrane remnant, superiorly over the labyrinth and posteriorly over the facial ridge. The graft is applied directly atop the stapes superstructure.

Continued on next page.

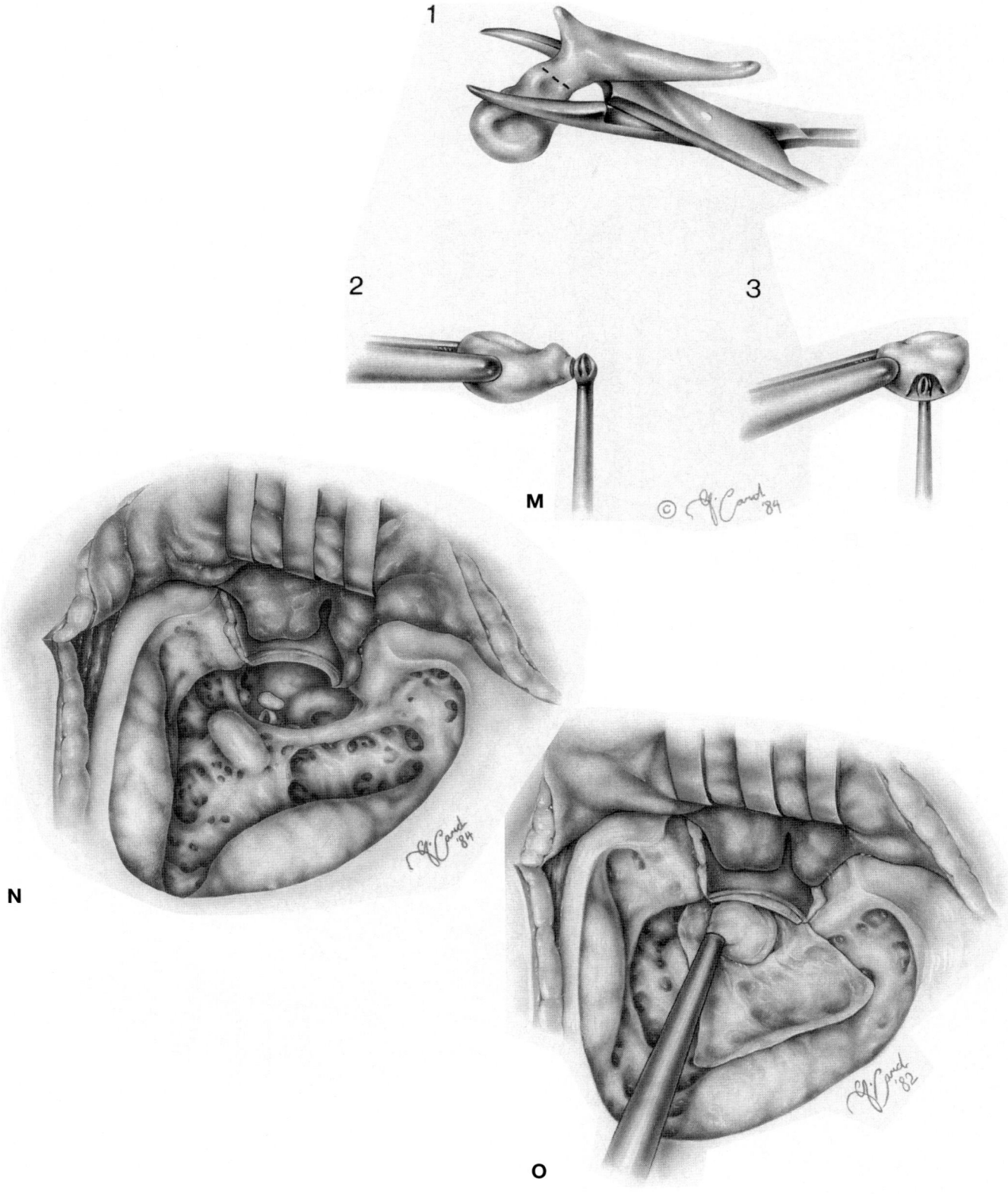

Figure 26–1 Continued. *M*, When the facial ridge is high, a sculpted homograft malleus head can be constructed to augment the height of the stapes superstructure. *N*, The sculpted homograft fits atop the stapedial capitulum, ready for grafting. *O*, Ointment "packing" fills the cavity.
Continued on next page.

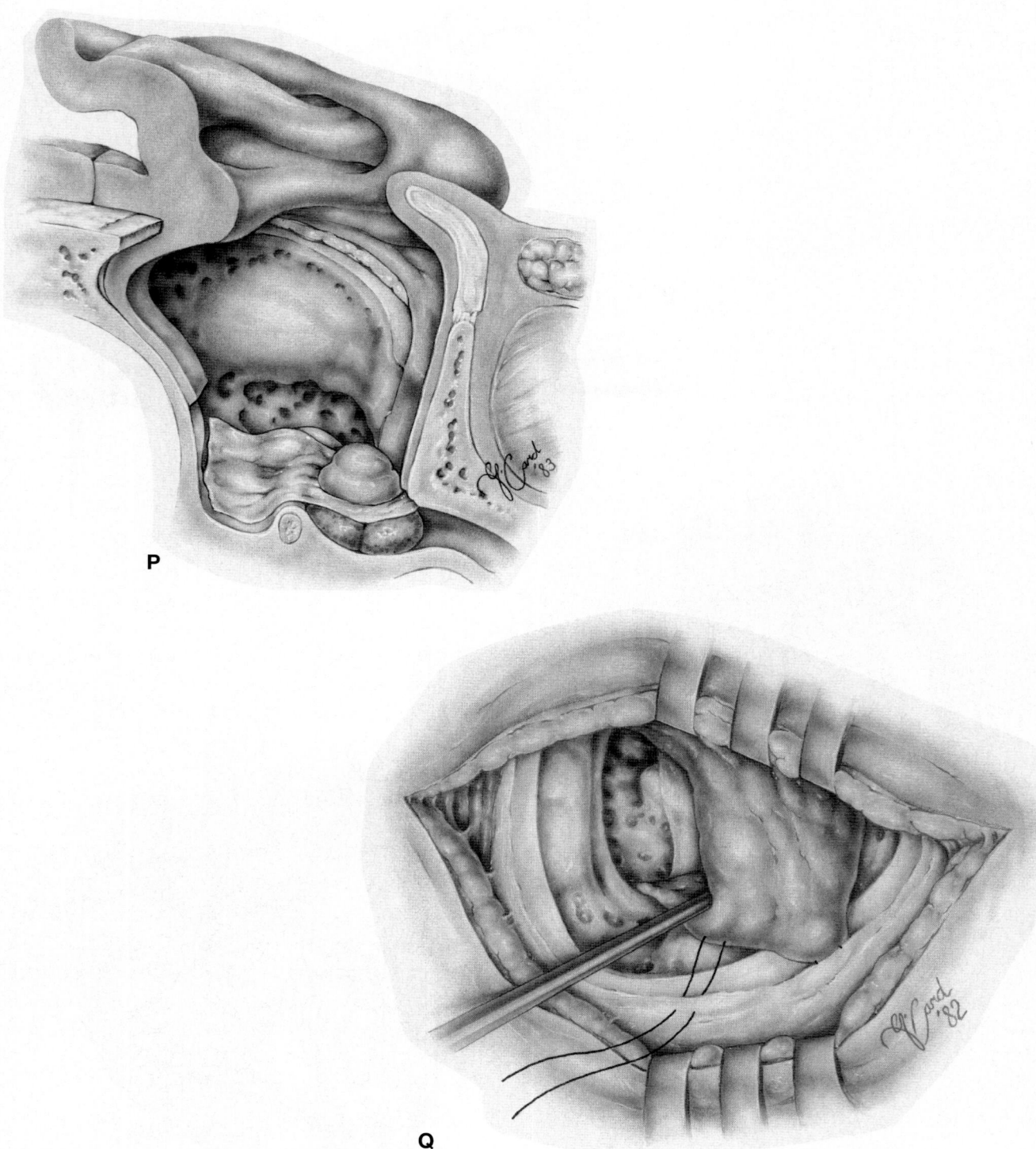

Figure 26–1 Continued. *P*, In cross-section, the low facial ridge, graft bed, with graft and initial ointment, is demonstrated. The posterior meatal flap is illustrated in the desired position. *Q*, The posterior flap is sewn to the posterior soft tissue margins of the incision. Tension on these sutures can then be tied.

to investigate. If disease extends into this region, and if the stapes is absent, the pyramidal eminence can be removed with a small diamond bur. Right angle hooks, whirlybird dissectors, micromirrors, and surgical telescopes can aid in cholesteatoma removal from this region. Tympanoplasty should not be performed if there is a question of residual cholesteatoma in the sinus tympani or hypotympanum.

At this point, the cavity should be smooth walled and free of active disease (Figure 26–1, H). Copious irrigation is used to lower the bacterial count and aid in hemostasis. The cavity should approach an ovoid or rectangular shape, with the facial ridge low. The stapes, if present, should be the only remaining ossicle. A portion of the anterior tympanic membrane may remain after removal of disease. The mastoid bowl has been saucerized and makes a gentle transition into the depths of the mastoid bone without ledges. This attention to detail helps ensure soft tissue obliteration of much of the cavity space.

Rarely, the mastoid is so contracted that the posterior canal wall is taken down as the antrum is exposed. This approach is potentially more dangerous to the facial nerve and ossicular chain and should be avoided whenever possible. Regardless of when the canal wall is removed, the remainder of the technique remains the same.

Meatoplasty

One percent lidocaine with 1:100,000 epinephrine is infiltrated into the conchal bowl. The entire posterior aspect of the conchal bowl is exposed using sharp dissection with an iris scissors through the fibrous periosteum and soft tissue. With a finger in the conchal bowl, a semilunar incision is made into the cartilage posteriorly until the knife tip is felt through the anterior skin. This crescent-shaped cartilage measures about 1.5 × 2 cm (Figure 26–1, I). A Körner flap is now developed by making incisions through the external auditory canal skin. An inferior incision is begun in the inferior canal at 6 o'clock, carried into the conchal bowl, and curved around the inferior margin of the bowl. A superior incision is made at 12 o'clock and carried between the tragus and the anterior helix. These incisions create a long (vascular strip) flap that is based in the posterosuperior aspect of the conchal bowl and will constitute the back wall of the mastoid cavity (Figure 26–1, J).

Grafting

The auricle and flap are retracted anteriorly to expose the mastoid and middle ear. Epinephrine-soaked absorbable gelatin sponge is removed and the middle ear and eustachian tube are packed with saline-moistened absorbable gelatin sponge to the level of the anterior annulus (Figure 26–1, K). The fascia graft is placed medial to the anterior annulus and drum remnant, extending over the stapes to the facial ridge into the mastoid bowl (Figure 26–1, L). As much of the mastoid bone as possible should be covered with fascia grafts to reduce granulations and speed epithelialization. In particular, perilabyrinthine, retrofacial, zygomatic, and peritubal cell tracts should be covered.

Ossicular reconstruction is limited in these cases. If the stapes is present, the fascia graft is placed directly onto the capitulum. If the stapes is lower than the facial ridge, the height can be augmented by using a malleus head goblet prosthesis atop the capitulum (Figure 26–1, M and N). With an absent stapes, ossicular reconstruction with autologous tissue is preferred over alloplastic prostheses. Once the fascia graft is in place, the surface is covered with polymixin B and bacitracin ophthalmic ointment (Figure 26–1, O and P).

The Körner flap must now be secured to the musculoperiosteum at the edge of the mastoid cavity. A 3.0 polyglactin 910 (Vicryl®) suture is placed subdermally at both edges of the base of the Körner flap and affixed posteriorly to the soft tissue. The tension of these sutures is adjusted until the meatus has the desired shape (Figure 26–1, Q). Overtightening of the sutures, especially the superior suture, will result in a protruding auricle. The postauricular incision is closed with a subcuticular absorbable suture. The mastoid bowl is filled with ointment or packed with gauze, and a mastoid dressing is applied.

Postoperative Care

The mastoid dressing is removed on the first postoperative day. A large piece of cotton is kept in the meatus, and a postauricular dressing is placed. Copious drainage occurs through the meatus for about 1 week, requiring frequent cotton changes. The postauricular dressing is removed on the second postoperative day, and antibiotic ointment is applied to the incision for 1 week. The patient is instructed to keep the ear dry and avoid nose blowing. Pain medication is prescribed, but oral antibiotics are not used routinely. The patient returns in 2 to 3 weeks. At the first postoperative visit, any area that has not been grafted is covered by a layer of granulation tissue. Exuberant granulation tissue should be débrided and treated with silver nitrate. Silver nitrate should not be used near an exposed facial nerve to avoid facial palsy. The granulation tissue should then be painted with 2% gentian violet and the patient instructed to use antibiotic otic drops two or three times per day until the next (at 2 to 3 weeks) visit. Drainage decreases with ensuing visits as re-epithelialization occurs. As epithelialization progresses, acetic acid irrigations can replace the use of antibiotic otic drops. Once the cavity is healed, the patient should return for a yearly visit and is given full water sport privileges.

COMPLICATIONS OF OPEN CAVITY PROCEDURES

The complications associated with open cavity mastoid operations are identical to those possible in any procedure in which the mastoid bone is removed and structures in the middle ear are manipulated. These include deafness or further hearing loss, facial paralysis, vestibular symptoms, cerebrospinal fluid leak, infection, and recurrent cholesteatoma or drainage. The incidence of certain complications may be higher, though, because of the nature of disease within the mastoid bone that requires a more extensive procedure such as an open cavity procedure.

Facial nerve paralysis is the most common major complication associated with open cavity procedures. Although facial nerve injury is at times unavoidable because of the extent of disease, most cases of postoperative facial paralysis are a result of unrecognized facial nerve trauma at the hands of an unskilled otologic surgeon. Normal surgical landmarks are often distorted in the diseased mastoid, and positive identification of vital structures is mandatory to perform a successful open cavity procedure. Surgical discipline must be maintained during the procedure to identify vital structures in a systematic fashion as the surgery progresses.

In particular, it is critical to identify the facial nerve throughout its course in the mastoid as soon as possible, which is best accomplished after the lateral semicircular canal and any ossicles within the posterior epitympanum have been identified. Especially in revision cases, the most effective way to locate the vertical segment of the facial nerve is to follow the digastric ridge to the stylomastoid foramen. The bony dissection may then proceed in a proximal direction to uncover the vertical segment as it approaches the second genu. This method also underscores the importance of preserving the posterior canal wall until late in the dissection since early identification of the nerve reduces the risk of injury as the canal wall is taken down. Early identification of the nerve also ensures that the facial ridge will be brought down appropriately (ie, until the nerve sheath can be identified through a thin layer of bone remaining on the fallopian canal). In cases of disease obliterating the stylomastoid foramen, the fallopian canal can be identified by following the chorda tympani nerve distally to the facial nerve trunk. This junction is approximately 5 mm from the stylomastoid foramen. Less specifically, the distal portion of the second genu of the facial nerve is found just inferior to the level of the lateral semicircular canal.

The management of postoperative facial paralysis bears brief mention. Facial nerve injury must be considered when any noticeable loss of facial nerve function has been identified. Eye closure is often inappropriately relied on as an indicator of total facial nerve paralysis. The tonus of the orbicularis oculi muscle appears to persist longer than that of the remaining facial musculature, and it is not unusual for eye closure to persist for several days after facial nerve injury has occurred. (Witness the fact that eye closure persists in the immediate postoperative period for patients with known facial nerve transection after removal of an acoustic tumor.) Unless facial nerve injury was noted at the time of the surgery, the axiom "Never let the sun set on a facial paralysis" should be followed. The patient should be returned to the operating room as soon as possible for exploration and decompression of the facial nerve. Especially in difficult cases, it is the author's policy to maintain sterility in the operating suite until the patient displays normal facial movement on emergence from general anesthesia.

The second most common complication of open cavity procedures is wound infection. This infection usually results in perichondritis of the auricle, manifested by a painful, swollen auricle with copious discharge. *Pseudomonas aeruginosa* is the causative organism, and treatment comprises high-dose fluoroquinolones and antibiotic-corticosteroid drops.

A "chocolate" or mucous retention cyst can occur in a healed mastoid cavity as a result of a collection of serum within a mucous membrane–lined pocket. Simple aspiration of the mucoid, brownish serum will reduce the size of the cyst, but recurrence is usually the case. Definitive management requires exposure of the cyst and complete removal of the mucoperiosteal pocket.

Cholesteatoma recurrence in open cavity procedures occurs in 4 to 28% of cases[18] and is usually caused by inaccessible disease or a remnant of matrix that was amputated at the time of surgery. Through routine follow-up, these "pearls" of recurrent cholesteatoma can be readily identified and removed in the office. Extensive recurrent disease, with its attendant complications, is more commonly found behind an intact canal wall rather than in an open cavity.

Recurrent aural drainage from a previously healed and dry cavity is usually the result of poor aural toilet. Breakdown of the epithelial lining and formation of granulation tissue occurs when epidermal debris is allowed to accumulate and becomes infected. Careful microscopic débridement of granulation tissue and application of gentian violet followed by antibiotic-corticosteroid otic drops will lead to re-epithelialization and a dry ear. It is critical that the patient understand the need for periodic, usually annual, examination to prevent such occurrences.

SUMMARY

Open cavity mastoid procedures are indicated when canal wall up procedures are inadequate to control disease. The vast majority of these procedures will result in a modified radical mastoidectomy. The creation of a dry mastoid cavity primarily depends on surgical technique. Identification of the facial nerve is critical in this procedure. Lowering of the facial ridge to the level of the facial nerve and development of a large external auditory meatus are mandatory for successful outcome. Grafting of the middle ear eliminates mucous discharge and may improve hearing. Long-term postoperative care is minimal, with patients returning to normal activity, including water exposure.

REFERENCES

1. Von Troltsch AF. Lehrbuch der Ohrenheilkunde mit Einschluss der Anatomicdes Ohres. Leipzig: Fogel; 1873.
2. Schwartz HH, Eysell CG. Ueber die Künstliche eroffnung des warzenfortsatzes. Arch Ohrenh 1873;7:157.
3. Von Bergmann E. Die chirurgische Behandlung von Hirnkrankheiten. Berlin: 1889.
4. Zaufal E. Technik der Trepanationdes Proc. Mastoid. Nach Kuster'schen Grundsatzen. Arch Ohrenh 1890;30:291.
5. Stacke L. Stacke's Operationsmethods. Arch Ohrenh 1893;35:145.
6. Körner O. Die eitrigen Erkrankungen des Schlafenbeins. Wiesbaden: Bergmann; 1899.
7. Bondy G. Totalaufmeisselung mit Erhaltung von Trommelfell und Gehorknochelchen. Monatsschr Ohrenheilk 1910;44:15.
8. Kopetsky SJ. Otologic surgery. 2nd ed. New York: Paul B. Hoeber; 1929.
9. Lempert J. Improvement of hearing in cases of otosclerosis: new one stage surgical technic. Arch Otol 1938;28:42.
10. Baron S. Modified radical mastoidectomy. Arch Otol 1949;49:280.
11. Zollner F. Die Radikal-Operatiion mit besonderem Bezug auf die Horfunktion. Ztschr Laryngol Rhinol Otol 1951;30:104.
12. Wullstein H. Funktionelle Operationen im Mitelohr mit Hilfe des freien Spaltlappen-Transplantates. Arch Ohren-Nasen-u Kehlkopfh 1952;161:422.
13. Jansen C. Ulur Radikaloperation Und Tympanoplastik. Sitz Ber Fontbild. Arztekamm. Ob. V. 18, February 1958.
14. Siebenmann F. Die Radical-operation des Cholesteatoma mittelst Anlegung breiter permanenter Oeffnungen gleihchzeitig gegen den Gehorgang und gegen die retroauriculare Region. Berl Klin Wochenschr 1893;30:12.
15. Shambaugh GE Jr, Derlacki EL. Primary skin grafting of the fenestra and fenestration cavity. Arch Otol 1956;64:46.
16. Guilford FR, Wright WK. Secondary skin grafting in fenestration and mastoid cavities. Laryngoscope 1954;64:626.
17. Jackson CG, Glasscock ME, Schwaber MK, et al. Open mastoid procedures: contemporary indications and surgical technique. Laryngoscope 1985;95:1037.
18. Hirsch BE, Kamerer DB, Doshi S. Single-stage management of cholesteatoma. Otolaryngol Head Neck Surg 1992;106:351.

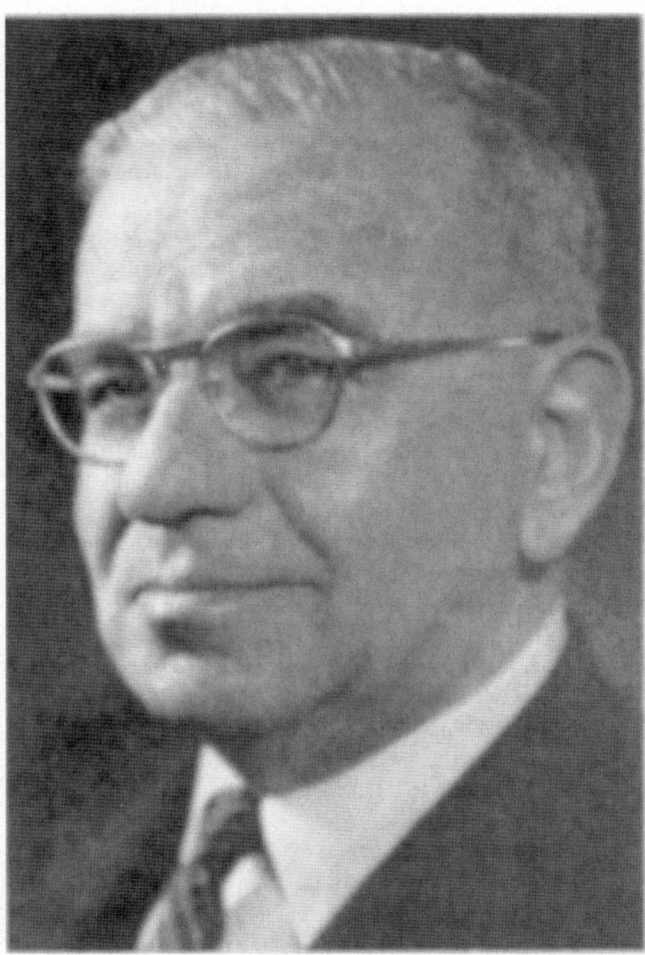

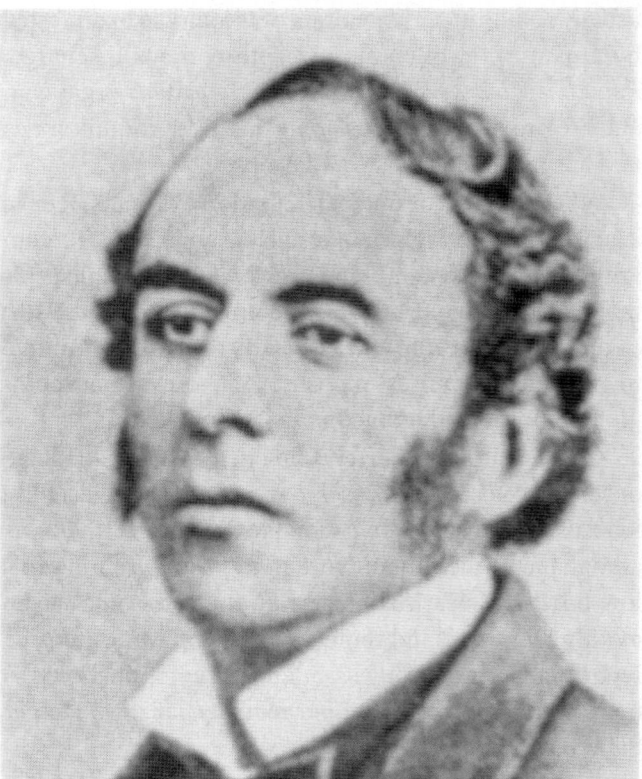

Joseph Toynbee (1815–1866). Demonstrated by anatomic dissection the common occurrence of stapes ankylosis as a cause of deafness.

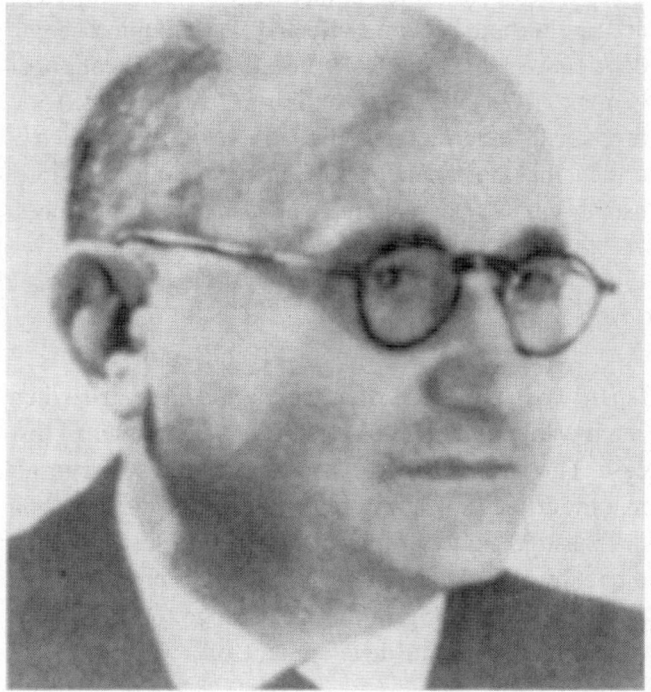

Samuel Rosen (born 1897). Had the vision to seize on a chance mobilization and thus revived the direct operation on the stapes. "The surgeon must ... go along ... step by step as the conditions unfold; trying ... to preserve or reconstitute the transformer action of the middle ear, with preference always for using the patient's own tissues..." (1960).

Maurice Sourdille (1885–1961). His ingenious tympanolabyrinthopexy permanently restored useful hearing for the first time in patients with otosclerosis and formed the basis for the one-stage fenestration operation of Lempert.

27

Stapedectomy for Otosclerosis

JOHN J. SHEA JR, MD
PAUL F. SHEA, MD
MICHAEL J. MCKENNA, MD

HISTORY

The first stapedectomy era began with great flourish in the last quarter of the nineteenth century, initiated by Johannes Kessel in Gras and then Jena, and stapes surgery was quickly taken up by other otologic surgeons in Europe. First mobilization of the stapes and then stapedectomy operations were done with the crude instruments available at the time. The earliest surgical attempts to improve hearing in stapes fixation were directed at the stapes itself. In 1878, Kessel incised the posterior part of the tympanic membrane, separated the incus from the stapes, and then tried to mobilize the stapes by applying pressure to its head in various directions.[1] When this was not successful, he removed the stapes.

In 1888, Boucheron reported 60 mobilizations, with the best results in cases of early ankylosis without involvement of the sound-perceiving apparatus.[2] Then in 1890, Miot, in a series of five articles, reported 200 stapes mobilizations with instruments, techniques, and results amazingly similar to those of Rosen's operation of 62 years later.[3] Miot observed the improvement in "cranial perception" (bone conduction) following successful mobilization owing, it is now known, to elimination of the bone conduction loss caused by stapes fixation (Carhart's notch). There were apparently no deaths or labyrinthine complications in Miot's series.

After completing his training at the Massachusetts Eye and Ear Infirmary in Boston, Frederick L. Jack went to observe the new operations for otosclerosis being performed in Europe, especially Vienna. Upon his return to the United States, he did mobilizations and stapedectomies, with mostly poor results. One patient operated on and reported by Jack became the link between the first successful stapedectomy and its revival in the middle of the twentieth century.

In 1892, Blake of Boston removed a stapes to improve hearing,[4] and in 1893, Jack reported a series of cases of extraction of the stapes.[5] Jack described one of these cases as having maintained quite good hearing 10 years later, noting that "The drums have healed. The portion covering the seat of the operation is somewhat sunken forming a moveable membrane on the oval window… Removal of the stapes does not destroy the hearing but sometimes improves it. The contrary statements in most textbooks… were incorrect."[5]

In 1899, Faraci published his results in 30 cases of stapes mobilization — the last recorded stapes operation to improve hearing for more than half a century.[6] In 1900 at the International Congress of Otolaryngology, Siebenmann was joined by Politzer and other leaders in otology in condemning Kessel and all others for the surgical attempts to improve hearing in otosclerosis as both useless and dangerous.[7] The reasons for the concerted and effective opposition are not clear, and one can only surmise that there were some unreported serious complications, and deaths, following stapedectomy. Kessel resigned from his position in Jena in disgrace and confined himself to research for the rest of his life.

The fenestration of the lateral semicircular canal operation began by accident, as often happens in medicine, when Holmgren, in Stockholm in the early 1920s, inadvertently made an opening in the lateral semicircular canal while removing infection from the mastoid and covered the opening with mucoperiosteum. The patient was able to hear better for a short while. After this success, Holmgren made the first deliberate effort at fenestration of the superior semicircular canal and covered the opening in the superior semicircular canal with mucoperiosteum through a postauricular incision, which buried the fenestra to the exterior. This "closed" fenestration operation resulted in temporary hearing gain, all of which was lost when the fenestra in the lateral semicircular canal closed. But it was a beginning, the first systematic step in the right direction.

To Maurice Sourdille, of Nantes, France, must go the credit for development of the modern exteriorized fenestra operation for otosclerosis. He visited Stockholm in 1924, observed one closed fenestra operation of Holmgren, and recognized the shortcoming of the Holmgren closed fenestra operation. He then developed his three-stage exteriorized fenestra operation. Many otologists came to study with Sourdille, including Juan Tato, who returned to Buenos Aires and did the first fenestration in the new world in 1934 (J Tato, personal communication, 1958). In 1937, Sourdille was invited to address the Otolaryngology Section of the New York Academy of Medicine, in the publication of which his address was published that same year.[8] Unfortunately for him, Julius Lempert was in the audience and recognized that he could improve on this three-stage postauricular operation with his new one-stage endaural approach to the middle ear and mastoid. He then quickly reported his results with his new one-stage endaural fenestration operation.[9] Others, including Shambaugh, came to study with Lempert and quickly reported their results.[10]

The second stapedectomy era began when Rosen (Figure 27–1) accidentally mobilized the stapes while trying to verify that the stapes was fixed prior to performing a fenestration.[11] When Rosen recognized what he had done — made the patient hear better by accidentally mobilizing the stapes — he mobilized the stapes in other patients and soon published his results in the *New York State Journal of Medicine*,[12] without giving credit to Miot[3] and others whose reports on mobilization of the stapes he must have read.

I (the first author) went to observe Rosen do mobilization of the stapes in the fall of 1953 and was much impressed. He arranged for me to go to Vienna to study at the First Ear Clinic of the University of Vienna and practice mobilization of the stapes on the abundant cadaver material available there. While there, I read the

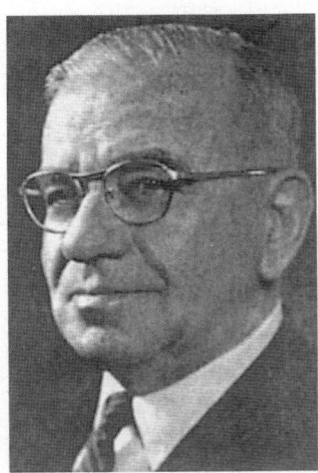

Figure 27–1 Samuel Rosen, MD. He had the vision to seize on a chance mobilization and thus revived the direct operation on the stapes.

1892 report of Frederick L. Jack, of Boston, whom I had met while I was a resident at the Massachusetts Eye and Ear Infirmary in 1949, on "Remarkable Improvement in Hearing by Removal of the Stapes."[13] What aroused my interest was a second report in 1902, "Supplemental Report on a Case of Double Stapedectomy Operated Upon Ten Years Ago."[14] In this patient, after removal of the stapes from both ears 3 weeks apart, the drums became adherent to the margins of the oval window in each ear, and the patient could hear well from both ears 10 years later. I realized at once what was needed, which — no one had realized up to then — was to reconstruct the sound-conducting mechanism of the middle ear after the stapes was removed, which no one had done. I (Figure 27–2) did the first such stapedectomy on May 1, 1956, covered the oval window with a thin slice of subcutaneous tissue, and reconstructed the sound-conducting mechanism of the middle ear with a Teflon (DuPont, Wilmington, Delaware) replica of the stapes (Figure 27–3). I reported this first stapedectomy at the First Symposium on Mobilization of Stapes in 1956.[15] Stapedectomy was gradually taken up by all otologists all over the world and has continued, with remarkably few changes, to the present.

By 1956, several developments had set the stage for the revival of operations on the fixed stapes in otosclerosis. The success of the fenestration operation had overcome the prejudice against operations for otosclerosis. Antibacterial drugs afforded added protection against infection. Electric illumination and magnification by

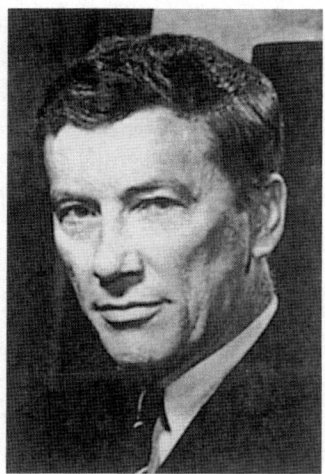

Figure 27–2 John J. Shea Jr, MD. He revived stapedectomy more than half a century after Blake and Jack, adding prosthetic restoration of ossicular continuity from the incus to tissue covering the oval window.

loupe and surgical microscopes made operations through the ear canal more practical. Audiometry to measure and report hearing results verified improvements. Finally, Lempert's transcanal approach to the middle ear without perforation of the tympanic membrane proved ideal for operations on the stapes.

The microscope made possible the use of microchisels and drills to loosen the footplate, the development of anterior crurotomy mobilization by Fowler,[16] and my revival of stapedectomy in 1956.[15] Unlike Blake and Jack, who failed to comprehend the need to reconstruct an ossicular chain and who left the oval window open, I closed the oval window after extraction of the stapes "with a thin slice of connective tissue" and inserted a prosthesis from the incus to the oval window to restore the normal mechanics of the middle ear.

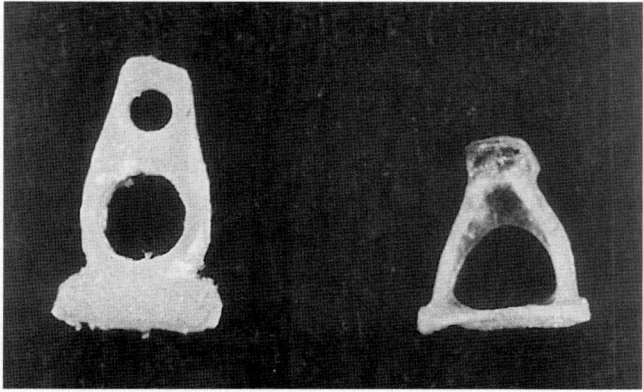

Figure 27–3 Teflon replica of the stapes.

Many modifications of the stapedectomy have been designed and employed, all following the principles firmly established by Shea, that the oval window needs to be sealed and that there must be ossicular continuity by using a prosthesis from the incus to the oval window. Among these modifications are a prosthesis of fat tied to a wire loop; a preformed wire loop against vein, fascia, or perichondrium to seal the oval window; and a piston-type prosthesis of stainless steel, tantalum, platinum, or Teflon. Most surgeons currently prefer a tissue graft rather than absorbable gelatin sponge Gelfoam (Pharmacia & Upjohn Company, Kalamazoo, Michigan) to seal the oval window as being less likely to result in perilymph fistula. The tendency for a preformed wire loop to become adherent to the edge of the oval window has prompted the use of a piston-type prosthesis of Teflon or stainless steel. In contrast to results obtained when removing the entire stapes footplate, or a major part of it, there appears to be less labyrinthine reaction when the prosthesis is inserted into a smaller opening in the footplate, using a very thin graft made from a pressed vein or from the dried loose areolar tissue superficial to the temporalis fascia. The latter technique is described in this text, although other methods may be equally satisfactory.

ETIOLOGY OF OTOSCLEROSIS

Otosclerosis is a common bone disorder of the bony labyrinth, unique to the endochondral layer of the temporal bone and known to affect only human beings.[17] It is among the most common causes of acquired hearing loss, with clinical manifestations occurring in approximately 1% of individuals in some populations. Histologic evidence of the disease process can be found in up to 10% of serially sectioned temporal bones. The most common clinical manifestation is a conductive hearing loss as a result of stapes fixation. In some cases, with large lesions that encroach on the cochlea, an irreversible sensorineural loss may occur. In most cases, the disease is bilateral.

Histologically, otosclerosis is characterized by a wave of abnormal bone remodeling with resorption of the otic capsule bone and replacement with a hypercellular woven bone that, over time, undergoes further remodeling, resulting in a sclerotic mosaic architecture. Ultrastructural characterization of the cellular components of the active remodeling phase reveals an absence of acute inflammatory cells and an abundance of histiocytes, osteoblasts, and osteoblast precursor cells, as well as other mononuclear cells.[18,19]

At the time of this writing, the cause of otosclerosis is undetermined. However, there is a well-established hereditary predisposition, with approximately half of all affected individuals having family members known to be affected. The remaining cases appear to be sporadic. Multiple genetic studies of otosclerosis have been reported to support an autosomal dominant mode of inheritance with penetrance in the range of 20 to 40.[20–24] There is also evidence to suggest that otosclerosis may be heterogenetic, with more than one gene defect giving rise to the otosclerosis phenotype.[25] The genes responsible for the development of otosclerosis have yet to be established. Linkage analysis of two large families with presumed otosclerosis and an unusually high degree of penetrance have revealed linkage to two separate foci.[26,27]

There is evidence to suggest that some cases of clinical otosclerosis may be related to the COL1A1 gene, which is one of the two genes that code for type I collagen, the predominant collagen of bone.[28] Some patients with clinical otosclerosis have been found to have abnormalities in COL1A1 expression similar to that observed in patients with type I osteogenesis imperfecta.[29]

Approximately 50% of patients with type I osteogenesis imperfecta develop hearing loss that is clinically indistinguishable from otosclerosis. Although only a few temporal bones from patients with type I osteogenesis imperfecta have been studied, the lesions within the otic capsule appear to be histologically indistinguishable from otosclerosis and in all likelihood represent the same fundamental underlying disease process.

During the last decade, there has been mounting evidence that some cases of otosclerosis may be related to a persistent measles virus infection of the otic capsule, perhaps similar to what is speculated to occur in Paget's disease of bone, where there is also mounting evidence for the presence of a defective paramyxovirus.[30–32]

Transmission electron microscopy of active otosclerotic stapes footplate fragments obtained at stapedectomy has revealed the presence of filamentous structures within the rough endoplasmic reticulum and cytosol of osteoblasts and preosteoblasts that are morphologically indistinguishable from measles nucleocapsid. These findings have been corroborated by immunohistochemical studies as well as molecular biologic studies that have demonstrated the presence of measles ribonucleic acid in active otosclerotic lesions.[33,34] In addition, there is evidence to suggest that the perilymph of patients with otosclerosis has elevated levels of antibody to measles virus.

One hypothesis that has been formulated from the culmination of these investigations is that otosclerosis may be initiated primarily by measles infection, which is capable of involving many different tissues and organs. Infections that occur within the unique embryonic rest areas of the temporal bone account for the sole predilection for the temporal bone. The establishment of persistent infection may be related to the relatively quiescent metabolic state or terminal differentiation of the osteocytes/chondrocytes within the embryonic rests, resulting in a restricted expression of the measles genome with little or no expression of late viral genes critical for complete viral assembly and escape.[34] Infected cells produce factors that destabilize the extracellular matrix and activate the remodeling process.[35–37] The progression and extension of the abnormal remodeling process are dependent on an underlying genetic defect in collagen metabolism. There may be multiple different mutations within the COL1A1 gene, as well as mutations in other genes within the collagen metabolism pathway, that result in the generation of an unusable extracellular matrix with a high propensity for remodeling.[38] In this model, the incomplete penetrance may be related to the occurrence, timing, and severity of the initial infection, which would also account for the development of small lesions (both histologic and small lesions with stapes fixation) in individuals without an underling genetic defect.

INDICATIONS FOR STAPEDECTOMY

The degree of footplate fixation is estimated by the size of the air–bone gap, whereas the degree of cochlear hearing loss is measured by the bone conduction curve, taking into account the variable Carhart's notch. In every patient, to confirm the presence and size of a genuine air–bone gap, the clinician should use the 256- or 512-Hz magnesium tuning fork to perform the Rinne test. Although the preoperative hearing tests indicate the degree of fixation, they do not predict the pattern and extent of oval window involvement by otospongiosis, which can be determined only when the oval window and stapes are exposed under the operating microscope.

Stapedectomy is indicated when the stapes is firmly fixed, as demonstrated by an air–bone gap of at least 30 dB for the speech frequencies and a negative Rinne test result for the 256- and 512-Hz magnesium tuning forks.

By contrast, fully successful stapes mobilization or successful stapedectomy not only corrects the entire conductive component of loss, it also removes Carhart's notch, often with overclosure of the preoperative air–bone gap. Stapedectomy can be useful for improving hearing aid use in the presence of stapes fixation with a profound cochlear loss, provided that there is sufficient speech discrimination, as determined by audiometry and a speaking tube. Poor speech discrimination and a history of vertigo in recent months are contraindications to stapedectomy because they indicate the possibility of endolymphatic hydrops, with the risk of further cochlear loss should the labyrinth be opened.

Operation on a patient's only hearing ear should be avoided because of the small but definite and unpredictable risk, about 1%, of a significant, permanent cochlear loss. In about 1% of ears, there is fibrous, not bony, fixation of the stapes, and mobilization of the stapes, not stapedectomy, should be done with good permanent hearing gain.

TECHNIQUE OF STAPEDECTOMY

Preoperative Preparation

Because the ideal patient for stapedectomy is also an ideal candidate for a hearing aid, he or she should be fully informed of this fact and of the uncertainties and risks of operation. Because verbal explanations are notoriously misinterpreted or forgotten by patients, a full written disclosure of the risks and likely results should be signed by the patient and a witness and kept in the record.

If the ear has not been operated on before and there is a large air–bone gap with good cochlear function, including excellent speech discrimination, the patient has at least 9 chances in 10 of a useful hearing improvement that will be maintained. There is, however, 1 chance in 100 that there may be a complete loss instead of a gain, rendering that ear unsatisfactory for a hearing aid.

Dizziness of some degree follows nearly every stapes operation, lasting a few hours to several days and, in rare cases, much longer. Taste may be affected, whether or not the chorda tympani nerve is torn or cut, gently pushed out of the way, or not visibly traumatized. Permanent loss or distortion of taste can occur. An unhealed perforation of the tympanic membrane, which is very rare, may require subsequent repair.

Paralysis of the facial nerve should be mentioned as a possible complication. It occurs in less than 1% of operations, usually begins 5 days to a week after operation, and is caused by edema of the nerve in the fallopian canal as a result of activation of a *Herpes* infection in the chorda tympani and facial nerves by the trauma of operation.[39] In cases in which the laser has been used, overheating of the nerve is an alternative etiology. Much more rarely, when a dehiscent or aberrant facial nerve protrudes over or crosses the footplate, especially in a repeat operation, the facial nerve may be injured during operation. The patient can plan to return to work 1 week after stapedectomy.

Following a successful stapes operation, the patient should return each year for hearing tests to detect beginning sensorineural hearing loss, owing to cochlear involvement by otosclerosis, which calls for sodium fluoride therapy. Should symptoms of endolymphatic hydrops, including imbalance, fullness in the ear, tinnitus, and hearing drop, occur at any time, the patient should return immediately because this may indicate a perilymph fistula, requiring repeat operation, or endolymphatic hydrops, which should respond to medical therapy.

The preoperative preparation of the patient includes inspection of the canal for any evidence of external or middle ear infection that necessitates postponement of the operation for treatment.

Anesthesia

The stapes operation can be performed under either local or general anesthesia. Local anesthesia causes slightly less bleeding and allows the patient's hearing to be assessed intraoperatively. General anesthesia is safer today than in the past and is usually preferred by the patient. With either type of anesthesia, the ear canal is infiltrated with lidocaine with epinephrine to obtain hemostasis. It is safer to use premixed carpules to ensure the correct concentration of epinephrine and lidocaine.

Custom dilution of stock (1:1,000) epinephrine is fraught with the potential for catastrophic cardiac complications as a consequence of dilutional error.

Obtaining the Tissue Graft

A number of autograft tissues can be used to cover the oval window, including vein, temporalis fascia, perichondrium, and fat. Vein is harvested from the back of the hand, all loose connective tissue is removed, and it is used adventitia side down, intima side up. Fat is obtained from the lobule of the ear. Temporalis fascia is harvested through a small incision above and behind the ear. The graft is dried and cut to shape. Perichondrium is harvested from the tragus and is pressed to make a thin sheet of tissue.

Exposure of the Oval Window

A speculum holder should be used to hold the largest speculum that can be inserted into the canal. A curved or triangular incision is made in the skin of the ear canal, beginning 1 mm and extending 6 mm lateral to the drum, with a pointed, disposable blade. The skin flap is elevated to the sulcus tympanicus with a blunt elevator. The fibrous annulus is elevated from the sulcus tympanicus with the same blunt elevator and is pushed down over the edge of bone sulcus (Figure 27–4). Special care is needed in separating the attachment of the posterior fold of the pars tensa to the midpoint of the sulcus posteriorly. If there is bleeding, light cautery may be needed to be applied to any bleeding point in the skin incision.

In most ears, to gain adequate exposure of the oval window and stapes, 2 to 4 mm of posterosuperior bony canal rim must be removed with the angled middle ear curet, taking care not to injure the chorda tympani nerve, which should be freed of filmy adhesions and gently displaced upward or downward to visualize the footplate fully. Enough bone is removed until the facial nerve and the pyramidal eminence can be seen (Figure 27–5).

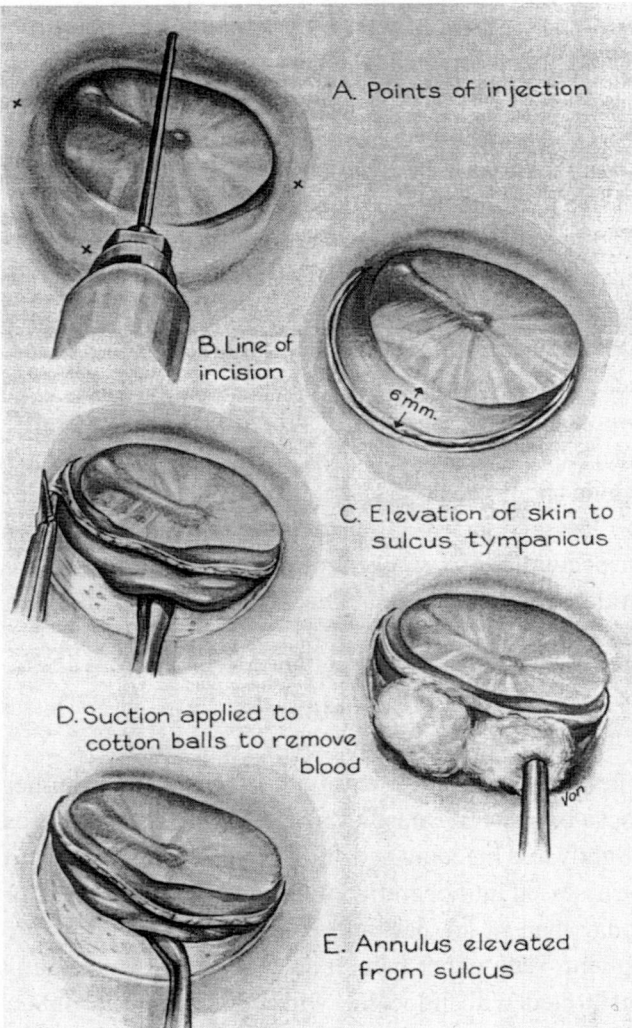

Figure 27–4   Creation of a meatal flap.

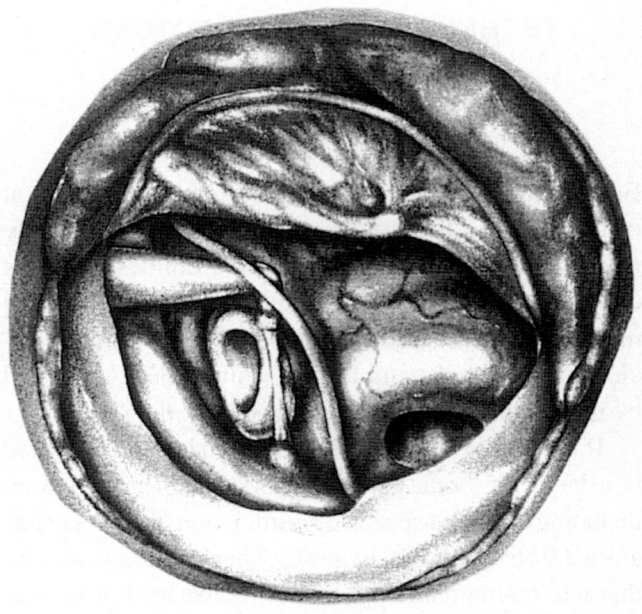

Figure 27–5   Exposure of an oval window following removal of bone from the posterosuperior bony meatal rim.

Removal of the Stapes Superstructure

A number of techniques are used to remove the stapes superstructure. First, the incudostapedial joint must be separated, using an angled joint knife. Next the stapes tendon is cut, using middle ear scissors.

Three techniques are used to remove the superstructure:

1. If the footplate is rigidly fixed, the superstructure can be fractured downward using a sharp pick in the cup in the head of the stapes. Usually, a fracture occurs at the base of the crura. Some surgeons prefer to create a "safety" hole in the footplate prior to fracturing the superstructure. This hole facilitates footplate removal should the footplate be mobilized in fracturing the crura.
2. The crura can be severed, using a microcrurotomy bur in a microdrill. This is a simple, atraumatic technique that has gained in popularity (Figure 27–6).
3. The superstructure can be vaporized using an argon or carbon-dioxide laser (Figure 27–7).[40] This technique is the least traumatic of the three, but, for most surgeons, an argon or carbon-dioxide laser is often not available.

Footplate Removal and Creation of a Fenestra

There are currently three options available to the otologic surgeon:

1. Total footplate removal is a proven method of creating this opening. First, mucosa is removed from the footplate and surrounding bone and bleeding is controlled using small pledgets of Gelfoam. A small hole in the thin, central portion of the footplate is made, using a fine pick or laser, and then the footplate is cut across. With small angled hooks, the pieces of the footplate are gently removed, taking great care to avoid dropping fragments into the vestibule or aspirating any perilymph. Any small fragments falling into the vestibule are left in place (Figure 27–8).
2. Posterior half footplate removal has gained in popularity. Less postoperative vertigo and better high-frequency hearing occur with this technique. The

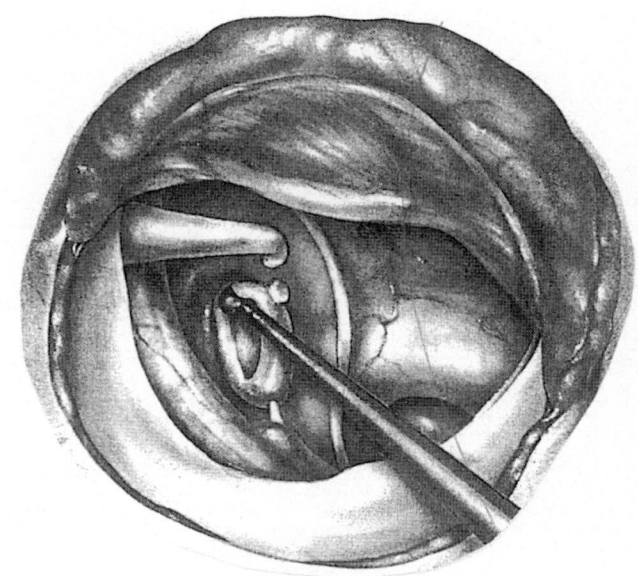

Figure 27–6 Use of a microcrurotomy bur to sever the crura.

footplate is cut across with a pick or laser as with total footplate removal, but only the posterior half is removed.

3. Similar to posterior half footplate removal, small fenestra stapedectomy gives less postoperative vertigo and better high-frequency hearing than total footplate removal. Small fenestra stapedectomy is a more precise method of creating a hole in the footplate than posterior half footplate removal. Several techniques are available, including use of an argon or a carbon-dioxide laser,[40] a micropick, or a micro-

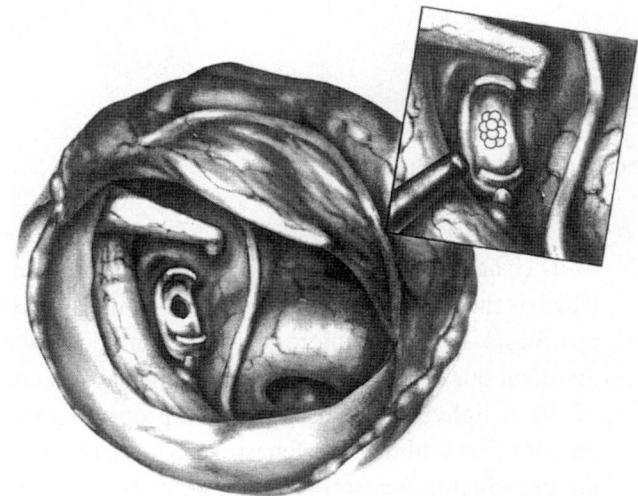

Figure 27–7 Argon laser used to remove the stapes superstructure. *Inset* shows the creation of a "rosette" in the stapes footplate.

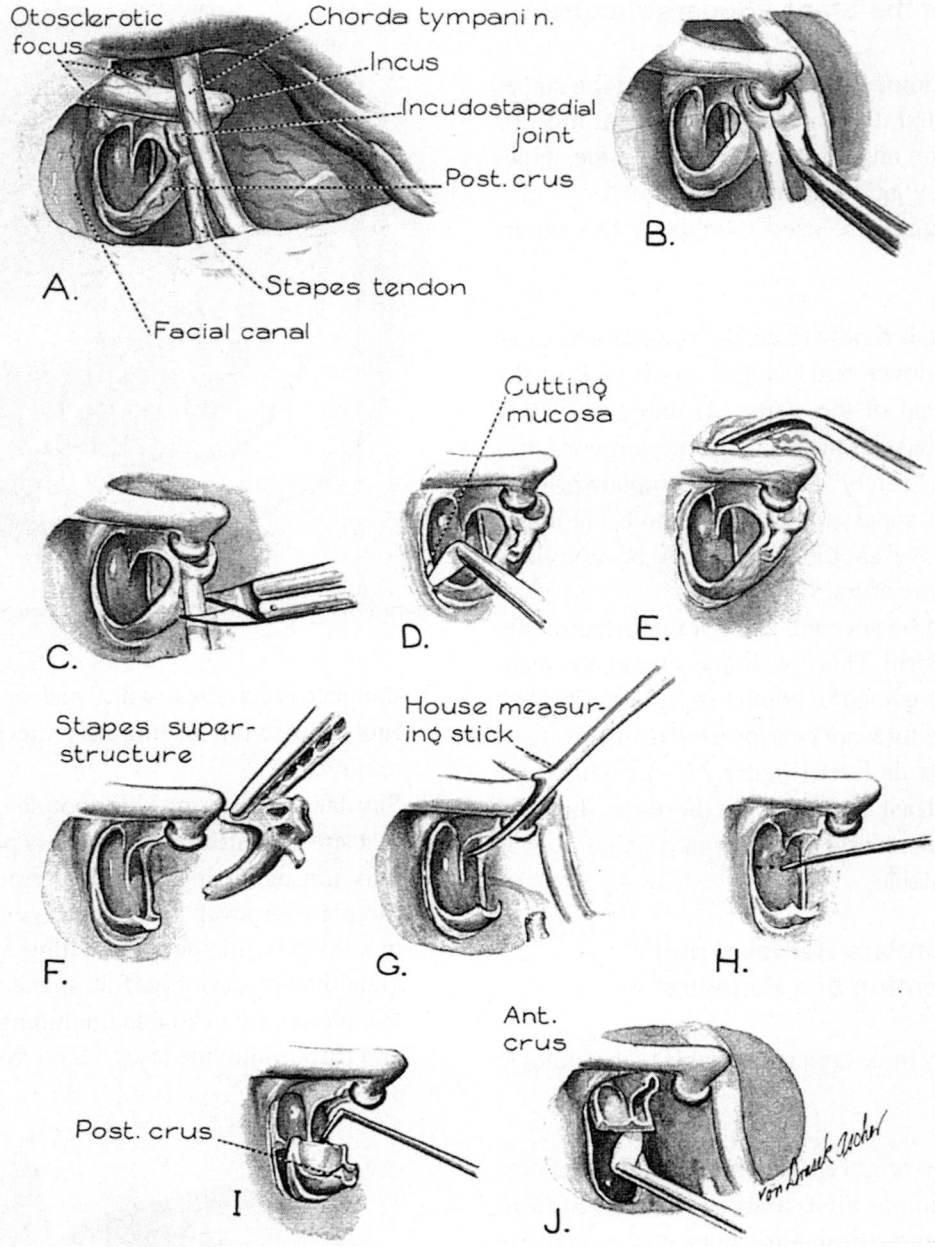

Figure 27–8 Stapedectomy.

drill. Usually a 0.7-mm diameter fenestra is made, which is the ideal size when using a 0.6-mm diameter prosthesis. In using a microdrill, a 0.7-mm diameter diamond bur is chosen to create the fenestra (Figure 27–9). A light touch is used to avoid protruding the bur into the vestibule. The fenestra can be sized using the bur. Such a fenestra can also be made with the argon or carbon-dioxide laser, creating a rosette of opening, and the center bone is removed with a pick.

Tissue Seal of the Oval Window

In the past, a tissue seal over the oval window was considered an essential part of the procedure. In most ears, vein or perichondrium or fascia graft is placed over the oval window opening, and a small margin of tissue is draped around the periphery. Although a tissue seal is certainly prudent, reports of successful stapedectomy with Gelfoam and no living tissue seal do exist. In these

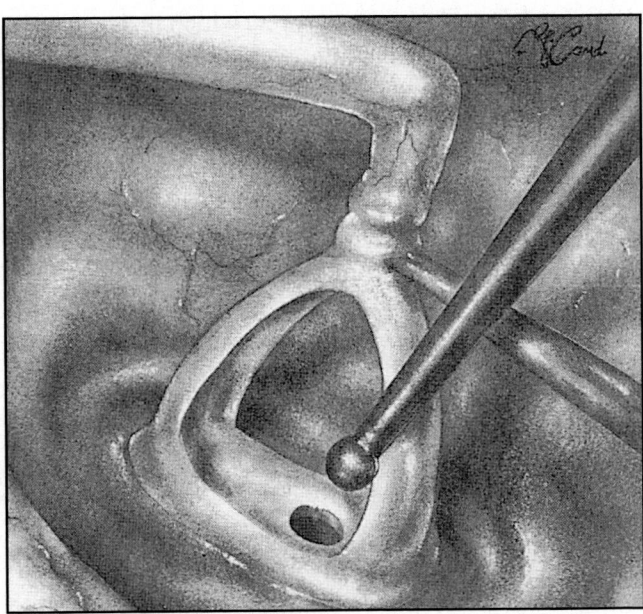

Figure 27–9 Footplate fenestration done with a microbur.

cases, blood from the operative field and/or Gelfoam are used to seal the oval window opening.

Prosthesis Placement

A variety of prostheses are available for stapes replacement, and these can be categorized into four main groups:

1. The cup piston prosthesis of Shea, made of Teflon (Figure 27–10), and the Robinson prosthesis, made of stainless steel (Figure 27–11), are the best prostheses by far. The prosthesis is measured from the undersurface of the lenticular process to the footplate and is usually 4 mm in length. This prosthesis is self-centering, that is, it tends to come to rest in the center of the oval window opening after insertion. The 0.6-mm diameter shaft is used most often. A narrow stem prosthesis, 0.4 or 0.5 mm in diameter, can be used when a small fenestra is created.

2. The original Shea Teflon piston prosthesis (Figure 27–12) was designed to attach to the long process of the incus when the lenticular process extends beyond the center of the oval window. This prosthesis can be used either with a small fenestra technique or with total footplate removal. The prosthesis length is measured from the undersurface of the long process of the incus to the footplate, plus 0.25 mm. The Teflon ring is spread open, and the prosthesis is pressed onto the incus. Because Teflon has "memory," the ring in the head of the Teflon piston will close without crimping. The prosthesis position can

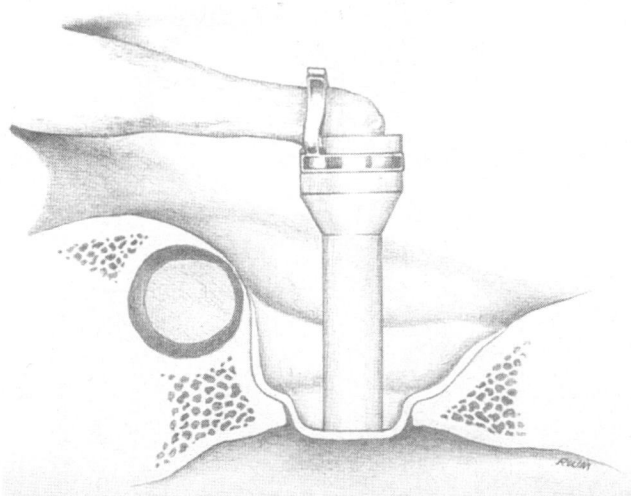

Figure 27–10 Shea platinum Teflon cup piston prosthesis.

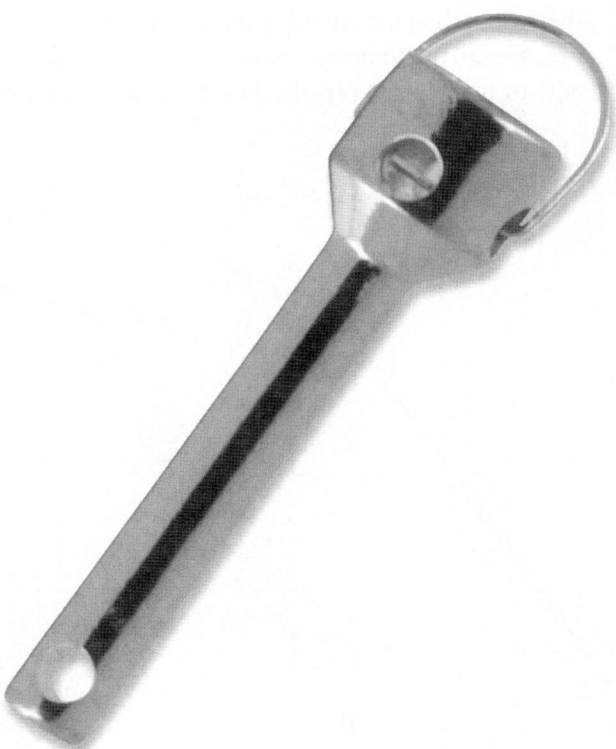

Figure 27–11 Robinson stainless steel prosthesis. (Courtesy of Gyrus, ENT Division, Memphis, Tennessee.)

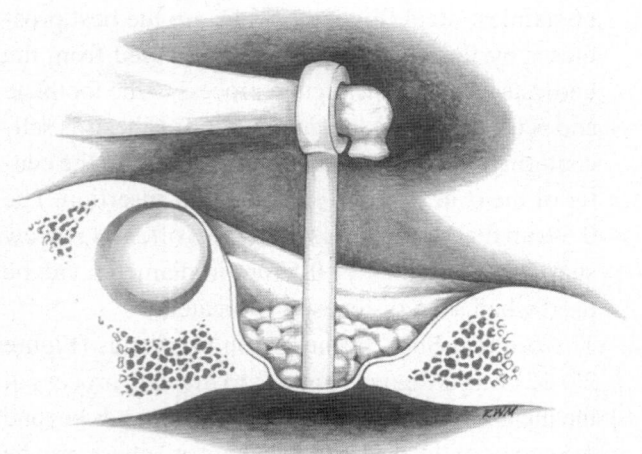

Figure 27–12   Shea Teflon piston prosthesis.

be adjusted easily. The prosthesis should protrude into the vestibule about 0.25 mm.

3. The McGee/Fisch-type piston prosthesis consists of a malleable ribbonlike crook connected to a metal or Teflon piston (Figure 27–13). The crook must be crimped onto the long process of the incus. The prosthesis can be used either with a small fenestra technique or with total footplate removal. The prosthesis length is measured from the undersurface of the incus to the footplate, plus 0.25 mm. One advantage of the McGee prosthesis is that the distal 0.25 mm of the prosthesis is scored, which makes checking the prosthesis length easier in a small fenestra stapedectomy.

4. The House wire prosthesis is made of a thin stainless steel wire (Figure 27–14). On one end is a shepherd's crook and on the opposite end is a small loop. The crook is attached and crimped onto the long process of the incus, and the small loop at the other end extends into the Gelfoam, sealing the oval window. A related prosthesis is the fat and wire prosthesis. Because the wire is attached to and stabilized by the fat, this prosthesis is more easily attached.

Following placement of the prosthesis, the malleus is palpated, and the movement of the prosthesis is verified. The tympanomeatal flap is then gently returned to its original position. Antibiotic powder is then blown into the ear canal, and the ear canal incisions are covered with narrow strips of moist Gelfoam.

Postoperative Care

Postoperatively, the patient is given adequate analgesics and instructed to avoid straining or blowing the nose. Antibiotics are not routinely prescribed. Nowadays most stapedectomy operations are done on an outpatient basis, and the patient is discharged in several hours when fully recovered. The patient is called the day after operation and is seen in 2 weeks to a month.

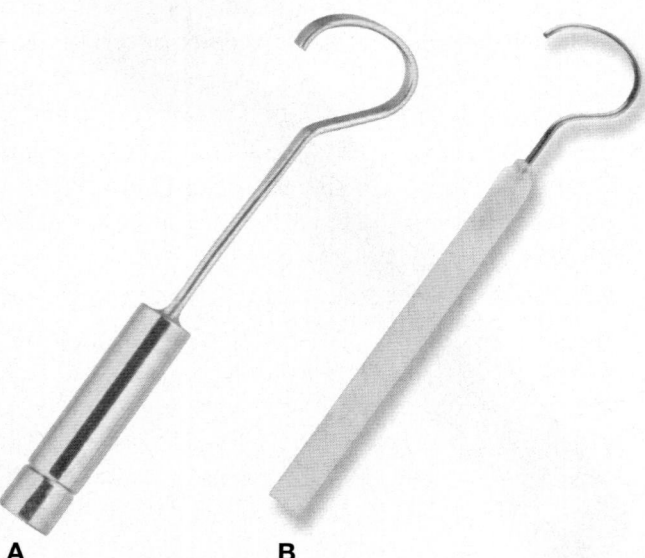

A   **B**

Figure 27–13   *A*, McGee piston prosthesis. *B*, Fisch platinum Teflon piston prosthesis. (Courtesy of Gyrus, ENT Division, Memphis, Tennessee.)

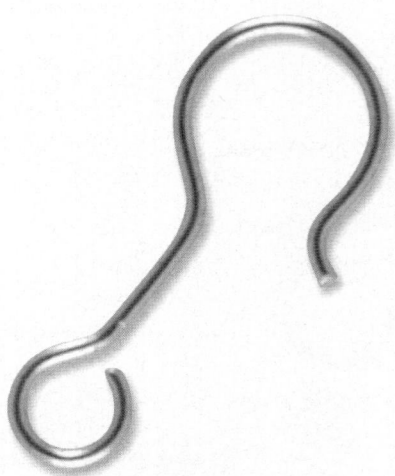

Figure 27–14   House wire prosthesis. (Courtesy of Gyrus, ENT Division, Memphis, Tennessee.)

Special Problems During Stapedectomy

Malleus fixation, floating footplate, obliterative otospongiosis, "biscuit footplate," dehiscent facial nerve obscuring the footplate, postoperative granuloma, fixed malleus, round window closure, fracture of the long process of the incus, otitis media, and perilymph "gusher" are special problems to be dealt with during and after operation.

Floating Footplate Problem

The "safety" hole helps in the extraction of a footplate with minimal trauma to the vestibular contents should the footplate mobilize and become "floating." If necessary, a very tiny hole may be made with a diamond drill or laser in the promontory edge of the oval window to help in removing a "floating footplate." In rare cases, the surgeon may elect to leave the "floating" footplate in place, seal the oval window opening with a vein or other tissue graft, and place the prosthesis over the "floating" footplate.

Obliterative Otospongiosis

When the margins of the oval window are found to be obliterated by otospongiosis, a "drill-out" is required. The approximate location of the oval window is established by the crura and the fallopian canal. With a small diamond drill or argon or carbon-dioxide laser, the bone in the oval window is carefully thinned down until a blue area appears, and then a round opening is made about twice the width of the 0.6-mm Teflon piston. The tissue graft is applied, and the prosthesis is positioned as before, extending 0.25 mm beyond the inner rim of the oval window.

"Biscuit Footplate"

The "biscuit footplate" is the thickened footplate with well-defined margins produced by a primary focus in the footplate. With a tiny diamond drill or argon or carbon-dioxide laser, the footplate is cut across the center, and the margins of the footplate are thinned until the footplate can be extracted in two pieces, removing the entire focus of otospongiosis and thus "curing" the disease, provided that other foci are not present. The tissue graft and prosthesis are applied as before.

Dehiscent, Prolapsed Facial Nerve

At a first operation, there is little difficulty in identifying and avoiding injury to a dehiscent, prolapsed facial nerve protruding down over the footplate. In most such ears, a small fenestra can be made in the footplate, which is covered with a thin tissue graft, and a 0.6-mm piston is inserted without trauma to the nerve.

A more difficult and dangerous problem arises when a revision stapedectomy is performed on such an ear when the dehiscent facial nerve has become embedded and pulled down by fibrous tissue covering the oval window niche. Even the most careful removal of the fibrous tissue may result in injury to the facial nerve, postoperative facial paralysis, and a subsequent malpractice lawsuit. Facial nerve injury in such ears cannot always be avoided and must be ascribed to anatomic anomaly, not to surgical negligence.

Postoperative Granuloma

Granuloma of the oval window is an uncommon complication of stapedectomy in which Gelfoam is used to seal the oval window. Granuloma usually develops soon (within the first 2 weeks) after operation and causes a sudden hearing loss and disturbance of balance. A grayish-red mass in the posterosuperior quadrant of the drum is the hallmark physical finding. The ear should be explored as soon as possible and the granuloma removed. A living tissue seal is required to cover the oval window. Early operation can usually save the hearing.

Fixed Incus and/or Malleus

Ankylosis of the incus and/or malleus head to the attic wall can occur by itself or more in combination with otosclerotic stapes ankylosis. Prolonged immobility of the stapes may predispose to incus and/or malleus ankylosis. In every stapedectomy, the mobility of the malleus and incus should be verified by palpation. Should the incus and/or malleus be fixed, this should be corrected prior to inserting the prosthesis.

If the body of the incus and not the malleus is fixed, the incus is separated from the head of the stapes and removed. If the head of the malleus and not the incus is fixed, the neck of the malleus is cut across and the head of the malleus is removed. If both the body of the incus and the head of the malleus are fixed, they are both removed. The entire or half of the stapes footplate is removed and the oval window is covered with a living oval window seal. We have had very good hearing improvement by inserting a total ossicular replacement prosthesis (TORP) with a porous hydroxyapatite head and a silver wire around the shaft protruding up to fit on the far side of the malleus. This holds the TORP in good contact with the drum, malleus, and incus if one is left in place (Figure 27–15).

If the incus and/or malleus are fixed, but not the stapes, the head of the incus and/or malleus are removed, and a partial ossicular replacement prosthesis is inserted from the head of the stapes to the undersurface of the drum (Figure 27–16).

Round Window Closure

Partial involvement of the margin of the round window niche by otospongiosis is common, next in frequency to oval window involvement, but unlike the oval window, there is no effect on hearing unless the niche is solidly closed. A tiny opening, no larger than a red blood cell, suffices for to and fro vibrations of the cochlear fluid column between the oval and round windows, with no loss of hearing. The round window can be occluded by fibrous tissue without impairment of its function.

Complete bone closure of the round window, associated with stapes ankylosis, is quite rare and causes a severe combined sensorineural and conductive loss. Stapedectomy in such a situation can result in some

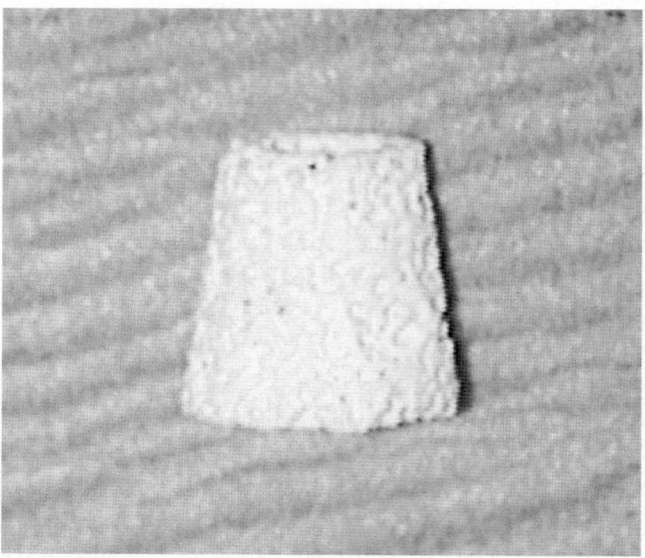

Figure 27–16 Porous hydroxyapatite partial ossicular replacement prosthesis.

hearing improvement.[41] Attempts to open the round window have been disappointing and should be avoided.

Fracture of the Long Process of the Incus

The best way to reconstruct the sound-conducting mechanism of the middle ear after fracture of the long process of the incus is with the porous hydroxyapatite TORP with wire as used with a fixed incus and/or malleus and is described above.

Acute Otitis Media

Acute otitis media in the immediate postoperative period usually presents no problem if a living oval window seal is used. Culture and the appropriate antibiotic are the treatment of choice.

Perilymph Gusher

A rare, alarming, and serious problem of stapes surgery is a profuse flow of perilymph the moment that the vestibule is opened, owing to abnormal patency of the cochlear aqueduct and/or internal auditory canal. Elevation of the head of the table to reduce cerebrospinal fluid pressure in the head usually stops the flow of perilymph. Sealing the oval window opening by a tissue graft held in place by a prosthesis, followed by bed rest of the patient while maintaining a 30-degree elevation of the head until the ear dressing remains dry for 24 hours, usually stops the perilymph leak. Sometimes it is necessary to place a

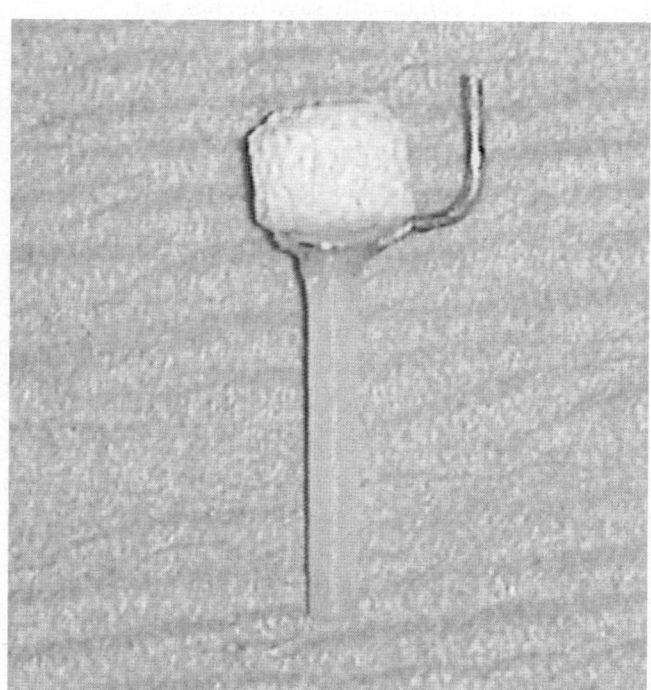

Figure 27–15 Porous hydroxyapatite total ossicular replacement prosthesis with wire.

lumbar drain to stop the leak.[42] A permanent cochlear loss may result after such a complication. Further operation on this ear or the other ear is contraindicated. A large cochlear aqueduct and/or internal auditory canal can usually be seen on a computed tomographic scan.

Postoperative Follow-up

The patient is seen after fully recovered. The ear canal and drum are inspected, and any complications are noted. Most patients are not dizzy, but there is usually some loss of balance. The patient is seen in 2 to 4 weeks after operation and nearly always shows a good gain in hearing and discrimination, but the best level of hearing is generally recorded 3 months to 1 year postoperatively.

Complications of Stapedectomy

Severance of or trauma to the chorda tympani nerve often but not always causes loss or distortion of taste on the side of the operation. Facial paralysis of the Bell's palsy type can occur 5 to 7 days after an uneventful stapedectomy, which is owing to the activation of *Herpes* infection dormant in the chorda tympani nerve or facial nerve. In most cases, recovery begins in one to several weeks and is complete, but in rare cases, recovery is delayed and incomplete with synkinesis and spasm. Postoperative facial palsy should be treated with large doses of corticosteroids, as in idiopathic Bell's palsy. Decompression of the nerve might be indicated in rare cases. Postoperative perforation of the drum should be treated by the appropriate antibiotic and rarely requires surgical repair.

Otitis media and suppurative labyrinthitis should not occur with careful sterile technique, and, as Miot pointed out as early as 1890, these complications indicate failure to maintain proper asepsis during operation.

Postoperative Perilymph Fistula

A rare cause for immediate and late cochlear loss after stapedectomy is a slow leak of perilymph from the oval window. The symptoms are those of postoperative endolymphatic hydrops. Exploration of the middle ear must be considered, with avoidance of entering the vestibule if a fistula is not found, because creating a fistula, no matter how tiny and how quickly sealed, makes hearing loss caused by hydrops worse. If a fistula is found, a connective tissue graft applied to the oval window opening is used to seal the fistula. The prognosis for relief of persistent vertigo caused by a perilymph fistula is favorable after such a revision, but recovery of useful hearing is rare and should not be promised to the patient.

Perilymph fistula is more common after wire and Gelfoam or wire fat stapedectomy. This type of fistula could also occur with a sudden change in air pressure during a plane flight.

Revision of Stapes Operations

Loss of initial gain in hearing after stapes mobilization or stapedectomy can be caused by refixation of a mobilized footplate, gradual adherence of the prosthesis to the edge of the oval window, osseous closure of the oval window, fixing the prosthesis, aseptic necrosis of the tip of the long process of the incus, slippage of the prosthesis from the long process, loosening of the wire attachment to the incus or ankylosis of the malleus, and, rarely, ankylosis of the incus and/or malleus to the attic wall. Air and bone conduction and discrimination testing, always confirmed by tuning forks, establish whether there is recurrence of a large air–bone gap without sensorineural loss or whether the loss of hearing is largely or entirely sensorineural. Tympanometry helps to define the type of conductive deficit. Revision is indicated for all genuine conductive losses, occurring early or late after stapedectomy, with the probability of a useful hearing improvement. However, the prognosis for maintaining satisfactory hearing after a revision is less favorable than after primary stapedectomy.

The technique of revision of a stapes operation is exactly the same as for the original operation except that the chorda tympani nerve is likely to be embedded in adhesions to the drum, so that injury to it is more probable to gain a satisfactory view of the oval window niche. Adhesions between tympanic membrane and incus and in the oval window niche are separated with a tiny right-angled hook or middle ear scissors, keeping in mind the possibility of a dehiscent facial nerve that may have prolapsed over the oval window subsequent to the first operation.

Recurrence of a conductive deficit after successful stapedectomy with wire prosthesis is often attributable to adhesion of the wire to the edge of the oval window. Substituting a Teflon or stainless steel piston prosthesis in such a case usually reduces or eliminates the conductive deficit.

Early and Late Sensorineural Hearing Loss Following Stapedectomy

Immediate, sometimes irreversible sensorineural loss after stapedectomy may occur following the most carefully performed, uneventful, and atraumatic operation, owing to endolymphatic hydrops, possibly with perilymph fistula or middle ear granuloma. The best treatment is with immediate large doses of corticosteroids, such as 40 to 60 mg of prednisolone or 4 mg of dexamethasone, for 10 to 14 days.

The possibility of a perilymph fistula must be kept in mind and exploration of the middle ear without opening the vestibule considered when medical therapy of hydrops fails to improve the hearing and control the vertigo and other symptoms of hydrops.

HISTORICAL PROCEDURES

Fowler Anterior Crurotomy Mobilization

Anterior crurotomy mobilization is rarely employed today and is presented for historical interest. Anterior crurotomy is accomplished in three steps:

1. The anterior crus is sectioned by applying a curved microchisel saw or laser to the anterior crus, close to the footplate of the stapes. The chisel is then pushed inward toward the footplate to remove thin shavings of bone until the crus fractures. The distal fragment of crus is pushed forward to leave a gap between it and the proximal fragment to prevent healing of the fractured crus. Sometimes the entire stapes and footplate become freely mobile before the anterior crus is sectioned, in which case nothing more need be done.
2. The footplate is cut across its center by repeated light pressure of a fine pick, or with a straight microchisel or laser.
3. The posterior half of the footplate, now separated from the anterior portion fixed by the anterior otospongiotic focus, is nearly always impacted against the posterior edge of the oval window and needs to be freed by gentle pressure on the posterior rim of the footplate. A tiny connective tissue graft is placed anteriorly at the site of footplate fracture to seal the vestibule.

Fenestration Operation of Holmgren, Sourdille, and Lempert

The fenestration operation, never employed today for stapedial otosclerosis, will remain forever as a mighty landmark in the evolution of surgery to restore hearing in otosclerosis. Clinical experience with thousands of fenestrated ears requiring annual or more frequent cleaning of the fenestrated cavity continues to provide a unique opportunity to follow the course of otospongiotic disease through hearing tests administered over many years. The one-stage endaural fenestration operation, introduced in 1938 by Lempert,[9] with the application to it of the operating microscope in 1940 by Shambaugh, marked the turning point from surgery for aural suppuration to microsurgery for otosclerosis in a clean field for the restoration of hearing.

REFERENCES

1. Kessel J. Über das mobilisieren des Steigbügels durch ausschneiden des Trommelfelles, Hammers und amboss bei Undurchgängigkeit der Tuba. Arch Ohrenh 1878;13:69.
2. Boucheron E. La mobilization de l'étrier et son procèdé opératoire. Union Méd Paris 1888;46:412.
3. Miot C. De la mobilization de l'étrier. Rev Laryngol 1890;10:113.
4. Blake CJ. Middle ear operations. Trans Am Otol Soc 1892;5:306.

5. Jack FL. Further observations on removal of the stapes. Trans Am Otol Soc 1893;5:474.

6. Faraci G. Importanza acustica e funzionale della mobilizzazione della staffa; resultati di una nuova serie di operazioni. Arch Ital Otol Rinol Laryngol 1899;9:209.

7. Siebenmann F. Sur le traitement chirurgical de la sclérose otique. Congr internat Méd Sect Otol 1900;13:170.

8. Sourdille M. New technic in the surgical treatment of severe and progressive deafness from otosclerosis. Bull N Y Acad Med 1937;13:673.

9. Lempert J. Improvement of hearing in cases of otosclerosis: new one-stage surgical technic. Arch Otol 1938;28:42.

10. Shambaugh GE Jr. Fenestration operation for otosclerosis; experimental investigations and clinical observations. Acta Otolaryngol Suppl (Stockh) 1949;79.

11. Rosen S. Palpation of stapes for fixation: preliminary procedure to determine fenestration suitability for otosclerosis. Arch Otol 1952;56:610.

12. Rosen S. Mobilization of the stapes to restore hearing in otosclerosis. N Y State J Med 1953;53:2650.

13. Jack FL. Remarkable improvement in hearing by removal of the stapes. Trans Am Otol Soc 1892;5:284.

14. Jack FL. Supplementary report on a case of double stapedectomy operated upon ten years ago. Trans Am Otol Soc 1902;8:99.

15. Meltzer PE, Lindsay JR, Goodhill V, et al. Symposium. The operation for the mobilization of the stapes in otosclerotic deafness. Laryngoscope 1956;66:729.

16. Basek M, Fowler EP Jr. Anatomical factors in stapes-mobilization operations. AMA Arch Otolaryngol 1956;63:589.

17. Wang PC, Merchant SN, McKenna MJ, et al. Does otosclerosis occur only in the temporal bone? Am J Otol 1999;20:162–5.

18 McKenna MJ, Mills BG, Galey FR, Linthicum FH Jr. Filamentous structures morphologically similar to viral nucleocapsids in otosclerotic lesions in two patients. Am J Otol 1986;7:25–8.

19. McKenna MJ, Gadre AD, Rask-Andersen H. Ultrastructural characterization of otospongiotic lesions in re-embedded celloidin sections. Acta Otolaryngol (Stockh) 1990;109:397–405.

20. Larsson A. Otosclerosis: a genetic and clinical study. Acta Otolaryngol Suppl (Stockh) 1960; Suppl 154:

21. Morrison AW, Bundey SE. The inheritance of otosclerosis. J Laryngol Otol 1970;84:921–32.

22. Gapany-Gapanavicius B. Otosclerosis: genetics and surgical rehabilitation. Jerusalem: Keter, 1975.

23. Donnell GN, Alfi OS. Medical genetics for the otorhinolaryngologist. Laryngoscope 1980;90:40–6.

24. Causse JR, Causse JB. Otospongiosis as a genetic disease. Early detection, medical management, and prevention. Am J Otol 1984;5:211–23.

25. Ben Arab S, Bonaïti-Pellĭ C, Belkahia A. A genetic study of otosclerosis in a population living in the north of Tunisia. Ann Genet 1993;36:111–6.

26. Tomek MS, Brown MR, Mani SR, et al. Localization of a gene for otosclerosis to chromosome 15q25-q26. Hum Mol Genet 1998;7:285–90.

27. van dan Bogaert, et al. A second gene for otosclerosis, OTSC2, maps to chromosome 7q34-36. Am J Hum Genet 2001;68:495–500.

28. McKenna MJ, Kristiansen AG, Bartley ML, et al. Association of COL1A1 and otosclerosis. Evidence for a shared genetic etiology with mild osteogenesis imperfecta. Am J Otol 1998;19:604–10.

29. McKenna MJ, Kristiansen AG, Tropitzsch AS. Similar COL1A1 expression in fibroblasts from some patients with clinical otosclerosis and those with type I osteogenesis imperfecta. Ann Otol Rhinol Laryngol 2002;111:184–9.

30. McKenna MJ, Mills BG. Immunohistochemical evidence of measles virus antigens in active otosclerosis. Otolaryngol Head Neck Surg 1989;101:414–21.

31. McKenna MJ, Adams JC. Immunohistochemical demonstration of measles fusion and phosphor protein antigens in active otosclerosis. In: McCabe BF, Veldman JE, Mogi G, editors. Immunology in otology, rhinology and laryngology. Amsterdam: Kugler; 1992. p. 101–7.

32. McKenna MJ, Mills BG, Galey FR, et al. Filamentous structures morphologically similar to viral nucleocapsids in otosclerotic lesions in two patients. Am J Otol 1986;7:25–8.

33. McKenna MJ, Kristiansen AG, Haines J. Polymerase chain reaction amplification of a measles virus sequence from human temporal bone sections with active otosclerosis. Am J Otol 1996;17:827–30.

34. Niedermeyer HP, Arnold W. Otosclerosis: a measles virus associated inflammatory disease. Acta Otolaryngol (Stockh) 1995;115:300–3.

35. Yamabe T, Dhir G, Cowan EP, et al. Cytokine-gene expression in measles-infected adult human glial cells. J Neuroimmunol 1994;49:171–9.

36. Schneider-Schaulies J, Schneider-Schaulies S, ter Meulen V. Differential induction of cytokines by primary and persistent measles virus infections in human glial cells. Virology 1993;195:219–28.

37. Schultz-Cherry S, Hinshaw VS. Influenza virus neuraminidase activates latent transforming growth factor ß. J Virol 1996;70:8624–9.

38. Iruela-Arispe ML, Vernon RB, Wu H, et al. Type I collagen-deficient Mov-13 mice do not retain SPARC in the extracellular matrix. Implications for fibroblast function. Dev Dyn 1996;207:171–83.

39. Shea JJ, Ge X. Delayed facial palsy after stapedectomy. Otol Neurotol 2001;22:465–70.

40. Perkins RC. Laser stapedectomy for otosclerosis. Laryngoscope 1980;90:880.

41. Shea JJ, Farrior JB. Stapedectomy and round window closure. Laryngoscope 1987;97:1:10.

42. Shea JJ. Management of perilymph leak. Laryngoscope 1976;86:255.

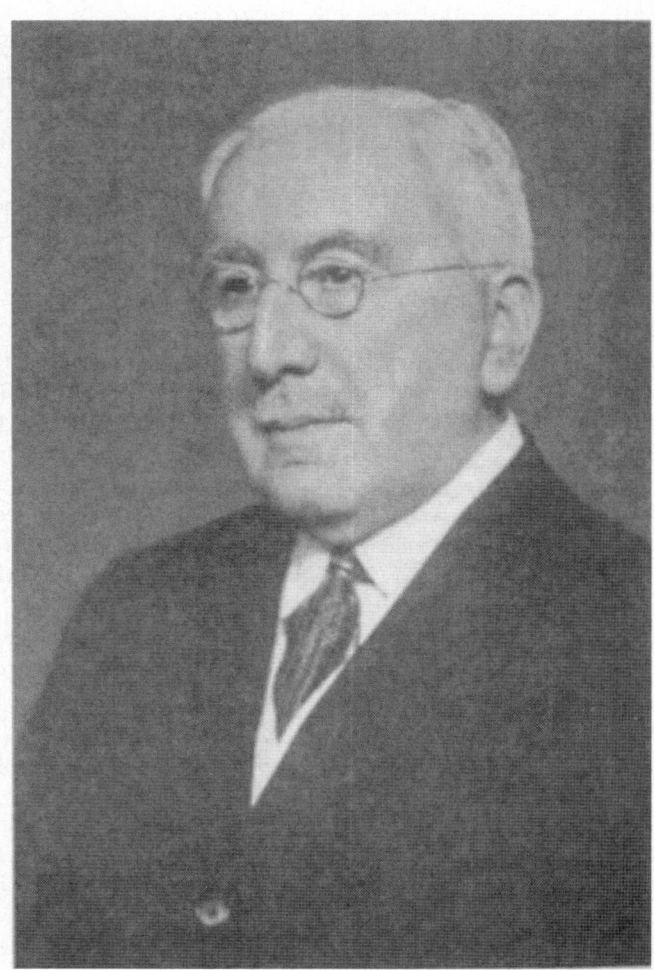

Sir Charles Ballance (1856–1936). Foremost pioneer aural surgeon of Great Britain; also founder and first president of the Society of British Neurological Surgeons. In experiments with Arthur B. Duel of New York, he established the superiority of intratemporal facial nerve grafts over anastomosis to other nerves.

28

Implantable Hearing Devices

RICHARD WIET, MD
CARLOS ESQUIVEL, MD
DICK HOISTED, MD

THE HEARING AID PROBLEM

It is estimated that over 22 million Americans suffer from hearing loss and that sensory hearing loss accounts for the majority of cases.[1] Throughout the United States, only a small percentage of patients are users of hearing aid devices, presumably owing to the problems of cosmetic appearance, discomfort, or sound distortion. Of these three problems, the most common complaints relate to sound distortion and lack of clarity. Older individuals have difficulty adjusting to the settings of an aid. In addition, as a general rule, the worse the hearing loss, the worse the ability to adjust the hearing aid to a satisfactory gain. These problems open the door for the development of new technologies, including middle ear implants.

Conventional hearing aids transform, amplify, and transform acoustic energy into an electrical signal that then becomes mechanical energy and is perceived as sound. Simply put, the hearing aid is a microphone, amplifier, and loudspeaker packaged in a plastic mold with a number of modifications that create a louder sound within the ear canal. Sound vibrates the tympanic membrane and ossicular chain. Conventional hearing aids have characteristics that limit their use in certain patients with hearing loss. The location of the microphone with respect to the receiver can increase the potential for feedback and distortion. Within the aid, sound takes a detour via a miniature loudspeaker, receiver, and tiny tube that act as a sound pressure conduit. The speaker/receiver is the main limiting factor to amplification. All of these factors contribute to reduce the quality and crispness of the sound of a conventional hearing aid.

The concept of driving the ossicular chain directly by a mechanical vibrator could avoid the discomfort of an in-the-canal device and the limitations of sound quality of a conventional hearing aid. All of the issues discussed above stimulated research that has culminated in the beginning of the era of implantable middle ear systems for hearing amplification.

DEVELOPMENT OF IMPLANTABLE HEARING DEVICES

The first published report of an implantable hearing device was by Wilska in 1935. He placed small pieces of iron on the tympanic membrane and a coil within the ear canal; the coil created a magnetic field, which, in turn, caused the iron and the tympanic membrane to vibrate.[2] The patient reported a gain in tone reception.

The use of a piezoelectric system was first investigated by Vernon and colleagues.[3] Yanagihara, Suzuki, and colleagues devised the first clinically applicable piezoelectric system.[4-6] They implanted piezoelectric vibrators into patients with mixed hearing loss and reported excellent results.

The use of middle ear electromagnetic devices has been investigated by several researchers, including Hough and colleagues,[7] Fredrickson and colleagues,[8] Goode and Glatke,[9] and Kartush and Tos.[10]

The devices in use today use either piezoelectric or electromagnetic drivers, and they can be either partially or totally implantable. A partially implantable system uses a microphone with a speech processor and a transmitting coil that are connected to the internal (implanted) device. Sound energy is converted to electrical energy by technology very similar to that used in cochlear implants. The driver (either piezoelectric or electromagnetic) converts electrical energy to mechanical energy; the driver is connected to the incus or the stapes. A totally implantable system differs by having a microphone (or receiver) that is placed under the skin, in the middle ear, or in the external auditory canal. The microphone is connected to a speech processor that converts sound energy to an electrical signal. The driver, which can be connected to the incus or stapes, converts the electrical signal to mechanical vibrations.

PRINCIPLES OF OPERATION OF CURRENT SYSTEMS

Piezoelectric Devices

Piezoelectric ceramics have been used in commercial devices (eg, buzzers, telephones, microphones, and loudspeakers) and in medical products (eg, flowmeters and ultrasonography equipment) for many years. Piezoelectric ceramics are hard, chemically inert, and completely insensitive to humidity or other atmospheric influences; they can be composed of many different materials — most commonly of lead, titanium, and zirconate crystal — and have both mechanical and electrical properties. Piezoelectric materials generate an electrical potential when mechanically strained; conversely, an electric potential causes physical deformation. These materials can function both as a microphone and as a loudspeaker.

Currently, there are two piezoelectric ceramic systems, one using a monomorph and the other a biomorph design. The monomorph crystal is made of a single layer of piezoelectric material, which can change its shape depending on the force applied to it. The biomorph crystal is composed of two layers of piezoelectric material of opposite polarities, which are separated by inert material. The power output is directly related to the size (length) of the crystal. Mathematical modeling has demonstrated that the power consumption of a piezo-

electric transducer is much less than that of electromagnetic devices.[11]

Electromagnetic Devices

An electromagnetic transducer comprises two elements: a transmitting coil and a receiving magnet. The current of the coil induces a magnetic flux, which varies according to the alternating current; the fundamental characteristic of magnets is that they vibrate in perfect synchrony with the frequencies within their field. A speech signal creates an alternating current field in the coil that is transduced by a magnetic field to the implanted magnet, which ultimately results in movement of the magnet.

The shape and size of the transmitting coil, as well as the composition and mass of the receiving magnet, can affect the sound delivered to the cochlea. Research has determined that any mass or object on the ossicular chain over 50 mg may cause a high-frequency hearing loss.[12] The magnetic field strength falls off as a cube of the distance between the coil and the magnet. That is, if the transmission coil is placed in the external ear canal (eg, as an in-the-ear shell), the magnetic field strength would be greater with the magnet on the umbo than on the stapes. Another inherent characteristic of electromagnetic induction systems is that the inductive resistance of a coil increases with frequency; accordingly, the amplifier must be designed to provide additional output in the high-frequency range.[13] It has been concluded that a better high-frequency response would be achieved if the magnet were placed on the stapes rather than on the more lateral umbo.[14]

CURRENT DEVICES

There are two US Food and Drug Administration (FDA)-approved middle ear implant devices: the Vibrant® Soundbridge™ and the Direct Drive Hearing System™. The remaining systems are under investigation in clinical trials, including the Envoy™ and the Middle Ear Transducer™. The Rion device is not under clinical investigation in the United States at the time of this writing (Table 28–1).

Table 28–1 CURRENT IMPLANTABLE HEARING DEVICES						
Manufacturer	Device	FDA Approved?	Type of Implantation	Implanted Transducer Type	Transducer Attachment	Audiometric Indication
Otologics LLS Boulder, CO	Middle Ear Transducer	No	Partial	Electromagnetic	Incus Intact chain	Sensorineural 15–19 dB, 250–4,000 Hz; discrimination > 20%
SOUNDtec, Inc Oklahoma City, OK	Direct Drive Hearing System	Yes	Partial	Electromagnetic	Stapes Intact chain	Sensorineural 10–100 dB, 250–6,000 Hz; discrimination > 60%
Symphonix Devices, Inc San Jose, CA	Vibrant Soundbridge	Yes	Partial	Electromagnetic	Stapes Intact chain	Sensorineural 30–85 dB, 500–4,000 Hz (PTA > 30 dB); discrimination > 50%
St. Croix Medical Minneapolis, MN	Envoy	No	Total	Piezoelectric	Stapes Disarticulated chain	Sensorineural 35–85 dB, 500–4,000 Hz; discrimination > 60%
Rion Co, Ltd Tokyo, Japan	Partially implantable hearing aid, E type	No	Partial/total	Piezoelectric	Stapes Disarticulated chain	Severe mixed HL, up to 50 dB (bone conduction)

Vibrant Soundbridge

The Vibrant Soundbridge (Symphonix Devices, Inc, San Jose, California) is the first partially implantable electromagnetic system to have received FDA approval (Figure 28–1). It is a direct drive electromagnetic system with a Floating Mass Transducer™ (FMT) that attaches to the incus.

The Soundbridge has two major components: the implanted Vibrating Ossicular Prosthesis (VORP) and an external amplification system (the Audio Processor™). The VORP consists of (1) a magnet, (2) a receiving coil, (3) a demodulator, (4) the VORP transition, (5) the conductor link, and (6) the FMT. The FMT, which is attached to the long process of the incus (Figure 28–2), comprises a magnet surrounded by two electromagnetic coils. The coils generate an electromagnetic field, causing the magnet to vibrate in a plane that is parallel to the plane of the stapes.

Subject selection criteria are age greater than 18 years; a stable, moderate to severe sensorineural hearing loss; and a minimum speech recognition score of 50% (Figure 28–3). Also, candidates must have failed an adequate

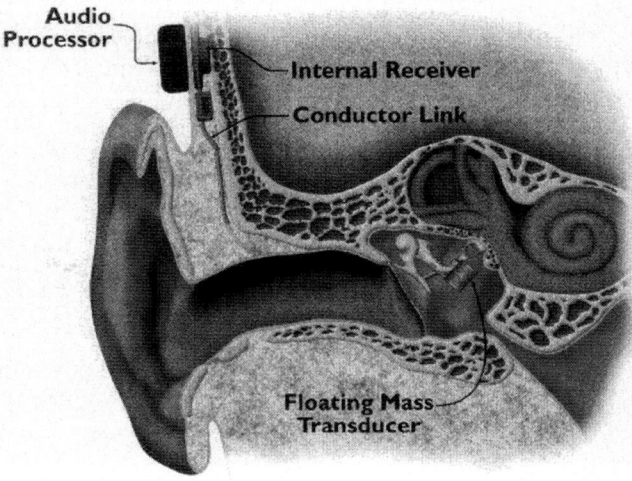

Figure 28–1 The Vibrant Soundbridge system.

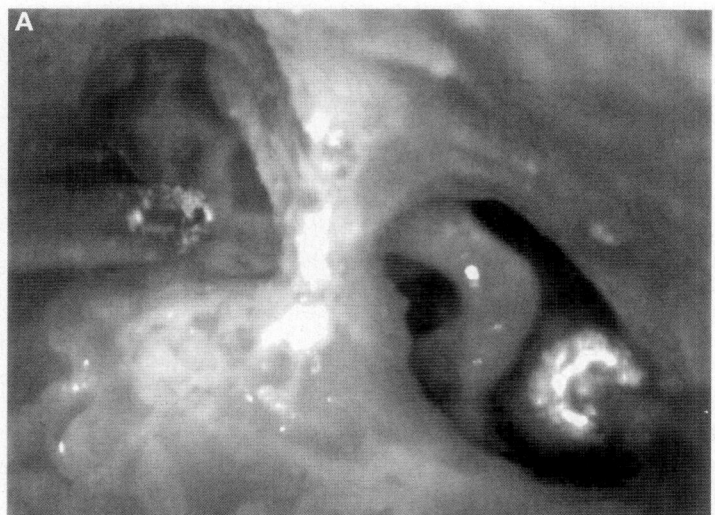

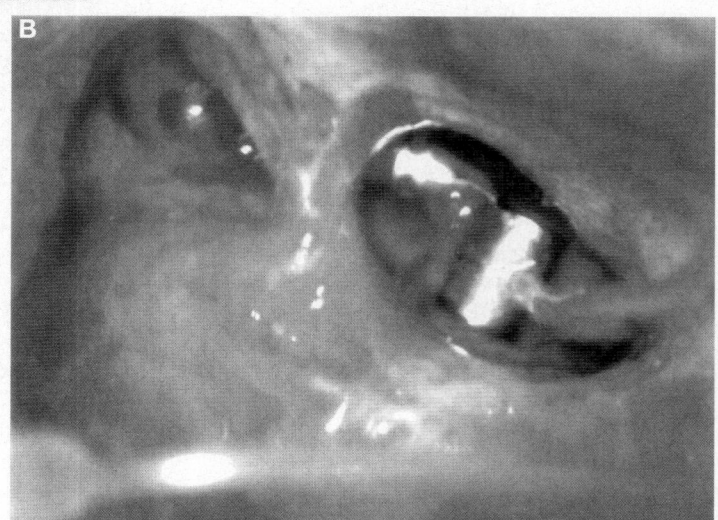

Figure 28–2 *A*, Intraoperative photograph of the widened tympanotomy. *B*, Intraoperative photograph of the Floating Mass Transducer secured to the incus.

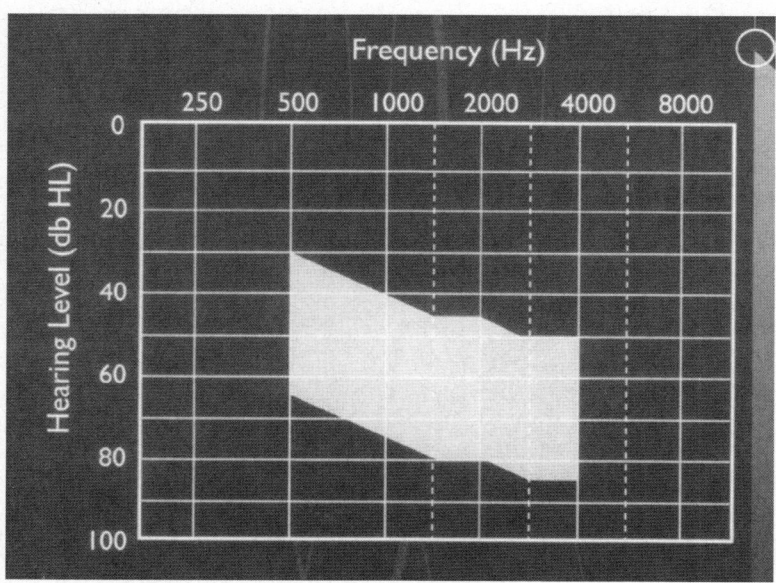

Figure 28–3 Current audiometric indications for the Symphonix Vibrant Soundbridge system.

trial of conventional hearing aids; they must have normal middle ear function and no history of chronic middle ear disease.

Implantation of the VORP uses techniques and approaches similar to those used in cochlear implantation and tympanomastoid surgery. The device can be implanted on an outpatient or overnight stay basis. The patient is prepped and draped as for tympanomastoid surgery. When deciding where to place the implant device, it is important to allow for the wearing of glasses or hats. The VORP is left in the package until the seat site is prepared and the surgeon is ready to implant the device. After the device is on the surgical field, only bipolar cautery should be used.

A myriad of incisions can be considered for placement of the device. We prefer a "reverse question mark" incision, as used in cochlear implant surgery. A simple mastoidectomy is performed in typical fashion, delineating the sigmoid sinus, tegmen, and posterior bony canal wall; the horizontal semicircular canal is identified and the fossa incudis is enlarged, enabling visualization of the short process of the incus through the aditus ad antrum. The device seat is created to stabilize the VORP and to allow for the pre-bent transition of the device conductor link to slope into the mastoidectomy so that the conductor link is as medial to the skull surface as possible. The facial recess (posterior tympanotomy) is

opened and may need to be extended posteriorly and inferiorly to allow for better visualization of the long process of the incus and incudostapedial joint (Figure 28–2, A). The facial nerve is identified, leaving a thin layer of bone over the nerve. The posterior tympanotomy should be large enough to allow for passage of the FMT (approximately the size of a 2.5- or 3.0-mm diameter bur). The buttress (posterior buttress) between the posterior tympanotomy and the aditus ad antrum should not be removed to avoid injury to the posterior incudal ligament.

Placement of the FMT requires the following steps. A small curve is "pre-bent" anteriorly/superiorly in the conductor link, a few millimeters from the FMT. This bend allows the conductor link to clear the bony wall of the facial recess so that it does not impede the movement of the FMT when it is crimped on the incus. Then the FMT is passed through the facial recess using a small suction tip (Figure 28–2, B). When the clip portion of the FMT is in position over the long process of the incus, it is gently pushed onto the incus with a suction tip or a right-angled hook. The clip should be as far superior on the incus as possible, and the axis of the FMT should parallel the axis of the motion of the stapes. Note that the FMT must be in intimate contact with the incudostapedial joint, which allows for contact with the stapes; however, the FMT must not contact the promontory, tympanic membrane, or pyramidal eminence. The

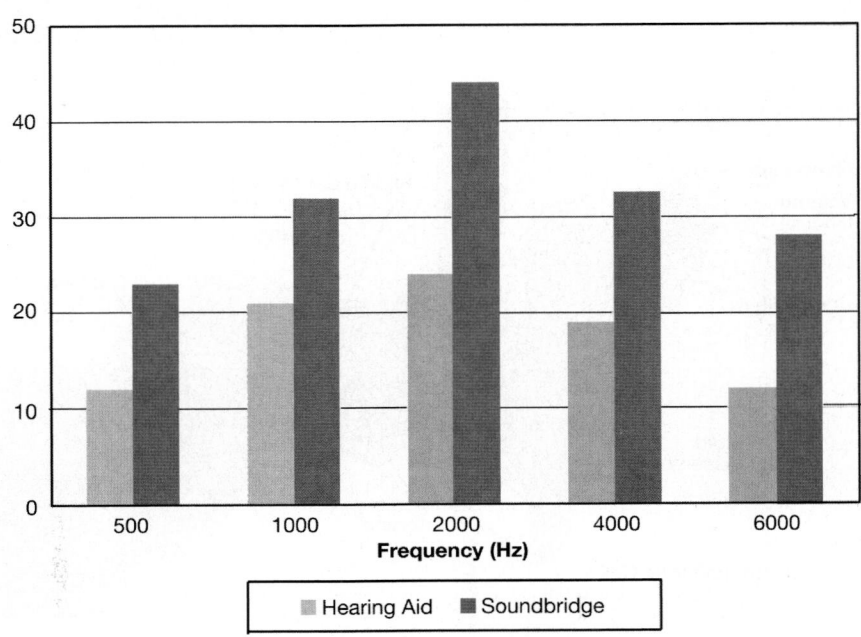

Figure 28–4 Functional gain (in decibels) in 50 patients 6 weeks postoperatively (data from Symphonix Devices, Inc).

FMT attachment clip is secured on the incus using "forming forceps" (Symphonix Devices, Inc), making sure that the jaws of the crimping tool are centered over both legs of the clip so that the attachment is secure.

The incision is closed in routine fashion, and 8 weeks postoperatively, the device is adjusted and activated.

According to data provided by Symphonix Devices,[15] all 54 patients who underwent implantation of the Vibrant Soundbridge noted significant improvement in overall sound clarity and quality. A small (4%) percentage of patients experienced a decrease in residual hearing. The Vibrant Soundbridge resulted in a statistically significant increase in functional gain from 500 through 6,000 Hz when compared to the patient's presurgery aided condition (Figure 28–4). The implant was associated with significantly reduced acoustic feedback, when compared with the patient's own hearing aid, in over 97% of patients. The Vibrant Soundbridge was noted to have enhanced overall fit and comfort in 98% of patients.

SOUNDtec™ Direct Drive Hearing System™

The SOUNDtec (Oklahoma City, Oklahoma) Direct Drive Hearing System (DDHS) consists of an external processing portion and an internally implanted portion. The external processor is located behind the ear (BTE) and consists of a microphone, a preamplifier, and a power amplifier (Figure 28–5). The power amplifier allows for excellent battery life — approximately 600 hours (2 to 4 weeks). The external processor has electrodes that are connected to an electromagnetic coil housed in a custom, deep ear mold, which holds the coil near the tympanic membrane. The implanted portion consists of a neodymium-iron-boron magnet, which is magnetized along its long axis and has a total weight of 27 mg (including its housing). The ideal location of the magnet, for both functional efficiency and surgical accessibility, has been determined to be the incudo-stapedial joint.

Subject selection criteria are (1) bilaterally symmetric, moderate to moderately severe sensorineural hearing loss (Figure 28–6); (2) bone conduction thresholds within 10 dB of air conduction thresholds; (3) discrimination scores greater than 60% (for the NU-6 word list) bilaterally; (4) stable hearing loss of at least 2 years duration; (5) failure of a trial of at least 6 months with an optimally fitted hearing aid; (6) age between 21 and 80 years; and (7) no history of chronic otitis externa/otitis media or of symptoms suggestive of retrocochlear pathology.

Implantation can be performed under local anesthesia, as for a transcanal stapedectomy. A tympanomeatal flap is elevated, and the posterior half of the tympanic cavity is exposed, removing the scutum as necessary to visualize the incudostapedial joint. The incudostapedial joint is separated atraumatically. The attachment ring is

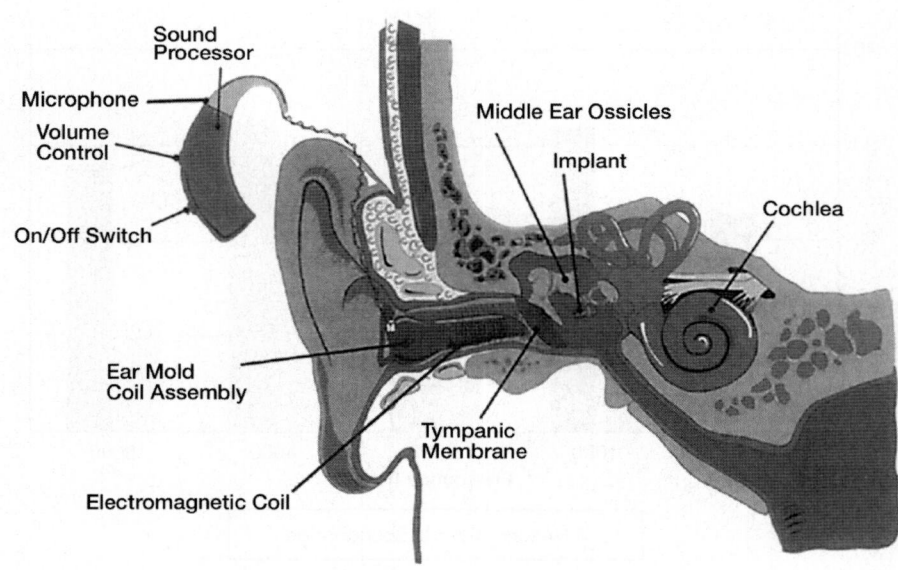

Figure 28–5 The SOUNDtec Direct Drive Hearing System showing the implant, coil assembly, and behind-the-ear processor.

Frequency in Hz

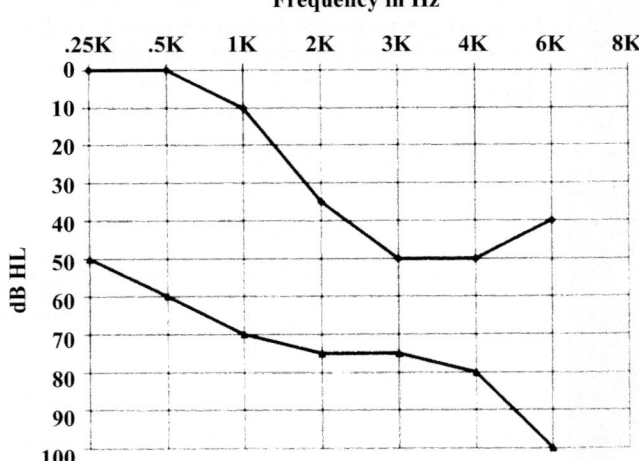

Figure 28–6 Current audiometric criteria for the SOUNDtec Direct Drive Hearing System (pure-tone air conduction thresholds). Upper and lower threshold boundaries are included.

placed around the joint using a suture retraction technique (Figure 28–7). The implant is placed in its desired position with respect to the tympanic membrane, and its axis is aligned with respect to the canal. The surgeon can accomplish this alignment by looking down the canal and maneuvering the cylinder so that its flat top is seen completely and its sides are barely visible around the rim top. A Gelfoam cast is placed around the entire prosthesis for stabilization. The tympanomeatal flap and the tympanic membrane are replaced and the canal is packed in the usual manner.

A 10-week healing period is allowed after implantation before the ear mold assembly is fitted. The ear mold is vented and tapered to be nonocclusive and comfortable.

The results (of the first 10 patients) of a 100-subject, multicenter clinical trial of the SOUNDtec DDHS have been recently reported.[16] There were no effects on residual hearing by loading the stapes with the implant. The SOUNDtec DDHS yielded a 52% improvement in hearing compared with their optimally fitted hearing aids (Figure 28–8). Subjects also noted improvement in ease of communication, ease of hearing in reverberant backgrounds, and ease of hearing in background noise, when compared with their optimally fitted hearing aid.[16] The results to date also suggest an improvement in the quality of life for many patients with hearing impairment.

The adverse effects have been minimal. The risk of additional sensorineural hearing loss was less than 1%; the average conductive loss owing to loading the ossicular chain was 2.6 dB. Owing to the design of the implant, there has been little to no ossicular chain erosion seen.

As with all electromagnetic devices, the interference from other electromagnetic devices can potentially result in extraneous auditory perceptions. Currently, the device must be removed prior to the patient undergoing a magnetic resonance imaging (MRI) scan, although Hough has presented data suggesting MRI compatibility.[16]

Middle Ear Transducer™

Otologics LLC (Boulder, Colorado) is the manufacturer of the Middle Ear Transducer (MET). The unit consists

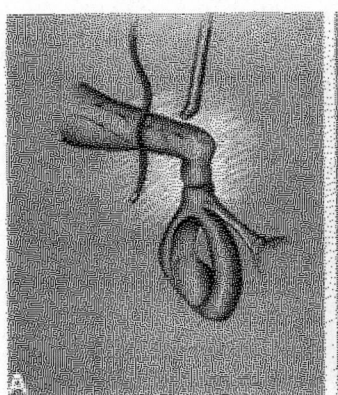 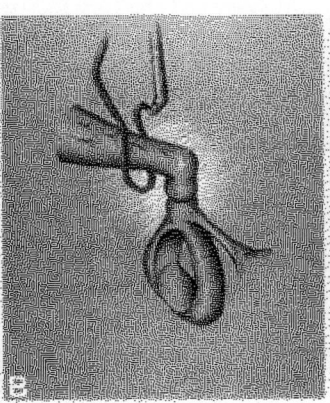 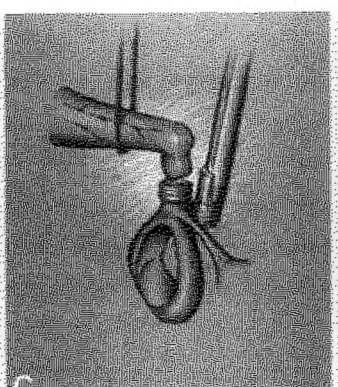 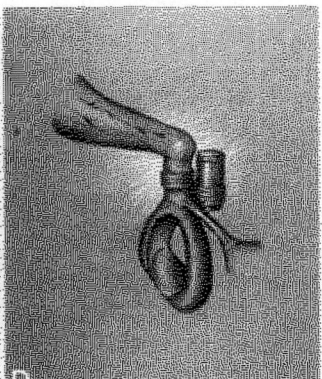

Figure 28–7 Suture retraction technique. *A*, Ball-tipped suture on one side of the incus with a magnetic suture retrieval instrument inserted on the opposite site. *B*, Suture loop formed around the incus to expedite joint incision and wireform insertion. *C*, Retraction of incus while inserting the SOUNDtec wireform ring using a suction insertion instrument. *D*, Magnet and wireform in position with reformation of the incudostapedial joint through the ring.

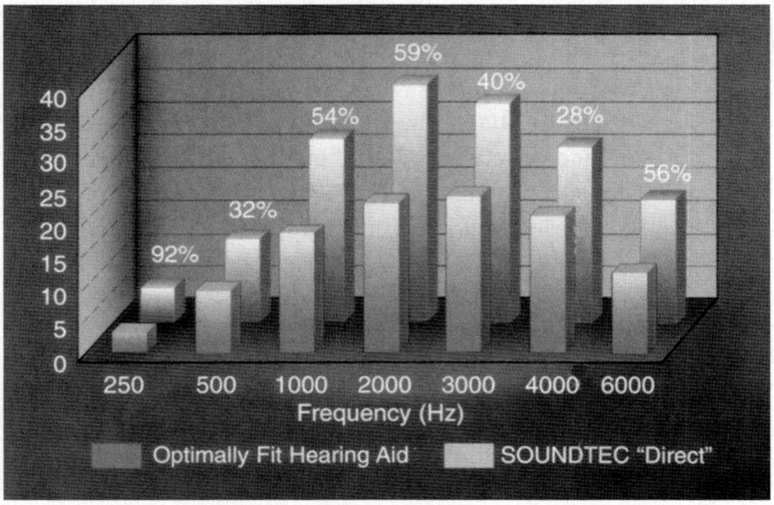

Figure 28–8 Comparison of average improvement in functional gain for the first 10 subjects in the SOUNDtec Direct Drive Hearing System phase II clinical trial.

of two parts: an external component and an implanted component. The external component comprises a microphone, speech processor, battery, and transmitter — all housed in a BTE hearing aid case (Figure 28–9). The implanted portion is composed of a subcutaneous electronic package with a transcutaneous receiver and the middle ear electromagnetic transducer. The transducer attaches directly to the body of the incus. The electromagnetic transducer has a probe, which is coupled to the body of the incus and vibrates the ossicular chain (Figure 28–10). The mechanical advantage of the device offers better impedance matching with more efficient transmission of sound. Outputs of up to 140 dB SPL have

been measured, and the frequency response curve is reported to be flat up to 1,000 Hz (Table 28–2).[17]

The MET is designed for patients with moderately severe to severe sensorineural hearing loss (Figure 28–11). Since the device uses a magnet, it is not MRI compatible and is prone to interference from electromagnetic fields.

The MET is implanted via a postauricular atticotomy. A hole is drilled in the mastoid cortex for the mounting ring, which secures the electromagnetic motor. A laser fenestration is created in the body of the incus for the

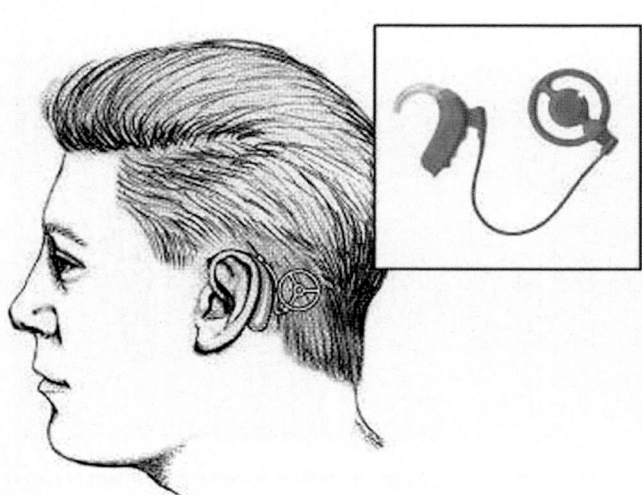

Figure 28–9 The external sound processor of the Middle Ear Transducer system.

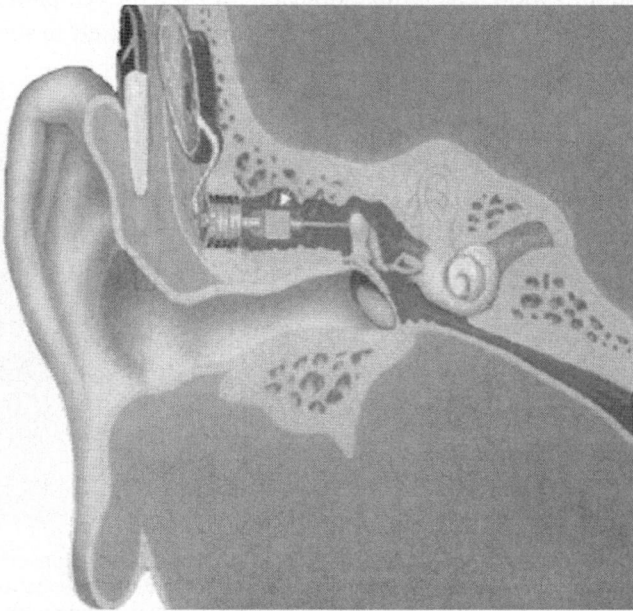

Figure 28–10 Implanted Middle Ear Transducer Ossicular Stimulator.

Table 28–2 AUDIOMETRIC THRESHOLDS FOR THE MIDDLE EAR TRANSDUCER						
	Frequency (kHz)					
Thresholds	0.25	0.5	1	2	4	8
Lower limit	15	15	45	45	45	55
Upper limit	80	85	95	100	105	115

probe tip. The external speech processor is attached and programmed approximately 6 weeks postoperatively.

Envoy™

The Envoy (St. Croix Medical, Minneapolis, Minnesota) is the first fully implantable device to use piezoelectric ceramics. The device consists of a speech processor and two piezoelectric ceramic units — one is a mechanical driver and the other is a sensor (Figure 28–12). The sensor attaches to the malleus, detecting movement of the malleus resulting from tympanic membrane vibration. The mechanical signal thus generated is transformed into an electric signal that is then amplified. The amplified electric signal is relayed to the driver, which is attached to the stapes, and causes the stapes to vibrate. This unique design allows a tremendous reduction in the amount of energy required to drive the system, with a potential battery life of greater than 5 years.

The surgical procedure required for implantation is similar to that used for other devices, that is, a postauricular mastoidectomy performed under general anes-thesia. An atticotomy is performed to allow attachment of the sensor — either to the head of the malleus or the body of the incus (Figure 28–13). The facial recess is opened to allow visualization of the stapes, facial nerve, and chorda tympani nerve. The incudostapedial joint is divided, and the long process of the incus is separated from the body. A considerable amount of space is required in the facial recess to allow for movement of the driver; at times, space limitation necessitates removal of the incus.

St. Croix Medical recently obtained FDA approval to begin testing the Envoy in clinical trials. The results are pending.

Rion

The work of Yanagihara and colleagues with the Rion Company culminated in the development of a partially implantable piezoelectric device (Figure 28–14); more recently, they have begun to investigate a totally implantable system.

The partially implanted device consists of an ossicular vibrator, a microphone, an amplifier, and a transcutaneous transmitter contained in a BTE unit. The microphone converts sound into electrical signals that are fed into the amplifier. After amplification, the electrical signals are transferred to the external link. The piezoelectric biomorph, which is connected to the stapes at one end and secured to the mastoid cortex at the other (Figure 28–15), transforms the electrical signals into vibrations, vibrating the stapes.

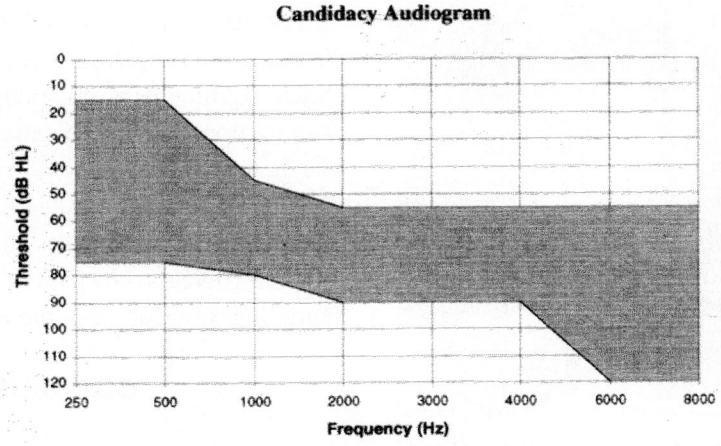

Figure 28–11 Current audiometric thresholds for the Middle Ear Transducer.

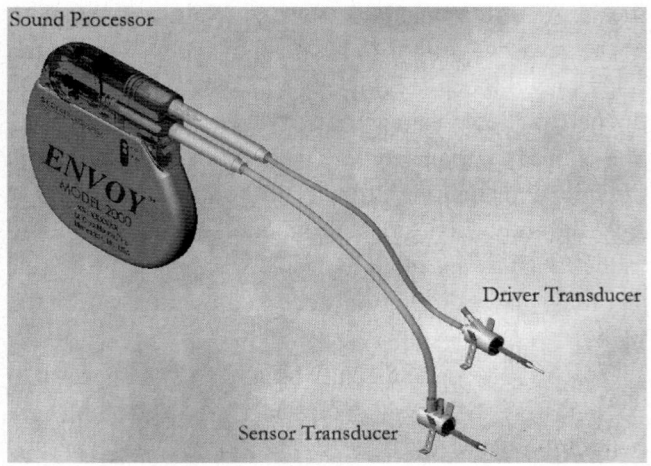

Figure 28–12 The Envoy implant. (Courtesy of St. Croix Medical, Minneapolis, Minnesota.)

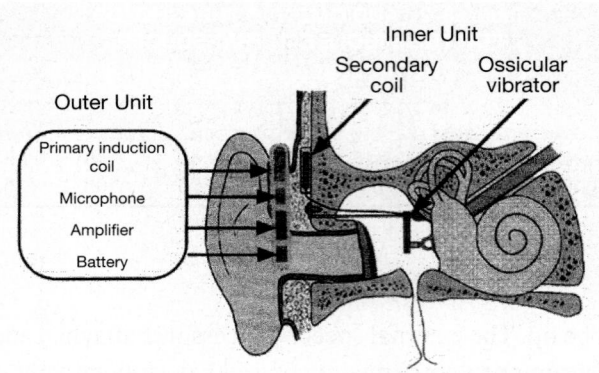

Figure 28–14 The Rion system, type E. A microphone, amplifier, battery, and magnetic coil are housed in an ear level container. Sound signals received by the microphone are amplified and transmitted to the ossicular vibrator by means of magnetic induction.

The device was designed for patients with a conductive hearing loss from chronic otitis media in whom conventional means had failed to restore hearing. Audiologic criteria include a mixed deafness with average bone conduction levels for the speech frequencies (500, 1,000, and 2,000 Hz) not exceeding 50 dB and speech discrimination scores better than 70%.

The device is implanted, using local anesthesia and a postauricular incision, into an individual who has previously undergone a canal wall down or intact canal

wall mastoidectomy (Figure 28–15). The mastoidectomy cavity is enlarged to allow access to the stapes and to accommodate the ossicular vibrator. Once the mastoidectomy is completed, the intraoperative vibratory test is performed.[18] The result of this test indicates the degree of hearing improvement likely to be gained with the device. The mastoid cortex is drilled to allow placement of the internal coil, and the ossicular vibrator is fixed to the temporal bone using screws. The tip of the vibrator element is attached to the head of the stapes. Implantation in a canal wall down mastoidectomy additionally requires removal of the skin lining the mastoid cavity and the external auditory canal with closure of the external auditory canal. An anteriorly based temporalis muscle flap is rotated over the fixing plate and the shaft of the vibrator.

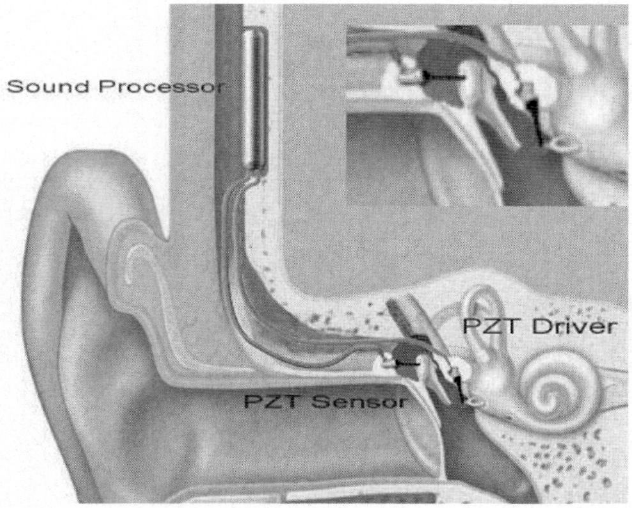

The device has been implanted in Japan over the last 20 years. Hearing level improvements of 36 dB were observed 3 months postoperatively, but at the most recent examination, the improvement decreased to 21 dB.[19] The device is reported to provide natural quality sound, very close to physiologic hearing, without discomfort and feedback.[19] In some cases, the device has functioned for over 10 years. No patient has developed a sensorineural hearing loss from the implantation.

CONCLUSIONS

Middle ear implants appear to enhance sound amplification and sound quality for patients with moderate to

Figure 28–13 Envoy implant coronal view showing the position of the sensor and driver. (Courtesy of St. Croix Medical, Minneapolis, Minnesota.)

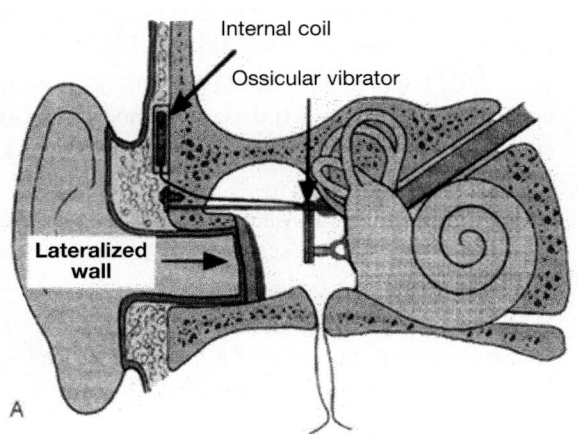
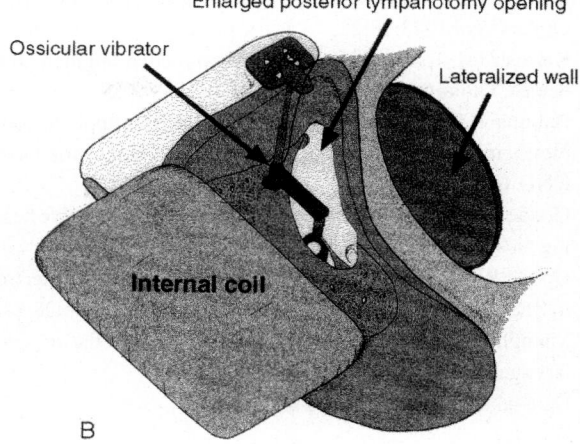

Figure 28–15 Canal wall up implantation procedure for the Rion system. *A*, Principle of the procedure. *B*, Surgical view. The internal component is implanted in the middle ear cavity via the enlarged posterior tympanotomy.

severe sensorineural hearing loss. However, as technology continues to improve, hearing aids may compete with middle ear implants. Similarly, improvements in cochlear implant technology (eg, speech encoding and simulation techniques) have the potential to capture an increasing number of patients who might otherwise be candidates for middle ear implants.

Potentially, there is a large population of patients who can benefit from middle ear implants. However, a careful screening process should be undertaken to identify appropriate candidates. When evaluating a patient for an implantable hearing device, it is imperative that the patient be fitted with a "state-of-the-art" hearing aid prior to electing implantation. The device selected must be matched to the patient's hearing loss because the devices available have differing amplification limitations.

Long-term results for many of the implants are still pending. One concern regards the potential for ossicular necrosis (eg, owing to FMT attachment to the incus or laser fenestration). With the ossicular movement generated by the implant, retrograde sound transmission may occur, necessitating the removal of the incus or the malleus head (as with the Envoy). Another concern is that stereophonic hearing is lost with implantation. Individuals may continue to use a conventional hearing aid in the unimplanted ear, eliminating some of the esthetic benefit gained from a totally implantable middle ear device.

Financial considerations may stand in the way of wide use of middle ear implants as they are not covered (to date) by insurance.

REFERENCES

1. Snik FM, Cremers WRJ. First audiometric results with the Vibrant Sound Bridge, a semi-implantable hearing device for sensorineural hearing loss. Audiology 1999;38:335.
2. Wilska A. Ein Mehtode Zur Bestimmung der horschwellenamplituden des Tarommelfells bei verschieden frequenzen. Skan Arch Physiol 1935;72:161.
3. Vernon J, Brummet R, Johnson B, et al. Evaluation of an implantable type hearing aid by means of cochlear potentials. Volta Rev 1972;1:20.
4. Suzuki J, et al. Problems and solutions in the implantion and acoustic characteristics of an implantable artifical middle ear. Artif Organs 1980;9:495.
5. Suzuki J, et al. Evaluation of a middle ear implant: a six month observation in cats.6 Acta Otolaryngol (Stockh) 1983;95:646.
6. Suzuki J, Kordera K, Yanagihara N. Middle ear implants in humans. Acta Otolaryngol (Stockh) 1985;99:313.
7. Hough J, Dormer K, Meikle M, et al. Middle ear implantable hearing device: ongoing animal and human evaluation. Ann Otol Rhinol Laryngol 1988;97:650.
8. Fredrickson JM, Tomlinson D, Davis ER, et al. Evaluation of an electromagnetic implantable hearing aid. Can J Otolaryngol 1973;2:53.

9. Goode R, Glattle T. Audition via electromagnetic induction. Arch Otolaryngol 1973;98:23.

10. Kartush JM, Tos M. Electromagnetic ossicular augmentation device. Otolaryngol Clin North Am 1995;28:155.

11. Balumann JW, Leysieffer H. Basics of energy supply to completely implantable hearing aids for sensorineural hearing loss. HNO 1998;46:121.

12. Goode RL. Current status of electromagnetic implantable hearing aids. Otolaryngol Clin North Am 1989;22:201.

13. Goode RL. Current status and future of implantable electromagnetic hearing aids. Otolaryngol Clin North Am 1995;28:141.

14. Maniglia AJ. Implantable hearing devices state of the art. Otolaryngol Clin North Am 1989;22:175.

15. Data taken from Vibrant Soundbridge.

16. Hough JVD, et al. Semi-implantable electromagnetic middle ear hearing device for moderate to severe sensorineural hearing loss. Otolaryngol Clin North Am 1989;22:175.

17. Fredrickson JM, Coticchia JM, Khosla S. Ongoing investigations into an implantable electromagnetic hearing aid for moderate to severe sensorineural hearing loss. Otolaryngol Clin North Am 1995;22:107.

18. Yanagihara N, Aritomo H, Yamanaka E, et al. Intraoperative assessment of vibratory-induced hearing. Adv Audiol 1988;4:124.

19. Yanagihara N, et al. Long-term results using a piezoelectric semi-implantable middle ear hearing device — the Rion Device E-type. Otolaryngol Clin North Am 2001;34:389.

VI

Surgery of the Inner Ear

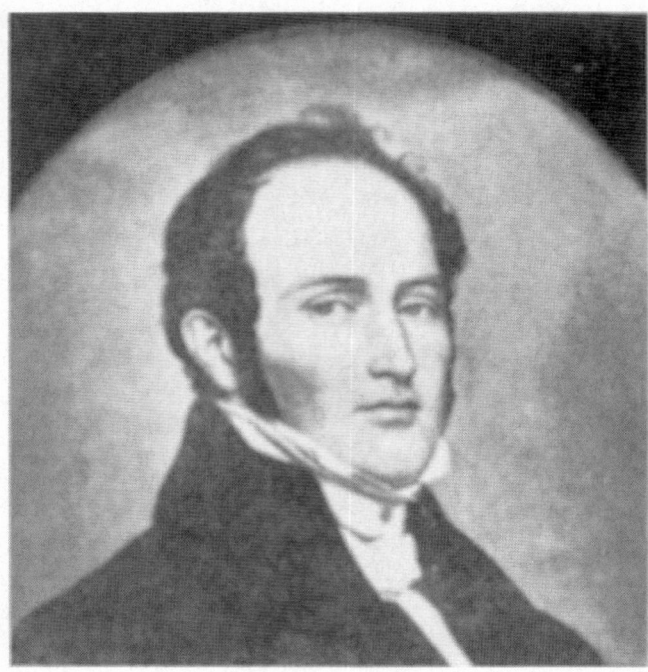

Prosper Meniere (1799–1862). Described the symptomatology and proved the labyrinthine origin of episodic vertigo with deafness.

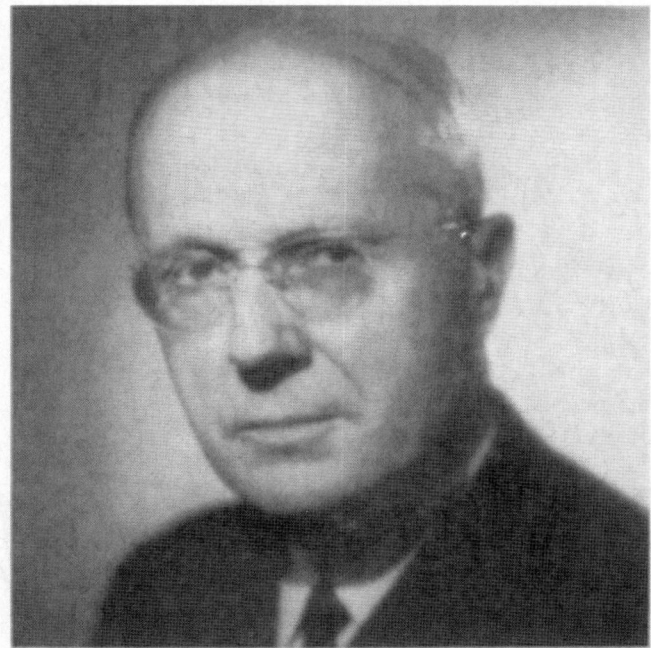

Georges Portmann (1890–1985). Proposed surgical drainage of the endolymphatic sac for Ménière's disease.

29

Surgical Treatment of Peripheral Vestibular Disorders

JOHN R. E. DICKINS, MD
SHARON S. GRAHAM, MS

HISTORICAL ASPECTS

The triad of clinical symptoms consisting of episodic vertigo, fluctuating hearing loss, and tinnitus was first attributed to a vestibular rather than a cerebral disorder by Prosper Meniere.[1] Thus, the disease, also referred to as idiopathic endolymphatic hydrops, now bears his name. In a series of articles in 1861,[2] Meniere noted the symptoms of repeated attacks of vertigo with nausea and vomiting that recurred frequently over a period of weeks, months, or years with long, asymptomatic periods except for hearing loss. Describing the hearing loss as ordinarily unilateral, sensorineural, and involving primarily the low frequencies, Meniere also described associated tinnitus. In 1923, Shambaugh and Knudson[3] described the symptom of diplacusis; Crowe[4] noted the tendency toward hearing fluctuation. Fowler[5] and Dix and colleagues[6] found recruitment to be characteristic of the sensorineural hearing loss; and Cawthorne[7] and Lindsay[8] confirmed pathologically that Meniere's disease produced marked distention of the endolymphatic labyrinth in the cochlea and vestibule. In 1871, Knapp[9] postulated that this distention was caused by increased endolymphatic pressure, comparing this inner ear hydrops with glaucoma. This theory was adapted in 1926 by Portmann,[10] who further theorized that decompression of the endolymphatic system should relieve the symptoms of this disorder. In 1938, Hallpike and Cairns[11] in England, and Yamakawa,[12] independently and simultaneously in Japan, reported the histopathologic finding of endolymphatic hydrops in Meniere's disease.

Over the past 30 years, endolymphatic hydrops has been documented to have many causes, including labyrinthine injury, inflammation, and congenital anomaly. Accordingly, Meniere's disease is the term applied to the symptoms of hydrops only when the cause remains enigmatic (ie, idiopathic endolymphatic hydrops).

Theories abound attempting to explain other disorders causing recurrent episodes of vertigo, without the associated symptoms of Meniere's disease. These disorders include benign paroxysmal positional vertigo (BPPV), which Schuknecht[13] attributed to cupulolithiasis; disabling positional vertigo, which Janetta and colleagues[14] believes arises from vascular compression of the eighth cranial nerve; and the myriad of vestibular symptoms related by Fee,[15] among others, to a perilymph fistula of the labyrinth.

The initial surgical procedures used for the treatment of vertigo were destructive. In 1904, Parry[16] reported intracranial section of the eighth cranial nerve, whereas Milligan[17] and Lake[18] published their techniques for opening the lateral semicircular canal and vestibule. In 1928, Dandy[19] advocated complete eighth cranial nerve section for relief of vertigo in Meniere's disease; however, 2 years earlier, Portmann[10] had performed the first endolymphatic sac decompression, beginning the trend for the conservative management of Meniere's disease.

In accordance with the theory that Meniere's disease is secondary to overproduction or underabsorption of endolymph, a variety of endolymphatic sac decompression procedures have been developed and used over the past several decades. Shambaugh[20] proposed that underabsorption was caused by ischemia of the endolymphatic sac and recommended decompression of the endolymphatic sac through the mastoid for treatment. Actual exposure and opening of the endolymphatic sac for drainage were proposed by House,[21] who used an endolymphatic subarachnoid shunt. Paparella[22] advocated drainage into the mastoid with an endolymphatic mastoid shunt, whereas Arenberg and colleagues,[23] believing endolymphatic hydrops to be analogous to glaucoma, used a unidirectional valve placed into the endolymphatic duct. Other drainage procedures included repetitive puncture of the saccule through the oval window by Fick[24] and Cody.[25] Creating a "permanent" connection (ie, a fistula) between the endolymphatic and perilymphatic compartments has also been attempted via the round window by disrupting the basilar membrane (House, the otic-periotic shunt)[26] or by fracture displacement of the osseous spiral lamina (Schuknecht, cochleosacculotomy).[27] Other conservative methods, including cryosurgery and application of ultrasonography to the labyrinth, also attempted to create a permanent fistula between the endolymphatic and perilymphatic systems. All conservative procedures have met with limited and variable success.

Destructive procedures are of proven efficacy in controlling vertigo of peripheral origin, but this efficacy carries with it the expense of total hearing loss in the operated ear. In 1957, Schuknecht[28] described transcanal labyrinthectomy for the control of vertigo secondary to peripheral dysfunction. Transmastoid labyrinthectomy, with or without eighth cranial nerve section, has been described as the surest method to destroy all labyrinthine neuroepithelium.[29] Section of the vestibular nerve via the suboccipital approach, first attempted by Parry,[16] was reported in 1941 by Dandy[30] to be effective in controlling Meniere's disease. During his career, Dandy performed over 600 retrosigmoid (suboccipital) vestibular neurectomies for Meniere's disease. In the 1950s, House[31] developed the middle cranial fossa route for exposure of the internal auditory canal and advocated its use for selective superior vestibular nerve section. Total middle fossa vestibular nerve section was later reported by Glasscock and associates[32] and Fisch[33]; this procedure afforded excellent control of vertigo, with a good possibility of hearing preservation. The retrosigmoid approach was first described by Pulec and Hitselberger[34] and was later popularized by Silverstein and Norrell for vestibular nerve section.[35] The retrosigmoid exposure allows improved visualization of the cleavage plane between the cochlear and vestibular nerves, thus allowing complete and selective sectioning of the vestibular nerve. Recently, intratympanic gentamicin injec-

tion has largely replaced the use of nerve section in the treatment of Meniere's disease.

ETIOLOGY OF MENIERE'S DISEASE

Despite the detailed description of the pathology of Meniere's disease, namely, endolymphatic hydrops, its cause remains unknown. It is thought that inadequate resorption, rather than abnormal production of endolymph, underlies the development of endolymphatic hydrops. Production of endolymphatic hydrops in experimental animals by blockage or destruction of the endolymphatic sac[36] implicates dysfunction of the sac in inadequate reabsorption. Shambaugh[37] postulated that dysfunction of the sac was caused by reduced vascularity and advocated sac decompression as a means to improve blood supply and therefore reabsorption by the sac. Later studies by Gussen[38] reinforced the theory of vascular insufficiency. In the face of continued endolymph production, functional failure of the sac results in distention of the endolymphatic system as endolymph slowly and progressively accumulates. This distention eventually culminates in membrane rupture, with release of endolymph into the perilymphatic system. The toxic effect of the high potassium concentration of endolymph on structures normally bathed in perilymph precipitates vertigo and hearing loss.

A variety of disorders can cause the symptoms of Meniere's disease. Metabolic disorders linked to Meniere's include thyroid dysfunction, elevated triglycerides, and diabetes mellitus. Immunologic disorders and allergy[39,40] have also been considered to play a role in the development of Meniere's. Autoimmune disorders have been implicated as etiologic by patient history, with only marginal laboratory findings.[41] Antecedent viral infection, bacterial infection, and syphilis have all been associated with the symptoms of Meniere's disease.

EVALUATION OF THE PATIENT WITH VERTIGO

In the evaluation of any patient, obtaining an accurate and complete history is the first and most important step. In patients with vertigo, two major factors complicate obtaining the history. One is the lack of a defined language for describing vestibular dysfunction. The symptom of vertigo is one of spatial disorientation.

Being out of touch with one's surroundings can manifest in a number of different ways. Vertigo may be described as a sense of rotation in relationship to the environment, where either the patient or the environment is moving. This sense of rotation may be in either the horizontal or vertical axis. Unsteadiness is characterized by loss of equilibrium, often with a sensation of falling to one side or the other or forward or backward. Lightheadedness is most commonly described as a sense of fainting or of impending syncope. Without a standard language to describe these sensations, not unlike trying to describe pain, the patient and physician may have difficulty communicating. For this reason, similar stimuli may evoke a much more intense reaction in one patient than another. The second complicating factor comprises the myriad of medical conditions that may be contributory. Neurologic problems such as multiple sclerosis or peripheral disease can present with dizziness. Cardiac arrhythmias, gastrointestinal problems, and endocrine problems all may have some degree of dizziness, lightheadedness, or presyncope as a symptom. One of the most common causes of dizziness is medication use, be it prescription, nonprescription, herbal, or recreational. Prescription medications can be of particular concern in the elderly.

As the patient describes the symptoms, careful attention to clues helps lead to a diagnosis. A detailed history of past otologic problems is important, particularly noting episodes of recurrent infections, prior ear surgery, or a history of cholesteatoma or chronic otitis media.

It is helpful to distinguish vertigo of spontaneous onset from that induced by positional changes. In the patient with spontaneous episodic vertigo, the frequency and duration of the spells are important, as is a description of the initial episode. Not uncommonly, sporadic spells may have occurred years in the past, only to recur at a later date with increased frequency. The severity of the spells is measured by disability related to vegetative symptoms such as nausea, vomiting, diaphoresis, and even diarrhea. The length of the spell extends from onset to the resumption of normal activity. Headache and neck discomfort are not uncommon; the severity and duration of the headache should be noted as the severity may be suggestive of central nervous system problems such as migraine. Any auditory symptoms that may precede the spell such as fullness, hearing loss, tinnitus, diplacusis, or recruitment should be noted.

If the vertigo is induced by positional changes, an accurate description of the provocative movement is critical. A prior history of head trauma or of episodes of acute, spontaneous vertigo prior to the onset of the movement-induced vertigo may help clarify the history.

Probing for neurologic symptoms accompanying the spells is important, as is a careful review of the past medical history, looking specifically for cardiac, neurologic, gastrointestinal, or endocrine disease. Inadequately controlled diabetes mellitus may present with dizziness. Patients who have known autoimmune disease may present with the symptoms of Meniere's disease. Their treatment is usually aided by control of their underlying autoimmune process.

Patients with vertigo frequently present with substantial psychiatric overlay. A recent study by Anderson and colleagues[42] has shown that episodic vertigo, when evaluated by a series of quality of life measures, is one of the most debilitating diseases not requiring hospitalization. Although outwardly appearing fairly normal, these patients are no longer capable of day-to-day activities. Being at risk of the sudden onset of vertigo, nausea, and vomiting diminishes the confidence to participate in many normal life activities. Stress tends to aggravate the spells. Because of this association between stress and episodes of vertigo, patients may be labeled as having psychiatric problems.

A thorough neurotologic examination, with special attention to evaluation of all of the cranial nerves, is mandatory. Microscopic examination of the ear should be performed to rule out evidence of otitis media, cholesteatoma, or middle ear mass. A general neurologic examination, including cerebellar testing, may be helpful in determining the site of the lesion.

A universal complement to the findings of the history and physical examination of the patient with vertigo is a complete audiogram including speech discrimination testing and impedance audiometry. On completion of the standard audiogram, there may be enough information for a tentative diagnosis and a trial of medical therapy. However, if standard audiometry is not strongly suggestive of an etiology or if medical therapy fails, then a more in-depth evaluation of the audiovestibular system is indicated. The auditory brainstem response, although not always sensitive to eighth nerve lesions, may be of substantial benefit in pinpointing the location of auditory pathway dysfunction, which may suggest a diagnosis.

Electrocochleography is employed in an attempt to identify hydrops, particularly in atypical cases. Whereas Coates[43] and Morrison and colleagues[44] reported that a prolonged summating potential is indicative of hydrops, Ferraro and coworkers[45] believe that a prolonged summating potential and an enlarged summating to action potential ratio are pathognomonic of hydrops. Although these changes occur predominantly in symptomatic ears, they may be helpful in evaluating the asymptomatic ear. Electrocochleography can be done either transtympanically or extratympanically with a canal leaf electrode, which is felt to be less accurate but easier to perform. Otoacoustic emissions, particularly distortion-product otoacoustic emissions, have been studied in patients with hydrops, but no consistent pattern has been detected.

Dehydration testing,[46] using either glycerol or urea, can cause a transient improvement in the sensorineural hearing loss, fullness, and tinnitus of Meniere's disease. Dehydration test results (decrease, no change, or, in rare cases, a worsening of hearing) can help to clarify therapeutic options. Glycerol testing is not commonly used today because of headaches as a frequent side effect. Urea causes fewer headaches but also less dehydration.

Vestibular testing should include electronystagmography with caloric and positional testing, which provides useful data for identifying the symptomatic ear and documents the functional status of the asymptomatic ear. Of some diagnostic help is the fact that the subjective symptoms induced by the caloric test are frequently very similar in character to, although usually less severe than, those experienced in a classic Meniere's attack. Computerized dynamic platform testing combines vestibulo-ocular and vestibulospinal information in an attempt to define a vestibular disorder; it also attempts to evaluate the coordination of the vestibulospinal responses to visual and proprioceptive input.[47] Rotary chair testing can help differentiate peripheral from central causes of vertigo by comparison of the gain and symmetry of the response. Although there is no single, definitive test, it appears that evaluation of the results of a combination of tests can lead to a more precise identification of site of lesion and degree of dysfunction in patients with vertigo.

Typically, laboratory evaluation for vertigo is not productive since most patients are referred after having been evaluated by an internist or family practitioner. For patients who have not previously undergone medical evaluation, tests to consider include a complete blood count, a lipid profile, and a fasting blood sugar. Should the fasting blood sugar be abnormal, a 5-hour glucose tolerance test is indicated. Serologic testing for syphilis should be considered as syphilitic otitis can mimic Meniere's disease. Evaluation for autoimmune disease is frequently omitted from a general medical evaluation. It is known that patients with rheumatoid arthritis, systemic lupus erythematosus, and other autoimmune diseases may manifest the symptoms of Meniere's disease, as may individuals with autoimmune inner ear disease (AIED). Routine screening of immune function is probably unnecessary but should be considered in atypical Meniere's (eg, Meniere's disease presenting bilaterally or Meniere's unresponsive to routine therapy).[48–52]

Radiologic evaluation of patients with vertigo is helpful. Magnetic resonance imaging (MRI) scans provide an adequate evaluation for skull base tumors, cerebellopontine angle lesions, vascular disease, multiple sclerosis, and vascular compression of the eighth nerve.

Computed tomographic (CT) scanning is preferred for the evaluation of chronic ear disease, cholesteatoma, an enlarged vestibular aqueduct,[53] or a dehiscent superior semicircular canal.[54]

DIFFERENTIAL DIAGNOSIS OF VERTIGO

Potential diagnoses for patients with vertigo are numerous. In spite of a thorough evaluation, as outlined above, it is not uncommon for the clinician to be unable to arrive at a precise diagnosis. At present, the inability to sample inner ear fluid pressures and analyze endolymphatic or perilymphatic chemical composition tends to make a precise diagnosis problematic at best. For this reason, most diagnoses of vertigo are tentative; only over a trial period of therapy is a correct diagnosis confirmed. It should be the intention of the clinician to constantly reassess whether the working diagnosis remains viable at follow-up appointments.

ACUTE, NONRECURRENT VERTIGO

The most common cause of acute vertigo is vestibular neuronitis. Evidence suggests that in the vast majority of cases there is a viral cause, which may often represent a reactivation of a *herpes simplex* virus infection.[55,56] However, ischemia, either of the peripheral labyrinth or of the brainstem, can present similarly and must be considered as indicated by associated medical conditions. Typically, vestibular neuronitis presents with the acute onset of vertigo, nausea, and vomiting. There may be a mild spell preceding the major episode by 1 to 2 days. The usual course begins with severe illness for 24 to 48 hours, followed by several days of moderate dysequilibrium and then a protracted period of weeks to months of movement-induced vertigo as the symptoms gradually resolve. Although most patients are free of symptoms after recovery from the acute episode, some go on to experience recurrent episodes of vertigo.[57]

EPISODIC VERTIGO

Meniere's Disease

The hearing loss of Meniere's disease is so characteristic that frequently the diagnosis is suggested simply by this portion of the history and examination. Patients frequently note fullness in one ear that may be intense enough to be described as pain. Tinnitus, or a change in baseline tinnitus, may accompany the fullness. Hearing loss, sound distortion, or recruitment then occurs; this prodrome is completed with an acute severe spell of vertigo. Not uncommonly, after the vertigo has passed, the hearing will temporarily improve, only to deteriorate with the onset of another episode. These episodes of vertigo may be separated by days, months, or even years. Between spells, there may be periods of dysequilibrium or movement-induced vertigo, depending on the severity of the damage to the vestibular system. The hearing loss may fluctuate and/or progress. Rarely, Meniere's disease may present with a sudden hearing loss. The majority of patients tend to have unilateral disease initially; however, with extended follow-up, the disease often becomes bilateral. Atypical forms of Meniere's disease include vestibular Meniere's and cochlear Meniere's. Vestibular Meniere's can be difficult to diagnose as episodic vertigo occurs without associated aural symptoms. Vestibular Meniere's tends to respond to the same medical therapy as typical Meniere's and frequently progresses to typical Meniere's disease. Cochlear Meniere's manifests with recurrent aural fullness, fluctuation in hearing (especially in the low frequencies), and tinnitus, without episodic vertigo or dysequilibrium. As with vestibular Meniere's, cochlear Meniere's responds to the medical management of typical Meniere's disease and tends to progress to full-blown Meniere's disease.

Estimates of the bilateral frequency of Meniere's disease vary widely. Paparella and Griebe[58] have suggested that approximately 50% of patients will develop Meniere's disease in the contralateral ear, and in the majority of cases, the second ear will become involved within 5 years. If the second ear becomes involved rapidly (within the first year), the possibility of AIED must be considered.

One of the major problems with the literature on Meniere's disease is the inconsistency of definition of data. In an attempt to clarify the reporting of treatment results, the American Academy of Otolaryngology-Head and Neck Surgery (AAO-HNS) has attempted to establish reporting criteria (Table 29–1).[59,60]

ACQUIRED ENDOLYMPHATIC HYDROPS

Classic Meniere's disease occurs in ears with no prior otologic disease. In other patients, the diagnosis can clearly be traced to a specific etiology or event. Schuknecht and Gulya[61] described a simple classification system for Meniere's disease that facilitates understanding of the disease. Classic Meniere's disease is classified as idiopathic symptomatic hydrops. Those cases that develop following infection (either viral or bacterial), trauma, AIED, or other causes are classified as symptomatic acquired hydrops. Those cases associated with congenital inner ear dysplasia are classified as symptomatic embryopathic hydrops. Over the years, many patients initially classified as idiopathic have been reclassified into the acquired or embryopathic group.

Autoimmune Inner Ear Disease

Autoimmune inner ear disease, described by McCabe,[48] Hughes and colleagues,[49] Harris,[50] and others, is believed to be an autoimmune disorder in which the inner ear is the sole target. Autoimmune inner ear disease appears more common than first described by McCabe. Patients

Table 29–1 AAO-HNS CRITERIA FOR MENIERE'S DISEASE*		

In 1996, the Committee on Hearing and Equilibrium reaffirmed and clarified the 1985 guidelines, adding initial staging and reporting guidelines.

Vertigo
a. Any treatment should be evaluated no sooner than 24 months
b. Formula to obtain numeric value for vertigo: average number of definitive spells/month in a 24-month period after therapy _____ × 100 = numeric value
c. Numeric value scale

Numeric Value	Control Level	Class
0	Complete control of definitive spells	A
41–80	Limited control of definitive spells	B
81–120	Insignificant control of definitive spells	C
>120 Worse		D
Secondary treatment initiated		E

Disability
a. No disability
b. Mild disability: intermittent or continuous dizziness/unsteadiness that precludes working in a hazardous environment
c. Moderate disability: intermittent or continuous dizziness that results in a sedentary occupation
d. Severe disability: symptoms so severe as to exclude gainful employment

Hearing
a. Hearing is measured by a four-frequency pure-tone average (PTA) of 500 Hz, 1 kHz, 2 kHz, and 3 kHz
b. Pretreatment hearing level: worst hearing level during 6 months prior to surgery
c. Post-treatment hearing level: poorest hearing level measured 18–24 months after institution of therapy
d. Hearing classification:
   i.   Unchanged = –10-dB PTA or –15% speech discrimination
   ii. Improved >10-dB PTA improved or > 15% discrimination improved
   iii. Worse > 10-dB PTA worsened or >15% discrimination worsened

In 1996, the Committee on Hearing and Equilibrium reaffirmed and clarified the guidelines, adding initial staging and reporting guidelines.

Initial Hearing Level

Stage	Four-tone average (dB)
1	≤ 25
2	26–40
3	41–70
4	> 70

Functional Level Scale

This is a subjective scale determined by the patients.
Regarding my current state of overall function, not just during attacks.
1 My dizziness has no effect on my activities at all.
2 When I am dizzy, I have to stop for a while, but it soon passes and I can resume my activities. I continue to work, drive, and engage in any activity I choose without restriction. I have not changed any plans or activities to accommodate my dizziness.
3 When I am dizzy I have to stop what I am doing for a while, but it does pass and I can resume activities. I continue to work, drive, and engage in most activities I choose, but I have had to change some plans and make some allowance for my dizziness.
4 I am able to work, drive, travel, and take care of a family or engage in most activities, but I must exert a great deal of effort to do so. I must constantly make adjustments in my activities and budget my energies. I am barely making it.
5 I am unable to work, drive, or take care of a family. I am unable to do most of the active things that I used to do. Even essential activities must be limited. I am disabled.
6 I have been disabled for 1 year or longer and/or I receive compensation because of my dizziness or balance problem.

*Adapted from the Committee on Hearing and Equilibrium.[59,60]

classically present with bilateral, rapidly progressing sensorineural hearing loss, with or without vertigo, that is unresponsive to the standard therapy for Meniere's disease but that almost universally responds to high-dose corticosteroids. Establishing the diagnosis of AIED remains problematic; response to a trial of corticosteroid therapy is often used as a diagnostic indicator. Western blot analysis for antibodies to heat shock protein 70 and lymphocyte transformation testing are being studied for use in the diagnosis and possible therapeutic monitoring of AIED.[51] At this writing, neither has achieved a level of accuracy to prompt widespread use.

Routine laboratory results for immune system function tend to be normal. Any patient with apparent bilateral Meniere's disease, at presentation or on a delayed (within 5 years) basis, should be evaluated for AIED.

Trauma

Oval and round window perilymph fistulae can present with fluctuating, progressive sensorineural hearing loss and episodic vertigo and may occur following closed head injury, significant barotrauma, or stapedectomy. The existence of spontaneous oval or round window fistulae has been a subject of continued debate over the years.[62,63] Most studies suggest that spontaneous fistulization is a rare event and is usually associated with an anomalous labyrinth. Certainly, any patient with a history of barotrauma or head injury should be evaluated for a perilymph fistula. Fistulae usually close spontaneously; however, continued symptoms after a period of bed rest for several days suggest the need for exploration of the middle ear.

Labyrinthine Concussion

Following head injury, with or without temporal bone fracture, some patients may develop symptoms mimicking Meniere's disease secondary to intralabyrinthine damage. Labyrinthine concussion may be difficult to distinguish from postconcussion syndrome; differentiation must be made as the therapeutic modalities are different.

Migraine

Basilar artery migraine can be very difficult to differentiate from Meniere's disease as it can present with fluctuating hearing loss, episodic vertigo, dysequilibrium, and tinnitus. Typically, the pain of a migraine headache is much worse than the typical muscle tension headache seen in patients with Meniere's disease. Johnson[64] has reviewed the diagnostic differences between Meniere's disease and migraine. For those patients who have the symptoms of Meniere's disease and are unresponsive to routine therapy, a therapeutic trial of migraine treatment may be considered. Vestibular and auditory testing, other than detecting a positive dehydration test or abnormal electrocochleography, is not beneficial in distinguishing the two entities.

Enlarged Vestibular Aqueduct

Patients presenting in their teens to early twenties with episodic vertigo and a fluctuating or progressive hearing loss should be evaluated for the presence of an enlarged vestibular aqueduct. As described by Emmett,[53] this congenital abnormality consists of an abnormally wide vestibular aqueduct. On CT scan, the duct is ≥ 1.5 mm wide in diameter. These patients have progressive/fluctuating hearing loss of variable severity, which may follow even a minor head injury; they may have episodic vertigo as well. The symptoms are thought to relate to the excessive transmission of cerebrospinal fluid (CSF) pressure to the inner ear. Current therapeutic modalities are limited, although many patients transiently respond to the medical therapy used for Meniere's disease. Welling and colleagues[65] reported their results in 10 patients who underwent occlusion of the enlarged aqueduct in an attempt to control progression of the hearing loss. Nine of the 10 patients suffered some hearing loss associated with the surgery and 5 had a loss exceeding 25 dB. These investigators cautioned against surgical occlusion of the enlarged aqueduct.

Infections

Syphilitic otitis can mimic Meniere's disease, still exists, and must be considered within the diagnostic possibilities.

POSITIONAL VERTIGO

Benign Paroxysmal Positional Vertigo

Vertigo is induced in BPPV by motion such as lying down, rolling over, or raising the head to look up. The spells usually occur 5 to 10 seconds following the movement, last 10 to 20 seconds, and may be particularly violent. Schuknecht and Ruby[66] theorized that BPPV reflected cupulolithiasis affecting the posterior semicircular canal on the basis of the temporal bone histopathologic finding of particles adhering to the ampulla of the posterior semicircular canal. According to this theory, otoconia from the utricle become dislodged and attach to the posterior semicircular canal ampulla, rendering it sensitive to gravity. Others have postulated that canalolithiasis (free-floating particles) underlies BPPV.[54]

Nonclassic Benign Positional Vertigo

Following vestibular neuronitis or head injury, patients often experience a period of movement-induced vertigo, which usually diminishes with time and exercise. Symptoms do not quite fit the criteria for classic BPPV as described by Dix and colleagues.[6] Other types of paroxysmal positional vertigo have been described, involving primarily the horizontal semicircular canal. Minor[54] has described vertigo brought on by head movement or loud noise that is related to dehiscence of the superior semicircular canal.

OTHER CAUSES OF VERTIGO

Eustachian Tube Dysfunction

Eustachian tube dysfunction can cause aural fullness, pressure, and, occasionally, vertigo. Usually, vertigo develops in association with myringostapediopexy or myringoincudopexy in which motion of the tympanic membrane impacts directly on the stapes, causing vertigo. Many patients with endolymphatic hydrops, simply because of fullness in the ear, have been subjected to a series of useless tubal inflations. To quote Hilger, "The eager and repetitious catheter has been a poor substitute for diagnosis much over-long."[68] The differentiation of early hydrops and eustachian tube dysfunction may not be easy.

Middle Ear and Mastoid Disease

If associated with cholesteatoma, chronic otitis media, and/or modified radical mastoidectomy, vertigo may reflect direct labyrinthine involvement, either through a fistula, serous labyrinthitis, or bacterial labyrinthitis. Infection in the surrounding tissue, such as an infected modified radical mastoidectomy cavity or an infected mastoid, can lead to vertigo via serous labyrinthitis. The diagnosis and treatment of these disorders are described elsewhere.

Vascular Compression Syndrome

Janetta and colleagues[14] have described a variety of syndromes secondary to large vessel and microvascular compression of cranial nerves as they exit the brainstem, including trigeminal neuralgia and hemifacial spasm. It is thought that cranial nerve compression may also precipitate intractable tinnitus, hearing loss, and vertigo and can be successfully treated with decompression. Brackmann[69] has reaffirmed that, in certain patients, vascular decompression can alleviate incapacitating positional vertigo. Brackmann uses air-contrast CT scanning to determine which patients might benefit from this procedure.

Cerebellopontine Angle and Skull Base Lesions

Tumors involving the eighth nerve or invading the otic capsule typically do not present with episodic vertigo but rather with progressive hearing loss and dysequilibrium. On occasion, however, such tumors may present with episodic vertigo. Benign tumors such as meningiomas, cholesterol granulomas, and glomus tumors can present at the skull base, causing otologic symptoms. In the cerebellopontine angle, the most common tumors are vestibular schwannomas and meningiomas; other tumors, such as lipomas and epidermoids, are encountered less frequently. Malignant tumors, most commonly breast, prostate, and lung cancers, can metastasize to the skull base or the cerebellopontine angle as well as spread along the meninges.

CENTRAL NERVOUS SYSTEM VERTIGO

A common cause of dysequilibrium and vertigo of central nervous system origin is microvascular disease, especially in patients over 60 years of age. Treatment appropriate for Meniere's disease, especially sedatives, tends to make these patients worse. Avoidance of labyrinthine sedatives, treatment of vascular insufficiency, and physical therapy may well help stabilize and improve the quality of life. Multiple sclerosis and cerebellar degeneration may mimic Meniere's disease and must be ruled out.

Patients with acute ischemia of the brainstem caused by small vessel disease may present similarly to vestibular neuronitis. The course tends to be much longer with much greater ataxia; also, these patients are in an older age group. For those who continue to have problems beyond the normal 4- to 6-week time frame, vestibular testing can aid in identifying the site of lesion. In addition to brainstem ischemia, occlusion of the labyrinthine artery can present with profound hearing loss and severe vertigo and has a course similar to that of viral neuronitis.

Dolichoectasia of the basilar artery may distort the eighth nerve, producing a Meniere's-like syndrome. The dilated and tortuous vessel not only distorts the eighth nerve, it also impinges on the brainstem. There is a significant risk for thrombosis and consequent embolic stroke.

MEDICAL MANAGEMENT OF VERTIGO

Vertigo is a medical disease and should be treated with medications. Surgical intervention is reserved for those patients who are refractory to medical intervention.

During the course of management of the patient with vertigo, it is not uncommon for symptoms to evolve and for the diagnosis to change. The patient may present with acute vestibular neuronitis and move through a phase mimicking BPPV before the symptoms finally resolve. Another patient may present with vestibular Meniere's progressing to full-blown Meniere's or may present with Meniere's disease only to be determined to have AIED.

Labyrinthine Sedatives

The treatment of an acute attack of vertigo or recurrent attacks of vertigo is based on the use of labyrinthine sedatives. Antiemetics are used to manage severe nausea and vomiting. At this time, the most effective suppressants of the negative symptoms associated with acute vertigo are promethazine, dolasetron, and prochlorperazine. For less severe vertigo, in which oral medications can be used, diazepam is particularly effective; McCabe and Bernstein[70] have shown that this drug is extremely effective in treating all types of vertigo of peripheral origin. Diazepam is such a powerful vestibular suppressant that it is almost impossible to obtain a caloric response in patients who have had the medication within 24 to 48 hours of electronystagmographic testing. The usual dose of diazepam is 2.5 to 5 mg orally three times a day. A major side effect of diazepam is depression. Lorazepam seems to be effective as a vestibular suppressant that is associated with less depression as a side effect; the usual dose is 0.5 to 1 mg orally two to three times a day. Diazepam and lorazepam, as well as other benzodiazepines, are effective in treating acute vertigo; however, because of their vestibular suppressive effects, they tend to prevent central vestibular compensation. Accordingly, it is recommended that they be used only in short courses, that is, no longer than 3 to 4 days. Other medications useful in the treatment of acute vertigo are meclizine and dimenhydrinate, both of which are more sedating than diazepam or lorazepam.

Anticholinergic Drugs

In conjunction with vestibular suppressants, anticholinergic drugs, such as atropine or glycopyrrolate, can be used to reduce nausea and vomiting. Scopolamine is a potent anticholinergic drug that is used to treat motion sickness. Scopolamine, conveniently available for transdermal use, is an excellent drug for motion sickness but is of limited use in acute vertigo.

Antiviral Medications

The herpes simplex virus is suspected to cause a number of cases of vestibular neuronitis. Oral antiviral drugs, such as valacyclovir and famciclovir, are effective against the *herpes simplex* and *herpes zoster* viruses and should be considered in the management of vestibular neuronitis. The dosage of valacyclovir is 500 to 1,000 mg three times a day for 7 to 10 days, whereas famciclovir is administered at a dosage of 500 mg three times a day for 7 to 10 days. There is no published placebo-controlled study of the efficacy of these medications in the treatment of vestibular neuronitis; however, clinical experience supports their use.

Diuretics

Diuretics are considered the first line of therapy for Meniere's disease. They may also be effective in the treatment of post-traumatic vertigo or mild AIED. The most commonly used diuretic is triamterene and hydrochlorothiazide (Maxzide®) in doses varying from 25 to 75 mg. If this diuretic is ineffective or if its efficacy diminishes with time, changing to chlorthalidone, bumetanide, or furosemide may be of benefit. Serum electrolytes must be monitored when using any diuretic, even the so-called "potassium-sparing" agents. Dietary supplementation with potassium-rich foods may be adequate, but it is not uncommon for patients to require potassium supplementation.

Corticosteroids

Response to prednisone therapy is one of the hallmarks of AIED. Because of the difficulty in diagnosing AIED, some clinicians, such as Harris and Ryan,[71] recommend a 30-day course of prednisone (1 mg/kg daily) for those patients in whom AIED is suspected. A positive response (improved hearing and/or diminished vertigo) serves as clinical evidence for AIED, following which the prednisone is slowly tapered until the minimal dose is reached that maintains the desired clinical response. Prednisone has many side effects and can be quite dangerous in long-term use; for these reasons, a number of alternative medications have been used to treat AIED. Methotrexate is the most widely used. Sismanis and colleagues[72] have described significant clinical response to a dose of methotrexate ranging from 10 to 20 mg per week given orally as a single dose. Folic acid (1 mg/day orally) is used in conjunction with methotrexate. Side effects seen with this dosage of methotrexate include liver dysfunction and pulmonary fibrosis; however, the incidence of problems with methotrexate is significantly lower than those of long-term prednisone therapy. Once the patient is begun on methotrexate, the prednisone is tapered and discontinued. In addition to methotrexate, cyclophosphamide has been used for the treatment of AIED. Cyclophosphamide has a number of potentially fatal side effects, such as the induction of malignancies, and therefore is not widely used.

Antidepressants

Antidepressants can be useful in the treatment of BPPV and chronic recurrent vertigo for several reasons. Tricyclic antidepressants, especially amitriptyline, seem to be useful in controlling some of the milder spells of dysequilibrium. Amitriptyline is also effective in alleviating the cervical muscle spasm that frequently occurs in patients with recurrent vertigo. Additionally, higher-dose amitriptyline, nortriptyline, or trazodone may be used to control migraine-associated vertigo. The effective dose of amitriptyline varies from 10 to 100 mg taken at night. Nortriptyline doses typically range from 10 to 75 mg. Trazodone is usually effective in doses of 50 to 150 mg taken at night. Selective serotonin reuptake inhibitor (SSRI) antidepressants are effective adjuncts in those patients with a significant depressive overlay caused by the recurrent vertigo. The use of SSRIs or other antidepressants may be necessary to help patients cope with their vertigo.

Antiseizure Medications

In the small number of patients suspected of having the vascular compression syndrome described by Janetta and colleagues,[14] it may be appropriate to use antiseizure drugs such as phenytoin, carbamazepine, or gabapentin.

Other Agents

Beta blockers (eg, propranolol) and calcium channel blockers (eg, verapamil) are useful in the treatment of migraine-associated vertigo and may be used in addition to high doses of tricyclic antidepressants or other medications used to control migraine.

ALLERGIC MANAGEMENT

In a number of patients with Meniere's disease, allergy appears to be etiologic. In such cases, the "shock organ" is the inner ear. Seasonal exacerbations can occur owing to inhalant/pollen allergies. A recent study by Derebery and Berliner[73] found a significant increase in allergy symptoms and findings in patients with Meniere's syndrome when compared to a control population. Management includes skin testing followed by desensitization injections of the specific allergen(s), according to Rinkel's skin titration technique.

A less easily managed problem involves food allergies causing Meniere's disease. In some patients, an attack of Meniere's disease can be precipitated by the ingestion of certain foods, for example, wheat, milk, corn, and egg. Elimination diets, as determined by provocative testing and cytotoxic studies,[74] can be helpful.

DIETARY MODIFICATION

In addition to diuretics, sodium restriction has long been a mainstay in the management of Meniere's disease, dating back to its initial description by Furstenberg and colleagues.[75] Their salt restriction diet was described prior to the availability of effective, well-tolerated diuretics. Although it is quite strict, the underlying concept remains valid today. Sodium restriction to an intake of approximately 2 g daily is a useful adjunct to the management of Meniere's disease. Smoking cessation, as well as a reduction in caffeine intake, is also recommended in the control of Meniere's disease.

STRESS

It is recognized that stress provokes decompensation in patients with vertigo. The exact mechanism is not understood, but whether the patient is suffering from Meniere's disease, BPPV, or other vestibular dysfunction, stress complicates control of the disease process. Patients should be counseled as to the role of stress in aggravating vestibular symptomatology, and every effort should be made to lower stress levels.

Table 29–2   CAWTHORNE'S HEAD EXERCISES*
Eye exercises
Looking up, then down—at first slowly then quickly; 20 times.
Looking from one side to other—at first slowly, then quickly; 20 times.
Focus on finger at arm's length, moving finger one foot closer and back again; 20 times.
Head exercises
Bend head forward then backward with eyes open—slowly, later quickly; 20 times.
Turn head from one side to other side—slowly, then quickly; 20 times.
As dizziness decreases, these exercises should be done with eyes closed.
Sitting
While sitting, shrug shoulders; 20 times.
Turn shoulders to right, then to left; 20 times.
Bend forward and pick up objects from ground and sit up; 20 times.
Standing
Change from sitting to standing and back again; 20 times with eyes open. Repeat with eyes closed.
Throw a small rubber ball from hand to hand above eye level.
Throw a ball from hand to hand under one knee.
Moving about
Walk across room with eyes open, then closed; 10 times.
Walk up and down a slope with eyes open, then closed; 10 times.
Walk up and down steps with eyes open, then closed; 10 times.
Any game involving stooping or turning is good.

*Exercises to be carried out for 15 minutes twice a day, increasing to 30 minutes.

PHYSICAL THERAPY

Most peripheral vestibular disorders respond to an exercise program such as simple outdoor walking with head movement. Cawthorne[76] described a set of exercises that remain useful for the treatment of vertigo (Table 29–2). These exercises help speed the recovery from a labyrinthine insult such as vestibular neuronitis, ablative surgery, or BPPV.

Telian and Shepherd,[77] Shumway-Cook and Horak,[78] and others have studied the role of central vestibular adaptation in the recovery from peripheral vestibular dysfunction. They have shown that an individualized course of physical therapy can alleviate symptoms and improve function in patients with a variety of vestibular disorders. Although, conceptually, the program is based on the precepts of Cawthorne,[76] it goes beyond them. Emphasis is placed on habituation exercises and postural control. The therapeutic program is most successful in uncompensated peripheral vestibular lesions; it has been shown to be effective in the treatment not only of BPPV but also unresolved vestibular neuronitis and post-traumatic vertigo and in aiding recovery from vestibular ablation surgery. Although less successful in vestibular dysfunction related to head injury and in dysequilibrium of aging, physical therapy may still be superior to medication. The fundamental concept of vestibular rehabilitation is that a reduction in the use of labyrinthine sedatives promotes, in most cases, a better long-term functional outcome.

EPLEY MANEUVER

In 1992, Epley[79] described a therapeutic maneuver—the canalolith repositioning procedure (CRP)—for BPPV, based on his theory of the etiology of BPPV. The theory espoused by Epley differs from that advocated by Schuknecht[13]; Epley's theory implicates free-floating debris (canalolithiasis) in the posterior semicircular canal in the vertigo of BPPV. It is thought that with the CRP, the debris can be moved from the posterior semicircular canal to the vestibule, thereby eliminating its effect on the canal. With only one CRP, some 75 to 80% of patients experience symptom resolution, at least temporarily. The CRP is summarized in Table 29–3.

Table 29–3 CANALOLITH REPOSITIONING PROCEDURE
1. The patient is placed in a seated position.
2. The patient is then laid supine, with the head hanging off the table in a modified Hallpike position with the head rotated 45 degrees to the affected ear.
3. While still in the head-hanging position, the head is rotated to 45 degrees to the opposite side.
4. The patient's head and body are rotated until facing downward 135 degrees from supine.
5. With the head still turned to the right, the patient is brought to the sitting position.
6. The head is turned forward with the chin down 20 degrees.
At each step, there is a pause while the induced nystagmus resolves. The procedure is repeated until no nystagmus is produced; the use of Frenzel lenses, video-oculography, or the use of a low-intensity vibrator over the mastoid may enhance effectiveness.

SURGICAL TREATMENT OF VERTIGO

Indications for Surgery

Surgical treatment of vertigo is reserved for those patients who fail maximal medical therapy. The overwhelming majority of patients respond to one of the medical therapies listed above; however, a small but significant number of patients continue to have incapacitating episodic vertigo. In these patients, invasive procedures are potentially indicated. There is no one standard procedure that will uniformly control episodic vertigo in all cases; the choice of procedure is dictated by a number of factors. First and foremost is the degree of disability caused by the vertigo, that is, the frequency and severity of the vertiginous episodes and how they impact the patient's life. Employment status, the presence of other disabilities, and other general health risks modulate the impact of the vertigo on the patient. The status of the hearing is also a tantamount consideration as a number of the surgical procedures cause irreversible and complete hearing loss in the operated ear. Historically, hearing has been sacrificed in surgical procedures for vertigo if deemed "nonserviceable." Historically, nonserviceable hearing has been defined as hearing no better than a 50-dB pure-tone average and a 50% speech discrimination. This definition is clearly inappropriate today. With ever-improving hearing aids and cochlear implantation, the definition of serviceable hearing is changing. There is no agreed-upon definition for what constitutes serviceable hearing. What is considered serviceable varies with patient needs, the hearing status of the contralateral ear, and the degree of tinnitus, recruitment, and sound distortion in the affected ear.

In addition to the degree of hearing loss and the severity and frequency of vertigo, age, comorbid medical conditions, and the likelihood of vestibular compensation after surgery factor into surgical decision making. The majority of the surgical procedures used to control vertigo ablate the affected peripheral vestibular system; therefore, the central vestibular system must compensate for the peripheral loss for postoperative recovery to occur.

A major dilemma arises when treating vertigo in an only hearing ear or the better hearing ear. In such cases, extreme caution should be exercised; only very conservative procedures should be considered. Medical therapy should be pursued intensively in anticipation of a spontaneous remission, thereby avoiding any destructive procedures.

Surgical Procedures of Historical Interest

In general, surgery for vertigo can be divided into auditory-sparing (conservative) and auditory-ablative (destructive) procedures. A multitude of different procedures have been devised over the years, especially to treat the vertigo of endolymphatic hydrops. There are several procedures of historical interest that are no longer in general use. These procedures are conservative in that they aim to preserve residual hearing. Overall, the vertigo control achieved by these procedures has not been sufficient to warrant their general use.

Sacculotomy
In 1964, Fick[24] hypothesized that rupture of the distended saccule seen in endolymphatic hydrops should equalize endolymph and perilymph pressures. Fick therefore recommended puncture of the stapes footplate with a sharp needle to rupture the underlying saccule. Cody[25] expanded on this idea by designing a stainless steel tack that would penetrate the footplate and remain in place; it was thought that the saccule would rupture itself on the sharp point of the tack every time it distended. Both procedures used a transcanal approach, with the elevation of a tympanomeatal flap. Long-term follow-up has revealed a considerable incidence of progressive hearing loss.

Cochleosacculotomy
Alternative approaches to the permanent fistulization of the endolymphatic and perilymphatic spaces were devised by House[26] (the otic-periotic shunt) and by Schuknecht[27] (cochleosacculotomy). Both procedures were performed via an exploratory tympanotomy approach. In the otic-periotic shunt procedure, a tube was placed through the round window membrane to perforate the basilar membrane. In the cochleosacculotomy, a right-angled hook was inserted through the round window membrane so as to cause a fracture/dislocation of the osseous spiral lam-

ina. Owing to the high incidence of sensorineural hearing loss, these procedures are rarely performed.

Ultrasonography
Although the effects of ultrasonography on the labyrinth are not well understood, Arslan[80] introduced its use on the labyrinth in Europe in 1954. The rate of facial nerve injury was unacceptably high with the early ultrasonic generators but has been reduced with the introduction of smaller, more readily calibrated machines. The procedure is performed under local anesthesia through the middle ear or mastoid. In the mastoid approach, a "blue line" is created in the horizontal semicircular canal. The probe is then placed on the "blue line" and ultrasound is applied until the initially visualized irritative nystagmus (beating toward the operated ear) reverses to a paralytic nystagmus (beating away from the operated ear). Ultrasonic treatment of the labyrinth can also be performed through a tympanotomy approach by applying the probe to the round window membrane.[81]

Cryosurgery
Wolfson and colleagues[82] described a procedure to ablate the vestibular apparatus by freezing the membranous labyrinth with a cryoprobe. This procedure was performed through a mastoidectomy and involved "blue lining" the horizontal semicircular canal. House[83] likewise applied a cryoprobe to the round window through a tympanotomy approach. Cryoprobe procedures have been abandoned because of the high incidence of facial paralysis.

Streptomycin Therapy

Although streptomycin therapy is not a surgical procedure, it is an ablative procedure and has been advocated as a useful treatment for vertigo for many years. It is indicated for the treatment of bilateral disease or vertigo arising from an only hearing ear. Intramuscular injection of streptomycin can alleviate episodic vertigo but carries with it the morbidity of increasing imbalance and possibly Dandy's syndrome. Many patients who would have been considered candidates for streptomycin injection therapy may now be diagnosed as having AIED and are treated with corticosteroids, methotrexate, or other drugs.

However, on rare occasion, a patient may be found who could benefit from streptomycin therapy.

First advocated by Fowler[84] and later by Schuknecht,[28] streptomycin therapy ablates the vestibular labyrinth while sparing the cochlea. One gram of streptomycin is given twice a day for 10 to 20 days by intramuscular injection. After the tenth day, caloric testing is done every other day and audiograms are obtained daily. The patient is instructed to report any increase in tinnitus or further decrease in hearing. When the caloric response has been completely ablated, the injections are discontinued. After streptomycin therapy, patients no longer experience episodic vertigo but are frequently left with residual ataxia that usually diminishes with time but may not disappear completely. To avoid permanent ataxia and oscillopsia, Graham and Kemink[85] proposed a "titration" streptomycin therapy. The initial dose of streptomycin is reduced from 20 to 10 g. Graham and Kemink recommended that streptomycin therapy be stopped when symptoms cease, if hearing declines, or if oscillopsia develops. If symptoms return, streptomycin can be administered in 5-g increments until symptoms again disappear.

Currently, streptomycin is very difficult to obtain in the United States.

CURRENT SURGICAL OPTIONS

Perilymph Fistula Repair

If there is a suspicion of a perilymph fistula underlying vertigo, perilymph fistula "repair" should be undertaken via an exploratory tympanotomy approach. A perilymph fistula should be considered particularly in patients with congenital labyrinthine anomalies or those who have had direct trauma to the ear, operative procedures at the oval window, or severe closed head trauma or barotrauma. A standard tympanomeatal flap is used, and care should be taken to reduce the infusion of local anesthetic into the middle ear space as it can be confused with perilymph. Both the oval and round windows should be inspected carefully with the operating microscope. Placing the patient in Trendelenburg's position and increasing CSF pressure by repeated Valsalva's maneuvers may help in the identification of small leaks. The mucosa of the oval and round window niches should be

scarified with a straight pick, and perichondrium, adipose tissue, or fascia should be placed in these regions even if no distinct fistula is recognized. The postoperative care of these patients includes bed rest for several days with avoidance of straining or heavy lifting for several weeks.

The results of fistula repair vary. Interpretation of the results is complicated by the difficulty of conclusively identifying a perilymph fistula, particularly one with low flow. It can be impossible to differentiate perilymph fluid from local anesthetic solution or tissue transudate. This minimally invasive procedure may be considered for those patients who have had substantial trauma and who continue to have persistent vertigo.

Endolymphatic Sac Surgery

Endolymphatic sac decompression or drainage has been espoused for the management of endolymphatic hydrops since Portmann's work in 1926.[10] A variety of procedures have been described, ranging from simple decompression or shunting the sac into the mastoid or subarachnoid space to cannulating the endolymphatic duct to drain the endolymphatic compartment.

The procedure begins with a simple mastoidectomy with identification of the middle and posterior fossa dural plates, sinodural angle, sigmoid sinus, and antrum (Figure 29–1); the horizontal semicircular canal and incus are then identified. Using a diamond bur, the facial nerve is identified, leaving intact a thin bony covering from the horizontal canal to the stylomastoid foramen. This step is important because the endolymphatic sac lies on the dura medial to the fallopian canal and the retrofacial air cells. Visualization of the facial nerve enables safe removal of the retrofacial cells and identification of the endolymphatic sac. The posterior semicircular canal is next identified; in a well-pneumatized temporal bone, identification is best accomplished by exenterating air cells superior to the canal and following the canal to the facial nerve. In a sclerotic bone, the exact location of the posterior canal can be determined by "blue lining." Once the posterior canal has been identified, the posterior fossa dural plate is removed between the sigmoid sinus and the posterior canal. The endolymphatic sac is located by tracing an imaginary (Donaldson's) line through the horizontal semicircular canal, perpendicular to and bisecting the posterior semicircular canal. The upper

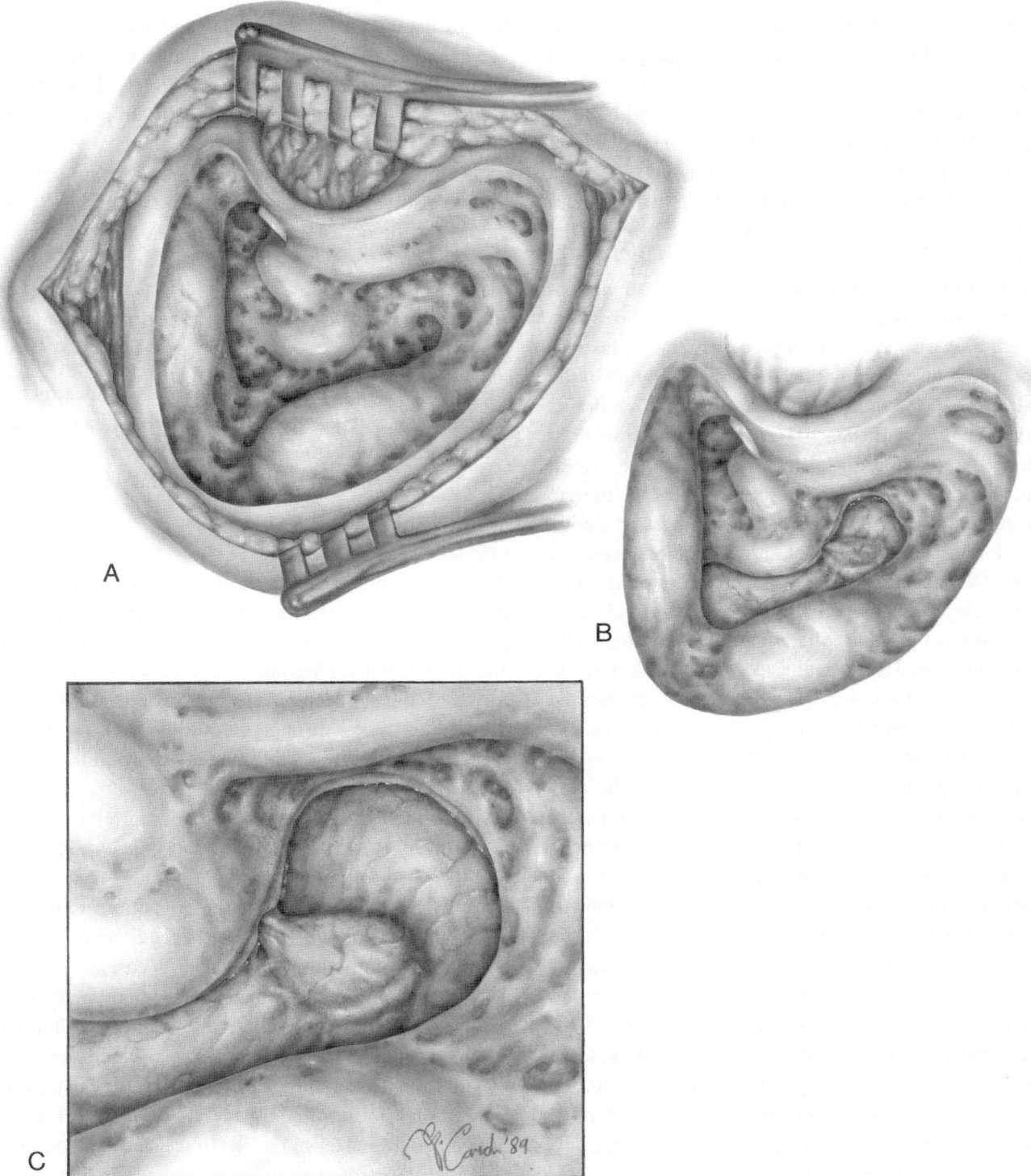

Figure 29–1 Endolymphatic sac procedure. *A,* A standard simple mastoidectomy is performed. The middle and posterior fossa dura plates, sinodural angle, sigmoid sinus, and antrum are identified. The horizontal canal and incus are then identified as well as the digastric ridge. The facial nerve is skeletonized from the horizontal canal to the stylomastoid foramen; copious irrigation is used to keep the nerve cool. Facial nerve monitoring can be beneficial. The retrofacial cell tract is opened. *B,* The posterior semicircular canal is identified and the posterior fossa dura plate is removed between the sigmoid sinus and the posterior canal. *C,* The upper edge of the endolymphatic sac is identified; it generally lies at or below Donaldson's line (a line extended posteriorly along the long axis of the horizontal canal that bisects the posterior semicircular canal).

edge of the endolymphatic sac is usually located just inferior to this line. The precise management of the sac subsequent to its identification varies according to which procedure is conducted.

In decompression of the sac, removal of all bone of the posterior fossa dural plate completes the procedure. Attempts to revascularize the decompressed sac with a temporalis muscle pedicle flap have been abandoned.

Shunting of the sac can be performed either into the mastoid or the subarachnoid space (Figure 29–2). House[21] developed the endolymphatic subarachnoid shunt procedure, in which both walls of the endolymphatic sac are incised, and a specially designed silicone (Silastic®) shunt tube is inserted into the lateral prolongation of the basal cistern. It is thought that endolymph then drains into the subarachnoid space. Because the subarachnoid space is entered, there is a risk of CSF leakage, which is prevented by suturing temporalis muscle over the sac or using adipose tissue to obliterate the mastoid cavity.

Endolymphatic mastoid shunting requires insertion of one of a number of variably shaped pieces of Silastic® into the sac, with Paparella and Hanson's[22] technique being the most popular. The edge of the sac is usually opened, all intraluminal adhesions are lysed, and the duct is probed. One or more pieces of Silastic are inserted into the sac and protrude through the incision to allow for permanent drainage (Figure 29–3).

Endolymphatic sac shunt procedures can be performed either in a hospital setting or on an outpatient basis. The morbidity of the procedure relates to the mastoidectomy; usually, patients can return to work and normal activities within a week. It is not uncommon to have some increased vestibular symptomatology for the first 2 to 3 weeks following surgery, but spontaneous resolution is anticipated. The endolymphatic subarachnoid shunt procedure entails the increased risk not only of CSF leakage but also the possibility of posterior cranial fossa hemorrhage if the shunt tube penetrates an arachnoid vein.

The efficacy of endolymphatic sac surgery is controversial. A review of sac procedures by Glasscock and colleagues[86] in 1984 reported control of vertigo after a minimum of 2 years in a group of sac surgery patients. With the Arenberg endolymphatic mastoid shunt, there was a 49% relief of vertigo. In the subarachnoid shunt, relief was obtained in 66%, whereas in the mastoid shunt, using a simple sheet of Silastic, 59% obtained relief. These were not reported in terms of the current AAO-HNS

criteria.[61] Silverstein and colleagues[87] have pointed out that the natural history of patients with medically treated Meniere's disease is the same or better than those who have undergone endolymphatic sac surgery. Jackson and colleagues[88] found that only some 30% of patients who underwent sac surgery avoided a secondary procedure within the first 5 years. The advantage of sac surgery lies in its conservation of hearing; its overwhelming disadvantage is the poor long-term control of symptoms.

Vestibular Nerve Section

Vestibular nerve section is considered a nondestructive procedure since it generally spares auditory function. Several approaches to the vestibular nerve medial to the labyrinth are possible, spawning several procedures.

Middle Fossa Approach

Although Dandy[19] first described vestibular nerve section via the suboccipital approach, the middle fossa approach, as popularized by House,[31] gained wide acceptance in the 1970s. The approach is the same as that used for vestibular schwannoma resection or decompression of the facial nerve through the middle fossa. There are some major differences once the internal auditory canal has been identified.

Once the House-Urban self-retaining retractor is in place, the temporal lobe elevated, the geniculate ganglion identified, and the superior semicircular canal "blue lined," a diamond bur and suction irrigation are used to follow the facial nerve to the internal auditory canal. The bone of the internal auditory canal is carefully drilled away so that only its dura remains. It is important to carry the dissection to the most lateral extent of the internal auditory canal to identify "Bill's bar," which separates the anteriorly located facial nerve from the posteriorly located superior vestibular nerve. A right angle hook is placed into the posterior portion of the canal and the dura is incised, thus protecting the facial nerve from unintended traction. The dura is removed from the canal, exposing its contents. At this point, the hook is placed into the superior vestibular nerve canal (using Bill's bar as a landmark), and the nerve is extracted (Figure 29–4; see also figures in Chapters 31 and 32) and retracted with a small-gauge suction. The vestibulofacial anastomosis is sectioned.

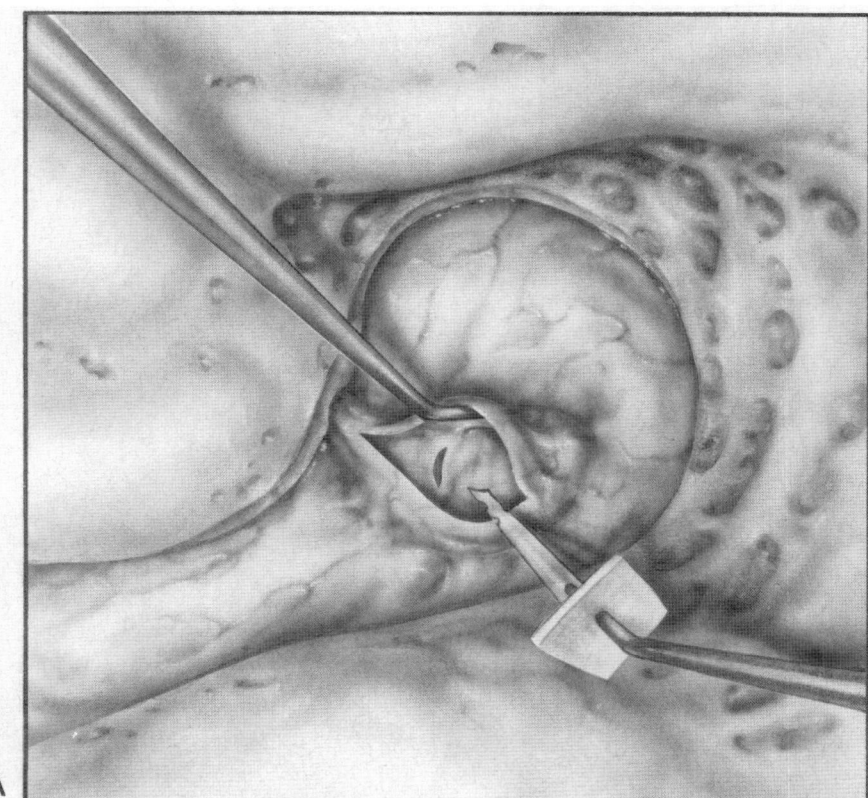

Figure 29–2 Endolymphatic subarachnoid shunt. *A,* After opening the lateral wall of the endolymphatic sac, an incision is made into the medial wall and the posterior fossa to open into the lateral prolongation of the basal cistern. Dissection in the cistern is carried out bluntly so as not to interrupt any bridging veins. *B,* A silicone (Silastic) shunt tube is inserted to maintain a drainage route between the endolymphatic sac and the basal cistern. A muscle plug is usually sutured over the lateral aspect of the endolymphatic sac to facilitate closure and prevent cerebrospinal fluid leak.

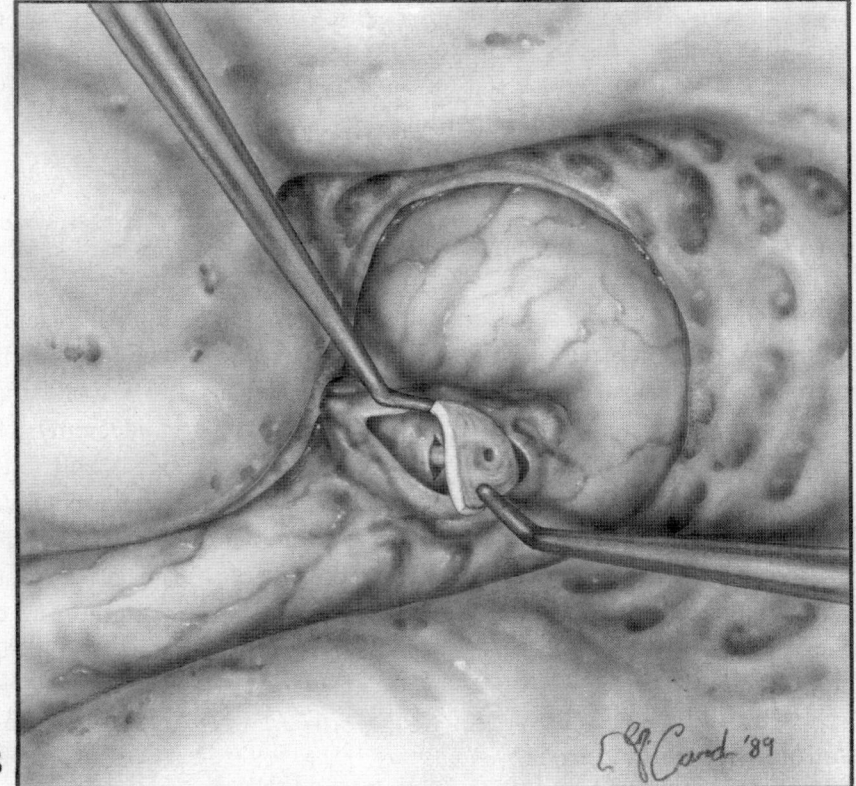

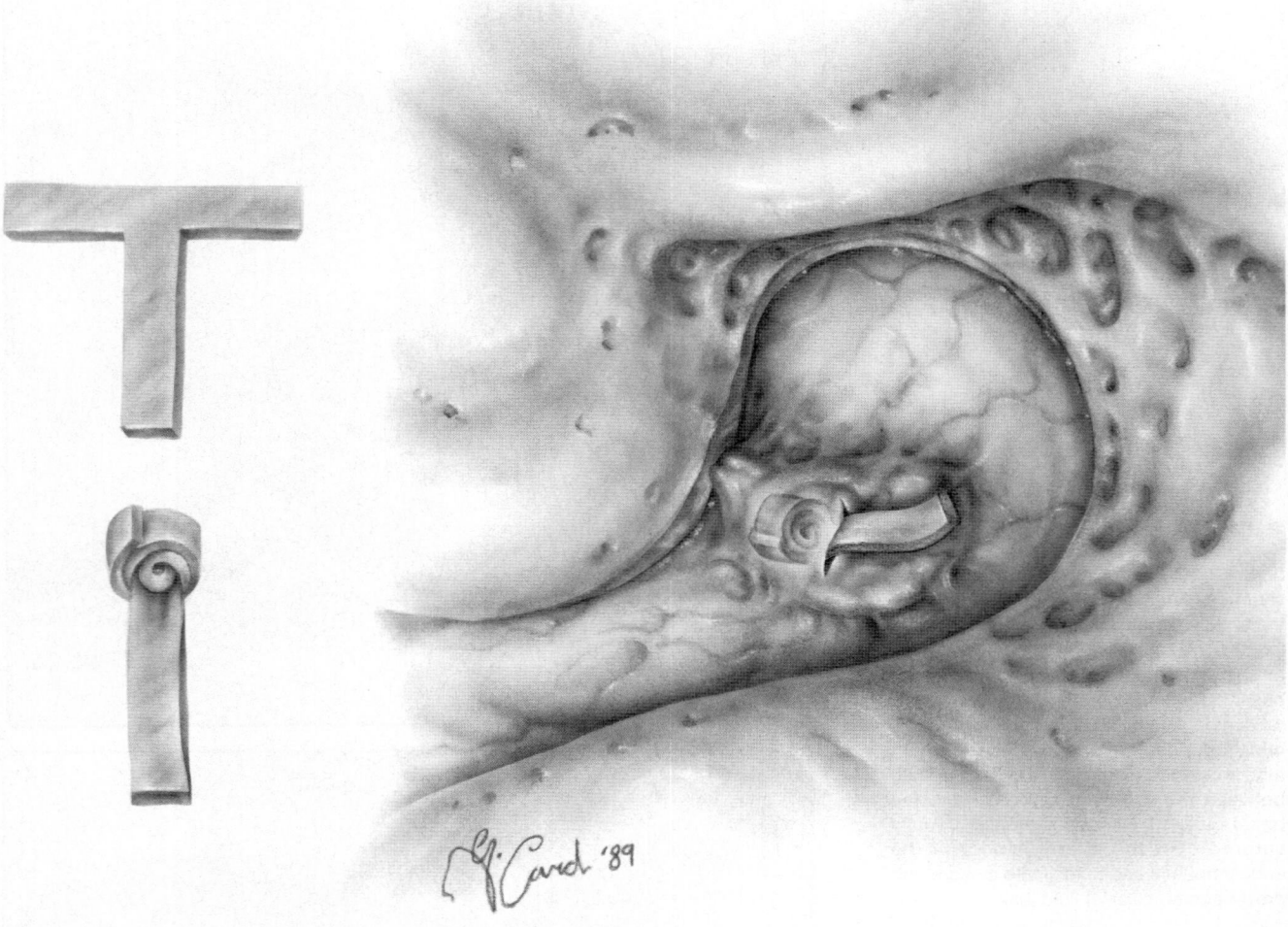

Figure 29–3 Paparella's technique of endolymphatic mastoid shunting. A "T"-shaped piece of silicone (Silastic) is inserted into the open endolymphatic sac to form a permanent fistula between the lumen of the sac and the mastoid cavity.

Continuing to retract the superior vestibular nerve, the surgeon reaches into the posteroinferior aspect of the internal auditory canal and extracts the inferior vestibular nerve, taking care to avoid the internal auditory artery and cochlear nerve. Once both vestibular nerves have been extracted, they are sectioned proximal to Scarpa's ganglion with sharp (eg, Yasargil) scissors. The internal auditory canal is covered with a pledget of absorbable gelatin sponge (Gelfoam®), followed by a plug of temporalis muscle.

Retrolabyrinthine Approach

The retrolabyrinthine approach to vestibular nerve section is technically less demanding than the middle fossa approach. The retrolabyrinthine approach takes advan-

tage of the ability to identify the vestibular nerve in the cerebellopontine angle before it enters the internal auditory canal through the mastoid. After simple mastoidectomy, the middle and posterior fossa dural plates are identified as well as the facial nerve, horizontal semicircular canal, and entire sigmoid sinus. The posterior semicircular canal is completely delineated and the posterior fossa dura is completely decorticated. Retrosigmoid air cells are exenterated for at least 1 cm posterior to the sigmoid sinus. The posterior fossa dura is incised just anterior to the sigmoid sinus from the sinodural angle to the jugular bulb. The dura is then reflected over the posterior semicircular canal. Through the dural window, the vestibulocochlear nerve can be identified at the brainstem. With high-power magnification, a cleavage plane can usually be identified and dissected,

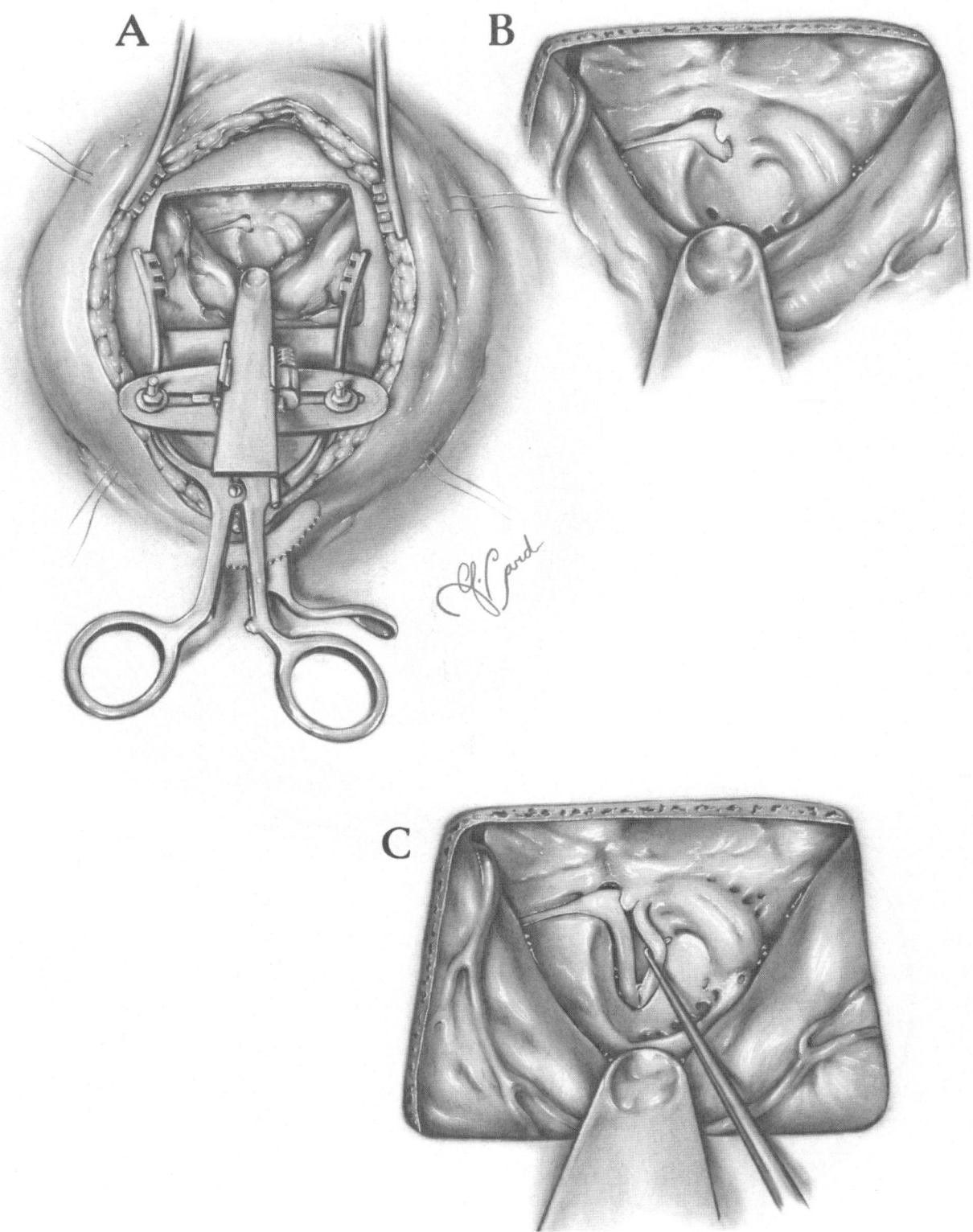

Figure 29–4 *A,* The temporal portion of the squamosa is identified through a standard vertical middle fossa incision. After the bone flap is removed, the dura is elevated from posterior to anterior, exposing the floor of the temporal fossa. *B,* Using suction irrigation and a diamond bur, the arcuate eminence is identified, as is the meningeal artery. *C,* The facial nerve has been identified and traced into the internal auditory canal. The superior semicircular canal has been "blue lined." The internal auditory canal has been skeletonized and opened; the superior and inferior vestibular nerves are then avulsed.

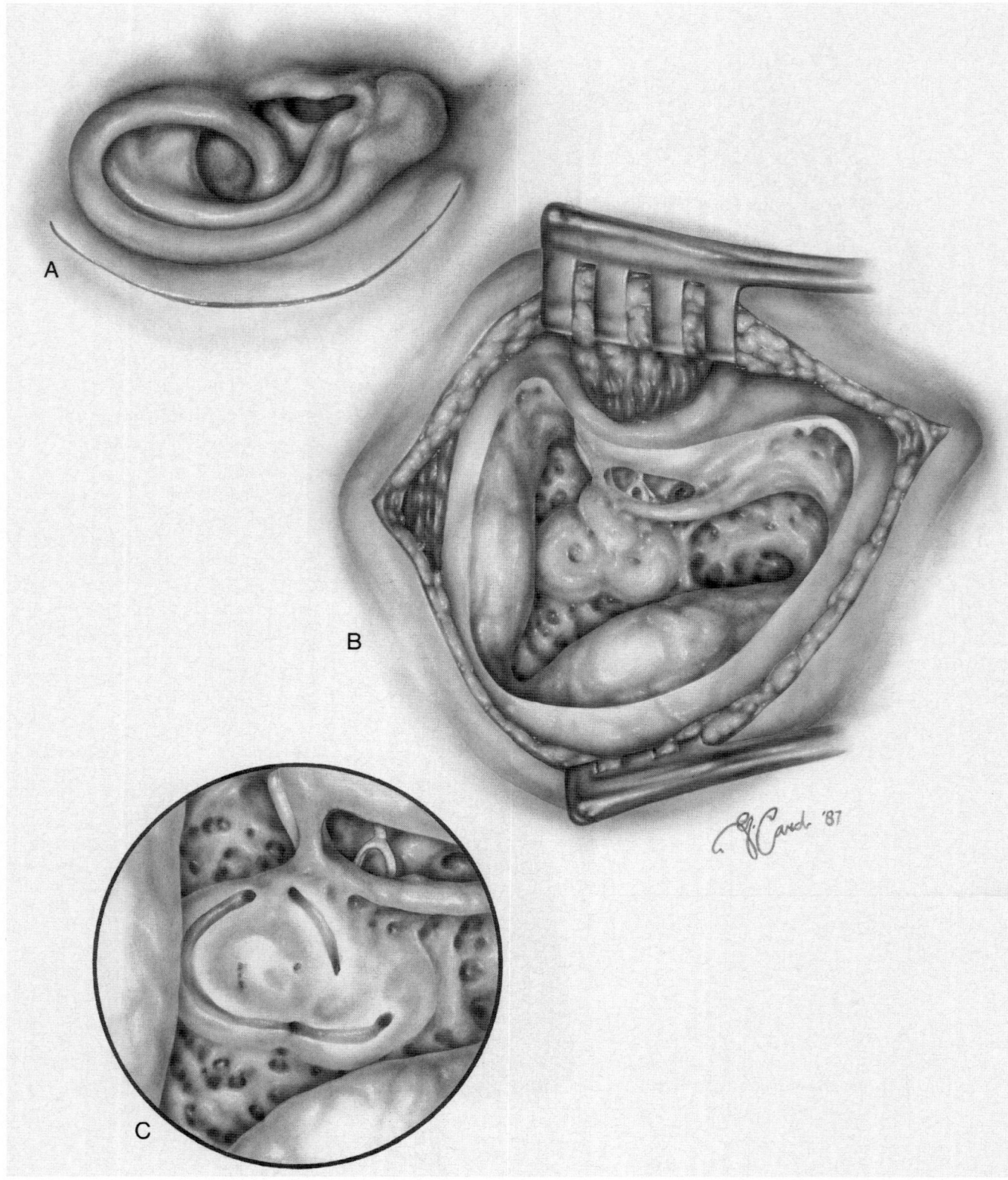

Figure 29–5 *A* and *B*, A curvilinear or vertical incision is made approximately 7 cm behind the postauricular crease. Note the relationship of the incision to the sigmoid sinus and cerebellum. The incision is made after the anterior flap is developed deep to the suboccipital pericranium. *C*, A suboccipital craniotomy is performed, exposing the sigmoid sinus anteriorly and the transverse sinus superiorly. Bone is removed inferiorly and posteriorly to a degree adequate to gain access to the posterior fossa. The amount of bone removal required varies somewhat with patient anatomy.

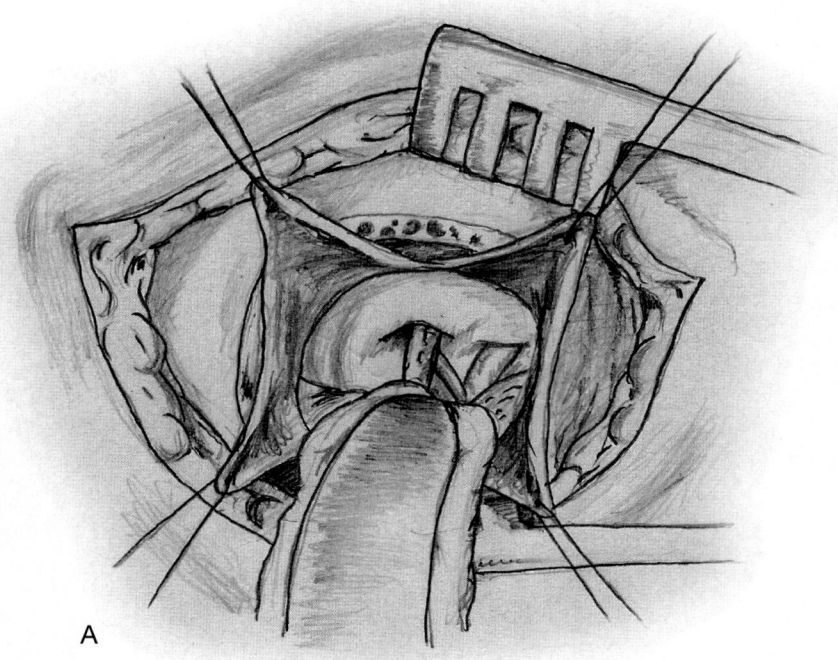

A

Figure 29–6   *A* and *B*, The posterior fossa dura is opened either in an H-shaped incision or in an incision that follows the sigmoid sinus. The basal cistern is entered and cerebrospinal fluid drained, allowing the cerebellum to drop away, exposing the angle. The seventh and eighth nerves and fifth, ninth, tenth, and eleventh nerve complexes are identified. *C*, Using a sharp #1 knife (or eye blade), the eighth nerve is split along its long axis between the cochlear and vestibular divisions. When a cleavage plane is not visible, the nerve is divided roughly down the middle.

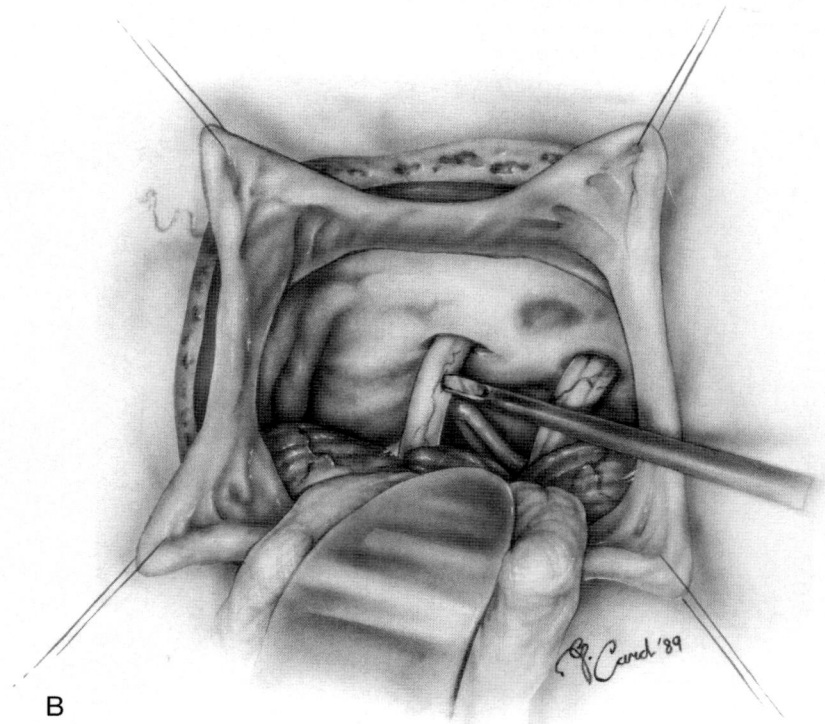

B

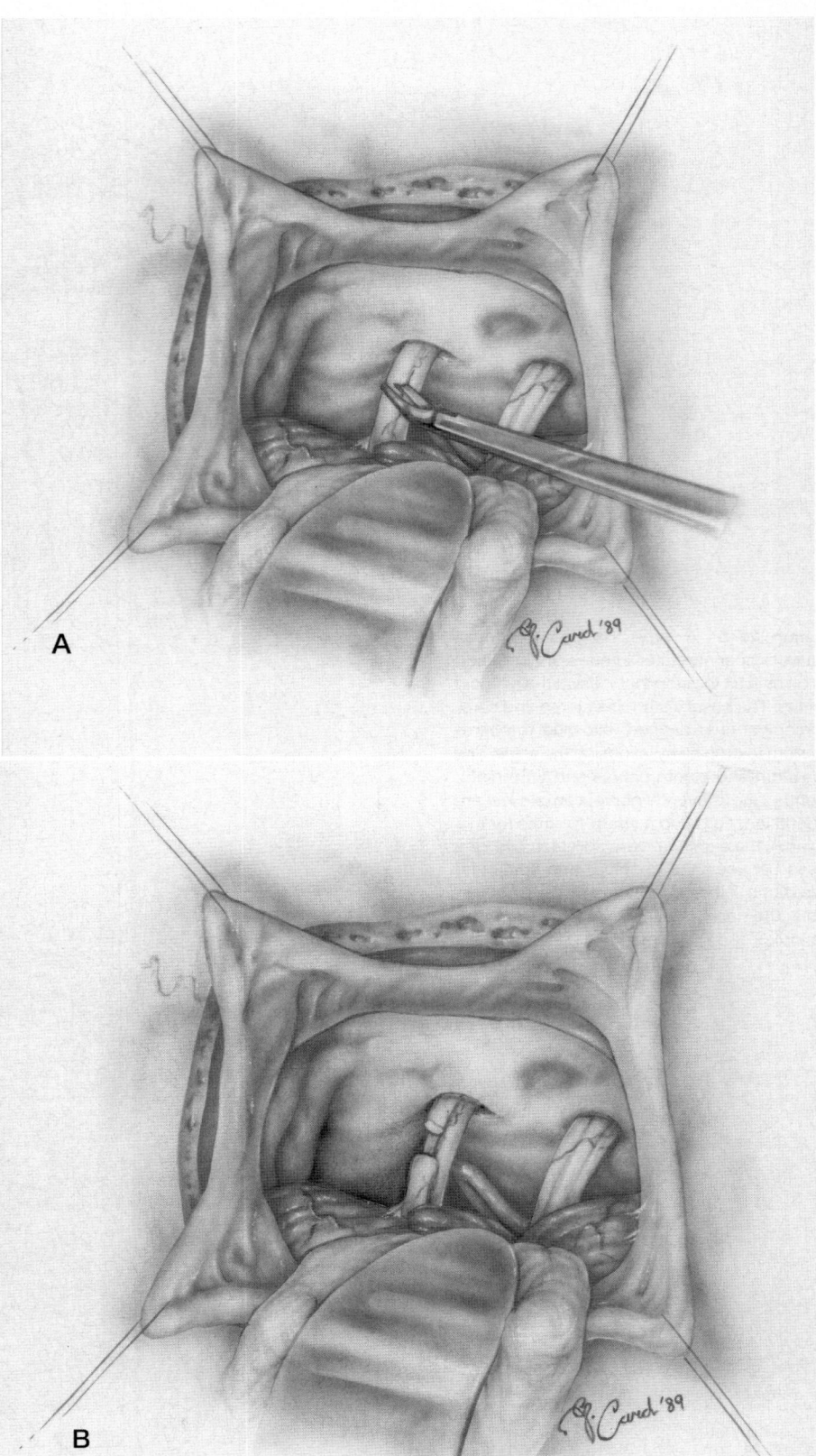

Figure 29–7   *A*, The vestibular nerve is then transected with fine-tipped microsurgical scissors. Intraoperative auditory brainstem response may be used during this dissection to help maintain auditory nerve continuity. *B*, Following the transection, the vestibular nerves pull apart.

separating the superiorly located vestibular nerve from the inferiorly located cochlear nerve. The vestibular nerve is then sectioned, with complete section confirmed by retraction of both ends of the nerve. The dural flap is reapproximated with 4-0 silk sutures, and the mastoid defect is obliterated with adipose tissue.

Retrosigmoid Transmeatal Vestibular Nerve Section

The major disadvantage of the retrolabyrinthine approach is that it affords only limited exposure of the posterior cranial fossa. The retrosigmoid (suboccipital) approach provides a much more generous exposure of the posterior fossa, allowing more room for manipulation of the blood vessels around the seventh and eighth cranial nerve complex and better access for hemostasis. A standard suboccipital exposure is employed in which the sigmoid sinus is the anterior limit of exposure. The posterior fossa dura is opened, and the cerebellopontine angle and petrous ridge are exposed by retraction of the cerebellum. Usually, once the cistern is entered inferiorly and CSF is drained, there is no need to retract the cerebellum as it falls medially. The vestibular, cochlear, and facial nerves are identified, and the vestibular nerve is sectioned as previously described (Figures 29–5 to 29–7). The dura is reapproximated, the bone flap replaced, and the wound closed.

Results

All nerve section procedures have similar risk factors, including a small chance of cerebrovascular accident associated with surgery, the possibility of CSF leakage, and meningitis. The incidence of CSF leak is the highest in the retrolabyrinthine approach.

Because of the intracranial nature of these procedures, the immediate postoperative period requires a surgical intensive care unit or the surgical recovery room. Hospitalization for 3 to 4 additional days is required to allow the patient to complete the initial steps of vestibular compensation.

With middle fossa neurectomy, Glasscock and colleagues[32] and Fisch[33] have reported relief of vertigo in 94% of the cases, with a significant hearing loss in only 4 to 9%. Retrolabyrinthine neurectomy[89,90] successfully

relieves vertigo in 75 to 88% of cases, with 70% of patients having no hearing loss. A hearing loss of less than 20 dB, most commonly conductive, was noted in 20% of patients. The hearing conservation rates achieved with vestibular nerve section by any route remain the standard for all hearing conservation procedures that destroy the peripheral vestibular system.

Gentamicin Perfusion

In the 1990s, gentamicin perfusion/injection emerged as a predominant therapy for the incapacitating vertigo of Meniere's disease. Gentamicin is an aminoglycoside antibiotic that is preferentially toxic to the hair cells and dark cells of the vestibular labyrinth. A variety of techniques[91–93] have been developed to ablate the diseased vestibular labyrinth with intratympanic gentamicin. Dosage schedules and routes of administration vary considerably according to technique, making direct comparison of results to derive the optimal regimen difficult.

The patient is placed in the Trendelenburg position with the affected ear turned up and the head turned at a 45-degree angle. The posterior aspect of the tympanic membrane is anesthetized using a drop of phenol and a gentamicin solution (either a solution buffered with sodium bicarbonate with a gentamicin concentration of 30 mg/cc or a nonbuffered solution with a gentamicin concentration of 40 mg/cc) is injected by fine needle. The entire posterior half of the tympanic cavity is filled with gentamicin; the creation of a pinpoint tympanic membrane perforation anterior to the malleus allowing air escape facilitates this process. The patient is left in position for 45 minutes and then discharged, with instructions to return in 1 week for a second injection.

The perioperative care in this outpatient procedure is minimal. Because of the pain associated with the injection, a small dose of midazolam (or another analgesic agent) intravenously may be useful to lessen the discomfort. In the days following the injection, there is usually minimal pain. Not uncommonly, several weeks after the second injection, there is a period of unsteadiness. In the majority of cases, two injections suffice to relieve episodic vertigo. If the vertigo persists and there is no evidence of hearing loss, additional injections may be performed.

Driscoll and colleagues,[92] using a treatment regimen consisting of a single gentamicin injection, reported short-term results of control of vertigo in 85 to 90% of the cases, with a 5 to 10% incidence of acute hearing loss related to the injection. Kaplan and colleagues,[93] using slightly higher doses of gentamicin and a longer follow-up, reported similar results.

The advantages of gentamicin injection are clear. At least in the first several years, the procedure seems to achieve a level of vertigo control similar to that of vestibular neurectomy without the associated morbidity or mortality. The long-term efficacy of gentamicin injection therapy is unknown, as is the number of patients who will require additional procedures for vertigo control.

Microvascular Decompression

Janetta and colleagues[14] and, more recently, Brackmann[69] have described an entity referred to as disabling positional vertigo, caused by vascular compression of the eighth cranial nerve. In a procedure similar to that used in microvascular decompression of the fifth cranial nerve for tic douloureux, the cerebellopontine angle is exposed via suboccipital craniotomy. Using microscopic visualization, the vessels surrounding the seventh and eighth cranial nerve root entry zones and the internal auditory canal are examined. Any vessels compressing the nerves are elevated and a piece of Teflon® felt (or similar sponge) is interposed between the nerve and the vessel.

The postoperative care of these patients is similar to that following vestibular neurectomy as it entails intracranial exposure. The results reported in the small series of Janetta and colleagues[14] and Brackmann[69] seem promising; however, disabling positional vertigo is somewhat difficult to diagnose and occurs infrequently.

Destructive Procedures

Destructive procedures are designed to rid the patient of vertigo by completely destroying vestibular and auditory function. As mentioned above, the level of hearing that constitutes serviceable hearing is impossible to generalize and can be determined only on a case-by-case basis.

Transcanal Labyrinthectomy

The middle ear is exposed through a tympanomeatal flap. The incus and stapes are disarticulated and extracted. Complete exposure of the oval window and round window is imperative (Figure 29–8). The footplate is removed and a right angle hook is inserted into the vestibule to remove all neuroepithelium. Schuknecht[28] advocates packing the vestibule with Gelfoam soaked in streptomycin. Another technique includes drilling off the promontory to connect the oval and round windows to ensure complete removal of the contents of the vestibule.

Transmastoid Labyrinthectomy

The advantage of the transmastoid labyrinthectomy is that all neuroepithelium is systemically removed under direct vision with the operating microscope. After a simple mas-

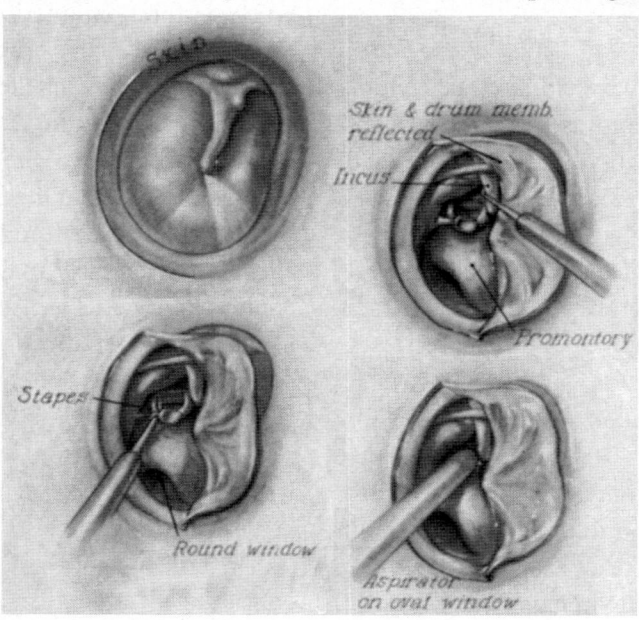

Figure 29–8   Schuknecht's transtympanic labyrinthotomy for Meniere's disease.

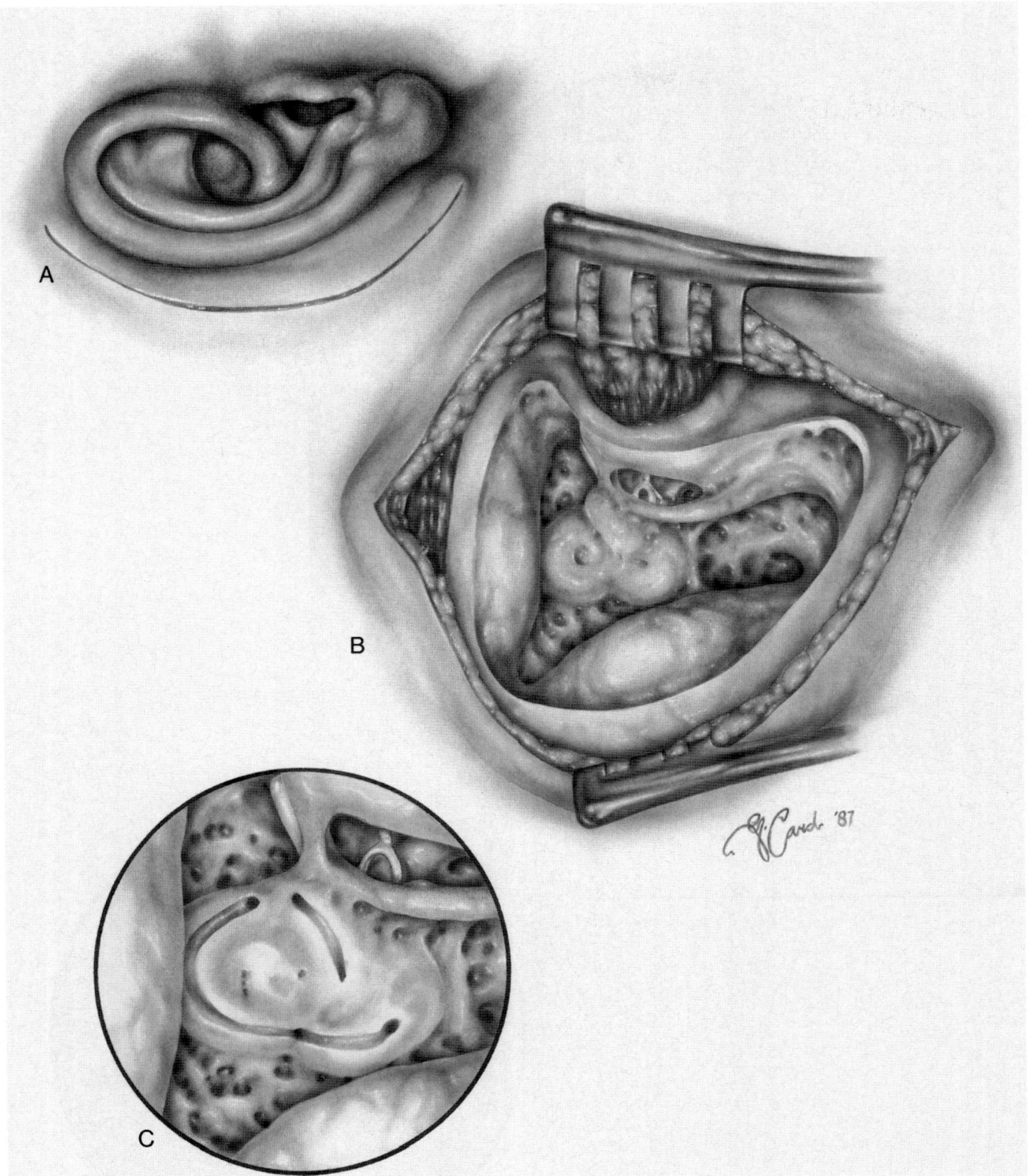

Figure 29–9   Transmastoid labyrinthectomy. *A*, A postauricular incision is made. *B*, A complete mastoidectomy is performed. The fossa incudis, digastric ridge, and vertical portion of the facial nerve are identified. The facial recess is opened. *C*, The incudostapedial joint is disarticulated and the incus removed. The semicircular canals are then opened, beginning with the horizontal canal and continuing to the posterior and finally the superior canals.

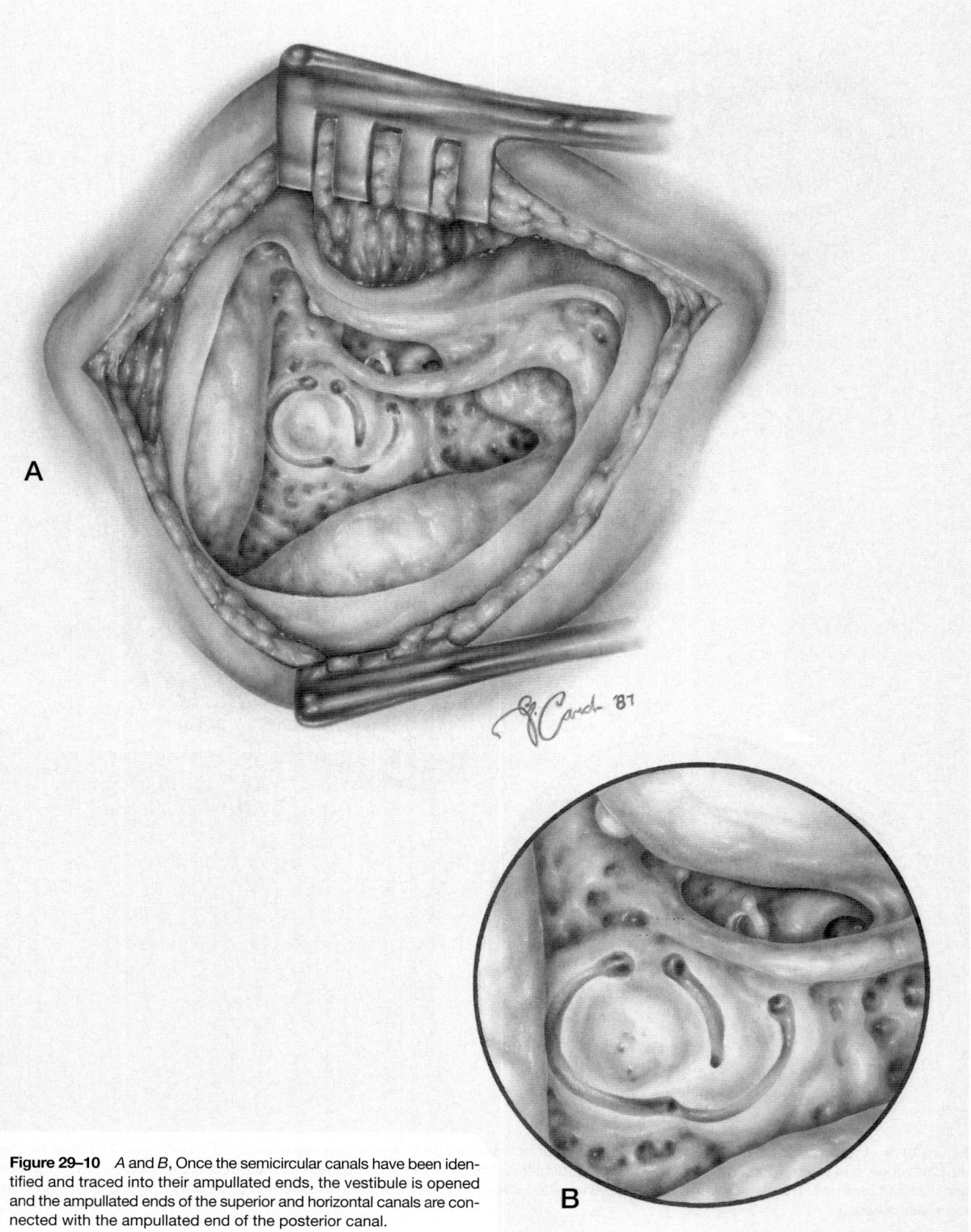

Figure 29–10   *A* and *B*, Once the semicircular canals have been identified and traced into their ampullated ends, the vestibule is opened
and the ampullated ends of the superior and horizontal canals are connected with the ampullated end of the posterior canal.

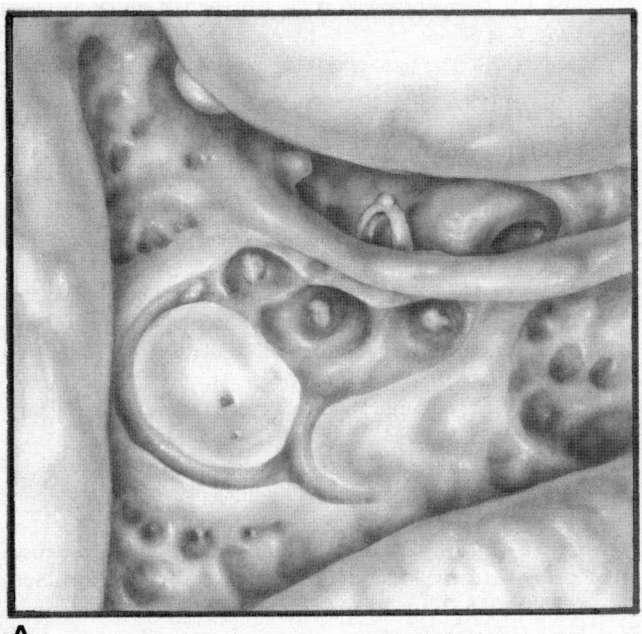 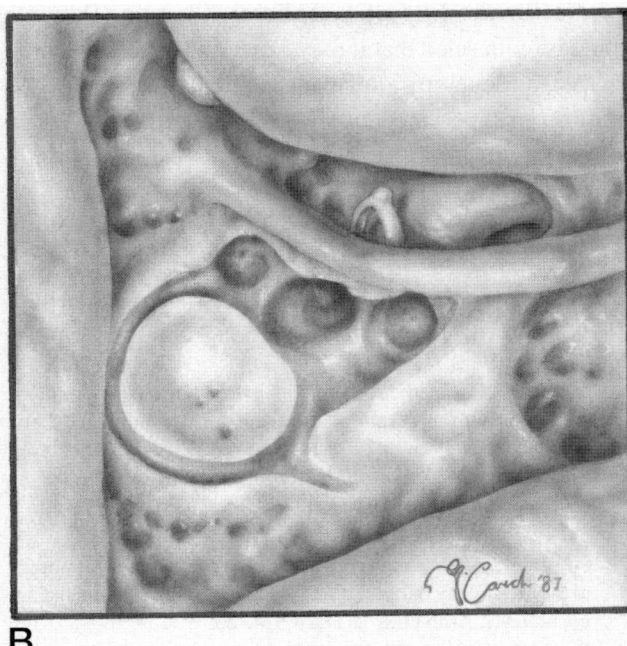

Figure 29–11 *A*, The ampullae and neuroepithelium of the three semicircular canals are exposed, as are the saccule and utricle. *B*, The neuroepithelium is removed under direct visualization.

toidectomy, the vertical segment of the facial nerve is identified. The semicircular canals are then drilled away in a systematic fashion, beginning with the horizontal, then the posterior, and, finally, the superior canal. Dissection is continued until all three ampullae have been exposed and their neuroepithelium extracted. Great care must be exercised while working around the second genu of the facial nerve. This area is at risk of either direct injury from a drill or thermal damage from the heat of dissection.

To visualize the entire vestibule, the horizontal segment of the facial nerve must be identified while leaving intact a thin bony covering. In this manner, all neuroepithelium can be extracted under direct visualization. The postauricular incision is routinely closed (Figures 29–9 to 29–11).

A translabyrinthine vestibular nerve section can be performed using the same approach and involves skeletonizing the internal auditory canal after the labyrinthectomy has been performed. The dura of the internal auditory canal is opened and the inferior and superior vestibular nerves are sectioned. The mastoid cavity must be obliterated with an adipose tissue graft as in translabyrinthine vestibular schwannoma removal.

Labyrinthectomy is generally performed in a hospital setting to accommodate management of anticipated postoperative vertigo. Not uncommonly, the postoperative vertigo is fairly limited as the underlying disease process has destroyed much vestibular function. The patient may be released as soon as independently ambulatory.

Transcanal labyrinthectomy is a comparatively noninvasive approach to labyrinthine destruction; however, there is a significant incidence of incomplete labyrinthectomy, especially in the hands of the inexperienced surgeon. Reaching the posterior semicircular canal ampulla is extraordinarily difficult. In general, transmastoid labyrinthectomy is preferred as it has the advantage of allowing the complete and systematic removal of all vestibular neuroepithelium under direct vision through the operating microscope.

Transmastoid labyrinthectomy has a 90 to 95% chance of controlling the episodic vertigo of Meniere's disease. Total hearing loss in the operated ear is an inevitable consequence of this procedure. There is limited, if any, additional gain in vertigo control by incorporating a cochleovestibular nerve section to the labyrinthectomy.

Any procedure that ablates the peripheral vestibular system depends on the central nervous system to compensate for the loss of peripheral function. Patients should be counseled that if they experience stress, become inactive, or develop significant medical illness, the dysequilibrium experienced in the postoperative period may recur.

REFERENCES

1. Williams HL. Meniere's disease. Springfield (IL): Charles C Thomas; 1952.

2. Meniere MP. Maladies de l'oreille interne offrant les symptoms de la congestion cerebrale apoplectiforme. Gaz Med Paris 1861;16:55–88.

3. Shambaugh GE, Knudson V0. Report of an investigation of ten cases of diplacusis. Trans Am Otol Soc 1923;16:397–412.

4. Crowe SJ. Meniere's disease. Medicine 1938;17:1–27.

5. Fowler EP. Measuring sensation of loudness: a new approach to the physiology of hearing and functional and differential diagnostic tests. Arch Otol 1937;26:514–20.

6. Dix MR, Hallpike CS, Hood JD. Observations upon loudness recruitment phenomenon. J Laryngol Otol 1948;62:671–8.

7. Cawthorne TE. Meniere's disease. Ann Otol Rhinol Laryngol 1947;56:18–34.

8. Lindsay JR. Labyrinthine dropsy. Laryngoscope 1946;56:325–38.

9. Knapp H. A clinical analysis of the inflammatory affections of the inner ear. Arch Ophthalmol 1871;2:204–83.

10. Portmann G. The saccus endolymphaticus and an operation for draining the same for the relief of vertigo. J Laryngol Otol 1927;42:809–19.

11. Hallpike CS, Cairns H. Observations on the pathology of Meniere's syndrome. J Laryngol Otol 1938;53:625–31.

12. Yamakawa K. The inner ear of a patient with Meniere's disease. J Otorhinolaryngol Soc Jpn 1938;44:2310–12.

13. Schuknecht HF. Cupulolithiasis. Arch Otol 1969;90:765–78.

14. Janetta PJ, Molter MB, Moller AR. Disabling positional vertigo. N Engl J Med 1984;310:1700–5.

15. Fee GA. Traumatic perilymph fistula. Arch Otol 1968;88:43–7.

16. Parry RH. A case of tinnitus and vertigo treated by division of the auditory nerve. J Laryngol Otol 1904;19:402–3.

17. Milligan W. Meniere's disease: a clinical and experimental inquiry. J Laryngol Otol 1904;19:440–1.

18. Lake R. Removal of the semicircular canals in a case of unilateral aural vertigo. Lancet 1904;1:1567–8.

19. Dandy WE. Meniere's disease: its diagnosis and method of treatment. Arch Surg 1928;16:1127–52.

20. Shambaugh GE Jr. Surgery of the endolymphatic sac. Arch Otol 1966;83:302–11.

21. House WF. Subarachnoid shunt for drainage of endolymphatic hydrops. Laryngoscope 1962;72:713–28.

22. Paparella MM, Hanson DG. Endolymphatic sac drainage for intractable vertigo (method and experiences). Laryngoscope 1976;86:697–703.

23. Arenberg IK, Stahle J, Glasscock ME, et al. Endolymphatic sac valve surgery: I. The technique. Laryngoscope 1979;89 Suppl 17:1–151.

24. Fick IA. Decompression of the labyrinth. Arch Otolaryngol 1964;79:447–56.

25. Cody DTR. The tack operation for endolymphatic hydrops. Laryngoscope 1969;79:1737–49.

26. House WF. Meniere's disease: management and theory. Otol Clin North Am 1975;8:515–37.

27. Schuknecht HF. Cochleosacculotomy for Meniere's disease: theory, technique and results. Laryngoscope 1982;92:853–7.

28. Schuknecht HF. Ablation therapy in Menière's disease. Acta Otolaryngol Suppl (Stockh) 1957;132:1–42.

29. Glasscock ME, Davis WE, Hughes GB, et al. Labyrinthectomy versus middle fossa vestibular nerve section in Meniere's disease: a critical evaluation of relief of vertigo. Ann Otol Rhinol Laryngol 1980;1:378–90.

30. Dandy WE. The surgical treatment of Meniere's disease. Surg Gynecol Obstet 1941;72:421–26.

31. House WF. Surgical exposure of the internal auditory canal and its content through the middle cranial fossa. Laryngoscope 1961;71:1363–85.

32. Glasscock ME, Kveton JF, Christiansen SG. Middle fossa vestibular nerve section: an update. Otol Head Neck Surg 1984;92:216–27.

33. Fisch U. Vestibular and cochlear neurectomy. Trans Am Acad Ophthalmol Otolaryngol 1974;78:252–60.

34. Pulec J, Hitselberger R. Retrosigmoid vestibular nerve section. Arch Otolaryngol 1972;96:412–5.

35. Silverstein H, Norrell H. Retrolabyrinthine surgery: a direct approach to the cerebellopontine angle. Otolaryngol Head Neck Surg 1980;88:462–9.

36. Kimura RS, Schuknecht HF. Membranous hydrops in the inner ear of the guinea pig after obliteration of the endolymphatic sac. Pract Otorhinolaryngol 1965;27:343–8.

37. Shambaugh GE Jr. Surgery on the endolymphatic sac. Arch Otol 1966;83:305–10.

38. Gussen R. Meniere's disease: new temporal bone findings in two cases. Laryngoscope 1971;81:1695–9.

39. Duke WW. Menière's syndrome caused by allergy. JAMA 1923;81:2179–88.

40. Derlacki EL. Non-surgical management of Meniere's disease. Laryngoscope 1954;64:271–82.

41. Hughes GB, Kinney SE, Barna BP, et al. Autoimmune reactivity in Meniere's disease: a preliminary report. Laryngoscope 1983;93:410–21.

42. Anderson JP, Harris JP. Impact of Meniere's disease on quality of life. 2002. [In press.]

43. Coats AC. The summating potential and Meniere's disease. Arch Otolaryngol 1981;107:199–211.

44. Morrison AW, Moffat DA, O'Connor AF. Clinical usefulness of electrocochleography in Menière's disease: an analysis of dehydrating agents. Otolaryngol Clin North Am 1980;13:703–10.

45. Ferraro JA, Arenberg IK, Hassanein RS. Electrocochleography and symptoms of inner ear dysfunction. Arch Otol 1985;3:22–31.

46. Kluckhoff I. Effect of glycerine on fluctuant hearing loss. Otolaryngol Clin North Am 1975;8:345–55.

47. Black FO. Vestibular function assessment in patients with Meniere's disease. Laryngoscope 1982;92:1419–36.

48. McCabe BF. Autoimmune sensorineural hearing loss. Ann Otol Rhinol Laryngol 1979;88(5 Pt 1):585–9.

49. Hughes GB, Kinney SE, et al. Autoimmune reactivity in Meniere's disease: a preliminary report. Laryngoscope 1983;93: 410–7.

50. Harris JP. Autoimmunity of the inner ear. Am J Otol 1989;10: 193–5.

51. Gottschlich S, Billings P, Keithley E, et al. Assessment of serum antibodies in patients with rapidly progressive sensorineural hearing loss and Meniere's disease. Laryngoscope 1995;96:1347–52.

52. Hirose K, Wener MH, Duckert LG. Utility of laboratory testing in autoimmune inner ear disease. Laryngoscope 1999;109: 1749–54.

53. Emmett JR. The large vestibular aqueduct syndrome. Am J Otol 1985;387–415.

54. Minor LB. Superior canal dehiscence syndrome. Am J Otol 21:9–19.

55. Adour KK, Hilsinger RL, Byl FM. Herpes simplex polyganglionitis. Otolaryngol Head Neck Surg 1980;88:270–4.

56. Arbusow V, et al. Distribution of herpes simplex type 1 in human geniculate and vestibular ganglia: implications for vestibular neuronitis. Ann Neurol 1999;46:416–9.

57. Schuknecht HF, Kitamura K. Second Louis H. Clerf Lecture: vestibular neuritis. Ann Otol Rhinol Laryngol 1981;90 Suppl 78:1–19.

58. Paparella MM, Griebe MS: Bilaterality of Meniere's disease, Acta Otolaryngol (Stockh) 1984;97:233–7.

59. Committee on Hearing and Equilibrium. Meniere's disease: criteria for diagnosis and evaluation of therapy for reporting. AAO-HNS Bull 1985;4:6–7.

60. Committee on Hearing and Equilibrium. Guidelines for the diagnosis and evaluation of therapy in Meniere's disease. Otolaryngol Head Neck Surg 1996;114:236–41.

61. Schuknecht HF, Gulya AJ. Endolymphatic hydrops: overview and classification. Ann Otol Rhinol Laryngol 1983;92 Suppl 106:1–20.

62. Selzer S, McCabe BF. Perilymph fistula: the Iowa experience. Laryngoscope 1986;94:37–44.

63. Daspit CP, Churchill D, Linthicum FH. Diagnosis of perilymph fistula using ENG and impedance. Laryngoscope 1980; 90:217–22.

64. Johnson GD. Medical management of migraine-related dizziness and vertigo. Laryngoscope 1998:108 Suppl 85:1–28.

65. Welling DB, Slater PW, Martyn MD, et al. Sensorineural hearing loss after occlusion of the enlarged vestibular aqueduct. Am J Otol 1999;20;338–43.

66. Schuknecht HF, Ruby RRF. Cupuloliathiasis. Adv Otorhinolaryngol 1973;2:434–43.

67. Hall S, Ruby R, McClure J. The mechanisms of benign paroxysmal positional vertigo. J Otolaryngol 1979;8:15–8.

68. Hilger JA. Otolaryngologic aspects of hypometabolism. Ann Otol Rhinol Laryngol 1956;65:395–408.

69. Brackmann D. In Press. Vascular decompression. American Neurotology Society Presentation, 2001. p. 267–71.

70. McCabe BF, Bernstein P. The effect of diazepam on vestibular compensation. Laryngoscope 1974;84:267–71.

71. Harris JP, Ryan AF. Fundamental immune mechanisms of the brain and inner ear. Otolaryngol Head Neck Surg 1995;112: 639–53.

72. Sismanis A, Salley LE, et al. Methotrexate in the management of immune mediated cochleovestibular disorders: clinical experience with 53 patients. J Rheumatol 2001;28:1037–40.

73. Derebery MJ, Berliner KL. Prevalence of allergy in Meniere's disease. Otolaryngol Head Neck Surg 2000;123:69–75.

74. Bryan WTK, Bryan MP. The application of vitro cytotoxic reactions to clinical diagnosis of food allergy. Laryngoscope 1960;70:810–7.

75. Furstenberg AC, Lashmet FH, Talbot F. Meniere's symptom complex: medical treatment. Ann Otol Rhinol Laryngol 1954; 43:1035–52.

76. Cawthorne TE. Positional nystagmus. Ann Otol Rhinol Laryngol 1954;65:481–7.

77. Telian SA, Shepherd NT. Update on vestibular rehabilitation therapy. Otolaryngol Clin North Am 1996;29:359–71.

78. Shumway-Cook A, Horak FB. Rehabilitation strategies for patients with vestibular deficits. Neurol Clin 1990;8;441–57.

79. Epley JM. The canalolith repositioning procedure: for treatment of benign paroxysmal positional vertigo. Otolaryngol Head Neck Surg 1993;107:399–404.

80. Arslan M. Direkt Applikathion des UltrashaHs auf das knockerne Labyrinth zur Therapieder Labyrinthose (Morbus Meniere). I-I. N. Ohrenh 1954;4:166–70.

81. Tabb HG, Norris CH, Hagan WE. Round window ultrasonic irradiation for Meniere's disease with ENG monitoring. Laryngoscope 1978;88:1460–7.

82. Wolfson RJ, Cutt RA, Ishiyama E, et al. Cryosurgery for Meniere's disease. Laryngoscope 1968;78:632–8.

83. House WF. Cryosurgical treatment of Meniere's disease. Arch Otol 1966;84:616–22.

84. Fowler EP Jr. Streptomycin treatment of vertigo. Trans Am Acad Ophthalmol Otolaryngol 1948;52:239–47.

85. Graham MD, Kemink JL. Titration streptomycin therapy for bilateral Meniere's disease: a progress report. Am J Otol 1984; 5:534–41.

86. Glasscock ME, Kveton JR, Christiansen SG. Current status of surgery for Meniere's disease. Otolaryngol Head Neck Surg 1984;92:67–82.

87. Silverstein H, Smouha E, Jones R. Natural history vs. surgery for Meniere's disease. Otolaryngol Head Neck Surg 1989;100: 6–16.

88. Jackson CG, Dickins JR, McMenomy SO, et al. Endolymphatic system shunting: a long-term profile of the Denver Inner Ear Shunt. Am J Otol 1996;17:85–8.

89. House JW, Hitselberger WE, McElveen Jr, et al. Retrolabyrinthine section of the vestibular nerve. Otolaryngol Head Neck Surg 1984;92:212–24.

90. Millen SJ, Meyer G. Retrosigmoid intracanalicular vestibular nerve section: an alternative surgical approach for Meniere's disease. Am J Otol 1986;7:330–41.

91. Youssef TF, Poe DS. Intratympanic gentamicin injection for the treatment of Meniere's disease. Am J Otol 1998;19:435–42.

92. Driscoll CL, Harner SG, et al. Low dose intratympanic gentamicin and the treatment of Meniere's disease: preliminary results. Laryngoscope 1997;197:83–9.

93. Kaplan DM, Nedzelski JM, et al. Intratympanic gentamicin for the treatment of unilateral Meniere's disease. Laryngoscope 2000;110:1298–305.

30

Cochlear Implants

PETER S. ROLAND, MD

Cochlear implants are the first true bionic sense organs. The human cochlea is, in effect, an electromechanical transducer. Cochlear implants, like the human hair cell, receive mechanical sound energy and convert it into a series of electrical impulses. This transformation is not trivial, and some of the brightest engineering minds have spent hundreds of thousands of hours determining how this transformation should be accomplished so as to provide the human auditory cortex with the most meaningful information. Cochlear implants are not hearing aids. Hearing aids merely amplify mechanical sound waves and increase their energy content. Hearing aids do not fundamentally alter the nature of the signal.

Cochlear implants are playing an increasingly important role in the management of both adults and children with hearing impairment. Although the results remain variable and unpredictable for a given individual, a substantial proportion of implant recipients now recover high levels of open-set speech understanding. Cochlear implants permit implant recipients to reintegrate with the hearing world.

In the early days of implantation, there was considerable concern that the constant electrical stimulation produced by the implant would injure residual neural elements within the cochlea. This concern has been laid to rest. The preponderance of available scientific evidence has demonstrated that dendrite stimulation either enhances spiral ganglion cell survival or, at worst, has no effect on spiral ganglial cell counts at all.[1–3]

Linthicum and Anderson demonstrated that of 46 temporal bones with total sensorineural hearing loss, 37 had more than 3,500 residual spiral ganglion cells and would be potential cochlear implant candidates based on that definition.[4] Nadol has shown that the highest num-ber of residual spiral ganglion cells are found following aminoglycoside toxicity and sudden sensorineural hearing loss. The lowest numbers of surviving spiral ganglion cells are seen in individuals with congenital/genetically mediated losses and following bacterial meningitis.[5] Nadol has shown a strong positive correlation between the diameter of the cochlear nerve and the total spiral ganglion cell count ($p \le .001$). This offers the possibility of indirectly assessing the spiral ganglion cell population by measuring the size of the auditory nerve.[5]

Although the history of cochlear implantation in adults goes back well over 20 years, cochlear implantation in children is more recent. Implantation was initially limited to postlingually deafened children because it was widely believed that the device would have little utility for children with severe to profound congenital hearing loss.

Project Hope, combining the results of three different types of survey instruments, has estimated that there are at least 464,000 and possibly as many as 738,000 severe to profoundly hearing-impaired persons among the 22 million Americans with hearing loss. On the basis of these estimates, about 5 of every 10,000 infants have severe to profound hearing loss and, using the US Bureau of the Census data from 1998, 5,600 children under 2 years of age are profoundly hearing impaired.[6] Cheng has estimated that cochlear implants may be useful in as many as 200,000 children in the United States.[7]

IMPACT OF HEARING LOSS

The impact on the US economy of severe/profound hearing loss is substantial. Estimates indicate that as much as 2.5 billion dollars may be lost in workforce productivity. Approximately 42% of individuals with severe/profound hearing impairment between the ages of 18 and 44 years are not working, compared to 18% of the general population.[8,9]

In addition to lost productivity, there are direct costs associated with severe/profound hearing loss. For example, approximately 2 billion dollars is spent to provide equal access for hearing-impaired individuals as required by law.

More than 120 billion dollars is spent in educational costs. Despite substantial resources invested in the education of severe/profoundly hearing-impaired individuals, 44% fail to graduate from high school as compared to 19% of normal-hearing populations. Only 5% of severe to profoundly deaf individuals graduate from college compared to 13% of normal-hearing children.[8] The cost of educating a severe to profoundly deaf child is vastly increased and approaches half a million dollars per child for kindergarten through grade 12. This is 50 times the cost of educating a normal-hearing child.[10,11] The cost of cochlear implantation and associated rehabilitative services (ranging from $29,000 to 46,000) is modest in comparison. If cochlear implantation can shift only 1 child in 10 into a normal, mainstream classroom, the savings in educational costs alone would pay all of the costs of implantation for all 10 implant recipients. Current evidence suggests that considerably more than 1 of 10 children would be able to function within mainstream classrooms, and there is justifiable optimism that the high unemployment rates seen currently in individuals with severe to profound hearing loss can be lowered substantially as a result of widespread implantation.[9] There are already studies indicating that cochlear implantation can improve earnings for adults.[12]

Deaf Culture

The National Association for the Deaf (NAD) is an organization of deaf individuals who believe in "deaf culture." According to the NAD, "deaf people like being deaf, want to be deaf and are proud of their deafness." They do not regard deafness as a disability.[11] Deaf culturalists believe that deaf individuals live and participate in a unique culture and that attempts to eliminate deafness are a form of cultural imperialism or even genocide.[13]

For the most part, deaf culturalists use American Sign Language (ASL). American Sign Language is a dis-

tinctively different language from English with an entirely different grammatical structure. Facility in ASL does not translate into facility with even written English. Deaf culturalists believe that ASL is a "natural" communication system (the basis for this claim of "naturalness" is unclear) for deaf children and that spoken, written, or even signed English is "unnatural." Deaf culturalists believe that deaf children are natural members of deaf culture, and to restore their hearing is to deny them their natural birthright.[8,13]

Deaf culturalists, while claiming on the one hand that deafness is not a disability, derive support and benefit from billions of dollars in disability benefits. Insofar as cochlear implants are effective, deaf individuals who decline to use them have an "elective disability." Tucker has questioned the extent to which individuals with elective disabilities may call on society to provide supportive services and accommodations.[11]

The strongest advocates of deaf culture are quite explicit about the implications of their views: hearing parents have no "right" to make decisions about their deaf children if those decisions might result in hearing restoration. That right, they claim, belongs to the culture to which they "naturally belong" and should be made by deaf culturists on their behalf.[11,13] Some of these deaf culture activists regard cochlear implants in children as a form of "child abuse." These issues have been carefully examined by Balkany and colleagues, with the following conclusion:

> However, the arguments of these leaders are internally contradictory: They hold that deafness is not a disability but support disability benefits for the deaf; they maintain both that cochlear implants do not work and that they work so well that they are "genocidal" (i.e., they will eliminate deafness). Their position opposes the ethical principles of beneficence and autonomy as they relate to self-determination and privacy. Ethical standards hold that the best interest of the child precedes the interest of a special interest group and that parents have the responsibility to determine their child's best interest.[10]

Cost Effectiveness

In 1996, two-thirds of US health care plans cited the absence of cost-effectiveness data as a reason to reject payment for cochlear implants.[7] Although data may have been lacking in the past, good cost-effectiveness data are now available from several sources. Among others, the UK Nottingham group, using conservative assumptions, has demonstrated that cochlear implantation is cost effective within the British health care system.[14–17]

Most cost-effectiveness studies compare efficacy using quality-adjusted life years (QALYs). A QALY is an additional year of life with perfect quality of health. If health is only "50% of perfect," then only half a QALY is awarded for that extra year of life. It would take 5 extra years of life to equal one QALY if health quality during these years was only 20% of perfect. Since the life expectancy of cochlear implant recipients is not anticipated to change as a result of implantation, any increase in QALYs must result directly from improved health utility. Health utility can be measured using a variety of different instruments, including a visual analog scale and a health utility index-2 (HUI-2). These scales have been used most commonly in assessing the cost effectiveness of cochlear implants. The time trade-off instrument has been used only recently to assess the quality of life for children.

Krabbe and colleagues compared 45 postlingually deafened adult multichannel cochlear implant users with 46 deaf candidates on the waiting list for cochlear implants. Three health-related quality of life instruments were used: a specially developed cochlear implant questionnaire, the SF-36 health status questionnaire, and the HUI-2. All three questionnaires detected improvements in health-related quality of life attributable to cochlear implant use.[18]

In 1999, Palmer and colleagues prospectively evaluated cost effectiveness in 62 adult cochlear recipients.[19] Adults who received the implant had a health utility gain (using HUI) of 0.2. Ninety percent of the gain occurred within 6 months of implantation. Using standard models, a 0.2 improvement in health utility resulted in a cost of $14,670 per QALY. Cheng and colleagues published a series of articles assessing the cost effectiveness of cochlear implants. In their studies, half of the substantial loss of health utility (0.6) is recovered by a cochlear implant.[20] Based on their estimates, the cost per QALY for a pediatric cochlear implant recipient varied between $5,197 and $9,029, depending on which survey instrument was used.[21] Generally speaking, a cost of $20,000 to $25,000 per QALY is considered a cost-effective intervention (ie, "a good deal"). For example, placement of a defibrillator has a cost of $34,836 per

QALY. A total knee replacement is $59,292 per QALY. Cochlear implantation has been demonstrated to have one of the highest cost-effectiveness ratings of any current intervention. Overall, including indirect costs such as reduced educational expenses, the cochlear implant provided a savings to society of $53,198 per child.[7,19–21]

PREOPERATIVE EVALUATION

Initial screening for cochlear implant candidacy in postlingually deafened adults begins with pure-tone audiometry and speech discrimination testing. As a general rule, potential cochlear implant candidates will have a pure-tone average greater than 70 dB and a standard speech discrimination score of less than 20 to 30%. The Ad Hoc Subcommittee of the Committee on Hearing and Equilibrium of the American Academy of Otolaryngology-Head and Neck Surgery has recommended that final candidacy determination be made using Hearing In Noise Test (HINT) sentence testing and consonant/nucleus/consonant (CNC) word testing. The HINT provides a reliable and efficient measure of speech recognition in quiet and noise. It is an adaptive test, and its difficulty can be varied to avoid ceiling effects.[22] The HINT is not used in an adaptive mode for pre-evaluation/surgical candidacy purposes, but the adaptive mode is useful to assess results and compare outcomes. The CNC test is an open-set word recognition test that has the same phonemic distribution as English. High-quality disks can be obtained to standardize performance measurements pre- and postoperatively and across institutions. Hearing In Noise Test sentence scores of less than 50% in quiet and CNC scores of less than 20% are used as general candidacy guidelines.

Postlingually deafened children are tested using the same measures as adults, but testing children with prelingual hearing loss is more difficult. Prelingually deafened children require special tests. Indeed, in the early years of cochlear implantation, adequate tests for assessing cochlear implant candidacy in prelingual children had to be developed. Existing tests were inadequate.

The Early Speech Perception (ESP) test assesses speech perception ability and is available in both a low verbal and a standard version. Speech perception ability is divided into three subtests to assess the child's capacity to (1) distinguish patterns in speech ("ball" versus "cookie" versus "airplane" versus "ice cream cone"), (2) identify spondee words ("hot dog," "cowboy," "airplane"), and (3) discriminate monosyllabic words ("ball," "boot," "boat," "bat"). It is useful for children who have developed such language skills. A number of other tests are also used in the evaluation of young and prelingually deafened children. These include the Craig Lip Inventory, Meaningful Auditory Integration Scale (MAIS), Infant-Toddler MAIS. This is a specialized area and requires a specialized clinician.

Medical Evaluation

Once it has been determined that a person is a good audiologic candidate, a medical evaluation is necessary. The medical evaluation should determine that a candidate can undergo the operative procedure with acceptable risks. Radiographic imaging of the temporal bone should be obtained to identify any potential anatomic variations that might contraindicate the operation or require alternations to the usual surgical procedure.

Traditionally, radiographic evaluation of cochlear implant candidates has been performed using high-resolution computed tomographic (CT) scanning. Recent refinements in magnetic resonance imaging (MRI) permit greatly enhanced resolution, and now MRI is also very useful in the preoperative assessment of cochlear implant candidates. There are pros and cons to both techniques (Table 30–1). Each technique is capable of providing important information not provided by the other. Some thought should be given to the individual patient's circumstance and the potential difficulties that may be encountered in that individual before the decision is made as to which type of scan should be requested. Sometimes both types of imaging will be needed.

It has become clear that MRI is the most sensitive technique for identifying early labyrinthitis ossificans. Even high-resolution CT scanning may miss cochlear obstruction in up to 50% of candidates. Computed tomographic scanning cannot detect labyrinthine obstruction until frank ossification has developed. On the other hand, MRI relies on the presence or absence of a fluid signal within the labyrinthine bone. Consequently, anything that displaces or eliminates fluid from within the cochlea or semicircular canals, notably unossified fibrous tissue, will result in a detectable abnormality.[23–26] Consequently, MRI has become the diagnostic modality of choice for the detection of postmeningitic endocochlear obstruction.

Magnetic resonance imaging can demonstrate an absent or hypoplastic cochlear nerve. Using currently available 1.5-T magnets, precise measurements of the size of the cochlear nerve are difficult, but higher-strength magnets may soon permit more exact quantification of cochlear nerve diameter. Since cochlear nerve diameter appears to correlate with the number of surviving spiral ganglion cells, quantification of the size of the cochlear nerve may allow more exact prediction of postoperative outcome after cochlear implantation.[27] An absent cochlear nerve is one of the few absolute contraindications to cochlear implantation. Although a small internal auditory canal on CT scan suggests an absent cochlear nerve, absence of the cochlear nerve can definitely be verified on MRI using parasagittal reconstructions through the internal auditory canal (Figure 30–1).

Defects in the cribriform area, which present the likelihood of an intraoperative "gusher," can be identified on MRI scanning and warn the surgeon about this potential difficulty. Central nervous system (CNS) abnormalities that could adversely affect the outcome of implantation can also be well identified on MRI.

High-resolution CT scanning, however, permits more complete characterization of hypoplasia, aplasia, incomplete partitioning defects (Mondini deformities) (Figures 30–2 and 30–3), and enlarged vestibular aqueducts. High-resolution CT scanning permits fairly precise mapping of the fallopian canal and facial nerve. A clear understanding of facial nerve anatomy is especially important in those persons with temporal bone developmental anomalies that increase the likelihood of anomalous facial nerve anatomy.

Table 30–1 CT OR MRI?		
	CT	MRI
Morphology of cochlea and semicircular canals	++	+++
Patency of cochlear duct	+	++
Status of cochlear nerve	–	+++
Anatomy of facial nerve and fallopian canal	++	+
Defect of the modiolus	+	+++–
Defect of cribriform area	+++	++
Enlarged vestibular aqueduct	++	+++
Enlarged cochlear aqueduct	+++	+
Presence of round or oval window	+++	–
CNS abnormalities		+++

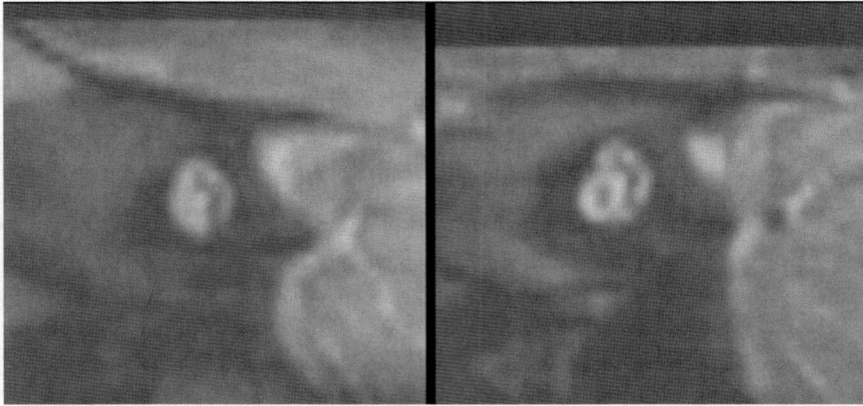

Figure 30–1   Sagittal reconstruction of the internal auditory canal showing normal configuration and orientation of the nerves in the internal auditory canal on the right and the absence of the cochlear nerve on the sagittal reconstruction to the left. Illustration courtesy of Dr. Timothy Booth.

Psychological Evaluation

A psychosocial evaluation is usually a part of the evaluation of the pediatric patient. The purpose of a psychosocial evaluation is to determine the intellectual ability of the child, establish the child's expectations for postimplant performance, and identify family issues that may affect implantation or post implant performance. If the child's intelligence is less than normal, the goals for the child, along with expectations, should be scaled back. Rehabilitative milestones for these recipients may be achieved more slowly. In severe to profoundly deaf children, nonverbal tests must be used. A revised form of the Wechsler Intelligence Scale is available for this purpose. Using these results, the psychologist, working with the speech pathologist and audiologist, will establish whether the child has developed the necessary cognitive and behavioral skills for successful programming. Success is much more likely if the implant can be effectively programmed. If the child has not yet developed these skills, it is in some instances worthwhile postponing the implant long enough for the appropriate behavior to emerge. Intensive therapy can be directed toward the child's particular deficits to help him/her develop the necessary skill set.

Family issues that may affect the success of the implant such as marital stress, depression, or abuse must

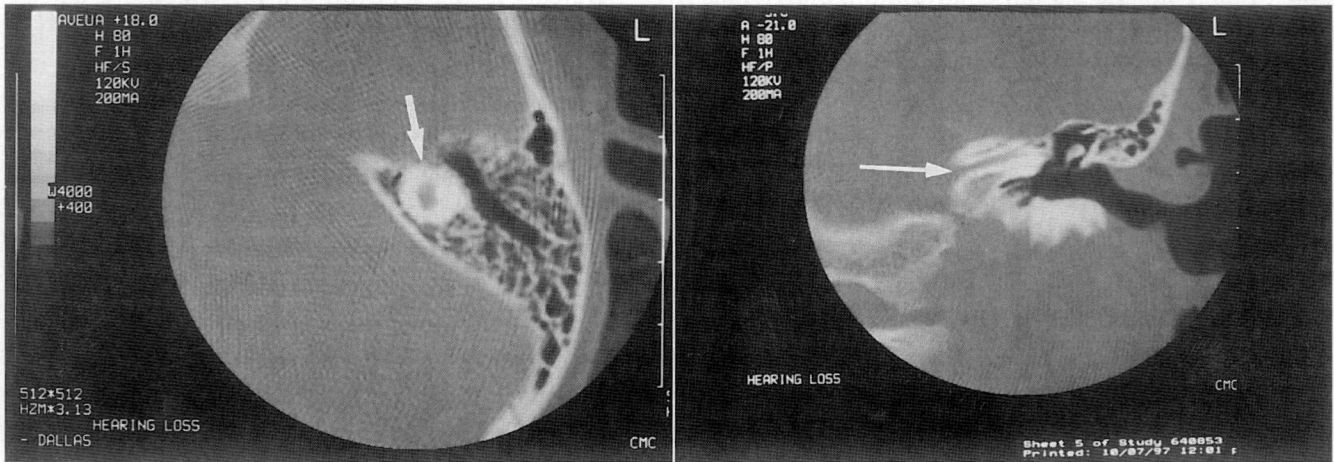

Figure 30–2   Axial section on the left demonstrates a severe cochlear malformation—in this case, a common cavity deformity (*white arrow*). There is no internal auditory canal visible through this section. The image on the right shows that there is a small canal present that is just large enough to accommodate the facial nerve. The cochlear and vestibular nerves are absent, as are the vestibule and semicircular canals.

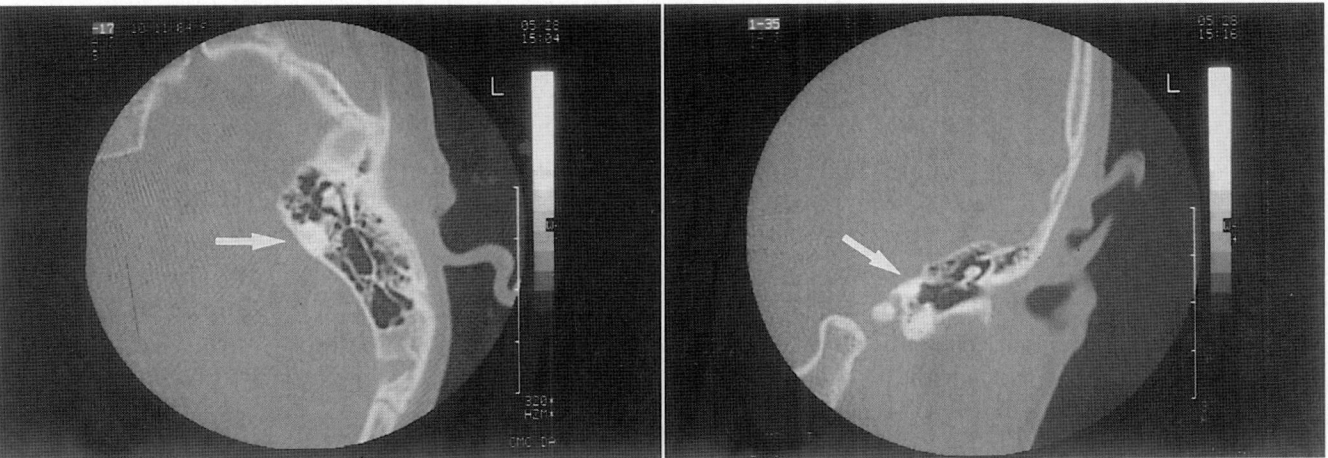

Figure 30–3 The axial section on the left shows the complete absence of the cochlea. There is only some sclerotic bone where the cochlea should be. There is a complete absence of the internal auditory canal on both the axial and the coronal sections (*right*). Although no evidence of the internal auditory canal is apparent on these films, the patient had normal facial nerve function, indicating that the facial nerve was in fact intact.

be identified and resolved. If the cochlear implant candidate is an adolescent, then special attention must be given to make sure that the parent's wishes and those of the adolescent are not substantially different. For example, an adolescent well integrated into a signing community may agree to an implant as a result of parental pressure when he/she really does not want one. If implanted, he/she is likely to become a nonuser.

Family dynamics are assessed during the psychosocial evaluation. Sometimes significant problems of family interaction are recognized that can be improved with appropriate therapy. Such therapy often continues long after the implant has been placed and successfully programmed. Improved family dynamics can significantly enhance a child's ability to become a successful implant user.

Perhaps the most important part of the psychosocial evaluation is to assess both the recipient's and his/her family expectations for the device. Almost nothing creates more trouble in the postoperative period as do unrealistic expectations on the part of cochlear implant recipients or their family members. The evaluating psychologist can accurately assess both the open and the "hidden" expectations of potential recipients and/or their families for the device. If expectations are unrealistic, they can be modified prior to implantation. When expectations are realistic, the chance of disappointment, anger, and rejection of the device is greatly diminished.

Multihandicapped Candidate

The assessment of multihandicapped individuals can be especially challenging. Handicaps most commonly associated with congenital hearing loss often include mental retardation, visual and motor delays, epilepsy, autism, cerebral palsy, attention-deficit disorder, and a variety of syndromic abnormalities including CHARGE association (coloboma of the eye, heart anomaly, choanal atresia, retardation, and genital and ear anomalies), Usher's syndrome, and Pendred's syndrome.

Lesinski and colleagues have evaluated 47 children who were implanted and had one or more associated handicaps. Eighty-two percent of these children were successfully programmed.[28] Isaacson and colleagues evaluated 5 children with significant disabilities matched to 5 children without such disabilities. Benefits were realized in the children with disabilities, but they did less well overall.[29] Waltzman and colleagues have evaluated 29 children between the ages of 2 and 12 years with significant handicaps. These children received significant benefit, but development was slower and less stable.[30]

Although associated handicaps are not in and of themselves a contraindication to cochlear implantation, children with multiple handicaps should be carefully evaluated by a team that understands not only the nature of their handicaps but the requirements for programming and successful use of a cochlear implant.

Which Ear to Implant

The selection of which ear to implant can be difficult. In the earliest days of cochlear implantation, the worse hearing ear was generally selected. It was argued that the implantation itself would destroy residual hearing (and it does in at least 50% of cases) and that the better hearing ear should be conserved in case the implant did not work.[31] Over the years, that philosophy has changed. As experience with cochlear implants has grown, confidence in them has increased. Experience to date indicates that the ability to eliminate patients who will not benefit from the implant has become quite good. Consequently, many programs currently select the better hearing ear. It is reasoned that the better hearing ear is likely to have a higher population of residual neural elements and hence offer the possibility of better performance. Most implant surgeons have had the experience of implanting the worse hearing ear, with the result that the patient has achieved no benefit. In such cases, one is inclined to wonder if the results would have been better if the better hearing ear had been implanted. Moreover, it is now often felt that if the residual hearing in the better hearing ear could provide significant benefit, then the patient would not be an appropriate implant candidate. Despite such reasoning, it has not been possible to verify, on the basis of quantitative outcome data, that implanting the better hearing ear produces superior results. Indeed, there is some evidence that results are just as good when the poorer ear is implanted, especially if the difference between them is small.[32] Although this may well be true when differences between ears are small, the question remains unanswered when differences between ears are large.

Outcome data on cochlear implantation have shown repeatedly and with a fairly high degree of reliability that the longer the duration of deafness, the worse the postoperative performance. Consequently, differences in length of deafness between ears are often used to select the ear to receive the implant. The most recently deafened ear is chosen. Anatomic considerations may guide side selection. If one ear is significantly dysplastic or hypoplastic, the contralateral ear may be selected.

Differences in cochlear patency are also often determinative. Although labyrinthitis ossificans is generally symmetric over long periods of time, it may initially progress more rapidly in one ear than in the other. The least obstructed labyrinth should be chosen.

Sometimes a previous procedure in one ear makes the other ear more desirable. Canal wall down mastoidectomy in one ear would make the contralateral side more appealing because the standard operative procedure would not require modification.

Occasionally, there is a marked difference in vestibular function between one ear and the other. Previous trauma (surgical or otherwise) may have significantly reduced labyrinthine function on one side. If so, that side should be chosen so as to preserve the ear with the better vestibular function. If, however, the ear with reduced labyrinthine function is also the worse hearing ear or the ear with the longer duration of deafness, the situation becomes more difficult. In such circumstances, it may be justified to implant the ear with better vestibular function if, in the opinion of the implanting surgeon, a significantly better hearing outcome is likely to be obtained.

Ultimately, auditory information must reach the cerebral cortex to be useful. Even when peripheral auditory function is identical, there may be significant differences in the amount of CNS activation obtained by stimulating one side as opposed to the other. New techniques in brain imaging such as single-photon emission CT, functional MRI, and refined cortical auditory electrophysiology may allow differences in CNS activation to be identified preoperatively.[33]

Age of Implantation

Cochlear implantation in children began in the second half of the 1980s under the close supervision of the US Food and Drug Administration (FDA). It was initially limited to postlingually deafened children because it was widely believed that the device would have little utility for children with congenital hearing loss. Over the decades, the indications have expanded based on documented outcomes submitted to and reviewed by the FDA.

The age of implantation has slowly been lowered from 2 years through 18 months to 1 year of age. Initial objections to implanting very young children were partially based on the perceived potential for electrode migration/extrusion secondary to skull growth. This concern was addressed by Roland and colleagues, who used computer graphic analysis to assess electrode position on serial postoperative radiographs. Children were followed from 1 to 75 months, and no change in electrode position was noted.[34]

Almost all experts in the area of speech and language development have believed, on an intuitive basis, that younger age of implantation will be associated with improved outcomes. Slowly, evidence to support their intuitions is accumulating. Researchers at the University of Michigan have demonstrated that the post implantation speech recognition scores of 48 7 year olds varied according to the length of time the child had been implanted. The longer the child had the implant, the better the speech recognition scores. They evaluated an additional 53 children 36 months after their implant had been placed. Holding the length of use fixed, they demonstrated that the children's performance improved as age at time of implant decreased. Moreover, at a fixed postimplant age, children implanted at younger ages demonstrated better performance.[35] Svirsky and colleagues have shown that postimplant, the rate of expressive and receptive language learning approaches that of normal-hearing children. However, catch-up effects are hard to show. Consequently, younger age at implantation would leave a narrower gap between normal-hearing and implanted children.[36] Moog and Geers have shown that normal levels of language and reading are associated with earlier age of implantation.[37] Cheng and colleagues's meta-analysis showed that more rapid gains in speech perception are associated with earlier age in implantation.[21]

Reservations have also been voiced about implanting older patients. Concerns about effectiveness and cost utility have been raised. Although ganglion cell loss is a feature of many forms of presbycusis, it rarely reduces ganglion cell populations below the 3,000 (about 10% of normal) cells necessary for speech recognition. Data on speech recognition scores in elderly patients who have received cochlear implants verify that the elderly are as likely to achieve successful hearing outcomes as are younger patients.

A number of other concerns have been raised about the geriatric population. It has been suggested that they are at greater risk for soft tissue complications because of decreased blood flow in scalp tissues, related not only to microvascular disease but also to an increasing incidence of diabetes. However, no such increase of soft tissue complications has been verified.[38] Because elderly individuals recover less promptly from vestibular injuries, it has

been hypothesized that the impact of cochlear implant on ambulation and falling could be disproportionately severe in an elderly population. No data have been produced to support this concern, and Labadie and colleagues have shown no differences in hospital stays between geriatric and younger patients.[38] If enough vestibular function was destroyed to affect ambulation, one would expect a delay in hospital discharge. It has been noted that depression, social isolation, and anxiety are more prevalent in both the deaf and the elderly, and it has been speculated that the combination of both could mitigate against successful rehabilitation. However, several studies have evaluated the effectiveness of cochlear implants in the elderly. Labadie and colleagues have demonstrated that both geriatric and younger patients have statistically significant increases in Central Institute for the Deaf (CID) and CNC scores (there was no difference between groups).[38] Satisfaction with the device has also been demonstrated as increased self-confidence and improved quality of life.[39]

Candidacy Guidelines

As cochlear implants have achieved documented improvements in open-set speech recognition scores, FDA guidelines for implantation have been expanded. Initially, FDA guidelines suggested that potential recipients should have pure-tone averages (PTAs) of 90 dB or greater. The guideline has been lowered to 70 dB in recent clinical trials. It was initially suggested by the FDA that appropriate implant candidates should have HINT sentence scores of less than 20% in quiet. This criterion has now been substantially relaxed, and individuals with less than 50% correct responses to HINT sentences in quiet are considered appropriate candidates. It is worth emphasizing that FDA-approved criteria are guidelines and do not constrain an experienced implant team from making thoughtful exceptions. There is a move toward using CNC words as a criterion, primarily to avoid ceiling effects during postoperative evaluation.

Auditory Neuropathy

Auditory neuropathy is a recently identified type of sensorineural hearing loss. It is defined as a condition in which otoacoustic emissions are present but auditory brainstem response (ABR) waveforms are absent in the context of normal middle ear functions. It is hypothesized that the condition occurs because cochlear hair cells are discharging dyssynchronously, such that no identifiable action potential develops in the cochlear nerve. Hearing loss in this condition is variable, perhaps because of variable degrees of dyssynchrony. Since hearing aids only increase sound intensity and do nothing to restore synchrony, they have not been effective. Cochlear implants, in theory, could restore synchrony by bypassing the cochlear hair cells and stimulating the auditory nerve directly and synchronously.

Labadie and colleagues have reported that the sound-field threshold improved from an average of > 70 dB preoperatively to better than 37 dB postoperatively in four patients with auditory neuropathy after cochlear implantation.[40] Electrical ABR showed detectable waveforms on apical, middle, and basal turn stimulation. Shallop and colleagues have shown good results for cochlear implantation in five children with auditory neuropathy at 1-year follow-up.[41] All had significant improvements in sound detection, speech perception, and communication skills. Shallop and colleagues interpreted the presence of a robust N1 on neural response telemetry (NRT) as an indication that synchrony was at least partially restored. Otoacoustic emissions remained in the contralateral ear but were eliminated in the operated ear after implantation.[41]

Bilateral Implantation

Some surgeons, most notably in Europe, have developed considerable enthusiasm for bilateral implantation. There are several potential benefits from using two implants.

Normal-hearing listeners benefit from the "head shadow effect." At any given time, in a normal listening environment, each ear receives signals with different signal-to-noise ratios (SNRs). Normal listeners can pick the ear with the best SNR and enhance their ability for speech understanding. This benefit becomes apparent in noisy environments, where individuals with unilateral hearing experience greater difficulty in speech understanding.

Unilateral hearing makes sound localization almost impossible. Normal-hearing listeners use both interau-ral time delays and interaural intensity differences to localize sound. Normal-hearing listeners can detect as little as 1 to 2 degrees of difference in the origin of a sound signal. It is speculated that cochlear implant users could gain significant sound localization ability using bilateral implants.

It has been documented that bilateral implant users can gain significant sound localization using both time discrimination and interaural intensity cues. It has been demonstrated that an average temporal resolution of 50 μs was achievable in four of eight bilaterally implanted patients, which should be adequate for 10 degrees of angle resolution in a free-field environment. One patient had a 25-μs resolution. Normal-hearing patients have, at best, 9 μs of resolution. On average, it is about 15 μs. The extent to which improved sound localization might enhance speech perception in noise remains to be determined.

D'Haese and colleagues have documented benefit in a group of 22 patients with bilateral implants.[42] Speech recognition in noise was improved when both implants were used simultaneously, and the difference was statistically significant. (Comprehension of monosyllables delivered in quiet was also significantly better when using both implants rather than using either implant alone.) D'Haese and colleagues were able to conclude that some of this benefit was attributable to factors other than merely the head shadow effect, including binaural unmasking ("squelch" effect) and diotic summation.[42]

Despite these potential advantages, bilateral implantation remains controversial. A number of questions remain to be answered, including the following:

1. Could a cochlear implant user achieve some of the same results from using two microphones feeding through a single implant?
2. Should one "use up" both ears, especially in a child? Although the recipient may adapt and obtain more benefit from bilateral cochlear implantation, it is reasonable to assume that over the period of a typical child's life (70+ years), significant improvements in technology will be made. Should the second ear be held in reserve to take advantage of such technological improvements? Will the nonstimulated ear suffer neural degeneration and/or neural pathway degeneration if left unstimulated for many years?
3. Will the increase in mapping difficulty obviate benefit? Dealing with the problems of binaural loudness

summation and pitch matching across ears may be difficult and require substantial increase in mapping time. If the maps are poorly coordinated, the conflict between maps may eliminate the potential benefit.

4. Can bilateral implantation produce significant bilateral vestibular injury?
5. Is bilateral implantation cost effective?

The move toward bilateral implantation is occurring slowly and with great caution in the United States. There appears to be an emerging consensus that the benefits of bilateral implantation should be clearly demonstrated in adult subjects before bilateral implantation is advocated for children.

Device Selection

Three devices are currently implanted in the United States (Table 30–2). Many programs offer all three devices. Each device has advantages and disadvantages, and choosing among them can be difficult. To date no systemic differences in performance between devices have been demonstrated. Consequently, the final decision is often made on the basis of patient preference.

Coding Strategy

A speech coding strategy defines the method by which pitch, loudness, and timing of sound are translated into a series of electrical impulses. There are a variety of coding strategies currently in use. All of the three devices available in the United States are capable of using more than one type of strategy. Strategies can be categorized into two types: simultaneous or nonsimultaneous.

Simultaneous Strategies

Simultaneous strategies permit the activation of more than one electrode at the same time.

Only the Clarion® (Advanced Bionics Corporation, Sylmar, Calif.) device is capable of simultaneous stimulation. The utility of simultaneous activation is contested, and the currently available outcome data are equivocal. Nonetheless, many implant professionals and potential recipients believe that simultaneous stimulation can improve speech outcomes and provide a more natural quality of sound.

When two electrodes are activated simultaneously, there is a potential that their signals will interfere with each other, a phenomenon known as "channel interaction." The lower the intensity of an emitted signal, the lower the likelihood that it will interact with a signal from a neighboring channel. When an electrode is close to the ganglion cells within the modiolus, it takes less energy to stimulate the cell. Consequently, simultaneous strategies appear to benefit from modiolus-hugging electrode arrays (see below).

Nonsimultaneous Strategies

Continuous interleaved sampling (CIS) strategies stimulate each active electrode serially. Every electrode is stimulated in turn, one after the other. No electrode is bypassed or stimulated out of order. Assuming that each electrode stimulates a different frequency within the cochlea, the cochlea receives complete information about the frequency composition of the incoming signal, even for frequencies that are not represented in the incoming signal. It is clear that, up to a certain point, the rapidity with which this sequential stimulation occurs affects speech recognition. Although there has been an inclination to believe that "the faster the better," it has not been possible to unequivocally demonstrate that "very fast" CIS strategies produce improved speech recognition.

All three currently available devices can be programmed using a CIS strategy. However, the rates at which stimulation occur are different.

Feature extraction strategies do not attempt to encode complete frequency information about the incoming signal; rather, they attempt to "extract" the frequency information that will be most useful to the CNS for the purposes of speech understanding. Once those features of the incoming signal believed to most important for speech understanding have been selected by the processor, they are presented to the electrodes. The electrodes are not activated sequentially because only those electrodes that represent frequencies "extracted" from the incoming signal are activated. These strategies are often called "roving strategies" because they "rove" around the

Table 30–2 COMPARISON DEVICES		
Nucleus 24 "Contour" **Denver, CO**	**Clarion C-II** **Sylmar, CA**	**MED-EL Combi 40+** **Innsbruck, Austria**
Manufacturer Cochlear Melbourne, Australia 20,000 implanted worldwide Nucleus 22 approved in 1982 First multichannel behind-the-ear device	Advanced Bionics Sylmar, California Over 8,000 implanted worldwide Makes other neurostimulators Clarion device approved in US in 1991	MED-EL Innsbruck, Austria Over 6,500 worldwide Developing implants since 1976 About 400 US implants
FDA approved age for each implant 12 mo	12 mo	18 mo
Length of electrode array 25 mm	24 mm	31 mm
Type of electrode Flexible "coiling" perimodiolar electrode array Focused stimulation	Straight array that can be placed into a perimodiolar position by use of an attached or separate electrode Focused stimulation	Soft, flexible straight array designed for lateral wall stimulation
Special electrode arrays Yes—a split array is available	No	Yes—both a split array and a compressed array are readily available
Number of electrodes 24 (2 are ground electrodes)	16	24 + 1 additional ground electrode
Number of channels 22	16 The addition of "virtual" channels could bring count up to 31	12 – each electrode pair = 1 channel
Processing speed: maximum potential stimulation rate in pulses per second 14,400	Pulsatile (sequential): Up to 250,000 nonsimultaneous biphasic pulses per second Digital-analog (simultaneous): up to 100,000 updates per second	18,180
MRI compatibility Not MRI compatible but the magnet is easily removable and replaceable as a simple minor procedure using local anesthesia	Standard device is not MRI compatible, but a special order "magnetless" device is available	Under investigation for 0.2 T in the US MRI safe at 0.2, 1.0, 1.5 T internationally Special scanning protocol must be followed
Speech processor and headpiece Both body worn and ear level available Directional (front-facing) microphone	Body-worn processor Ear level planned Omnidirectional microphone	Both body-worn and ear level processor Omnidirectional microphone
Accessory equipment Telephone adapter FM cable Personal audio cable Lapel microphone Monitor earphones Television/high-fidelity cable Battery charger Pouch or harness for children Spare cable in a variety of lengths and colors	Telephone adapter Auxiliary microphone Telecoil Belt clip for adults Battery charger Battery charger car adapter Variety of pouches or harnesses for children Spare cable in a variety of lengths and colors	Body worn processor: 2 belt clip options, 2 battery chargers, pouch or harness for children, spare cable in a variety of lengths and colors BTE processor: 4 battery packs for BTE that can be worn in a variety of ways, numerous attachment options for BTE, FM cables, personal audio cable, telephone adapter, lapel microphone, dry-aid kit, battery charger
Program storage capacity Body-worn processor can store 4 Ear-level processor can store 2	Body-worn processor can store 3 Ear-level processor can store 2–3	Body-worn processor can store 3 Ear-level processor can store up to 9 programs (mostly 3 programs with 3 volume settings for each program are chosen)
Speech coding strategies Can use SPEAK, CIS, and ACE	Can use SAS, CIS, and MPS CII can use high-resolution mode processing	Body-worn processor can use CIS and high rate N of M Ear-level processor uses high-rate CIS+ (implemented the Hilbert transformation)
Warranty Implanted components: 10 yr External component: 3 yr Accidental damage and loss coverage is available for all devices for < $200/yr Speech processor covered for loss one time in the initial 3-year warranty	Implanted components: 10 yr External components: 3 yr Accidental damage and loss coverage is available for all devices for < $200/yr	Implanted components: 10 yr External components: 3 yr Limited accidental damage and loss coverage is available for all devices for < $400/yr Unlimited accidental damage and loss coverage is available for all devices for $675/yr Accidental damage and loss coverage is available for all devices for < $385/yr (unlimited)

MRI = magnetic resonance imaging; BTE = behind the ear; SPEAK = spectral peak; CIS = continuous interleaved sampling; ACE = above combination encoders; SAS = simultaneous analog stimulation; MPS = multiple pulsatile; CII = Clarion 2.

electrode array, activating only those electrodes needed to supply the relevant information. Only late-generation feature extraction strategies are currently used. The MED EL COMBI 40® (MED EL Co., Innsbruck, Austria) can be programmed using an "N of M" feature extraction strategy, whereas the Nucleus 24® (Cochlear Corporation, Melbourne, Australia) device can be programmed using spectral peak (SPEAK) or above combination encoder (ACE). The ACE is, in effect, a fast form of SPEAK. The programming audiologist can adjust the number of frequencies selected from a given incoming signal (called "maxima") and the rate at which those features are presented to the electrode array.

Although there are theoretical reasons to believe that one strategy may be superior to another, no systematic differences between the most advanced strategies for any device have yet been demonstrated.

Styling

Other features that may be important for patients in device selection are appearance and styling. Each device looks different, and one may be more attractive to a given individual than another. Since compelling differences in performance cannot be demonstrated, the use of esthetic criteria in deciding between devices is not entirely irrational.

Modiolus-Hugging Electrode

It is widely believed that if the stimulating electrodes are closer to the auditory nerve cells, then stimulation will be more efficient and more efficacious. The ganglion cells reside in the core of the cochlear spiral, an area termed the modiolus. Consequently, there has been an ongoing effort to move the stimulating electrodes as close to the modiolus as possible. Electrodes that are in close approximation to the modiolus are referred to as modiolus-hugging electrodes. Two strategies are currently being implemented to move the electrodes close to the modiolus. Clarion has developed the use of a positioner. The positioner is a small, carefully shaped Silastic obturator that slides into the scala tympani lateral to the electrode array and pushes it inward toward the modiolus. The Nucleus device has a self-coiling electrode array with

"memory." The electrode array comes with a stylette, which keeps the electrode array relatively straight and relatively stiff so that it can be easily inserted. Once the electrode is inserted, the stylette is withdrawn and the electrode array "springs back" into its original, coiled configuration. Coiling wraps the electrode array tightly around the modiolus. Both techniques appear to be effective.

It has been convincingly demonstrated that the amount of electrical energy necessary to stimulate cochlear neurons is reduced when the electrodes are in close proximity to the modiolus.[43] Both threshold level and comfort level are lowered. Since channel interaction is a potentially significant problem with simultaneous strategies, it is not surprising that the number of cochlear implant recipients who prefer to use the simultaneous strategy has significantly increased since Clarion has started using a modiolus-hugging array. Since the amount of current required to stimulate cochlear neurons is significantly reduced in modiolus-hugging array, battery life is extended when such arrays are used. Battery life is an important issue in the emerging competition for a totally implantable device. It has not been demonstrated, however, that modiolus-hugging electrodes produce improved speech recognition compared to nonmodiolus-hugging arrays.

Ear-Level Processor

The availability of an ear level processor is very important for many patients. Most implant surgeons have cared for individuals who simply rejected cochlear implantation out of hand until the ear-level processor became available. An ear-level processor is now available for all of the devices available in the United States. The MED-EL ear-level processor is unique in that performance is demonstrably better using the ear-level device than the body-worn processor.

There are significant differences between behind-the-ear hearing aids with respect to processor capacity and battery life, which may help guide a patient's choice.

Magnetic Resonance Imaging

Although concerns about postoperative MRI scanning are not a major issue for most patients, they are a very important issue for a select minority. Individuals with CNS disorders that have traditionally been followed using MRI techniques are the most likely to be concerned. Magnetic resonance imaging has traditionally been considered contraindicated in cochlear implant recipients because of the potential for interaction between the two magnets. There are four possible interactions that could occur between the implanted magnet and a strong external magnetic field: movement of the stimulator/receiver or electrode array, generation of noxious or even injurious auditory stimuli, generation of heat, and demagnetization. These interactions have been investigated and are partially understood:

1. It seems clear that the energies produced by even a relatively strong magnetic field will not produce sufficient heat to be troublesome.
2. Those few patients who have had MRI scans with cochlear implants in place have not reported injurious or disturbing auditory sensations.
3. Although there is some concern about movement in stronger magnetic fields, it does not appear to be a problem in magnetic fields of lower strengths (< 0.5 T) (most "open" MRI units are of this strength), and it may be that external stabilization of the device can limit the potential for movement of the stimulator/receiver even in stronger fields.
4. Demagnetization does occur, in vitro, with as much as 10% of the magnetic strength lost with each scan. The degree of demagnetization depends on the length of time the device is scanned and the strength of the magnetic field.[44]

Several solutions have been offered by different manufacturers.

Advanced Bionics® (Sylmar, Calif.) manufactures a special version of the Clarion implant that has no magnet. It needs to be specially ordered in advance. The external headpiece is held to the magnetless stimulator/receiver with a special earpiece. To function correctly, the stimulator/receiver must be implanted closer to the auricle, so special care needs to be taken during the operative procedure. Weber and colleagues have reported on 11 individuals with magnetless Clarion devices, and the headpieces were stable and worked well.[45] A single patient has been reported who was implanted in England again with success.[46]

The Cochlear Corporation (Melbourne, Australia) manufactures the Nucleus device with a removable magnet. The magnet can be extracted through an incision made directly over the stimulator/receiver and then replaced later. The required incision is small, and it appears that the magnet can be easily removed as an outpatient procedure using only local anesthesia.

The electromagnetic interference between the MED-EL device and a 1.5-T scanner was within acceptable limits except for torque, which was questionable. Scanning at 0.2 T was clearly safe, and the MED-EL device has received the FDA's permission in an investigative setting for use in a low-strength magnetic resonance scanner. However, there is a "blackout zone" extending 2 to 4 cm around the device in every direction. Consequently, magnetic resonance scanning, even though it can be performed safely, will not provide meaningful information about those areas of the skull base and brain close to the implant.[44]

Investigators at the University of Vienna evaluated 11 patients in a 1-T magnet. Each patient was evaluated 1 day before planned explantation. Auditory perception was evaluated before and after examination, and all explanted devices were assessed for function. There was no detectable movement of the electrode or the receiver coil in any of the patients, and there was no measured temperature change. There were no adverse stimuli reported by any subject. They concluded that the presence of a MED-EL cochlear implant was not a firm contraindication to MRI.[47]

Special Electrode Arrays

For a number of years, Med-EL has manufactured special electrode arrays for special clinical situations. A "compressed array" is available that includes the same number of electrodes as the standard array but compressed into about 60% of the distance. The compressed array is useful for patients with labyrinthitis ossificans when only a portion of the cochlear duct is available for implantation. If a "drill out" procedure is performed, it is usually possible to get the entire compressed array into the accessible portion of the cochlea. The compressed array is also useful for common cavity deformities of the cochlea. Electrode arrays placed in a single, common cavity tend to "curl up" so that the distal portion of the electrode curls over on itself and the electrodes overlap. There is less overlap of electrodes using the compressed electrode array.

A second special electrode array divides the electrodes and puts about half of the electrodes on each of two separate leads. Double arrays are also designed for subjects with labyrinthitis ossificans. Separate cochleostomies are performed into the inferior and superior portions of the basal turn of the cochlea, and the electrode arrays are then passed separately into the superior and inferior portions of the basal turns. This design allows a greater number of electrodes to be inserted than could be inserted using a technique limited to drilling out only as much of the basal turn as can be reached through a single, round window cochleostomy.

Cochlear Corporation also makes a split or double array and continues to manufacture the straight (noncontour) array. The Nucleus double array is designed for use in patients with labyrinthitis ossification. The straight array has electrode placement that is closer together than even the MED-EL compressed array, but because there are more electrodes, the length of the entire array is longer than MED-EL's compressed array.

THE SURGICAL PROCEDURE

Preoperative Consideration

Roughly half of the cochlear implants performed in children in the United States are performed as outpatients and half as inpatients. Liu and colleagues have shown that outpatient cochlear implantation is safe.[48] However, its acceptance by parents is less than universal. It is tolerated but not necessarily desired. Follow-up surveys have shown that the later in the day the operation finishes and the further away the patients live, the less likely parents and recipients are to be satisfied with the outpatient setting.

Prophylactic Antibiotics

Although no double-blind studies have been conducted to justify the efficacy of perioperative antibiotics, they are administered by almost all surgeons. Intravenous antibiotics should be given at least 20 minutes before the incision is made. Antibiotics should be continued for the first 24 hours postoperatively.

Incision and Skin Flap

A variety of incisions have been used. Initially, cochlear implants were almost always performed using the same type of C-shaped incision used for routine mastoidectomy but significantly enlarged so that the incision line did not overlap the implanted stimulator/receiver (Figures 30–4 and 30–5). It is widely believed that the incision should not cross the edges of the device. If the incision must cross over the stimulator/receiver, it should cross it at right angles and not parallel one of its edges. Although this admonition is widely promulgated in descriptions of surgical technique, it is frequently violated in practice.

In the mid-1990s, the inverted U–shaped incision became increasingly more common. The inverted U had several advantages. Theoretical considerations suggest that most of the blood flow to the skin of the postauricular area comes from inferiorly upward and that the blood supply to an inverted U–shaped flap is better. It is hard to incorporate a previous mastoidectomy incision into a postauricular C-shaped flap without producing a potentially avascular area between the two incisions. A few cases of flap necrosis are known to have occurred when an enlarged postauricular C-shaped incision was placed behind a previous mastoidectomy incision. It is much easier to incorporate a previous mastoidectomy incision into an inverted U; the previous mastoidectomy incision simply becomes the anterior limb of the inverted U.

As ever more experience in implantation was obtained, the posterior limb of the inverted U was abandoned, and an incision that looked a bit more like an inverted L or an inverted J became more common. Over the last decade or so, incisions have become progressively shorter and more cosmetically acceptable.

Once the incision has been completed, the flap is elevated. The flap can be elevated either as a single layer or in two layers. If two layers are separately elevated, the superficial layer should be elevated first and the deep tissues, which include the periosteum of the mastoid, temporalis fascia, and temporalis muscle, should be left intact. The periosteum of the mastoid should then be ele-

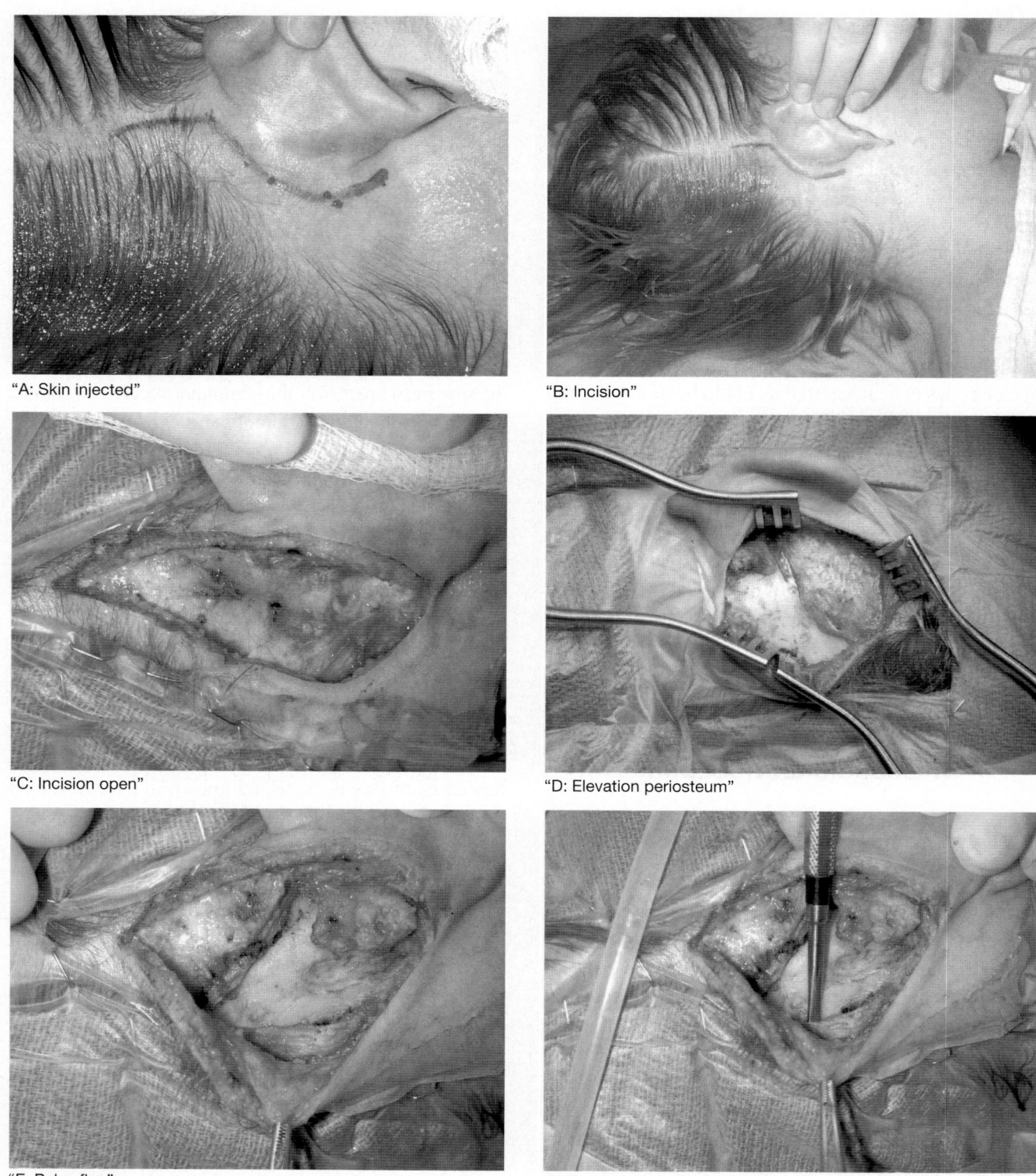

"A: Skin injected"

"B: Incision"

"C: Incision open"

"D: Elevation periosteum"

"E: Palva flap"

"F: Superperiosteal pocket"

Figure 30–4   A series of photographs indicating the steps in cochlear implantation.

Continued on next page.

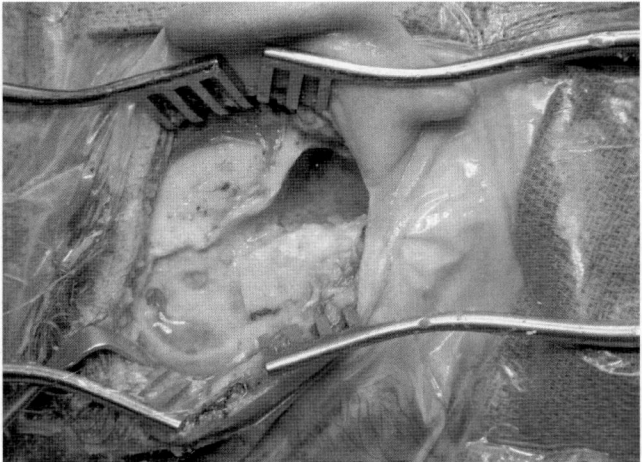

"G: Mastiodectomy and well"

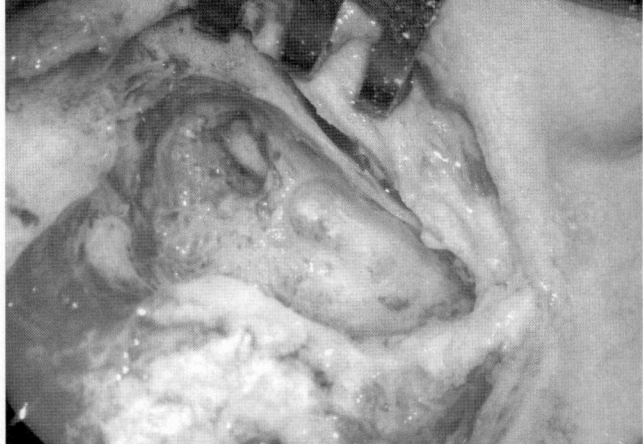

"H: Facial recess begun"

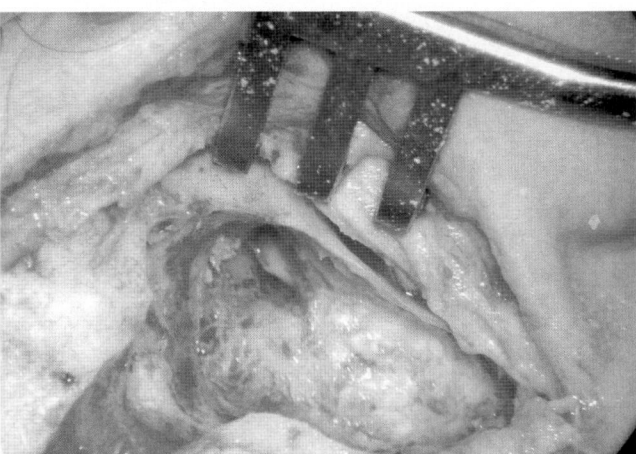

"I: Facial recess complete"

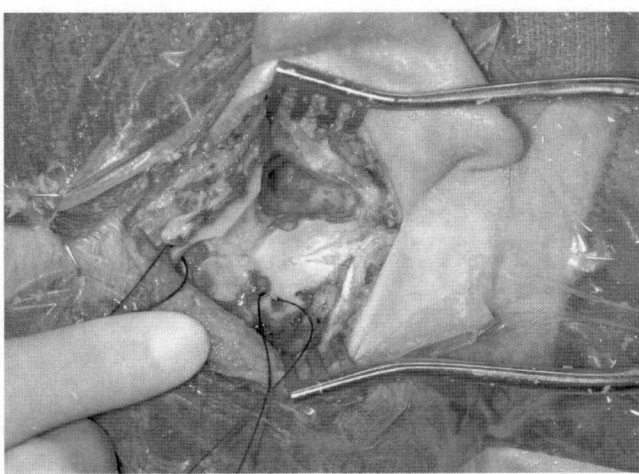

"J: Suture ready"

Figure 30–4 Continued. A series of photographs indicating the steps in cochlear implantation.

Continued on next page.

vated as an anteriorly based Palva flap, which can then be sutured back into position at the end of the case to protect the electrode array in the mastoid cavity. The Palva flap is made by elevating the deep tissue overlying the mastoid cortex but leaving it attached to the posterior canal skin. The Palva flap should be as large as possible and, hopefully, will cover the takeoff point of the electrodes for the Nucleus and Clarion devices (Figure 30–6).

The area on the skull that will receive the stimulator/receiver should then have the deep tissues removed from it.

Thought should be given to flap thickness. It is difficult for the external device to be held to the implanted stimulator/receiver if the skin thickness overlying the stimulator/receiver is greater than 6.0 mm. Thinning

should be done cautiously, however. Excessive thinning can lead to flap necrosis and exposure of the device. If the surgeon is faced with the choice of having the flap too thick or too thin, he/she should opt to leave the flap a little bit thicker. The flap can be thinned separately as a secondary procedure if necessary, and this is much easier than trying to deal with an exposed device.

The Well

A portion of the skull as flat as possible should be selected for placement of the stimulator/receiver, especially for those devices sealed in ceramic containers (MED-EL and Clarion) (Figure 30–7). In small children, this may necessitate placement a bit more superiorly, in

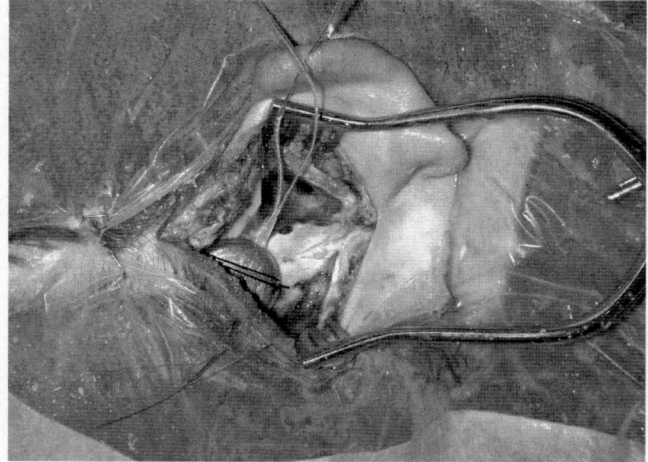

"K: Stim_Rec in"

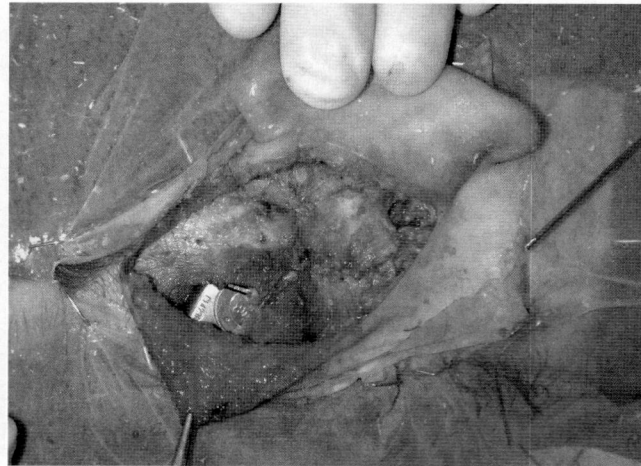

"L: Deep closure"

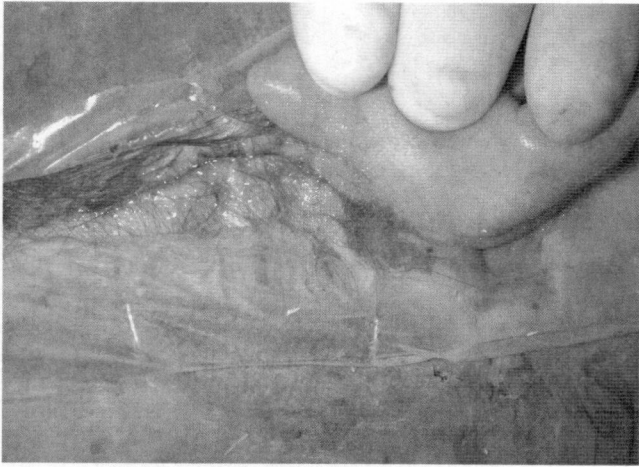

"M: Skin closure"

Figure 30–4   Continued. A series of photographs indicating the steps in cochlear implantation.

the area of the temporal squama, than in adults, where reasonably flat spots can often be found over the occipital portion of the skull base. If an ear-level processor is to be used, the stimulator/receiver should be placed 2.5 cm posterior to the posterior border of the external auditory canal to avoid interfering with placement of the ear-level processor. Once the site has been selected, the surgical drill is used to create a defect in the skull contoured to fit the implanted device exactly.

The skull of small children, especially children between 1 and 2 years of age, may be only 2 and 3 mm in thickness. For these children, the implant often rests on exposed dura. Some surgeons seek to leave an "island" of bone in the center of the area of exposed dura, whereas other surgeons are comfortable removing all of the bone from the dura.

A channel in the bone must be formed so that the electrode leads can pass freely from the stimulator/receiver into the mastoid cavity. There should be no sharp edges or constraints at the point of takeoff of the electrode leads from the stimulator/receiver.

Mastoidectomy

Once a site has been created to accommodate the stimulator/receiver, a mastoidectomy is performed (see Figure 30–7). The mastoidectomy cavity should not be saucerized. The edges should be left as acute as possible. These edges will help retain the electrode leads within the confines of the mastoid cavity. Once the mastoidectomy is complete, the facial recess is identified and widely opened. The most inferior portion of the

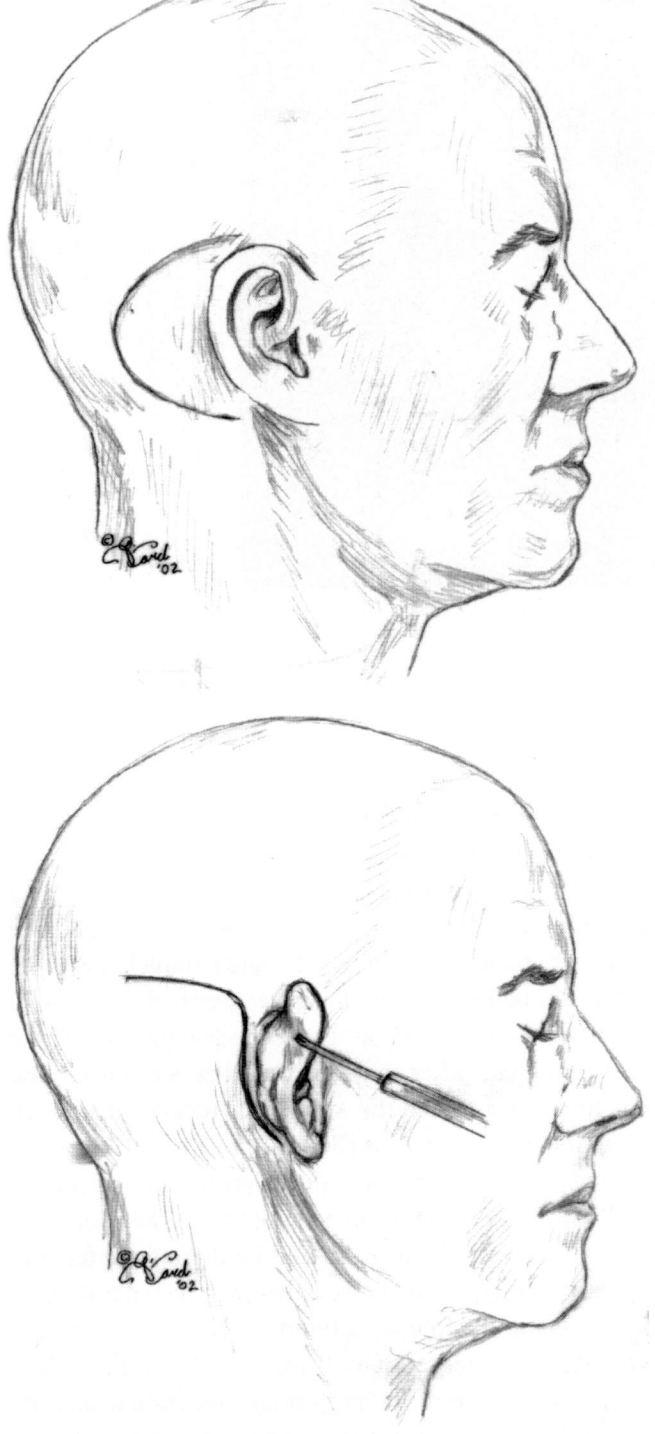

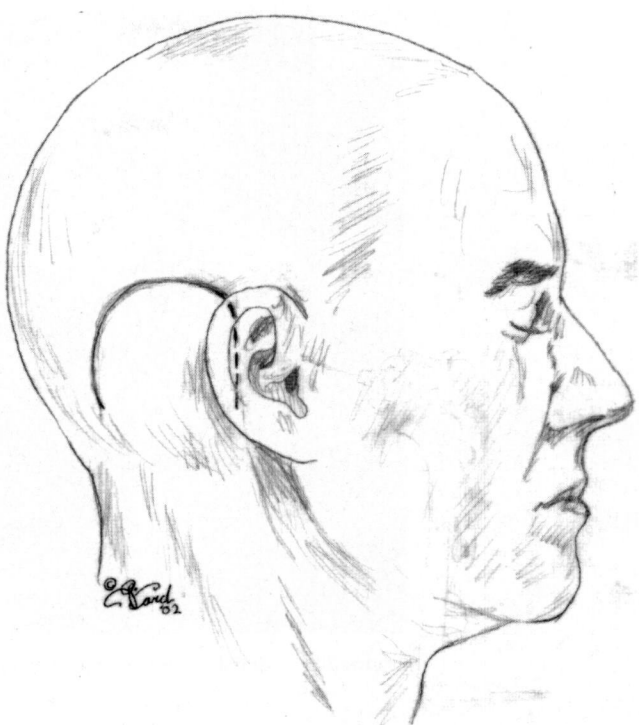

Figure 30–5 The three types of cochlear implant incisions used or illustrated, including the "C" incision, the inverted "U," and the "hockey stick" incision.

ble to see even the anterior boundary of the round window niche.

Almost all anomalous facial nerves are displaced anteriorly and medially. Just distal to the oval window, they turn directly into the hypotympanum and run just inferior to or directly over the round window area. Consequently, when the facial nerve is absent from its usual position, it does not form the posterior boundary of the facial recess. If, as the facial recess is opened, it seems that the recess is unusually large, a facial nerve anomaly should be suspected. The recess will be large because its usual posterior medial boundary, the facial nerve, is missing from its normal position and has been displaced medially and a bit anteriorly.

Cochleostomy

Once the facial recess has been widely opened, the round window niche can be clearly seen. It is often useful to remove the anterior lip of the round window niche so that the anterior attachment of the round window membrane

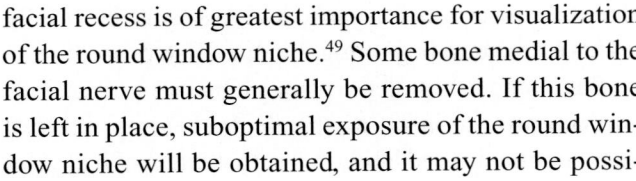

facial recess is of greatest importance for visualization of the round window niche.[49] Some bone medial to the facial nerve must generally be removed. If this bone is left in place, suboptimal exposure of the round window niche will be obtained, and it may not be possi-

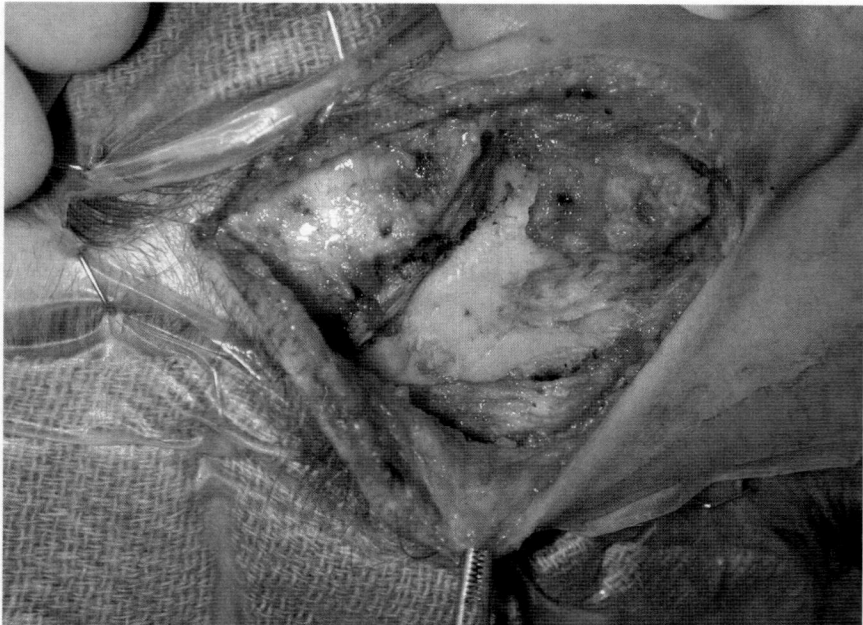

Figure 30–6   Skin flaps have been elevated and the mastoid exposed.

itself can be visualized. Almost all surgeons now make the cochleostomy somewhat anterior to the anterior attachment of the round window membrane to avoid the "hook" of the cochlea. This allows a straighter, more direct insertion of the electrode array into the scala tympani (Figure 30–8).

The size of the cochleostomy will vary between devices. Earlier generations of Clarion devices required a cochleostomy of 2 mm or more. Most currently available devices can be easily inserted through a cochleostomy of between 1.0 and 1.5 mm in diameter. Many surgeons prefer to make the cochleostomy sufficiently large so that they can see clearly down the basal turn of the scala tympani and be certain that the device is being inserted into the cochlea.

Insertion of the Electrode Array

As soon as the actual device is brought into the operative field, the monopolar cautery should be removed. Use of the monopolar cautery near the device risks damaging it and rendering it nonfunctional. Bipolar cautery can be used safely.

Opinions vary as to whether the electrode array should be inserted before or after fixation of the stimulator/receiver. Some very experienced surgeons feel that they can manipulate the electrode array more easily and have a greater chance of an atraumatic and complete insertion if the stimulator/receiver is not yet attached to the skull and can be moved freely as the electrode is passed into the scala tympani. Other surgeons find it easier to insert the electrode array once the stimulator/receiver has been fixed into its bony recess (Figure 30–9).

The electrode array should be inserted as atraumatically as possible, and force should never be used. The tip of the electrode array should be directed anteriorly upward so that it will slide easily along the lateral (antimodiolar) wall of the scala tympani. Each manufacturer provides a special set of tools for insertion of their electrode, and directions for appropriate insertion technique are different for every device. These directions change from time to time, and the recommended technique for electrode insertion for each device should be briefly reviewed prior to beginning the operative procedure.

Some surgeons prefer to place a lubricant into the scala tympani prior to inserting the electrode array. The two most commonly used lubricants are a mixture of half glyc-

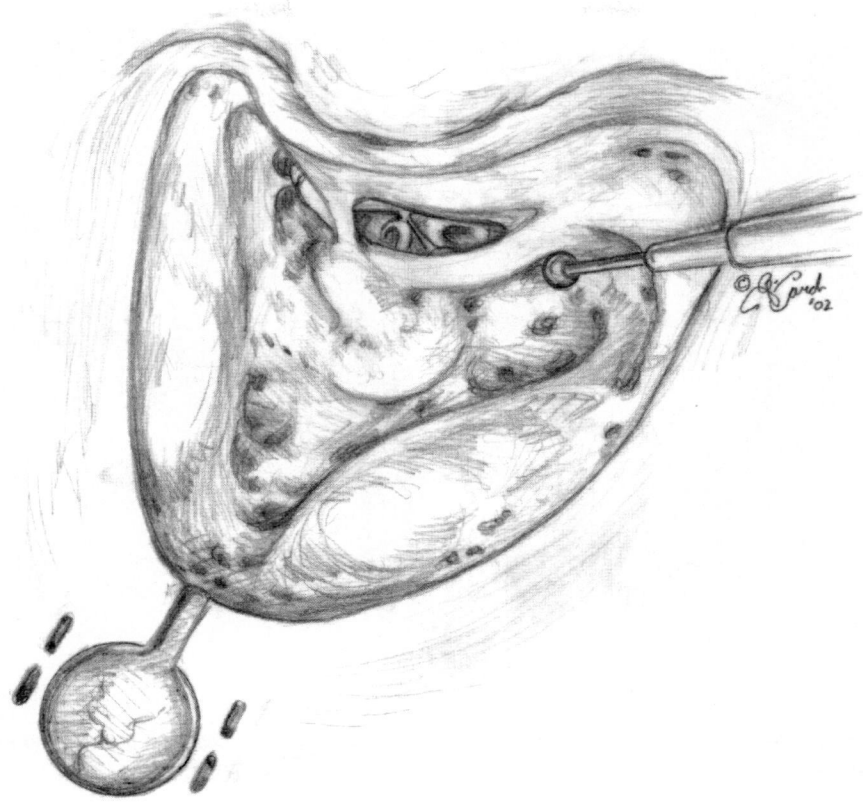

Figure 30–7 A well has been drilled to accommodate the electronics package of the cochlear implant, and a mastoidectomy with facial recess has been performed.

erin and half water and a viscoelastic material such as Healon® or Provisc®. Lubricants may allow easier passage of the electrode array into the cochlea. Lubricants also encourage bone dust and other debris to "float out" of the scala tympani prior to electrode insertion and perhaps minimize the development of postoperative osteoneogenesis.

Incomplete insertions are now uncommon except when there is an anomaly of cochlear morphology or labyrinthine ossification.

Once the electrode array has been satisfactorily inserted, the cochleostomy should be sealed with a small piece of soft tissue.

Fixation

If the stimulator/receiver has not yet been fixed to the skull base, its fixation should now be accomplished. The traditional way of securing the stimulator/receiver is by sutures. Drill holes are made above and below the receptacle site, and sutures are passed through these

holes and over the implant. Drill holes must be made very cautiously. It is easy, especially in a young child, to penetrate the dura with the sharp end of a perforating bur and create a cerebrospinal fluid leak. More worrisome is the possibility of injury to a subdural vein resulting in postoperative intracranial hemorrhage. The number, type, and position of the sutures have varied substantially. Most commonly, a single suture is placed across the device (Figure 30–10).

Alternatively, a strip of material is placed over the stimulator/receiver to hold it firmly in its well. The strip is secured with mini-plates or screws. Nonabsorbable materials such as Gortex® and absorbable materials such as AlloDerm® have been used. Some implant surgeons prefer this technique because it provides secure fixation and is quick. However, the materials involved are expensive and add considerably to the amount of foreign body placed into the wound. European surgeons have long used glues and cements to fix both the stimulator/receiver and the electrode array. Some surgeons no longer use any type of fixation, espe-

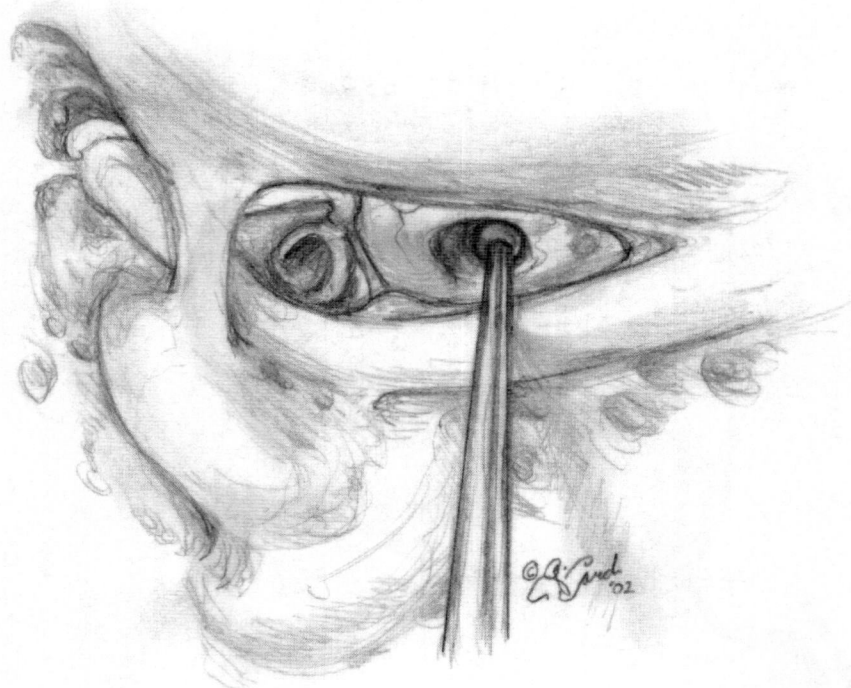

Figure 30–8   The cochleostomy is performed through the facial recess just anterior and a bit superior to the interior attachment of the round window membrane.

cially in an adult in whom the receptacle site in the skull is relatively deep. Few surgeons in the United States fix the electrode leads in any way.

Two implant systems have a second, separate lead leaving the stimulator/receiver and ending as a ground electrode. This ground electrode needs to be placed beneath the temporalis muscle, directly on the squamous portion of the temporal bone. If placed directly into the muscle, repeated muscle contraction will result in breakage of the ground electrode.

Closure

Closure should be accomplished in layers. A three-layer closure begins with separate, interrupted sutures used to close the deep layer and to return the Palva flap to its usual position over the mastoid cavity. If possible, the Palva flap should cover the takeoff of the electrode leads from the stimulator/receiver. Inverted, interrupted sutures are then used to approximate the subcuticular layer of the skin closure. Staples, fast-absorbing suture, nonabsorbable sutures, and tissue adhesive have all been used for the final closure layer.

Middle Cranial Fossa Approach

Colletti and colleagues have advocated a middle cranial fossa approach to cochlear implantation as an alternative to the traditional transmastoid approach.[50] They have implanted 11 postlingually deafened adults through the middle cranial fossa approach. They believe that by opening the basal turn of the cochlea at its most superior point and by using a double electrode array, they have been able to place electrodes both antegrade toward the apex and posteriorly toward the round window. They assert that they have achieved deeper penetration with more extended coverage of the length of the cochlear duct in this fashion.

In addition to the potential for stimulating larger areas of the cochlea, Colletti and colleagues noted that this technique would avoid ossification limited to the basal turn of the cochlea, the most common area of ossification.[50] Although the middle fossa technique

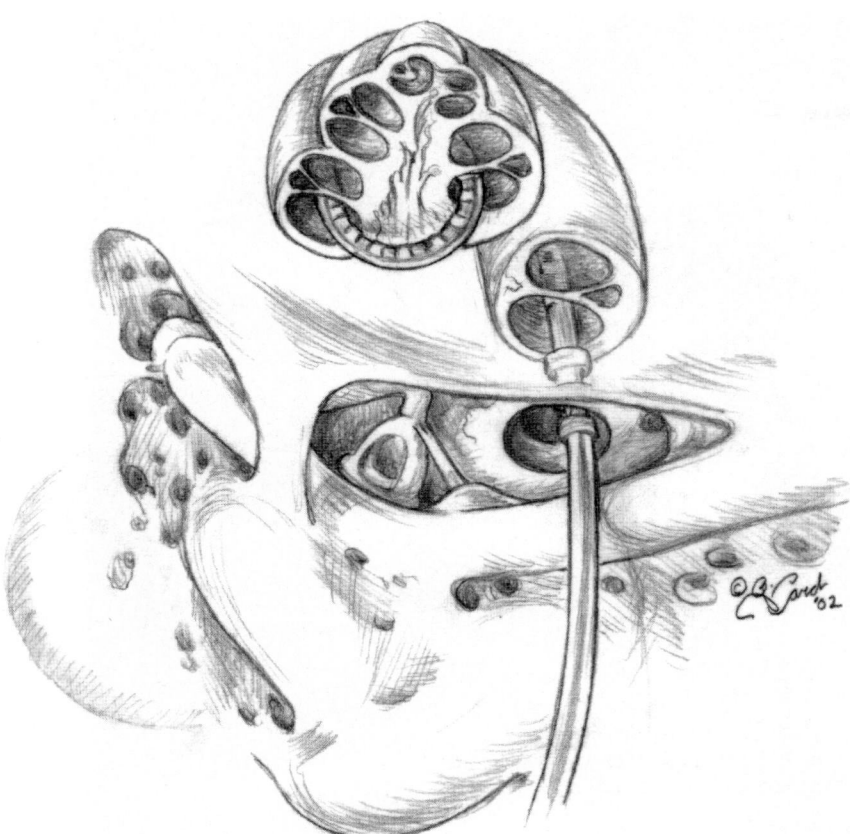

Figure 30–9 This cross-sectional drawing shows that the electrodes are next to the modiolus, which contains the ends of the cochlear nerve.

would clearly bypass isolated ossification of the basal turn near the round window, it is unclear how one would deal with extensive ossification through a middle fossa approach. Moreover, deep insertion is not necessarily better. The spiral ganglion cells that subserve the most apical turn of the cochlea may actually reside closer to the middle turn, with only their dendrites extending out apically.

Colletti and colleagues are especially enthusiastic about a middle cranial fossa technique in individuals who have open, canal wall down mastoidectomy cavities.[50] They discussed at some length the difficulties in placing an implant in such cavities. They believe that staged procedures, months apart, should be used and that, even so, there is considerable risk of contamination and postoperative infection. Colletti and colleagues appear to overestimate the difficulties in dealing with an open cavity. Although many surgeons prefer to use a staged procedure in such circumstances, others are comfortable placing the implant and closing the external auditory canal at the same operation.[51]

The number of surgeons capable of performing a middle cranial fossa operation and placing a cochlear implant by that route is certainly limited, and the operation has at least theoretical risks not associated with the typical transmastoid technique. It is worth noting that hospitalization for Colletti and colleagues's 11 patients ranged from 5 to 13 days! This would substantially increase cost and would be unattractive to most patients and surgeons in the US.[50]

The technique is intriguing and may offer some advantages in special situations. It should be studied further.

POSTOPERATIVE COMPLICATIONS: EARLY COMPLICATIONS

Intraoperative facial nerve injury is feared by both patients and surgeons alike. Fortunately, this complication is rare. The incidence of temporary postoperative weakness is unknown, but probably even a transient paresis is uncommon and occurs in less than 1 to 2% of cases. Although isolated case reports verify that permanent facial paralysis has occurred, its rate of occurrence appears to be less than 1%. Preoperative CT

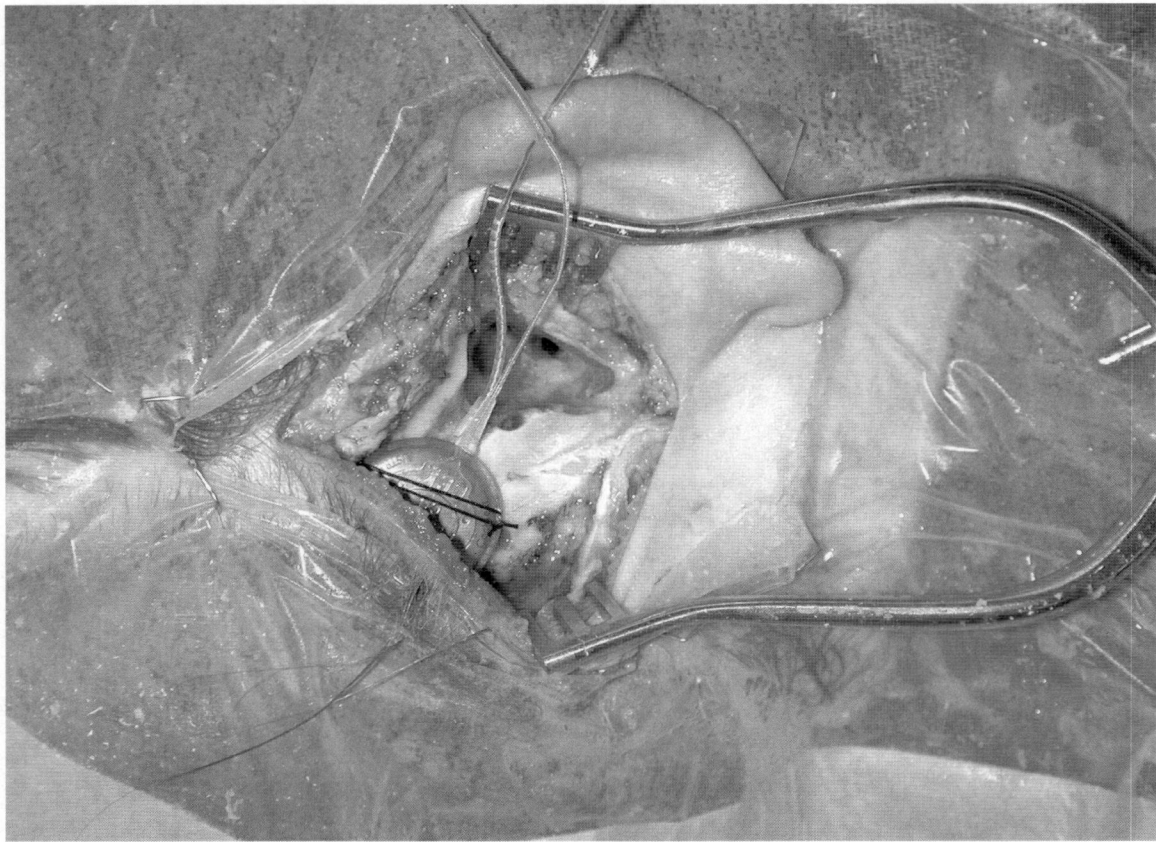

Figure 30–10 The implant is in position.

scanning is performed routinely for most cochlear implant recipients, and, consequently, the anatomy of the facial nerve is generally known prior to starting the operative procedure. Extra care must be taken when implanting patients with cochlear dysplasia because the incidence of facial nerve anomalies is higher in this group of patients. Some surgeons who do not use facial nerve monitoring routinely do use it if a cochlear anomaly has been identified.

Postoperative alteration of taste is quite common after cochlear implant surgery. The chorda tympani is occasionally divided and often irritated because the facial recess must be opened widely enough to get a good look at the round window niche. Taste disturbance is generally transient, and cochlear implant recipients rarely complain about it 6 months after surgery.

The incidence of postoperative bleeding or hematoma formation after cochlear implant surgery is quite low but does occur occasionally. A hematoma of more than 4 or 5 cc probably requires evacuation to prevent its becoming organized and fibrotic or infected. If possible, it should be drained by opening an inferior portion of the incision. If that cannot be accomplished, it can be cautiously aspirated. Care must be taken to make sure that the needle does not in any way injure the cochlear implant. Repeated aspiration is sometimes necessary.

Infection

Postoperative wound infection is generally trivial and can be handled by gently opening the wound in the area of the infection and treating the patient with appropriate antibiotics. A broad-spectrum antibiotic should be used initially. In adults, a quinolone is perhaps the best choice. In children, the use of a second- or third-generation cephalosporin is a good initial selection. The antibiotic can then be changed if necessary based on culture and sensitivity results. Almost all perioperative wound infections respond to appropriate antibiotic therapy, and it is rarely necessary to remove the device because of postoperative wound infection.[52,53]

Wound Dehiscence

Wound dehiscence can occur and is more likely in an active child than in an adult. If the area of dehiscence is small, the wound can be left to heal by secondary intention or the child can be returned to the operating room for secondary closure. Again, simple postoperative wound dehiscence is unlikely to result in a device exposure and is unlikely to require device removal.

Flap necrosis, on the other hand, is a most serious complication and frequently will require device removal.[54] Flap necrosis can occur as the result of overly aggressive thinning of the flap, as the result of a flap design that has not given adequate consideration to previous incisions, or as a consequence of infection. At minimum, flap necrosis requires recovering the device. Temporoparietal fascial flaps, along with various scalp rotation flaps, can be used for this purpose, depending on the circumstances.

Early Device Failure

Device failure can occur immediately: an "out of the box" failure. Unless intraoperative device telemetry is performed, out of the box failures will not be recognized until programming is attempted. A telemetry feature that allows the integrity of the device to be checked in the operating room is available on some late-generation devices.

Out of the box failures may be the result of factory defects or a consequence of damage during surgical manipulation. Buckled, broken, or exposed electrodes can result in failure of the entire electrode array or may leave only one or several electrodes nonfunctional. To prevent such failures, cochlear implants should always be handled gently. One must remember to discard the monopolar cautery once the implant is brought into the field. If the operating surgeon, for any reason, believes

that the device is not going to function perfectly, the implant should be returned to the factory and a backup device should be used.

If the electrode array is not within the cochlea, the device will appear to function properly when it is checked by device telemetry but, of course, will not program because the electrodes are not in the vicinity of the auditory nerve (Figures 30–11 and 30–12). One advantage of NRT (see below) is that it can be used to assess physiologic efficacy and thereby verify placement. Extracochlear implantation can occur when hypotympanic air cells are mistaken for scala tympani. This mistake is easier to make than one might think. It can be prevented by taking great care to be sure that one has the expected view of the antimodiolar wall of the scala tympani and of the inferior surface of the basilar membrane prior to inserting the device. Unless the surgeon is sure he/she has inserted the device into the cochlea, interoperative radiographs should be obtained.

The electrodes can come to rest in a position outside the cochlea because the electrode array has moved or migrated after an initial correct placement. As every cochlear implant surgeon has noted, the electrode leads have some "spring" to them. Depending on the position of the proximal portions of the electrode leads in the mastoid, the array may tend to "spring back" out of the cochlea after each attempt to advance it. If the proximal portion of the electrode leads is not properly positioned in the mastoid cavity, these recoil forces can result in partial or complete withdrawal of the electrode array from the scala tympani. The most common cause of displaced electrodes, however, is movement of the electrode array after a "drill out" procedure (see below). Unless the electrode array is securely fixed, it will tend to become displaced; see below for further discussion of a method for preventing this type of movement.

If the implanting surgeon has any reason to believe that the electrode is not in a good position, a lateral skull film to ascertain its placement should be obtained before the procedure is terminated.

Cerebrospinal Fluid Leak

A CSF leak can occur as the result of penetration of the dura when placing the stimulator/receiver. This is most likely in young children in whom the skull is very thin. It is perhaps more likely to occur with placement of the

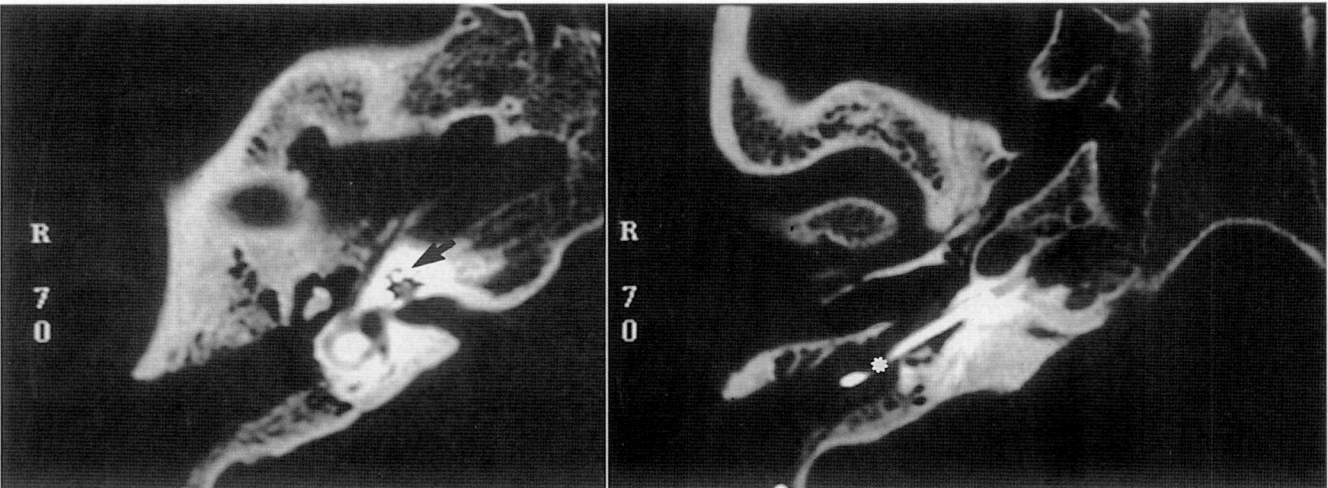

Figure 30–11 A computed tomographic (CT) scan showing the well-positioned electrode array. The axial scan on the left shows the individual electrodes within the lumen of the cochlea (*black arrow*). The image on the right is also an axial CT scan. The *asterisk* indicates the electrode lead, which can be followed into the vestibule.

drill holes for the tie-down sutures than with any other portion of the operation.

Cerebrospinal fluid gushers can occur when the scala tympani is opened to place the electrode array. Gushers are most likely to occur in the presence of modiolar defects. Modiolar defects are one of the most common forms of congenital anomaly seen within the cochlear implant population. Cerebrospinal fluid gushers are more the rule than the exception in severe cochlear dysplasia, such as common cavity deformity. Generally, the CSF leak can be controlled by packing the common cavity or vestibule with muscle. Drill out procedures for severe labyrinthitis will also occasionally result in CSF leak. The hard bone of the fully ossified otic capsule leaves few landmarks, and a surgeon may inadvertently wander into the middle fossa, posterior fossa, or inter-

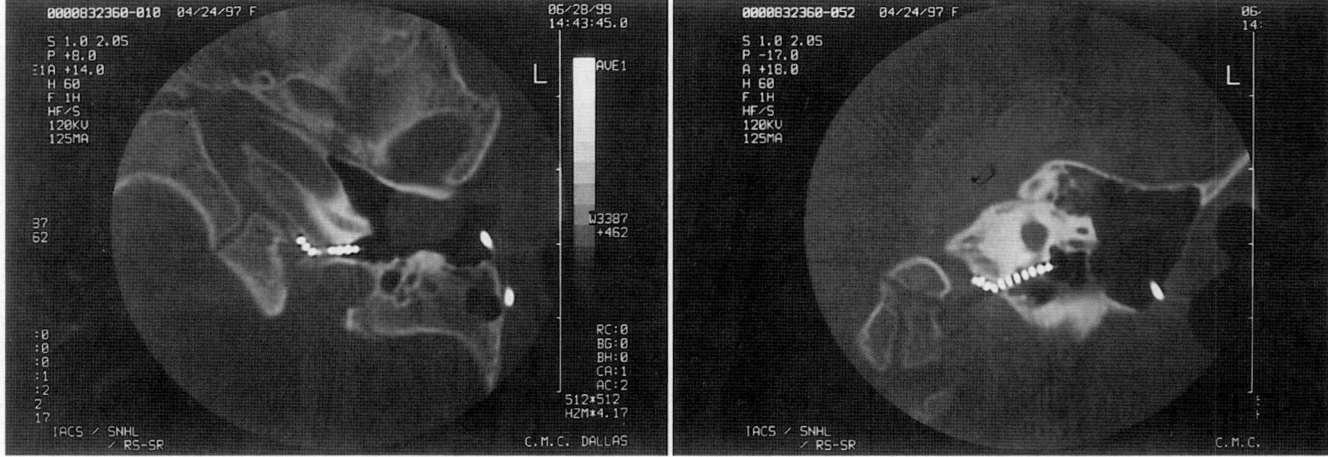

Figure 30–12 A malpositioned electrode array. The patient has a common cavity deformity. The axial computed tomographic scan on the left shows that the electrode array is posterior and medial to the common cavity and not within it. The coronal image on the right indicates that it also passes inferiorly to the common cavity deformity.

nal auditory canal in attempting to create a trough in the presumed position of the scala tympani.

If occluding the vestibule or common cavity does not control the leak, the ear must be closed by plugging the eustachian tube, filling the middle ear and mastoid with fat, and oversewing the external auditory canal.

From time to time, the operating surgeon will think that he/she has adequately controlled the egress of CSF only to find that there is CSF otorrhea or rhinorrhea postoperatively. Spinal drainage will often reduce CSF pressure and allow these areas to heal without a second operation, but reoperation is occasionally necessary.

Balance Disturbance

The incidence of vertigo and dizziness postoperatively is surprisingly low. Overall, fewer than 10% of patients experience significant dizziness. There is some reason to believe that the incidence of postoperative vertigo may vary a bit according to the extent to which the implant fills the scala tympani. When recipients do experience significant postoperative vertigo, it usually resolves within a few weeks. A few geriatric patients have had postoperative ataxia that resolves only over a period of several months.

Central Nervous System Complications

Postoperative meningitis can occur but appears to be no more common after cochlear implantation than after other otologic procedures. Clearly, individuals who have perioperative CSF leak are at higher risk. If meningitis is suspected, a lumbar puncture should be performed after a CT scan has eliminated the risk of herniation. Antibiotics should be withheld until cultures have been obtained. As soon as the diagnosis has been verified by lumbar puncture, broad-spectrum antibiotic therapy can be initiated.

POSTOPERATIVE COMPLICATIONS: LATE COMPLICATIONS

One of the most feared late complications of cochlear implantation is extrusion or exposure of the device. As mentioned above, it is widely believed that keeping suture lines as far as possible from the edge of the implant significantly reduces the incidence of excursion or exposure, although data to support this claim are not available. Once exposure has occurred, it is not always necessary to remove the implant. Parkins and colleagues have listed two criteria for successful salvage of an exposed prosthesis:

1. Repair must remove enough skin and cicatrix to avoid suture lines that parallel the implant edge closer than $1\frac{1}{2}$ cm.
2. A paracranial flap should be rotated to fully cover the device with or without a temporoparietal flap as the initial layer of closure.[55]

Pain

Occasionally, patients will complain of postoperative pain at the site of the implant for months after the operation. This appears to be a form of periosteitis. It is generally well managed by long-term use of nonsteroidal anti-inflammatory agents (3 to 6 weeks).

Displacement

Late device migration or displacement is uncommon. Displacement can occur as a result of physical injury—especially if the stimulator/receiver has not been sutured into position. Electrodes can be displaced as the result of scar tissue formation. Device displacement and migration can best be assessed on fine-cut CT scans of the temporal bone, which will often allow visualization of individual electrodes and the stimulator receiver.

Late Device Failure

Late failure of stimulation is usually the result of internal device failure. Some of these failures are the result of trauma, but others appear to happen spontaneously. The external components of the device should first be replaced with loaner components. If that solves the problem, then the problem lies in the external component. If, however, replacement of external components results in no improvement, then a fine-cut CT scan should be obtained to make sure that the stimulator/receiver is still appropriately positioned, the electrodes have not migrated, and no wires are broken. If the CT scan offers no explanation, then a company representative should be contacted for an "integrity check." Integrity checks seek to determine the electrical integrity of the device. Unfortunately, they are often inconclusive. One is then left unsure as to whether there has been some dramatic change in the patient's auditory system or if there has been an internal device failure. Often the only way to resolve this dilemma is to replace the device and see if performance is improved. Most commonly, it is.

Otitis Media

Prior to experience in implanting children, there was a great deal of concern that otitis media would present serious problems to children with cochlear implants. It was feared that every episode of otitis media would lead to infection of the implant and that chronic infection would require frequent device removal. This has not turned out to be the case. Luntz and colleagues have evaluated 60 children, 74% of whom had had at least one episode of otitis media prior to implantation. All postoperative infections resolved with routine systemic antibiotic therapy without any additional complications. All children who had acute otitis media postoperatively (16%) had had it preoperatively.[56] Luntz and colleagues's experience is representative of the experience of others, and no case reports of acute otitis media leading to long-term device infection and/or requiring explantation have been published.

SPECIAL PROBLEMS

Cochlear Dysplasia

An important percentage of children with severe to profound hearing loss suffer from malformations of the cochlea. Malformations range from very mild incomplete partitioning defects through common cavity deformities to complete aplasias (see Figures 30–2 and 30–3). The most commonly seen defects are enlarged vestibular aqueducts and defects of the modiolus. These defects do not necessarily prejudice the outcome of cochlear implantation, nor do they necessarily require an alternation of surgical technique or the use of special electrode arrays.

More severe defects require some alternation of technique.[57]

Common cavity deformities present special challenges because the extent and position of residual neuroepithelium are unknown. Common cavity deformities are more than usually likely to be associated with a defective cribriform area, allowing abnormal communication between the common cavity and the internal auditory canal. The defect not only makes the CSF gusher more common, it also potentially allows the electrode array to slide directly into the internal auditory canal.

Some types of common cavity deformities make entrance through the round window area difficult or impossible. If the usual points of access to the cochlea are not available, the electrode array can be inserted directly through the lateral semicircular canal into the common cavity defect, as has been described by McElveen and colleagues.[58]

Facial nerve anomalies are more common in children who have significant cochlea dysplasia than in children who do not. The facial nerve is much more likely to be abnormal if the cochlea and semicircular canals are both involved in the malformation (Figure 30–13).[45] Most facial nerve anomalies involve anterior displacement of the nerve. The facial nerve may pass directly over the oval window niche (or where the oval niche should have been). Occasionally, the nerve will pass anterior to the oval window niche over the promontory.

Although there have been a number of case reports and two questionnaire-based surveys on the results of cochlear implantation in children with cochlear dysplasia, no large series of patients with dysplasia has been reported. Graham, after reviewing the available information, believes that the range of potential outcomes is similar for children with cochlear dysplasia as for children without cochlear dysplasia.[46] Nonetheless, most experienced implant centers warn the parents of children with significant cochlear deformities that the chances of success are somewhat reduced and that their expectations should be scaled back.

Labyrinthitis Ossificans

About 5% of children who have had bacterial meningitis suffer profound hearing loss (Figure 30–14). Up to

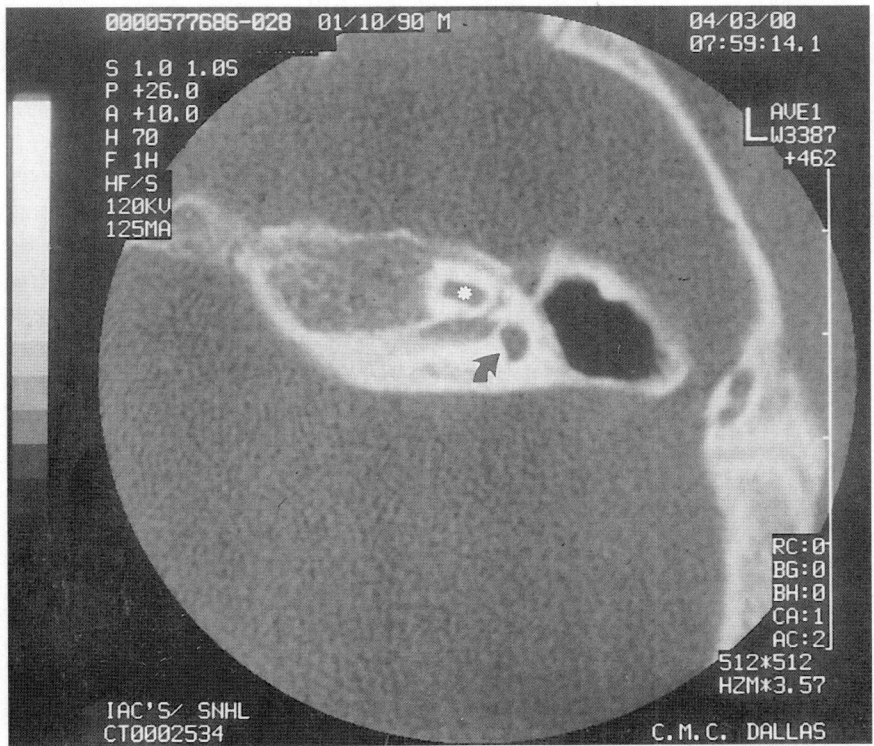

Figure 30–13 The *asterisk* lies in the common cavity of a markedly dysplastic cochlea. The *black arrow* points to the only vestigial remnant of the semicircular canal: a single sac.

80% of those children develop some degree of ossification. It appears that the infection spreads from the subarachnoid space to the labyrinth via the cochlear aqueduct. Consequently, labyrinthine ossification occurs first and is worst where the cochlear aqueduct enters the labyrinth: at the scala tympani in the area of the round window.[59] Three stages of labyrinthitis ossificans can be identified: acute, fibrous, and ossification. The ossification process begins as early as 3 weeks after the initiation of meningitis and may progress for as long as 9 months.[60,61] Fortunately, the auditory nerve is preserved despite even advanced levels of ossification. Nadol has shown that the number of spiral ganglion cells decreases with increasing ossification and duration of deafness.[5]

Children who have lost hearing as the result of meningitis need to be closely monitored for the development of ossification. Since the earliest form is fibrous, CT scanning may not demonstrate it. An MRI scan is more sensitive because it can detect the absence of fluid within the obstructed cochlear duct and does not depend on the formation of new bone (Table 30–2).

There are several ways of managing a cochlea obstructed with fibrous tissue or new bone formation. Occasionally, ossification is limited to the basal turn of the cochlea in the area of the round window and persistent drilling through the usual cochleostomy will penetrate the area of ossification until an open scala tympani can be identified. In such cases, the electrode array can be inserted as usual.

The earliest method of handling more extensive cochlear ossification was simply to continue drilling straight into the basal turn of the cochlea as far as possible—generally a distance of 6 to 8 mm. The surgeon then had to settle for as much of the electrode array as could be placed into this short segment of drilled out, inferior basal turn. Four to eight electrodes were usually the most that could be inserted.

If there appears to be relatively extensive ossification of the basal turn of the scala tympani, an attempt should

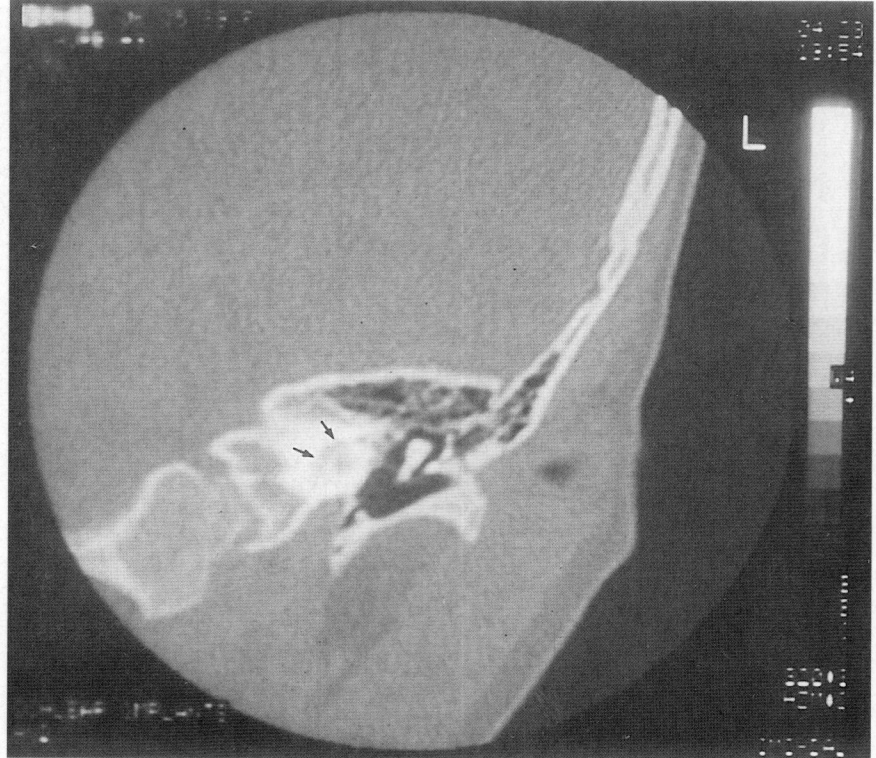

Figure 30–14 Coronal section through the cochlea. The *arrows* indicate haziness in the lumen of the membranous cochlear labyrinth, indicating early ossification.

be made to insert the electrode array into the scala vestibuli. Although the scala vestibuli is somewhat smaller than the scala tympani, the combined cross-sectional area of scala tympani and scala media is about the same as the area of the scala tympani.[62] Consequently, there is enough room to accommodate the electrode array if Reissner's membrane is sacrificed. To access the scala vestibuli, the original cochleostomy should be extended posteriorly and superiorly toward the inferior limit of the oval window. If the scala vestibuli is also obliterated, a classic "drill out" procedure should be considered.

The classic drill out procedure was first described by Balkany and colleagues and allowed placement of many more electrodes into the ossified cochlea.[63] The posterior wall of the external auditory canal is removed, the soft tissue of the external auditory canal is excised, and the ear is closed. The entire lateral wall of the basal turn of the cochlea is then systematically removed, creating a trough in what had been the basal cochlear turn. Care must be taken to avoid the carotid artery anteriorly and to avoid penetrating the floor of the middle cranial fossa

superiorly. As much as 300 to 360 degrees at the basal turn of the cochlea can be opened in this way. These early drill out procedures had a 50% failure rate because the electrode "pulled away" from the cochlea in the immediate postoperative period. Balkany and colleagues have recently described three modifications to this drill out procedure, two of which are designed to eliminate displacement of the electrode array.[64] The operation begins by identifying the round window and drilling anteriorly into the basal turn as usual. Drilling is continued approximately 6 to 8 mm anteriorly directly into the basal turn. A tympanomeatal flap is then designed, incised, and elevated, and the middle ear space is entered through the external auditory canal. The tympanomeatal flap should be superiorly based. The incus is removed, and the drum is separated from the malleus. After identifying the middle ear landmarks, the previously drilled tunnel in the cochlea is entered approximately 4 mm anterior to the round window niche. This leaves a "bridge" of that bone intact that will secure the electrode array. The trough is then continued anteriorly and superiorly up the ascending bend of the basal turn to the level of the semicanal for the tensor tympani. It is then followed posteriorly to the anterior edge of the oval window and then inferiorly to complete the opening of the basal turn. Great care must be taken to avoid the carotid artery anteriorly and the facial nerve posteriorly. The electrode array is then passed into the original cochleostomy, and the tip is retrieved in the open basal turn. The residual intact "bridge" of bone helps prevent electrode migration. Pieces of the incus are then used to wedge the tip of the electrode array into the trough. The cochlea around the electrode array is packed with fat.

A final option for management of the ossified cochlea is to use a split- or double-electrode array. To place the double array, a cochleostomy is made anterior to the round window membrane as usual. It is extended anteriorly superiorly directly into the ossified basal turn for about 8.0 mm. Care must be taken to avoid the internal carotid artery. The incus is removed along with the incus buttress. The stapedial crura are carefully cut and removed so as not to avulse the stapes footplate. A second cochleostomy is then performed immediately above the oval window. It is drilled to a depth of 7.0 mm paralleling the tympanic portion of the facial nerve. The two electrode arrays are then placed into the two cochleostomies separately. The cochleostomies are sealed with soft tissue.

REVISION SURGERY

There are several reasons for reoperating in the area of an existing cochlear implant:

1. There has been device failure.
2. A technologically outdated device needs to be removed and an updated device inserted.
3. The device becomes extruded or exposed. Revision operation may or may not require explantation and/or reimplantation.
4. The skin flap must be revised, usually because it is too thick.
5. An additional procedure is being performed in the area of the implant, for example, auricular reconstruction.

If the surgery in the area of the implant does not involve explanting the device, then great care must be taken to maintain its integrity and functionality. First, the monopolar cautery must not be used. In its stead, the Shaw® knife (a heated scalpel blade) has been found useful.[65] Caution should be exercised to avoid injury to the electrodes. It is important to know the type of device that has been implanted if one is to have some idea of where the electrodes will be located. For example, the Clarion device has the electrode takeoff at its anterior-most portion. The electrode takes off as a single lead. On the other hand, the MED-EL device has two electrodes that leave from the side of the device. The takeoff of the electrodes will be inferiorly positioned when the implant is placed on one side of the head and superiorly when the implant is placed on the contralateral side.

The electrode leads generally take a fairly straight path from the device into the mastoid and through the facial recess. The flying ground electrode, however, may lie in an unpredictable position, often looping back on the stimulator/receiver in an unpredictable fashion. It is sometimes useful to obtain a plain, lateral, skull radiograph to be sure of exactly where the stimulator/receiver is located and where the various electrode leads lie.

The stimulator/receiver is usually found in a mesothelium-lined pouch that is relatively easy to identify. There is usually little scar tissue formation between the stimulator/receiver and the surrounding soft tissues. Consequently, soft tissues are easy to separate from the stimulator/receiver. In the case of children, there will often be substantial amounts of bony regrowth. Bony regrowth may cover the lateral portions of the implant. Not infrequently, some drilling must be performed to release the stimulator/receiver from its bony niche.

The amount of scarring and the density of mucosal adhesions found in the area of the facial recess and middle ear are variable. It is generally possible to carefully follow the electrode leads from the stimulator/receiver through the facial recess into the cochlea. However, even very gentle traction on the electrode leads will withdraw the electrode array from the cochlea. Its utility as a guide through the facial recess and into the previous cochleostomy is then lost.

If the revision operation is designed to recover an existing device after exposure or infection, then long-term postoperative antibiotics are necessary. If skin organisms are involved in the infection, as much as 6 weeks of therapy may be required (John Niparko, personal communication, 2001).

Reimplantation is generally successful. Balkany and colleagues[66,67] have reported on 16 patients who underwent reimplantation. The most common reason was device failure. After the results with the new device have been compared with the results with the old device, the reimplantation procedure was compared with the initial operation in terms of length of insertion, number of electrodes programmed, and postoperative audiometric results. Among these 16 subjects, there were no significant differences between the initial implant and the reimplanted device.[31,66,67]

Henson and colleagues reviewed 28 patients who had been reimplanted. Both the initial devices and the reimplanted devices were Nucleus 22s. Thirty-seven percent had improved performance, 26% showed no significant change in performance, and 37% showed poor performance. Subjectively, 57% felt that their hearing was better, and 43% thought it was poorer. There was no correlation between performance and cause of device failure, length of use of the old device, surgical complications, change of electrode insertion depth, or preoperative variables such as age, etiology, or duration of deafness.[68]

Parisier and colleagues retrospectively analyzed 27 consecutive multichannel cochlear implant reinsertions. Open-set speech recognition scores and speech perception ability remained stable or improved compared with the results before implantation.[69]

POSTOPERATIVE CONSIDERATIONS FOR SURGEONS

Device Activation

Two to 4 weeks postoperatively, when the wound is well healed, the cochlear implant is activated. This is a process frequently referred to as "hook-up." The first decision that must be made during the hook-up process is to determine the stimulation mode. Every "channel" requires an active electrode paired with a ground electrode. It was initially believed that greater frequency specificity and therefore improved speech recognition would result from narrow band, highly specific stimulation of the cochlea. It was believed that widespread dispersion of current would result in activation of a large number of neurons and obscure frequency specificity. Consequently, each active electrode was paired with another electrode on the intracochlear electrode array, which served as its ground electrode. The active electrode can be coupled to any other electrode on the array: the electrode next to it or the electrode furthest away. When the active electrode is grounded to another intracochlear electrode, stimulation mode is referred to as "bipolar." The distance of the ground electrode to the active electrode is expressed as "bipolar + 1," "bipolar + 2," etc.

Although intuition suggested that narrow bands of stimulation (ie, bipolar mode) would be most effective, experience has challenged that assumption. Monopolar modes of stimulation are now frequently used. Each electrode within the cochlea is grounded to an extra-cochlear electrode, resulting in wide current spread throughout the cochlea with every stimulation. Monopolar stimulation requires the availability of an electrode outside the cochlea. All currently available receivers have such electrodes. The ground electrode may be a separate electrode attached to a separate lead, may be built into the back of the stimulator/receiver, or both.

Initial programming of the device also requires that the threshold level, most comfortable loudness level, and uncomfortable loudness level be determined for each active electrode. This is a laborious process, taking several hours in adults. Together, measures of threshold level and comfortable loudness levels set the electrical dynamic range inside which all auditory signals will fall. Frequency bands are then assigned to each electrode pair by the software program. In the young, prelingually deaf child, this can be a very complicated matter requiring many days. Use of objective assessment of threshold can be especially helpful in these younger, prelingual deafened subjects. A recent improvement in the area of cochlear implantation is the development of objective methods to assess threshold. These include NRT, estimation of stapedial reflex, and electrical ABR.

Neural response telemetry uses radio frequency telemetry to measure the action potential in the auditory nerve. It differs from the older device telemetry (which evaluated only the internal electronics of the implant itself) because it can objectively evaluate the physiologic response to the device. Neural response telemetry can be obtained both intraoperatively and postoperatively. The stimulus intensities necessary to generate an action potential in the auditory nerve can be determined and then used to provide target settings for the speech processor. Shallop and colleagues have confirmed a particular relationship between comfort settings and NRT thresholds in children.[70] Behavioral thresholds and comfort levels correlate well with NRT thresholds when the appropriate correction factor is applied.[71] The correction factor needed to program all electrodes is consistent across the electrode array and, consequently, can be determined from behavioral programming of a single electrode. Once the correction factor has been accurately determined, it can be applied to all electrodes in the NRT-generated map. Programming of young children can be done more accurately and more quickly using NRT.

An electrical ABR can be used in a similar fashion. The mean ABR threshold was predictive of the average comfort level in a study by Brown, but there was a fair amount of intersubject variability.[72]

A third method by which an objective estimate of comfort levels can be obtained is using the stapedius reflex. Intraoperatively, the stapedius muscle can be seen contracting in response to high stimulus intensities. When the stimulus used to elicit the reflex is electrical, the response is referred to as an electrical stapedius reflex. When the electrical stapedius reflex is performed intraoperatively to test the implant and contraction of the stapedius muscle is noted visually, the test is referred to as a visual electrical stapedius reflex test. Although the usual understanding of the protective nature of the stapedius reflex would lead one to believe that the presence of the stapedius reflex would correlate best with uncomfortable loudness levels, it has now been shown that it actually correlates better with most comfortable loudness level.[41,70,73–75]

Facial Nerve Stimulation

Facial nerve twitching as a consequence of activated cochlear implant electrodes is not uncommon. Bigelow and colleagues noted this in 8% of 58 patients implanted at the University of Pennsylvania.[76] Kelsall and colleagues evaluated 14 patients (7% of implant recipients) at their institution.[77] Both investigators found that the electrodes in the mid basal turn were the most common electrodes involved—presumably because of the anatomic proximity to the labyrinthine portion of the

facial nerve. Both studies and others have noted otosclerosis to be a particular risk factor. Bigelow and colleagues reported that the preoperative CT scanning can often identify those potential cochlear implant recipients at greatest risk. In all cases, facial nerve stimulation was eliminated by deactivating the provoking electrodes.[76,77] Gold and colleagues have suggested that sodium fluoride may reduce the risk and incidence of facial nerve stimulation in otosclerotic patients.[78]

Postoperative Rehabilitation

Postoperative rehabilitation is an important part of cochlear implantation. In children, especially prelingually deafened children, it is absolutely critical and makes the difference between a successful transition to implant use and a failure. The topic will be significantly slighted in this chapter written principally for surgeons. However, it is imperative that every implant surgeon recognizes that for many implant recipients, aggressive and intensive rehabilitation is absolutely essential. Rehabilitation focuses on making sure that the recipient can adequately use the information provided by the implant. The rate at which rehabilitation is accomplished varies substantially between one recipient and another. Clearly, the postlingually deafened individual with deafness of brief duration will progress much more quickly than the prelingually deafened adult. Most rehabilitative services are provided by specially trained speech-language pathologists. It should be recognized that this is a relatively specialized area, and the general speech-language pathologist may not be able to adequately meet the needs of the cochlear implant recipient. Parents play a critical role in rehabilitating children, and their active involvement in the rehabilitation process greatly accelerates the development of both expressive and receptive language skills.

RESULTS

Postlingually Deafened Adults

It is now recognized that postlingually deafened adults will achieve open-set word recognition in most cases. Because the efficacy of cochlear implants in postlingually deafened adults is no longer disputed, few results have been published recently.

In the recently completed Nucleus 24 Contour® trial, substantial improvement was seen after only 6 months of use. The average HINT sentence score rose from < 5% to almost 50%.[79]

Gstoettner and colleagues have evaluated the benefit reached by 21 consecutive postlingually deafened adults who received the MED-EL COMBI 40+ device. At 12 months postimplant, sentence understanding averaged > 85%.[80] Whereas overall hearing results have improved dramatically in the last decade, individual hearing results remain variable and unpredictable.

Children

Waltzmann and colleagues evaluated 36 prelingually deaf children who received Nucleus® devices and were less than 5 years old. All children developed significant open-set speech recognition, and 37 of the 38 children use oral language as their sole means of communication.[81] Blamey and colleagues evaluated 47 prelingually deafened children with a mean unaided PTA of 106 dB using a cochlear implant and compared those children with 40 children with a mean PTA of 78 dB who used hearing aids. Both groups were treated in an oral/aural rehabilitation setting. They were closely followed and repeatedly evaluated over a 3-year period. Their results suggest that all children will reach 90% open-set speech recognition but that they will all enter secondary school about 4 to 5 years delayed unless they receive intensive language therapy.[82] Tomblin and colleagues have shown that grammatical development is significantly enhanced in prelingually deafened children who receive cochlear implants compared with those who do not.[83]

An important, practical way to assess the effectiveness of cochlear implantation is to establish use versus nonuse rates. Presumably, children who find cochlear implants useful will use them. Those children who do not find cochlear implants useful will not use them. Archbold and colleagues followed 161 children for 3 years. All were users. Parents rated 89% of the children as full-time users and 11% "most of the time users." Teachers rated the children slightly higher: 95% were rated full-time users and only 4% were rated "most of the time users." Neither parents nor teachers rated any child an occasional users or a nonuser.[84]

A number of variables have been considered in trying to account for the variability in outcome. Cheng and colleagues have shown that hearing outcomes are independent of the cause of deafness in children.[21] The length of the electrode array and the number of active electrodes do not appear to be important beyond a certain threshold number. Once 8 to 10 electrodes have been successfully inserted into the cochlea, the number of electrodes no longer correlates with postoperative performance. It has been hypothesized, and seems logical, that greater depth of insertion will increase performance, but no validation of this hypothesis has been forthcoming. Hodges and colleagues have shown that insertion of the Nucleus 22 device beyond 22 rings did not improve performance in 31 patients.[31]

Length of deafness appears to be an important variable and has had predictive value in a number of studies. Together with preoperative CID sentence scores, Rubinstein and colleagues have shown that duration of deafness accounts for 70% of the variance seen in cochlear implant recipients.[52,53]

Cheng and Niparko have demonstrated that postoperative performance appears to be independent of age of onset after 1 year of implant use.[85] There is increasing evidence that younger age of implantation leads to better outcomes, as discussed above.

Mode of communication appears to have a significant impact on outcome. Hodges and colleagues have shown that children using oral-only modes of communication experience better outcomes than children using total communication. Indeed, in their study, it was the most important predictor of success.[31] Geers and Nicholas, in an evaluation of 180 cochlear implant recipients, found that children in an environment that required them to depend on spoken language (rather than sign language) received more benefit from their cochlear implants.[86]

On the other hand, Robbins and colleagues evaluated 23 profound prelingually deaf children and found no difference between those using oral communication and those using total communication.[87]

Speech and Language Acquisition

Not only has improved speech perception (hearing) as the result of cochlear implantation been clearly demonstrated, but an improved ability to develop expressive speech and language skills has also been documented. But evidence to support dramatically improved expressive language skills in cochlear implant recipients is accumulating a bit more slowly. Moog and Geers evaluated 22 prelingually deaf children who received cochlear implants. They all had speech intelligibility scores that were statistically better than children managed with hearing aids, and half had language scores that fell within the average range for normal-hearing children.[37] Tobey and colleagues have shown that speech intelligibility correlates with the level of speech recognition and is better if children have received auditory verbal therapy than if they have been managed in a total communication environment.[88] Robbins and colleagues compared 23 prelingually deafened cochlear implant children to 89 deaf children treated without a cochlear implant (not with ossification) using the Reynell Developmental Language scale. Cochlear implant recipients exceeded by 7 months the gains predicted on the basis of previous maturation studies. Language development rate was about the same as in normal-hearing children.[87] Svirsky and colleagues compared 43 cochlear implant children to 52 children who used hearing aids. Cochlear implant users had better speech intelligibility than did the hearing aid users, and auditory verbal children had better speech intelligibility than children managed with total communication.[36] Miyamoto and colleagues reported that children with cochlear implants had much higher reported gains in expressive language skills after implantation than would have been predicted on the basis of an observed cohort of 89 unimplanted deaf children.[89]

Cochlear implants, in summary, allow a child to recover a normal ability to acquire speech and language once the implant has been placed but do not fully overcome the detrimental effects of early auditory deprivation. Thus, the gap between chronological age and language age, which progressively increases in unimplanted children, remains constant after cochlear implantation (see Figure 30–14).

ACKNOWLEDGMENTS

The following individuals have made important contributions to this chapter and are deserving of special recognition: Emily Tobey, PhD; Tim Booth, MD; Melissa Waller, MS CCC/A; and Pamela Kruger, MS CCC/A. Special thanks is extended to Sue Knight, my administrative assistant, whose tireless efforts saw this chapter through multiple revisions. Without her cheerful collaboration, the task could not have been completed.

REFERENCES

1. Miller AL. Effects of chronic stimulation on auditory nerve survival in ototoxically deafened animals. Hear Res 2001;151:1–14.

2. Leake PA, Hradek GT, Snyder RL. Chronic electrical stimulation by a cochlear implant promotes survival of spiral ganglion neurons after neonatal deafness. J Comp Neurol 1999;412:543–62.

3. Shepherd RK, Matsushima J, Martin RL, Clark GM. Cochlear pathology following chronic electrical stimulation of the auditory nerve: II. Deafened kittens. Hear Res 1994;81:150–66.

4. Linthicum FH Jr, Fayad J, Otto SR, et al. Cochlear implant histopathology. An J Otol 1991;12:245–311.

5. Nadol JB Jr. Patterns of neural degeneration in the human cochlea and auditory nerve: implications for cochlear implantation. Otolaryngol Head Neck Surg 1997;117(3 Pt 1):220–8.

6. Blanchfield BB, Feldman JJ, Dunbar JL, Gardner EN. The severely to profoundly hearing-impaired population in the United States: prevalence estimates and demographics. J Am Acad Audiol 2001;12:183–9.

7. Cheng AK, Rubin HR, Powe NR, et al. Cost-utility analysis of the cochlear implant in children. JAMA 2000;284:850–6.

8. Blanchfield BB, Feldman JJ, Dunbar J. Severely to profoundly hearing impaired population in the United States: prevalence and demographics. Project HOPE Center for Health Affairs 1999;284(7).

9. Mohr PE, Feldman JJ, Dunbar J. The societal costs of severe to profound hearing loss in the United States. Policy Anal Brief H Ser 2000;2:1–4.

10. Balkany T, Hodges AV, Goodman KW. Ethics of cochlear implantation in young children. Otolaryngol Head Neck Surg 1996;114:748–55.

11. Tucker BP. Deaf culture, cochlear implants, and elective disability. Hastings Cent Rep 1998;28:6–14.

12. Francis HW, Koch ME, Wyatt JR, Niparko JK. Trends in educational placement and cost-benefit considerations in children with cochlear implants. Arch Otolaryngol Head Neck Surg 1999;125:499–505.

13. Haimowitz S. Deaf culture. Hastings Cent Rep 1999;29:5.

14. O'Neill C, O'Donoghue GM, Archbold SM, Normand C. A cost-utility analysis of pediatric cochlear implantation. Laryngoscope 2000;110:156–60.

15. Hutton J, Politi C, Seeger T. Cost-effectiveness of cochlear implantation of children. A preliminary model for the UK. Adv Otorhinolaryngol 1995;50:201–6.

16. Summerfield AQ, Marshall DH, Archbold S. Cost-effectiveness considerations in pediatric cochlear implantation. Am J Otol 1997;18 Suppl 6:S166–8.

17. Summerfield AQ, Marshall DH, Davis AC. Cochlear implantation: demand, costs, and utility. Ann Otol Rhinol Laryngol Suppl 1995;166:245–8.

18. Krabbe PF, Hinderink JB, Van Den Broek P. The effect of cochlear implant use in postlingually deaf adults. Int J Technol Assess Health Care 2000;16:864–73.

19. Palmer CS, Niparko JK, Wyatt JR, et al. A prospective study of the cost-utility of the multichannel cochlear implant. Arch Otolaryngol Head Neck Surg 1999;125:1221–8.

20. Wyatt JR, Niparko JK, Rothman M, deLissovoy G. Cost utility of the multichannel cochlear implants in 258 profoundly deaf individuals. Laryngoscope 1996;106:816–21.

21. Cheng AK, Grant GD, Niparko JK. Meta-analysis of pediatric cochlear implant literature. Ann Otol Rhinol Laryngol Suppl 1999;177:124–8.

22. Luxford WM. Minimum speech test battery for postlingually deafened adult cochlear implant patients. Otolaryngol Head Neck Surg 2001;124:125–6.

23. Arriaga M, Carrier D. MRI and clinical decisions in cochlear implantation. Am J Otol 1996;17:547–53.

24. Ellul S, Shelton C, Davidson HC, Harnsberger HR. Preoperative cochlear implant imaging: is magnetic resonance imaging enough? Am J Otol 2000;2:528–33.

25. Phelps PD, Proops DW. Imaging for cochlear implants. J Laryngol Otol Suppl 1999;24:21–3.

26. Maxwell AP, Mason SM, O'Donoghue GM. Cochlear nerve aplasia: its importance in cochlear implantation. Am J Otol 1999;20:335–7.

27. Nadol JB Jr, Hsu WC. Histopathologic correlation of spiral ganglion cell count and new bone formation in the cochlea following meningogenic labyrinthitis and deafness. Ann Otol Rhinol Laryngol 1991;100(9 Pt 1):712–6.

28. Lesinski A, Hartrampf R, Dahm MC, et al. Cochlear implantation in a population of multihandicapped children. Ann Otol Rhinol Laryngol Suppl 1995;166:332–4.

29. Isaacson JE, Hasenstab MS, Wohl DL, Williams GH. Learning disability in children with postmeningitic cochlear implants. Arch Otolaryngol Head Neck Surg 1996;122:929–36.

30. Waltzman SB, Scalchunes V, Cohen NL. Performance of multiply handicapped children using cochlear implants. Am J Otol 2000;21:329–35.

31. Hodges AV, Dolan AM, Balkany TJ, et al. Speech perception results in children with cochlear implants: contributing factors. Otolaryngol Head Neck Surg 1999;121:31–4.

32. Chen JM, Shipp D, Al Abidi A, et al. Does choosing the "worse" ear for cochlear implantation affect outcome? Otol Neurotol 2001;22:335–9.

33. Roland PS, Tobey EA, Devous MD. Pre-operative functional assessment of auditory cortex in adult cochlear implant users. Laryngoscope 2001;111:77–83.

34. Roland JT Jr, Fisherman AJ, Waltzman SB, et al. Stability of the cochlear implant array in children. Laryngoscope 1998;108(8 Pt 1):1119–23.

35. Kileny PR, Zwolan TA, Ashbaugh C. The influence of age at implantation on performance with a cochlear implant in children. Otol Neurotol 2001;22:42–6.

36. Svirsky MA, Robbins AM, Kirk KI, et al. Language development in profoundly deaf children with cochlear implants. Psychol Sci 2000;11:153–8.

37. Moog JS, Geers AE. Speech and language acquisition in young children after cochlear implantation. Otolaryngol Clin North Am 1999;32:1127–41.

38. Labadie RF, Carrrasco VN, Gilmer CH, Pillsbury HC III. Cochlear implant performance in senior citizens. Otolaryngol Head Neck Surg 2000;123:419–24.

39. Buchman CA, Fucci MJ, Luxford WM. Cochlear implants in the geriatric population: benefits outweigh risks. Ear Nose Throat J 1999;78:489–94.

40. Labadie R. Cochlear implant performance in children with auditory neuropathy. In: Annual Meeting of the American Otological Society, Palm Desert, CA, May 12–13, 2001.

41. Shallop JK, Peterson A, Facer GW, et al. Cochlear implants in five cases of auditory neuropathy: postoperative findings and progress. Laryngoscope 2001;111(4 Pt 1):555–62.

42. D'Haese PS, Hochmair I, Garnham C, Nopp P. First results in bilateral cochlear implantation according to the BilCIA Protocol. In: Wullstein Symposium - Bilateral Cochlear Implantation Wurzburg. Wurzburg (Germany): 2001.

43. Frijns JH, Briaire JJ, Grote JJ. The importance of human cochlear anatomy for the results of modiolus-hugging multichannel cochlear implants. Otol Neurotol 2001;22:340–9.

44. Teissl C, Kremser C, Hochmair ES, Hochmair-Desoyer IJ. Magnetic resonance imaging and cochlear implants: compatibility and safety aspects. J Magn Reson Imaging 1999;9:26–38.

45. Weber BP, Lenarz T, Dillo W, et al. Malformations in cochlear implant patients. Am J Otol 1997;18 Suppl 6:S64–5.

46. Graham J, Lynch C, Weber B, et al. The magnetless Clarion cochlear implant in a patient with neurofibromatosis 2. J Laryngol Otol 1999;113:458–63.

47. Youssefzadeh S, Baumgartner W, Dorffner R, et al. MR compatibility of Med EL cochlear implants: clinical testing at 1.0 T. J Comput Assist Tomogr 1998;22:346–50.

48. Liu JH, RP, Waller MA. Outpatient cochlear implantation in the pediatric population. Otolaryngol Head Neck Surg 2000;122:19–22.

49. Hamamoto M, Murakami G, Kataura A. Topographical relationships among the facial nerve, chorda tympani nerve and round window with special reference to the approach route for cochlear implant surgery. Clin Anat 2000;13:251–6.

50. Colletti V, Fiorino FG, Carner M, et al. New approach for cochlear implantation: cochleostomy through the middle fossa. Otolaryngol Head Neck Surg 2000;123:467–74.

51. Gray RF, Ray J, McFerran DJ. Further experience with fat graft obliteration of mastoid cavities for cochlear implants. J Laryngol Otol 1999;113:881–4.

52. Rubinstein JT, Gantz BJ, Parkinson WS. Management of cochlear implant infections. Am J Otol 1999;20:46–9.

53. Rubinstein JT, et al. Residual speech recognition and cochlear implant performance: effects of implantation criteria. Am J Otol 1999;20:445–52.

54. Kumar A, Mugge R, Lipner M. Surgical complications of cochlear implantation: a report of three cases and their clinical features. Ear Nose Throat J 1999;78:913–9.

55. Parkins CS, Metzinger SE, Marks HW. Management of late extrusions of cochlear implants. 1998;768–73.

56. Luntz M, Hodges AV, Balkany T, et al. Otitis media in children with cochlear implants. Laryngoscope 1996;106:1403–5.

57. Luntz M, Balkany T, Telischi FF, Hodges AV. Surgical techniques for cochlear implantation of the malformed inner ear. Am J Otol 1997;18 Suppl 6:S66.

58. McElveen JT Jr, Carrasco VN, Miyamoto RT, Linthicum FH Jr. Cochlear implantation in common cavity malformations using a transmastoid labyrinthotomy approach. Laryngoscope 1997;107:1032–6.

59. Bhatt S, Halpin C, Hsu W, et al. Hearing loss and pneumococcal meningitis: an animal model. Laryngoscope 1991;101(12 Pt 1):1285–92.

60. Brodie HA, Thompson TC, Vassilian L, Lee BN. Induction of labyrinthitis ossificans after pneumococcal meningitis: an animal model. Otolaryngol Head Neck Surg 1998;118:15–21.

61. Nabili V, Brodie HA, Neverov NI, Tinling SP. Chronology of labyrinthitis ossificans induced by *Streptococcus pneumoniae* meningitis. Laryngoscope 1999;109:931–5.

62. Gulya AJ, Steenerson RL. The scala vestibuli for cochlear implantation. An anatomic study. Arch Otolaryngol Head Neck Surg 1996;122:130–2.

63. Balkany T, Gantz BJ, Steenerson RL, Cohen NL. Systematic approach to electrode insertion in the ossified cochlea. Otolaryngol Head Neck Surg 1996;114:4–11.

64. Balkany T, Bird PA, Hodges AV, et al. Surgical technique for implantation of the totally ossified cochlea. Laryngoscope 1998;108:988–92.

65. Roland JT Jr, Fisherman AJ, Waltzman SB, Cohen NL. Shaw scalpel in revision cochlear implant surgery. Ann Otol Rhinol Laryngol Suppl 2000;185:23–5.

66. Balkany TJ, Hodges AV, Gomez-Marin O, et al. Cochlear reimplantation. Laryngoscope 1999;109:351–5.

67. Balkany T, Hodges AV, Goodman K. Ethics of cochlear implantation in young children. Otolaryngol Head Neck Surg 1999; 121:673–5.

68. Henson AM, Slattery WH 3rd, Luxford WM, et al. Cochlear implant performance after reimplantation: a multicenter study. Am J Otol 1999;56–64.

69. Parisier SC, Chute PM, Popp AL, Suh GD. Outcome analysis of cochlear implant reimplantation in children. Laryngoscope 2001;111:26–32.

70. Shallop JK, Facer GW, Peterson A. Neural response telemetry with the nucleus CI24M cochlear implant. Laryngoscope 1999; 109:1755–9.

71. Abbas PJ, Brown CJ, Shallop JK, et al. Summary of results using the Nucleus C124M implant to record the electricity evoked compound action potential (EAP). Ear Hear 1999;20:45–59.

72. Brown CJ, Hughes ML, Lopez SM, Abbas PJ. Relationship between EABR thresholds and levels used to program the CLARION speech processor. Ann Otol Rhinol Laryngol 1999; 177:50–7.

73. Shallop JK, Ash KR. Relationships among comfort levels determined by cochlear implant patient's self-programming, audiologist's programming, and electrical stapedius reflex thresholds. Ann Otol Rhinol Laryngol Suppl 1995;166:175–6.

74. Clark GM. Cochlear implants in the third millennium. Am J Otol 1999;20:4–8.

75. Cohen NL. Surgical techniques to avoid complications of cochlear implants in children. Adv Otorhinolaryngol 1997;52: 161–3.

76. Bigelow DC, Kay DJ, Rafter KO, et al. Facial nerve stimulation from cochlear implants. Am J Otol 1998;19:163–9.

77. Kelsall DC, Shallop JK, Brammeier TG, Prenger EC. Facial nerve stimulation after Nucleus 22-channel cochlear implantation. Am J Otol 1997;18:336–41.

78. Gold SR, Miller V, Kamerer DB, Koconis CA. Fluoride treatment for facial nerve stimulation caused by cochlear implants in otosclerosis. Otolaryngol Head Neck Surg 1998;119:521–3.

79. Parkinson AJ, Parkinson WS, Tyler RS, et al. Speech perception performance in experienced cochlear-implant patients receiving the SPEAK processing strategy in the Nucleus Spectra-22 cochlear implant. J Speech Lang Hear Res 1998;41: 1073–87.

80. Gstoettner WK, Hamzavi J, Baumgartner WD. Speech discrimination scores of postlingually deaf adults implanted with the Combi 40 cochlear implant. Acta Otolaryngol (Stockh) 1998; 118:640–5.

81. Waltzman SB, Cohen NL, Gomolin RH, et al. Open-set speech perception in congenitally deaf children using cochlear implants. Am J Otol 1997;18:342–9.

82. Blamey PJ, Sarant JZ, Paatsch LE, et al. Relationships among speech perception, production, language, hearing loss, and

age in children with impaired hearing. J Speech Lang Hear Res 2001;44:264–85.

83. Tomblin JB, Spencer LJ, Tye-Murray N. A preliminary study of grammatical development in prelingually deaf children with and without cochlear implant experience. Cochlear Implants 2001;290–1.

84. Archbold S, O'Donoghue G, Nikolopoulos T. Cochlear implants in children: an analysis of use over a three-year period. Am J Otol 1998;19:328–31.

85. Cheng AK, Niparko JK. Cost-utility of the cochlear implant in adults: a meta-analysis. Arch Otolaryngol Head Neck Surg 1999; 125:1214–8.

86. Geers AE, Nicholas J, Tye-Murray N, et al. Effects of communication mode on skills of long-term cochlear implant users. Ann Otol Rhinol Laryngol 2000;109(12 Pt 2):89–92.

87. Robbins AM, Svirsky M, Kirk KI. Children with implants can speak, but can they communicate? Otolaryngol Head Neck Surg 1997;117(3 Pt 1):155–60.

88. Tobey EA. Factors associated with speech intelligibility in children with cochlear implants. Ann Otol Rhinol Laryngol 2000;109 Suppl 185:28–9.

89. Miyamoto RT, Svirsky MA, Robbins AM. Enhancement of expressive language in prelingually deaf children with cochlear implants. Acta Otolaryngol (Stockh) 1997;117:154–7.

VII

Surgery of the Internal Auditory Canal/ Cerebellopontine Angle/Petrous Apex

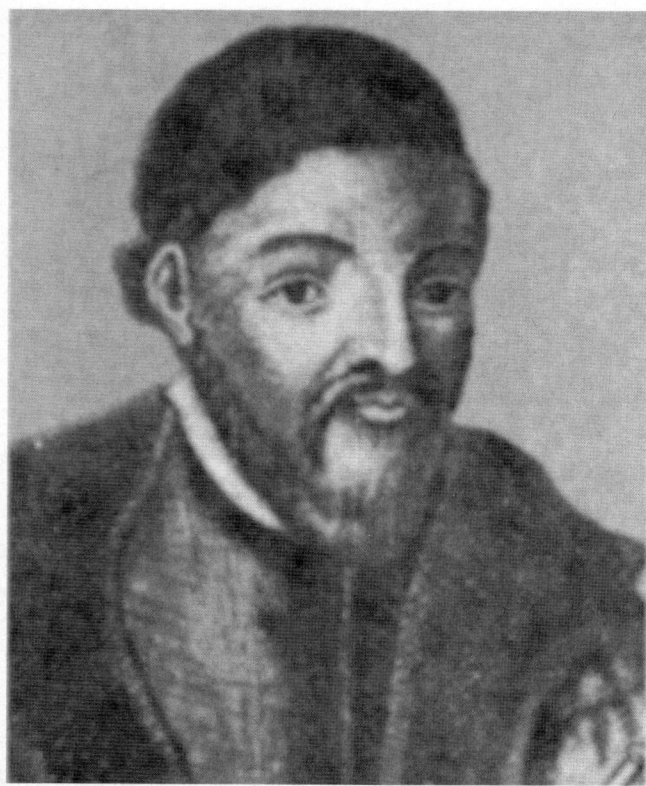

Gabriel Fallopius (1523–1562). Described the fallopian canal for the intratemporal portion of the facial nerve.

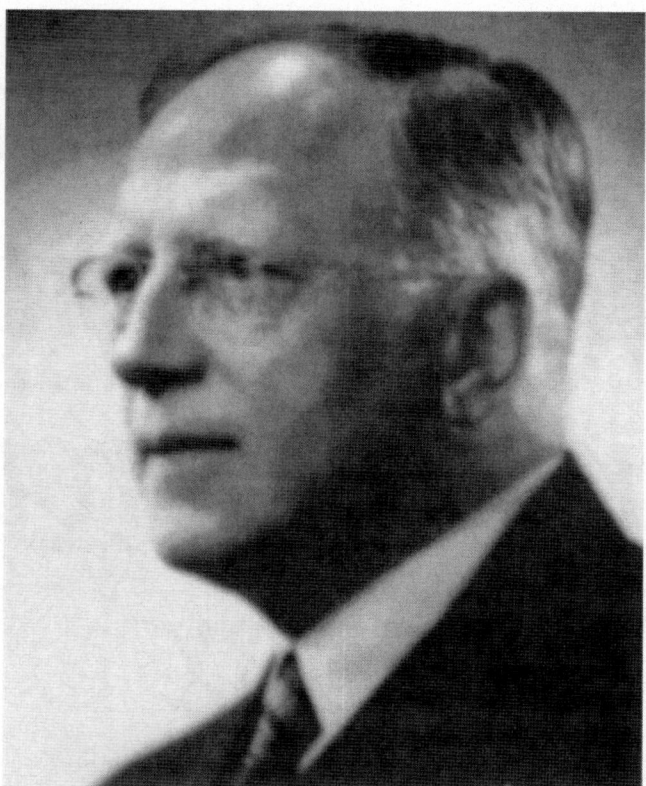

Sterling Bunnell (1882–1957). In 1927 performed the first successful intratemporal suture of the facial nerve and in 1930 the first successful facial nerve graft within the temporal bone.

31

Surgery of the Facial Nerve

RAVI N. SAMY, MD
BRUCE J. GANTZ, MD

Facial nerve dysfunction causes noticeable disfigurement and emotional distress to those suffering from it. Facial paresis and paralysis affect both voluntary and involuntary motion and can be a detriment to social interaction. More than any other cranial nerve, the facial nerve affects nonverbal humanistic expression, which is a significant component of communication. Facial palsy may also interrupt normal daily functions, such as eating and drinking; more importantly, it may disrupt the protective function of the eye. Before discussing the diagnosis and treatment of facial nerve disorders, one must understand the nerve's complex anatomy, physiology, and function. Management of facial nerve dysfunction is individualized and may include observation, administration of pharmacologic agents, surgical intervention, physical therapy, and psychological counseling.[1] These will be discussed in detail later in the chapter.

ANATOMY

An understanding of the anatomy of the facial (seventh cranial) nerve is essential to diagnose and treat facial nerve dysfunction. The nerve contains approximately 7,000 to 10,000 fibers.[2,3] The facial nerve originates from the facial motor nucleus, which lies in the lateral portion of the anterior pons[4] and is composed of four cell groups. Facial nerve function is highly organized at the central nervous system level. Some level of topographic organization probably continues as the nerve courses peripherally. The facial nerve hooks around the nucleus of the sixth cranial (abducens) nerve. As a result, brainstem lesions involving the seventh nerve also usually involve the sixth nerve.

The facial nerve exits the brainstem at the pontomedullary junction caudal to the fifth cranial (trigeminal) nerve and approximately 1.5 mm anterior, medial, and superior to the eighth cranial (vestibulocochlear) nerve (Figure 31–1).[4,5] The facial nerve is smaller in diameter than the vestibulocochlear nerve (1.8 mm versus 3 mm). The facial nerve then crosses the cerebellopontine angle (CPA) (a distance of 15 to 17 mm) with the eighth cranial nerve and the nerve of Wrisberg (nervus intermedius).[6] The nervus intermedius not only carries secretory fibers to the lacrimal, sublingual, and submaxillary glands, but it also carries afferent fibers conveying taste from the anterior two-thirds of the tongue and sensation from the posterior wall of the external auditory canal (EAC) (see Figure 31–1).[7]

The facial nerve passes through the porus of the internal auditory canal (IAC). The superior and inferior vestibular nerves lie immediately posterior and inferoposterior to the facial nerve, respectively. The cochlear nerve lies caudal to the facial nerve in the IAC. By the lateral end (fundus) of the IAC, the facial nerve has merged with the nervus intermedius. The length of the IAC portion of the nerve is approximately 8 to 10 mm.[6] The facial nerve enters the labyrinthine segment of its fallopian canal through the meatal foramen, which is the narrowest portion of the entire canal and measures approximately 0.68 mm in diameter. The labyrinthine segment (4 mm in length) makes up the first segment of the bony fallopian canal and is the narrowest and shortest portion of the canal.[8] In addition to the small diameter of the meatal foramen, a dense arachnoid band encircles the nerve at the lateral end of the IAC. This band contributes to the anatomic "bottleneck" that can constrict

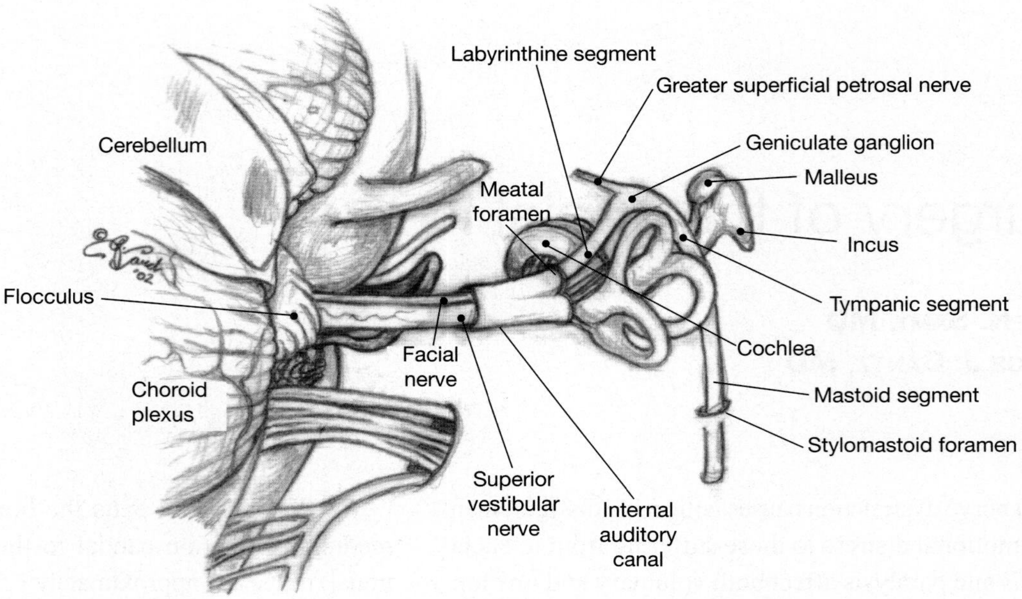

Figure 31–1 The course and relationships of the left facial nerve from the pontomedullary junction to the intratemporal course.

the nerve in disorders that induce edema of the nerve, such as Bell's palsy. Thus, the meatal foramen and labyrinthine segment of the nerve play a pivotal role in the pathophysiology of facial paralysis, as will be discussed later in this chapter. The labyrinthine segment is posterocephalad to the cochlea, anteromedial to the ampulla of the superior semicircular canal, and posterior to the vestibule.[3] Subsequently, the fallopian canal takes a long (approximately 30 mm), tortuous course through the temporal bone.[9] The fallopian canal provides a bony covering for the facial nerve that is longer than that of any other nerve. This bony encasement protects the nerve but also renders it vulnerabe to certain diseases and disorders (Figure 31–2).[7]

At the geniculate ganglion (GG), the facial nerve takes a sharp (75 degree) posterior turn at the first (internal) genu. The GG contains bipolar ganglion cells for the sensory functions of the nervus intermedius. The greater superficial petrosal nerve (GSPN) arises from the GG and emerges through the hiatus of the fallopian canal (facial hiatus) onto the floor of the middle fossa. The GSPN contains secretory fibers to the lacrimal gland that synapse in the pterygopalatine ganglion; postganglionic fibers then innervate the lacrimal gland.[3]

From the GG, the facial nerve courses in its tympanic (horizontal) segment, which is the second segment of the fallopian canal and measures 11 mm in length. The nerve runs posteriorly, becoming the cephalad margin

of the oval window niche. The nerve then makes a second turn (the second or external genu). At this point, the facial nerve gives off a branch to the stapedius muscle. The facial nerve then proceeds vertically in the mastoid cavity (vertical/mastoid segment), which measures 13 mm in length. Approximately midway in its mastoid segment, the facial nerve gives off the chorda tympani nerve (Figure 31–3). However, the points of origin of the nerve to the stapedius muscle and the chorda tympani nerve can be quite variable—anywhere between the second genu and the stylomastoid foramen.[10] The preganglionic, parasympathetic fibers present in the chorda tympani nerve synapse in the submandibular ganglion; postganglionic fibers innervate the submandibular and sublingual glands.[3] The facial nerve leaves the temporal bone and the fallopian canal via the stylomastoid foramen, lying between the mastoid tip and the styloid process. As the nerve approaches the stylomastoid foramen, it becomes encircled by the fibrous tendon of the digastric muscle, which becomes part of the nerve sheath and firmly attaches the nerve to surrounding structures. Surgical release of the nerve requires sharp dissection of the surrounding muscle to avoid neural injury. At the pes anserinus in the parotid gland, the extratemporal portion of the nerve divides into the temporofacial and cervicofacial trunks. The major peripheral branches arising from the trunks are the temporal, zygomatic, buccal, marginal mandibular, and cervical.

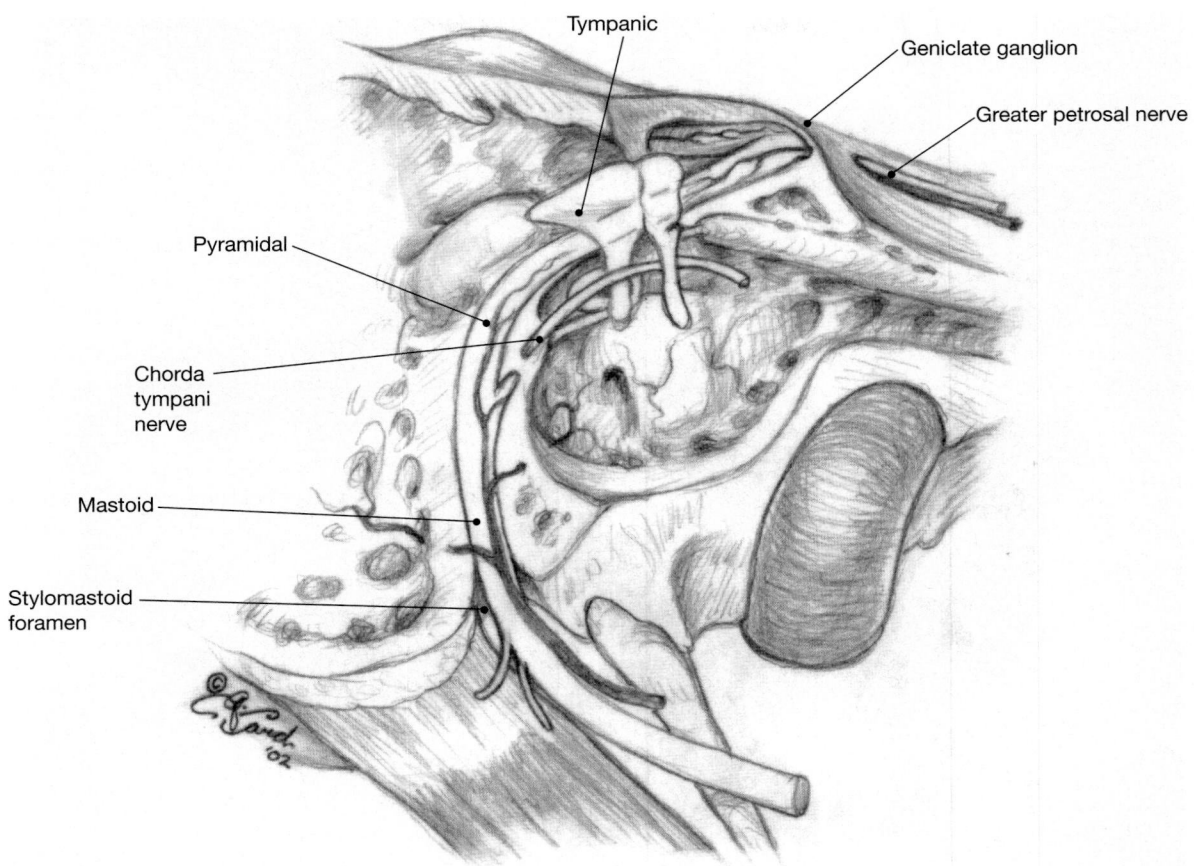

Tympanic

Geniclate ganglion

Greater petrosal nerve

Pyramidal

Chorda tympani nerve

Mastoid

Stylomastoid foramen

Figure 31–2 Overview of the facial nerve in its intratemporal course.

Minor variations and major anomalies often occur in the course of the facial nerve, predisposing the nerve to inadvertent surgical injury. The most common variation is a dehiscence of the fallopian canal, found in over 50% of temporal bones.[7] The most frequent site of dehiscence is the horizontal segment (91%). An uncovered nerve may herniate inferiorly and obscure the stapes.[11] During embryologic development, the fallopian canal originates from the primordial otic capsule and Reichert's cartilage (second branchial arch). Although ossification of these structures normally begins during gestation and is completed by the end of the first year of life, incomplete ossification often occurs, resulting in exposure (dehiscence) of the nerve.[12] More serious anomalies of the different segments of the intratemporal facial nerve are seen in congenital malformations of the middle and outer ear.[13] The discussion of specific malformations and the relative risk to the facial nerve is beyond the scope of this chapter.

HISTOLOGY

Each nerve fiber, consisting of a nerve cell body and an axon, is surrounded by an insulating layer of myelin secreted by Schwann cells. A single nerve fiber is surrounded by numerous Schwann cells, which also provide metabolic support. The axon relies upon its parent neuron for nutrient replenishment through axoplasmic flow, which proceeds at the rate of 1 mm/day. Each nerve fiber is surrounded by multiple connective tissue layers, endoneurium, forming a tubule. Multiple tubules are bound together in bundles by additional connective tissue (perineurium). Additional connective tissue (epineurium) forms the nerve sheath.[7] The three connective tissue layers are complex in function and anatomy. They play important functions, including resisting stretching, maintaining tensile strength and intraneural pressures, providing insulation and circulation, and minimizing functional deterioration even in the presence

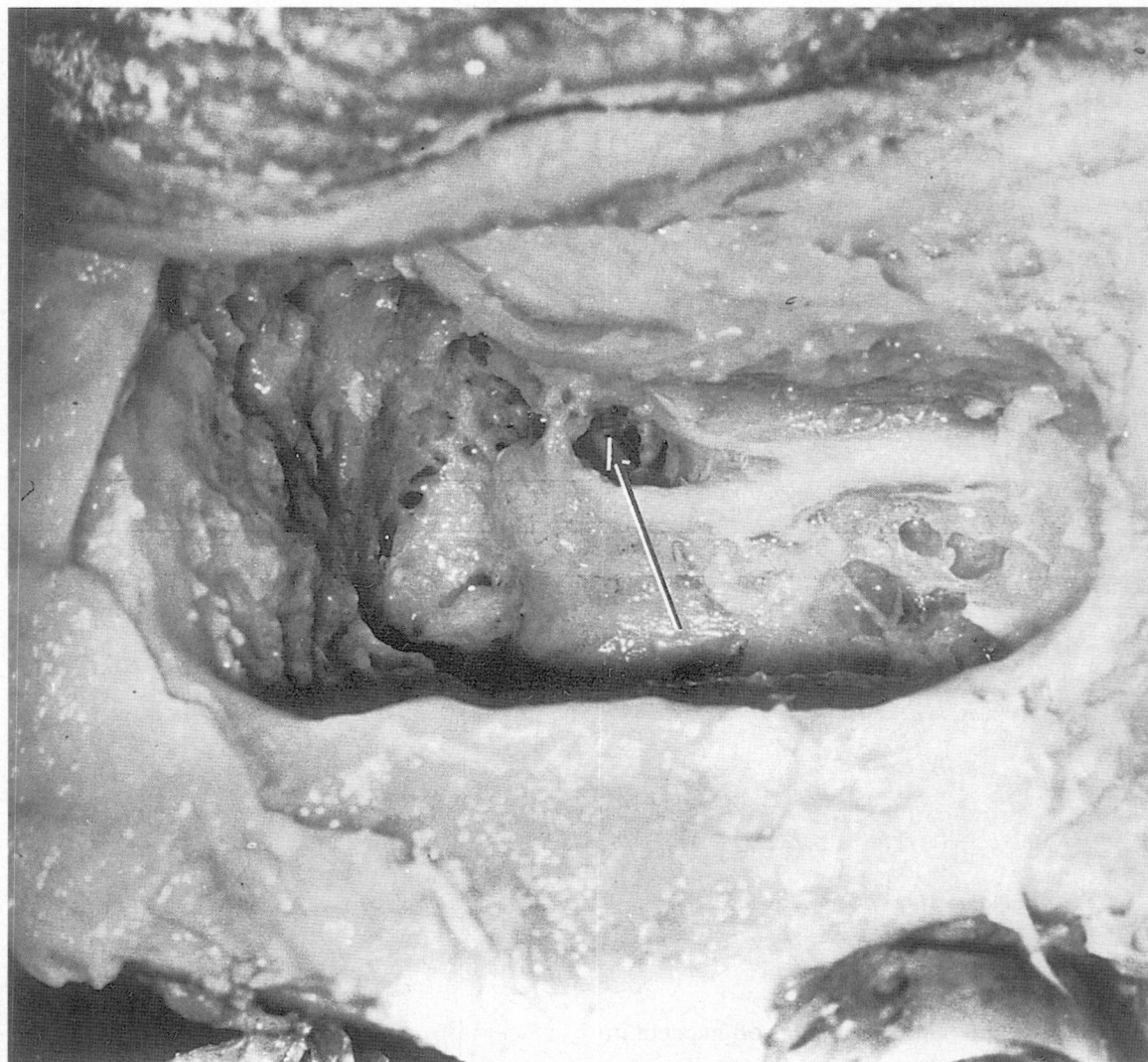

Figure 31–3   The facial recess (*arrow*) lies between the facial and chorda tympani nerves. The incudostapedial joint is visible just to the right of the arrowhead. Reproduced with permission from Gulya AJ, Schuknecht HF. Anatomy of the temporal bone with surgical implications. 2nd ed. Pearl River (NY): Parthenon Press; 1995.

of gradually applied deforming forces (eg, vestibular schwannomas or cholesteatomas).[3,7] Unfortunately, the facial nerve has no protective layer until it reaches the labyrinthine segment, leaving the nerve highly vulnerable during procedures in the CPA or IAC.

VASCULAR SUPPLY

The principal arterial supply of the facial nerve is provided by three main sources: (1) the labyrinthine artery, a branch of the anterior inferior cerebellar artery (AICA) (the AICA may lie anterior to cranial nerves VII and VIII or between them in the IAC or CPA); (2) the superior petrosal artery, a branch of the middle meningeal artery; and (3) the stylomastoid artery, a branch of the postauricular artery.[4] These three branches have numerous anastomoses and constitute the extrinsic vascular system, which runs in the epineurium. Veins accompany the arteries in the fallopian canal. An intraneural vascular plexus (intrinsic system) originates from the extrinsic system. This plexis can support segments of the nerve when it is mobilized from the fallopian canal, even when the extrinsic system is disrupted.[7] Lymphatic vessels are located in the epineurial layer.[3,7,14]

PATHOPHYSIOLOGY

In 1943, Seddon described three types of progressive nerve injury: neuropraxia, axonotmesis, and neurotmesis.[15] When pressure is placed on a nerve, the transmission of nerve impulses may be blocked. If the pressure is not sustained for long, release of the pressure usually results in a rapid and complete recovery of function with no residual dysfunction and no distal wallerian degeneration.[16] This type of injury is known as neuropraxia. Axonotmesis is a more severe injury and involves sectioning of an axon or sufficient pressure to block axoplasmic flow.[7] Although endoneurial tubules are preserved, distal wallerian degeneration occurs. Neurotmesis describes total nerve transection (all three protective sheaths are involved). In actuality, there is usually a mixture of the different types of injury unless there has been complete nerve transection. Wallerian degeneration usually occurs over a 72- to 96-hour period following injury. Distal nerve excitability is therefore usually maintained for 3 to 4 days following severe injury.[3,7,16]

A more detailed classification of neural injury was proposed by Sunderland in 1951.[17] He proposed five progressively severe degrees of nerve injury, as opposed to the three types of nerve injuries described by Seddon. However, the Sunderland classification pertains only to traumatic injuries of the peripheral nerve and not to viral, inflammatory, or infiltrative lesions.[18] A first-degree injury is reversible and allows complete recovery. In second-degree injury, wallerian degeneration occurs, but endoneurial architecture is preserved; recovery is usually complete. In third-degree injury, wallerian degeneration and disruption of endoneurial architecture occur. There

is incomplete recovery, usually complicated by functional sequelae. Second- and third-degree injuries are approximately equivalent to axonotmesis. Fourth-degree injury reflects significant nerve injury. Only the epineurium is intact, and recovery tends to be poor.[7] Fifth-degree injury involves complete and total disruption of nerve continuity; recovery cannot occur without surgical intervention. In general, the quality of the return of facial movement is inversely proportional to the amount of neural degeneration caused by injury.[19] As facial nerve function returns, most patients and physicians first notice a return of tone to the facial musculature that precedes a return of gross movement.[7]

If the injury is third degree or worse, there is disruption of the endoneurium, perineurium, and/or the epineurium. If recovery does occur, the axon develops a growth cone that begins to bring nutrients to the cell body. Branching of a regenerating axon with protoplasmic threads entering several empty neural tubules usually occurs. In other words, regenerating axon sprouts can enter the endoneurial tube of another axon, resulting in innervation of an inappropriate muscle.[7] Thus, a single axon can innervate widely separated facial muscles, resulting in synkinesis—simultaneous movement of different facial muscles.[3,7] Synkinesis may be cosmetically disfiguring and has been treated temporarily by chemodenervation with botulinum toxin. Animal studies using vincristine have shown a delay in reinnervation of selected muscles. Vincristine may someday be used in patients to prevent the development of synkinesis.[20,21]

Although the rate of axon regeneration is generally thought to be 1 mm/day, the rate of regeneration and overall recovery depend on several variables, including the etiology and severity of the paralysis, the degenerative process, and individual neuronal factors (eg, the longer the duration of degeneration, the poorer the quality of facial nerve recovery). Numerous cellular and systemic factors also affect the recovery process. Patient age, level of nutrition, blood supply, comorbidities (eg, diabetes mellitus), and concurrent wound infection also influence the quality of regeneration.[3,7]

CARE OF THE EYE

Before turning to a discussion of facial nerve disorders and their treatment, the most important function of the facial nerve, protection of the eye, must be reviewed. Although facial paralysis is cosmetically displeasing, causes functional discomfort, and impairs communication, the most significant associated complication involves the eye. If the eyelids do not function well, the conjunctiva is not lubricated properly,[7] and the eye becomes dry. If eye dryness occurs in conjunction with other abnormalities, such as decreased lacrimation (eg, owing to GSPN disruption) and/or decreased corneal sensation (because of trigeminal nerve dysfunction), corneal complications are likely to occur, including exposure keratitis, ulceration, and blindness. Thus, one must instruct the patient in proper eye care.

The ultimate objectives in management of the eye are, in order, (1) corneal protection with preservation of vision and eye function, (2) comfort, and (3) cosmetic restoration.[22] If the facial nerve has been severed and an interposition graft inserted, it may take 6 months or longer for orbicularis oculi function to return. During this long period of time, lid loading with gold weight placement, an easily reversible procedure, may be performed. Some surgeons prefer a lateral tarsorrhaphy, which can be either temporary or permanent.

For patients whose facial function is likely to return in a short period of time, care of the eye can be accomplished using conservative measures. The patient is instructed to instill artificial tears frequently, even every hour if needed. The patient and his/her family member should monitor for conjunctival injection, a sign of irritation and dryness. The complaint of a foreign body sensation also indicates dryness. The patient should use a long-lasting ophthalmic lubricant at night or during the day if asleep. (Some patients prefer routine use of ointment during the day as well.) The patient may consider using a moisture chamber or taping of the eye whenever asleep. Wind protection, through the use of glasses, is recommended. If concerns of impending ocular damage arise, an urgent ophthalmologic consultation is required. Thus, treatment is highly individualized and is affected by the expected duration of paralysis.[3]

EVALUATION OF FACIAL NERVE FUNCTION

Numerous methods of grading facial nerve palsy have been developed since the 1940s.[1] Although no gold standard or universally accepted system exists, the most commonly used scale is the House-Brackmann (HB)

facial nerve grading system, which differentiates six grades of facial function (I to VI).[23] The American Academy of Otolaryngology-Head and Neck Surgery has adopted this system to standardize the reporting of disorders of the facial nerve and treatment results. Prior to the adoption of this scale, scientific analysis of data lacked a uniform and objective measure.[3,24] The use of this scale represents a major stride in the objective analysis of facial nerve data (Table 31–1). However, the HB scale is not a perfect grading system because of the problems of interobserver and intraobserver variability. Also, the grading system is applicable only to disorders of the nerve proximal to the pes anserinus.[4] The scale is not appropriate for single-branch injuries, such as a penetrating injury to the face affecting only the buccal branch. Future improvement in grading the status of facial nerve function may involve the use of dialized images or computerized dynamic functional analysis.[25] Additionally, others have suggested the inclusion of a patient-based system to measure overall impairment and disability, which would assist in evaluating quality-of-life issues affected by facial disfigurement.[1]

At the University of Iowa, we use a different grading system, known as the repaired facial nerve recovery scale (RFNRS), for nerve resections repaired by neurorrhaphy or interposition grafting (Table 31–2).[26] Like the HB scale, the RFNRS has six grades but uses letters instead of numbers (grades A to F). There is some correlation between the two grading systems, with grade A approximately equivalent to grade I, grade B to grade II, and so on.[26] The HB scale is not useful in assessing transected or repaired nerves for three reasons: (1) all repairs cause mass movement; (2) most patients can eventually close their eyes and have good oral sphincter function; and (3) almost no patients are able to raise their eyebrow or forehead. The HB system works well as long as there is an intact nerve sheath or incomplete nerve injury (ie, Sunderland grades I to IV).[26]

EVALUATION OF PATIENTS WITH FACIAL NERVE DISORDERS

There is no substitute for a thorough history and physical examination in the evaluation of a patient with a facial nerve disorder. Factors that are assessed include date of onset, rapidity of progression, comorbidities, risk factors, duration of symptoms, and associated symptoms.

Table 31–1   HOUSE-BRACKMAN NERVE GRADING SYSTEM

Grade	Description	Characteristics
I	Normal	Normal facial function in all areas
II	Mild dysfunction	Gross: slight weakness noticeable on close inspection; may have very slight synkinesis
		At rest: normal symmetry and tone
		Motion: forehead—moderate to good function; eye—complete closure with minimum effort; mouth—slight asymmetry
III	Moderate dysfunction	Gross: obvious but not disfiguring difference between two sides; noticeable but not severe synkinesis; contracture and/or hemifacial spasm
		At rest: normal symmetry and tone
		Motion: forehead—slight to moderate movement; eye—complete closure with effort; mouth—slightly weak with maximum effort
IV	Moderately severe dysfunction	Gross: obvious weakness and/or disfiguring asymmetry
		At rest: normal symmetry and tone
		Motion: forehead—none; eye—incomplete closure; mouth—asymmetric with maximum effort
V	Severe dysfunction	Gross: only barely perceptible motion
		At rest: asymmetry
		Motion: forehead—none; eye—incomplete closure; mouth—slight movement
VI	Total paralysis	No movement

Adapted from House JW and colleagues.[23]

For example, a description of otalgia associated with auricular vesicles is a sign of Ramsay Hunt syndrome and not of Bell's palsy. The physical examination includes a thorough head and neck examination, with an assessment for cervical lymphadenopathy and parotid gland pathology, which is suggestive of a malignant process. The auricle and external ear are examined closely for lesions consistent with Ramsay Hunt syndrome. The tympanic membrane and mesotympanum are examined with an otomicroscope (with pneumatic evaluation). All branches of the facial nerve are examined. If the forehead branches are intact but all other branches are paralyzed, a central etiology is likely. Involvement of a single branch tends to indicate a lesion distal to the pes anserinus in the parotid. Evaluation of the cerebellum and other cranial nerves is also performed. Other components of the general physical examination are performed as warranted by symptomatology.

Laboratory studies are performed as warranted. For bilateral facial palsy, additional testing includes the following: a complete blood count (looking for infection, leukemia), erythrocyte sedimentation rate (vasculitis), blood chemistry (diabetes mellitus), human immunodeficiency tests, fluorescent treponemal antibody tests (syphilis), or a lumbar puncture with cerebrospinal fluid (CSF) examination (Lyme disease, multiple sclerosis, Guillain-Barré syndrome).[18,27]

Audiometry plays an important role in the evaluation of facial paralysis. Every patient undergoes a pure-tone air and bone conduction audiogram, testing of speech reception threshold and speech discrimination, and tympanometry. Findings on the audiogram should be symmetric; if they are not, a retrocochlear workup is performed. For example, a unilateral sensorineural hearing loss on the same side of the facial paralysis may indicate a tumor in the IAC or CPA (or possibly Ramsay Hunt syndrome).[18] Additional audiometric studies, such as

Table 31–2   REPAIRED FACIAL NERVE RECOVERY SCALE

Score	Function
A	Normal facial function
B	Independent movement of eyelids and mouth, slight mass motion, slight movement of forehead
C	Strong closure of eyelids and oral sphincter, some mass motion, no forehead movement
D	Incomplete closure of eyelids, significant mass motion, good tone
E	Minimal movement in any branch, poor tone
F	No movement

Adapted from Gidley PW and colleagues.[26]

acoustic reflex decay or auditory brainstem response testing, can also be used to detect retrocochlear lesions. If vestibular complaints or abnormalities are detected, an electronystagmogram (ENG) and rotary chair testing are performed.

If the patient presents with the classic findings and history of Bell's palsy, radiographic imaging is not performed. However, if symptoms, signs, audiometry, or any additional testing is abnormal, imaging studies are obtained. Radiographic studies are also performed if no return of facial function is noted within 6 months of the onset of Bell's palsy, which is suggestive of a tumor. Plain films and polytomography no longer play a role in diagnosis. Fine-cut computed tomographic (CT) scans of the temporal bone (in the axial and coronal planes) and magnetic resonance imaging with gadolinium (Gd-MRI) play complementary roles. Gadolinium MRI of the brain and brainstem is useful in establishing the presence of lesions in the CPA or IAC, such as a facial nerve neuroma or vestibular schwannoma. The soft tissue detail of the MRI complements the CT scan's high-resolution views of the osseous structures of the temporal bone, including the fallopian canal and its anatomic relations. Computed tomographic evaluation of the temporal bone is helpful in determining the presence of intratemporal tumors, cholesteatomas, and fractures. In some instances, MR angiograms and/or conventional arteriography are indicated if there is a concern about the presence of a vascular lesion, such as a glomus tumor.

Topodiagnostic testing (eg, taste and saliva testing, Schirmer's tear test, stapedial reflex) is of historical significance only and, because of questionable accuracy and clinically imprecise administration, has been replaced by more objective and accurate investigations. Topodiagnostic tests evaluate different functions of the nerve to determine the site of the abnormality or lesion. However, since the loss of nerve impulse propagation is an electrophysiologic event, an electrodiagnostic test is employed to determine the site of injury and prognosis, helping separate which patients will fully recover from those likely to exhibit incomplete return of function.[28,29]

ELECTROPHYSIOLOGIC TESTING

Electrical testing evaluates the condition of the nerve and establishes the degree of dysfunction. Electroneurography (ENOG) and electromyography (EMG) are the two most precise and objective electrical diagnostic tests

used to assess facial paralysis. They have replaced maximal stimulus and nerve excitability testing and other subjective electrical tests. Electrical testing is not employed if a patient exhibits paresis since the presence of even minimal voluntary motion indicates minor injury with a high probability of full recovery.

Electroneurography can estimate the amount of severe nerve fiber degeneration. It is most useful between 4 and 21 days after the onset of complete paralysis.[28] Since it takes 3 days for wallerian degeneration to occur after a severe injury, ENOG is not performed until the fourth day. The interpretation of much of the initial diagnostic information gathered with ENOG was based on the observation of patients with Bell's palsy. Subsequently, ENOG has been used in a variety of other conditions, including trauma and acute otitis media; however, it does not appear to be as useful in Ramsay Hunt syndrome owing to the multiple sites of injury in this disorder.[16]

Electroneurography uses an evoked electrical stimulus to activate the facial nerve as it exits the temporal bone at the stylomastoid foramen. The technique of performing ENOG can influence the results.[19] The technical aspects of test performance must be standardized if ENOG is to provide relevant clinical information regarding prognosis of facial nerve function and recovery.[30] Electroneuronography provides an objective recording of the evoked biphasic compound muscle action potential (CMAP), which occurs with facial movement. The CMAP is measured with surface electrodes. Supramaximal stimulation is used to obtain the maximum amplitude of the CMAP, which correlates with the number of remaining fibers that can be stimulated. The CMAP from the paralyzed side is compared with the CMAP of the normal side, which serves as control (mean CMAP of healthy nerves is approximately 5,320 μV).[30] A percentage of degenerated nerve fibers is calculated. Degeneration of greater than 90% occurring within the first 14 days of complete paralysis indicates poor recovery in > 50% of patients.[28] In addition to the percentage of degeneration, the rate of degeneration is important. Patients who reach a severe level of degeneration in 5 days have a poorer prognosis than those who reach it in several weeks. In other words, if 90% degeneration does not occur by 3 weeks after the onset of Bell's palsy, a good prognosis is indicated.[19] Electroneurography is not useful in long-standing (> 3 weeks) facial paralysis or as a diagnostic test for tumors because concurrent degeneration and regeneration may be occurring—a phenomenon termed desynchronization. Because all nerve fibers must depolarize synchronously to generate a CMAP, no response may be seen on ENOG, even when polyphasic potentials (a favorable sign of regenerating nerve fibers) are noted on the EMG.

Voluntary EMG testing is performed in conjunction with ENOG when 90% or greater neural degeneration is recorded. This test measures voluntary motor activity using needle electrodes placed in the orbicularis oris and orbicularis oculi muscles. The patient is asked to make forceful contractions. The finding of active motor unit potentials in the presence of paralysis means that deblocking is occurring and that the prognosis for return of normal facial motion is good. In cases of long-standing facial paralysis, one looks for defibrillation potentials that suggest wallerian degeneration or for polyphasic potentials that suggest reinnervation.

COMMON DISEASES AND DISORDERS OF THE FACIAL NERVE

Facial nerve dysfunction can stem from a variety of causes and may involve the supranuclear tract to the brainstem (intracranial course), the intratemporal segments, or the extratemporal portions. The disorder may even involve multiple segments of the nerve. The paralysis can be idiopathic or caused by trauma, systemic infection, acute or chronic otitis media, metabolic disorders, toxins, vasculitides, neurologic disorders, neoplasms (both benign and malignant), radiation therapy, and numerous other causes.[18] Owing to the limited space in this chapter, only the most commonly associated causes will be presented. The diagnosis and management of Bell's palsy, as discussed below, will serve as a paradigm in the treatment of other facial nerve disorders.

IDIOPATHIC FACIAL PARALYSIS (BELL'S PALSY)

Bell's palsy is named after the British physician Sir Charles Bell, who described the onset, physical findings, and course of the disease in 1821. However, some historical records have shown that Nicolaus A. Friedrich of Wurzburg published an account of three patients with idiopathic peripheral facial nerve paralysis 23 years before Bell's report (1798).[31] Although Bell's palsy is the most common cause of facial palsy (80%), with an inci-

dence of 20 to 30 cases per 100,000 individuals, it is still a diagnosis of exclusion.[28]

Bell's palsy is an acute, unilateral, peripheral facial paralysis. Although frequently called idiopathic facial paralysis, a viral etiology is the most likely cause; numerous studies have identified herpes simplex virus 1 (HSV-1) as the causative agent, and it has been found in patients who have undergone decompression for Bell's palsy.[32] In an animal model of Bell's palsy, it has been demonstrated that HSV inoculation can cause a transient facial paralysis.[33] Polymerase chain reaction (PCR) assays have been performed on fresh and stored geniculate ganglions obtained from temporal bone specimens and have detected HSV-1.[29,34,35] (In a similar fashion, the presence of varicella-zoster virus [VZV] DNA has been shown in patients affected by herpes-zoster oticus, also called Ramsay Hunt syndrome).[36]

There is no sex predilection for Bell's palsy. A person of any age may be affected, with those in the fifth and sixth decades of life most at risk. The age of the patient is also important because older patients tend to have a poorer recovery. Right- and left-sided disease occur equally. Recurrence is seen in up to 10% of patients; however, recurrence should heighten suspicion for another etiology, such as a tumor involving the facial nerve. Pregnancy increases the risk owing to hormonal changes. Approximately 10% of patients have a family history of Bell's palsy. A substantial proportion of patients has an upper respiratory tract infection preceding (by 7 to 10 days) the onset of paralysis.

The facial paralysis in Bell's palsy may be abrupt in onset or gradually worsen over 2 to 3 days. However, the paralysis is not slowly progressive (over weeks to months), which is consistent with a primary facial nerve tumor or malignant process. Other symptoms that tend to rule out Bell's palsy include facial twitching, hearing loss, vestibular dysfunction, otorrhea, and severe, unrelenting otalgia.[28]

The pathophysiology of Bell's palsy involves nerve swelling within the inelastic fallopian canal. The edema and inability to expand beyond the bony confines inhibit the flow of axoplasm, which creates a conduction block. The site of inhibition of nerve impulse propagation is at the narrowest portion of the fallopian canal, the meatal foramen. This area constricts axoplasmic flow (Figure 31–4).

The natural history of Bell's palsy dictates recovery, usually beginning within 3 weeks. Full recovery typically occurs within 6 months. Unfortunately, approximately 15% of patients experience severe deformity, with minimal return of facial movement. Another 15% of patients experience asymmetric movement and/or synkinesis.[37] Thus, despite a good prognosis for 70% of patients, there are approximately 8,000 people in the United States each year with permanent and disfiguring facial weakness.[38] Identification of patients at risk of poor recovery must be accomplished within 2 weeks of onset of complete paralysis if surgical intervention is to be an option.

The management of the patient with idiopathic facial paralysis depends on a number of variables. Treatment within the first 2 weeks of onset is important to minimize the chance of ocular complication or residual, permanent facial dysfunction, such as synkinesis. Patients presenting with facial palsy within the first 2 to 3 weeks are treated with high-dose oral corticosteroids (prednisone 1 mg/kg or 60 to 80 mg orally, each day) for 10 days. Corticosteroids have been shown to improve recovery of facial function.[38,39] Patients with a history of diabetes mellitus or hypertension or those at risk for these corticosteroid-induced complications are advised to monitor their blood sugar and blood pressure. An oral medication is also given to decrease the chance of gas-

trointestinal ulceration from the corticosteroids (eg, histamine$_2$ blocker or proton pump inhibitor).

Owing to the probable viral nature of Bell's palsy, valacyclovir (500 mg orally, three times a day) is also recommended. Valacyclovir is the prodrug of acyclovir and is more rapidly and extensively absorbed than acyclovir. Use of an antiviral agent in addition to corticosteroid treatment has been shown to improve the recovery of facial function when compared to corticosteroid treatment alone.[40] Care of the eye, as previously discussed, is instituted as needed. Treatment (other than eye care) is probably unnecessary if facial function is improving on its own at the time of presentation; the patient is then seen in 1 month.

Intermittent (every 2 to 3 days) examinations are also performed to assess for progression of the disease process to complete facial paralysis. If the patient either progresses to complete paralysis or presents with complete paralysis, an ENOG is obtained 4 days after occurrence of complete paralysis. If degeneration is less than 90%, the corticosteroids and the antiviral agent are continued for the full treatment course. Electroneurographic testing is repeated every 1 to 3 days until > 90% degeneration is detected and no voluntary motor unit

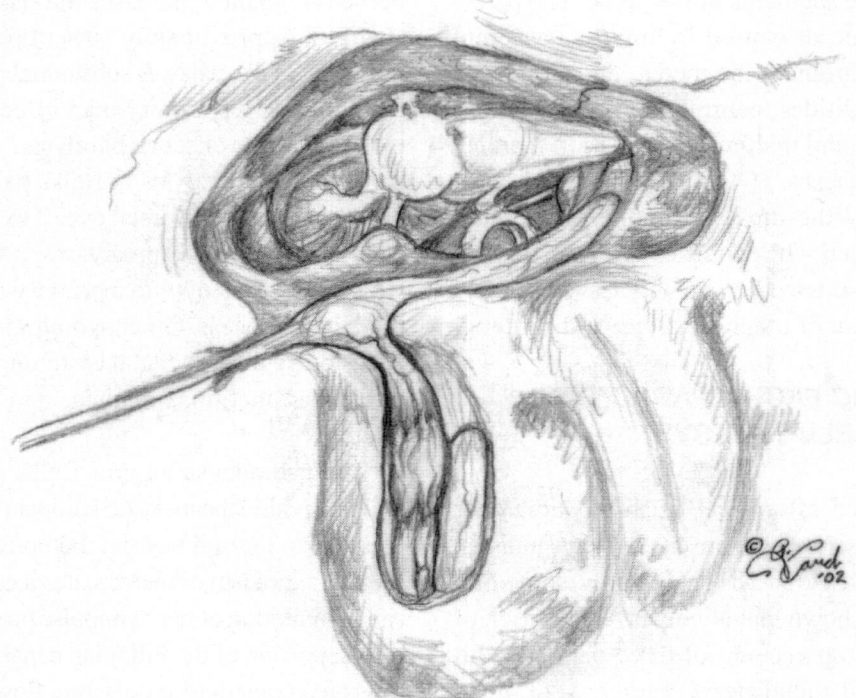

Figure 31–4   Diagram of the labyrinthine segment and meatal foramen. This unique anatomy predisposes the nerve to injury by the pathophysiologic process (edema) of Bell's palsy.

potentials are noted on EMG; at that time, surgical decompression is an option. However, if > 90% degeneration occurs after the 2-week window, surgery is not an option.[41] After 14 days of paralysis, surgical decompression does not alter the outcome, and its potential risks outweigh any potential benefit. Electromyographic testing, but not ENOG testing, is performed if patients present more than 3 weeks after the onset of paralysis and have no facial movement.

Surgical management of Bell's palsy has evolved along with the understanding of the pathophysiology of the disease.[4] Facial nerve decompression was first suggested in 1923 but not performed until 1931.[42] Since that time, surgical decompression has been very controversial.[43] A landmark multicenter, prospective study was published by the senior author.[41] In this study, middle cranial fossa (MCF) decompression more than doubled the chances of good facial nerve recovery (HB grade I or II) compared to medical treatment alone. The findings were highly statistically significant ($p = .0002$). Thus, at the University of Iowa, all patients with more than 90% neuronal degeneration within 2 weeks of onset, who are under 65 years of age, are counseled to undergo MCF surgical decompression of the meatal foramen, labyrinthine segment, GG, and proximal tympanic portion and without any medical contraindications. However, facial nerve decompression is a very technically challenging procedure and should be performed only in centers experienced in the MCF approach.[4] Transmastoid decompression does not have any value in this disease process, which affects the meatal foramen and labyrinthine segment. Our algorithm for management of Bell's palsy is outlined in Figure 31–5.

TRAUMATIC FACIAL PARALYSIS

Temporal bone fractures, blunt or penetrating head and neck trauma, and iatrogenic surgical injury are all com-

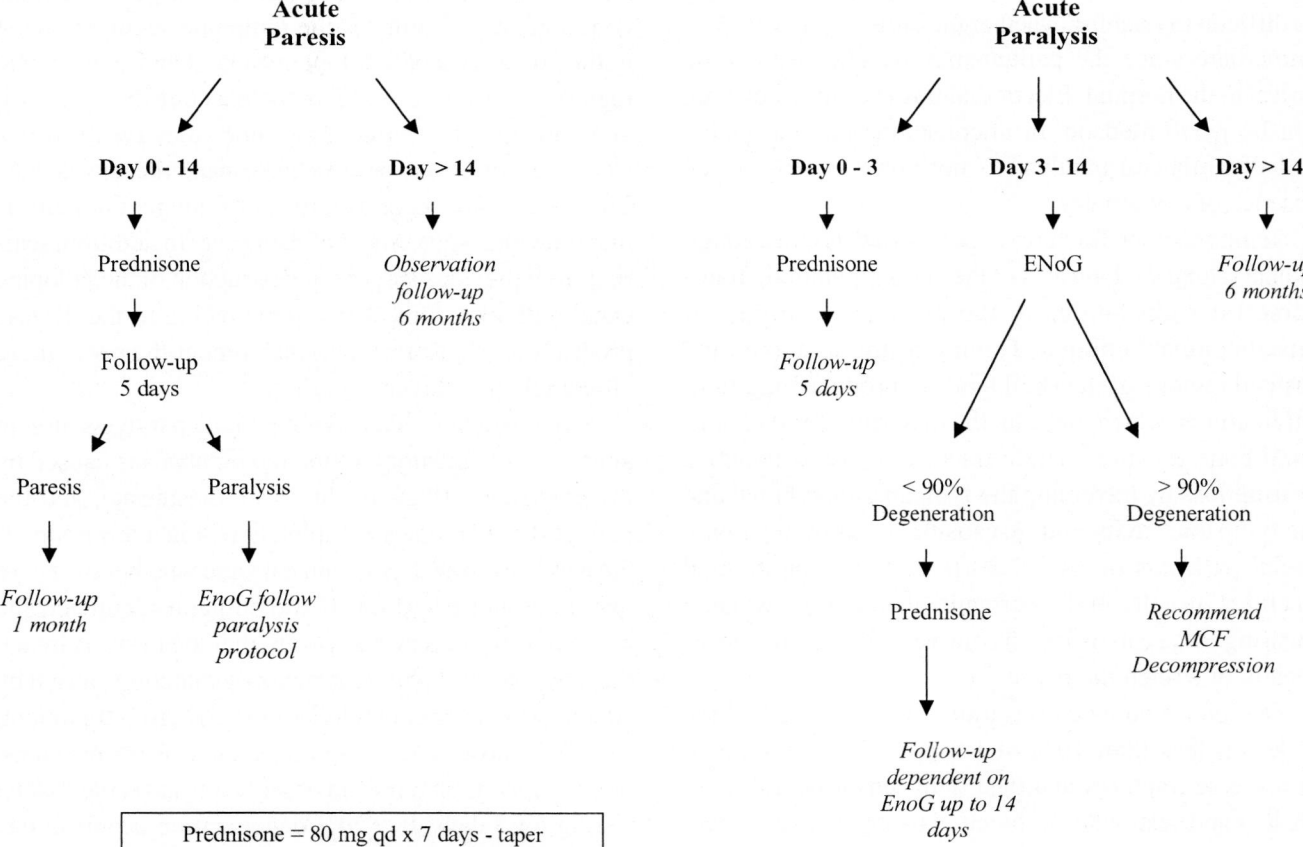

Figure 31–5 Bell's palsy management algorithm. ENOG = electroneurography; MCF = middle cranial fossa. Adapted from Gantz BJ and colleagues.[41]

mon causes of facial nerve injury. Motor vehicle accidents account for a substantial proportion of the injuries, although the incidence of post-traumatic facial palsy is decreasing owing to the use of seat belts and airbags.[44] The treatment of trauma-related dysfunction depends on many of the same factors listed above for Bell's palsy. After a thorough history and physical examination, an audiogram and electrodiagnostic tests are performed. Additionally, radiologic studies (temporal bone CT scans —fine-cut, axial, and coronal planes, bone window) assist in the determination of the site of the injury, which may involve multiple segments; unfortunately, imaging may not always be able to pinpoint the area of injury.

Animal experiments have shown that traumatic injuries requiring surgical repair exhibit 90% or greater neural degeneration within 1 week after the onset of the injury. In addition, the timing of the onset of the paralysis gives a clue as to the mechanism of injury; delayed paralysis most likely reflects nerve edema from the trauma (or viral reactivation), whereas immediate paralysis suggests nerve disruption or a severe compression injury, such as a bone fragment.[19] In some cases, it may be difficult to establish whether the onset of paralysis was immediate since the patient may be unconscious on arrival to the hospital. Electrodiagnostic testing, however, can be performed on an unconscious patient. Occasionally, bilateral paralysis is not noted because of an absence of asymmetry.[7]

Temporal bone fractures are classified as either longitudinal (along the long axis of the petrous pyramid), transverse (at right angles to the petrous pyramid), or mixed/complex/oblique. Trauma to the temporal and parietal regions of the skull tends to produce longitudinal fractures, which make up the majority (90%) of temporal bone fractures. These fractures cause conductive hearing loss by traversing the tympanic membrane and the tympanic cavity and by causing a hemotympanum. Facial paralysis occurs in 20 to 25% of longitudinal fractures, usually in the perigeniculate region, where a shearing force can disrupt the nerve, penetrate the nerve sheath, or stretch the nerve.[19]

Occipital trauma causes transverse fractures, which make up less than 10% of temporal bone fractures. Transverse fractures manifest with sensorineural hearing loss and vestibular dysfunction owing to involvement of the otic capsule or the IAC. Although less common than longitudinal fractures, they are more likely to cause facial nerve damage, occurring in up to 50% of fractures.[19] In transverse fractures, the facial nerve is usually injured at its labyrinthine segment.

In general, the indications for facial nerve decompression and exploration are similar to those discussed in the Bell's palsy section of this chapter.[6] However, if the paralysis is immediate in onset, surgical exploration after 2 weeks should be preceded by neurosurgical clearance. Delayed-onset paralysis is managed similarly to Bell's palsy.

Iatrogenic injury to the facial nerve may occur even in the hands of the most qualified surgeons. The best way to prevent iatrogenic injury to the facial nerve is to identify it early and use it to find other structures. Injury can occur in the absence of direct trauma, such as the friction of a diamond bur heating the nerve. Removing surrounding disease can affect the vascular supply of the nerve and result in ischemia with temporary paralysis.[7] During mastoid surgery, the facial nerve is most commonly injured at the second genu. If the nerve is known to have been disrupted, it should be repaired immediately (ie, intraoperatively).[45] In middle ear surgery, the most common site of injury is the tympanic segment owing to the prevalence of a fallopian canal dehiscence in that region. There are several factors that contribute to iatrogenic facial nerve injury. The injury may result from a lack of technical skill or inadequate anatomic knowledge.[7] The injury may occur as a result of congenital malformation with displacement of the nerve. In addition, scarring from previous surgery or destruction of the fallopian canal with exposure of the nerve owing to the disease process (eg, cholesteatoma) may render the nerve more vulnerable to inadvertent injury.[7]

If the patient awakens with a facial paralysis, urgent attention is mandatory. Often the paralysis is caused by the persistent effects of the local anesthetic, and the patient should recover completely within a few hours. If the paralysis persists, one must decide whether the nerve may have been injured. If the surgeon identified the nerve during surgery and is sure that the nerve is intact, the paralysis probably represents dysfunction caused by edema. Management includes corticosteroid treatment, electrodiagnostic testing, and serial clinical examinations. Some surgeons recommend observation and serial ENOG testing for 3 days. If > 90% degeneration occurs at day 3, then exploration is performed. If on exploration it is found that injury disrupted more than 50% of the nerve diameter, the injured portion is resected and either end-to-end anastomosis or interpositional grafting is performed.

All surgery involving, or near to, the facial nerve has the potential to injure the nerve. Thus, intraoperative neurophysiologic monitoring (EMG) plays a significant role. Available monitors have both visual and auditory real-time feedback for use by the operating team.[46] In addition, surgical draping with a clear plastic drape allows the nurse to monitor facial movement. The endotracheal tube is positioned on the side of the mouth opposite to the surgery.[47] During neurotologic/skull base surgical procedures (eg, removal of CPA tumors such as vestibular schwannomas), the facial nerve can be injured easily, especially if the tumor is large or adheres to the nerve. Although neurophysiologic monitoring is the "standard of care" in skull base surgery, studies have shown that facial nerve monitoring can aid in the surgical decision-making process and help avert potential injury to the nerve in tympanomastoid surgery as well. Although monitoring is no substitute for experience gained in the temporal bone laboratory or operating room, it is a valuable tool that can be useful to surgeons at all levels of experience. Monitoring may help in identification and localization of the facial nerve, guide in safer dissection and drilling, and minimize nerve irritation from direct trauma and traction.[46,48] Monitoring is also useful in locating the site of nerve conduction block in acute facial paralysis as the block is located between the area that responds and the area that does not respond to electrical stimulation.[47] Electrical stimulation at the end of the procedure can be used to confirm the integrity of the nerve.[46] Research has shown that intraoperative electrophysiologic measures of the CMAP correlate with postoperative facial function after vestibular schwannoma resection.[49]

In general, traumatic injury to the facial nerve often requires exploration and nerve repair. As will be discussed later in this chapter, grafts are used frequently in nerve repair, although grafting in a traumatized temporal bone may be difficult. The surgical approach is determined by the portion of the facial nerve affected and the amount of residual hearing. Potential surgical routes include the MCF, transcanal, transmastoid, or translabyrinthine, (which may be used singly or in combination).[44] The facial nerve may be explored safely from the IAC to the stylomastoid foramen. When possible, repair should be performed within 72 hours of an injury, allowing identification of distal segments electrically before wallerian degeneration occurs.[19] Owing to the propensity for patients with temporal bone fractures to have concomitant intracranial or systemic injuries, repair is performed only when the patient has been stabilized and is able to withstand a general anesthetic. If possible, the repair is performed within the first week of injury because it is technically easier. The further the time of repair from the time of injury, the greater the amount of granulation tissue, fracture healing, scarring, and bleeding complicating the repair of the nerve.[19]

TUMORS INVOLVING THE FACIAL NERVE

Both benign and malignant tumors can affect the facial nerve—in the intracranial cavity, within the temporal bone, and in the parotid gland. Approximately 5% of facial nerve dysfunction is caused by the presence of a tumor.[7] One must differentiate intrinsic from extrinsic facial nerve tumors (eg, a primary facial nerve tumor versus tumor contiguous to the facial nerve or metastatic disease). Extrinsic tumor involvement is much more common than intrinsic; numerous benign and malignant neoplasms occur in and around the temporal bone. Within the temporal bone itself, skull base neoplasms and metastasis from breast and lung cancer are common neoplasms causing facial paralysis in adults, whereas hematologic malignancies (leukemia, lymphoma) are usually etiologic in children.[18] Management of all of these lesions is beyond the scope of this chapter, as is a complete listing; however, some of the more common tumors are facial schwannomas, congenital cholesteatomas, hemangiomas, glomus tumors, vestibular schwannomas, squamous cell carcinoma, and parotid gland neoplasms. This chapter focuses on lesions of the facial nerve proximal to the stylomastoid foramen.

The most common sign of tumor involvement is a slow progressive facial paralysis. A facial palsy progressive beyond 3 weeks of onset and with no return of function by 6 months is considered to be caused by tumor unless proved otherwise.[7] Benign tumors compress the facial nerve, whereas malignant lesions invade the nerve. Thus, it is sometimes possible to dissect a benign tumor from the nerve without damaging the nerve. However, with malignant neoplasms, the nerve is resected with the tumor.

Early diagnosis of facial palsy caused by tumor relies on a high index of suspicion. In addition to a slowly progressive paralysis, several other clinical features should heighten suspicion of a tumor involving the facial nerve. Twitching of the facial nerve in association with palsy is not seen in Bell's palsy. In addition, recurrent palsy may reflect the presence of a tumor. Pain, although seen in Bell's palsy or Ramsay Hunt syndrome, is also seen with tumors involving the facial nerve. Involvement of other cranial nerves in addition to the facial nerve is also suggestive of a neoplasm.[7] Evaluation for a neoplastic etiology of a facial palsy includes radiologic imaging (both CT and MRI scans).

Vestibular schwannomas are benign tumors and are the most common lesions of the IAC and CPA. Facial paralysis is an unusual manifestation of these tumors and generally signifies an advanced stage of tumor growth. Vestibular schwannomas rarely invade the facial nerve. It is possible for a patient with a vestibular schwannoma and facial palsy to have a concomitant Bell's palsy as the true etiology of facial nerve dysfunction. In the absence of nerve sheath invasion, the facial nerve generally appears to tolerate gradual compression well. Facial nerve dysfunction may also occur owing to local vascular compromise.[50]

Nerve sheath and vascular neoplasms make up the greatest percentage of intrinsic facial nerve tumors (although they are relatively rare as a group). These tumors, including facial schwannomas (neuromas), meningiomas, hemangiomas, and glomus tumors,[18] may present with facial weakness relatively early in their course.[50] In general, facial nerve schwannomas are uncommon, slow-growing neoplasms that arise from the nerve sheath anywhere from the CPA to the peripheral branches of the facial nerve.[51] Most facial nerve schwannomas are intratemporal and most often involve the labyrinthine segment and GG.[51,52] A recent retrospective review demonstrated that facial nerve schwannomas were more likely to involve multiple segments than a single segment.[52] Management decisions are based on the patient's desires, age, degree of facial function, tumor location, and hearing status.[4] The goal in the management of these tumors is to maximize long-term facial nerve function while minimizing morbidity. At most centers, management typically entails tumor resection with grafting. However, at our institution, a review of 21 patients with primary/intrinsic facial nerve tumors showed that

observation is possible, especially for patients with HB grade I or II facial function. Surgical decompression is an option for patients with HB grade II to III facial function. Resection and grafting are recommended for grade IV or worse. Conservative management with either observation or decompression is often an appropriate option since the best facial nerve function result after resection and grafting is an RFNRS grade C, owing to the presence of mass motion. Nonetheless, treatment is individualized; a patient with brainstem compression from a facial neuroma but with HB grade I function would still undergo resection with grafting.

The most common malignant tumor involving the facial nerve is squamous cell carcinoma of the head and neck. The tumor may be a primary tumor of the temporal bone (squamous cell carcinoma of the auricle), an extension from a regional tumor (squamous cell carcinoma of the skin), or a metastatic lesion (eg, from the oral cavity, nasopharynx, etc). Basal cell carcinoma is a locally invasive lesion that usually occurs on the auricle and, if left untreated, can involve the facial nerve. Other malignant neoplasms include sarcomas, melanomas, and adenoid cystic carcinomas of the parotid gland, which have a significant propensity for neural invasion.

INFECTION

Many infections can cause facial paralysis, such as mumps, mononucleosis, and poliomyelitis.[6] Besides Bell's palsy, the most common infectious causes of facial nerve paralysis are acute otitis media (sometimes complicated by mastoiditis), chronic otitis media (with or without cholesteatoma), Lyme disease, necrotizing otitis externa, and herpes-zoster oticus.

Facial paralysis as a complication of otitis media has become rare owing to ready access to medical care and antibiotics.[6] Hospital admission with close observation and institution of systemic antibiotics (initially intravenous followed by oral) are necessary to bring the infection under control. A myringotomy with tympanostomy tube placement is required to allow for drainage and to prevent the development of further complications, such as a mastoiditis or intracranial spread. Fluid is obtained for Gram stain, culture, and pathology (if so desired). Antibiotic selection is then tailored to culture results. Systemic corticosteroids are probably helpful, and their use is based on the premise that at least some of the dysfunction is caused by edema. In some cases, the paralysis is due to a congenital dehiscence of the fallopian canal. A CT scan is performed to determine whether there is an associated coalescent mastoiditis, in which case, a mastoidectomy is required. Fortunately, in most instances, recovery of facial nerve function is complete. Electrodiagnostic testing should be performed to document the degree of neural injury. If greater than 90% neural degeneration occurs within 2 weeks, the mastoid and tympanic segments are decompressed. Decompression in the face of acute infection is extremely difficult and should be performed only by very experienced surgeons.

Facial paralysis complicating chronic otitis media is rare, even if the disease destroys the fallopian canal and compresses the facial nerve. Occasionally, granulation tissue can cause irritation of the nerve, edema, and dysfunction. Treatment is surgical; topical or systemic antibiotics are used as adjunctive modalities to control otorrhea and bacterial superinfection. As with acute otitis media, other complications of chronic otitis media include hearing loss, vestibular dysfunction, and intracranial sequelae.

Lyme disease is caused by a spirochete *Borrelia burgdorferi* and has been reported in many parts of the world. Infection by this spirochete can cause a myriad of systemic complications and disorders. However, the most common neurologic manifestation of this disease is facial nerve paralysis. One study showed that patients suffering from Lyme disease who presented with facial palsy had longer-lived neurologic symptoms than other patients with Lyme disease, especially if antibiotic treatment was delayed.[53] Serologic diagnosis, possibly supplemented by a lumbar puncture and CSF analysis, is followed by antibiotic therapy (doxycycline, amoxicillin). An infectious disease consultation is recommended in view of the potential of this spirochete to cause widespread systemic damage.[6]

Necrotizing otitis externa (NOE) classically occurs in elderly patients with poorly controlled diabetes mellitus or in patients who are immunosuppressed (eg, human immunodeficiency virus). Necrotizing otitis externa begins in the EAC and, if left untreated, progresses to involve the temporal bone (causing facial paralysis) and skull base, eventually involving the lower cranial nerves and intracranial cavity. If not dealt with quickly and effectively, NOE can be fatal. It is most commonly caused by *Pseudomonas aeruginosa* but may be caused by other bacteria and fungi as well. Diagnosis includes radiologic imaging (CT and MRI as the situation dictates) and nuclear imaging studies (gallium and technetium bone scans). Dry ear precautions, EAC débridement, topical antibiotics, and long-term intravenous antibiotics are used in treatment. Antibiotics are continued until the gallium scans show no evidence of infection. For those cases that fail to improve with medical therapy, hyperbaric oxygen therapy has shown promise. Surgery (radical débridement of the temporal bone and skull base) is used only in recalcitrant cases and is performed in an attempt to save the patient's life.

Herpes-zoster (VZV) oticus (Ramsay Hunt syndrome) underlies approximately 3 to 12% of facial paralyses in adults and 5% in children.[6] Polymerase chain reaction assays have been used for the early diagnosis of VZV infection and to differentiate it from Bell's palsy.[54] Ramsay Hunt syndrome, the second most common cause of facial paralysis, has a much poorer prognosis than Bell's palsy and represents reactivation of the virus in the geniculate ganglion. Varicella-zoster virus infections without skin lesions (zoster sine herpete) can occur and can be mistaken for Bell's palsy. Varcella-zoster virus–infected patients may have a viral prodrome followed by severe otalgia. Vesicles appear in the ear canal and on the auricle. Patients may also develop sensorineural hearing loss and vestibular dysfunction. The facial paralysis is usually rapidly progressive and other cranial nerves, including V and IX through XII, can be involved.

Unfortunately, in nearly half of the cases, Ramsay Hunt syndrome leaves the patient with significant residual facial nerve dysfunction. However, early treatment with antiviral medication has reduced the long-term sequelae. Owing to "skip" regions of facial nerve involvement, surgical decompression is not recommended. In immunocompetent patients, corticosteroid therapy is indicated, and intravenous acyclovir or oral valacylovir is used as well. Antiviral therapy, in combination with corticosteroid treatment, has been shown to be more effective than corticosteroids alone.[54] Since the active phase of Ramsay Hunt syndrome persists for a longer period of time than that of Bell's palsy, the duration of corticosteroid and antiviral is longer than for Bell's palsy (3 weeks versus 2 weeks). Bacterial superinfection of the vesicles may occur and is treated with oral antibiotics.[18]

FACIAL PARALYSIS IN CHILDREN

Although facial nerve abnormalities in children include congenital and acquired pathologies, the principles of management are essentially the same as those for adults.[6] Bell's palsy is a common cause of facial palsy in children, as in adults; however, the spontaneous recovery rate for children is higher than for adults. The incidence of neonatal facial palsy is approximately 1 to 2 per 1,000 deliveries, most of which (80%) are related to birth trauma. Forceps delivery or cephalopelvic disproportion can injure the nerve in its vertical segment or as it exits the stylomastoid foramen; the lack of development of the mastoid tip predisposes the facial nerve to injury during delivery and during mastoid surgery in neonates and infants.[6] The facial paralysis is usually unilateral and partial. Other causes of acquired facial paralysis in children include birth weight exceeding 3.5 kg, intracranial hemorrhage, intrauterine trauma, primiparity, prolonged second stage of labor, and maternal exposure to teratogens (eg, thalidomide).[4] Signs of traumatic paralysis include periauricular ecchymosis and hemotympanum. Most of the acquired facial palsies (90%) recover without treatment.[6,55]

In the newborn, the differentiation of acquired versus congenital facial paralysis must be made. Congenital facial paralysis has a poor prognosis and does not require urgent treatment. The evaluation and management of the palsy include physical examination for other anomalies or neurologic dysfunction, ENOG, EMG, and radiologic imaging. Electroneurography should be performed within the first 48 hours of life. If the distal nerve is stimulable, the paralysis is most likely caused by trauma; recovery of function is highly likely. One etiology of congenital paralysis is Möbius' syndrome, which can be unilateral or bilateral and involves cranial nerves VI and VII. Möbius' syndrome probably stems from nuclear agenesis.[6] Other congenital disorders associated with facial nerve palsy are hemifacial microsomia and its variant, Goldenhar's syndrome (oculoauriculovertebral dysplasia). Additional congenital syndromes, especially those involving first and second branchial arch abnormalities, can be associated with facial palsy. Miscellaneous causes of facial palsy include bony dysplasia (osteopetrosis: Albers-Schönberg disease) and Melkersson-Rosenthal syndrome (idiopathic recurrent facial palsy associated with fissured tongue and recurrent facial/labial edema).[4]

Facial nerve function that fails to recover after birth, a family history of craniofacial abnormality, other abnormalities (especially neurologic), bilateral palsy, absence of electrical response, and a silent EMG are all consistent with congenital paralysis. A muscle biopsy may be indicated to determine prognosis and management.

SURGERY OF THE FACIAL NERVE

The entire length of the facial nerve, from the brainstem to the parotid segments, is amenable to surgical intervention. When discussing anticipated results with the patient prior to surgery, it is extremely important that the patient have realistic expectations. Unfortunately, the restoration of normal facial motion (in particular, involuntary movement) is beyond the capabilities of modern techniques. The restoration of a dynamic smile with symmetry at rest is an achievable goal[19]; however, such a successful outcome demands that the surgeon have detailed knowledge of the three-dimensional anatomy of the temporal bone,[6] which requires many hours of practice in the temporal bone dissection laboratory.

There are two general surgical methods for rehabilitating a paralyzed face, dynamic and static.[7] Facial reanimation has the best outcome when facial nerve integrity can be re-established and directed by the facial nucleus. Even when this can be accomplished, the wide range of possible results must be clearly explained to the patient. The choice of procedure depends on the circumstances of each individual case. Dynamic rehabilitation may involve multiple procedures, performed singly or in combination: surgical exposure of the nerve with decompression, grafting, end-to-end anastomosis, and nerve or neuromuscular transfers.

Facial nerve electrophysiologic monitoring and visual monitoring (through a clear drape by the scrub nurse) are used intraoperatively. The importance of visual observation—with visualization of the entire profile, including the forehead, eye, mouth, and chin—cannot be overemphasized and serves as a back-up to intraoperative EMG. To facilitate visual observation, the endotracheal tube is taped to the side of the mouth opposite the surgical procedure.[31]

Proper instrumentation is critical to the conduct of a successful procedure. An operating microscope offers unparalleled visualization. When working in the immediate vicinity of delicate structures such as the facial nerve, the largest diamond bur that the operative site can safely accommodate is used. Copious irrigation clears the operative area of debris and dissipates friction-induced heat, which can induce temporary and permanent facial palsy. Although diamond burs are generally safer than cutting burs near the facial nerve (especially for surgeons in training), diamond burs generate more heat.[56] The final eggshell layer of bone overlying the nerve is removed with a blunt elevator to prevent direct, bur-induced damage to the nerve.[6] If neurolysis (incision of the sheath) is planned, disposable microblades are used. Cauterization near the nerve is done sparingly (if at all) with bipolar electrocautery at a low current level.

Regardless of what must be done to the facial nerve, the basic exposure in the temporal bone involves opening the fallopian canal without disruption of nearby neurovascular, intracranial, or inner ear structures. Depending on the site of the lesion and preoperative hearing, the nerve may be exposed via the MCF, translabyrinthine, and/or transmastoid approaches.

For the MCF approach, the patient lies supine with the involved ear facing the ceiling. The surgeon sits at the head of the operating table while the anesthesiologist is at the foot. Prior to induction, antithromboembolic stockings and pneumatic compression devices are placed on the legs to minimize the occurrence of deep venous thrombosis or pulmonary embolism. Facial nerve and auditory brainstem monitoring leads are applied. The anesthesiologist is not allowed to use long-acting paralytic agents. An arterial line, temperature probe, and urinary catheter are placed. The patient is given a dose of prophylactic antibiotics and corticosteroids. The end-tidal carbon dioxide level is dropped to approximately 25 mm Hg by hyperventilation. The side of the head is shaved and the proposed incision site is infiltrated with local anesthestic with epinephrine. The operative site is prepared and draped.

A posteriorly based skin flap measuring approximately 6 × 8 cm is created within the hairline above the ear (Figure 31–6). This flap can be extended into the postauricular area if a transmastoid approach is also needed. The incision is carried down to the level of the temporalis fascia, a large piece of which is harvested for later use to cover the MCF floor. An anteriorly based temporalis muscle flap is elevated from the outer cortex of the skull. Care is taken to prevent injury to the frontal branch of the facial nerve, which lies on the undersurface

of the superficial temporalis (temporoparietal) fascia. At this time, the patient is given 250 cc of 20% mannitol over 30 minutes to induce a diuresis, reducing intracranial pressure and facilitating retraction of the temporal lobe. A 4 × 5 cm craniotomy, centered on the zygomatic root, is created with a cutting bur, which allows visualization of dura at all times and minimizes the risk of a dural tear, as can more easily happen with a craniotome. The bone flap is dissected from the temporal lobe dura; care is taken to protect the middle meningeal artery that is sometimes encased within the bone. Dura is elevated from the MCF floor in a posterior to anterior and a lateral to medial direction. Posteromedially, the petrous ridge is identified. The ridge is the medial limit of dissection as the dura is elevated anteriorly to the foramen spinosum, which is traversed by the middle meningeal artery. The microscope is then brought in to view the surgical field. The greater superficial petrosal nerve is identified. Any open air cells are occluded with bone wax to prevent a postoperative CSF leak.

The House-Urban retractor is placed to maintain extradural retraction of the temporal lobe (Figure 31–7). The retractor blade tip is carefully placed at the medial

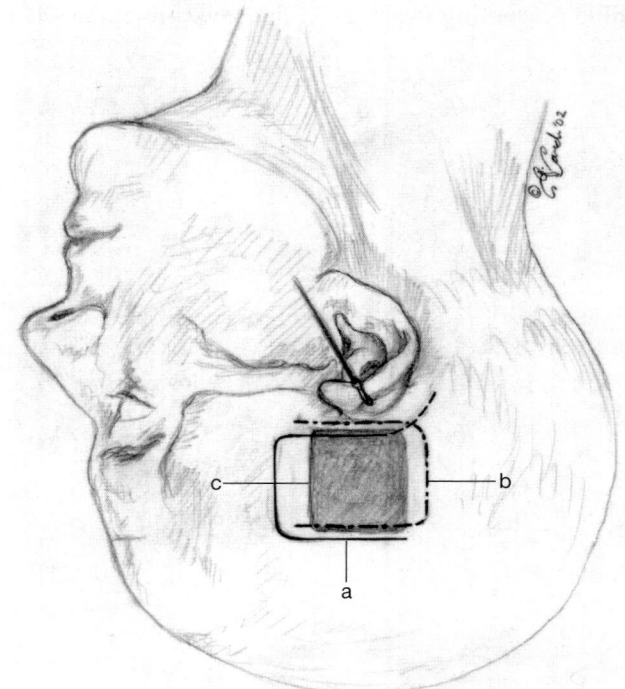

Figure 31–6 The incisions used in the skin and muscle for the middle cranial fossa approach. *a*, Posteriorly based skin flap; *b*, anteriorly based temporalis muscle flap; *c*, bone flap.

margin of the petrous ridge. The superior semicircular canal (SSC) is identified by slowly removing bone over the arcuate eminence; identifying the yellow-white dense bone of the otic capsule is helpful. If the arcuate eminence is not evident, mastoid air cells are opened posteriorly. Drilling progressively anteriorly reveals the dense otic capsule bone. The otic capsule is slowly removed to "blue line" the SSC. Otic capsule drilling should be done in the direction of the SSC, which is perpendicular to the petrous ridge. Locating the SSC allows identification of the rest of the vital structures of the temporal bone: the IAC, cochlea, GG, and tympanic cavity. A preoperative Stenver's view helps to determine the depth of the SSC from the MCF floor.[6]

The IAC is located by removing bone at a 45- to 60-degree angle anteromedial to the SSC (Figure 31–8) and is followed laterally to the meatal foramen and labyrinthine segment of the facial nerve. The labyrinthine segment and GSPN are used to locate the GG. The thin bone of the tegmen tympani is removed to expose the ossicles lying in the attic. The facial nerve is followed laterally from the GG into the middle ear as far as its tympanic segment at the cochleariform process. The MCF approach is the only route that can gain the necessary exposure of the labyrinthine segment, IAC, and CPA while preserving hearing. At the same time, the MCF approach affords access to the tympanic segment. The MCF approach can be used in combination with the transmastoid approach for access to the entire intratemporal course of the facial nerve; it can be used for facial nerve decompression in longitudinal fractures of the temporal bone and in Bell's palsy, the removal of vestibular schwannomas that do not impinge on the brainstem, and the removal of facial nerve tumors limited to the areas listed above.

Once the surgical procedure is completed, the IAC defect is covered with a temporalis muscle plug; a bone chip can be used to cover any large MCF floor defects to prevent a postoperative dural herniation or encephalocele. The retractor is removed and temporalis fascia is placed on the MCF floor. Hyperventilation is stopped. The bone flap is replaced and the wound is closed in layers. A bulky mastoid dressing is applied. The patient is monitored in the intensive care unit overnight with hourly neurologic checks and is transferred to a routine surgical ward the following day. Antibiotics and corticosteroids are administered for 48 hours postoperatively. In addition, the patient is kept on fluid restrictions for 72 hours postoperatively to minimize the risk of a CSF leak. If a CSF leak does occur, a lumbar drain is placed and used for 5 days. If the CSF leak still continues, the wound is re-explored to locate the site of the leak.

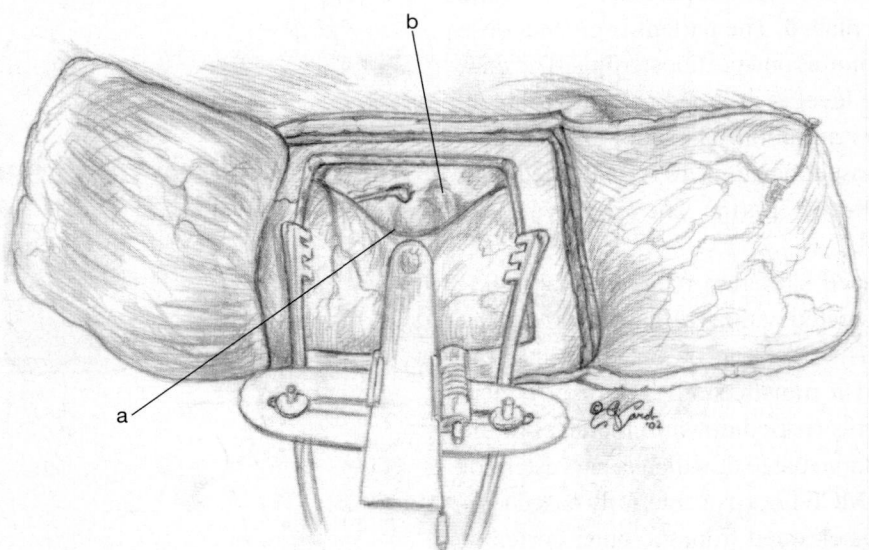

Figure 31–7 Placement of the House-Urban retractor to view the middle cranial fossa floor. *a*, Petrous ridge; *b*, arculate eminence.

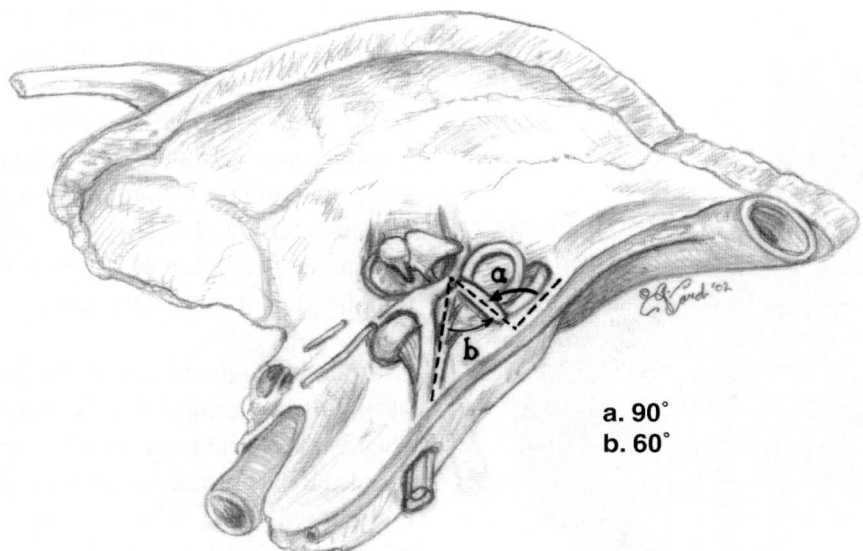

a. 90°
b. 60°

Figure 31–8 View of the middle cranial fossa floor and the relationships between the superior semicircular canal, internal auditory canal, cochlea, and middle ear. *a,* Relationship between superior semicircular canal and petrous ridge; *b,* relationship between superior semicircle canal and internal auditory canal.

Patients are encouraged to ambulate early in the postoperative period to minimize the risk of a pneumonia or deep vein thrombosis/pulmonary embolism. Patients are discharged home when they are stable, ambulating well, tolerating oral intake, and without evidence of CSF leak. The length of stay in the hospital averages 3 days postoperatively.

To approach the facial nerve via the translabyrinthine or transmastoid approach, the initial set-up of the patient and the operating room is basically the same. However, a routine postauricular incision is made in the hairline and a 2- to 3-cm-wide Palva flap is created. A self-retaining retractor holds the ear forward. A large cutting bur and continuous suction-irrigation are initially used. A complete mastoidectomy is initially performed, with exposure of the middle and posterior fossa dural plates, sinodural angle, sigmoid sinus, digastric ridge, incus, and lateral semicircular canal. The landmarks for the vertical segment of the facial nerve are the horizontal semicircular canal, fossa incudis, chorda tympani nerve, and the digastric ridge. The facial recess (the region bounded by the facial and chorda tympani nerves and the fossa incudis) is opened. This exposure gives access to the tympanic segment of the nerve. A diamond bur is used to delineate the course of the nerve by leaving only an eggshell layer of bone (Figure 31–9). Occasionally, the incus and head of the malleus must be removed to obtain adequate exposure, and ossicular reconstruction with a partial ossicular reconstruction prosthesis decreases the resulting conductive hearing loss. Once the exposure has been completed, the eggshell bone over the facial nerve is gently removed and the sheath can be opened.

The translabyrinthine approach begins with the transmastoid exposure described above but additionally incorporates a labyrinthectomy to access the IAC, labyrinthine segment, and GG. This approach can also allow complete mobilization of the facial nerve from the brainstem to the stylomastoid foramen.

HEMIFACIAL SPASM

Hemifacial spasm can be debilitating and makes it difficult for the patient to eat, talk, and interact socially. Usually, the entire face is affected by spasms and contractures. Hemifacial spasm is distinct from simple blepharospasm or neurologic disorders such as the myokymia of multiple sclerosis.[7] Some cases of hemifacial spasm are caused by a loop of AICA or another artery or vein pressing on the facial nerve; treatment involves placing a Teflon® sponge between the offending vessel and the nerve via the posterior fossa (retrosigmoid) approach. In other cases, the facial nerve spasm reflects irritation by a CPA

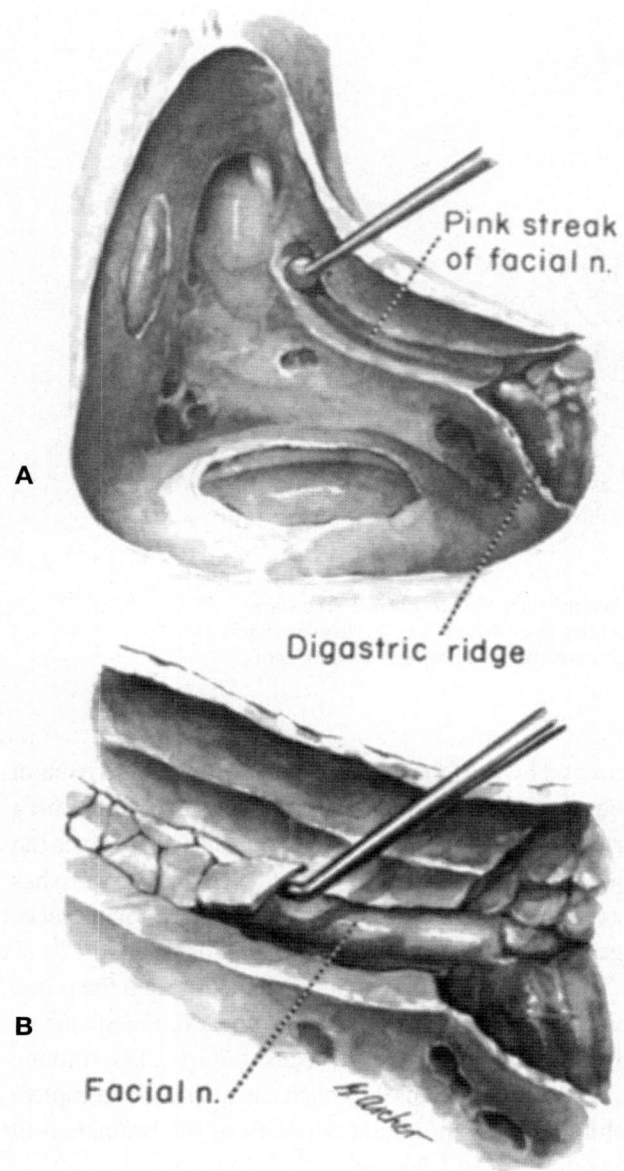

Figure 31–9 *A,* Diamond bur used to delineate course to facial nerve. *B,* Eggshell pieces of bone taken off the facial nerve to allow access to the nerve for grafting, rerouting, or decompression.

tumor. Thus, evaluation includes a thorough neurotologic examination and imaging. At our institution, patients undergo Gd-MRI and an magnetic resonance angiogram to assess for a CPA lesion or a vascular loop.

NERVE REPAIR AND GRAFTING

Restoration of the continuity of the facial nerve by a primary neurorrhaphy is always preferred over nerve grafting if it can be accomplished without tension. Primary neurorrhaphy and nerve grafting alone can restore involuntary emotional expression because control by the facial nucleus is retained. Primary repair or grafting can be performed on the intracranial, intratemporal, and extratemporal portions of the facial nerve; however, there are limitations, and perfect restitution of facial movement cannot be achieved. There are two main limitations: proliferation of connective tissue at the anastomotic sites and nondirected growth of regenerating fibers.[57]

When a segment of the facial nerve is disrupted (eg, by tumor or trauma), the best functional results are obtained with cable grafting. Grafting is also recommended if there is tension at the anastomotic site of a primary nerve repair. Immediate neurorrhaphy optimizes results. The time beyond which nerve repair or grafting is abandoned in favor of other reconstructive methods is approximately 18 to 24 months.[7] Electromyography helps determine whether any muscle function remains and thus provides information about the advisability of dynamic versus static rehabilitation.

The surgical approach chosen is based on the site needing repair and whether hearing is present. The interposed graft is aligned with the severed ends of the facial nerve (Figure 31–10). The anastomosis is performed under the operating microscope for the best results; atraumatic technique is required. When available, a surgically exposed and enlarged fallopian canal can help secure the anastomosis. When anastomosis is performed between the labyrinthine and the tympanic segments, the GG is bypassed to shorten the gap (possibly permitting an end-to-end anastomosis) and to prevent misdirected growth of the regenerating nerve fibers along the GSPN.[57] It is best to "freshen" the ends of both the nerve and graft by making an oblique (45 degrees) cut with a sharp knife, increasing the surface area for the anastomosis.[26] Epineurium is removed in the region of the anastomosis to minimize the formation of fibrous tissue. The nerve ends are secured with three sutures (in a tripod arrangement) of 8-0 to 10-0 monofilament suture (eg, nylon or polypropylene) in the epineurium.[19] Additional sutures cause additional trauma and connective tissue proliferation.[57] In grafting the intracranial portion of the nerve (owing to the absence of epineurium, as well as brain and CSF pulsation and overall technical difficulty), only one to three sutures are placed. Sutureless anastomosis, using tissue adhesive or even blood, has been advocated.[5,57] Some surgeons have proposed using collagen tubules or splints, whereas others believe that they cause additional fibrosis and negatively affect the final result. When grafting is performed, the graft should be approximately 25% longer than needed to allow for a tension-free anastomosis (in a lazy-S configuration). A silk suture can be used to measure the gap between the nerve ends.[5]

A retrospective review has been performed of 27 patients who underwent facial nerve grafting associated with a neurotologic procedure at our institution.[26] Fourteen patients had grafts at the brainstem. Over 90% of patients had some facial function by 8 months follow-up. Patients who had grafts performed distal to the meatal foramen seemed to have better function overall, although the difference was not statistically significant.

The effect that radiation has on the function of nerve grafts is unknown. Some believe that radiotherapy is so detrimental to the outcome of facial nerve graft function that dynamic or static sling procedures should be performed, instead of grafting, in all patients who are to undergo postoperative radiation therapy. However, the outcome achieved with such sling procedures is usually inferior to nerve grafting. In a recent retrospective study of patients who underwent nerve grafting followed by radiation therapy to approximately 6,000 cGy, no difference was noted in facial nerve function that could be attributed to the radiation therapy.[58] In addition, the use of a nerve graft followed by radiation therapy does not preclude the use of other reconstructive techniques if the graft fails.

Two sensory nerves are used primarily in facial nerve grafting: the greater auricular and the sural (Figure 31–11). The greater auricular nerve is used most frequently. It approximates the size of the facial nerve, is in the field of surgery, and provides a graft of up to 12 cm in length. The greater auricular nerve is located by drawing a line perpendicular to a line drawn between the mastoid tip and the angle of the mandible[6]; it lies immediately beneath the platysma muscle, on the sternocleidomastoid muscle. Extreme care is used in handling the graft. Once the graft has been harvested, it is placed in a physiologic solution. The graft should be removed only after the preparatory work on the facial nerve stumps is complete, improving the survival of the Schwann cells of the donor nerve.[57]

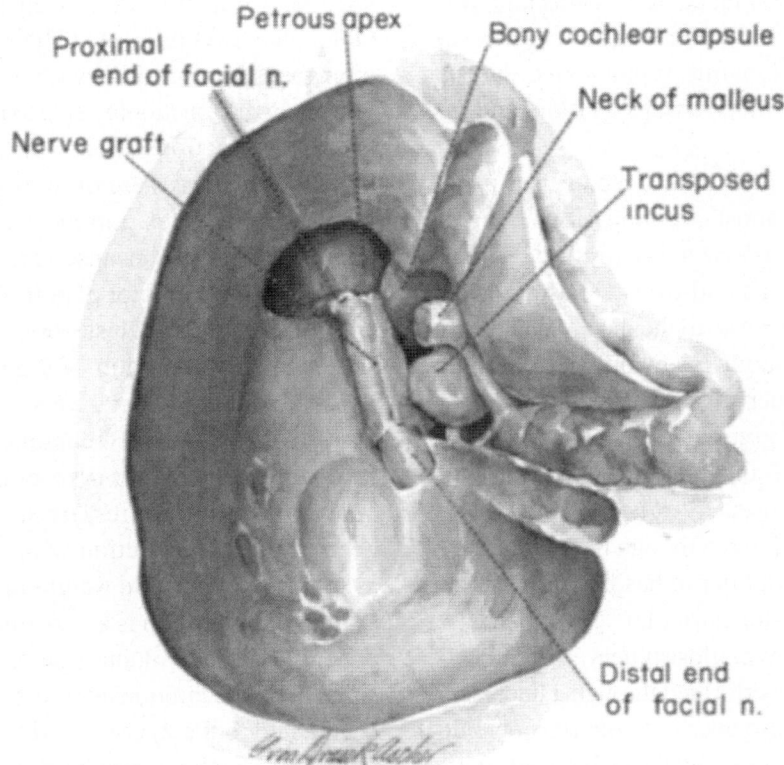

Figure 31–10 View of nerve graft as performed via a transmastoid approach.

The sural nerve, which supplies sensation to the lateral lower leg and foot, is also used for grafting. This nerve can provide a graft of up to 35 cm in length and has branches that can be used to reconstruct the branching pattern of the facial nerve.[6] Owing to its length, the sural nerve is particularly useful in cross-facial anastomosis.[57] The sural nerve is found posterior to the lateral malleolus, adjacent to the saphenous vein.

FACIAL REANIMATION

There are many factors important in reanimation: cause and degree of paralysis, timing/duration of paralysis, and patient factors (age, general health, patient expectations, life expectancy, nerve condition, healing capacity). The ultimate goals of reanimation include eye closure, oral competence, muscle tone/facial symmetry at rest, voluntary movement/symmetry with animation, minimal synkinesis, and involuntary (mimetic) movement. Although no technique is considered ideal, neurorrhaphy or nerve grafting is thought to be the best currently available. Occasionally, however, neither is feasible nor preferable (eg, lack of proximal nerve for anastomosis). For primary repair or grafting to be successful, an intact peripheral facial nerve trunk and functioning facial musculature are needed. However, additional options for dynamic repair exist, such as nerve transfer/crossover, muscle transposition, and free muscle transfer.

An alternate method of dynamic repair uses a substitution nerve graft, the most common of which is the hypoglossal to facial (XII-VII) nerve graft. Originally, the procedure comprised an end-to-end anastomosis of the proximal hypoglossal nerve to the distal facial nerve. The procedure has been modified by only partially sectioning the hypoglossal nerve and interposing, by end-to-side anastomoses, a greater auricular nerve graft between the hypoglossal and facial nerves. Since the hypoglossal nerve is transected only halfway, tongue function can be preserved. Even though the risk of injuring the grafted hypoglossal nerve has been minimized with the use of the greater auricular "jump" graft, a functional, contralateral hypoglossal nerve still must be present. This procedure is performed through a linear incision placed in a neck crease overlying the sternocleidomastoid muscle. The facial nerve is located at the stylomastoid foramen; the hypoglossal nerve is identi-fied as it crosses the external carotid artery and is dissected proximally and distally. A greater auricular nerve graft longer than the gap is harvested.[7] The remainder of the procedure is similar to the nerve repair and grafting described above. Recovery of facial movement begins at approximately 6 months. Seventh to twelfth nerve grafting is a relatively simple procedure that provides strong neural input and results in acceptable dynamic function. The disadvantages of this technique include mass movement and potential tongue hemiatrophy, which rarely results in chewing, swallowing, or speech difficulties. The VII-XII anastomosis is preferable to the facial to spinal accessory nerve anastomosis.

If there is no functional neuromuscular system, surgical reconstruction involves muscular transposition rather than primary nerve repair, grafting, or XII-VII grafting. A variety of transposition procedures have been described, including transposition of both pedicled (temporalis) and free muscle (gracilis, rectus abdominus, abductor hallucis, pectoralis minor, latissimus dorsi) grafts.[18] In adults, the pedicled grafts are most commonly used. Free muscle transfer with a neurovascular anastomosis (using the contralateral facial nerve for innervation) is the mainstay of treatment of children with congenital disorders (such as Möbius' syndrome or Goldenhar's syndrome).[18] The cross-face graft usually interposes the sural nerve between the distal buccal branch on the functioning side to the nonfunctioning side; however, variations exist. Unfortunately, free muscle transfer procedures are of limited effectiveness.

Muscle transposition most commonly employs the temporalis muscle because of its good location, length, contractility, and vector of pull. The masseter and digastric muscles are used less often. The temporalis muscle is good for reanimation of the mouth in patients with long-standing (at least 1 year in length) paralysis.[45] It is a proven and useful technique for facial reanimation in patients in whom nerve grafting or cranial nerve substitution procedures are not possible. It has also been used in conjunction with other procedures, such as placement of a gold weight in the upper eyelid. Temporalis transposition is a dynamic technique that allows patients to have a voluntary smile. Static (adynamic) versions of this technique use Gortex® or fascia lata, which is attached to the zygoma and then run subcutaneously to the corner of the mouth to support the sagging facial musculature. Overcorrection is required at first owing

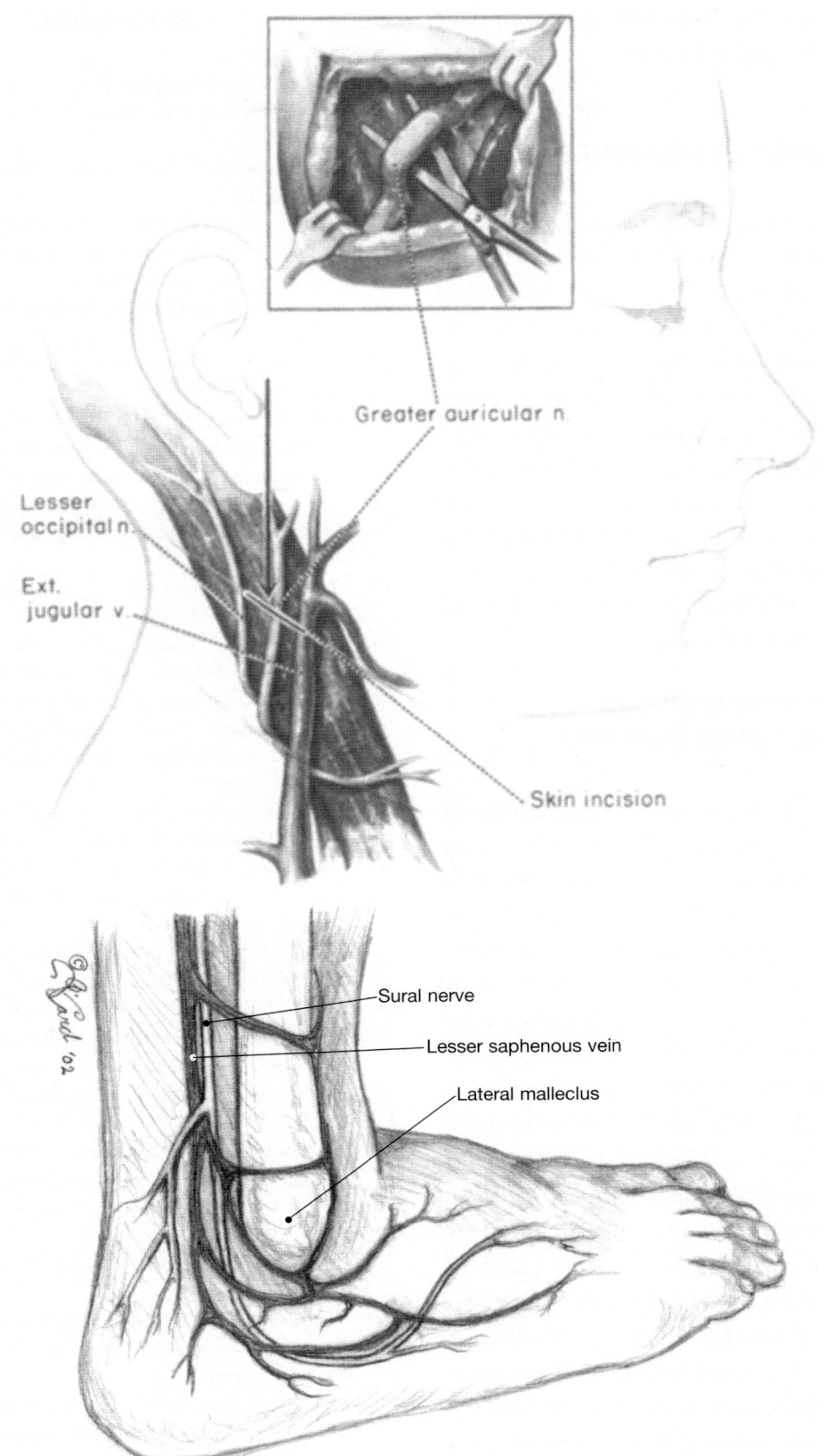

Greater auricular n.

Lesser occipital n.

Ext. jugular v.

Skin incision

Sural nerve

Lesser saphenous vein

Lateral malleclus

Figure 31–11   The two most commonly used nerves for nerve grafting: the greater auricular nerve (*A*) and the sural nerve (*B*).

to relaxation of the tissues with time. Although static slings afford relative symmetry at rest, they provide no movement.

ADJUNCTIVE MEASURES

The patient and the surgeon must realize that, unfortunately, even the best postoperative result does not achieve perfection in cosmesis and facial symmetry. This lack of perfection provides a stimulus for continued basic and clinical research. In the meantime, there are additional steps that may be taken to further enhance the patient's appearance, including facial reconstructive procedures (eg, facelift, browlift, blepharoplasty), makeup, prostheses, hairstyles, and the use of glasses to mask incisions. Facial nerve rehabilitation, with the use of biofeedback, has also shown some promise, giving the patient a sense of hope, control, and participation in the ultimate outcome of facial nerve function and appearance.

COMPLICATIONS OF FACIAL NERVE SURGERY

Before embarking on surgery of the facial nerve, the patient must be educated in detail regarding the disease process, the surgeon, and the expected results to obtain a truly informed consent. The surgeon must discuss potential risks, complications, hazards, and alternatives. However, the patient must be made aware that these potential problems are rare if the surgery is performed by a well-trained and skilled otologic, neurotologic, and skull base surgeon. The complications of surgery in general are first discussed (ie, anesthetic complications, bleeding, pain, myocardial infarction, etc). The major complications unique to facial nerve surgery are injury to the nerve itself and injury to the surrounding structures (semicircular canals, ossicles, cochlea, sigmoid sinus, etc). Depending on the approach, conductive and/or sensorineural hearing loss and vestibular dysfunction can occur. Additional risks posed by neurotologic/skull base approaches include intracranial hematoma, neurologic deficit (stroke or cranial nerve injury), CSF leak, seizures, meningitis, death, deep venous thrombosis, and pulmonary embolism.

REFERENCES

1. Kahn JB, et al. Validation of a patient-graded instrument for facial nerve paralysis: The FaCE scale. Laryngoscope 2001; 111:387–98.
2. Van Buskirk C. The seventh nerve complex. J Comp Neurol 1945;82:303–33.
3. Jackson CG. Facial nerve paralysis: diagnosis and treatment of lower motor neuron facial nerve lesions and facial paralysis. AAOHNSF. Rochester, 1986.
4. Rubinstein JT, Gantz BJ. Facial nerve disorders. Clinical otology. p. 367–80.
5. Fisch U, et al. Intracranial facial nerve anastomosis. Am J Otol 1987;8:23–9.
6. Gantz BJ, Wackym PA. Facial nerve abnormalities. In: Smith JD, Bumsted R, editors. Pediatric facial plastic and reconstructive surgery. Raven Press; 1993. p. 337–47.
7. Glasscock-Shambaugh. Facial nerve surgery. p. 434–65.
8. Lindeman H. The fallopian canal. Acta Otolaryngol (Stockh) 1960;158:204–11.
9. Sunderland S, Cosar DF. The structure of the facial nerve. Anat Rec 1953;116:147–65.
10. Haynes OR. The relations of the facial nerve in the temporal bone. Ann R Coll Surg Engl 1963;16:175.
11. Baxter A. Dehiscence of the fallopian canal. An anatomical study. J Laryngol Otol 1971;85:587–94.
12. Anson BJ, et al. Surgical anatomy of the facial nerve. Ann Otol Rhinol Laryngol 1963;72:713–34.
13. Nager GT, Proctor B. The facial canal: normal anatomy varieties and anomalies: II. Trans Am Otol Soc 1983;70:61–77.
14. Lundborg G. Ischemic nerve injury. Experimental studies on intraneural microvascular pathophysiology and nerve function in a limb subjected to temporary circulatory arrest. Scand J Plast Reconstr Surg Suppl 1970;6:3–113.
15. Seddon HJ. Three types of nerve injury. Brain 1943;66:237.
16. Gantz BJ. Evaluating acute facial paralysis using electroneurography and intraoperative evoke electromyography. Course 3514, 1983 Instruction Session. American Academy of Otolaryngology-Head and Neck Surgery, Inc.
17. Sunderland S. A classification of peripheral nerve injuries producing loss of function. Brain 1951;74:491.
18. Perry BP, Gantz BJ. Diagnosis and management of acute facial palsies. Adv Otolaryngol Head Neck Surg 1999;13:127–62.
19. Gantz BJ. Traumatic facial paralysis. In: Current therapy in otolaryngology-head and neck surgery 1984–1985. BC Decker; 1987. p. 112–5.
20. Yian CH, Paniello RC, Spector JG. Inhibition of motor nerve regeneration in a rabbit facial nerve model. Laryngoscope 2001;111:786–91.
21. Paydarfar JA, Paniello RC. Functional study of four neurotoxins as inhibitors of post-traumatic nerve regeneration. Laryngoscope 2001;111:844–50.
22. Jelks GW, et al. The evaluation and management of the eye in facial palsy. Clin Plast Surg 1979;6:397–419.

23. House JW, Brackmann DE. Facial nerve grading system. Otolaryngol Head Neck Surg 1985;93:146–7.

24. House JW. Facial nerve grading systems. Laryngoscope 1983; 93:1056–69.

25. Neely JG, et al. Computerized quantitative dynamic analysis of facial motion in the paralyzed and synkinetic face. Am J Otol 1992;13:97–107.

26. Gidley PW, et al. Facial nerve grafts: from cerebellopontine angle and beyond. Am J Otol 1999;20:781–8.

27. Birkmann C, Halber M, Bamborschke S, et al. Bell's palsy: electrodiagnostics are not indicative of cerebrospinal fluid abnormalities. Ann Otol Rhinol Laryngol 2001;110:581–4.

28. Gantz BJ. Idiopathic facial paralysis. In: Current therapy in otolaryngology-head and neck surgery. BC Decker; 1987. p. 62–6.

29. Carreno M, et al. Amplification of herpex simplex virus type 1 DNA in human geniculate ganglia from formalin-fixed, non-embedded temporal bones. Otolaryngol Head Neck Surg 2000; 123:508–11.

30. Gantz BJ, Holliday M, Gmuer AA, Fisch U. Electroneurographic evaluation of the facial nerve. Method and technical problems. Ann Otol Rhinol Laryngol 1984;93:394–8.

31. Bird TD, Nicolaus A. Friedrich's description of peripheral facial nerve paralysis in 1798. J Neurol Neurosurg Psychiatry 1979;42:56–8.

32. Murakami S, et al. Bell's palsy and herpes simplex virus: identification of viral DNA in endoneurial fluid and muscle. Ann Intern Med 1996;124:27–30.

33. Toshiaki S, et al. Facial nerve paralysis induced by herpes simplex virus in mice: an animal model of acute and transient facial paralysis. Ann Otol Rhinol Laryngol 1995;104:574–81.

34. Burgess RC, Michaels L, Bale JF Jr, Smith RJ. Polymerase chain reaction amplification of herpes simplex viral DNA from the geniculate ganglia of a patient with Bell's palsy. Ann Otol Rhinol Laryngol 1994;103:775–9.

35. Takasu T, Furuta Y, Sato KK, et al. Detection of latent herpes simplex virus DNA and RNA in human geniculate ganglia by the polymerase chain reaction. Acta Otolaryngol (Stockh) 1992;112:1004–11.

36. Wackym PA. Molecular temporal bone pathology: II. Ramsay-Hunt syndrome (herpes zoster oticus). Laryngoscope 1997;107: 1165–75.

37. Peitersen E. The natural history of Bell's palsy. Am J Otol 1982;4:107–11.

38. Grogan PM, Gronseth GS. Practice parameter: steroids, acyclovir, and surgery for Bell's palsy (an evidence-based review): report of the Quality Standards Subcommittee of the American Academy of Neurology. Neurology 2001;56:830–6.

39. Ramsey MJ, Dersimonian R, Holtel MR, Burgess LP. Corticosteroid treatment for idiopathic facial nerve paralysis: a meta-analysis. Laryngoscope 2000;110(3 Pt 1):335–41.

40. Adour et al. Bell's palsy treatment with acyclovir and prednisone compared with prednisone alone: a double-blind, randomized, controlled trial. Ann Otol Rhinol Laryngol 1996;105:371–8.

41. Gantz BJ, Rubinstein JT, Gidley P, Woodworth GG. Surgical management of Bell's palsy. Laryngoscope 1999;109:1177–88.

42. Adour KK, Diamond C. Decompression of the facial nerve in Bell's palsy: a historical review. Otolaryngol Head Neck Surg 1982;90:453–60.

43. Friedman RA. The surgical management of Bell's palsy: a review. Am J Otol 2000;21:139–44.

44. Darrouzet V, Duclos JY, Lignoro D, et al. Management of facial paralysis resulting from temporal bone fractures. Our experience in 115 cases. Otolaryngol Head Neck Surg 2001;125: 77–84.

45. May M, Sobol SM, Brackmann DE. Facial reanimation: the temporalis muscle and middle fossa surgery. Laryngoscope 1991; 101:430–2.

46. Kwartler JA, Luxford WM, Atkins J, Shelton C. Facial nerve monitoring in acoustic tumor surgery. Otolaryngol Head Neck Surg 1991;104:814–7.

47. Gantz BJ. Intraoperative facial nerve monitoring. Am J Otol 1985;Suppl:58–61.

48. Noss RS, Lalwani AK, Yingling CD. Facial nerve monitoring in middle ear and mastoid surgery. Laryngoscope 2001;111: 831–6.

49. Axon PR, Ramsden RT. Assessment of real-time clinical facial function during vestibular schwannoma resection. Laryngoscope 2000;110:1911–5.

50. Wexler DB, Fetter TW, Gantz BJ. Vestibular schwannoma presenting with sudden facial paralysis. Arch Otolaryngol Head Neck Surg 1990;116:483–5.

51. Chiang CW, Chang YL, Lou PJ. Multicentricity of intraparotid facial nerve schwannomas. Ann Otol Rhinol Laryngol 2001;110: 871–4.

52. Kertesz TR, Shelton C, Wiggins RH, et al. Intratemporal facial nerve neuroma: anatomical location and radiological features. Laryngoscope 2001;111:1250–6.

53. Kalish RA, Kaplan RF, Taylor E, et al. Evaluation of study patients with Lyme disease, 10–20 year follow-up. J Infect Dis 2001;183:453–60.

54. Furuta Y, Ohtami F, Mesuda Y, et al. Early diagnosis of zoster sine herpete and antiviral therapy for the treatment of facial palsy. Neurology 2000;12;55:708–10.

55. Falco NA, Eriksson E. Facial nerve palsy in the newborn: incidence and outcome. J Plast Reconstr Surg 1990;85:1–4.

56. Abbas GM, Jones RO. Measurements of drill-induced temperature change in the facial nerve during mastoid surgery: a cadaveric model using diamond burs. Ann Otol Rhinol Laryngol 2001;110:867–70.

57. Fisch U. Facial nerve grafting. Otolaryngol Clin North Am 1974;7:517–29.

58. Brown PD, Eshleman JS, Foote RL, Strone SE. An analysis of facial nerve function in irradiated and unirradiated facial nerve grafts. Int J Radiat Oncol Biol Phys 2000;48:737–43.

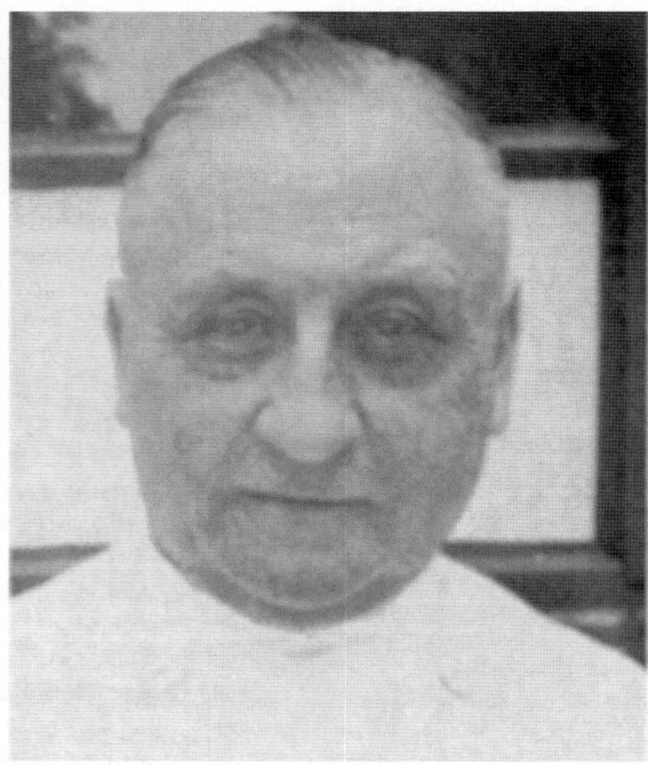

F. H. Quix (1874–1946). Professor of otolaryngology in Utrecht. He was the first to remove a vestibular schwannoma by the translabyrinthine approach.

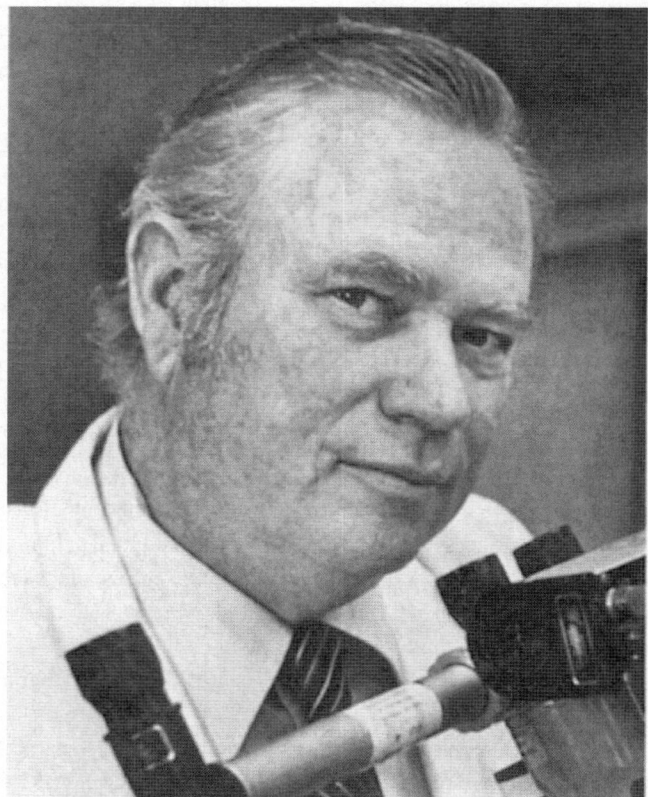

William F. House (born 1923). Developed and demonstrated the advantages of transtemporal bone microsurgical removal of vestibular schwannomas.

32

Vestibular Schwannoma

D. Bradley Welling, MD
John M. Lasak, MD

HISTORICAL ASPECTS

The entity now referred to as a vestibular schwannoma (previously acoustic neuroma, neurinoma, or neurilemmoma) was first observed at autopsy in 1777. Sir Charles Bell published the first clinical case report of a vestibular schwannoma in 1833.[1] His patient had a large tumor in the left cerebellopontine angle that had caused unilateral deafness, facial paralysis, temporal and masseter muscle paralysis (fifth cranial nerve), difficulty in speech and swallowing (tenth cranial nerve), and respiratory difficulty (brain stem) that led to the patient's demise.

At first deemed inoperable because of surgical inaccessibility, a vestibular schwannoma was successfully removed for the first time in 1894 by the pioneer otologic and neurologic surgeon Sir Charles A. Ballance.[2] The occasional operations that followed in the next two decades carried a mortality rate of around 80%. By the early 1900s, the diagnosis of brain tumors had progressed to the point that patients with particular symptoms were definitely found to have brain tumors.[3] Supratentorial lesions could be differentiated from infratentorial ones, but it was not possible to differentiate cerebellar from extracerebellar lesions at this time.[3] Gradually, however, the various distinguishing characteristics of posterior fossa tumors were appreciated, and in 1902, Henneberg and Koch introduced the term cerebellopontine angle tumor.[4]

Cushing, in his classic monograph *Tumors of the Nervus Acusticus and the Syndrome of the Cerebellopontine Angle*, carefully described and defined the clinical features of cerebellopontine angle tumors.[5] He categorized the progressive symptoms seen with gradually enlarging lesions into six stages:

[It] can be gathered that the symptomatic progress of the average acoustic tumor occurs more or less in the following stages: First, the auditory and labyrinthine manifestations; second, the occipitofrontal pains with suboccipital discomforts; third the incoordination and instability of the cerebellar origin; fourth, the evidence of involvement of adjacent cerebral nerves; fifth, the indications of increase in intracranial tension with a choked disc (papilledema) and its consequences; sixth, dysarthria, dysphagia, and finally cerebellum crises and respiratory difficulties.[5]

Cushing emphasized that unilateral hearing loss is the initial manifestation of a vestibular schwannoma and that the examiner must ascertain the status of the patient's hearing. The majority of Cushing's early patients had large (stage 4 or 5) tumors; he foresaw the need for early diagnosis to avoid the sequelae of tumor enlargement. In his 1917 publication describing the outcomes of his first 30 operations,[5] Cushing reported a surgical mortality rate of 30% — a dramatic reduction. In his 1932 publication, Cushing reported a further decrease in mortality rate to 4%[6]; however, most patients underwent subtotal, intracapsular tumor removal, and many subsequently required additional surgery to manage recurrences.

Dandy modified Cushing's techniques and in 1925 reported his series of patients, in whom complete tumor removal was accomplished with a further reduction in the mortality rate.[7] Dandy developed the unilateral cerebellar approach to the cerebellopontine angle, removing the lateral third of the cerebellum to improve exposure of the angle. Dandy also applied the Halstedian principles of meticulous hemostasis and gentle handling of tissues. However, Dandy made no effort to preserve the facial nerve, nor, apparently, did he appreciate the consequences of ligating the anterior inferior cerebellar artery.

The next significant advance in vestibular schwannoma surgery occurred in 1949, the year in which Atkinson published his autopsy studies documenting that occlusion of the anterior inferior cerebellar artery was the principal cause of operative mortality in vestibular schwannoma surgery.[8]

By World War II, most otolaryngologists were aware of the appropriate evaluation of a unilateral hearing loss. Using radiographs and vestibular studies, tumors typically were identified in Cushing stage 2 or 3.

In the 1950s, as noted by House, the nationwide operative mortality rate for acoustic neuroma surgery in the United States remained high, approaching 40% in many locales.[3] This high mortality rate prompted House to investigate the translabyrinthine approach to vestibular schwannomas.

Early in the history of surgery for vestibular schwannoma, Panse proposed an approach through the labyrinth.[9] However, Quix, who chiseled away the entire labyrinth with a mallet and gouge after a radical mastoidectomy approach, was the first to actually use this approach.[10] Although bleeding from the superior petrosal sinus necessitated termination of the operation, it was completed 4 days later, when the walls of the internal auditory canal were chiseled away, the carotid artery was exposed, and the tumor was removed. Quix predicted that this translabyrinthine approach would bring the small vestibular schwannoma within the realm of the otologist. Cushing warned that "while the otologist doubtless will be the first to recognize and diagnose these cases…there is no possible route more dangerous or difficult than this one…proposed by Panse."[6] His warning effectively dampened enthusiasm for the translabyrinthine approach to vestibular schwannoma removal for several decades.

In 1961, House,[11] using the middle fossa approach to the internal auditory canal described 7 years earlier by Clerc and Battise,[12] successfully removed a small, intracanalicular vestibular schwannoma. Soon House realized that the translabyrinthine approach was preferable for all but the smallest tumors in patients with serviceable hearing. In 1964, House reported 47 consecutive translabyrinthine complete or subtotal microsurgical removals without a fatality—a record never before achieved for these common and eventually lethal tumors.[13] The preser-

vation of facial nerve function in the majority, the virtual absence of cerebellar trauma, and the amazingly brief convalescence compared with posterior fossa operations led to a remarkable series of more than 1,000 operations for vestibular schwannomas of all sizes by House and his associates. Glasscock and others have duplicated these extremely low morbidity and mortality rates.[14]

House's great interest in vestibular schwannomas, coupled with his early diagnosis and improved surgical techniques, prompted other otologists and neurosurgeons to attempt new procedures. In 1973, Smith and colleagues[15] advocated a microscopic suboccipital approach similar to that proposed by Rand and colleagues[16] for preservation of hearing in vestibular schwannoma excision. Several neurosurgeons have reported their considerable experience with the suboccipital approach and the microscope, for example, MacCarty.[17]

Rhoton advocated the suboccipital approach for hearing preservation.[18] Wade and House later reported their results with 20 vestibular schwannoma patients in whom hearing preservation, via the middle fossa approach, had been attempted[19]; hearing was preserved in 35% of patients.

The morbidity and mortality rates of vestibular schwannoma surgery continue to improve. The operating microscope, first used by Nylén and introduced to the United States by Shambaugh, revolutionized neurotologic and neurosurgical microsurgery, enabling better visualization and preservation of neural structures. More recently, intraoperative monitoring and stimulation of the facial nerve have enabled better identification, dissection, and preservation of the facial nerve during vestibular schwannoma removal.[20,21] Furthermore, the advent of sophisticated diagnostic techniques, such as magnetic resonance imaging (MRI), has enabled the diagnosis of tumors in stage 1, that is, while still confined to the internal auditory canal. Such early diagnosis has improved the likelihood of hearing preservation with tumor removal. As predicted by Cushing,[5,6] early diagnosis has resulted in decreased morbidity and mortality rates.

The clinical characteristics of, and diagnostic strategies for, vestibular schwannomas are discussed in this chapter. Additionally, the molecular biology of these tumors, as currently understood, is reviewed. Lastly, the therapeutic options, surgical approaches for removing vestibular schwannomas, and operative complications are described.

PATHOLOGY

Vestibular schwannomas are benign, encapsulated tumors that arise from the Schwann cells of the vestibular nerve—hence the term vestibular schwannoma or vestibular neurilemmoma. The superior vestibular nerve fibers most often are the site of origin, giving rise to nearly two-thirds of tumors.[22] The inferior vestibular nerve is the site of origin in the remaining one-third. Rarely, the cochlear portion of the eighth cranial nerve or the facial nerve is the site of schwannoma origin.

Vestibular schwannomas arise at the junctional zone of the vestibular nerve, the region at which the Schwann cells and neuroglial supporting cells meet. Schwann cells tend to accumulate at the junctional zone, their progression to the brainstem slowed by neuroglial supporting cells. In addition to Schwann cell nests, "whorl-like formations," eosinophilic bodies, and ganglion cells are found at the junctional zone, as described by Prisig and colleagues in their study of serially sectioned temporal bones; they considered the Schwann cell nests to be the forerunners of vestibular schwannomas.[23] The events that led to the development of schwannomas are further discussed below. Interestingly, vestibular schwannomas have been reported to occur in 2.4 to 3.5% of temporal bones examined.[22,24] This high incidence likely reflects the selection bias as incidental schwannomas are not found on MRI in asymptomatic patients nearly as often.

Most vestibular schwannomas originate in the region of the internal auditory canal, enlarging the porus and extending into the cerebellopontine angle.[25] The color and the consistency of the schwannomas depend on the size of the tumor and the degree of tumor degeneration. Typically, tumors are either yellow or pinkish gray and have a rubbery consistency. Large tumors more often are mottled, owing to hemorrhage and fibrosis, and may have cystic regions, owing to necrosis and degeneration within the tumor. However, some tumors appear to have an intrinsic cystic nature, not reflective of necrosis.

Microscopic examination of a vestibular schwannoma reveals an encapsulated tumor, with the nerve of origin compressed at its periphery.[25] Vestibular schwannomas are composed of two histologic types: Antoni A and Antoni B. Antoni A tumors are compact and cellular, with elongated spindle cells and whorling or pal-isading nuclei aligned in rows (Verocay bodies). Antoni type B histology is loose and much less cellular, with a spongy appearance (Figure 32–1). Most vestibular schwannomas are predominantly type A, intermingled with areas of type B. Vascularity is prominent, and thickened or hyalinized vessel walls are typical. As the tumor grows, myxoid areas, histiocytic infiltration, necrosis, and fibrosis are also seen.

Initially, a tumor confined to the internal auditory canal produces no symptoms as it slowly fills the canal; however, with continued growth, it begins to press on the cochlear, vestibular, and facial nerves and the labyrinthine vessels. Tinnitus and sensorineural hearing loss appear as the cochlear nerve is compressed, and sudden sensorineural loss may occur with labyrinthine vessel compression. Loss of vestibular nerve function occurs slowly with tumor growth, and vestibular symptomatology usually is subtle because of the compensatory ability of the contralateral labyrinth. With continued tumor enlarge-

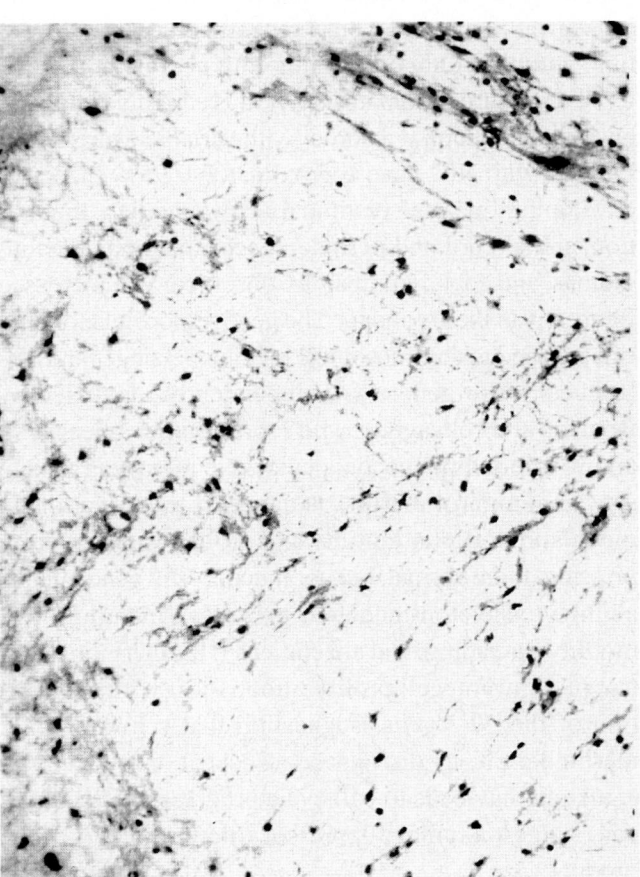

Figure 32–1 Typical vestibular schwannoma histopathology (low power; hematoxylin and eosin stain).

ment, the internal auditory canal gradually expands. The (motor) facial nerve is more resistant to tumor compression; accordingly, facial weakness is generally seen only with large tumors. The facial nerve may even be stretched to a gossamer band on the tumor surface without impairment of function.

With protrusion of the tumor into the cerebellopontine angle, it may assume a pear shape. Continued enlargement leads to compression of the superiorly located fifth cranial nerve, which results in ipsilateral anesthesia (eg, absent corneal reflex). Large tumors may also compress the lower cranial nerves, resulting in neuropathy of the ninth, tenth, eleventh, and even twelfth nerves. If the tumor is not detected and removed, hydrocephalus, visual disturbance, and death owing to tonsillar herniation may ensue.

MOLECULAR BIOLOGY

The molecular events underlying the formation of vestibular schwannomas have been recently elucidated beginning with the study of families with neurofibromatosis 2 (NF2). Neurofibromatosis type 2 is a highly penetrant, autosomal dominant disorder with variable expressivity. Patients with NF2 have approximately a 95% chance of developing bilateral vestibular schwannomas. In addition, spinal cord and peripheral schwannomas, meningiomas, and ependymomas are observed with increased frequency in these patients. The gene responsible for NF2 was mapped to chromosome 22q12 by Seizinger and colleagues.[26] The gene was independently identified by Rouleau and colleagues[27] and Trofatter and colleagues[28] and was found to encode a cytoskeletal protein named schwannomin (or merlin) that appears to have a role in modulating cellular motility and proliferation. Overexpression of the normal, but not mutant, NF2 gene inhibits actin-cytoskeleton-mediated processes including cell motility, spreading, and attachment.[29] Furthermore, control of Schwann cell proliferation is lost with inactivation of the NF2 gene, suggesting that schwannomin/merlin deficiency disrupts some aspect of intracellular signaling that leads to cell cycle progression.[30,31] These data suggest a tumor suppressor role for the NF2 gene product.

Vestibular schwannomas are usually sporadic, resulting from Schwann cell transformation within the vestibular division of the eighth cranial nerve. It is believed that mutations inactivating both alleles of the NF2 gene are responsible for the development of sporadic tumors. Patients with NF2 inherit one defunct copy of the NF2 gene through a germline mutation. Inactivation of the second allele in the Schwann cell results in the loss of NF2 tumor suppressor function and schwannoma formation.

Interestingly, mutations within the NF2 gene have been identified in the majority of, but not all, vestibular schwannomas. In a recent series, NF2 gene mutations were identified in 66% of unilateral tumors and 33% of bilateral tumors.[32] Analysis of the NF2 gene promoter has revealed that there are regulatory elements in the NF2 5′ flanking regions.[33] It has been hypothesized that mutations in these NF2 regulatory regions may be responsible for some cases of vestibular schwannoma. Furthermore, complementary deoxyribonucleic acid (cDNA) microarray expression patterns between schwannoma tissue and normal vestibular nerve have revealed that approximately 0.5% of genes within the schwannoma are deregulated when compared with the normal nerve.[34] Several of these genes are known to associate with schwannomin/merlin, and others include growth regulatory genes controlling intracellular signaling pathways and cell cycle progression. Therefore, vestibular schwannoma tumorigenesis may involve deregulation of several other genes in addition to NF2.

DIAGNOSIS

The early diagnosis of vestibular schwannomas may depend on the exact location of the tumor along the vestibular nerve. If the tumor arises in the internal auditory canal, it produces tinnitus and hearing loss early in its course. Should the lesion have its origin in the cerebellopontine angle, tinnitus and hearing loss might not become evident until the tumor has attained a larger size. Occasionally, patients and physicians are not as aggressive in the evaluation as may be ideal. Thus, relatively large tumors continue to be found, even in an era in which the diagnosis of small tumors is possible.

The differential diagnosis of a vestibular schwannoma includes any entity that produces a unilateral sensorineural hearing loss and/or tinnitus. Vestibular schwannomas are the most common lesions of the cerebellopontine angle. The next three most common lesions are meningiomas, primary cholesteatomas, and arachnoid cysts. Internal auditory canal lipomas also enter the differential diagnosis. Any of these lesions may mimic a vestibular schwannoma and can be differentiated by MRI and/or computed tomography (CT).

Early diagnosis depends on a high index of suspicion by the physician. A patient with unilateral sensorineural hearing loss and/or unilateral tinnitus, with or without balance disturbance, should be suspected of having a vestibular schwannoma. The patient presenting with these symptoms should have a basic neurotologic evaluation consisting of a thorough history, physical examination, and routine audiometric studies. If the basic neurotologic evaluation reveals any suspicious findings, special audiometric and vestibular studies may be obtained. However, as will be discussed below, MRI is the most sensitive modality to diagnose vestibular schwannomas; therefore, imaging is required for these patients.

HISTORY

The typical patient with a vestibular schwannoma experiences a unilateral tinnitus followed by a slowly progressive sensorineural hearing loss. However, patients may present with a sudden sensorineural loss. Seldom does the patient complain of true vertigo. Mild imbalance is not uncommon because as the tumor grows, it slowly destroys vestibular function. Although the contralateral labyrinth generally compensates for the vestibular loss, patients may complain of mild unsteadiness. The family history should be assessed for NF2.

NEUROTOLOGIC EXAMINATION

In addition to the routine head and neck examination, all patients suspected of having a vestibular schwannoma require a complete neurotologic examination. Neurotologic screening includes an evaluation of vestibular, cerebellar, and cranial nerve function. The examiner first notes the presence or absence of any spontaneous nystagmus, gaze nystagmus, and vertical nystagmus. Frenzel lenses are helpful and prevent the patient from visually fixating and suppressing a nystagmus of peripheral origin. Horizontal gaze nystagmus is occasionally observed, and the quick component usually is directed away from the affected ear. Rotary nystagmus and positional nystagmus can also be seen with the affected ear in the dependent position. Vertical nystagmus is always pathologic and suggests a central vestibular disorder, such as brainstem compression or cerebellar involvement by a tumor. Romberg testing is used to evaluate for a tendency to drift to the side of the lesion. Dysmetria, fine movements, gait, and heel-shin tests are performed to detect cerebellar involvement.

Multiple cranial nerves may be affected by a cerebellopontine angle tumor, and the number of nerves involved is usually directly proportional to the size of the tumor. Eighth nerve dysfunction is suggested by tinnitus, vestibular symptoms, and hearing loss. The tuning fork examination helps detect a sensorineural hearing loss on the suspect side. With larger tumors, the corneal reflex may be diminished, and there may be hypesthesia on the involved side of the face. Although large tumors frequently affect fifth cranial nerve sensory function, they seldom cause paresis or paralysis of the (motor) seventh cranial nerve. The more vulnerable sensory (to the posterior external auditory canal wall) seventh nerve fibers are more often affected; Hitzelberger's sign — anesthesia of the posterior wall of the external auditory canal — reflects this involvement of the sensory component of the facial nerve. It is unusual for vestibular schwannomas to affect cranial nerves other than the fifth, seventh, and eighth; however, large cerebellopontine angle tumors may affect neighboring nerves, so a complete cranial nerve examination is advised.

AUDIOMETRIC STUDIES

Audiometric studies — pure-tone air and bone conduction threshold assessment with speech discrimination testing — are very important in early diagnosis because the audiogram is what catches the examining physician's attention, first raising suspicion for a vestibular schwannoma. An asymmetric sensorineural hearing loss with disproportionately poor speech discrimination is the audiometric finding most suggestive of a vestibular schwannoma. A patient with a vestibular schwannoma may have very little or no hearing loss if the tumor is very small or if the tumor originates beyond the internal auditory canal in the cerebellopontine angle, thus not causing neural compression. Occasionally, a large cerebellopontine angle tumor can be found in a patient who has normal hearing and a 100% discrimination score.

A number of special audiometric tests historically have been used in the evaluation of a patient with a suspicious audiogram to aid in detecting a retrocochlear lesion. The stapedial reflex decay test is an easily performed audiometric study. By means of an impedance bridge, the stapedial reflex is elicited at the suprathreshold level, and decay to half-amplitude in 5 seconds or less is suggestive of retrocochlear pathology. Of historical interest is the Performance Intensity Function for Phonetically Balanced Words (PIPB) test, which evaluates speech discrimination at progressively higher sensation levels. As the presentation level increases, the speech discrimination score should also increase until a maximum score is obtained. Discrimination should not decrease with additional increases in presentation level. Should a decrease occur, the phenomenon is known as "rollover" and is consistent with a retrocochlear lesion. As Burkey and colleagues have suggested, patients with abnormal special auditory tests should be imaged to further assess for retrocochlear pathology.[35] The stapedial reflex decay and PIPB tests are not routinely used in screening currently because more sensitive and specific tests are available.

One of the most sensitive audiometric tests available is the auditory brainstem response (ABR) (for detailed information, see Chapter 8). Early studies with ABR reported better than 90% sensitivity for the diagnosis of vestibular schwannomas.[36,37]

An interaural wave V latency difference of greater than 0.2 msec, or a prolonged I–V interwave time interval, suggests a retrocochlear disorder such as a vestibular schwannoma (Figure 32–2). Additionally, the complete absence of wave V is suggestive of retrocochlear pathology.

A major limitation in the utility of ABR in the evaluation of vestibular schwannomas is that the patient must have no greater than a 70-dB threshold. Recent reports have indicated that the sensitivity of the ABR to intracanalicular acoustic tumors less than 1 cm ranges from 58 to 89%. We, and other authors, in an attempt to improve the cost effectiveness of patient evaluation, have recommended using MRI to screen for vestibular schwannomas in patients with suspicious histories and audiometric findings.[38–40] Others have recommended ABR as the initial screening study in low- to intermediate-risk patients.[41,42]

Don and colleagues reported a modification of the standard ABR, called the stacked ABR.[43] This measure calculates the wave V amplitude by temporally aligning the wave V of each derived-band ABR and then summating the time-shifted responses. The stacked ABR is reported to be sensitive to the presence of small intracanalicular tumors and to have excellent specificity for the absence of tumors in patients with normal hearing. These authors recommend stacked ABR for vestibular

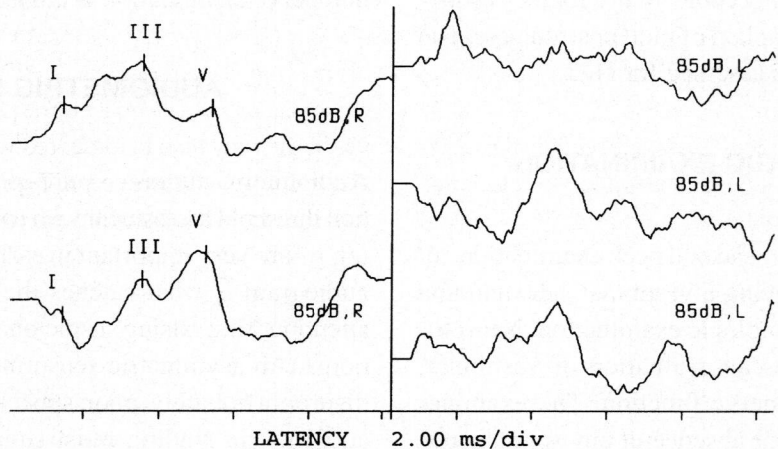

Figure 32–2 Auditory brainstem response tracing of a left ear with a vestibular schwannoma compared with the contralateral (*right*) normal hearing ear. Note the delayed latency of wave V compared with the normal ear (*right*) and the poor waveform morphology.

schwannoma screening when MRI is unavailable or not tolerated by the patient.

VESTIBULAR STUDIES

As a vestibular schwannoma slowly destroys vestibular function in the affected ear, gradual compensation takes place.[44] Therefore, patients with vestibular schwannomas rarely complain of vertigo but often note slight unsteadiness or clumsiness. Although the finding of decreased vestibular function on caloric testing ipsilateral to a sensorineural hearing loss historically has been useful in suggesting the diagnosis of a vestibular schwannoma, at present, it is not sensitive enough to be helpful diagnostically.[38] Caloric testing measures the response of the lateral semicircular canal, which is innervated by the superior vestibular nerve; accordingly, a small inferior vestibular nerve schwannoma might not cause an abnormal caloric response.

Linthicum and Churchill described a simple method for examining the caloric response without sophisticated equipment.[45] The patient's head is placed at a 30-degree angle, and a small amount of ice water is placed in the external auditory canal for 20 seconds. The eyes are examined for nystagmus, usually with Frenzel lenses. Absent or diminished nystagmus suggests a reduced vestibular response.

A more sophisticated method of determining vestibular function and one that is more widely used is electronystagmography (ENG) (see Chapter 9 for additional information), including bithermal caloric testing, according to the technique of Hallpike and Cairns.[46] Eye tracking tests can reveal central vestibular dysfunction in the presence of a large tumor. Spontaneous nystagmus not observed with Frenzel lenses or the naked eye can be detected by ENG.

With the development of sophisticated imaging techniques (eg, MRI) and ABR testing, ENG is no longer used in the initial evaluation of patients in whom a vestibular schwannoma is suspected. Magnetic resonance imaging (discussed later) often can even differentiate the nerve of origin of small intracanalicular tumors. The significance of this fact is that hearing preservation may be more difficult in the removal of a tumor that arises from the inferior vestibular nerve, perhaps owing to the close proximity of the cochlear and inferior vestibular nerves.

During tumor dissection, an interruption of the cochlear nerve blood supply can result in postoperative hearing loss. When MRI cannot determine the nerve of origin of a small vestibular schwannoma, ENG may provide useful data. A reduced vestibular response in the involved ear suggests a superior vestibular nerve tumor. Therefore, the ENG examination may influence the surgical approach selected and provide useful information regarding the likelihood of hearing preservation.

IMAGING

Although audiometric and vestibular testing raise suspicions for a vestibular schwannoma, imaging studies provide the definitive diagnosis. Since the previous edition of this text, more sophisticated and less invasive imaging techniques have become available (see Chapter 11 for additional details). Fortunately, painful techniques carrying significant morbidity, such as posterior fossa myelography and gaseous or opaque contrast CT, are rarely necessary today. These imaging studies have been replaced by MRI and are used only when MRI is contraindicated.

Computed Tomography

One-millimeter CT scanning in both the axial and coronal planes provides excellent detail of the temporal bone and internal auditory canals. Erosion of the internal auditory canal from expansion of a vestibular schwannoma is well visualized by the exquisite bony detail provided by CT.[47] Subtle bone erosion in the cochlea or vestibule may also be detected with an intralabyrinthine schwannoma. However, CT provides less soft tissue detail than MRI. In addition, to visualize most tumors, CT must be performed with the administration of an intravenous contrast agent. Small tumors (less than 1 cm) are often missed by CT, even when contrast is used. Larger tumors, such as those causing brainstem compression, displacement of the fourth ventricle, and hydrocephalus, are readily appreciated by CT; therefore, CT may be considered for use in patients to whom intervention will be offered only if the tumor is exerting significant pressure on the brainstem. For a patient who cannot tolerate an MRI, or for one in whom it is contraindicated, air-contrast CT can often reveal an intracanalicular tumor.[48] Air is inserted into the lumbar spine by way of a lumbar puncture following the removal of cerebrospinal fluid (CSF). Seven to 10 cm³ of air (or oxygen) are injected into the subarachnoid space, and the patient is positioned so that the air rises into the posterior fossa, where it can outline a small tumor in the internal auditory canal. Both sides are studied to rule out bilateral lesions. Most patients complain of headache, which is usually temporary, after the procedure.

Magnetic Resonance Imaging

Magnetic resonance imaging is the imaging modality of choice to detect vestibular schwannomas of all sizes — when available and when a moderate or high level of suspicion exists, based on the patient's history and audiometric findings. Magnetic resonance imaging yields exceptional definition of the full course of the seventh and eighth cranial nerves from the brainstem to the periphery, including their course through the internal auditory canal.

Magnetic resonance images are obtained before and after administration of the paramagnetic contrast agent, gadolinium. On T_1-weighted images, a vestibular schwan-

noma is hyperintense compared to CSF and isointense to gray matter (Figure 32–3). On T_2-weighted images, the tumor appears isointense to CSF and hyperintense to gray matter. Additionally, the fluid-filled inner ear and CSF of the internal auditory canal are bright and clearly visualized on T_2-weighted sequences. Cystic tumors often have high signal intensity on T_2-weighted sequences because fluid fills the cystic components of the tumor. Gadolinium-enhanced, T_1-weighted images of a vestibular schwannoma reveal marked tumor enhancement and are considered to be the gold standard for imaging vestibular schwannomas (Figure 32–4). The sensitivity of gadolinium-enhanced MRI permits detection of schwannomas as small as 1 to 2 mm.[49]

Magnetic resonance imaging using the fast spin echo (FSE) technique is the most recent advance in the imaging of vestibular schwannomas. Excellent contrast between bone, neural structures, and CSF is achieved with these heavily T_2-weighted images, and the internal auditory canal contents are clearly visualized, with no need for costly contrast agents. Vestibular schwannomas are hypointense compared to CSF on T_2-weighted FSE sequences, and an intracanalicular tumor appears as a filling defect in the internal auditory canal (Figure 32–5). Investigators comparing gadolinium-enhanced, T_1-weighted MRI with T_2-weighted FSE sequences have reported that the latter modality can reliably detect mass lesions within the internal auditory canal and cerebel-

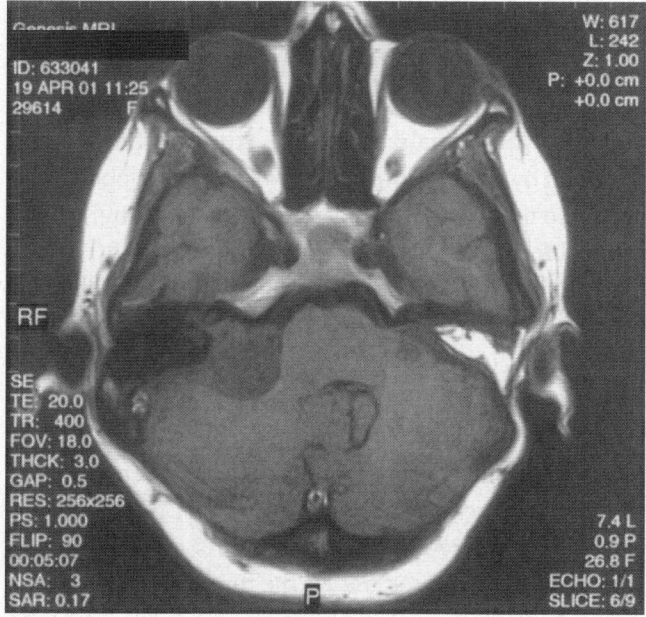

Figure 32–3   Vestibular schwannoma as seen with T_1-weighted magnetic resonance imaging. The tumor is isointense with gray matter.

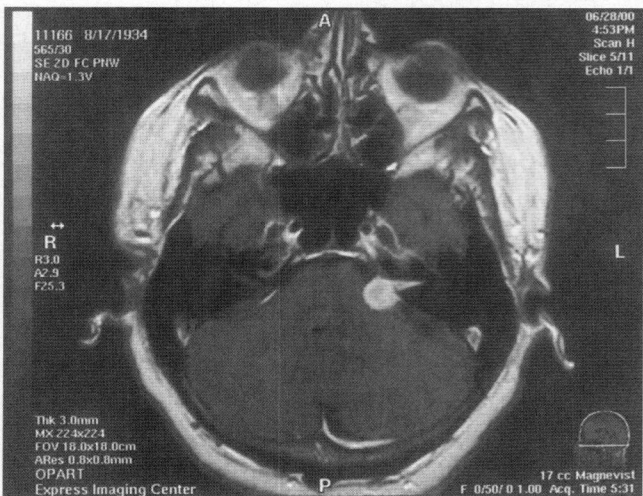

Figure 32–4   Vestibular schwannoma, as seen with gadolinium-enhanced, T_1-weighted magnetic resonance imaging. The vestibular schwannoma enhances brightly.

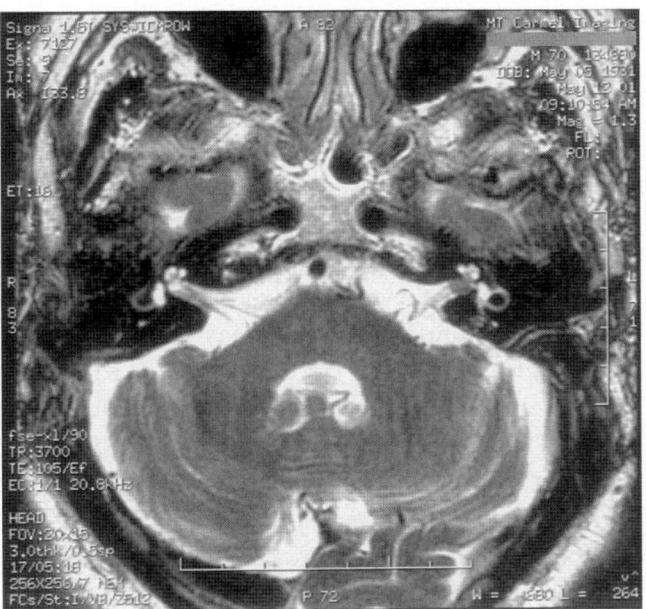

Figure 32–5 Fast spin echo magnetic resonance image of an intracanalicular vestibular schwannoma. The tumor is hypointense to cerebrospinal fluid and appears as a filling defect within the internal auditory canal.

lopontine angle and efficiently screen patients with sensorineural hearing loss.[50,51] It has been suggested that gadolinium may be needed only to confirm suspected tumors and that FSE MRI could be used as a highly sensitive and specific, yet cost-effective, screening method. Additionally, a FSE T_2-weighted sequence study can be completed much more quickly than a full MRI.

Patients with claustrophobia may not tolerate the confinement required for MRI; however, mild sedatives or open MRI units make the study tolerable for most patients. Owing to the strong magnetic field, patients with metallic prostheses, such as cardiac pacemakers and cochlear implants, cannot undergo MRI. Most stapes prostheses can tolerate the 1.5-Tesla magnet of MRI; however, these prostheses are likely to contraindicate MRI with more powerful magnets.[52]

In summary, MRI is the diagnostic test of choice for patients in whom a vestibular schwannoma is suspected. Fast spin echo MRI is a cost-efficient screening tool. Stacked ABR may be a useful screening tool when the degree of suspicion is not as high.

TREATMENT OPTIONS

The three options for the management of vestibular schwannomas are surgical excision, stereotactic radiation, and observation. Each treatment has its advantages and disadvantages. To a great extent, the decision is based on patient preference and the findings of observational studies. There is no randomized, controlled clinical trial that has objectively assessed outcomes of these treatment options. Consequently, clinical decision making can be difficult and on occasion is subject to biased opinion rather than being evidence based. Fortunately, in comparison with the morbidity and mortality of past decades, the outcomes of all three treatment options are quite good.

Observation

The indolent nature of many vestibular schwannomas has long been recognized, leading some physicians to recommend observation without immediate intervention as a reasonable treatment option.[53–58] The number of tumors that will grow over time is unknown, but ranges from 30 to 82% have been reported.[53,59,60] In a recent study, growth occurred in 66% of patients followed over a 5-year period.[60] The advantages of nonintervention for patients whose vestibular schwannoma does not exhibit growth are evident. No therapy may be necessary over the life span of the patient if no growth occurs.

Even with this conservative treatment option, there are inherent dangers. For example, although tumor growth rates average 2 mm per year, some tumors may grow up to 25 mm per year. As discussed below, the literature contains conflicting reports regarding the ability to predict future growth based on past growth patterns. A tumor may grow more quickly than the norm, compromising the ability to preserve hearing and facial nerve function with intervention, and may even endanger the patient's life.[59] Charabi and colleagues reported a 6% death rate owing to tumor-induced brainstem herniation in patients with vestibular schwannomas managed by observation.[61] Such a mortality rate has not been reported in other large series.[62,63] Patients who enter the observation period with salvageable hearing may lose hearing if the tumor grows. In one study, 28 patients were classified as candidates for a hearing preservation operation; 21 (75%) of the patients fell out of this classification during the observation period owing to tumor growth and/or deterioration of hearing.[61]

Typically, an MRI is obtained 6 months after the initial MRI and yearly thereafter if there is no imminent danger of brainstem compression. Observation is more likely to be considered a treatment option in patients over the age of 65 years.

When deciding among the treatment options, another consideration is the status of the contralateral ear. A watch-and-wait approach for patients with a vestibular schwannoma in their only-hearing ear is recommended when serviceable hearing remains and brainstem function is not at immediate risk.[63]

Growth Rate Prediction

The ability to predict accurately schwannoma growth rates by evaluating a set of factors such as tumor size at discovery, association with NF2, patient age, or growth in the first 6-month observation period would be helpful in making treatment decisions. Unfortunately, it is disputed which factors are predictive of growth rate. Growth rate within the first year has been reported to be predictive of subsequent growth by Bederson and colleagues,[64] but Charabi and colleagues reported that growth patterns were not static[59]; they changed during an extended observation period. Ogawa and colleagues found the growth rate of unilateral vestibular schwannomas to be slower than that of the bilateral vestibular schwannomas of NF2.[65] The growth rate of recurrent tumors was faster than that of unoperated tumors. The relationships between patient age, tumor growth rate, and tumor size also have been analyzed. The younger the patient or the larger the tumor, the greater the growth rate.[65] In counterpoint, Levo and colleagues found unilateral schwannomas to grow more rapidly than schwannomas associated with NF2.[58] The average tumor growth rate among unilateral vestibular schwannoma patients was 3.5 mm per year and among bilateral tumors 1.5 mm per year.[58] Study of the indicators of cellular proliferation showed a slightly higher proliferation labeling index (0.4 to 17.6%; mean = 2.7%) in NF2-associated schwannomas than in unilateral vestibular schwannomas (0 to 9%; mean = 2.2%).[66]

Stereotactic Radiation Therapy

In 1951, the Swedish neurosurgeon Leksell developed the first open stereotactic instrument by focusing multiple radiation beams on a single target. He reported his experience with closed cranial treatment of a variety of lesions over the next several years.[67] Currently, stereotactic radiation is the principal alternative active treatment for vestibular schwannomas (as opposed to microsurgical resection). The term "Gamma Knife®" is an often applied misnomer that may be confusing to patients. "Stereotactic radiation" is the preferred term as it is more descriptive of the treatment.

The goals of stereotactic radiation therapy are the long-term prevention of tumor growth, maintenance of neurologic function, and prevention of new neurologic deficits. Noren reported growth control, usually with shrinkage, in 95% of unilateral tumors.[68] The development of cranial neuropathies shows a direct relation to radiation dose. Miller and colleagues reported a facial neuropathy rate of 38% for a protocol delivering 20 Gy to the tumor periphery and an 8% facial neuropathy rate for a reduced dose of 16 Gy ($p = .006$).[69] Multivariate analysis revealed that the only factor associated with increased risk of post-treatment facial neuropathy was a tumor margin dose greater than or equal to 18 Gy. Facial nerve preservation rates up to 98% have been reported as radiation dosage to the tumor periphery have been reduced to less than 16 Gy.[68–72] Similarly, the incidence of trigeminal neuropathy was 29% for a protocol delivering 20 Gy and 15% for the reduced-dose 16-Gy protocol. Preservation of hearing is reportedly achieved in 65 to 70% of patients when 12 Gy or less are used, and tinnitus is rarely made worse.[68] Although delayed-onset cranial neuropathies can occur, in one study, no new neurologic deficits appeared more than 28 months after stereotactic radiation.[70]

Stereotactic Radiation Advantages
Potential advantages of stereotactic radiation over microsurgical resection include decreased hospitalization time, a quicker return to work, and, in some countries, a reduced cost of treatment.[73] Additionally, stereotactic radiation may be considered for elderly or medically infirm patients in whom tumor growth has been docu-

mented. The risks associated with microsurgical dissection, including infection and CSF leak, are avoided because of the minimally invasive nature of the treatment. Patients who demonstrate tumor recurrence after surgical removal may undergo salvage radiation therapy.[74] However, such tumor recurrence occurs only in 0.3 to 0.8% of patients treated in centers with considerable microsurgical experience.[75,76]

Stereotactic Radiation Disadvantages

Potential disadvantages of stereotactic radiation include radiation-induced hydrocephalus, even after treatment of tumors as small as 18 mm.[77] This complication, which is associated directly with tumor size,[71] was much more common in early reports; its occurrence has been reduced recently to 1.4 to 9.2%.

Some surgeons have reported great difficulty preserving the facial nerve in the surgical salvage of schwannomas that have failed radiation[78]; however, this difficulty has been disputed by others.[79,80]

The risk of a previously benign schwannoma undergoing malignant degeneration is a concern, especially in the younger patient with a schwannoma. Of 8,000 vestibular schwannomas treated with stereotactic radiation since 1969 worldwide, Noren reports an estimated 0.1% rate of malignant change.[68] Patients whose tumors underwent malignant transformation died despite microsurgical excision. Histopathologic analysis revealed a malignant, spindle cell neoplasm with numerous mitotic figures. The detection of rhabdoid elements by immunohistochemical analysis confirmed the diagnosis of a malignant triton tumor or sarcoma.[81,82] Other schwannomas surgically removed after stereotactic radiation failure have shown delayed radiation changes such as nucleolar and cytoplasmic enlargement and proliferation of endothelial cells,[83] as well as viable cells typical of schwannomas.[84] Although the incidence of malignant transformation is low, the follow-up time has been relatively short in the majority of studies. Also, it must be recognized that malignant schwannomas or triton tumors may occur spontaneously in the absence of a prior history of irradiation.[85,86]

Another consideration in stereotactic radiation therapy is the potential for sudden hearing loss, likely owing to swelling that occurs soon after radiation.[87] Additional decline in cranial nerve function may occur over several years following radiation. In one study, useful hearing was preserved in 10 of 10 patients immediately after radiation treatment but declined to 8 of 10 patients at 6 months, 6 of 10 patients at 1 year, and 5 of 10 patients at 2 years.[88]

Linear accelerators also have been used to deliver stereotactic radiation to vestibular schwannomas and are reported to achieve results similar to the Gamma Knife.[71,89]

Stereotactic Radiation in Neurofibromatosis 2

Patients with vestibular schwannomas associated with NF2 represent a special challenge because of the risk of complete deafness. Subach and colleagues reported an overall tumor control rate of 98% in 45 NF2-associated vestibular schwannomas treated with stereotactic radiation; the mean tumor margin dose was 15 Gy (range 12 to 20 Gy). During the median follow-up period of 36 months, 16 tumors (36%) regressed, 28 (62%) remained unchanged, and 1 (2%) grew. Useful hearing was preserved in 6 (43%) of 14 patients, and this rate improved to 67% after the radiation dose was reduced. Normal facial nerve function (House-Brackmann grade I) was preserved in 25 (81%) of 31 patients. Normal trigeminal nerve function was preserved in 34 (94%) of 36 patients.[90] A study by Ito and colleagues suggested that NF2 and tumor diameter were the common risk factors associated with increased hearing loss following stereotactic radiation but that larger populations and longer follow-up were necessary to draw rigorous conclusions.[80]

Radiation-Induced Malignancy

In a study of 2,311 patients with a history of childhood irradiation for enlarged tonsils and adenoids, Shore-Freedman and colleagues found 29 schwannomas, 2 neurofibromas, and 1 ganglioneuroma, representing a 1.4% incidence of tumors. Because of the frequency of tumor development and the strict localization of the tumors to the area of treatment, it was concluded that they were radiation induced. Analysis of the latency of these tumors indicates that they continue to occur for at least 30 years after the radiation exposure. In the same group of individuals, there have been 54 confirmed salivary gland tumors (40 benign and 14 malignant).[91]

Stereotactic radiation may be less likely to induce neoplastic change than fractionated radiation, and glandular tissue, which is prone to radiation-induced neoplasia, is not in the radiation field used for vestibular schwannomas. Thus, the overall risk of malignancy is less than for fractionated radiation. The overall risk of neoplastic change would appear to be less in patients over the age of 60 years; therefore, some clinicians, in keeping with the National Institutes of Health Consensus Development Conference report,[92] do not recommend radiation unless patients are elderly or otherwise medically infirm. The ultimate answer to the question of the long-term safety of stereotactic radiation will require at least a 30-year follow-up period. The risk of malignant degeneration must be weighed against the risk of complications of surgery, such as stroke or death.

Radiation versus Observation

Shirato and colleagues reported a comparative study of observation versus stereotactic radiotherapy in the management of vestibular schwannomas.[93] The study group consisted of 27 patients who underwent observation as initial treatment (observation group) and 50 who received stereotactic radiation. The stereotactic radiotherapy consisted of small-field, fractionated radiotherapy (36 to 44 Gy in 20 to 22 fractions over 6 weeks) with or without a subsequent 4-Gy boost. The tumor control rate in the radiation group, when delivered at these high levels, was significantly better than that of the observation group. Mean tumor growth was 3.87 mm per year in the observation group and −0.75 mm per year in the stereotactic radiation group. Forty-one percent of the observation group and 2% of the stereotactic radiation group required salvage therapy. They concluded that stereotactic radiotherapy provided better tumor control and a similar rate of hearing deterioration than did observation.[93] Intervention assignment was not randomized, however, representing an important bias in the study. Also, the number of tumors that were growing at the time of patient entry into the study was not defined.

In summary, although acceptable short-term outcomes have been reported with stereotactic radiation therapy for the treatment of vestibular schwannomas, long-term outcomes at current levels of radiation have not been well documented.[68–72] The average dose of radiation to the tumor margin has been progressively reduced since the technique was initially described, resulting in improved cranial nerve function and fewer brainstem complications. Unfortunately, these studies do not account for tumors that would not have grown without any treatment. We believe that longitudinal follow-up is required before definitive conclusions can be drawn regarding the ultimate rate of tumor control using reduced stereotactic radiation doses.[69]

Microsurgery

Historically, microsurgical excision has been the treatment of choice for vestibular schwannomas. There are four popular microsurgical approaches for vestibular schwannoma removal: the middle cranial fossa, the translabyrinthine, the suboccipital (retrosigmoid), and the combined. Over the last two decades, a multidisciplinary approach to the microsurgical removal of vestibular schwannomas has developed in tertiary referral centers. This amiable working relationship between the neuro-otologist and the neurosurgeon has led to improved hearing preservation rates and facial nerve outcomes in many patients.

Approach Selection

The middle fossa approach is used when hearing preservation is to be attempted. In our practice, hearing preservation is attempted when the pure-tone average is 30 dB or less and the speech discrimination is greater than 70%. However, in patients with poor hearing in the contralateral ear or with NF2, the criteria need not be so stringent. Small tumors restricted to the internal auditory canal are best accessed with the middle fossa approach. Generally, tumors of 1 to 1.5 cm can be successfully exposed and removed through the middle fossa route. The middle fossa approach affords excellent access to the fundus of the internal auditory canal while preserving the otic capsule and is ideal for tumors with lateral internal auditory canal extension. However, tumors with substantial extension into the cerebellopontine angle can be removed through the middle fossa approach if the superior petrosal sinus is ligated and the temporal lobe is further retracted.

The translabyrinthine approach directly traverses the temporal bone and otic capsule and is therefore preferred for patients without useful hearing preoperatively. This approach can be used for tumors of all sizes, provides excellent exposure of the cerebellopontine angle, and affords the widest exposure of the facial nerve, extending from the horizontal section within the temporal bone to the route entry zone at the brainstem. Furthermore, visualization of adjacent cranial nerves is facilitated by the wide exposure of the translabyrinthine approach. Cerebellar retraction is usually unnecessary, except with very large tumors. A relative advantage of the translabyrinthine approach over the middle fossa and suboccipital approaches is the avoidance of cerebellar or temporal lobe retraction. The fragility of blood vessels increases with age, thus increasing the likelihood of intraparenchymal bleeding with brain retraction.

The suboccipital (retrosigmoid) approach accesses the posterior fossa through a craniotomy inferior to the transverse sinus and posterior to the sigmoid sinus. Generally, the neuro-otologist views the suboccipital approach as a hearing preservation approach for medially located tumors. This approach affords superior exposure of the cerebellopontine angle when compared with the middle fossa approach. The posterior wall of the internal auditory canal is drilled away to expose the contents of the canal; however, the fundus of the canal cannot be visualized fully without drilling into the otic capsule, and the tumor can be left behind. Tumors of all sizes can be removed through the suboccipital approach, and this is the traditional technique used by neurosurgeons. Cerebellar retraction is required for most cases.

The combined approach is used for vestibular schwannomas greater than 4 cm. Hearing preservation is generally not an issue with tumors of this size, and the main concern is brainstem decompression and the prevention of increased intracranial pressure. Glasscock and Hays described a one-stage approach for the treatment of giant tumors, combining the translabyrinthine approach and the suboccipital approach, which enables additional cerebellar retraction and enhanced exposure of very large tumors.[44] The combined approach can be staged, performing tumor debulking, medial facial nerve identification, and brainstem decompression through the suboccipital approach, and then, at a later date, completing tumor removal with the addition of a translabyrinthine dissection. Identification of the lateral aspect of the facial nerve during the translabyrinthine dissection may facilitate facial nerve preservation with the removal of large tumors.

Special Considerations in Neurofibromatosis 2

Surgical removal of the vestibular schwannomas associated with NF2 presents increased complexity because of the more rapid growth rates, the more aggressive tumor behavior with respect to the facial nerve, and the importance of preserving hearing in at least one ear if at all possible. Likewise, the bilateral brainstem compression seen in NF2 poses a greater threat to vital brainstem function. There is controversy in the literature regarding the difficulty of surgical removal of unilateral vestibular schwannomas as opposed to NF2-related schwannomas. Samii and Matthies reported microsurgical results in 120 tumors removed from 82 NF2 patients through a suboccipital approach. Overall, hearing was preserved in 36% of ears, and anatomic facial nerve preservation was achieved in 85%. Two deaths occurred.[94] They concluded that the chances of anatomic and functional nerve preservation are lower for patients with NF2 than for patients with unilateral tumors.

Slattery and colleagues reported the outcomes of 18 NF2 patients (23 tumors) who underwent surgical excision of vestibular schwannomas. Measurable hearing was preserved in 65% of patients. House-Brackmann grade I or II facial function was maintained in 100% of patients with normal preoperative facial nerve function. Unlike Samii and Matthies, they concluded that in patients with NF2, hearing and facial nerve function outcomes are similar to those for patients with sporadic, unilateral vestibular schwannomas. They agreed that early intervention was crucial in obtaining favorable outcomes.[95] Early detection with aggressive screening is strongly associated with favorable outcomes.[96,97]

MICROSURGICAL RESECTION

Middle Cranial Fossa Approach

The surgeon is seated at the head of the bed during middle fossa surgery (Figure 32–6). The head is turned opposite the side of the lesion, and the operative site is shaved. Facial nerve electrodes are placed in the obicularis oris and oculi muscles, and the facial nerve monitor is tested to ensure that it is functioning appropriately. Mannitol (1 g/kg) is given intravenously at the start of the case to decrease CSF pressure. If there is no con-

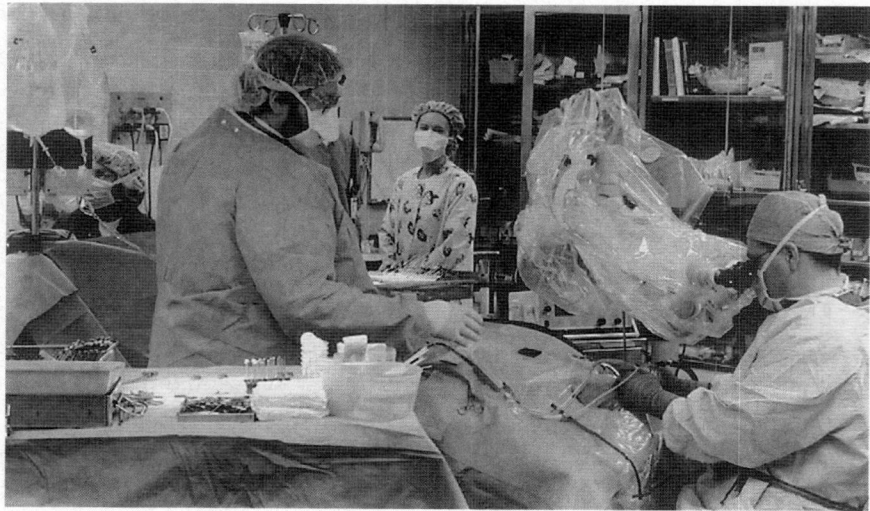

Figure 32–6 The operating room setup for middle fossa surgery. Note that the surgeon is seated at the head of the bed and the anesthesiologist at the foot.

traindication, the patient is also given 10 mg of dexamethasone intravenously. Antibiotic prophylaxis covering skin pathogens is given prior to the skin incision. The surgical site is prepared and draped for neurotologic surgery in the usual fashion.

The skin incision is made with a #10 scalpel and extends 1 cm anterior to and approximately 12 cm superior to the tragus. The superior limb of the incision is angled (approximately 15 degrees) anteriorly. The temporalis fascia is divided sharply, and the temporalis muscle is incised with electrocautery to the skull. A periosteal (Lempert) elevator is used to elevate the musculoperiosteum anteriorly and posteriorly. Dura hooks are placed to retract the temporalis muscle. The root of the zygoma is identified at this point as it serves as the center of the inferior limit of the craniotomy. The anesthesia team should be instructed to hyperventilate the patient to a CO_2 level of 25 mm Hg to further facilitate dural relaxation.

A 4 × 4 cm craniotomy is drilled using a 5-mm cutting bur or craniotome. The craniotomy window should extend 2 cm anterior and 2 cm posterior to the zygomatic root and be approximately 4 cm in the vertical dimension. The surgeon should switch to a diamond bur when the dura is approached to prevent dural tears. The bone flap is gently elevated off the dura and placed in antibiotic solution. Bleeding dural vessels are controlled with bipolar cautery. Exposed air cells within the zygomatic root should be sealed with either muscle or bone wax prior

to the completion of the case to prevent a potential passage for CSF egress.

Using the operating microscope and a dural elevator, the temporal lobe and dura are gently elevated off the skull base. Elevation should proceed carefully in a posterior to anterior direction to avoid injuring a dehiscent geniculate ganglion. Elevation proceeds to the anterior extent of the craniotomy, taking care not to lacerate the middle meningeal artery. Should the artery be lacerated, it is controlled with bipolar cautery. The temporal lobe and dura are elevated medially until the superior petrosal sinus and petrous pyramid are identified. As full exposure is accomplished, the arcuate eminence and greater petrosal nerve are identified. The greater petrosal nerve can be stimulated (at approximately 0.1 to 0.3 milliamps) to "back-stimulate" the facial nerve; this maneuver helps to avoid confusion with the lesser petrosal nerve, which is located laterally and parallels the course of the greater petrosal nerve along the floor of the middle cranial fossa.

The House-Urban middle fossa retractor is placed to facilitate retraction of the temporal lobe. Cottonoid sponges should be placed between the blade of the retractor and the dura for protection. Using a #4 diamond bur and suction irrigation, drilling begins in the region of the arcuate eminence, and the superior semicircular canal is "blue-lined." Bisecting the angle between the greater superficia petrosal nerve and the superior semicircular canal gives the approximate location of the meatal plane and underlying internal auditory canal. Using successively smaller diamond burs, the internal auditory canal is identified medially near the porus. Bone is removed more laterally, taking care to avoid fenestrating the cochlea or superior semicircular canal. Laterally, the vertical crest (Bill's bar) separating the anteriorly located facial nerve from the posteriorly located superior vestibular nerve is identified. The labyrinthine section of the facial nerve is identified as the nerve exits the lateral end of the internal canal and heads toward the geniculate ganglion.

Once the bone work is completed, the surgical site is irrigated to remove any bone dust that might obscure visualization. The dura of the internal auditory canal is incised along its posterior border, avoiding the facial nerve. The dural margins are reflected anteriorly and posteriorly, and the facial nerve is identified on the superior surface of the tumor (Figure 32–7, A). The nerve should be positively identified using the facial nerve stimulator set at 0.05 milliamps. As a result of the mass effect of the tumor, the facial nerve may occasionally be displaced anterior, inferior, or, rarely, even posterior to the tumor. Should this be the case, it is recommended that the nerve be positively identified at its lateral and medial limits prior to tumor dissection.

Using a sickle or Fisch knife, the facial nerve and tumor are gently separated. Often the tumor can be gently retracted away from the facial nerve with the suction tip, facilitating exposure of the plane between the nerve and the tumor (Figure 32–7, B). Once the facial nerve has been completely separated from the tumor, a 0.5-mm hook can be used to avulse the superior vestibular nerve laterally where it enters the temporal bone. The tumor is then carefully dissected free from the facial and cochlear nerves in a lateral to medial direction. The inferior vestibular nerve is usually intimately associated with the tumor and should be included with the specimen. Once the tumor is free from the internal auditory canal, the medial stalk of the vestibular nerve is sectioned with sharp microscissors (Figure 32–7, C), leaving the facial and cochlear nerves exposed and intact in the internal auditory canal (Figure 32–7, D). A plug of temporalis muscle is placed over the internal auditory canal, and the temporal lobe is allowed to expand. The bone flap is replaced, and the wound is closed in layers in a watertight fashion. A compression dressing is applied.

During hearing preservation surgery, the surgeon must remember that several important structures must be preserved. In addition to preserving the cochlea, labyrinth, and cochlear nerve, the labyrinthine artery within the internal auditory canal should be preserved. The surgeon should be aware of the fact that the anterior inferior cerebellar artery may loop into the internal auditory canal. Should this be the case, it is vital to dissect the vessel gently, free of surrounding structures, and maintain its integrity to prevent postoperative stroke.

Translabyrinthine Approach

The patient is placed in the supine position with the head turned away from the operative site. The hair is shaved above and behind the ear and the facial nerve monitor is attached along with other appropriate anesthetic monitors. Additionally, the left lower quadrant of the abdomen is prepared and draped to harvest an abdominal adipose graft. The left lower quadrant is used to avoid creating the appearance of an appendectomy scar.

A postauricular, C-shaped incision is made approximately 4 cm behind the postauricular crease (Figure 32–8, A). Dura hooks retract the edges of the skin flap anteriorly, and the musculoperiosteum is incised with electrocautery in a T- or C-shaped fashion. An elevator is used to elevate the musculoperiosteum, making sure not to tear the skin of the external auditory canal. Initially, a complete mastoidectomy is performed, exposing the middle and posterior fossa dural plates, sigmoid sinus, sinodural angle, antrum, and digastric ridge (Figure 32–8, B). Next the vertical portion of the facial nerve is identified with a fine-grit diamond bur and the facial recess is opened (Figure 32–8, C). The incudostapedial joint is separated and the incus is removed. In addition, the anterior attic is opened to remove the head of the malleus and facilitate exposure of the eustachian tube. A cylindrical piece of polytetrafluoroethylene/alumna compound (Proplast™) or a similar firm material is compressed and pushed into the eustachian tube orifice to prevent postoperative CSF rhinorrhea.

All bone is removed from the middle fossa dural plate, sinodural angle, and the sigmoid sinus at this point to provide ample working room to complete the labyrinthectomy and identify the internal auditory canal. Additionally, it is important to carry bone removal approximately 1 cm posterior to the sigmoid sinus so that the sinus can be retracted during subsequent tumor

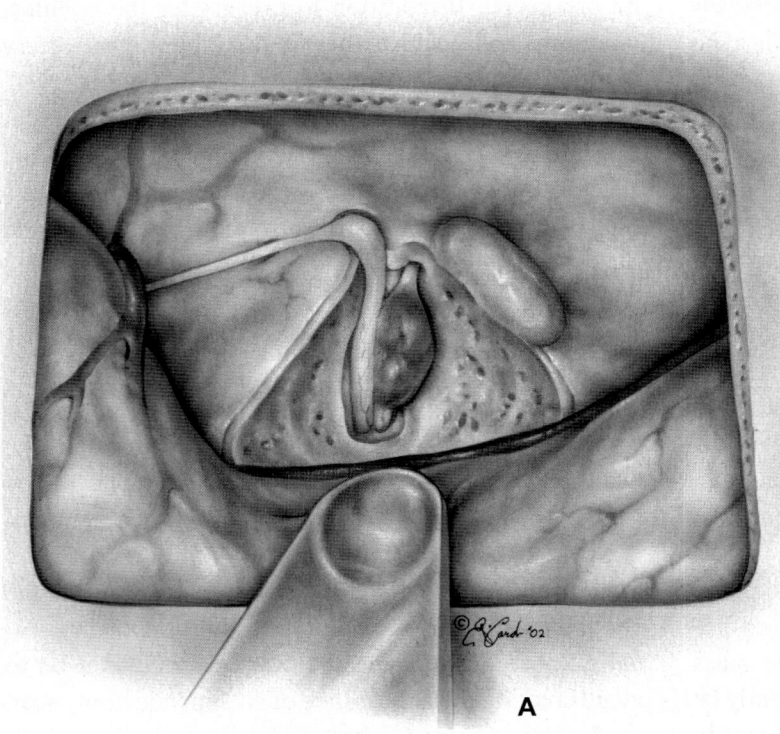

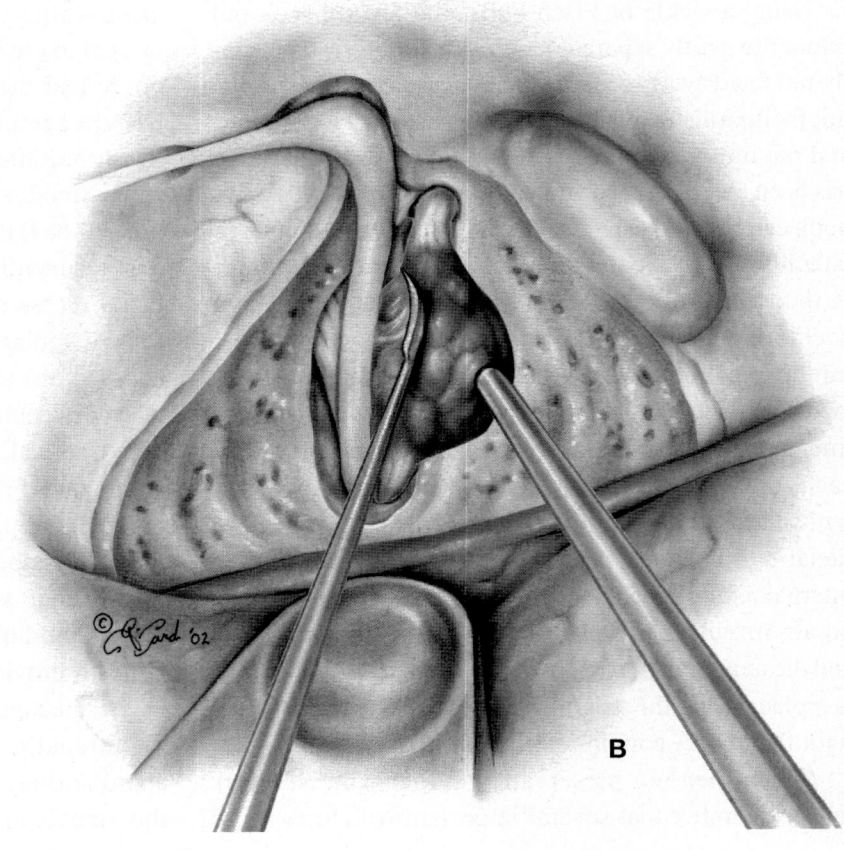

Figure 32–7 *A*, Middle fossa exposure of a right vestibular schwannoma. The internal auditory canal and its dura have been opened. The facial nerve is identified on the superior surface of the tumor. *B*, A suction tip is used to retract the tumor, and the plane between the facial nerve and tumor is developed. The facial nerve must be completely separated from the tumor prior to avulsing the superior vestibular nerve and dissecting the tumor from the cochlear nerve.

Continued on next page

Figure 32–7 (Continued) *C,* Once the tumor is dissected free from facial and cochlear nerves, the medial stalk of the vestibular nerve is sectioned with microscissors. *D,* The facial and cochlear nerves remain in the internal auditory canal after tumor dissection.

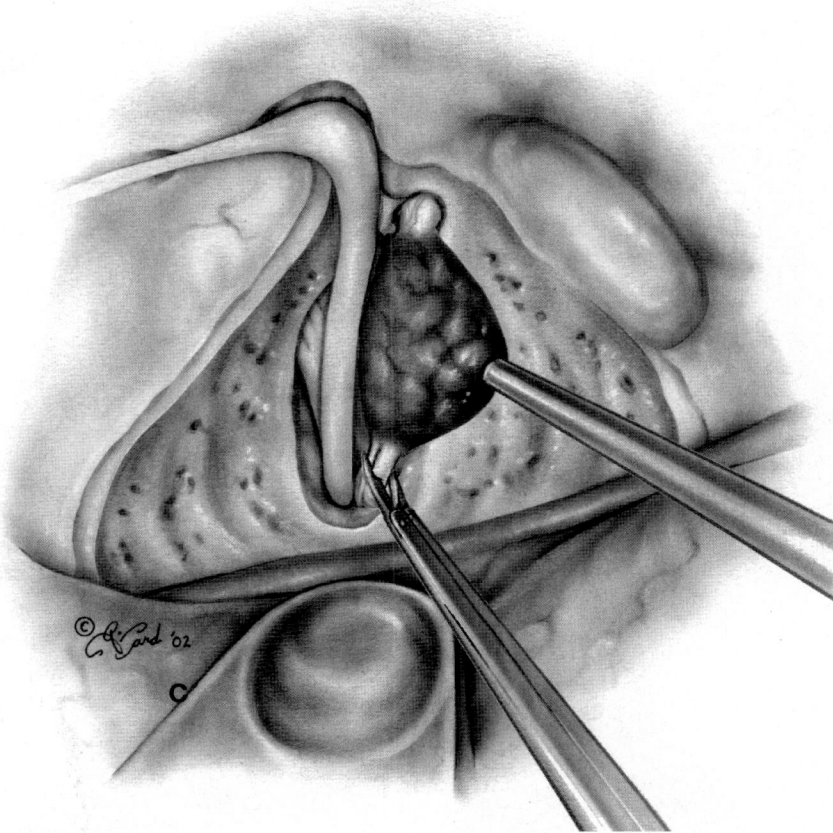

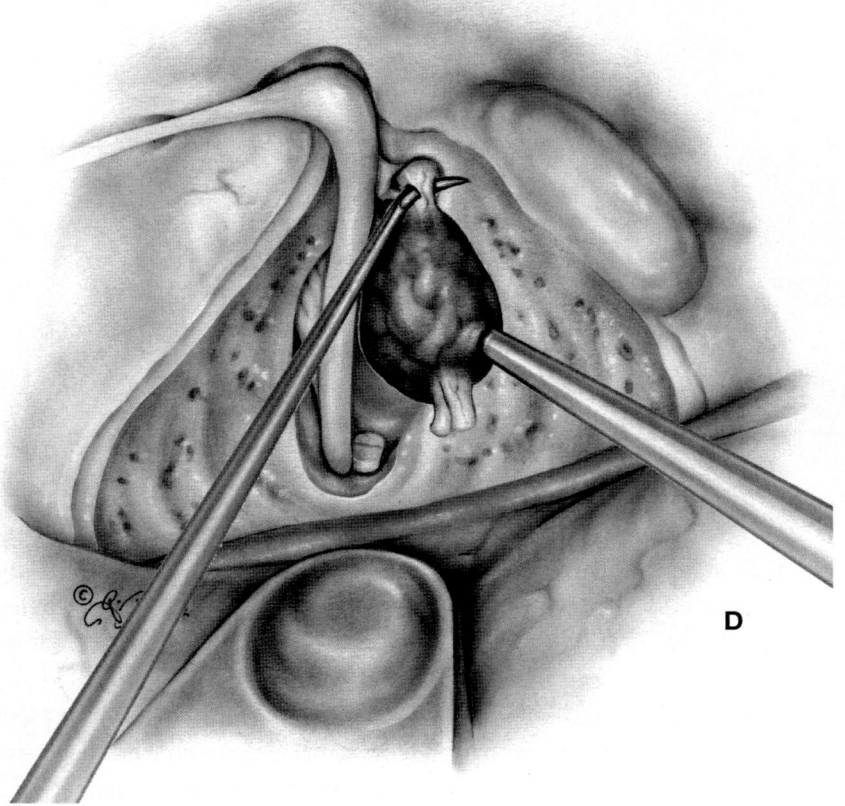

A

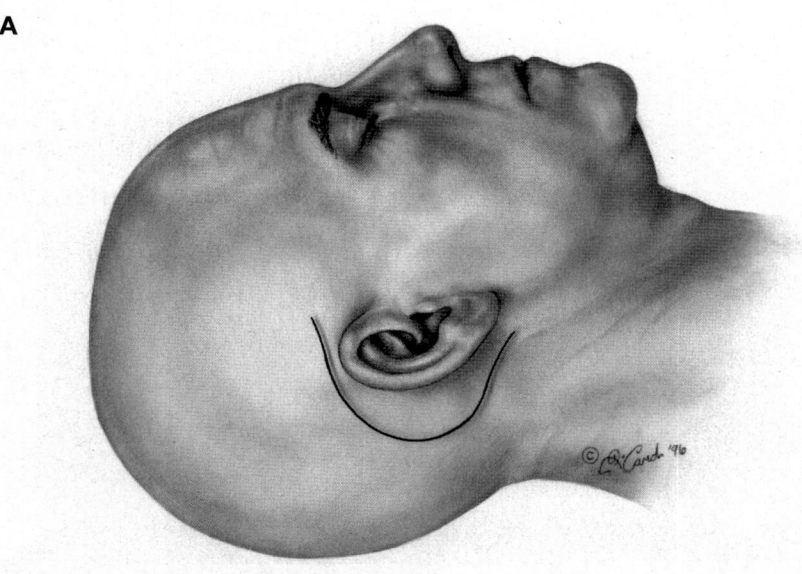

Figure 32–8 *A*, Translabyrinthine removal of a vestibular schwannoma. The postauricular incision is made approximately 4 cm posterior to the postauricular crease. *B*, A complete mastoidectomy is performed.

Continued on next page

B

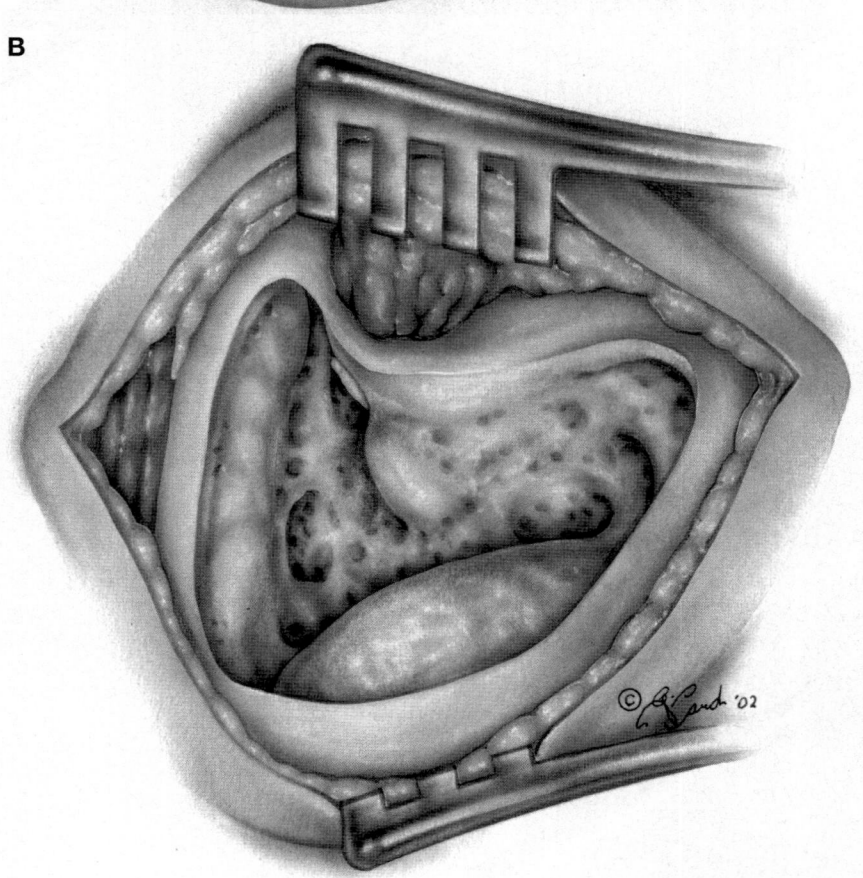

removal. Using a diamond bur and suction irrigation, the three semicircular canals are systematically removed, starting with the horizontal, moving to the posterior, and finishing with the common crus and superior canal (Figure 32–8, D). After the horizontal canal is removed with a fine-grit diamond bur to avoid injuring the horizontal segment of the facial nerve, a coarse diamond bur

may be used to complete the labyrinthectomy. The jugular bulb should be well defined; however, it is best to leave a thin shell of protective bone over this structure to prevent bleeding. Once the canals have been drilled away, the bone from the superior, inferior, and posterior aspects of the internal auditory canal is removed with successively smaller diamond burs and using copious irrigation. At

C

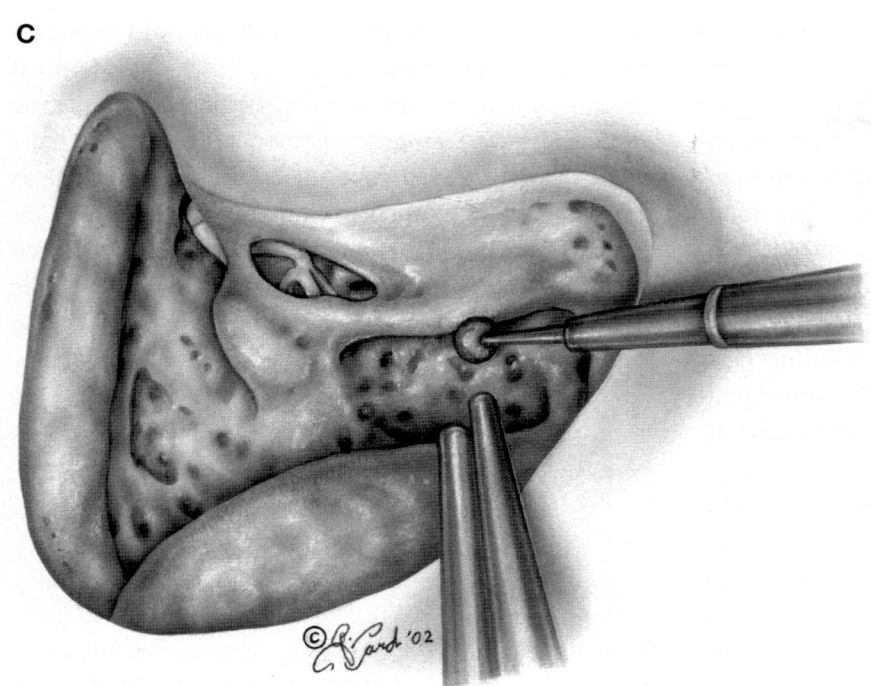

Figure 32–8 (Continued) *C*, The vertical portion of the facial nerve is identified and the facial recess is opened to gain access to the eustachian tube. *D*, The incudostapedial joint is separated and the incus removed. The malleus head is nipped, and the eustachian tube is occluded. The bone remaining over the sigmoid sinus and middle fossa dura is removed. A labyrinthectomy is performed.

Continued on next page

D

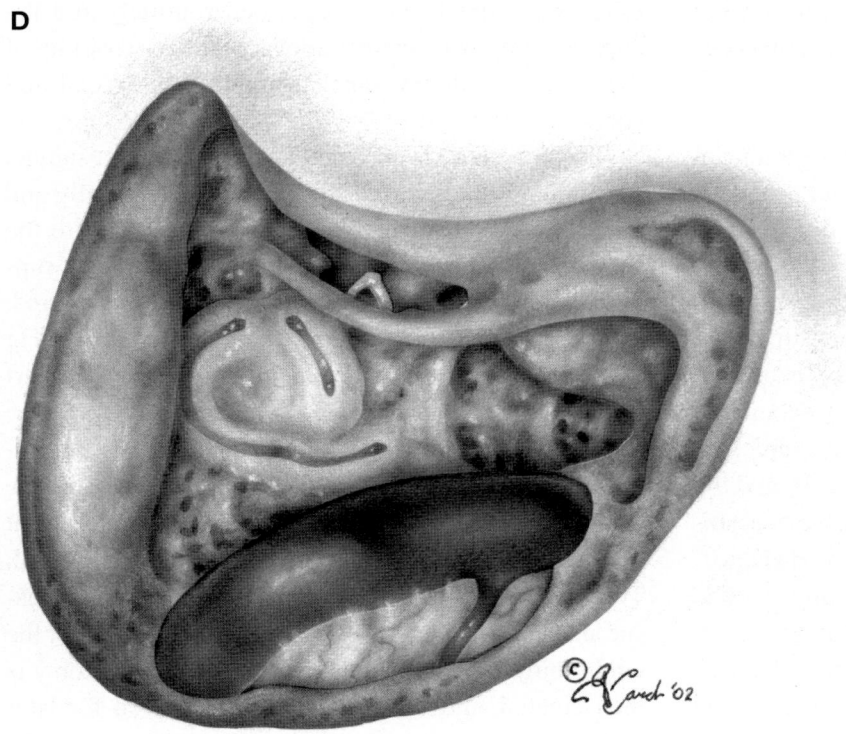

the fundus, the transverse crest, which separates the superior and inferior vestibular nerves, is identified. The macula cribosa superior (Mike's dot) facilitates identification of the lateral-most extent of the internal auditory canal and the facial and superior vestibular nerves. Figure 32–8, E, depicts the operative exposure at the completion of bone removal.

The posterior fossa dura is incised with a sharp knife blade or microscissors and a collagen sponge is placed under a cottonoid strip to protect the cerebellum. Microscissors are used to cut away the dura from the upper and lower edges of the internal auditory canal, connecting the incisions with the posterior fossa dura incisions, further exposing the cerebellum, tumors, and cerebellopontine angle. Small tumors are removed at this point without reducing them in size (Figure 32–8, F). Large lesions require reduction before they can be extracted (Figure 32–8, G), which begins with coagulating the tumor capsule vessels with a bipolar cautery and incising the capsule. Care should be exercised to cauterize only tumor capsule vessels. Larger vessels, such as the anterior inferior cerebellar artery, are gently swept off the tumor surface and preserved. The center of the tumor can be gutted using a variety of techniques, including laser vaporization, aspiration with the CUSA® (Cavitron Ultrasonic Surgical Aspirator, Valleylab, Boulder, Colorado), or simply microcup forceps extraction.

Once the tumor has been reduced in size, the posterior, superior, inferior, and medial aspects of the tumor capsule are dissected from the surrounding arachnoid, cerebellum, and brainstem. As the tumor is mobilized, cottonoid strips are gently placed between the tumor capsule and surrounding structures. Reducing the tumor capsule may facilitate identifying its medial relationship to the brainstem. The medial end of the facial nerve is identified at the brainstem with the aid of the facial nerve stimulator.

The remainder of the tumor is removed beginning at the fundus of the internal auditory canal and progressing medially. The vertical crest is identified. The superior vestibular nerve is gently displaced to allow visualization of the anteriorly located facial nerve, which is positively identified with the facial nerve stimulator (set at 0.05 milliamps). A right-angled hook is used to avulse the superior vestibular nerve and fully expose the facial nerve. The inferior vestibular and cochlear nerves are also released from their lateral attachments, and the plane between the tumor and the facial nerve is established. Tumor is removed from the canal in a medial direction, dissecting it away from the facial nerve. The House-Hough facial nerve dissector facilitates separating the anterior tumor capsule from the nerve. Dissection continues until the facial nerve is seen entering the brainstem and the tumor is free from the nerve. At this point, microscissors are used to sever the eighth nerve from the brainstem, and the tumor specimen is removed. The facial nerve is stimulated at the brainstem to determine its integrity, and the cerebellopontine angle is irrigated to identify any bleeding. Hemostasis is controlled with bipolar cautery and topical hemostatic agents as necessary.

The middle ear is packed with pieces of temporalis muscle, and approximately 1-inch strips of abdominal fat are used to fill the surgical defect. Care must be exercised when filling the dural opening adjacent to the facial nerve to prevent its avulsion. Tissue glues such as Tisseel® (Baxter Healthcare Corporation, Glendale, California) can be used. The musculoperiosteum is closed with absorbable suture in an interrupted fashion, and the skin is closed with a running-locking, continuous nylon suture. Every effort is made to ensure a watertight closure to prevent postoperative CSF leak. A mastoid-type compression dressing is placed, and the patient is observed overnight in the neurologic intensive care unit.

Suboccipital Approach

The suboccipital (retrosigmoid) approach to the cerebellopontine angle was first advocated by Dandy.[7] The microscope has been incorporated routinely and the approach improved on by removal of the posterior lip of the internal auditory canal to identify the facial and cochlear nerves.

The procedure is performed with the patient supine, chin slightly tucked, and the head turned laterally and placed in Mayfield pinions. Two disadvantages to the seated position are air embolism and lumbar disk rupture; therefore, the supine or lateral position is preferred. Hyperventilating the patient to a CO_2 level of 25 mm Hg and the use of intravenous mannitol (1 g/kg) at the start of the case help reduce intracranial pressure.

A curvilinear incision is made approximately four fingerbreadths behind the postauricular crease (Figure 32–9, A and B). The musculoperiosteum and cervical musculature are incised vertically down to the skull. The Lempert periosteal elevator is used to sweep this tissue anteriorly and posteriorly to provide exposure for the craniotomy. An approximately 4 × 4 cm craniotomy is then created, and the bone flap is preserved for later replacement. The superior limit of the craniotomy is the transverse sinus, and the anterior extent is the sigmoid sinus. The dura is initially incised with a #15 blade, and a cottonoid sponge is placed through the dural opening to protect the cerebellum. The remainder of the incision is made with microscissors, and the dura is retracted with stay sutures (Figure 32–9, C). Moistened microgelatin foam is placed on the outer surface of the retracted dura

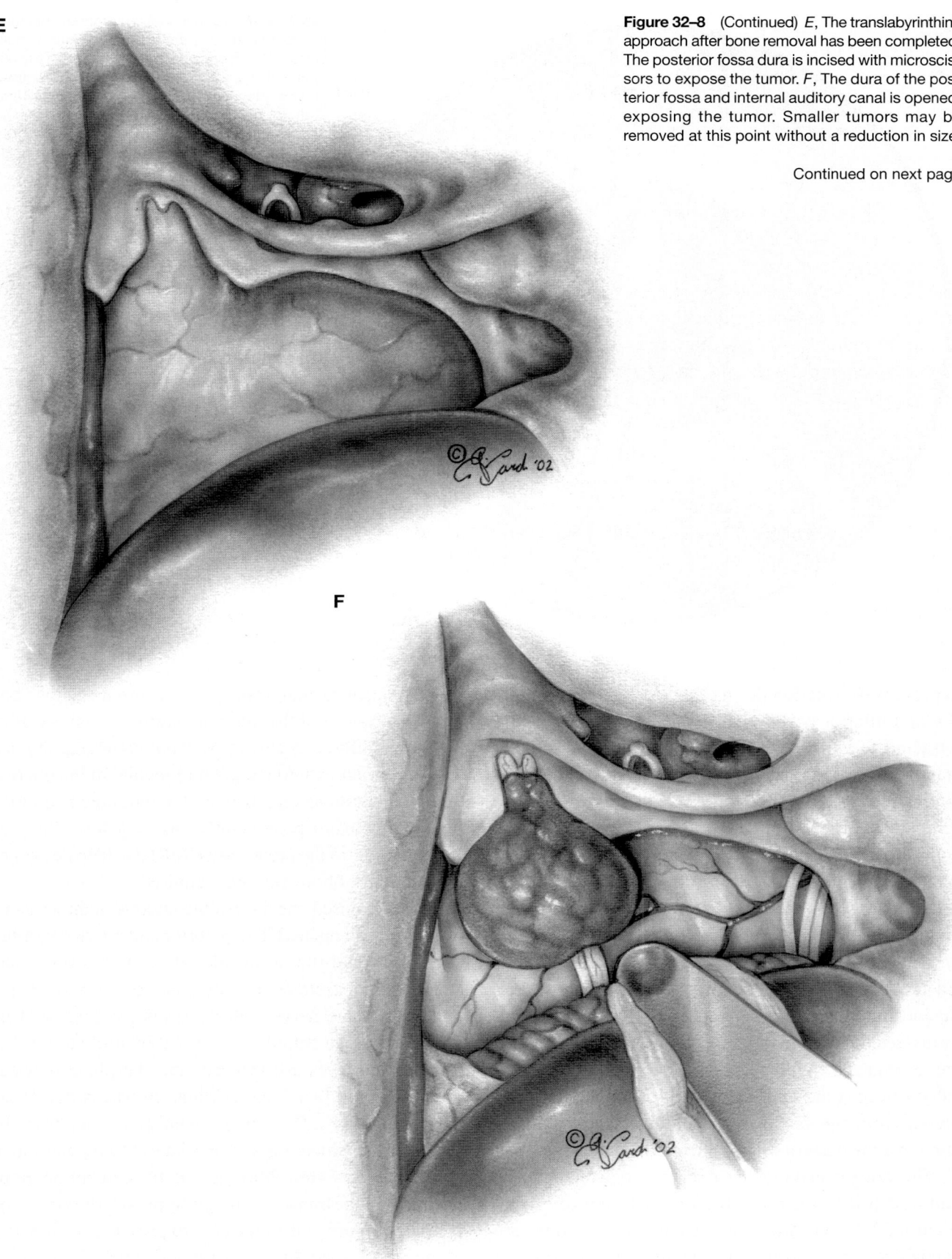

Figure 32–8 (Continued) *E,* The translabyrinthine approach after bone removal has been completed. The posterior fossa dura is incised with microscissors to expose the tumor. *F,* The dura of the posterior fossa and internal auditory canal is opened, exposing the tumor. Smaller tumors may be removed at this point without a reduction in size.

Continued on next page

E

F

G

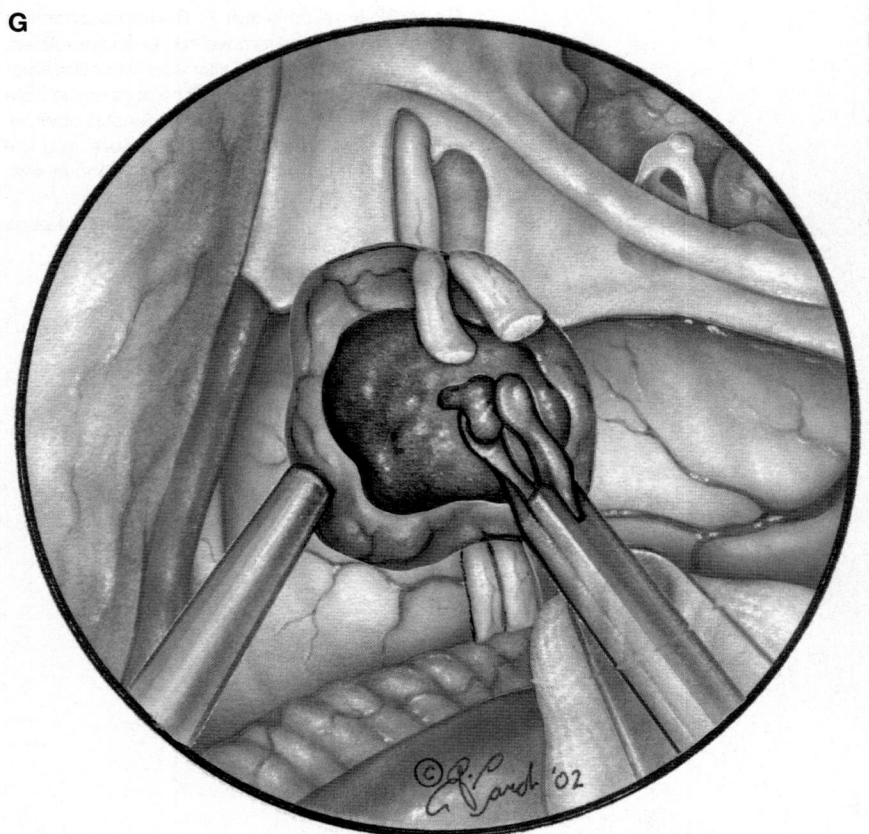

Figure 32–8 (Continued) *G*, Larger tumors must be reduced in size prior to removal. After debulking, the tumor capsule is separated from the surrounding structures. The vertical crest is identified, and the superior vestibular nerve is retracted inferiorly to identify the facial nerve. The vestibular nerves are avulsed, and the facial nerve is dissected free from the tumor in a lateral to medial direction.

to prevent desiccation during the procedure. The anterior and inferior portions of the cerebellum are gently retracted to expose the cerebellopontine cistern. An arachnoid knife is used to pierce the arachnoid, promoting the egress of CSF and cerebellar relaxation. The cerebellum is gently retracted to expose the cerebellopontine angle and tumor (Figure 32–9, *D*). Cottonoid sponges are placed over a biologic collagen sponge between the cerebellum and retractor to decrease trauma to the surface of the cerebellum.

The tumor capsule is incised, and the tumor is gutted and reduced, as previously described. The posterior, superior, inferior, and medial aspects of the tumor are gently dissected free from the cerebellum and brainstem, and the seventh and eighth nerves are identified at their root entry zones. If the tumor is small, it is completely dissected from the facial and cochlear nerves prior to removing the posterior lip of the internal auditory canal.

The dura overlying the posterior petrous apex is removed prior to drilling the internal auditory canal (Figure 32–9, *D*). Additionally, cottonoid sponges are placed around the porus to keep bone from entering the

cerebellopontine angle. Then, using a 3-mm diamond bur, the posterior lip of the internal auditory canal is drilled as far laterally as necessary without damaging the otic capsule structures. Staying 2 mm medial to the operculum and not advancing beyond the blue-lined common crus helps avoid postoperative hearing loss. Furthermore, review of the preoperative MRI can help determine the amount of bone removal required.

Once exposed, the dura of the internal auditory canal is incised and opened. The superior and inferior vestibular nerves and tumor are identified within the canal. Gentle inferior retraction of the superior vestibular nerve reveals the facial nerve, which is positively identified with the facial nerve stimulator (set at 0.05 milliamps). The vestibular nerves are avulsed, and the plane between the tumor and facial and cochlear nerves is developed (Figure 32–9, *E*). The tumor is gently dissected from the facial and cochlear nerves in a lateral to medial direction. The nerves are followed into the cerebellopontine angle, as in the translabyrinthine approach (Figure 32–9, *F*). The surgeon must take care to preserve the labyrinthine artery in hearing preservation cases.

A

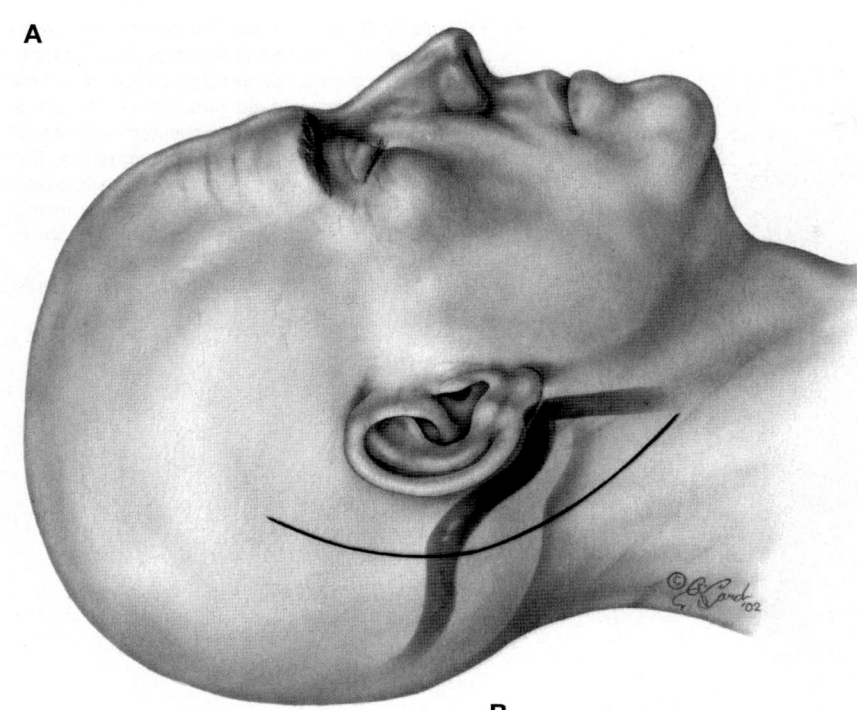

Figure 32–9 *A*, Suboccipital removal of a vestibular schwannoma. A curvilinear incision is made approximately four fingerbreadths behind the postauricular crease. Note the relationship of the incision to the sigmoid sinus, transverse sinus, and cerebellum. *B*, The incision margins are retracted, and a 4 × 4 cm craniotomy is created. The superior limit of the craniotomy is the transverse sinus, and the anterior limit is the sigmoid sinus.

Continued on next page

B

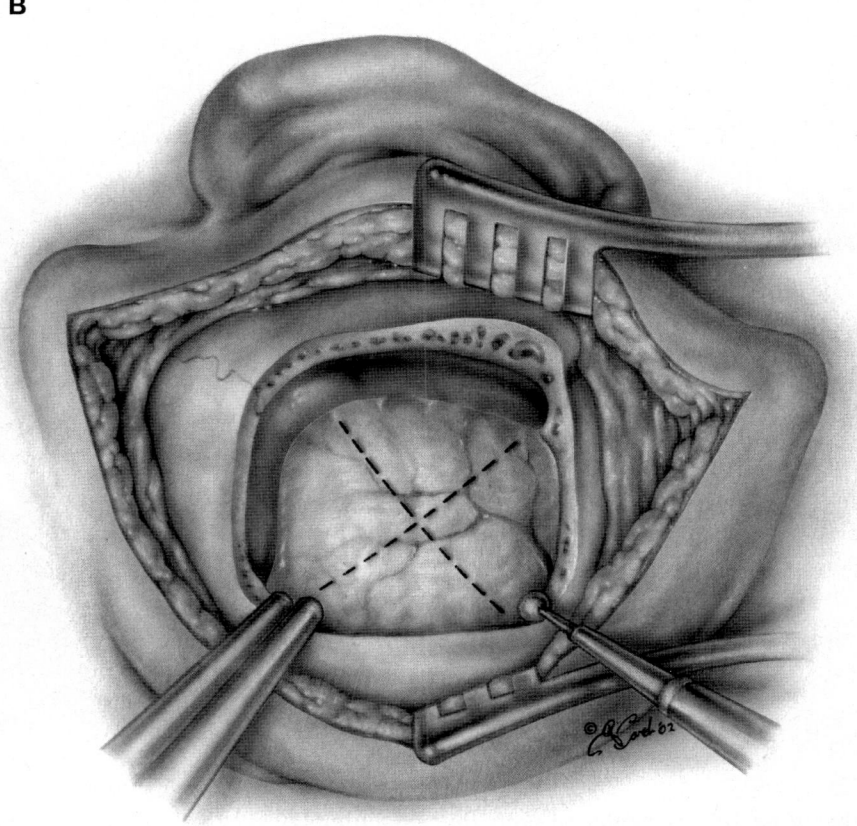

Once the tumor has been completely removed, all cottonoid sponges are removed. The surgical field is copiously irrigated and hemostasis obtained. The bone of the internal auditory canal is carefully inspected for air cells, and if any are visualized, they are occluded with bone wax. A piece of muscle is placed into the internal auditory canal to help prevent postoperative CSF leakage. The dura is closed in a running fashion with 3-0 silk,

C

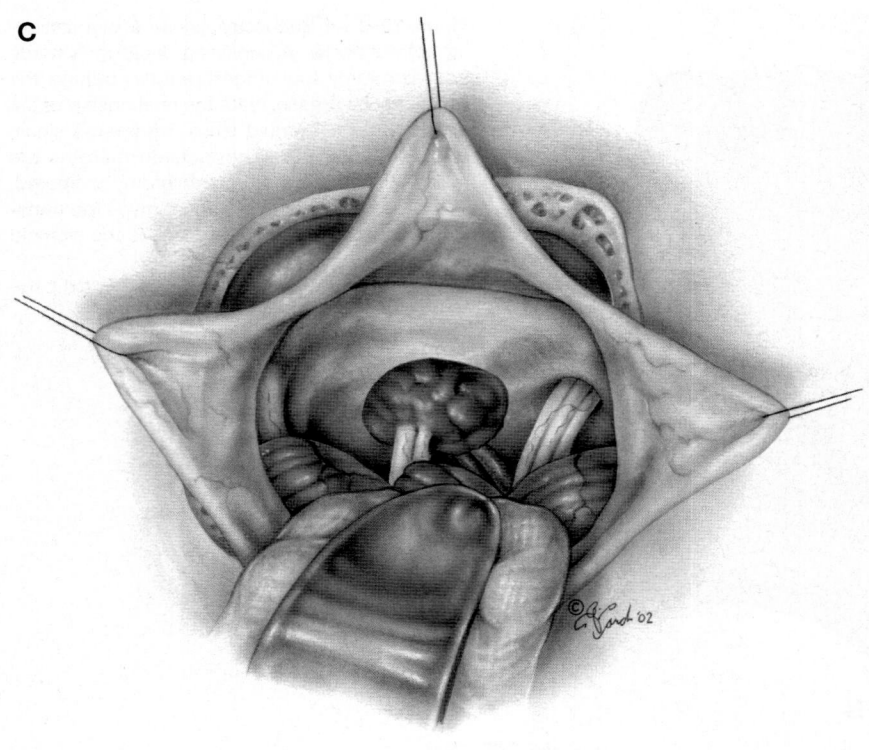

Figure 32–9 (Continued) *C*, Mannitol and hyperventilation provide brain relaxation, and the posterior fossa dura is opened. The cerebellopontine cistern is decompressed and the cerebellum is retracted to expose the cerebellopontine angle and tumor. *D*, Using a 3-mm diamond bur, the posterior lip of the internal auditory canal is drilled away. Staying 2 mm medial to the operculum and not advancing beyond the blue-lined common crus helps avoid violating otic capsule.

Continued on next page

D

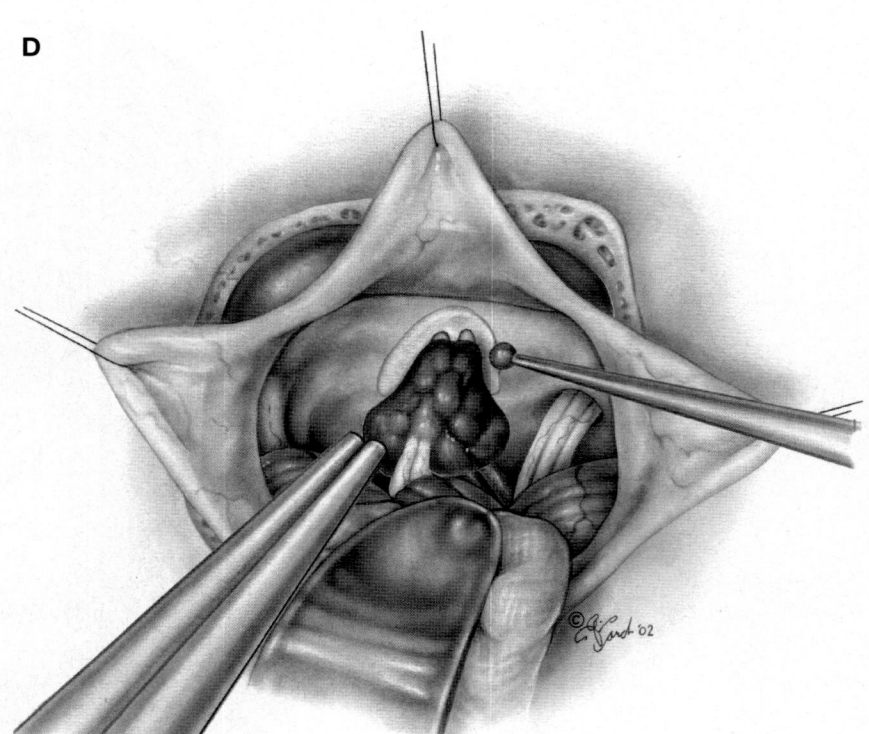

the bone flap is replaced, and the muscular layer is closed in layers with an absorbable suture. The skin is closed with a running 3-0 nylon suture (or stainless steel surgical clips), and a sterile pressure dressing is applied. The patient is monitored overnight in the neurologic intensive care unit.

One recent advance that has improved the visualization of the fundus of the internal auditory canal and hence has reduced the likelihood of leaving tumor behind is the intraoperative use of a 30-degree endoscope. The use of the endoscope eliminates blind dissection in the fundus and decreases the risk of residual disease.[98]

E

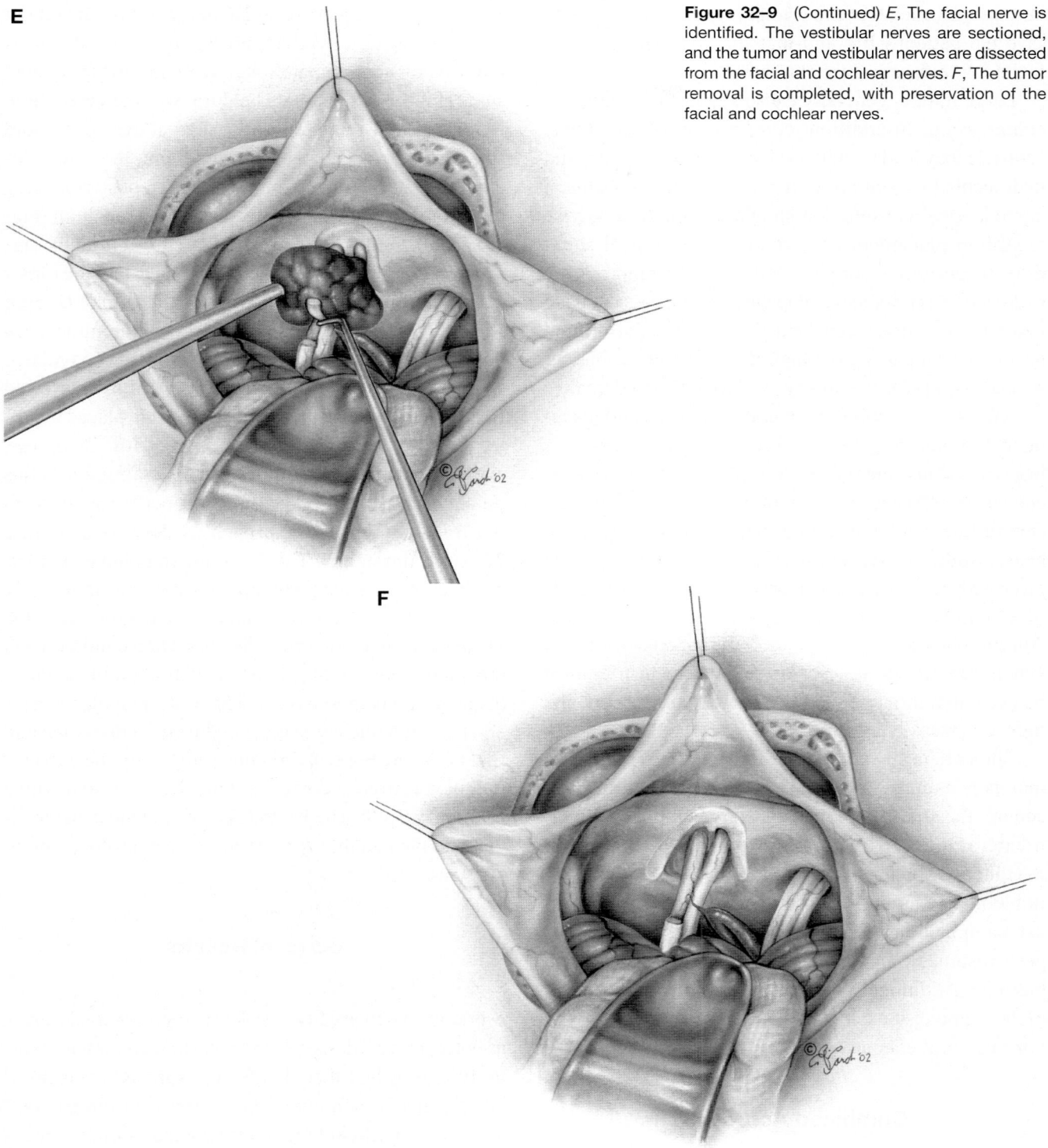

Figure 32–9 (Continued) *E*, The facial nerve is identified. The vestibular nerves are sectioned, and the tumor and vestibular nerves are dissected from the facial and cochlear nerves. *F*, The tumor removal is completed, with preservation of the facial and cochlear nerves.

F

Management of Large Vestibular Schwannomas

Giant (4.0 cm or larger) vestibular schwannomas require special perioperative, intraoperative, and anesthetic pre-cautions to prevent serious complications. As with any surgery, existing medical conditions are optimally managed prior to surgery. Furthermore, the consulting internist is informed that the operative, and hence anesthetic time, may be prolonged. Patients and their families are informed that the primary goal of surgery is to save the patient's life and that the chances of saving facial nerve function are extremely poor.

Large tumors generally cause significant brainstem compression. In addition, compression of the fourth ventricle may lead to increased intracranial pressure and hydrocephalus. Therefore, if there is hydrocephalus, a neurosurgical consultation should be sought to advise regarding placement of a ventriculoperitoneal shunt prior to definitive surgery. Failure to decompress the hydrocephalus prior to opening the posterior fossa or placing a lumbar drain can lead to brain herniation and death. The patient is given high-dose dexamethasone for several days prior to surgery to reduce brain edema.

After the induction of general anesthesia and placement of monitoring devices, a central venous catheter is inserted because the risk of air embolism may be heightened by the presence of a ventriculoperitoneal shunt; the central line can be used to evacuate air from the right heart. Additionally, intravenous mannitol (1 g/kg) is given early in the case, and hyperventilation to a CO_2 level of 25 mm Hg is used to decrease intracranial pressure. Additional diuresis can be accomplished with intravenous furosemide as necessary. Blood chemistries must be evaluated intraoperatively to detect and correct any induced electrolyte disturbances.

The patient's head is placed in Mayfield pinions to maintain stability throughout the case. During the procedure, the anesthesiologist and surgeon must communicate and be cognizant of the signs of brainstem dysfunction, such as an alteration in heart rate or a rise in blood pressure. If brainstem signs appear, all surgical manipulation near the brainstem is stopped, and surgery resumes only after vital signs have returned to baseline. Additionally, care is taken to avoid occlusion of the sigmoid sinus; loss of this venous channel can provoke cerebral edema.

Combined Approach

The one-stage, combined translabyrinthine-suboccipital approach described by Glasscock and Hays[44] was developed for the removal of giant vestibular schwannomas. The postauricular flap is larger than the one used for the translabyrinthine approach to expose more of the occipital bone and is retracted forward by dura hooks (Figure 32–10, A). A translabyrinthine approach is carried out as previously described (Figure 32–10, B). Next bone is removed for approximately 4 cm posterior to the sigmoid sinus (Figure 32–10, B). The dura over the cerebellum is incised and retracted with stay sutures. Cottonoid sponges are placed over the cerebellum, the cerebellopontine cistern is decompressed, and a posterior fossa retractor is inserted to gently retract the cerebellum (Figure 32–10, C). The tumor margins are freed from the surrounding tissues with cottonoid sponges, and the tumor center is removed to decompress the tumor (Figure 32–10, D). The capsule is cut away as the tumor size decreases. All vessels entering the tumor are coagulated with bipolar cautery. The capsule is carefully dissected free from the brainstem, and cottonoids are placed to protect the brainstem. The tumor is reduced to 2 cm or less, and the facial nerve is identified at the brainstem. At this point, the remainder of the surgery is performed through the translabyrinthine approach as described (Figure 32–10, E through I). The facial nerve is identified laterally in the internal auditory canal and traced medially toward the brainstem. The tumor is separated from the facial nerve and removed as the dissection continues. On complete tumor removal, the cerebellopontine angle is irrigated and hemostasis is obtained with bipolar cautery and topical hemostatic agents. The eustachian tube and middle ear are packed, abdominal adipose tissue is placed within the surgical defect, and the dura is closed with a running 3-0 silk. The wound is closed in the usual manner, and the patient is observed in the neurologic intensive care unit.

Surgical Results

Mortality and morbidity rates have progressively declined, as noted above. Glasscock and colleagues reported a mortality rate of less than 1% for the surgical excision of vestibular schwannomas.[99] Our series is in agreement.[76] The most significant factor influencing mortality rate is early tumor diagnosis through heightened physician and patient awareness. Early detection leads to decreased morbidity as well, with improved postoperative facial nerve function and hearing preservation. Preservation of facial nerve function is, to a great extent, size dependent,[100–102] although the tumor type also plays a role. Cystic tumors have a distinctly poorer facial nerve outcome.[103] Our series,

A

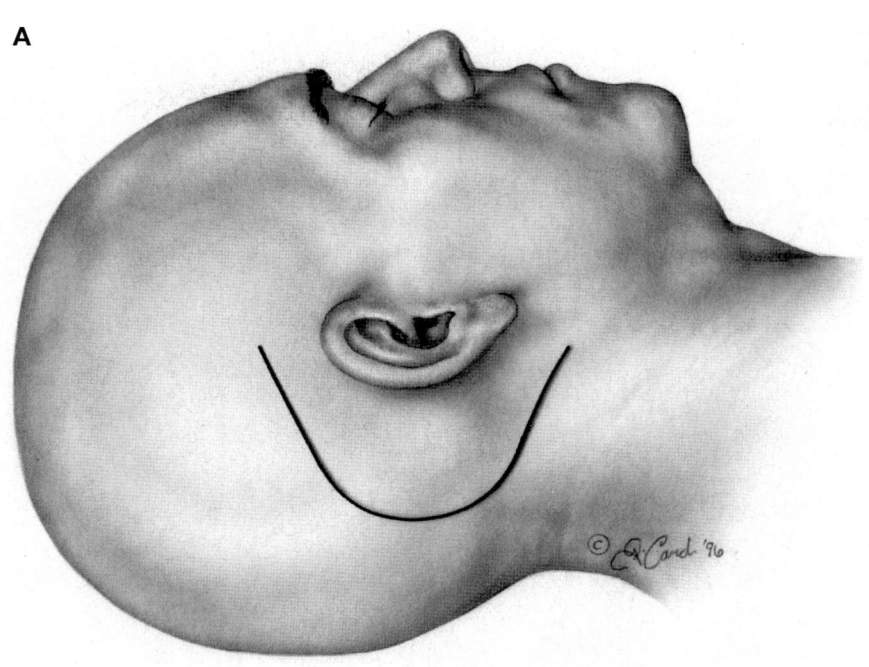

B

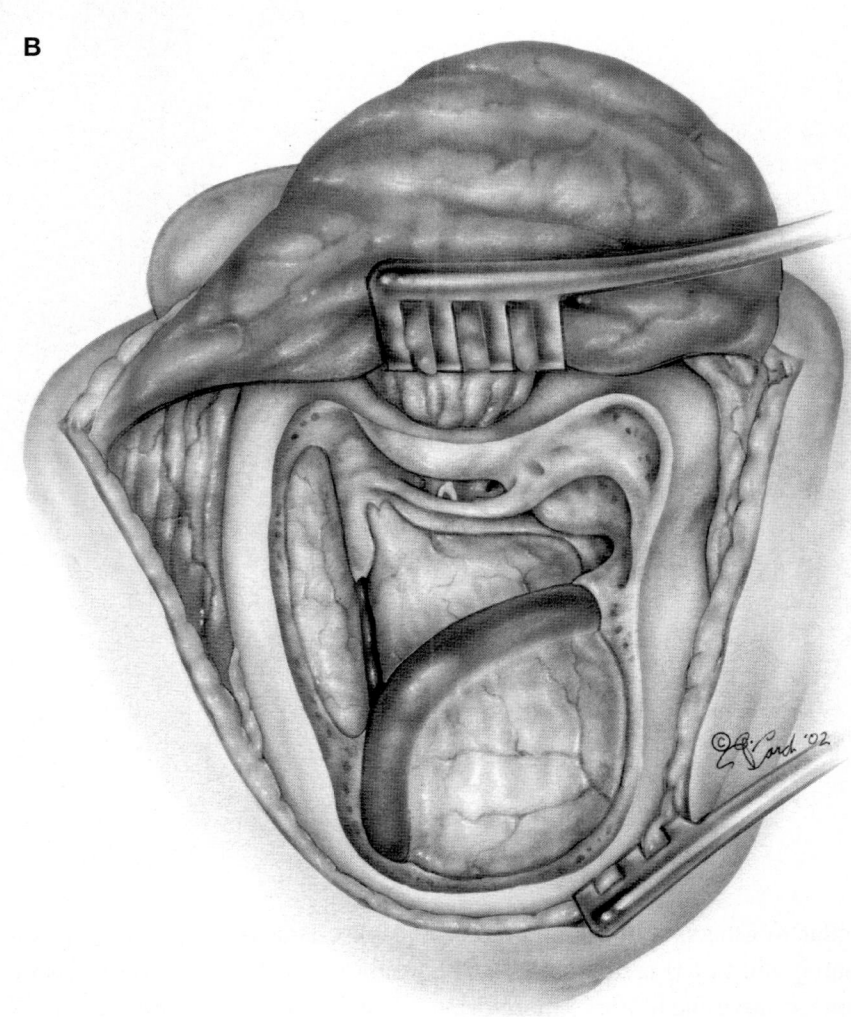

Figure 32–10 *A,* The combined approach for removal of giant vestibular schwannomas. A large postauricular flap is created. *B,* The translabyrinthine approach is accomplished first. Continued on next page

Figure 32–10 (Continued) *C*, A 4 × 4 cm area of bone is removed posterior to the sigmoid sinus and inferior to the transverse sinus to enable exposure of the posterior portion of the tumor. *D*, Once brain relaxation has been obtained, the posterior fossa dura is opened, the cerebellopontine cistern is decompressed, and the cerebellum is retracted. The tumor is gutted to reduce its size.

Continued on next page

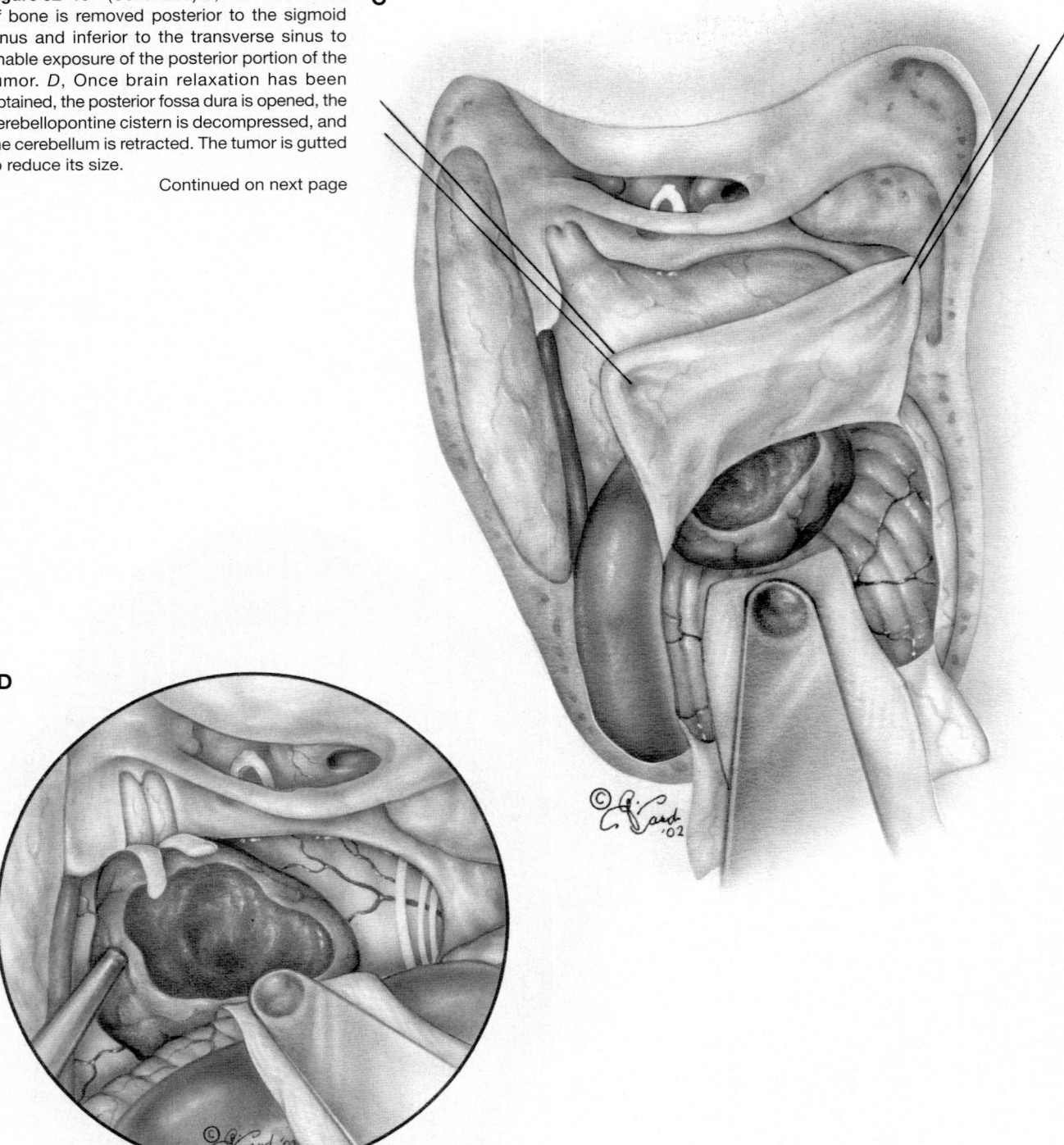

similar to others, shows preservation of House-Brackmann grade I or II results in 88% of all tumors.[76,104,105] Intraoperative facial nerve monitoring, which over the past decade has become "standard of care" for vestibular schwannoma surgery, has been associated with improved postoperative function.[104,105] Hearing preservation is also directly related to early detection, with preservation rates ranging from 26 to 60%.[76,100,101,106] Cerebrospinal fluid leak rates have declined to less than 10% with improved wound closure technique.[107] The

E

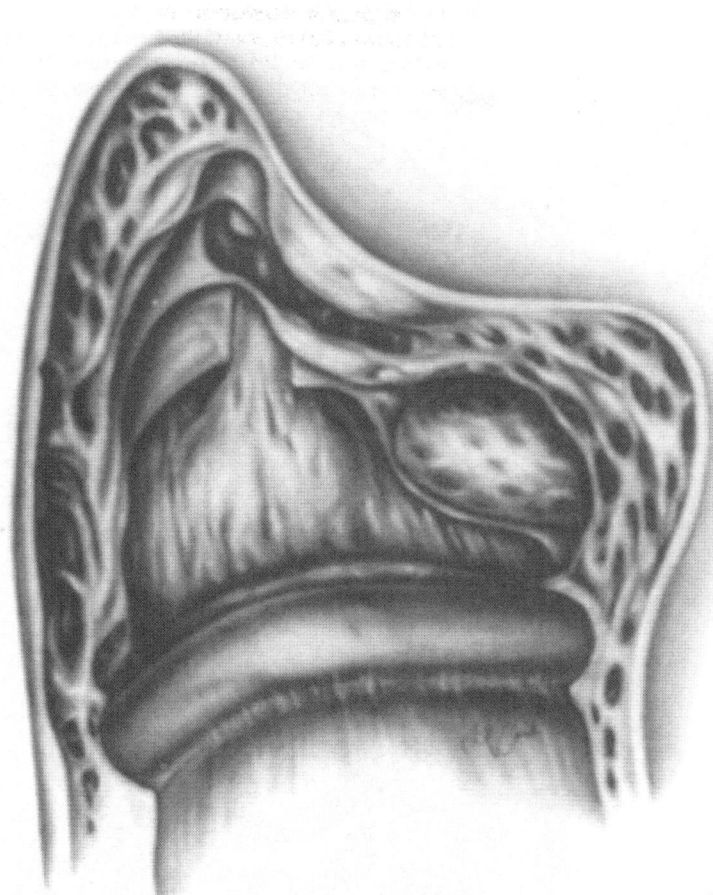

Figure 32–10 (Continued) *E*, Once the tumor has been reduced in size, the table is rotated back toward the surgeon, and the dura of the posterior fossa and internal auditory canal is opened. *F*, The vertical crest is identified, and the superior vestibular nerve is avulsed from its canal, revealing the facial nerve anterior to Bill's bar.

Continued on next page

F

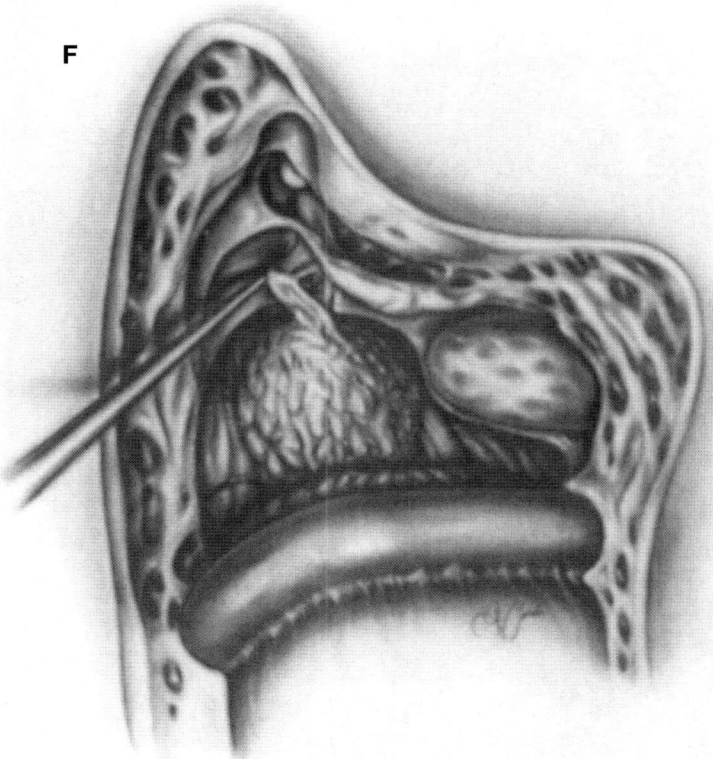

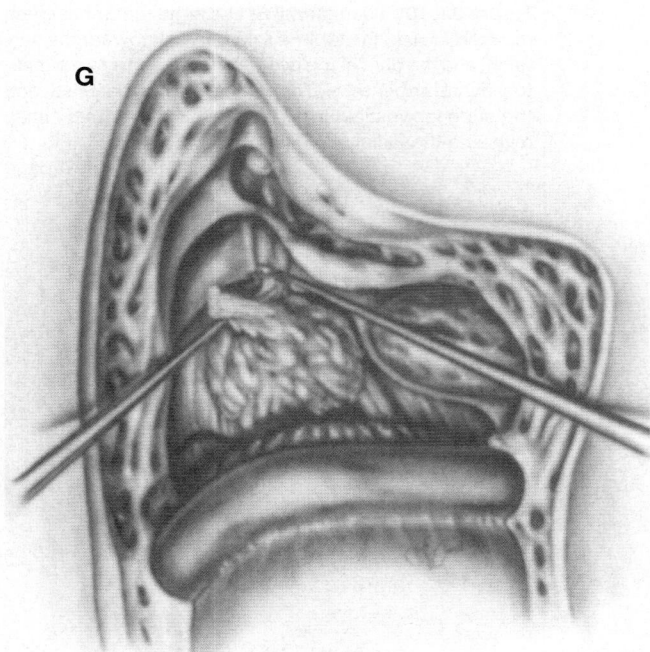

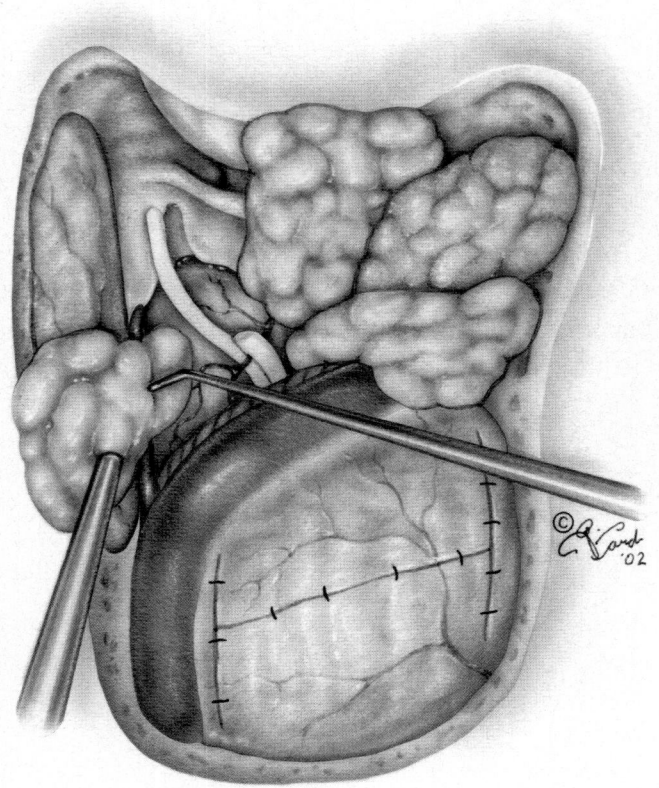

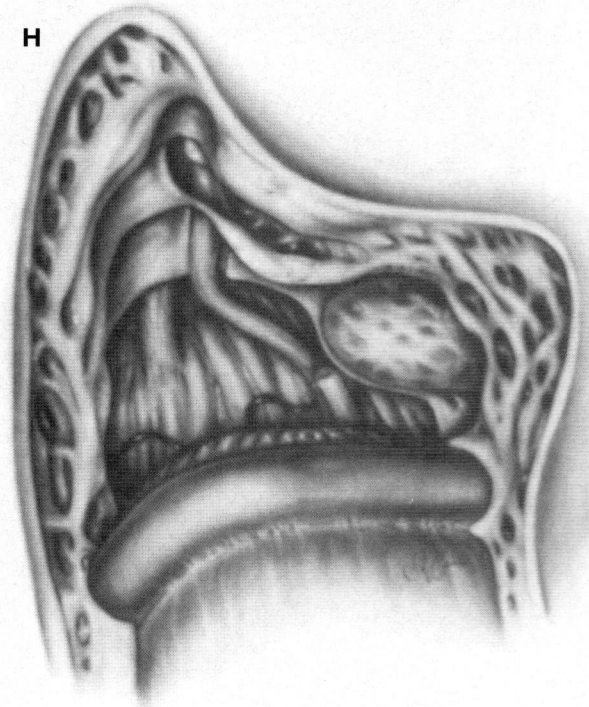

Figure 32–10 (Continued) *G*, The plane between the tumor and facial nerve is established, and the tumor is dissected free. *H*, The dissection is complete. The facial and superiorly located trigeminal nerves are seen in the cerebellopontine angle.

use of autologous fibrin glue has not been shown to significantly reduce CSF leak rates[108,109]; however, pooled fibrin glue may have some advantages.[110]

MENINGIOMA OF THE TEMPORAL BONE

Meningiomas are the second most common neoplasm in the cerebellopontine angle and therefore deserve brief discussion. Meningiomas are nonmetastasizing but often locally invasive benign neoplasms. They arise from the endothelial lining cells of the arachnoid villi found in the walls of the cranial venous sinuses and their tributary veins. Although meningiomas constitute approximately 18% of primary brain tumors, only about 3% of meningiomas arise from the petrous pyramid, about equally from its middle and posterior fossa surfaces.[111] Occasionally, it may be difficult at presentation to differentiate a meningioma from a vestibular schwannoma.

Symptoms produced by meningiomas are most often secondary to adjacent cranial nerve and brain compression. Tumors arising from the middle fossa surface of the petrous pyramid cause facial or eye pain and sensory and motor changes in the distribution of the fifth cranial nerve. Involvement of the fourth cranial nerve manifests with diplopia. As the lesion enlarges, seizures and sensory and motor aphasia may occur. The otolaryngologist is rarely the initial physician consulted by these patients. Meningiomas arising from the posterior surface of the petrous pyramid may present with the cerebellopontine angle syndrome, clinically mimicking a vestibular schwannoma. A meningioma arising within the internal auditory canal produces symptoms indistinguishable from those of a vestibular schwannoma; however, a meningioma usually originates outside the canal and involves adjacent cranial nerves and the cerebellum before affecting the eighth cranial nerve.

It is difficult to distinguish between vestibular schwannomas and meningiomas by audiovestibular testing. Imaging can often differentiate the two tumors. On contrast CT, meningiomas tend to have more marked and homogeneous enhancement than vestibular schwannomas and characteristically contain areas of calcification. Meningiomas are usually isointense or slightly hypointense to gray matter on T_1-weighted MRI sequences, with variable intensity on T_2-weighted images.

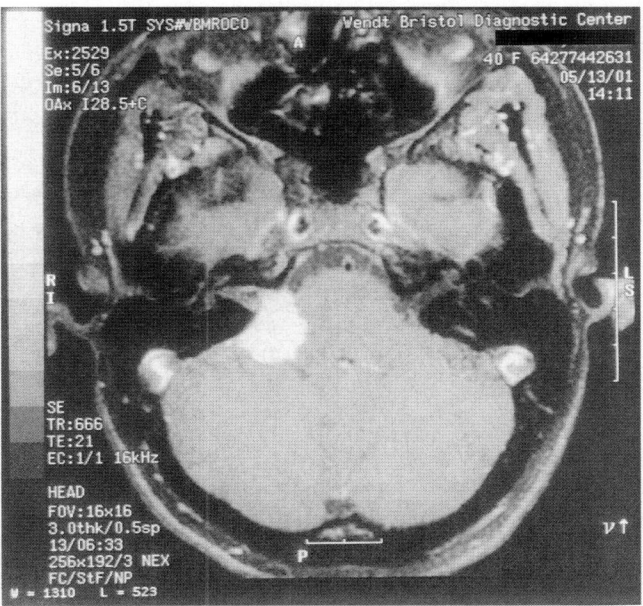

Figure 32–11 A cerebellopontine angle meningioma as seen on a gadolinium-enhanced, T_1-weighted magnetic resonance image. Note the broad-based attachment to the posterior fossa dura and the small posterior dural "tail."

Both vestibular schwannomas and meningiomas enhance on gadolinium-enhanced T_1-weighted images, but the vestibular schwannoma usually enhances more markedly. The shape of the lesion is also very useful in differentiating these tumors. Radiographically, meningiomas have a broad base of attachment to the posterior petrous pyramid and demonstrate a dural "tail," whereas vestibular schwannomas do not (Figure 32–11).

Meningiomas confined to the cerebellopontine angle are managed identically as described for the suboccipital approach to vestibular schwannomas. In cases in which hearing is severely impaired, the translabyrinthine approach may be used. Interestingly, the facial nerve is often splayed over the posterior aspect of the tumor, in contrast to vestibular schwannomas, in which the nerve is most often found anteriorly. This finding is likely related to the differing origin of these tumors. Meningiomas are typically slow-growing tumors, and surgical resection usually relieves symptoms. Long-term follow-up is necessary to validate complete removal.

Meningiomas that are located in the far anterior reaches of the cerebellopontine angle can be approached in a number of ways. The transcochlear approach has been used to gain access to this portion of the angle (Figure 32–12, A through E).[112] Traditionally, on completion of

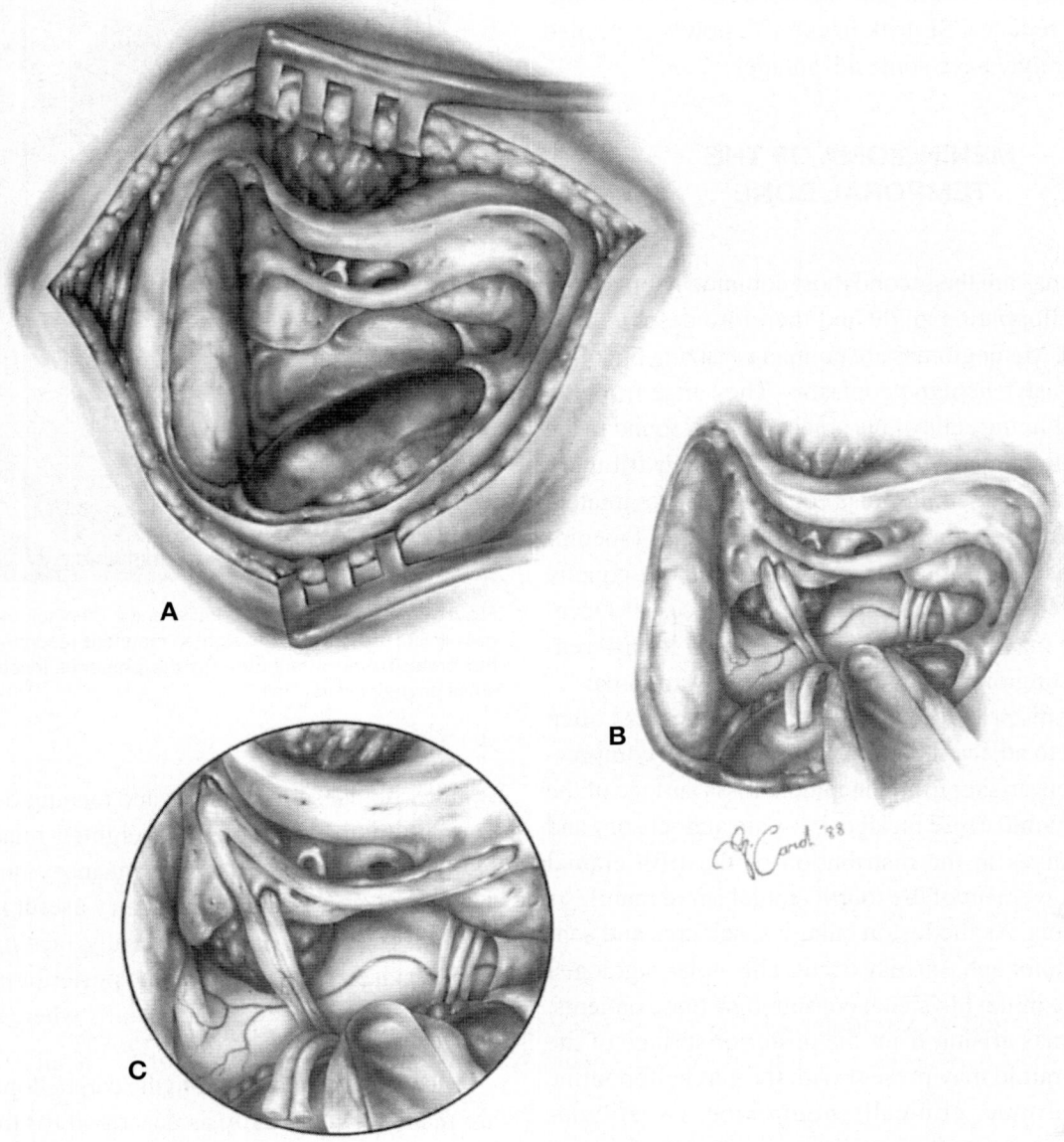

Figure 32–12 *A*, Transcochlear approach to the anterior cerebellopontine angle. The internal auditory canal has been exposed using the standard translabyrinthine approach. *B*, The posterior fossa and internal auditory canal dura have been opened. The superior and inferior vestibular nerves have been released from their lateral attachments, enabling visualization of the superiorly located facial nerve and the inferiorly located cochlear nerve. The meningioma can be seen within the confines of the anterior cerebellopontine angle, anterior to the facial and cochlear nerves. *C*, The labyrinthine segment of the facial nerve is identified, and the entire intratemporal course of the facial nerve is exposed. The nerve is skeletonized prior to mobilization.

Continued on next page

a translabyrinthine approach, the facial nerve is dissected from its fallopian canal and translocated posteriorly. The bone of the cochlea is drilled away, as is the bone medial to the carotid artery in the petrous apex. This bone removal expands access for tumor dissection anteriorly along the clivus.

Another approach to far anterior tumors is accomplished without facial nerve transposition. A transcochlear approach is still used; however, the cochlea is accessed after the canal wall has been taken down and the tympanic membrane removed. Wound closure includes closure of the external auditory canal.

In addition, House and colleagues have described an adapted middle fossa approach to lesions of the far anterior cerebellopontine angle.[113] In this approach, the internal carotid artery and the cochlea are delineated. The bony space between these two structures is opened, providing

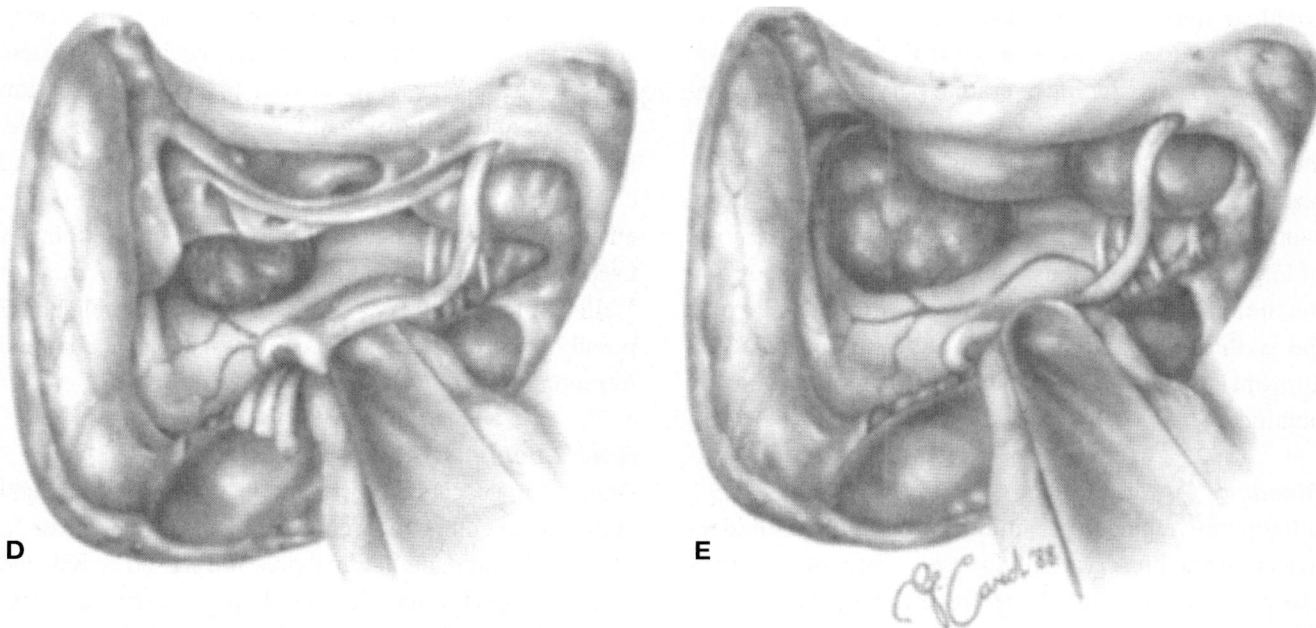

Figure 32–12 (Continued) *D and E*, The greater petrosal nerve is transected anterior to the geniculate ganglion, and the facial nerve is mobilized posteriorly. The otic capsule is drilled away with a diamond bur, and the internal carotid artery is delineated. Bone removal proceeds anteriorly to the internal carotid artery, giving access to the petrous tip and clivus.

access to the anterior portion of the cerebellopontine angle as well as control of the carotid artery.

COMPLICATIONS

Knowledge, avoidance, and identification of the possible complications of vestibular schwannoma surgery, and appropriate management should they occur, enable the best possible surgical outcome. Not surprisingly, the larger the tumor, the greater the morbidity and mortality.

Intraoperative Complications

Cranial Nerve Injury

As pointed out by Glasscock and colleagues, there is a positive correlation between tumor size and facial nerve injury.[99] Facial nerve outcome is poorest with large tumors. Understanding facial nerve anatomy and identifying the nerve as one proceeds through the dissection aid facial nerve preservation. As in any temporal bone procedure, the nerve is identified and skeletonized with a diamond drill during the translabyrinthine approach. Nerve trauma during labyrinthectomy is avoided by appreciating the relationship between the nerve and the lateral and posterior semicircular canals. During the

middle fossa approach, the surgeon must be cognizant that the facial nerve is most often located superficial to the tumor, and care must be exercised when incising the internal auditory canal dura. Furthermore, the plane between the tumor and the nerve should be established early during middle fossa surgery to avoid traction on the nerve as the tumor is removed. During all approaches, reducing the size of large tumors decreases traction on the nerve. Furthermore, use of the facial nerve integrity monitor greatly facilitates nerve preservation.

In the event of facial nerve transection, immediate repair, if possible, should be accomplished. Primary neurorrhaphy is likely to yield the best postoperative functional results. Rerouting the facial nerve or placing a greater auricular nerve interposition graft may be necessary to provide a tension-free anastomosis. Nerve transection in the cerebellopontine angle can be very difficult to repair, and, when impossible, a facial-hypoglossal anastomosis is performed at a later date. Postoperative eye care including artificial tears, ocular lubricants, and eye humidity chambers is instituted, and early upper lid gold weight placement is encouraged.

During hearing preservation cases, intraoperative ABR may be used to monitor wave V. Alterations in the ABR should result in immediate cessation of any surgical manipulation until the tracing returns to baseline. The cochlear nerve must be dissected carefully, and the labyrinthine artery must be preserved. During the removal of larger tumors, the lower cranial nerves must be identified and preserved. Excessive surgical manipulation of these nerves may lead to difficulties with deglutition postoperatively, requiring the institution of aspiration precautions. The fifth nerve is also at risk during the removal of larger tumors and must be atraumatically freed from the tumor. Tumors extending far anteriorly may involve the sixth nerve, and should an abducens palsy occur, appropriate ophthalmologic consultation should be obtained.

Bleeding

Intraoperative bleeding is minimized with careful identification and preservation of vessels. Care must be exercised when removing bone from the sigmoid sinus. Diamond burs are much less likely to cause laceration, and the use of a Freer elevator to remove the thin layer of bone from the sigmoid and superior petrosal sinus after drilling causes less trauma. When the sigmoid sinus is lacerated, bipolar cautery is usually ineffective unless the laceration is very small. When the sinus is lacerated, immediate compression and measures to stop the bleeding decrease the risk of air embolus. Placement of a piece of Gelfoam or Surgicel directly over the bleeding site, followed by pressure with a cottonoid, usually stops the bleeding. If this approach fails, extraluminal sinus occlusion is preferrable to intraluminal occlusion. A thin shell of bone should always be left covering the delicate jugular bulb to avoid bleeding. Should bleeding occur, the same techniques are used as for the sigmoid sinus.

Caution should be exercised if intraluminal occlusion is used near the jugular bulb because compression of the pars nervosa can cause neuropathy of the lower cranial nerves.

Arterial bleeders from the tumor surface are controlled with bipolar cautery, and bleeding from the center of the tumor during reduction is managed with Surgicel packing. Small veins within the cerebellopontine angle are preserved to prevent venous congestion; however, they can be bipolar cauterized if necessary. All arteries within the cerebellopontine angle are treated with respect and carefully dissected from the tumor surface. Cautious, deliberate dissection is carried out in this region, and arteries to the brainstem are never intentionally sacrificed.

A full grasp of the intratemporal carotid artery anatomy is a must when using the transcochlear approach. The carotid artery is identified to enable dissection within the anterior portion of the cerebellopontine angle. Diamond burs are used when removing the cochlea and delineating the carotid artery. Should laceration occur, an assessment of vessel backflow in the distal stump is used to estimate collateral flow through the circle of Willis. Shunting and primary repair are accomplished if possible, and a vascular surgeon's assistance is obtained intraoperatively.

Brain Edema

Brain edema occurs most commonly with the suboccipital approach secondary to cerebellar retraction. Prior to opening the dura, intracranial pressure should be reduced with intravenous mannitol and hyperventilation. Intravenous dexamethasone is used to prevent the development of edema. The cerebellopontine cistern must be accessed to allow the egress of CSF and provide further cerebellar relaxation prior to any surgical manipulation. Protecting the surface of the cerebellum from the retractor with a layer of cottonoid sponges also decreases trauma. Should significant edema occur, exposure will be limited, and the procedure may need to be terminated. In extreme cases, a portion of the cerebellum may need to be resected to decrease the rise in intracranial pressure. It is important to remember that the retracted temporal lobe is also at risk of becoming edematous in the course of middle fossa surgery.

Venous Air Embolism

Venous air embolism occurs when air is sucked into a venous sinus, emissary vein, or diploic vein. A large air embolus may travel to the right heart and ultimately the pulmonary circulation, causing cor pulmonale, insufficient gas exchange, and death. When a patient's head is above the heart, the intraluminal pressure of the head and neck venous system is subatmospheric, and an air embolus is more likely to occur. Therefore, the sitting position, once favored for the suboccipital approach, is discouraged. Preferably, the patient is in the supine position.

When a venous sinus is lacerated, immediate compression and measures to stop the bleeding decrease the risk of air embolism. Likewise, bleeding diploic spaces and mastoid emissary veins should be sealed immediately with bone wax. Air embolism is diagnosed by fluctuating blood pressure and a characteristic churning heart murmur. Once identified, the patient is placed in the left lateral decubitus position, and the air embolus is aspirated from the right heart through a Swan-Ganz catheter. Slightly lowering the patient's head encourages return of venous flow and decreased air entry through the wound. Additionally, nitrous oxide administration is discontinued, replaced by 100% oxygen.

Cardiac Arrhythmias

Tumor dissection from the brainstem can cause cardiac rhythm disturbances and altered hemodynamics. Typically, tachycardia and hypertension are observed with brainstem stimulation, and if either develop, the surgeon must cease tumor dissection immediately and not proceed again until vital signs have stabilized. The vagus nerve may be manipulated during the removal of large tumors, resulting in bradycardia and hypotension. Again, all surgical manipulation must stop until vital signs have returned to baseline.

Brain Herniation

Giant vestibular schwannomas may cause obstructive hydrocephalus (owing to compression of the fourth ventricle), leading to intraoperative herniation. It is essential that hydrocephalus be identified preoperatively. Increased intracranial pressure secondary to hydrocephalus presents with nausea, vomiting, headache, and visual disturbance. Funduscopic examination reveals papilledema. Prior to surgery, the neuro-otologist and neurosurgeon should determine the potential risk of herniation. Should the risk appear high, a ventricular drain should be placed prior to tumor removal. Ventriculoperitoneal shunts have inherent complications as well, such as infection and bleeding. Accordingly, the shunt is placed only in the high-risk patient.

Postoperative Complications

Hemorrhage

Regardless of approach, copious irrigation must be employed prior to wound closure to ensure that all clots are removed, and all bleeding sources must be identified and controlled. Bipolar cautery and topical hemostatic agents are used as necessary, and wound closure is begun only when there is no evidence of bleeding. Hemorrhage may be epidural, subdural, or intraparenchymal, the last of which is usually owing to overzealous retraction. Preferably, the patient is awakened and extubated at the completion of the procedure so that a neurologic examination can be accomplished. Neurologic status is frequently checked in the intensive care unit.

Postoperative hemorrhage is usually accompanied by altered mental status and vital signs within the first 24 hours after surgery. Deterioration may occur quickly, and prompt attention is critical. Patients in stable condition may be imaged, but time should not be wasted obtaining a CT scan if the patient's status is rapidly deteriorating. Opening the incision at the bedside under sterile conditions can decompress the brain and can be life saving. The source of hemorrhage is then identified and controlled in the operating room.

Brain edema may present early in the postoperative period with increased intracranial pressure, confusion, and altered mental status similar to hemorrhage. Often the edema is a consequence of cerebellar retraction in the suboccipital approach or of temporal lobe retraction in the middle fossa approach. Computed tomographic scanning can make the diagnosis if the patient's condition is stable, and intravenous mannitol and steroids are administered to decrease intracranial pressure. Early operative intervention may be required to control postoperative brain edema. Severely edematous cerebellar tissue may require resection. In addition, a ventricular drain may be necessary to manage hydrocephalus.

Infarction

Infarction may be secondary to arterial or venous occlusion. Mechanisms of occlusion include vessel division, coagulation, compression and thrombosis, and vasospasm.[114] Overzealous bipolar cautery can disrupt the blood supply to the brainstem; therefore, only vessel branches directly feeding the tumor may be coagulated. The anterior inferior cerebellar artery is a major contributor to pontine and cerebellar circulation and is often intimately associated with vestibular schwannomas and the eighth nerve. Interruption of this vessel causes extensive infarction of the pons and the "lateral pontomedullary syndrome," consisting of unilateral labyrinthine infarction, cerebellar infarction, ipsilateral facial and contralateral body sensory loss, contralateral hemiparesis, and, often, death. Therefore, when encountered, this vessel must always be gently swept off the tumor and preserved. If vasospasm occurs during manipulation, topical papaverine should be applied to promote vasodilatation.

Intraparenchymal infarction of the cerebellum or temporal lobe is usually related to brain retraction. Cerebellar infarction presents with brain edema, confusion, mental status changes, and cerebellar signs. Temporal lobe infarction may present with an expressive aphasia. To avoid infarction, it is essential to ensure brain relaxation. Intravenous mannitol should be given early in the procedure and an adequate diuresis confirmed. In addition, intravenous furosemide may be given if necessary. Hyperventilation to a pCO_2 of 25 mm Hg can further decrease intracranial pressure. Dural opening and brain retraction should only be accomplished once proper brain relaxation has been established.

Occlusion of the vein (or veins) of Labbé can precipitate temporal lobe venous infarction, cerebral edema, seizure, altered mentation, expressive aphasia, and even death. These veins drain into the distal transverse sinus and are therefore rarely encountered in vestibular schwannoma surgery. However, intraluminal packing of a lacerated transverse or proximal sigmoid sinus should be avoided to prevent injury to these veins.

Cerebrospinal Fluid Leak

The incidence of CSF leakage after vestibular schwannoma resection has been reported to be between 10 and 15%.[115] A CSF leak presents as clear, watery rhinorrhea, otorrhea, or leakage through the incision. Postoperative meningitis occurs more often in the presence of CSF leak, emphasizing the importance of its prevention. Patients with well-pneumatized temporal bones are at an increased risk; therefore, any open air cells must be sealed with muscle, fascia, or bone wax at the end of the case. A compression dressing is left in place for the first 72 hours after surgery.

In the course of the translabyrinthine approach, the middle ear is entered, creating a potential route for CSF rhinorrhea. Therefore, the eustachian tube should be identified by partially opening the facial recess and removing the incus and head of the malleus. The eustachian tube is packed with Proplast, muscle, or fascia and the middle ear space is obliterated with muscle. Care should be exercised when opening the facial recess and packing the middle ear to prevent damage to the tym-

panic annulus or membrane because such injury can lead to CSF otorrhea. Strips of abdominal fat are used to fill the posterior fossa dural defect. These strips are gently placed into the cerebellopontine angle, with the lateral two-thirds protruding into the mastoid cavity. The remainder of the cavity is filled with fat, and the incision is closed in a layered, watertight fashion.

At the close of a middle fossa procedure, a muscle or fascia graft is placed over the internal auditory canal and is covered in turn with a layer of Gelfoam. The weight of the temporal lobe holds the packing in place. During the suboccipital approach, the dural flaps must be kept moist throughout the procedure to facilitate later closure. If a watertight closure cannot be achieved, a pericranial graft is used to bridge the remaining gap. The incision is closed in multiple, watertight layers. Again, any open air cells must be sealed with tissue or bone wax.

Should CSF leakage occur through the incision, the site of leakage is oversewn sterilely at the bedside with a running-locking suture, and the compression dressing is replaced. Head of bed elevation, bed rest, and stool softeners are instituted. Insertion of a lumbar drain is necessary if these measures fail.

The management of CSF rhinorrhea depends on the surgical approach used. Re-exploring the surgical site and ensuring that the eustachian tube is occluded may most quickly address CSF rhinorrhea after translabyrinthine surgery. Lumbar drainage for 3 to 5 days may also be successful. Cerebrospinal fluid rhinorrhea after the middle fossa approach usually responds to lumbar drainage, with surgical intervention less frequently necessary. A CT scan is obtained prior to the insertion of a lumbar drain to rule out hydrocephalus, and no more than 10 to 15 cc of CSF is drained each hour. Additionally, sterile technique is paramount in placing and caring for a lumbar drain to prevent meningitis. A CSF sample for cell count, glucose, and protein should be examined if infection is suspected.

With persistent CSF rhinorrhea, a CT scan should be obtained to evaluate for the presence of an air cell tract that extends from the petrous apex to the medial aspect of the eustachian tube; this tract may have to be obliterated via a transcochlear approach.[116]

Meningitis

The third most common complication of vestibular schwannoma surgery (after facial nerve paralysis and CSF leakage) is meningitis. Meningitis presents with fever, headache, neck and back stiffness, photophobia, and mental status changes. A concomitant CSF leak is not uncommon. After a CT scan has been obtained to rule out hydrocephalus, a lumbar puncture should be performed and broad-spectrum, intravenous antibiotics (with good CSF penetration) started. The CSF is sent for Gram stain, cell count, protein and glucose content, and culture and sensitivity. A marked white cell count elevation, decreased glucose, and increased protein content are typical of bacterial meningitis. The Gram stain results can be obtained quickly and enable antibiotic adjustment. Consultation with an infectious diseases specialist is recommended, and ototoxic antibiotics are avoided if possible. In addition, wound infections should be cultured and the appropriate antibiotics started to prevent progression to meningitis.

Aseptic (or chemical) meningitis may occur and is more common than its bacterial counterpart.[117] The meningeal inflammation may be secondary to bone dust, blood, or other irritants. Regardless of the cause, headache and fever are present, and chemical meningitis may closely mimic bacterial meningitis. Therefore, bacterial meningitis is ruled out as previously described, and antibiotics are started. In aseptic meningitis, CSF analysis reveals an elevated white cell count and protein; however, the glucose level usually is normal. No organisms are identified by Gram stain and culture. Bacterial meningitis must be absolutely ruled out prior to cessation of antibiotic therapy. The addition of a corticosteroid or a nonsteroidal anti-inflammatory agent may help alleviate the symptoms.

Tension Pneumocephalus

Postoperative pneumocephalus is often seen on scans obtained early in the postoperative period and resolves without treatment. In contrast, the rare complication of tension pneumocephalus results from air trapping within the cranial cavity and may present with symptoms of increased intracranial pressure and mental status changes.[118,119] A CT scan can make the diagnosis and rule out other causes of increased intracranial pressure. This complication is much more likely when a ventriculoperitoneal shunt has been placed to manage the hydrocephalus of a large tumor blocking the fourth ventricle. If there is a communication with the mastoid air cell system, air can be drawn into, and trapped within, the cra-

nium, causing tension pneumocephalus. If discovered, appropriate treatment consists of occlusion of the eustachian tube and mastoid, which may also require transcochlear obliteration of air cells in the petrous apex. Rarely, it may be necessary to evacuate the excessive accumulation of air.

Miscellaneous Complications

Appropriate measures should be taken to prevent the complications inherent to all surgical procedures. Pneumatic compression boots are routinely placed prior to starting the surgical procedure and are left in place until the patient is ambulatory to prevent deep venous thrombosis formation and pulmonary embolism. Histamine$_2$ blockers should be instituted when corticosteroids are used to prevent gastrointestinal bleeding. Incentive spirometry and chest physiotherapy help avert postoperative pneumonia. Furthermore, indwelling intravenous catheters are replaced every 72 hours, and urinary catheters are removed as soon as possible to avoid iatrogenic infection.

REFERENCES

1. Bell C. The nervous system of the human body. Washington (DC): Green; 1833.
2. Ballance C. Some points in the surgery of the brain and its membranes. London: Macmillan & Co.; 1907.
3. House WF. A history of acoustic tumor surgery, 1900–1917: the Cushing era. In: House WF, Luetje CM, editors. Acoustic tumors. Vol 1. Diagnosis. Baltimore: University Park Press; 1979.
4. Henneberg, Koch. Uber "Centrale" Neurofromatese und die Geschwultse des kleinhirnbruckenwinkels (Acusticus neurome). Arch F Psychiat 1902;36:251.
5. Cushing H. Tumors of the nervus acusticus and the syndrome of the cerebellopontine angle. Philadelphia: WB Saunders; 1917.
6. Cushing H. Intracranial tumors. Springfield (IL): Charles C. Thomas; 1932.
7. Dandy WE. An operation for the total removal of cerebellopontine (acoustic) tumors. Surg Gynecol Obstet 1925;41:29.
8. Atkinson WJ. Anterior inferior cerebellar artery. J Neurol Neurosurg Psychiatry 1949;12:137.
9. Panse R. Clinical and pathological observations. IV. A glioma of the akusticus. Arch Ohrenh 1904;61:251.

10. Quix F. Ein Fall von operierter Acusticus-Geschwulst mit Darstellung mikrophotographischer Lichtbilder und Besprechung der Operationstechnik. Monatsschr Ohrenh 1915;717.

11. House WF. Surgical exposure of the internal auditory canal and its contents through the middle cranial fossa. Laryngoscope 1961;71:1363.

12. Clerc P, Battise R. Access to the intrapetrous structure from the intracranial aspect. Ann Otolaryngol 1954;21:20.

13. House WF. Report of cases, monograph. Transtemporal bone microsurgical removal of acoustic neuromas. Arch Otolaryngol 1964;80:617.

14. Glasscock ME, Hays JW. The translabyrinthine removal of acoustic and other cerebellopontine angle tumors. Ann Otol Rhinol Laryngol 1973;82:415.

15. Smith MF, Miller RN, Cox DJ. Suboccipital microsurgical removal of acoustic neuromas of all sizes. Ann Otol Rhinol Laryngol 1973;82:407.

16. Rand RW, Dirks DD, Morgan DE, et al. Acoustic neuromas. In: Youmans JR, editor. Neurological surgery. Vol 3. Philadelphia: WB Saunders; 1973.

17. MacCarty CS. Acoustic neuroma and the suboccipital approach (1967–1972). Mayo Clin Proc 1975;50:15.

18. Rhoton AL. The suboccipital approach to removal of acoustic neuromas. Head Neck Surg 1979;1:313.

19. Wade PJ, House WF. Hearing preservation in patients with acoustic neuromas via the middle fossa approach. Otolaryngol Head Neck Surg 1984;92:184–93.

20. Delgado TE, Bucheit WA, Rosenholtz HR, Chrissian S. Intraoperative monitoring of facial muscle evoked responses obtained by intracranial stimulation of the facial nerve: a more accurate technique for facial nerve dissection. Neurosurgery 1979;4:418–21.

21. Silverstein H, Smouha E, Jones R. Routine identification of the facial nerve using electrical stimulation during otological and neurotological surgery. Laryngoscope 1988;98:726–30.

22. Henschen F. Concerning the history and pathogenesis of cerebellopontine angle tumors. Arch Psychiatry 1915;56:21.

23. Prisig W, Eckermeier L, Mueller D. As to the origin of vestibular schwannomas. Seminar on the diagnosis and management of acoustic tumors and skull base tumors. Ear Research Institute, Los Angeles, CA (February 28 – March 3, 1978). Cited in Bebin J. Pathophysiology of acoustic tumors. In: House WF, Luetje CM, editors. Acoustic tumors. Vol 1. Diagnosis. Baltimore: University Park Press; 1979. p. 52.

24. Hardy M. Crowe SJ. Early asymptomatic acoustic tumor: report of 6 cases. Arch Surg 1936;32:292.

25. Gruskin P, Craberry J. Pathology of acoustic tumors. In: House WF, Luetje CM, editors. Acoustic tumors. Vol 1. Diagnosis. Baltimore: University Park Press; 1979.

26. Seizinger BR, Martuza RL, Gusella JF. Loss of genes on chromosome 22 in tumorigenesis of human acoustic neuroma. Nature 1986;322:644–7.

27. Rouleau GA, Merel P, Lutchman M, et al. Alteration in a new gene encoding a putative membrane-organising protein causes neurofibromatosis 2. Nature 1993;363:515–21.

28. Trofatter JA, MacCollin MM, Rutter JL, et al. A novel moesin-ezrin-radixin-like gene is a candidate for the neurofibromatosis 2 tumor suppressor. Cell 1993;72:791–800.

29. Gutmann DH, Sherman L, Seftor L, et al. Increased expression of the NF2 tumor suppressor gene product, merlin, impairs cell motility, adhesion, and spreading. Hum Mol Genet 1999;8:267–75.

30. Gussela JF, Ramesh V, MacCollin M, et al. Merlin: the neurofibromatosis 2 tumor suppressor. Biochim Biophys Acta 1999;1423:29–36.

31. Gutmann DH, Haipek CA, Burke SP, et al. The NF2 interacter, hepatocyte growth factor-regulated tyrosine kinase substrate (HRS), associates with merlin in the 'open' conformation and suppresses cell growth and motility. Hum Mol Genet 2001;10:825–34.

32. Welling DB. Clinical manifestations of mutations in the neurofibromatosis type 2 gene in vestibular schwannomas (acoustic neuromas). Laryngoscope 1998;108:178–89.

33. Welling DB, Akhmametyeva EM, Daniels RL, et al. Analysis of the human neurofibromatosis type 2 gene promoter and its expression. Otolaryngol Head Neck Surg 2000;123:413–8.

34. Welling DB, Lasak JM, Chang LS, et al. cDNA microarray analysis of vestibular schwannomas. Otol Neurotol 2002. [In press]

35. Burkey JM, Rizer FM, Schuring AG, et al. Acoustic reflexes, auditory brain stem response, and MRI in the evaluation of acoustic neuromas. Laryngoscope 1996;106:839–41.

36. Selters WA, Brackmann DE. Acoustic tumor detection with brainstem electric response audiometry. Arch Otolaryngol 1977;103:181.

37. Glasscock ME, Jacksom GJ, Josey AF, et al. Brainstem evoked response audiometry in a clinical practice. Laryngoscope 1979;89:1021.

38. Welling DB, Glasscock ME, Woods CI, et al. Acoustic neuroma: a cost-effective approach. Otolaryngol Head Neck Surg 1990;103:364–70.

39. Ruckenstein MJ, Cueva RA, Morrison DH, et al. A prospective study of ABR and MRI in the screening for vestibular schwannomas. Am J Otol 1996;17:317–20.

40. Schmidt RJ, Sataloff RT, Newman J, et al. The sensitivity of auditory brainstem response testing for the diagnosis of acoustic neuromas. Arch Otolaryngol Head Neck Surg 2001;127:19–22.

41. El-Kashlan HK, Eisenmann D, Kileny PR. Auditory brainstem response in small acoustic neuromas. Ear Hear 2000;21:257–62.

42. Robinette MS, Bauch CD, Olsen WO, et al. Auditory brainstem response and magnetic resonance imaging for acoustic neuromas: cost by prevalence. Arch Otolaryngol Head Neck Surg 2000;126:963–6.

43. Don M, Masuda A, Nelson R, Brackmann D. Successful detection of small acoustic tumors using the stacked derived-band auditory brain stem response amplitude. Am J Otol 1997;18:608–21.

44. Glasscock ME, Hays JW. A one-stage combined approach for the management of large cerebellopontine angle tumors. Laryngoscope 1978;88:1563.

45. Linthicum FH, Churchill D. Vestibular test results in acoustic tumor cases. Arch Otolaryngol 1968;88:56.

46. Hallpike CS, Cairns H. Observations on pathology of Meniere's syndrome. J Laryngol 1938;53:56.

47. Valvassori GE. Cerebellopontine angle tumors. Otolaryngol Clin North Am 1988;21:337–48.

48. Lipkin AF, Jenkins HA. Role of contrast computed tomography in the diagnosis of small acoustic neuromas. Laryngoscope 1984;94:890.

49. Valvassori GE, Palacios E. Magnetic resonance imaging of the internal auditory canal. Top Magn Reson Imaging 2000;11: 52–65.

50. Daniels RL, Swallow C, Shelton C, et al. Causes of unilateral sensorineural hearing loss screened by high-resolution fast spin echo magnetic resonance imaging: review of 1,070 consecutive cases. Am J Otol 2000;21:173–80.

51. Annesley DJ, Laitt RD, Jenkins JP, et al. Magnetic resonance imaging in the investigation of sensorineural hearing loss: is contrast enhancement still necessary? J Laryngol Otol 2001; 115:14–21.

52. William MD, Antonelli PJ, Williams LS. Middle ear prosthesis displacement in high-strength magnetic fields. Otol Neurotol 2001;22:158–61.

53. Fucci MJ, Buchman CA, Brackmann DE, et al. Acoustic tumor growth: implications for treatment choices. Am J Otol 1999;20: 495–9.

54. Glasscock ME 3rd, Papps DG Jr, Manolidis S, et al. Management of acoustic neuroma in the elderly population. Am J Otol 1997;18:236–41; discussion 241–2.

55. Nedzelski JM, Schessel DA, Pfleiderer A, et al. Conservative management of acoustic neuromas. Otolaryngol Clin North Am 1992;25:691–705.

56. Yamamoto M, Hagiwara S, Ide M, et al. Conservative management of acoustic neurinomas: prospective study of long-term changes in tumor volume and auditory function. Minim Invasive Neurosurg 1998;41:86–92.

57. Silverstein H, McDaniel A, Norrell H, et al. Conservative management of acoustic neuroma in the elderly patient. Laryngoscope 1985;95(7 Pt 1):766–70.

58. Levo H, Pyykko I, Blomstedt G. Non-surgical treatment of vestibular schwannoma patients. Acta Otolaryngol Suppl (Stockh) 1997;529:56–8.

59. Charabi S, Thomsen J, Tos M, et al. Acoustic neuroma/vestibular schwannoma growth: past, present and future. Acta Otolaryngol (Stockh) 1998;118:327–32.

60. Massick DD, Welling DB, Dodson EE, et al. Tumor growth and audiometric change in vestibular schwannomas managed conservatively. Laryngoscope 2000;110:1843–9.

61. Charabi S, Thomsen J, Mantoni M, et al. Acoustic neuroma (vestibular schwannoma): growth and surgical and nonsurgical consequences of the wait-and-see policy. Otolaryngol Head Neck Surg 1995;113:5–14.

62. Hoistad DL, Melnik G, Mamikoglu B, et al. Update on conservative management of acoustic neuroma. Otol Neurotol 2001;22:682–5.

63. Bhatia S, Karmarkar S, Taibah A, et al. Vestibular schwannoma and the only hearing ear. J Laryngol Otol 1996;110:366–9.

64. Bederson JB, von Ammon K, Wichmann WW, et al. Conservative treatment of patients with acoustic tumors. Neurosurgery 1991;28:646–50; discussion 650–1.

65. Ogawa K, Kanzaki J, Ogawa S, et al. The growth rate of acoustic neuromas. Acta Otolaryngol Suppl (Stockh) 1991;487: 157–63.

66. Aguiar PH, Tatagiba M, Samii M, et al. The comparison between the growth fraction of bilateral vestibular schwannomas in neurofibromatosis 2 (NF2) and unilateral vestibular schwannomas using the monoclonal antibody MIB 1. Acta Neurochir 1995;134:40–5.

67. Leksell L. A note on the treatment of acoustic tumours. Acta Chir Scand 1971;137:763–5.

68. Noren G. Long-term complications following Gamma Knife radiosurgery of vestibular schwannomas. Stereotact Funct Neurosurg 1998;70 Suppl 1:65–73.

69. Miller RC, Foote RL, Coffey RJ, et al. Decrease in cranial nerve complications after radiosurgery for acoustic neuromas: a prospective study of dose and volume. Int J Radiat Oncol Biol Phys 1999;43:305–11.

70. Kondziolka DS, Lusford LD, McLaughlin MR, et al. Long-term outcomes after radiosurgery for acoustic neuromas. N Engl J Med 1998;339:1426–33.

71. Martens F, Verbeke L, Piessens M, et al. Stereotactic radiosurgery of vestibular schwannomas with a linear accelerator. Acta Neurochir Suppl 1994;62:88–92.

72. Ogunrinde OK, Lusford LD, Kondziolka DS, et al. Cranial nerve preservation after stereotactic radiosurgery of intracanalicular acoustic tumors. Stereotact Funct Neurosurg 1995;64 Suppl 1:87–97.

73. van Roijen L, Nijs HG, Avezaat CJ, et al. Costs and effects of microsurgery versus radiosurgery in treating acoustic neuroma. Acta Neurochir 1997;139:942–8.

74. van Roijen L, Nijs HG, Avezaat CJ, et al. Costs and effects of microsurgical versus radiosurgical treatment of vestibular schwannoma. In: Third International Conference on Acoustic Neurinoma and Other CPA Tumors. 1999. Rome, Italy.

75. Shelton C. Unilateral acoustic tumors: how often do they recur after translabyrinthine removal? Laryngoscope 1995;105(9 Pt 1):958–66.

76. Welling DB, Slater PW, Thomas RD, et al. The learning curve in vestibular schwannoma surgery. Am J Otol 1999;20:644–8.

77. Thomsen J, Tos M, Borgesen SE. Gamma Knife: hydrocephalus as a complication of stereotactic radiosurgical treatment of an acoustic neuroma. Am J Otol 1990;11:330–3.

78. Slattery WH 3rd, Brackmann DE. Results of surgery following stereotactic irradiation for acoustic neuromas. Am J Otol 1995;16:315–9; discussion 319–21.

79. Pollock BE, Lunsford LD, Kondziolka DS, et al. Vestibular schwannoma management. Part II. Failed radiosurgery and the role of delayed microsurgery. J Neurosurg 1998;89:949–55.

80. Ito K, Kurita H, Sugasawa K, et al. Analyses of neuro-otological complications after radiosurgery for acoustic neurinomas. Int J Radiat Oncol Biol Phys 1997;39:983–8.

81. Comey CH, McLaughlin MR, Jho HD, et al. Death from a malignant cerebellopontine angle triton tumor despite stereotactic radiosurgery. Case report. J Neurosurg 1998;89:653–8.

82. Thomsen J, Mirz F, Wetke R, et al. Intracranial sarcoma in a patient with neurofibromatosis type 2 treated with Gamma Knife radiosurgery for vestibular schwannoma. Am J Otol 2000;21: 364–70.

83. Sangueza OP, Requena L. Neoplasms with neural differentiation: a review. Part II: malignant neoplasms. Am J Dermatopathol 1998;20:89–102.

84. Bonetti B, Panzeri L, Carner M, et al. Human neoplastic Schwann cells: changes in the expression of neurotrophins and their low-affinity receptor p75. Neuropathol Appl Neurobiol 1997;23:380–6.

85. Crandon IW, et al. Malignant triton tumour of the spine: a case report. West Indian Med J 1995;44:143–5.

86. Han DH, Kim DG, Chi JG, et al. Malignant triton tumor of the acoustic nerve. Case report. J Neurosurg 1992;76:874–7.

87. Chang SD, Poen J, Hancock SL, et al. Acute hearing loss following fractionated stereotactic radiosurgery for acoustic neuroma. Report of two cases. J Neurosurg 1998;89:321–5.

88. Ogunrinde OK, Lunsford LD, Flickinger JC, et al. Cranial nerve preservation after stereotactic radiosurgery for small acoustic tumors. Arch Neurol 1995;52:73–9.

89. Kwon Y, Kim JH, Lee DJ, et al. Gamma Knife treatment of acoustic neurinoma. Stereotact Funct Neurosurg 1998;70 Suppl 1:57–64.

90. Subach BR, Kondziolka DS, Lunsford LD, et al. Stereotactic radiosurgery in the management of acoustic neuromas associated with neurofibromatosis type 2. J Neurosurg 1999;90:815–22.

91. Shore-Freedman E, Abrahams C, Recant W, et al. Neurilemomas and salivary gland tumors of the head and neck following childhood irradiation. Cancer 1983;51:2159–63.

92. Acoustic neuroma. NIH Cons Statement 1991;9(4):11–3.

93. Shirato H, Sakamoto T, Sawamura Y, et al. Comparison between observation policy and fractionated stereotactic radiotherapy (SRT) as an initial management for vestibular schwannoma. Int J Radiat Oncol Biol Phys 1999;44:545–50.

94. Samii M, Matthies C. Management of 1000 vestibular schwannomas (acoustic neuromas): the facial nerve—preservation and restitution of function. Neurosurgery 1997;40:684–94; discussion 694–5.

95. Slattery WH 3rd, Brackmann DE, Hitselberger W. Hearing preservation in neurofibromatosis type 2. Am J Otol 1998;19: 638–43.

96. Welling DB. Clinical manifestations of mutations in the neurofibromatosis type 2 gene in vestibular schwannomas (acoustic neuromas). Laryngoscope 1998;108:178–89.

97. Glasscock ME, Hart MJ, Vrabec JT. Management of bilateral acoustic neuroma. Otolaryngol Clin North Am 1992;25:449–69.

98. Wackym PA, King WA, Poe DS, et al. Adjunctive use of endoscopy during acoustic neuroma surgery. Laryngoscope 1999;109:1193–201.

99. Glasscock ME, Kveton JF, Christianson S, et al. A systematic approach to the surgical management of acoustic neuroma. Laryngoscope 1986;96:1088.

100. Kaylie DM, Gilbert E, Horgan MA, et al. Acoustic neuroma surgery outcomes. Otol Neurotol 2001;22:686–9.

101. Wiet RJ, Mamikoglu B, Odom L, et al. Long-term results of the first 500 cases of acoustic neuroma surgery. Otolaryngol Head Neck Surg 2001;124:645–51.

102. Lanman TH, Brackmann DE, Hitselberger WE, et al. Report of 190 consecutive cases of large acoustic tumors (vestibular schwannoma) removed via the translabyrinthine approach. J Neurosurg 1999;90:617–23.

103. Fundova P, Charabi S, Tos M, et al. Cystic vestibular schwannoma: surgical outcome. J Laryngol Otol 2000;114:935–9.

104. Lalwani AK, Butt FY, Jackler RK, et al. Facial nerve outcome after acoustic neuroma surgery: a study from the era of cranial nerve monitoring. Otolaryngol Head Neck Surg 1994;111: 561–70.

105. Lenarz T, Ernst A. Intraoperative facial nerve monitoring in the surgery of cerebellopontine angle tumors: improved preservation of nerve function. ORL J Otorhinolaryngol Relat Spec 1994;56: 31–5.

106. Slattery WH 3rd, Brackmann DE, Hitselberger W. Middle fossa approach for hearing preservation with acoustic neuromas. Am J Otol 1997;18:596–601.

107. Leonetti J, Anderson D, Marzo S, et al. Cerebrospinal fluid fistula after transtemporal skull base surgery. Otolaryngol Head Neck Surg 2001;124:511–4.

108. Lebowitz RA, Hoffman RA, Roland JT Jr, et al. Autologous fibrin glue in the prevention of cerebrospinal fluid leak following acoustic neuroma surgery. Am J Otol 1995;16:172–4.

109. Hoffman RA. Cerebrospinal fluid leak following acoustic neuroma removal. Laryngoscope 1994;104(1 Pt 1):40–58.

110. Gillman GS, Parnes LS. Acoustic neuroma management: a six-year review. J Otolaryngol 1995;24:191–7.

111. Rubenstein LJ. Tumors of the central nervous system. In: Firminger HI, editor. Atlas of tumor pathology. Washington (DC): Air Force Institute of Pathology; 1972.

112. House WF, Hitselberger WE. The transcochlear approach to the skull base. Arch Otolaryngol 1976;102:334–42.

113. House WF, Hitselberger WE, Horn KL. The middle fossa transpetrous approach to the anterior superior cerebellopontine angle. Ann J Otol 1986;7:1.

114. Almeida GM, Bianco E, Sousa AS. Vasospasm after acoustic neuroma removal. Surg Neurol 1985;23:38–40.

115. Brennen JW, Rowed DW, Nedzelski JM, et al. Cerebral spinal fluid leak after acoustic neuroma surgery: influence of tumor size and surgical approach on incidence and response to treatment. J Neurosurg 2001;94:217–23.

116. Grant IL, Welling DB, Oehler MC, et al. Transcochlear repair of persistent cerebrospinal fluid leaks. Laryngoscope 1999; 109:1392–96.

117. House WF, Hitzelberger WE. The neuro-otologist's view of the surgical management of acoustic neuroma. Clin Neurosurg 1985;32:214–22.

118. Kithata LM, Katz JD. Tension pneumocephalus after posterior fossa craniotomy: report of four additional cases and review of postoperative pneumocephalus. Neurosurgery 1983;12: 164–8.

119. Miller CF, Furman WR. Symptomatic pneumocephalus after translabyrinthine acoustic neuroma excision and nitrous oxide anesthesia. Anesthesiology 1985;58:281–3.

33

Auditory Brainstem Implant

STEVEN R. OTTO, MA
DERALD E. BRACKMANN, MD
WILLIAM E. HITSELBERGER, MD
ELIZABETH H. TOH, MD
ROBERT V. SHANNON, PHD
LENDRA M. FRIESEN, MS

Frequently, loss of integrity of the auditory nerve after removal of vestibular schwannomas in neurofibromatosis type 2 (NF2) leaves patients completely deafened. Other communication methods such as signing and lipreading have provided some assistance but obviously cannot restore useful hearing sensations. The auditory brainstem implant (ABI) was developed to bypass the auditory nerve and directly stimulate the cochlear nucleus complex. Useful auditory sensations have resulted,[1,2] and the multichannel version of the ABI (Nucleus®, Cochlear Corporation, Englewood, Colorado) successfully completed US Food and Drug Administration (FDA) clinical trials in July 2000 and received approval for commercial release.

This chapter summarizes the history, surgical, and clinical aspects of ABI implantation and perceptual performance. The techniques have been refined in over 120 patients implanted with various implementations of the ABI since 1979 at House Ear Institute (HEI, Los Angeles, California). Since 1992, 92 patients have received multichannel devices: 71 with 8 electrode arrays and 21 with the most recent 21-electrode version (Nucleus ABI24).

Also in development is a multichannel penetrating electrode system designed to increase the precision of auditory neuron stimulation within the cochlear nucleus matrix. This is nearing the stage for limited clinical trials in humans.

General technical and theoretical considerations regarding ABI implantation and management of patients with NF2 have been summarized elsewhere.[3–5]

HISTORY OF DEVELOPMENT

In 1979, William House and William Hitselberger (Figure 33–1) first implanted an electrode to stimulate the cochlear nucleus of a patient with NF2 facing deafness

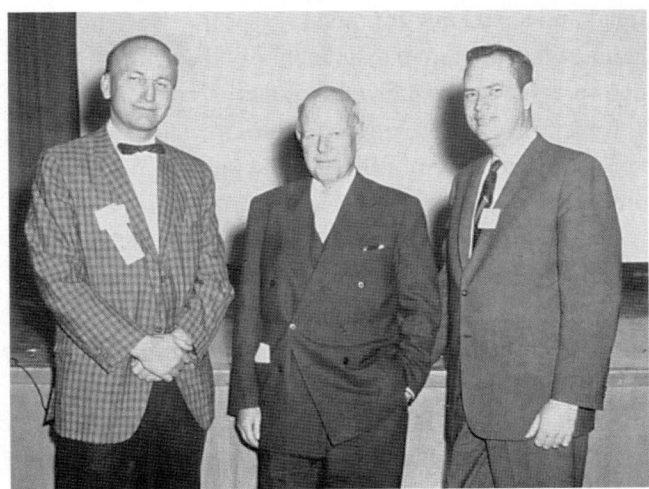

Figure 33–1 Pioneers in auditory brainstem implantation. William E. Hitselberger (*left*) and William F. House (*right*) with early supporter and colleague Herbert Olivecrona (*middle*) of Sweden.

after removal of a vestibular schwannoma. The patient was persistent in her requests that this be tried in the hope that it would allow her to continue to have some hearing sensations. The electrode was a simple ball type, and electrical stimulation was supplied by a modified body-worn hearing aid. Useful auditory sensations resulted, but the electrode proved somewhat unstable and was shortly removed. A two-electrode (later three) mesh-type array was subsequently developed by Huntington Medical Research Institute (HMRI, Pasadena, California) and was used successfully in 25 recipients until 1992. The speech processors were modified 3M/House-type cochlear implant processors that provided patients with sound awareness, ability to discriminate some environmental sounds, and significantly improved understanding of speech in conjunction with lipreading. Experiments also suggested that multichannel stimulation was feasible and would be potentially beneficial with a multiple-electrode array. This led to the development and successful use of the present multichannel ABI.

PATIENT SELECTION

At least 90% of individuals with NF2 exhibit bilateral vestibular schwannomas.[6] Treatment of these and other tumors associated with NF2 has significantly prolonged the life span of such patients. Although performance with the ABI has not reached cochlear implant levels, the auditory information provided can significantly enhance quality of life and the ability to function in occupational and social environments.

The ideal goal in management of NF2 remains hearing preservation through early diagnosis and treatment. However, the ABI provides an alternative to a desperate attempt to preserve nonserviceable hearing when large tumors are present and hearing conservation is unlikely.

The multichannel ABI is approved for use in individuals with NF2 who are at least 12 years of age. There are no preoperative audiologic criteria because the surgical procedure for tumor excision and electrode array placement eliminates any remaining hearing. Implantation may occur during first- or second-side vestibular schwannoma removal or in patients with previously removed tumors bilaterally. A small but significant number of patients (8% at HEI) have failed to experience auditory responses from the implant, mostly because of anatomic difficulties. First-side implantation can provide a second opportunity (if necessary) to achieve a functioning system when the second acoustic tumor is removed.

Since completion of the clinical trials phase, the ABI is now available to a wider range of potential recipients. Realistically, however, the ABI may not be for everyone. A number of non–implant-related factors including general health, vision, social activity, and anatomic status (as seen on magnetic resonance imaging [MRI]) can influence ABI benefit. Patient age can also be a factor. For example, teenage implantees in general have been less successful regular and enthusiastic users than older recipients. Patients with limited vision also may show relatively less benefit since the ABI works best in conjunction with lipreading. Candidates for ABIs should be apprised of the potential effects of these factors on their ability to benefit from the device.

PREOPERATIVE EVALUATION AND COUNSELING

Preoperative determination of informed consent regarding the ABI is extremely important to the success of an ABI program. The goal of preoperative evaluation and counseling is to help prepare patients for the loss of hearing after tumor removal and lay the groundwork that will help them acclimate to a new way of hearing with the ABI. Prospective recipients and their families should have appropriate expectations regarding the potential benefits and limitations of the device. A frank and thorough explanation of what is involved in using and improving with an ABI is necessary. Inadequate preparation can significantly delay and complicate acceptance and use of the implant.

A major criterion for successful integration and use of the device is a high level of motivation and determination to make maximal use of whatever auditory sensations the ABI provides. Willingness to participate in the postoperative follow-ups is also very important in optimizing device function. Preoperative counseling provides an opportunity to explore motivation issues and to explain the need for judicious compliance with the follow-up protocol. Special counseling may also be helpful in patients having difficulties coping with deafness and other disabilities related to NF2. Such difficulties can distract patients from learning to use an ABI.

Patients should also be counseled preoperatively about the likelihood that they will experience mild nonauditory sensations such as tingling or dizziness on some electrodes, as well as the slight but significant possibility that the ABI may not provide any auditory sensations. Our focus has been to maintain a tone of hopeful and cautious optimism in preoperative counseling of our patients. This has worked well in eliminating unpleasant surprises and properly setting the stage for postoperative rehabilitation.

The participation of an experienced, skilled, and coordinated multidisciplinary team is necessary for the successful treatment and management of patients with NF2. Each team member is essential to the success of an ABI program. Chief among these is the surgeon's skill and experience in removing acoustic tumors, preserving necessary structures, and accurately placing the electrode array. Electrophysiologic monitoring expertise contributes to proper identification of the implant site. Postoperatively, implant audiology expertise is required to program the speech processor and optimize perceptual performance. Even under ideal circumstances, adapting to and learning to use an ABI is an ongoing process that typically extends over a longer period than in cochlear implantation. New recipients should be encouraged that performance almost always improves greatly with experience.

DEVICE

Hitselberger and colleagues originally used a cochlear implant ball-type electrode in their first ABI recipient.[7] Subsequently, patients received a 2 × 8-mm fabric mesh array with two or three platinum ribbon electrodes. In 1992, HEI collaborated with Cochlear Corporation and Huntington Medical Research Institute (Pasadena, California) in the development of an eight-electrode multichannel ABI system. This was further upgraded to the present 21-electrode (Nucleus ABI24) system and receiver/stimulator shown in Figure 33–2, A. The electrode array comprises a flexible perforated silicone and mesh substrate with 0.7-mm platinum disk electrodes. This facilitates conformation of the array to the surface of the cochlear nucleus and promotes long-term stability. The ABI24 receiver/stimulator allows up to 2,400

pulse/second/electrode (ppse) of pulsatile stimulation and advanced sound-processing encoders.

The ABI24 system includes the Nucleus SPRINT™ sound processor, a microphone headset, and a transmitter coil (Figure 33–2, B). The processing strategy is the Nucleus SPEAK™ (spectral peak) strategy. This processor, also used in cochlear implantation, uses circuitry that analyzes input sound frequencies and codes the salient acoustic information to sequentially activate electrodes on the array. There is flexibility in the number of spectral maxima that can be transmitted, in the sequence and number of electrodes that can be activated, in the stimulus rate, and in available speech-processing strategies (including the Nucleus Advanced Combination Encoder™ [ACE]).

Basic function of the SPRINT processor is as follows. The processor incorporates a series of 21 contiguous-input analysis filters. These filters split the input sound spectra, and the resulting output is linked to selectable electrodes on the array. A major part of processor setup involves determining (via scaling and ranking of electrode-specific pitch) what an appropriate linking arrangement should be for individual patients. This varies greatly, but the general goal is to link low-frequency sounds with electrodes that sound lower in pitch and likewise with higher-frequency sounds. This strategy also optimizes speech and environmental sound perception in cochlear implants, but the process is relatively straightforward with this device because of the highly consistent tonotopic arrangement of neural processes in the cochlea. With an ABI, individual variations in cochlear nucleus anatomy, neuronal survival, and electrode placement result in a much more complex relationship. Therefore, programming ABI speech processors can take more time than programming cochlear implant recipients.

ANATOMIC CONSIDERATIONS

The dorsal and ventral cochlear nuclei are the targets for placement of the ABI electrode array. Although the nuclei are hidden by the cerebellar peduncle, surface landmarks are useful in identifying this region. Frequently, however, these structures may be distorted by tumor. Figure 33–3 shows the major structures of the pontomedullary junction and the translabyrinthine approach

A

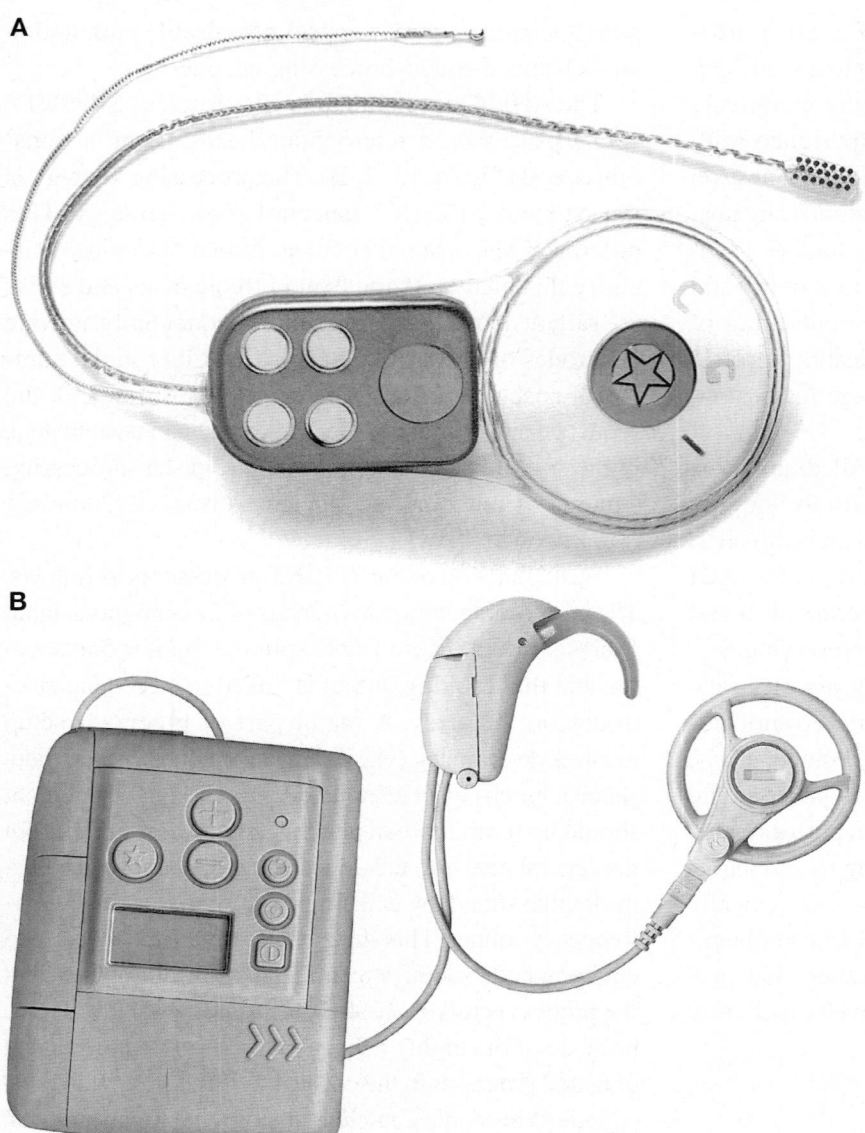

B

Figure 33–2 *A*, The Nucleus ABI24 auditory brainstem implant receiver/stimulator with 21-electrode surface array (and remote ball ground electrode) for the cochlear nucleus complex. *B*, Auditory brainstem implant Sprint (Nucleus) speech processor and ear-level microphone headset with transmitter coil.

surgical field of view. Important landmarks include the terminus of the sleevelike lateral recess forming the foramen of Luschka, inferiorly the root of the glossopharyngeal (ninth) nerve, and superior to the foramen the vestibulocochlear and facial nerve roots.

Normally, the intact choroid plexus marks the entrance to the lateral recess (foramen of Luschka), and the taenia obliquely traverses the roof of the lateral recess, marking the surface of the ventral cochlear nucleus. These structures may not be clearly identifiable when a large tumor distorts the lateral surface of the pons and medulla. In such cases, the stump of the eighth nerve may be traced to the opening of the lateral recess. The ninth

cranial nerve can also be used as a reference point for the lateral recess. A concavity sometimes visualized between the eighth and ninth nerves should not be confused with the introitus of the recess.

Within the lateral recess and on its superior aspect are found the dorsal and ventral cochlear nuclei. The electrode array is positioned well within the recess to provide positional stability. Electrical stimulation of the ventral cochlear nucleus, the main relay for eighth nerve input and the major portion of the ascending auditory pathway, is probably the primary source of auditory sensations even though some part of the array also lies adjacent to the dorsal cochlear nucleus.

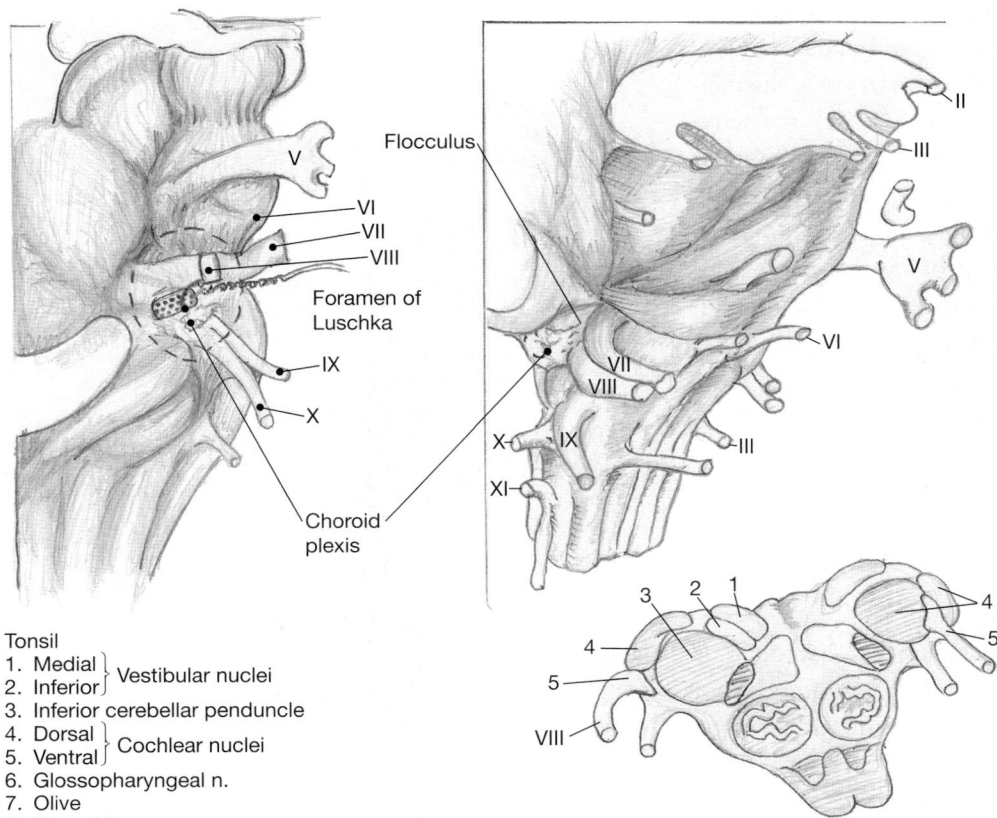

Figure 33–3 Schematic of the cochlear nuclei region demonstrating relative location of various landmarks. *Dashed area* represents approximate surgical view. Electrode array is fully inserted into proper position. Adapted from Otto SR, Hitselberger WE, Telischi FF, et al. Auditory brainstem implant. In: Brackmann DE, Shelton C, Arriaga MA, editors. Otologic surgery. 2nd ed. Philadelphia: WB Saunders; 2001. p. 594–603.

Tonsil
1. Medial ⎫ Vestibular nuclei
2. Inferior ⎭
3. Inferior cerebellar penduncle
4. Dorsal ⎫ Cochlear nuclei
5. Ventral ⎭
6. Glossopharyngeal n.
7. Olive
8. Pyramid

SURGICAL CONSIDERATIONS

The translabyrinthine craniotomy provides the best access for tumor removal and exposure of the lateral recess of the fourth ventricle. A typical translabyrinthine acoustic tumor removal process is followed except that recording electrodes are placed for monitoring electrically evoked auditory brainstem responses (EABRs) and any activity from cranial nerves VII and IX. Also, a standard postauricular incision is used initially but later extended superiorly and posteriorly to provide exposure for placing the receiver/stimulator. The incision margin should extend at least 1 to 2 cm beyond the device contour (Figure 33–4).

Monitoring of the EABR assists with confirmation that the electrode array is properly positioned. Slight adjustments of the array may be necessary to minimize responses that suggest activation of nonauditory neural structures. For EABR monitoring, subdermal needle electrodes are inserted at the vertex of the head, over the seventh cervical vertebrae, and at the hairline of the

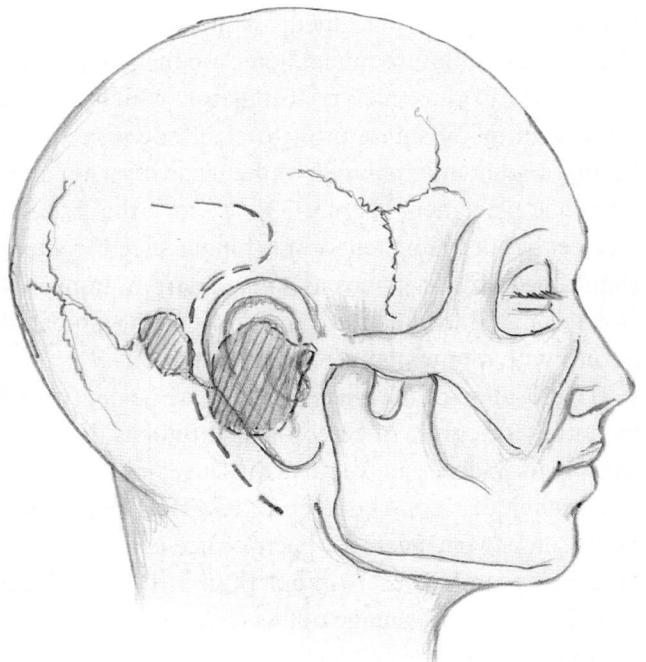

Figure 33–4 Location of the incision with respect to the planned site of receiver/stimulator.

occiput. For electromyographic recording of nonauditory activation, the facial nerve is monitored in the standard fashion,[8] and bipolar electrodes are inserted in the ipsilateral pharyngeal (soft palate) muscles to monitor activity from cranial nerve IX. After the receiver/stimulator has been secured and the array placed, a transmitter coil is placed over the receiver antenna. The ABR obtained with biphasic pulsatile stimulation of the cochlear nucleus differs from responses obtained using acoustic stimulation and from electrical stimulation using cochlear implants.[9] An experienced electrophysiologist interprets these waveforms intraoperatively and provides feedback to the neurosurgeon regarding placement.

IMPLANTATION PROCEDURE

Tumor dissection proceeds in the normal fashion via a translabyrinthine craniotomy. After complete tumor removal and adequate hemostasis, the site for the internal receiver posterosuperior to the mastoid cavity is determined, and temporalis muscle in this area is elevated off the parietal skull and excised. Using a replica of the receiver/stimulator as a guide, a circular area of bony cortex in this area is flattened using cutting burs, and a trough is created between the implant seat and the mastoid cavity for placement of the electrode wires (Figure 33–5). Suture tunnel holes are then created on either side of the receiver/stimulator, which is then fixed with nylon suture prior to electrode array positioning so that manipulation of the leads does not alter electrode placement (Figure 33–6). Once the internal receiver has been implanted, only bipolar electrocautery should be used for hemostasis since current transmission through the implant to the brainstem is a potential hazard with monopolar electrocautery.

The location of the lateral recess may be confirmed by noting the egress of cerebrospinal fluid as the anesthesiologist induces the Valsalva maneuver in the patient. This technique should be reserved as a final check after the opening to the recess has been located using standard landmarks since cerebrospinal fluid will be drained quickly, and the advantage of this technique is lost with multiple Valsalva maneuvers.

After identifying the foramen of Luschka, the electrode array is mounted on a Rosen needle and inserted

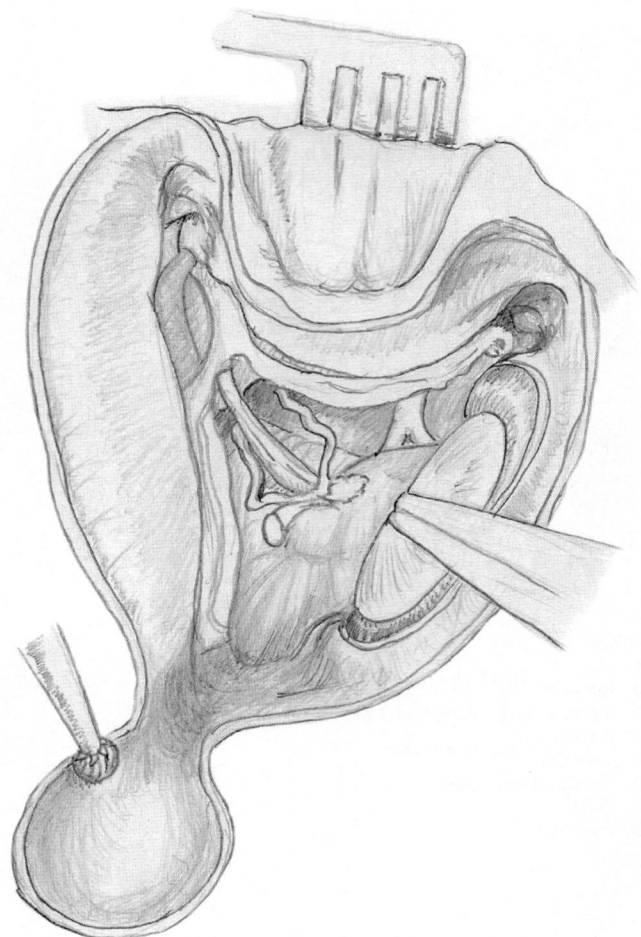

Figure 33–5 Schemmatic surgical view of the completed translabyrinthine craniotomy, trough for receiver/stimulator wires, and receiver/stimulator seat being drilled.

into the lateral recess with the electrodes oriented superiorly (Figure 33–7). With experience, we have found that the implant functions better, with fewer nonauditory side effects, when the electrodes are placed fully within the lateral recess.[4] After placement, selected electrodes in the array are activated to confirm their position over the cochlear nucleus. They are tested for the presence of EABRs, stimulation of adjacent cranial nerves (VII and IX), and changes in vital signs. The position of the electrode array usually needs very slight adjustment to maximize auditory stimulation and minimize electromyographic responses from the other nerves.

The electrode array is secured using a small piece of Teflon felt packed into the meatus of the lateral recess. Subsequent ingrowth of fibrous tissue eventually stabilizes the array in position. The electrode wiring is posi-

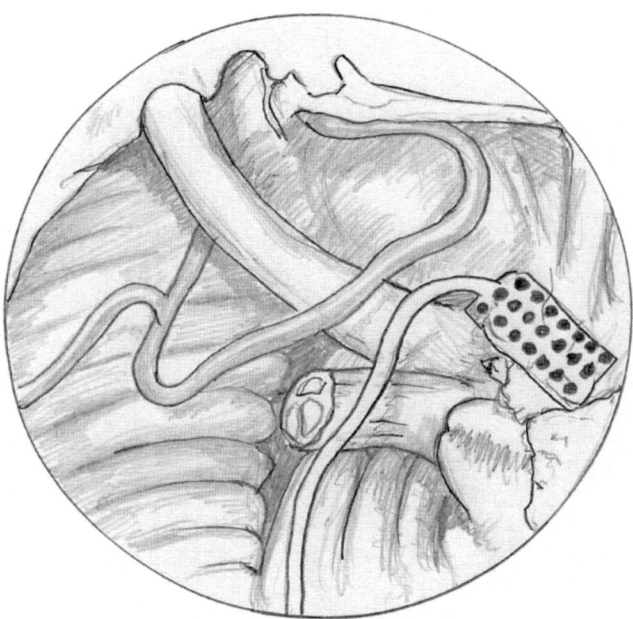

Figure 33–7 Schematic urgical view of the auditory brainstem implant electrode array being passed into the lateral recess (magnified view from Figure 33–5).

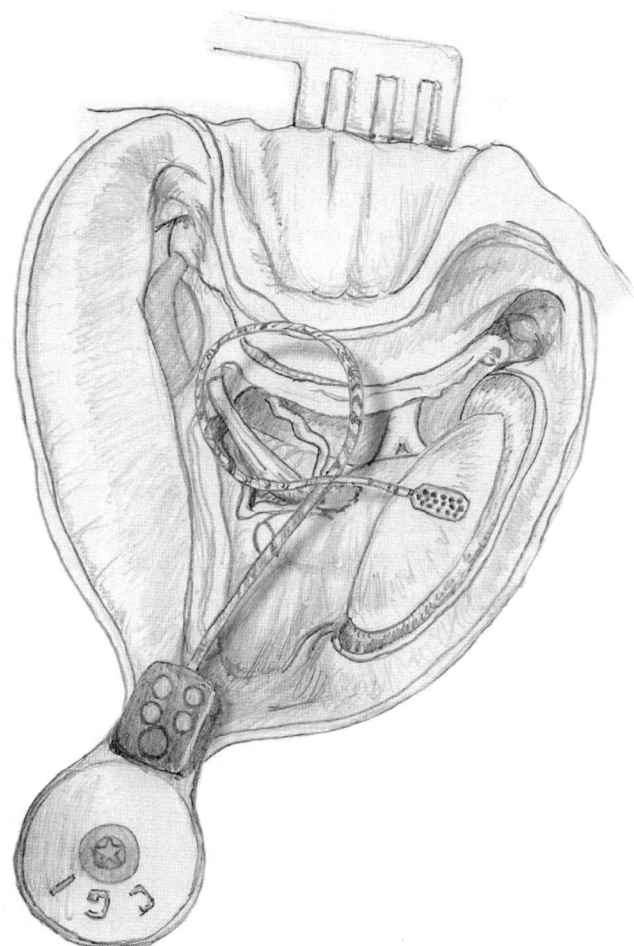

Figure 33–6 Schematic view of the receiver/stimulator in place.

tioned within the mastoid cavity and bony trough (Figure 33–8). The eustachian tube and middle ear are then packed with oxidized cellulose (Surgicel®) and muscle. Abdominal fat is used to obliterate the mastoid defect.

At this time, the magnet in the receiver/stimulator is removed to allow for future surveillance MRI. Since the magnet is typically removed from the receiver/stimulator at the time of implantation, there may be difficulty in identifying the location of the receiver/stimulator at the time of initial stimulation. Improper positioning of the external transmitter coil in such cases may lead to the false impression of device failure or stimulation failure on the part of the patient. We now routinely tattoo the center location of the circular receiver/stimulator antenna at the time of surgery to facilitate its location postoperatively. The incision is then closed in layers without drainage.

POSTOPERATIVE CARE

Postoperative care after auditory brainstem implantation is similar to that following routine craniotomies for acoustic tumor removal. A large mastoid-type dressing is left in place for 4 days. Careful attention to any moisture on the bandages allows prompt identification of cerebrospinal fluid leak through the postauricular wound. Intravenous antibiotics, for example, cefuroxime (Zinacef®, GlaxoSmithKline) 3 g, are administered prophylactically on induction of anesthesia.

The device is typically activated for the first time 4 to 8 weeks after implantation. This allows resolution of edema in the skin flap overlying the receiver/stimulator, which would otherwise prevent an adequate signal from reaching the implant. In actual use, implant patients must shave this area and apply a thin tape and metal disk ("retainer" disk), to which the magnetic transmitter coil adheres. The patient, or a companion, must be trained to ensure proper and consistent positioning of the transmitter coil over the implant receiver/stimulator. Many complaints about poor signal or deterioration in sound quality can be traced to improper positioning of the retainer disk.

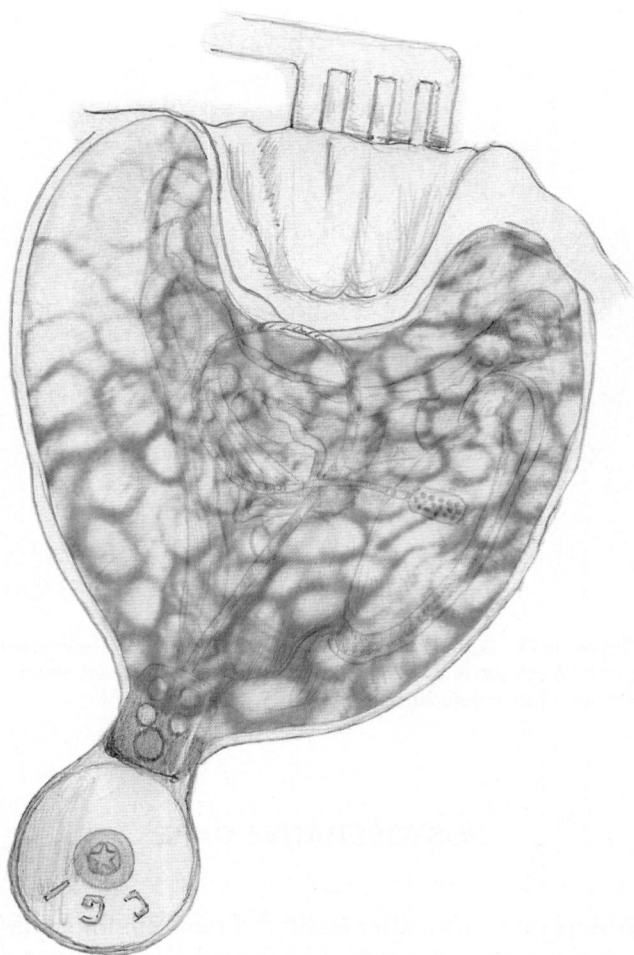

Figure 33–8 Schematic view of the implant, electrode wires, and fat in place prior to skin closure.

POSTOPERATIVE COMPLICATIONS

The most significant complication in the immediate postoperative period is cerebrospinal fluid leak. Unlike routine translabyrinthine surgery, in which the fluid usually takes the nasal route via the eustachian tube, the ABI electrode and wires provide a pathway along which cerebrospinal fluid can travel under the skin flap. We have noted a marked reduction in the leak rate after transitioning to the fully implantable receiver from the percutaneous connector used with the single-channel ABI. Prevention of a leak begins with meticulous dural approximation. Although the dural opening cannot be closed in a watertight manner, it should be approximated as closely as possible and strips of abdominal fat used to plug the residual dural defect. Muscle and oxidized cellulose

(Surgicel®) are commonly employed for eustachian tube closure and autologous fat for the mastoid cavity. Finally, a multilayered closure of the wound reduces the risk of cerebrospinal fluid leak through the incision.

Despite these precautions, patients with ABIs appear more prone to cerebrospinal fluid leak than those undergoing translabyrinthine procedures without implantation. Leaks from the nose and wound usually respond to reapplication of a mastoid pressure dressing and bed rest. A lumbar-subarachnoid drain is inserted for persistent leaks. When these maneuvers fail to control a leak, surgical exploration and repacking of the wound are necessary.

Meningitis can occur either spontaneously or as a result of postoperative cerebrospinal fluid leak. This unusual complication, when identified promptly, responds to antibiotics and control of the leak.

RESULTS

Comprehensive performance results from the initial group of multichannel ABI recipients have been reported elsewhere.[2] With some notable exceptions, speech perception with the ABI typically does not reach the very high levels generally attained with modern cochlear implants. However, the auditory sensations in combination with lipreading can be highly beneficial in facilitating oral communication. With regular and continued use of the ABI, recipients typically show substantial improvements in performance over time that may continue for many years. Regular use of the device greatly enhances performance, and patients should be counseled about this necessity preoperatively.

Fourteen percent of our multichannel ABI recipients scored at least 20% correct on sound-only sentence recognition tests. Several of these individuals were also able to communicate on the telephone to a limited extent. Three of 88 multichannel ABI recipients achieved sentence recognition scores of more than 50% in the first year[2]; however, it took several years for some other patients to show significant "open-set" ability.

Figure 33–9 shows mean speech perception scores on a number of tests for two groups of ABI recipients: those with less than 2 years experience versus those with 2 years experience or more. These results from the

FDA clinical trials were obtained from patients using the previous eight-electrode array. The group with longer duration of use shows substantial improvement in scores. This indicates that performance continues to improve at least up to 2 years after ABI connection. Several patients continued to improve even after 7 years. Patients with unrealistic expectations or those with useful hearing remaining on their second tumor sides often did not use their ABIs regularly and typically did not show improvements. When remaining hearing was lost, such as after second-side tumor removal, regular use of the ABI increased, and improvements usually occurred. First-tumor side implantation was beneficial in that it allowed patients to adjust to ABI sound gradually before becoming completely reliant on it.

Speech perception with the ABI, as with cochlear implants, may be related to the presence of electrode-specific pitch sensations.[10] The majority of ABI recipients experienced these percepts; however, the range, magnitude, and relative ranking varied greatly.[2] This may be attributable to variations in anatomy, neuronal survival, and proximity of the surface electrodes to auditory neurons. The number of electrodes available for use is also patient dependent. It is influenced in part by the presence of mild nonauditory sensations caused by the spread of activation to other nearby nonauditory brainstem sites. Nonauditory sensations typically have included tin-gling, dizziness, and a slight sensation of jittering of the visual field. By altering stimulus pulse duration and selecting other ground electrodes, it was usually possible to eliminate these side effects. In most cases, nonauditory sensations also decreased in magnitude over time. Primarily because of anatomic difficulties (eg, a large lateral recess, distortion or damage caused by large tumors, or inadequate adherence of the array to the brainstem surface), about 8% of our patients did not receive useful hearing after implantation. In a few such cases, we implanted another multichannel ABI when second-side tumors were removed, and this was successful.

Programming ABI speech processors requires experience. Pitch percepts, number of useable electrodes, and other factors can influence performance. The goal was to optimize the reception of important spectral cues. As part of the process, pitch sensations on available electrodes were scaled and ranked using classic psychophysical methods. An attempt was made to align the electrodes in proper pitch rank order relative to the frequency analysis bands in the sound processor. Such processor "maps" were considered to be properly "pitch ranked." Pitch percepts and nonauditory sensations fluctuated to some degree over time, and periodic reprogramming contributed to maintaining and improving performance. Patients who for some reason missed an appointment for this purpose often soon complained

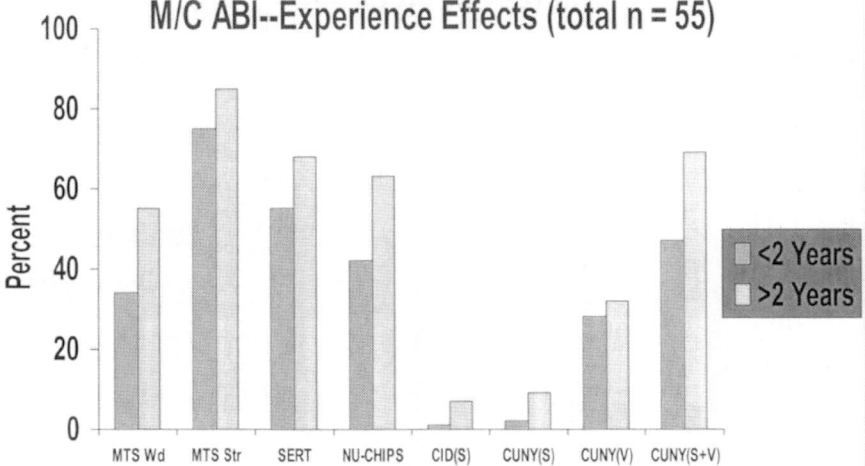

Figure 33–9 Mean speech perception scores from patients with less than 2 years experience versus those with 2 years or more experience. MTS Wd = monosyllable, trochee, spondee word recognition; MTS Stress = monosyllable, trochee, spondee stress recognition; SERT = sound effects recognition test; NU-CHIPS = Northwestern University Children's Recognition of Speech Test; CID = Central Institute for the Deaf sentences; CUNY = City University of New York sentences; S = sound only; V = vision only; S+V = sound plus vision.

that their ABI did not seem as helpful. "Tuning up" the ABI usually immediately rectified this difficulty.

We recently reviewed the relationship between the number of useable electrodes, electrode pitch, and performance. With the present surface electrode array, a strong relationship was not found,[11,12] suggesting that other cues such as temporal information may also be important. With the relatively large (0.7- to 1-mm diameter) surface electrodes, it was probably difficult to activate tuned neurons within the body of the cochlear nucleus with high specificity. Nevertheless, patients generally did better if they had at least three or four available electrode "channels" and if these electrodes were correctly assigned to speech processor analysis bandwidths. All of the best performers also experienced a wider range of pitch sensations (> 30 pitch scale units, 100-point scale) across electrodes.

Data relevant to this issue are presented in Figure 33–10. We tested vowel and consonant recognition in sound only with four different processor configurations in one of our best and most experienced (7 years) patients. She had an overall pitch scale range of approximately 35 units. In one processor configuration, all nine of her electrodes were used, but they were incorrectly (randomly) pitch ranked. Additionally two-, four-, and nine-electrode configurations were programmed in which the electrodes were correctly pitch ranked. Vowel and consonant recognition was poorest with the randomly pitch ranked nine-electrode configuration. Even the configuration using only two properly ranked electrodes resulted in better scores than the nine-electrode random configuration. Scores were nearly equivalent (52 to 55%) with the four- and nine-electrode processors. We subsequently tested two other good performers and found a similar pattern of scores.

Programming ABI sound processors can be more time consuming than cochlear implants,[10] but streamlining the process by de-emphasizing pitch ranking may be deleterious. The best configuration that could be relatively quickly obtained for the above patient was the four-electrode version. Qualitatively, she commented that this version sounded simpler—"like individual notes rather than chords." She further remarked that learning to use an ABI is an ongoing process, and that the four-electrode configuration might be easier for beginning users.

Cochlear implants can provide high levels of performance relative to the ABI, in part because of closer proximity to the tonotopic distribution of axonal processes in the modiolus. Microstimulation of brainstem auditory neurons in animals, such as with prototype needle electrodes, has been shown to be effective in accessing the tonotopic gradient.[13]

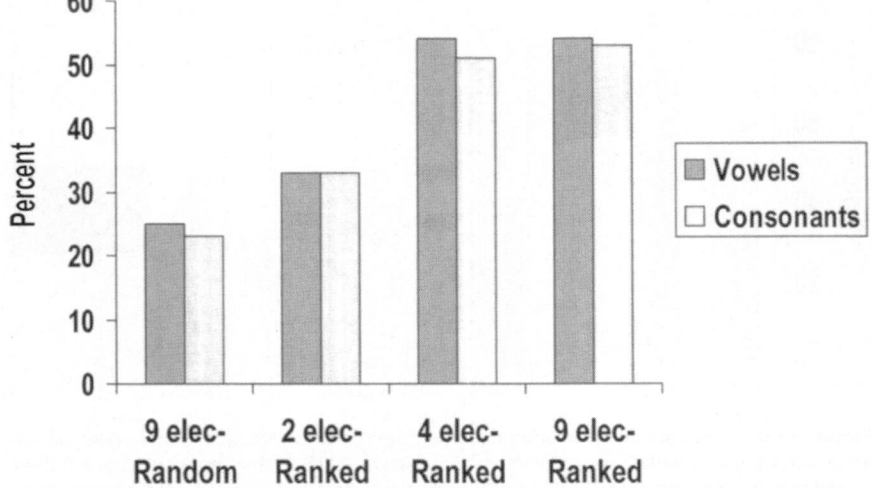

Figure 33–10 Effect of electrode pitch ranking and number of electrodes (elec) on vowel and consonant recognition (sound only) in a top-performing auditory brainstem implant recipient.

Application of this technology in humans with a six-electrode penetrating ABI array is planned and may lead to improved speech recognition with the ABI.

OTHER RESEARCH: EFFECTS OF STIMULATION RATE

The 21-electrode ABI allows higher stimulation pulse rates than the earlier 8-electrode version. In cochlear implants, stimulation rate has received considerable attention, with some investigators finding significant improvements in performance as the stimulation rate was increased.[14,15] Speech recognition results were measured in one ABI patient with the 21-electrode ABI as a function of the stimulation rate. One objective was to determine if immediate performance gains were possible with higher-rate speech-processing strategies.

One female adult, 58 years old and with 10 months of implant experience, was tested in this study using the Nucleus ACE processor. She had nine electrodes programmed in her processor for everyday use. These electrodes were 2, 3, 4, 5, 6, 7, 8, 9, and 10. Since she had very little range in pitch perception among these electrodes, they were simply arranged in ascending numer-ical order with progressively higher-frequency analysis bandwidths.

Speech perception tests consisted of medial vowel and consonant discrimination (with and without lipreading) and the Northwestern University Children's Perception of Speech test (NU-CHIPS).

Three conditions were selected using two, four, and eight electrodes (electrodes used in the two-electrode processor: 2, 6; four-electrode processor: 2, 4, 6, 8; eight-electrode processor: 2, 3, 4, 5, 6, 7, 8, 9). Processors were programmed with the fastest and slowest rates available, plus at least one intermediate rate. In the two-electrode conditions, only the fastest and slowest rates were tested because of time constraints. Stimulation rates ranged from 250 to 2,400 ppse, depending on the number of electrodes used.

Figure 33–11 shows consonant, vowel, and word recognition results from the ABI recipient as a function of the stimulation rate for two-, four-, and eight-channel continuous interleaved sampling processors. The lower open symbols present results using the ABI alone, and the filled symbols present results using the ABI plus lipreading. The dotted line in each panel presents the performance achieved by this patient with her own everyday SPEAK™ (Nucleus) processor (ie, a nine-electrode processor with which she had more than

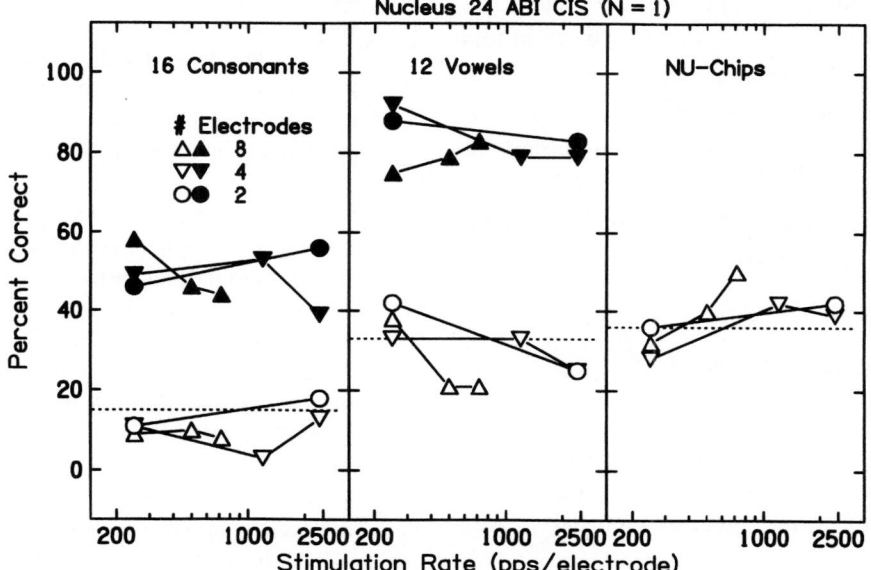

Figure 33–11 Consonant, vowel, and word recognition scores for one auditory brainstem implant (ABI) recipient as a function of stimulation rate for two-, four-, and eight-electrode continuous interleaved sampling (CIS) sound processors. *Open symbols* = ABI alone; *filled symbols* = ABI plus lipreading; *dotted line* = patient's own nine-electrode processor.

6 months experience). Little difference in performance was observed between the two-, four-, and eight-electrode processors, and no clear pattern was evident as a function of stimulation rate.

Consonant recognition was relatively constant as a function of stimulation rate and was similar to the low performance level obtained with the patient's own everyday processor. There appears to be a slight decrease in vowel recognition as stimulation rate was increased. Word recognition on the NU-CHIPS test also appears to be relatively unchanged as a function of stimulation rate. Subjectively, the subject did not report any clear preferences for fast or slow rates. Thus, the results from short-term experiments in this single patient do not provide any incentive to pursue high-rate stimulation strategies.

SUMMARY

The multichannel ABI has received FDA approval for commercial release as a viable means of providing useful hearing sensations to individuals deafened by bilateral vestibular schwannomas (NF2). The sound information provided by the device facilitates sound awareness, recognition, and spoken communication when used in conjunction with lipreading. A small number of ABI recipients also experience significant degrees of speech understanding even without lipreading. Methods of programming ABIs and processing speech sounds can influence performance and benefit, and further work in this area is ongoing. In the future, the ABI may be useful in treating deafness from other causes affecting the peripheral auditory neural pathway. Evaluation in humans of new microstimulation techniques with an ABI array designed to probe the matrix of the auditory brainstem will soon begin and may improve performance.

ACKNOWLEDGMENTS

The authors are grateful to Michael Waring for editorial assistance on electrophysiology and to the patients and staff of House Ear Clinic for their time and effort on behalf of ABI research.

REFERENCES

1. Eisenberg LS, Maltan AA, Portillo F, et al. Electrical stimulation of the auditory brainstem structure in deafened adults. J Rehabil Res Dev 1987;24:9–22.
2. Otto SR, Shannon RV, Brackmann DE et al. The multichannel auditory brainstem implant (ABI): results in 20 patients. Otolaryngol Head Neck Surg 1998,118:291–303.
3. Brackmann DE, Hitselberger WE, Nelson RA, et al. Auditory brainstem implant: I. Issues in surgical implantation. Otolaryngol Head Neck Surg 1993;108:624–33.
4. Shannon RV, Fayad J, Moore JK, et al. Auditory brainstem implant: II. Postsurgical issues and performance. Otolaryngol Head Neck Surg 1993;108:634–42.
5. Briggs RJ, Popovic EA, Brackmann DE. Recent advances in the treatment of neurofibromatosis type II. Adv Otolaryngol Head Neck Surg 1995;9:227–45.
6. Riccardi VM. Neurofibromatosis. Neurol Clin 1987;5:337–49.
7. Hitselberger N, House WF, Edgerton BS, Whitaker S. Cochlear nucleus implant. Otolaryngol Head Neck Surg 1984;92:52–4.
8. Niparko JK, Kileny PR, Kemink JL, et al. Neurophysiologic intraoperative monitoring: II. Facial nerve function. Am J Otol 1989;10:55–61.
9. Waring MD. Refractory properties of auditory brain-stem responses evoked by electrical stimulation of human cochlear nucleus: evidence of neural generators. Electroencephalogr Clin Neurophysiol 1998;108:331–4.
10. Otto SR, Ebinger K, Staller SJ. Clinical trials with the auditory brain stem implant. In: Waltzman S, Cohen N, editors. Cochlear implants. New York: Thieme Medical Publishers; 2000. p. 357–65.
11. Kuchta J, Otto SR, Shannon RV. The number of electrodes and perceptual performance in auditory brainstem implants. Abstract of presentation at 2001 Conference on Implantable Auditory Prostheses, Pacific Grove, CA, August 2001.
12. Kuchta J, Otto SR, Shannon RV. Pitch perception and perceptual performance in auditory brainstem implants. Abstract of presentation at 2001 Conference on Implantable Auditory Prostheses, Pacific Grove, CA, August 2001.
13. McCreery DG, Shannon RV, Moore JK, et al. Accessing the tonotopic organization of the ventral cochlear nucleus by intranuclear microstimulation. IEEE Trans Rehabil Eng 1998;4:1–9.
14. Brill SM, Hochmair I, Hochmair ES. The importance of stimulation rate in pulsatile stimulations strategies in cochlear implants. Presented at the XXIV International Congress of Audiology, Buenos Aires, August 1998.
15. Brill SM, Schatzer R, Nopp P, et al. JCIS:CIS with temporally jittering stimulations pulses: effect of jittering amplitude and stimulation rate on speech understanding. Presented at the 4th European Symposium on Paediatric Cochlear Implantation, s-Hertogenbosch, The Netherlands, June 1998.

34

Radiation Treatment for Acoustic Neuroma

JOHN C. FLICKINGER, MD

Radiosurgery and fractionated radiotherapy are alternatives to microsurgical resection of acoustic neuromas (vestibular schwannomas) with lower patient morbidity and seemingly comparable long-term tumor control rates.[1–11] For many years, surgery was generally regarded as the only effective treatment for vestibular schwannomas, based on the belief that these tumors were insensitive to radiation. Little consideration was given to using radiation for managing acoustic neuromas prior to the report by Wallner and colleagues on postoperative fractionated radiotherapy of acoustic neuromas and the early reports on radiosurgery from Sweden and Pittsburgh.[7,12,13]

Some head and neck surgeons, familiar with responses of malignant head and neck tumors to radiotherapy, may not fully appreciate the radiation responses of benign tumors. As a rule, benign tumors shrink slowly, if at all, after radiotherapy. Unlike malignant tumors, for which a complete response is needed after radiotherapy for long-term tumor control, the goal in irradiating benign tumors is to stop further tumor growth by either killing or inactivating all clonogens, which may comprise only a small proportion of the tumor. Long-term control of benign tumors with radiotherapy (despite little shrinkage) has been extensively documented for meningiomas, pituitary adenomas, and, only relatively recently, vestibular schwannomas.[5,7,14] Malignant tumors usually start shrinking and may disappear by the end of a course of radiotherapy, whereas benign tumors may take 3, 6, or even more than 12 months to even begin to shrink. The two most likely reasons for the slow rate of shrinkage are that the rate of cell death after radiation relates to the cell-cycle times (which are long in benign tumors) and that

some of the response may be attributable to late radiation effects on the tumor's supporting vasculature. If radiation were ever tried in patients with large acoustic tumors in urgent need of relief from brainstem compression and hydrocephalus, it would never shrink the tumors fast enough to show any benefit. Another understandable reason for the early lack of faith in radiation for vestibular schwannomas is that benign tumors such as vestibular schwannomas can be observed sometimes for years without any tumor growth. This fact makes it imperative that the effectiveness of radiotherapy of a benign tumor like a vestibular schwannoma is assessed in large series with long-term follow-up.

STEREOTACTIC RADIOSURGERY

Radiosurgery is the term coined by Leksell in 1951 to describe the closed-skull destruction of a stereotactically defined intracranial target using sharply defined, external beam ionizing radiation. In benign tumor radiosurgery, the destruction is mostly limited to the proliferative capacity of the tumor, as previously mentioned.[7] Leksell started with orthovoltage radiation in 1951 but switched to proton beam irradiation around 1960 before switching to cobalt 60 beams in his design for the gamma knife. Early successful reports on the successful use of gamma-knife radiosurgery in the treatment of arteriovenous malformations and acoustic neuromas spurred the development of linear accelerator (LINAC) radiosurgery techniques to produce similar radiation distributions.

The Radiosurgical Procedure

The radiosurgical procedure begins with application of a stereotactic frame that is compatible with the planned imaging. The frame application results in four small puncture wounds in the scalp to allow the tips of the fixation pins to touch the skull. In adults and children over the age of 12, the frame can be applied using local anesthesia and conscious sedation. Magnetic resonance imaging (MRI) is used by most gamma-knife groups in preference to computed tomography (CT) because of MRI's better tumor definition. Stereotactic MRI requires extensive quality control measures to avoid image distortion. A number of LINAC radiosurgery groups use image fusion to correlate prior nonstereotactic (without a head frame) MRI with stereotactic CT images, thereby sidestepping any potential MRI-related distortion or incompatibility problems with their stereotactic frames.

Once stereotactic MRI or CT images are acquired, sophisticated treatment planning programs are used to design treatment volumes to match the tumor. Gamma-knife and multiple-arc LINAC techniques produce relatively spherical dose distributions around each treatment center (isocenter) irradiated. Multiple isocenters are normally treated to match the nonspherical shapes of most vestibular schwannomas. Irradiating different portions of a tumor at a time with different doses of radiation to conform the radiation distribution more closely to the tumor is termed intensity-modulated radiotherapy. Conventional radiotherapy techniques irradiate the entire tumor with each treatment beam used (usually two to four beams).

Early Radiosurgery Results

In the 1980s and early 1990s, acoustic neuroma radiosurgery was performed with less sophisticated treatment plans than are available today.[2] Lower-resolution CT scans were used for treatment planning, making it harder to precisely define the tumor volume. Treatment planning software and hardware were slow and inflexible, which made it cumbersome to make sophisticated multiple isocenter treatment plans to closely match the irregular tumor shapes. Most treatment plans used two or three isocenters. Based on the limited initial Swedish experience, with some uncertainties in the dosimetry of their early treatment plans, it was believed in the 1980s that minimum tumor doses of 16 to 20 Gy were necessary to control acoustic neuromas.

The early radiosurgical experience in treating acoustic neuromas is best represented by Kondziolka and colleagues' analysis of the University of Pittsburgh experience from 1987 to 1992.[5] From 1987 to 1992, 162 patients with an acoustic neuroma underwent gamma-knife radiosurgery to a marginal dose of 12 to 20 Gy (median 16 Gy). Patients were surveyed after 5 to 10 years of follow-up; 98% of tumors were controlled with no further surgery. Tumors shrunk in 62% of patients. Temporary or permanent facial weakness developed in 21%, trigeminal neuropathy in 27%, and decrease in hearing in 49%.

Recent Radiosurgery Results

Radiosurgery results with current treatment techniques are well represented by the University of Pittsburgh experience from 1992 to 1997.[2] Unlike the early experience with CT-based treatment planning, MR-based treatment stereotactic imaging was used for more precise tumor imaging. More conformal treatment plans were possible through the use of more sophisticated treatment planning software. A total of 192 patients with previously untreated unilateral acoustic neuromas underwent gamma-knife radiosurgery during this time period. The median follow-up was 19 months (65 months maximum follow-up). Marginal tumor doses were 11 to 18 Gy (median 13 Gy), and treatment volumes were 0.1 to 33 cc (median 2.7 cc). Counting 1 mm temporary increases in average diameter as failures, the strict radiographic tumor control rate was 91.0%. Only one patient required surgical resection for sustained tumor growth for a 5-year actuarial clinical tumor control rate (no requirement for surgical intervention) for the entire series of 99.4%. The 5-year actuarial rate for developing any new facial weakness was 1.2%, facial numbness was 3.4%, decreased hearing was 27.1%, and complete loss of speech discrimination was 12.1%. For the 103 patients whose tumors were treated with a marginal dose of ≤ 13 Gy, the rate of developing any new facial weakness was 0%, any facial numbness was 3.1%, any decrease in hearing was 24.8%, and loss of any speech discrimination was 11.8%. No patient treated with marginal doses of < 15 Gy (n = 163) developed facial weakness. Hearing improved in 9 of 143 patients (6%) with decreased (Class II–V) hearing before radiosurgery. Thus, radiosurgery using modern techniques with MRI-based, highly conformal, multiple-isocenter treatment planning and marginal tumor doses of 12 to 13 Gy is associated with low risk of facial weakness (< 0.5%), trigeminal neuropathy (3%), hearing loss (12% complete loss of speech discrimination, 25% with any decrease in hearing), and high rates of tumor control (99% avoiding surgical resection).

Foote and colleagues found similar results in the University of Florida LINAC acoustic neuroma radiosurgery experience.[3] In 108 patients treated after 1994, the actuarial rates of facial and trigeminal neuropathy were 2% and 5%, respectively, as compared with a 29% risk for both facial and trigeminal neuropathy in 41 patients treated before 1994. Their 5-year actuarial tumor control rate was 87%. They found a nonsignificant trend toward poorer tumor control below a marginal dose of 10 Gy (p = .207) and recommended using a marginal dose of 12.5 Gy.

STEREOTACTIC FRACTIONATED RADIOTHERAPY

Radiobiologic Rationale

Although the early results with radiosurgery for acoustic neuromas such as the early University of Pittsburgh results (with a median marginal dose of 16 Gy) had lower rates of facial neuropathy and better hearing level than in most surgical series, there was obvious room for improvement. Most large-field conventional radiotherapy (which is usually performed to treat malignant tumors) is fractionated. Fractionation selectively protects late-reacting normal tissue (like cranial nerves and brain) compared with most malignant tumors. This advantage of fractionation has not been clearly established for benign tumors because they are difficult to study in the laboratory. Recent studies have found that some slow-growing malignant tumors, such as prostate cancer, are spared more by fractionation than the surrounding normal tissue.[12] Fractionated stereotactic radiotherapy has therefore been advocated as a way of lowering the risk of radiation injury to cranial nerves V, VII, and VIII in

the treatment of acoustic neuromas. Because of the high tumor control rates seen with the early experience in radiosurgery for acoustic neuromas and the fact that surgical salvage is still possible if tumors fail to be controlled by radiation, it is also reasonable to lower the dose of radiation administered to try to lower complications (whether single-fraction radiosurgery of fractionated radiotherapy is used). Because of this, most stereotactic fractionated radiosurgery schedules has used dose-fractionation schedules that appear to have lower expected biologic effects than early radiosurgery series.

Although different formulas can be used to extrapolate from different biologic effects of fractionated radiotherapy to single-fraction radiation, these extrapolations are generally regarded as unreliable. The equivalent effect of a single-fraction dose of 13 Gy on central nervous tissue (eg, cranial nerve) would be 88 Gy at 2 Gy per fraction as calculated with the Neuret formula (approximately equivalent to $\alpha/\beta = 0$) and 48.7 Gy at 2 Gy per fraction with the linear-quadratic formula ($\alpha/\beta = 2$). In comparison, hypofractionated schemes of 20 Gy in four and five fractions have equivalent central nervous system effects of 42 and 52 Gy predicted by the Neuret formula and 30 and 35 Gy with ($\alpha/\beta = 2$). There is presently no way to accurately determine parameters for estimating tumor control with these formulas for acoustic neuromas owing to the high tumor control rates seen with radiation treatment. Advocates of radiosurgery believe that fractionation affects benign tumor control and normal tissue complications equally, whereas groups treating acoustic neuromas with fractionated radiotherapy believe that fractionation will lead to a lesser effect on the normal tissue than the tumor.

Stereotactic Radiotherapy Results

Table 34–1 compares the results of several fractionated radiotherapy series for acoustic neuromas with the recent University of Pittsburgh and University of Florida radiosurgery results. Hearing loss and trigeminal nerve effects continue to be seen in large fractionated series in rates that are roughly comparable to recent radiosurgery experience. It is important to appreciate that larger series with longer follow-up are needed to adequately analyze differences in tumor control between techniques.

Table 1–1   COMPARISON OF ACOUSTIC NEUROMA TUMOR CONTROL AND COMPLICATIONS WITH DIFFERENT RADIOSURGERY AND FRACTIONATED RADIOTHERAPY SERIES

Institution	Minimum Tumor Dose/No. of Fractions	Patients (n)	Tumor Control (%)	Cranial Nerve Complications
University of Pittsburgh[2]	12–13 Gy/1 fr	103	99	V 3%, VII 0%, VIII 25%
Harvard Joint Center[11]	54 Gy/27–30 fr	12	100	V 8%, VII 0%, VIII 8%
Stanford University[8]	21 Gy/3 fr	33	97	V 16%, VII 3%, VIII 23%
Staten Island, New York[6]	20 Gy/4–5 fr	38	100	V 0%, VII 3% VIII 23%
Jefferson, Philadelphia[1]		56	86	V 7%, VII 2%, VIII 32%*
Sapporo, Japan[10]	40–48 Gy/20–23 fr	50	86	V 12%, VII 5%, VIII 53%

*Actuarial at 3 years.

RARE SEQUELAE OF RADIOSURGERY AND RADIOTHERAPY

The most common delayed effects of radiosurgery (facial weakness, numbness, or hearing loss) are rarely detected more than 2 to 3 years after radiosurgery. Radiation-induced tumors can arise 5 to 30 years after radiotherapy. The actuarial incidence of radiation-induced tumors after fractionated conventional radiotherapy for pituitary adenomas appears to be 1 to 2% in series with 20- to 30-year follow-up.[14] Similar doses of 40 to 60 Gy have been used in these series (usually 45 to 50 Gy in 25 to 28 fractions), with treatment volumes averaging 5 cm in diameter and a skull base target volume not very dissimilar from that used in the treatment of acoustic neuromas. The most common radiation-induced tumors in these series are meningiomas and primary gliomas (glioblastoma, anaplastic astrocytoma, etc). There are case reports of secondary tumors arising after radiosurgery, but the true incidence is not known. There are no good data on the effect of fractionation on second tumor formation. Since tumor induction appears to involve multiple mutations, it is reasonable to guess that it increases the risk of second tumor formation. Taking into account the smaller tumor volumes treated in radiosurgery and the use of single-fraction radiation, it is estimated that the risk of second tumor formation after radiosurgery is in the range of 1 in 500 (0.2%) with 30-year follow-up. With the effect of fractionation and slightly larger treatment volumes used with fractionated stereotactic radiosurgery as compared with radiosurgery, it is assumed that the risk of developing a second tumor should be more than 0.2% but less than 2%.

Primary acoustic neuroma radiosurgery is performed without first verifying tissue diagnosis. Rarely, a clinically diagnosed "acoustic neuroma" can progress after radiosurgery and is found to be a malignant tumor when a salvage surgical resection is performed. The likelihood of this occurring is expected to be in the range of 1 in 500 to 1 in 1,000. This event raises the question of whether the tumor initially was benign and underwent malignant transformation or whether the tumor was malignant to start with and was simply not controlled by radiosurgery.

Routine pregnancy tests should be performed prior to radiosurgery on any female patient of childbearing capability because even a low dose of scatter radiation to the pelvis can increase the risk of birth defects if the patient is pregnant.

Salvage Surgery after Failed Radiosurgery

It appears to be more difficult to preserve facial nerve function in patients requiring salvage surgery after failing radiosurgery. Facial nerve preservation seems most difficult for recurrent tumors that have first failed surgery and then fail radiation because of the effects of prior surgery and radiation. Arguing that initial surgical resection is a better strategy than initial radiosurgery because of difficulty preserving the facial nerve with reoperation may not be reasonable if one focuses on the low recurrence rates with radiosurgery or radiotherapy and the greater facial nerve injury rates with initial surgery. With only 2% of radiosurgery patients needing salvage surgery, the maximum rate of facial paralysis would be no more than 2% in the entire series if all resected patients developed facial weakness and 1% if it occurred in half.

REFERENCES

1. Andrews DW, Suarez O, Goldman HW, et al. Stereotactic radiosurgery and fractionated stereotactic radiotherapy for the

treatment of acoustic schwannomas: comparative observations of 125 patients treated at one institution. Int J Radiat Oncol Biol Phys 2001;50:1265–78.

2. Flickinger JC, Kondziolka D, Niranjan A, Lunsford LD. Results of acoustic neuroma radiosurgery: an analysis of 5 years' experience using current methods. J Neurosurg 2001;94:1–6.

3. Foote KD, Friedman WA, Buatti JM, et al. Analysis of risk factors associated with radiosurgery for vestibular schwannoma. J Neurosurg 2001;95:440–9.

4. Hanabusa K, Morikawa A, Murata T, Taki W. Acoustic neuroma with malignant transformation. Case report. J Neurosurg 2001; 95:518–21.

5. Kondziolka D, Lunsford LD, McLaughlin MR, Flickinger JC. Long-term outcomes after radiosurgery for acoustic neuromas. N Engl J Med 1998;339:1426–33.

6. Lederman G, Lowry J, Wertheim S, et al. Acoustic neuroma: potential benefits of fractionated stereotactic radiosurgery. Stereotact Funct Neurosurg 1997;69(1–4 Pt 2):175–82.

7. Noren G, Greitz D, Hirsch A, Lax I. Gamma knife surgery in acoustic tumors. Acta Neurochir Suppl (Wien) 1993;58:104–7.

8. Poen JC, Golby AJ, Forster KM, et al. Fractionated stereotactic radiosurgery and preservation of hearing in patients with vestibular schwannoma: a preliminary report. Neurosurgery 1999;45:1299–305.

9. Pollock BE, Lunsford LD, Kondziolka D, et al. Outcome analysis of acoustic neuroma management: a comparison of microsurgery and stereotactic radiosurgery. Neurosurgery 1995;36: 215–25.

10. Shirato H, Sakamoto T, Sawamura Y, et al. Comparison between observation policy and fractionated stereotactic radiotherapy (SRT) as an initial management for vestibular schwannoma. Int J Radiat Oncol Biol Phys 1999;44:545–50.

11. Varlotto JM, Shrieve DC, Alexander E 3rd, et al. Fractionated stereotactic radiotherapy for the treatment of acoustic neuromas: preliminary results. Int J Radiat Oncol Biol Phys 1996;36: 141–5.

12. Brenner DJ, Hall EJ. Fractionation and protraction for radiotherapy of prostate carcinoma. Int J Radiat Oncol Biol Phys 1999;43:1095–101.

13. Wallner KE, Sheline GE, Pitts LH, et al. Efficacy of irradiation for incompletely excised acoustic neurilemomas. J Neurosurg 1987;67:858–63.

14. Breen P, Flickinger JC, Kondziolka D, Martinez AJ. Radiotherapy for nonfunctional pituitary adenoma: analysis of long-term tumor control. J Neurosurg 1998;89:933–88.

35

Surgery for Cystic Lesions of the Petrous Apex

GORDON B. HUGHES, MD
JOUNG LEE, MD
PAUL M. RUGGIERI, MD

Cholesterol granuloma, cholesteatoma (epidermoid cyst), and mucocele account for 99% of primary cystic lesions of the petrous apex, with cholesterol granuloma being the most common (Table 35–1).[1] These lesions can be confused with normal bone marrow in a poorly pneumatized petrous apex, trapped fluid (effusion) within an apical cell,[2] and an arachnoid cyst.[3] Magnetic resonance imaging (MRI) and computed tomography (CT) can usually distinguish among these lesions. Rare primary lesions of the petrous apex include unifocal Langerhans' cell histiocytosis (eosinophilic granuloma),[4] chordoma, chondrosarcoma, and osteoclastoma. Secondary lesions include osteomyelitis, direct tumor spread, metastatic tumor, sphenoid mucocele, and aneurysm of the internal carotid artery.[5] Because primary and secondary neoplasms, encephaloceles, middle ear cholesteatoma, and osteomyelitis extending to the apex have been covered in previous chapters, this chapter will concentrate on diagnosis and management of primary "cystic" lesions of the petrous apex: cholesterol granuloma, cholesteatoma (epidermoid cyst), and mucocele.

PATHOLOGY

Cholesterol granuloma results from obstruction of and hemorrhage into a previously aerated space and may also arise from rapid fluctuation of air pressure within the narrow air channels leading to the petrous apex.[6,7] An expansile cyst fills the obstructed cells, lined by fibrous tissue and containing chocolate brown or black fluid filled with chronic granulation tissue and cholesterol crystals (Figure 35–1). As the cyst expands, the involved air cells dilate and the surrounding bone erodes.

Cholesteatoma (epidermoid cyst) consists of an epithelial wall, fibrous subepithelium, and keratin debris (Figure 35–2). The presence of epithelium distinguishes cholesteatoma from cholesterol granuloma. Epidermoid rests are thought to arise near the foramen lacerum[8] and can be distinguished from dermoid cysts that have skin adnexae (eg, sweat glands). As the cholesteatoma expands, bone erosion may result from osteolytic enzymes at the junction of the epithelium and fibrous subepithelium.

A mucocele results from obstruction of drainage from a highly pneumatized petrous apex and also can produce an expansile cystic lesion. The mucocele can be distinguished from cholesteatoma by the absence of keratinizing epithelium and from the cholesterol granuloma by the absence of cholesterol crystals and dense fibrous capsule (Figure 35–3). Some clinicians consider

Table 35–1 LESIONS OF THE PETROUS APEX
Primary
Cholesterol granuloma
Cholesteatoma (epidermoid cyst)
Mucocele
Trapped fluid (effusion)
Eosinophilic granuloma
Mesenchymal tumor (chondroma, chondrosarcoma,
osteoclastoma, fibrous dysplasia)
Secondary
Direct spread of neoplasm (nasopharyngeal carcinoma,
vestibular or jugular foramen schwannoma, trigeminal
neuroma, glomus tumor, clival chordoma, meningioma)
Metastasis or hematogenous spread (metastatic tumor,
lymphoma)
Infection (osteomyelitis, necrotizing external otitis)
Other (arachnoid cyst, aneurysm of internal carotid artery,
sphenoid mucocele)

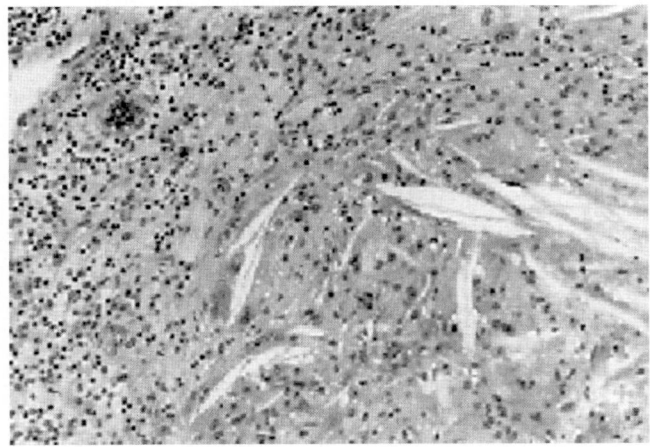

Figure 35–1 Cholesterol granuloma. The oblong, needle-shaped clefts contain crystals of cholesterol esters that have been dissolved during histologic processing of the specimen. Foreign body–type giant cells have formed about some of the crystals, and many lymphocytes and histiocytes also are present. (Hematoxylin and eosin stain; ×200 original magnification.)

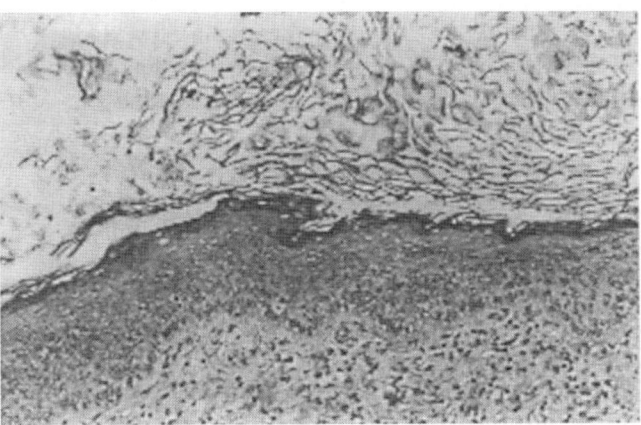

Figure 35–2 Cholesteatoma. This cross-section of cholesteatoma shows keratin debris, keratinizing epithelium, and fibrous subepithelium. (Hematoxylin and eosin stain; ×200 original magnification.)

chronic trapped effusion, mucocele, and cholesterol granuloma to represent varying stages of severity of the same pathologic entity. The same reasoning implies that chronic, symptomatic, trapped fluid may not represent a benign "leave me alone"[2] lesion but instead may require surgery.

CLINICAL PRESENTATION

Symptoms

Petrous apex findings ("lesions") can be asymptomatic and discovered coincidentally on MRI. Leonetti and colleagues performed a retrospective chart review to categorize a group of petrous apex findings that were noted incidentally on MRI in 88 patients.[9] These incidental findings, which were unrelated to the presenting clinical manifestations, included asymmetric fatty bone marrow (n = 41), inflammation (n = 19), cholesterol granulomas (n = 14), cholesteatomas (n = 9), and neoplasms (n = 5). Follow-up imaging and clinical surveillance of these patients did not demonstrate any significant change in the incidentally detected lesions. In all cases, the incidental MRI findings represented benign pathology. Therefore, the clinician should bear in mind that a petrous apex "lesion" noted on MRI may or may not directly relate to the patient's presenting signs and symptoms; the physician should not overreact to an MRI finding that may, in fact, be coincidental.

Most published reports of symptomatic petrous apex lesions include primary and secondary neoplasms and list hearing loss as the most common presenting symptom.[1,5,7] Non-neoplastic, primary cystic lesions of the apex, however, more often present with headache, head pain, or aural pressure. Headache is usually ipsilateral and retro-orbital or temporoparietal but also can be referred to the occiput or vertex. Hearing loss occurs when the eustachian tube is compressed (conductive loss) or the internal auditory canal or inner ear is invaded

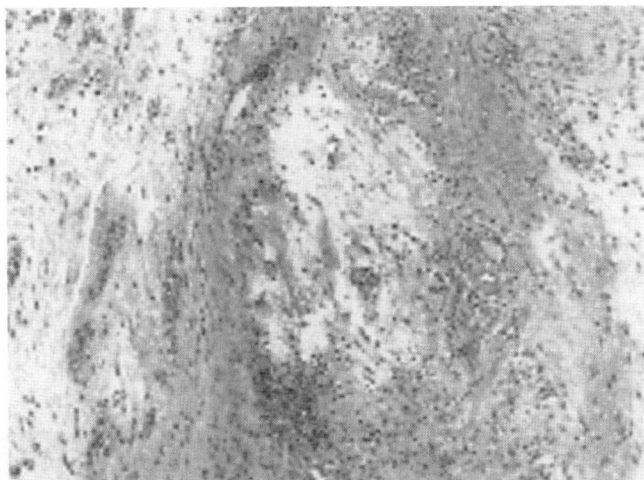

Figure 35–3 Mucocele. The mucocele consists of extravasated mucous ("mucous release reaction") with a surrounding inflammatory infiltrate. The mucocele can be distinguished from cholesteatoma by the absence of keratinizing epithelium and from cholesterol granuloma by the absence of cholesterol crystals. (Hematoxylin and eosin stain; ×200 original magnification.)

(sensorineural hearing loss) and can be accompanied by tinnitus. Less often, inner ear involvement can produce light-headedness or true vertigo. Trigeminal nerve compression can produce hypesthesia or paresthesia, especially along the distribution of the mandibular branch (V3). Facial palsy and spasm from seventh cranial nerve compression and diplopia from sixth cranial nerve compression are uncommon. Ophthalmoplegia from anterior extension into the cavernous sinus is rare. Syncope also is rare and suggests carotid artery compression. Otorrhea can result from secondary infection and drainage of the cystic lesion.

Signs

Otoscopy is usually normal but can reveal drum retraction, middle ear effusion, or drainage. Hypesthesia of cranial nerve V and palsy of cranial nerves VI or VII are uncommon. The patient may have imbalance in performing the Romberg test or tandem gait. Often the head and neck examination is completely normal.

AUDIOMETRIC AND VESTIBULAR EVALUATION

The audiogram can be normal or reveal conductive, sensorineural, or mixed hearing loss. Vestibular testing can detect canal paresis from inner ear involvement. We usually obtain an audiogram but rarely an electronystagmogram.

RADIOLOGIC EVALUATION

Cholesterol granuloma is not only the most common cystic lesion of the petrous apex, it is also the only one that is invariably hyperintense on both T_1- and T_2-weighted images on MRI (Table 35–2, Figure 35–4). Both

cholesteatoma and mucocele are hypointense on T_1 views (Figure 35–5).[6] Magnetic resonance imaging, however, lacks bone detail. A CT scan can show whether the cyst is expansile. An expansile cyst usually requires surgery; a nonexpansile cyst usually does not. A CT scan also differentiates potentially surgical cysts of the apex from nonsurgical, asymmetric fatty marrow and trapped fluid (effusion). Trapped fluid (effusion) will have low signal intensity on T_1-weighted image and high signal intensity on T_2-weighted image on MRI and nonexpansile fluid attenuation (opacification) within a pneumatized petrous apex on CT (Figure 35–6).[2] Asymmetric fatty marrow will have high signal intensity on T_1-weighted images and intermediate intensity on T_2-weighted images on MRI and a nonexpansile, nonpneumatized petrous apex on CT (Figure 35–7).[2]

CLINICAL EVALUATION

Ipsilateral retro-orbital pain is relatively specific for petrous apex disease, but some patients present with ear pain or pressure and temporoparietal headache. Because headache from petrous apex cystic lesions is the most common presenting symptom and otoscopy is often normal, the differential diagnosis of referred "ear" pain should be considered, especially when a small, nonexpansile petrous apex cyst is present on MRI but may not be the primary cause of the symptoms.

The facial nerve refers pain to the external ear canal and postauricular region. The second and third cervical nerves refer pain to the postauricular and mastoid regions. Trigeminal referred otalgia arises from lesions involving the oral cavity and floor of the mouth, teeth, mandible, temporomandibular joint (TMJ), palate, and preauricular skin. Glossopharyngeal referred otalgia arises from the tonsil, base of the tongue, soft palate, nasopharynx, eustachian tube, and pharynx. Vagal referred otalgia arises from the hypopharynx, larynx, and trachea. Dif-

Table 35–2 RADIOGRAPHIC FEATURES OF PETROUS APEX CYST, TUMOR, FLUID, AND MARROW				
Lesion	MRI (T_1)	MRI (T_2)	Enhancing	Expansile
Cholesterol granuloma	High	High	No	Yes
Cholesteatoma	Low-medium	High	No	Yes
Trapped fluid	Low/variable	High	No	No
Tumor	Low-medium	High	Yes	Yes

MRI = magnetic resonance imaging.

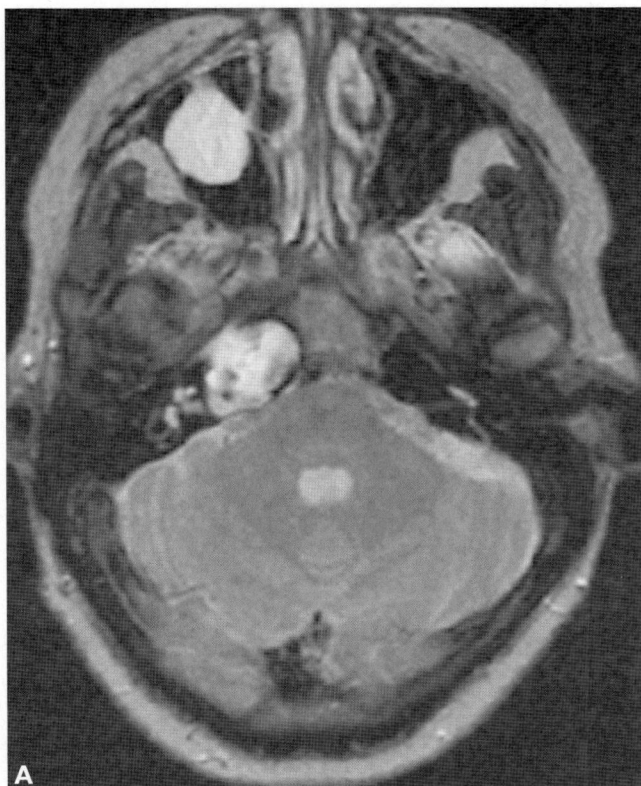

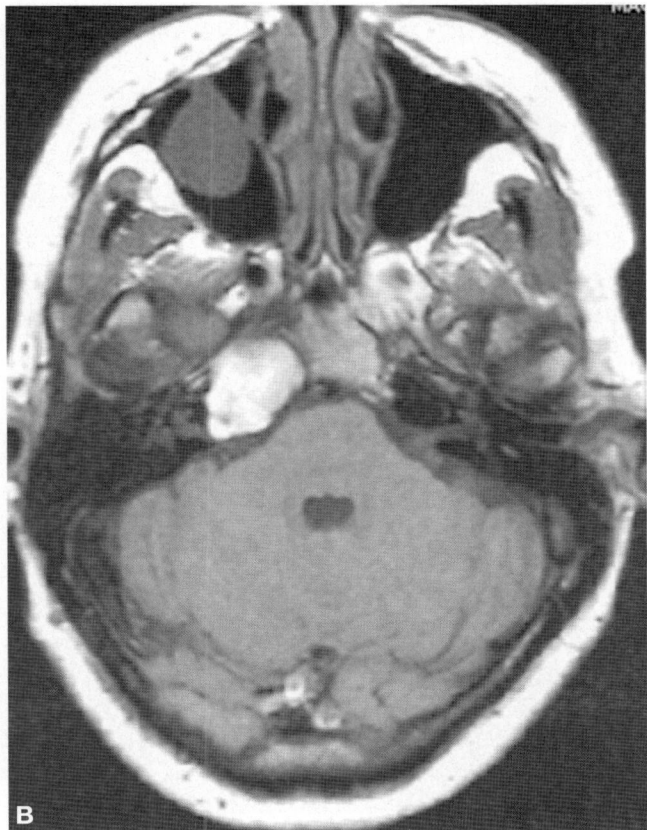

Figure 35–4   Cholesterol granuloma. *A*, Axial T$_2$-weighted fast spin-echo magnetic resonance image demonstrates a large, well-defined heterogeneously hyperintense mass in the right petrous apex that appears to be mildly expansile and impinges on the right carotid canal. A right maxillary sinus mucocele or polyp is noted coincidentally. *B*, The mass is also prominently hyperintense on the corresponding axial T$_1$-weighted spin-echo image. The signal intensity characteristics on T$_1$ and T$_2$ are quite typical for a cholesterol granuloma, presumably caused by prior hemorrhage.

Figure 35–4 continued on next page

ferential causes of referred otalgia include migraine, TMJ syndrome, cervical myalgia, fibromyalgia, dental abscess, head and neck malignancy (particularly occult neoplasm of the nasopharynx, sinus, tonsil, base of the tongue and hypopharynx), temporal arteritis, inflammatory sinusitis, carotidynia, trigeminal neuralgia, glossopharyngeal neuralgia, and gastroesophageal reflux disease.

Patients with ear pain and/or temporoparietal headache should have careful examination of the auricle and otoscopic examination of the external and middle ear. If the ear is normal, the anterior nares, oral cavity, oropharynx, laryngohypopharynx, neck, and scalp should be examined. The TMJ, temporal artery, tonsillar fossa, base of the tongue, carotid artery, and neck muscles should be carefully palpated for tenderness, mass, or spasm. The teeth can be percussed for tenderness. In selected cases, radiographic examination of the teeth, jaw, and sinuses can be obtained. If no cause is identified at this point, we recommend MRI of the brain and base of the skull (including infratemporal fossa) in both axial and coronal views, with and without gadolinium contrast enhancement.

Magnetic resonance imaging can reveal a petrous apex cystic lesion, encephalocele, or arachnoid cyst. Computed tomographic scanning can be obtained to identify bone destruction or bone marrow fat in asymmetric pneumatization. Computed tomography can also be useful in delineating hypotympanic air cells in situations for which an infracochlear drainage procedure is considered (see below). A cystic lesion of the petrous apex may be the only abnormality on clinical and radiographic evaluation. If other causes of ear pain and headache have been excluded (sometimes a treatment trial for migraine is warranted), then the relative benefits and risks of surgery of the cyst are explained to the patient. These depend on the type and size of the cyst, surgical excision or drainage, level of hearing, and approach selected.

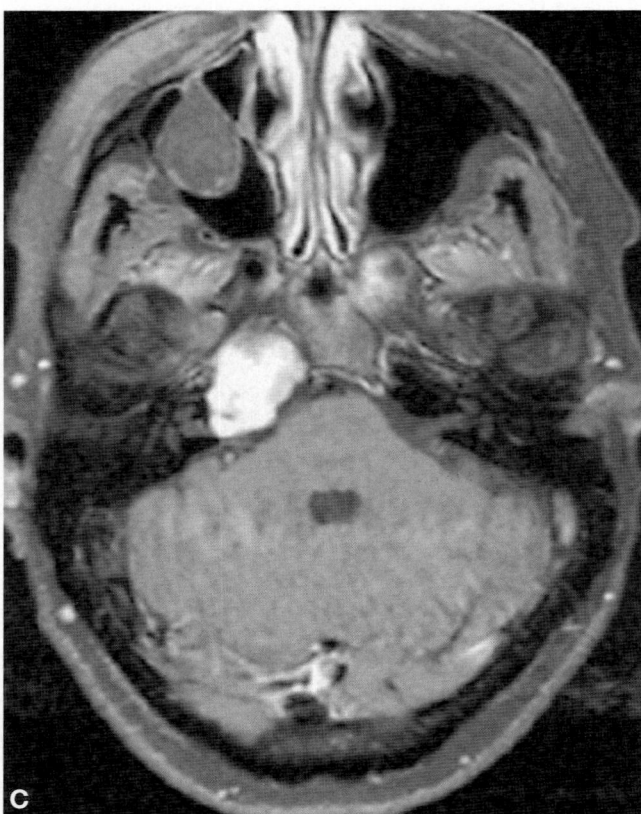

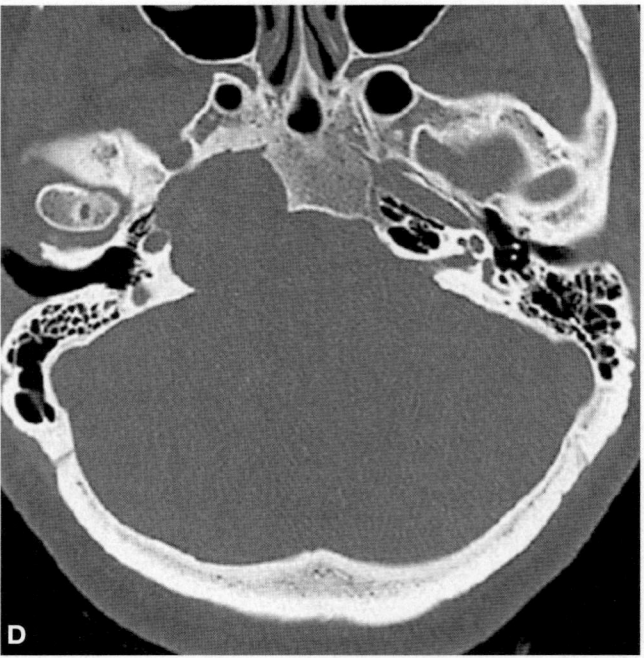

Figure 35–4 Cholesterol granuloma. *C,* Fat suppression eliminates the high signal intensity of the fat in the normal petrous apex to make the lesion more obvious but has no impact on the signal of the cholesterol granuloma itself. No enhancement can be appreciated along the periphery of the mass because of the degree of hyperintensity of the contents on the unenhanced T_1-weighted images. *D,* On the axial computed tomographic image, the mass is more obviously expansile and protrudes into the cerebellopontine angle cistern. There is a thin rim of surrounding, reactive sclerosis as would be expected with a slowly growing process.

SURGICAL APPROACH

For hearing preservation, the middle cranial fossa and infracochlear (hypotympanic) approaches are used for management of benign, non-neoplastic, cystic lesions of the petrous apex. For very large lesions, when additional exposure and control of the carotid artery are required, the transcochlear approach can be used with extension into the infratemporal fossa if necessary.[10] Because MRI provides very sensitive, early detection of smaller apical lesions, the transcochlear-infratemporal fossa approach is rarely needed. Surgical management of cholesteatoma differs from that of cholesterol granuloma and is covered more fully in the Discussion section.

The middle cranial fossa (transpetrosal) approach (Figure 35–8) to the petrous apex[11] is used to excise rather than simply drain the cyst and is the procedure of choice when the cyst location and lack of hypotympanic pneumatization make the infracochlear approach difficult. The middle cranial fossa approach provides good access to the cyst for total excision in most cases except those cysts that extend inferiorly or those that encircle the carotid artery. After general anesthesia is administered, a subarachnoid drain is placed, and 80 cc of cerebrospinal fluid (CSF) are removed slowly to relax the temporal lobe during elevation to expose the middle fossa floor. The drain is then clamped and removed at the end of surgery. The patient is placed supine with the head in points, and facial and auditory monitoring electrodes are placed. A subtemporal, 6-cm vertical incision extends superiorly from the zygomatic process, 1 cm anterior to the external auditory canal (Figure 35–8). A 3 × 2.5 cm bone flap is removed, and the temporal lobe is elevated extradurally to reveal the foramen spinosum anteriorly, arcuate eminence posteriorly, and superior petrosal sinus medially. Temporal lobe traction is gently maintained with a Greenberg retractor. The greater superficial petrosal nerve (GSPN) is identified and followed posteriorly to the geniculate ganglion, which is confirmed with the facial nerve stimulator. The basal turn of the cochlea lies just anterior and medial to the gan-

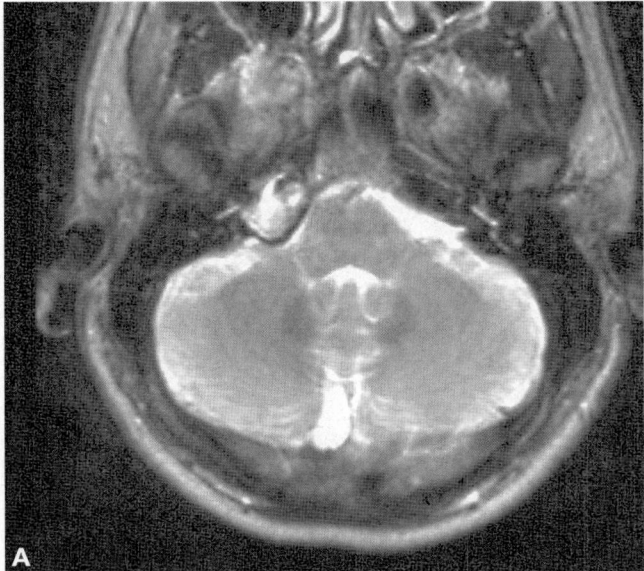

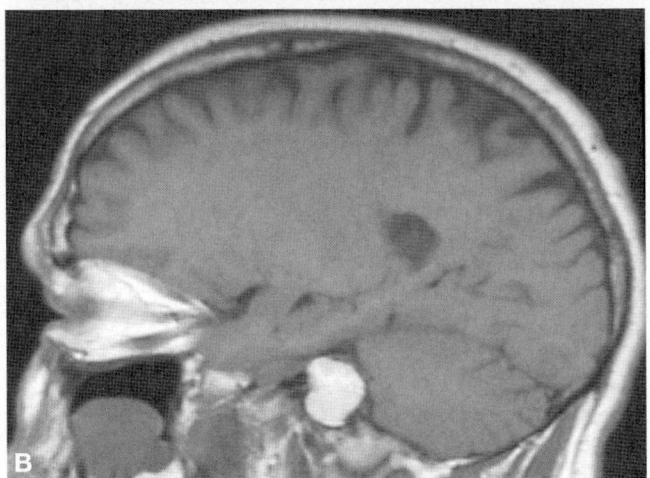

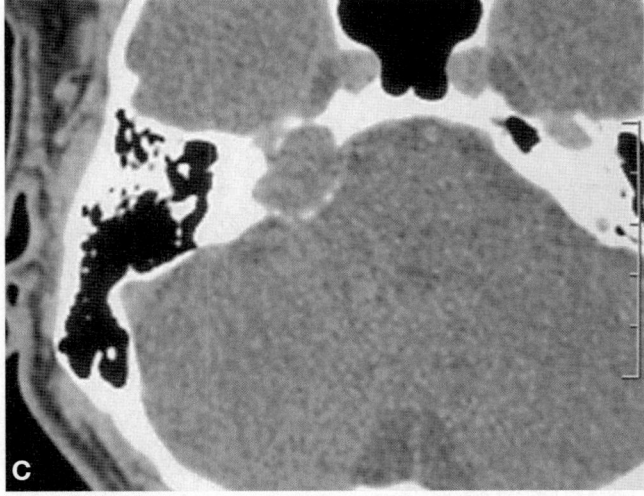

Figure 35–5   Cholesteatoma. *A*, Magnetic resonance image (MRI), axial view, fast-spin T_2 image without contrast demonstrates a hyperintense, homogeneous, expansile lesion of the right petrous apex. *B*, MRI sagittal view; T_1 image with contrast shows no enhancement. *C*, High-resolution computed tomographic scan, axial view, shows an expansile mass of the right petrous apex with a thin peripheral rim of bone extending into the cerebellopontine angle cistern.

glion and must be avoided to minimize the risk of postoperative hearing loss.

Between the foramen spinosum and arcuate eminence, the GSPN divides the petrous apex into the lateral Glasscock's triangle and the medial Kawase's triangle.[11] Glasscock's triangle is formed laterally by a line from the foramen spinosum toward the arcuate eminence, ending at the facial hiatus, medially by the GSPN, and at the base, the mandibular division of the trigeminal nerve. Kawase's triangle is formed laterally by the GSPN, medially by the petrous ridge (superior petrosal sinus), and at the base, the arcuate eminence. Both triangles provide access to the apex and preserve the GSPN to avoid postoperative dry eye; however, in large lesions, the GSPN can be sacrificed to provide greater exposure. Manipulation of the GSPN should be minimized to

avoid potential postoperative facial weakness. Just deep to the GSPN is the petrous carotid artery, which can be distinguished from cyst wall by its location, pulsation, and more reddish color. Just lateral to the artery is the eustachian tube, which also must occasionally be sacrificed. Any entry (intentional or accidental) into the eustachian tube must be recognized and appropriately repaired or packed to prevent postoperative CSF otorhinorrhea in the event that the dura is violated during craniotomy or during extradural middle fossa floor dissection.

Removal of bone proceeds anterior to the basal turn of the cochlea, down to the cyst wall with identification and preservation of the GSPN, carotid artery, and eustachian tube. The wall of the most common cystic lesion, cholesterol granuloma, is usually bluish and nonpulsatile but can be fibrotic and surprisingly thick. The cyst wall is fully exposed and then opened. Thick, brownblack fluid fills the cholesterol granuloma and is suctioned out. The walls of the cyst are gently probed with a blunt dissector to identify the anatomic extent of the cyst. Exposure for total or near-total excision may require sectioning the GSPN and eustachian tube at this point. Traversing the center of larger cysts is the carotid artery, which must be carefully preserved. The cyst wall is removed by blunt dissection as much as the artery will

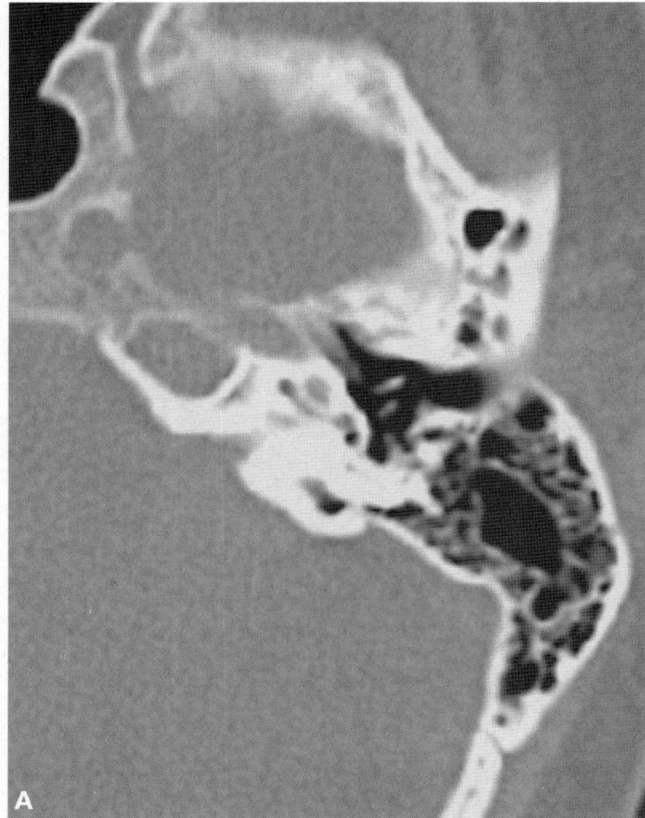

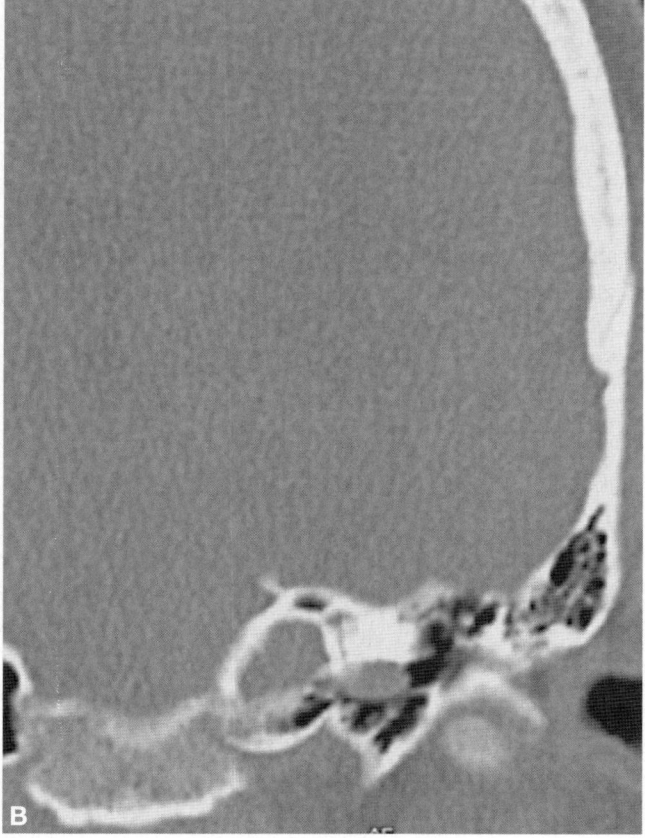

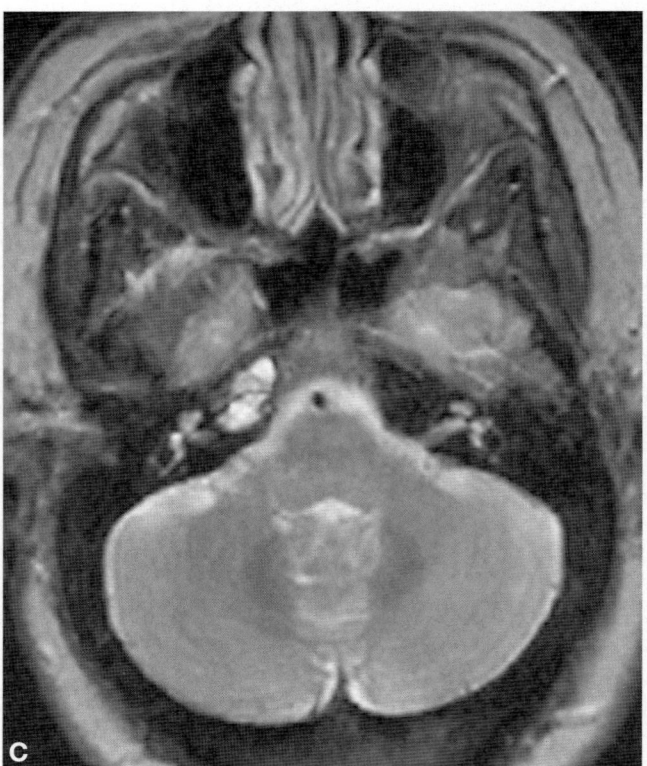

Figure 35–6   Retained fluid (effusion). *A,* Axial high-resolution computed tomographic (CT) scan demonstrates a sharply marginated mass in the left petrous apex. There is a thin rim of sclerosis that is best appreciated along the anterior margins, suggesting a slow-growing lesion. Although confluent in nature, there is no apparent bony expansion into the epidural space. Magnetic resonance imaging (MRI) could be done to confirm the cystic nature of the lesion. *B,* Corresponding coronal CT scan confirms the confluent nature without apparent expansion. *C,* Axial T$_2$-weighted MRI from a different patient with retained fluid in the air cells of the right petrous apex. This lesion does not have the same cystic appearance as the lesion in the patient in Figure 35–6, A and B. The linear hypointense foci in the large bright lesion represent visible septae and/or inflammatory reactive changes in the air cells that contrast against the long T$_2$ of the fluid.

permit. The posterior extension of the cyst may encroach on the cochlea and internal auditory canal; here also the cyst wall can be preserved to minimize postoperative sensorineural hearing loss.

The retractor is removed, and the temporal lobe is allowed to re-expand onto the middle fossa floor. The bone flap is refixed with miniplates and screws. The temporalis muscle-fascia layer is closed with #2-0 Neuralon suture, the subcutaneous tissues with #3-0 Vicryl suture, and the skin with running (not locked) #3-0 Dermalon suture. A local drain is not needed. A large, sterile compression dressing is applied over the ear and side of the head. If the lesion is a cholesterol cyst or mucocele

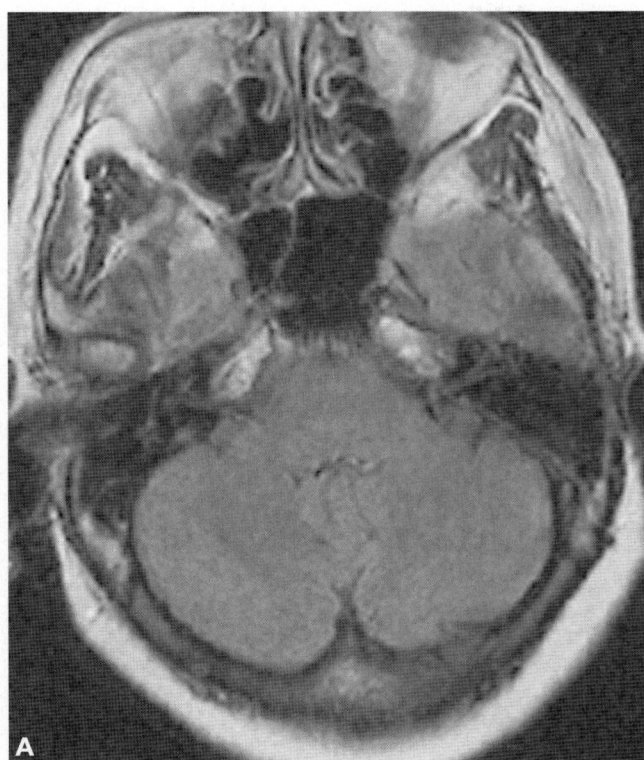

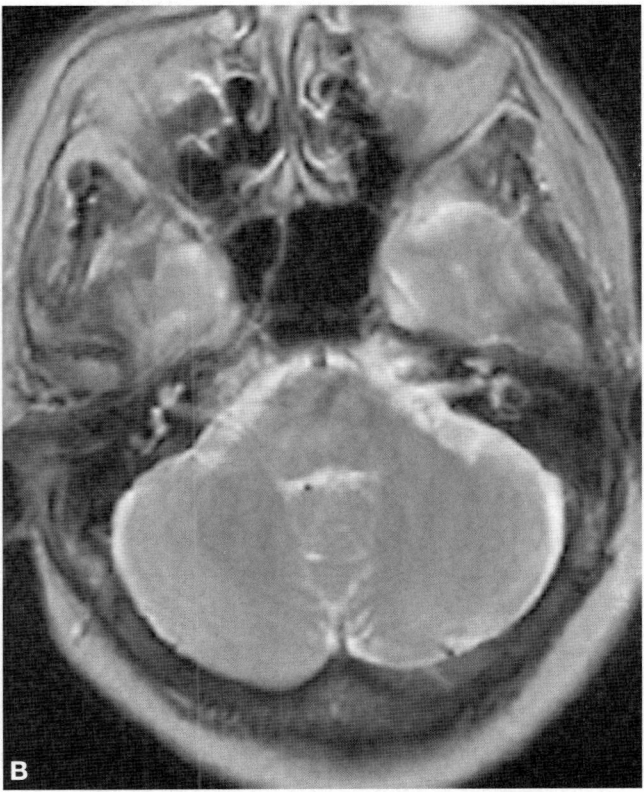

Figure 35–7 Fatty bone marrow. *A*, Axial fast fluid-attenuated inversion recovery image with mildly hyperintense signal in each petrous apex that is symmetric and identical in signal to the subcutaneous fat and the fat in the marrow of the occipital bone. *B*, On the axial fast T₂-weighted image, the petrous apices are mildly hyperintense but relatively symmetric and comparable to the signal of the marrow in the occipital bone.

caused by inadequate ventilation through the air cells (or if the eustachian tube is packed), a pressure-equalized (PE) tube can be placed in the drum. If it is an epidermoid cyst, a PE tube is not placed. The subarachnoid drain is removed in the operating room. Systemic antibiotics are not needed. The patient usually is ready for discharge after 2 or 3 days, at which time the dressing is removed. Postoperatively at 10 days, the skin sutures are removed, and an audiogram can be obtained.

The infracochlear-hypotympanic approach (Figure 35–9) to the petrous apex[12] is a more conservative procedure to provide drainage, decompression, and/or ventilation of a cholesterol cyst, mucocele, or trapped fluid (effusion), but not excision, and would not be used for an epidermoid cyst (cholesteatoma). This procedure is relatively safer and simpler than the middle fossa approach because it avoids dissection and possible injury to the GSPN, facial nerve, and eustachian tube and has less risk to the carotid artery and inner ear. Preoperatively,

a CT scan should be obtained to reveal adequate pneumatization between the cyst wall and the hypotympanum. General anesthesia is administered, and the patient is placed in the supine position with the operated ear upward, as in chronic ear surgery. Points, monitoring leads, and subarachnoid drainage are not needed. A superiorly based, radial incision is made in the ear canal approximately 8 mm lateral to the annulus. A postauricular incision is then carried down to temporalis areolar tissue and fascia, and a 2 × 2.5 cm piece of either tissue is obtained and dehydrated on a block for later use. The mastoid periosteum is incised in a standard "T" fashion, and the anterior flap is elevated toward and down the posterior canal wall until the radial incision is reached. The auricle and lateral external auditory canal skin are retracted anteriorly. The inferior three-quarters of the medial canal skin are then elevated to enter the middle ear but are left attached to the umbo of the malleus. A drill is used to remove additional inferior tympanic ring to enlarge the hypotympanic exposure. Drilling then proceeds inferior and medial to the cochlea, between the anterior carotid artery and the posterior jugular bulb. As the cholesterol granuloma is entered, dark fluid is

A

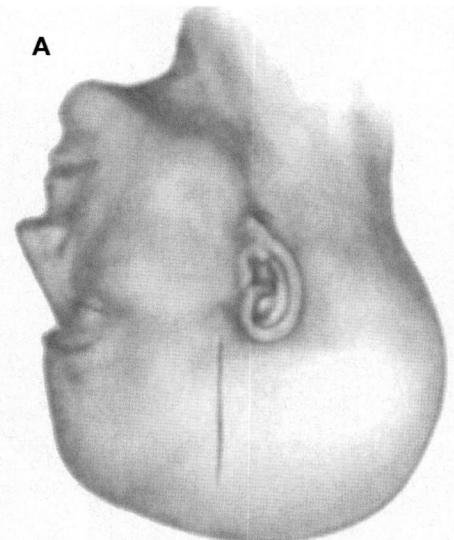

Figure 35–8 Middle cranial fossa approach, right ear, surgical position. A 6-cm vertical incision is made 1 cm anterior to the external auditory canal and superior to the zygoma. A temporal craniotomy is performed one-third posterior and two-thirds anterior to this line. Dura is elevated to the middle meningeal artery anteriorly, arcuate eminence posteriorly, and superior petrosal sinus medially to expose Kawase's and Glasscock's triangles. Bone of the floor of the middle cranial fossa is removed anterior to the basal turn of the cochlea and internal auditory canal (see text for cyst removal and wound closure).

B

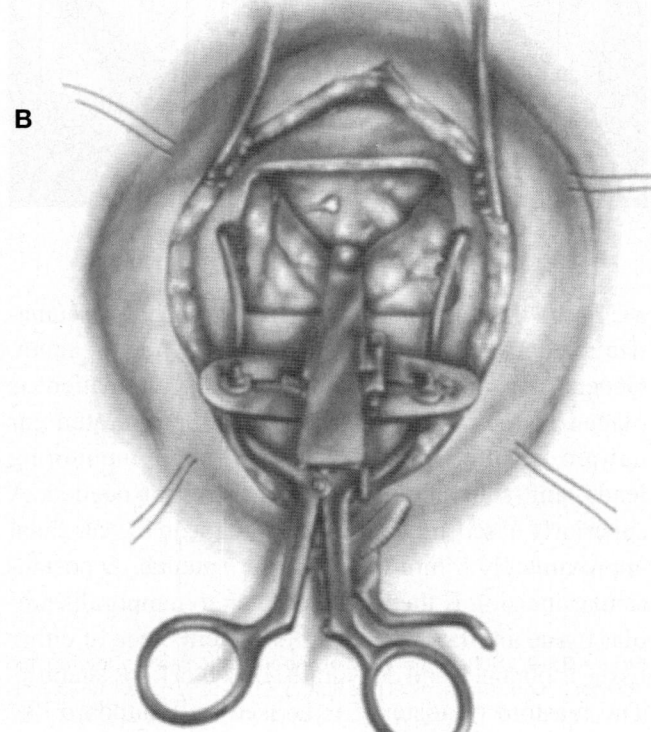

in its normal position. A PE tube can be placed and the canal filled with antibiotic ointment. The postauricular tissues are closed in two layers using absorbable suture. A sterile mastoid dressing is left on for one night, and the patient can be discharged home later that day or in the morning the next day. Systemic antibiotics are not needed.

The transcochlear approach (Figure 35–10) to the petrous apex[10] provides greater exposure and control of the carotid artery for large lesions but is rarely required for benign primary apical cysts when they are detected early by MRI. The translabyrinthine-transcochlear approach (subtotal petrosectomy, Figure 35–11) is a variation that combines transmastoid and cervical approaches. In both the transcochlear and translabyrinthine approaches, the patient is positioned supine with the head turned to the side. Facial nerve monitor leads are placed. Points, auditory monitoring, and subarachnoid drainage are not needed. The lower left quadrant of the abdomen is prepared for a fat graft. First, the skin of the lateral ear canal is incised radially. Then an anteriorly based, gently curved "C"-shaped incision is carried from the temporoparietal area down two fingerbreadths behind the auricle and then continued into a natural skin crease of the neck. As the flap is elevated to the ear canal at the level of the temporalis fascia superiorly and periosteum inferiorly, a small flap of mastoid perios-

removed. The air cells connecting the middle ear with the apex can be gently curetted or drilled to enhance postoperative drainage. A short, Silastic® catheter is placed into the connecting air cells. Temporalis fascia or areolar tissue is used to line and reinforce the enlarged inferior annular ring, and the tympanic membrane is replaced

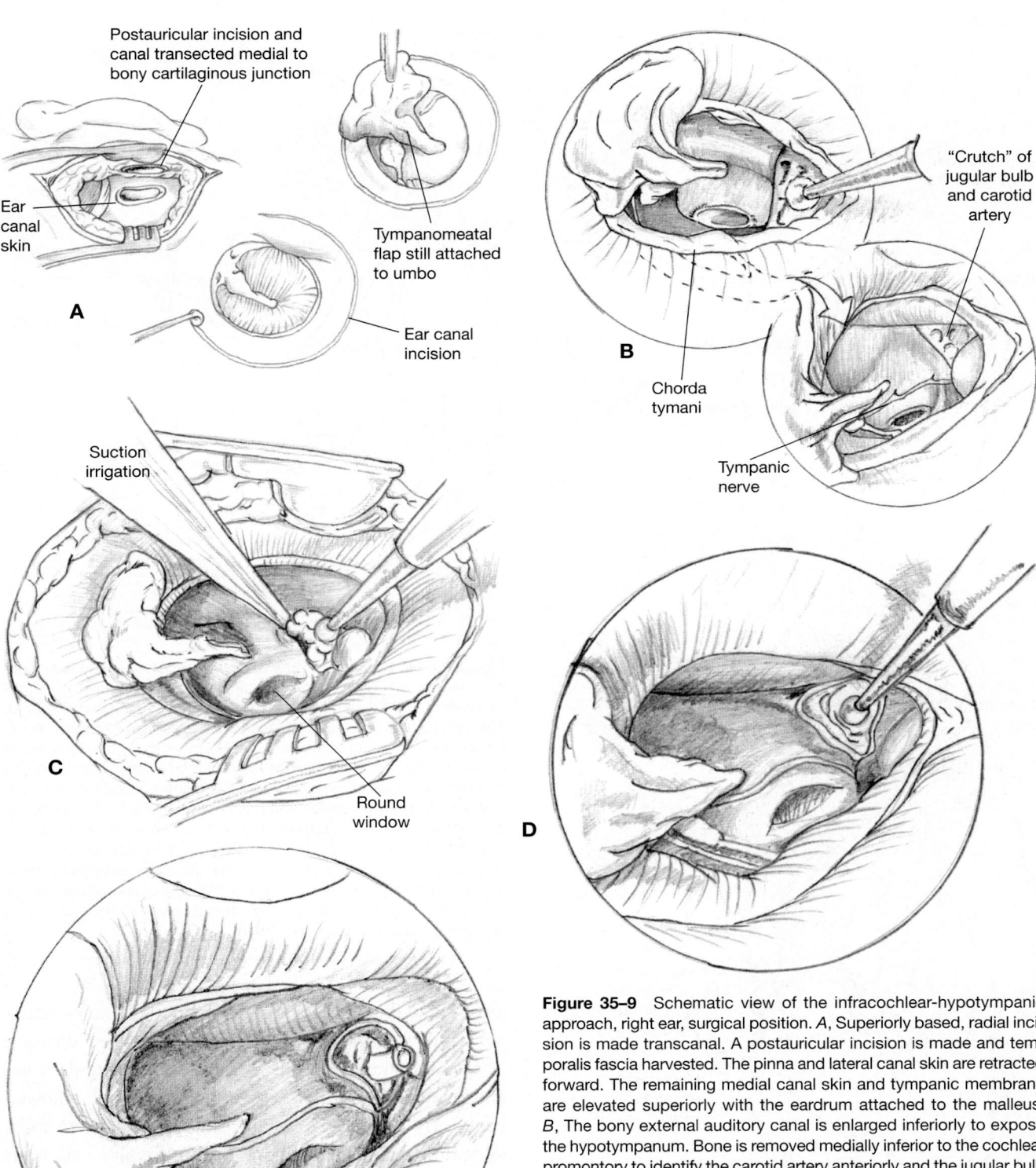

A, Postauricular incision and canal transected medial to bony cartilaginous junction

Ear canal skin

Tympanomeatal flap still attached to umbo

Ear canal incision

B, "Crutch" of jugular bulb and carotid artery

Chorda tymani

Tympanic nerve

C, Suction irrigation

Round window

D

E

Figure 35–9 Schematic view of the infracochlear-hypotympanic approach, right ear, surgical position. *A*, Superiorly based, radial incision is made transcanal. A postauricular incision is made and temporalis fascia harvested. The pinna and lateral canal skin are retracted forward. The remaining medial canal skin and tympanic membrane are elevated superiorly with the eardrum attached to the malleus. *B*, The bony external auditory canal is enlarged inferiorly to expose the hypotympanum. Bone is removed medially inferior to the cochlear promontory to identify the carotid artery anteriorly and the jugular bulb posteriorly. *C*, Hypotympanic bone removal proceeds medially between the carotid artery and jugular bulb into the anterior petrous apex air cells (*D* and *E*). The cholesterol granuloma cyst is reached and drained. A Silastic catheter is placed into the cyst to maintain drainage. Temporalis fascia is used to reinforce the inferior canal defect in an underlay grafting technique, the tympanic membrane is returned to its normal position, and the ear canal is filled with antibiotic ointment (if eustachian tube function has returned to normal, a PE tube may not be required). The postauricular incision is closed.

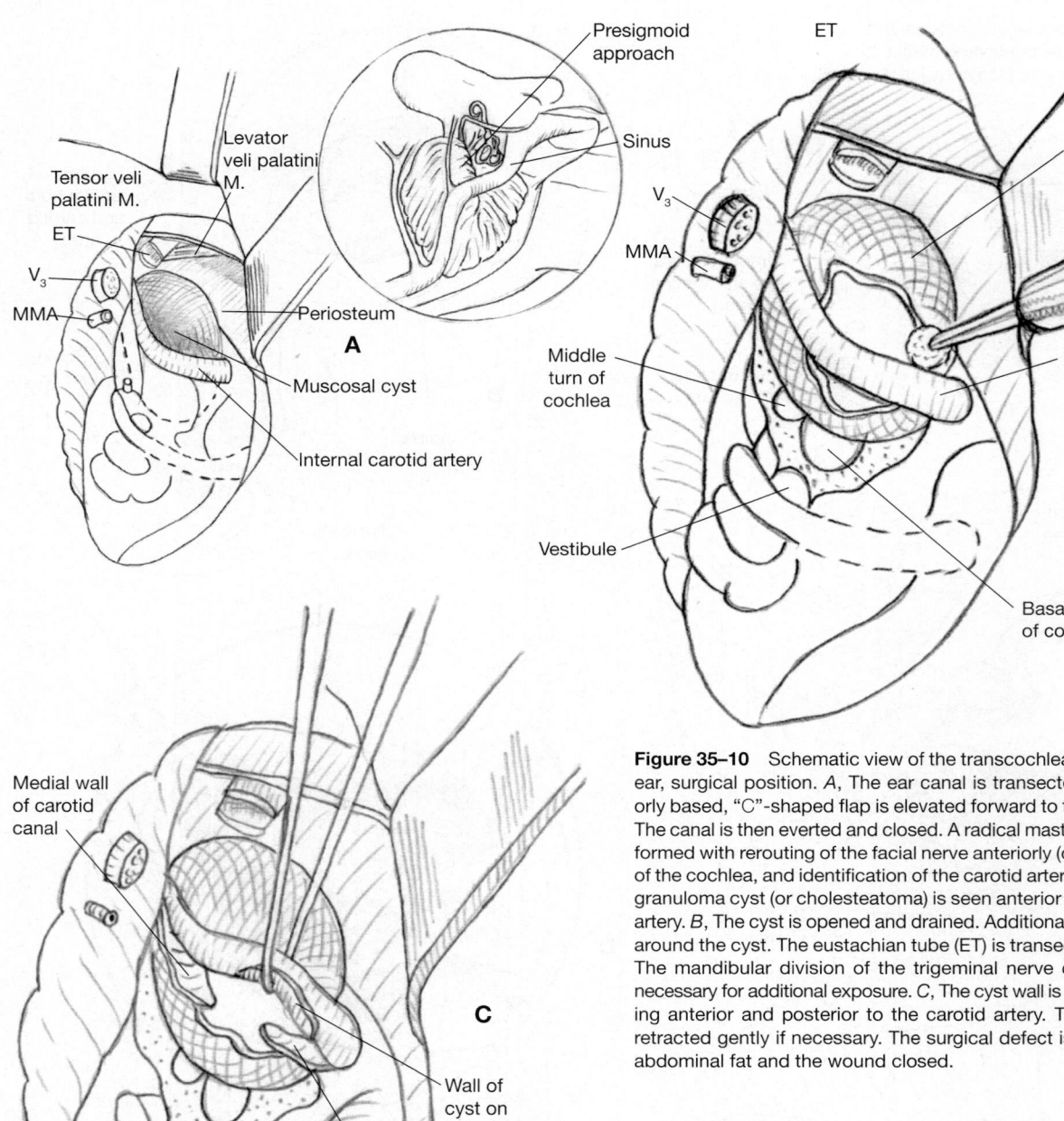

Figure 35–10   Schematic view of the transcochlear approach, right ear, surgical position. *A,* The ear canal is transected and an anteriorly based, "C"-shaped flap is elevated forward to the parotid gland. The canal is then everted and closed. A radical mastoidectomy is performed with rerouting of the facial nerve anteriorly (optional), removal of the cochlea, and identification of the carotid artery. The cholesterol granuloma cyst (or cholesteatoma) is seen anterior and medial to the artery. *B,* The cyst is opened and drained. Additional bone is removed around the cyst. The eustachian tube (ET) is transected and packed. The mandibular division of the trigeminal nerve can be divided if necessary for additional exposure. *C,* The cyst wall is resected by working anterior and posterior to the carotid artery. The artery can be retracted gently if necessary. The surgical defect is obliterated with abdominal fat and the wound closed.

teum anteriorly based on the ear canal also is elevated with the flap. The skin flap, periosteal flap, auricle, and lateral ear canal are elevated to the anterior border of the parotid gland. The cartilaginous canal is everted and closed, and the periosteal flap is sutured medially across the canal remnant to provide a second layer closure. Through the neck incision, the carotid artery, jugular vein, and related cranial nerves are identified and followed superiorly to the base of the skull. A complete mastoidectomy is performed, and the bony canal wall, tympanic membrane, and ossicles are removed. Middle ear mucosa is removed, and the eustachian tube is obliterated. The facial nerve is removed from its canal from the geniculate ganglion proximally to the stylomastoid foramen distally and is rerouted anteriorly to enhance transcochlear exposure to the apex. As the cochlea is removed, the carotid artery is carefully exposed and fol-

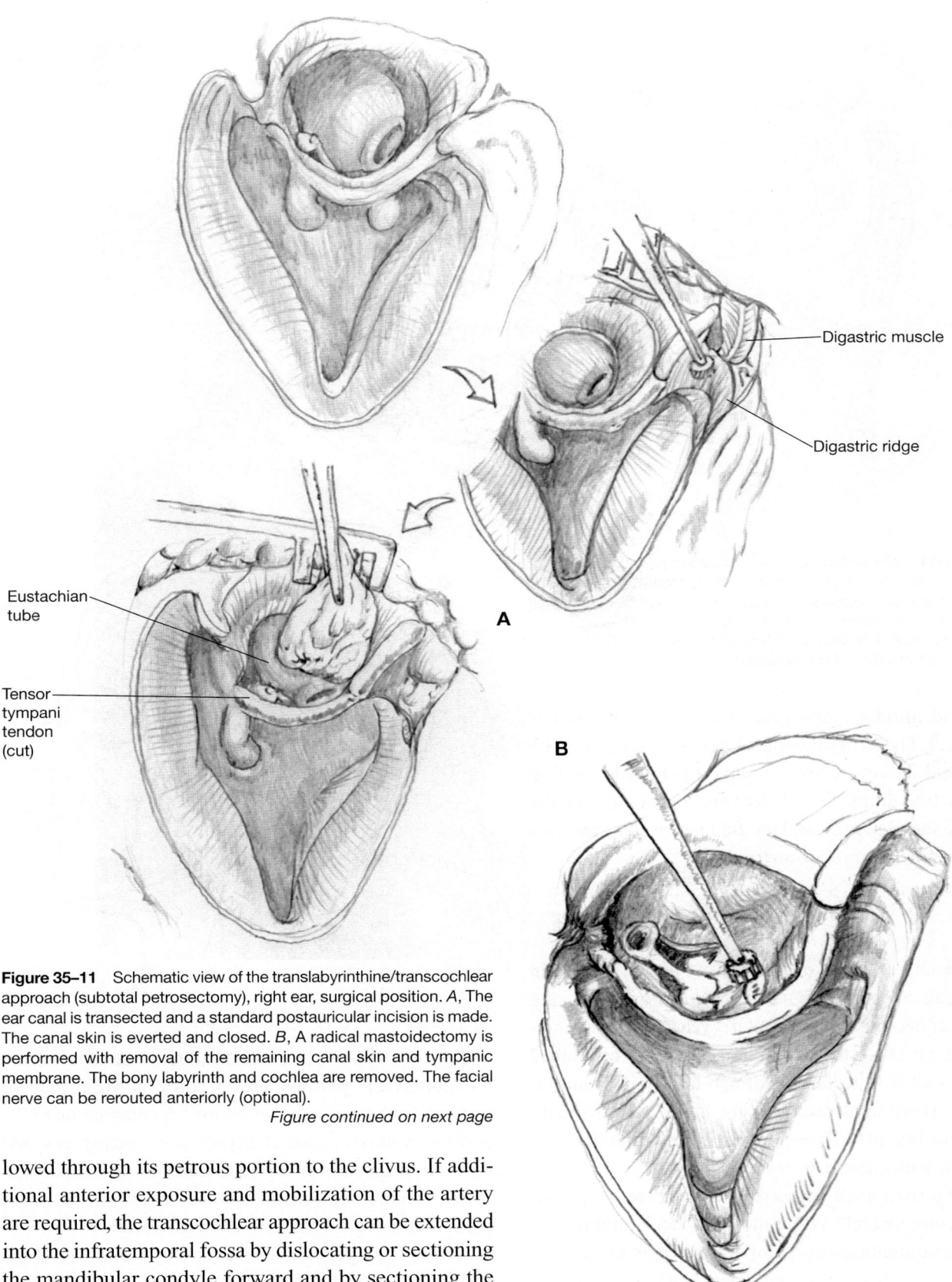

Figure 35–11 Schematic view of the translabyrinthine/transcochlear approach (subtotal petrosectomy), right ear, surgical position. *A,* The ear canal is transected and a standard postauricular incision is made. The canal skin is everted and closed. *B,* A radical mastoidectomy is performed with removal of the remaining canal skin and tympanic membrane. The bony labyrinth and cochlea are removed. The facial nerve can be rerouted anteriorly (optional).

Figure continued on next page

lowed through its petrous portion to the clivus. If additional anterior exposure and mobilization of the artery are required, the transcochlear approach can be extended into the infratemporal fossa by dislocating or sectioning the mandibular condyle forward and by sectioning the mandibular branch of the trigeminal nerve, eustachian

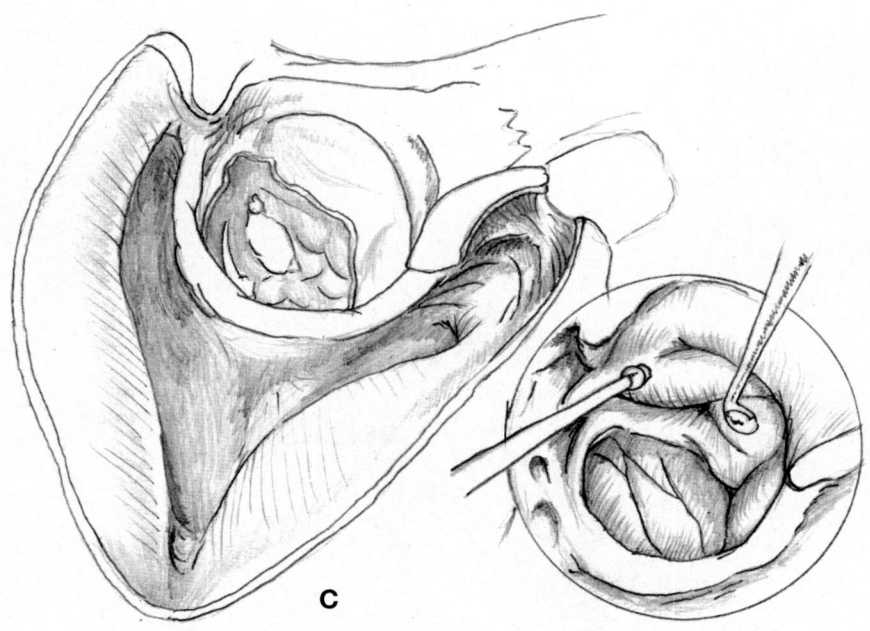

Figure 35–11 (*Continued*.) *C*, The cholesterol granuloma cyst (or cholesteatoma) is resected posterior to the carotid artery. The eustachian tube is obliterated and the remaining middle ear mucosa is removed. *D*, The defect is obliterated with abdominal fat and a flap of temporalis muscle is rotated inferiorly and secured laterally to the fat. The postauricular incision is closed.

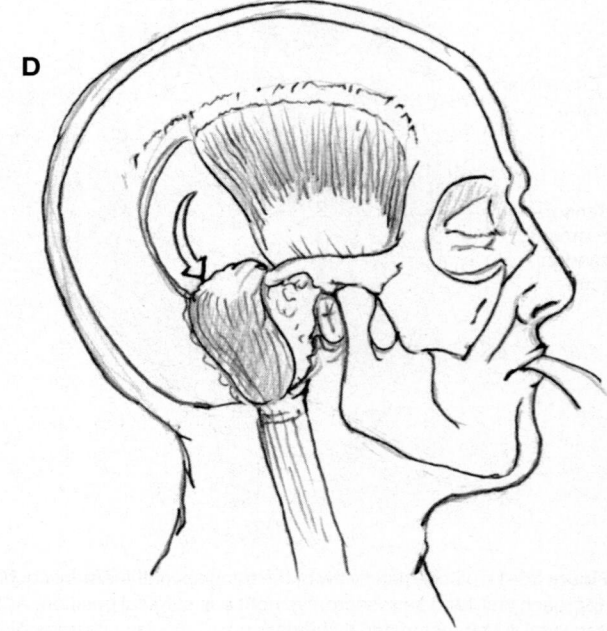

tube, and middle meningeal artery. Cyst removal is extradural. The temporal bone defect is obliterated with abdominal fat covered by a temporalis muscle rotation flap. Suction drainage catheters are left in place (away from the facial nerve), and the flap is closed in two layers. Systemic antibiotics are optional.

DISCUSSION

Management of a cystic lesion of the petrous apex can be difficult and controversial.[1,2,5–7,9,13] Is the cyst causing the symptoms, or is it coincidental?[9] When is surgery indicated? If it is cholesterol granuloma, should it be drained or resected? If it is cholesteatoma, is subtotal removal helpful? Does total resection for either lesion justify the morbidity of a transcochlear/infratemporal fossa approach with carotid artery dissection?

Is the petrous apex abnormality causing the symptoms, or is it coincidental? When the head, neck, and neurotologic examinations in the office are normal, we recommend a gadolinium-contrasted MRI of the brain, base of the skull, and infratemporal fossa in both axial and coronal views. The clinician should bear in mind that an "abnormal" petrous apex finding on MRI may or may not be the cause of symptoms.[9] A comparison of T_1- and T_2-weighted images often provides the diagnosis, and the size of the lesion suggests whether it is expansile. When in doubt, however, the clinician also should order a CT scan to further characterize the lesion.

When is surgery indicated for a cystic lesion of the apex? Surgery is indicated when the patient is symptomatic, when other causes are excluded, and particularly when CT also shows that the lesion is expansile and eroding bone. Patients with small lesions often have no symptoms; they should be treated conservatively. Magnetic resonance imaging or CT can be repeated in 6 or 12 months for comparison or sooner if the patient develops symptoms. Patients with expansile lesions present most often with headache or head pain and less often with middle ear effusion, sensorineural hearing loss, and/or dizziness. If the history and examination do not indicate another cause, surgery should be recommended.

General principles of surgical management are to (1) adequately drain or resect the lesion, (2) preserve hearing when possible, and (3) minimize the risk of cranial nerve and carotid artery injury and CSF leak. Should cholesterol granuloma be drained or resected? Drainage through the hypotympanic/infracochlear approach is fast, safe, and simple but, in our experience, may not provide long-term control of symptoms. Resection (total or near total) through the middle fossa has more risk to hearing if the surgeon inadvertently enters the cochlea or internal auditory canal, more risk to the facial nerve, and more risk to the carotid artery, which may be surrounded by cyst. We carefully identify and protect the carotid artery, leaving small remnants of cyst wall on the artery when necessary to minimize risk. Conservative, near-total removal offers good long-term control with minimal morbidity from surgery. Therefore, we recommend that the surgeon present both middle fossa and infracochlear/hypotympanic options to the patient and then help guide the final decision depending on the preference of the patient and the specifics of each case. If symptoms recur after a hypotympanic drainage procedure, then resection should be recommended through the middle cranial fossa.

Is total removal of cholesteatoma necessary to provide long-term relief? Simple drainage is not helpful since the pathogenesis of (solid) cholesteatoma is different from that of (fluid) cholesterol granuloma. Total resection is frequently possible when the lesion is small and separate from the carotid artery; however, small lesions usually are not symptomatic. Large, expansile lesions warrant surgery but surround the carotid artery and tend to recur if not totally removed. The risk to the carotid artery can be minimized by increasing exposure through the transcochlear/infratemporal fossa approach, which allows gentle manipulation and circumferential dissection of the petrous carotid artery but sacrifices hearing. However, the morbidity of this combined approach is not justified unless the ear is already deaf and the cholesteatoma is massive. We generally recommend subtotal resection of cholesteatoma through a middle fossa approach when the expansile lesion is still confined to the temporal bone and when hearing is good. Residual cholesteatoma may not grow because of interruption of its blood supply, can be followed by serial MRI, and can later be reoperated. Presenting symptoms can be controlled and morbidity minimized by this more conservative approach.

REFERENCES

1. Muckle RP, De La Cruz A, Lo W. Petrous apex lesions. Am J Otol 1998;19:219–25.

2. Moore KR, Harnsberger HR, Shelton C, Davidson HC. 'Leave me alone' lesions of the petrous apex. AJNR Am J Neuroradiol 1998;19:733–8.

3. Cheung SW, Broberg TG, Jackler RK. Petrous apex arachnoid cyst: radiographic confusion with primary cholesteatoma. Am J Otol 1995;16:690–4.

4. Goldsmith AJ, Myssiorek D, Valderrama E, Patel M. Unifocal Langerhans' cell histiocytosis (eosinophilic granuloma) of the petrous apex. Arch Otolaryngol Head Neck Surg 1993;119:113–6.

5. Amedee RG, Gianoli GJ, Mann WJ. Petrous apex lesions. Skull Base Surg 1994;4(1):10–4.

6. Curtin HD, Som PM. The petrous apex. Otolaryngol Clin North Am 1995;28:473–96.

7. Flood LM, Kemink JL. Surgery in lesions of the petrous apex. Otolaryngol Clin North Am 1984;17:565–74.

8. Gacek RR. Diagnosis and management of primary tumors of the petrous apex. Ann Otol Rhinol Laryngol Suppl 1975;84(18):1–20.

9. Leonetti JP, Shownkeen H, Marzo SJ. Incidental petrous apex findings on magnetic resonance imaging. Ear Nose Throat J 2001;80:200–6.

10. Fisch U, Mattox D. Pyramid apex: mucosal cyst and epidermoid cyst. In: Fisch U, Mattox D, editors. Microsurgery of the skull base. New York: Thieme; 1988. p. 304–13.

11. Miller CG. Transpetrosal approach to the petrous apex. Neurosurgery 1993;33:461–9.

12. Brackmann DE, Giddings NA. Drainage procedures for petrous apex lesions. In: Brackmann DE, Shelton C, Arriaga MA, editors. Otologic surgery. Philadelphia: WB Saunders; 1994. p. 572–7.

13. Franklin DJ, Jenkins HA, Horowitz BL, Coker NJ. Management of petrous apex lesions. Arch Otolaryngol Head Neck Surg 1989;115:1121–5.

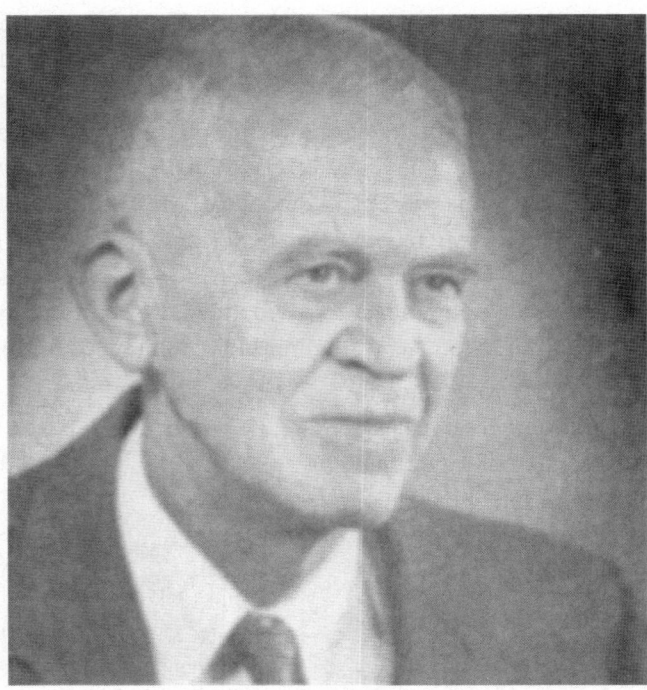

Stacy Rufus Guild (1890–1966). Discovered the glomus jugularie, the site of origin of the most common neoplasm of the middle ear.

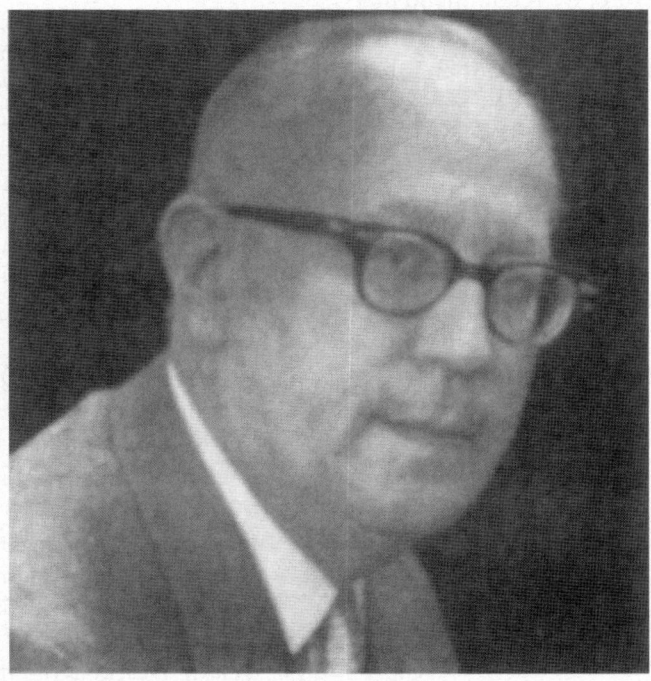

Harry Rosenwasser (born 1902). First described a vascular tumor of the middle ear as arising from the glomus jugularie.

VIII

Surgery of the Skull Base

36

Surgery for Benign Tumors of the Temporal Bone

C. Gary Jackson, MD, FACS

The evolution of surgery of the temporal bone (TB) has been based on and derived from technological advances concerned with the eradication of inflammatory disease of the middle ear (ME) and mastoid. Antibiotics, microsurgery, and amazing developments in neuroangiography and imaging have paced an astonishing neurotologic capacity.

Even so, tumors of the TB continue to confound advanced management strategies and capacities. As part of the skull base, the TB is relatively inaccessible. Furthermore, regional consequences of TB pathology usually occur late. The deepest recesses of the TB appear to be anatomically privileged sites with pathology clinically betrayed only when it reaches the ME or the complex anatomy, which directly relates to its position at the lateral cranial base.

The embryology of the TB is complex, reflecting the contribution of all germ layers. Consequently, a great variety of tumor cell types is possible, including both benign and malignant variants. Each is often unique and quite rare, disallowing any clinical familiarity with their diagnosis and/or management. Contemporary surgical protocols for benign lesions, notably glomus tumors (GTs), have led the way to a capacity that consistently emphasizes total tumor removal as well as maximization of postsurgical quality of life through minimization of cosmetic and neurologic loss. With neurosurgeons, head and neck surgeons, reconstruction specialists, and neuroradiologists, a collaborative approach to benign lesions has evolved; nonetheless, TB malignancy continues to be a formidable problem. Patients still die with progressive local disease, intolerable pain, neurologic loss, and all of the attributes of inanition so characteristic of the patient with terminal head and neck cancer.

This chapter examines tumors of the TB, cataloging rarer lesions and focusing on the most common benign lesion, the GT. The management concepts for GTs can be applied to rarer lesions.

ANATOMIC OVERVIEW

The four elements of the TB are the petrosa (the petrous portion), the squama (the squamous portion), the mastoid bone, and the tympanic bone. It constitutes the inferolateral skull base and is nearly completely formed at birth, completing development by age 3 years. In addition to its osseous structure, the TB contains almost every type of human tissue—epithelial, neural, epidermal, vascular, cartilaginous, and glandular.[1] Almost any tumor conceivable can arise within the TB. On its lateral-inferior surface lies the bony and cartilaginous external auditory canal (EAC). Lymphatics from the auricle and EAC drain into the parotid and pre- and retroauricular lymph nodes. Venous drainage is into the internal jugular vein.

The middle fossa dura overlies the superior surface. Anteromedially, the TB relates to the eustachian tube (ET), internal carotid artery (ICA), and the petrous ridge, with its superior petrosal sinus. The petrous apex houses the geniculate ganglion, an embryologically diverse structure, which is a common site of origin of a variety of neoplasms. The nasopharynx has an important anatomic relationship to the TB. Posterior-medially is the petrous portion housing the internal auditory canal (IAC) and its contents. Anteriorly lie the glenoid fossa, the semi-canal of the tensor tympani muscle, and canal for the ICA. The infratemporal fossa (IFTF) is further anterior.

The pneumatized spaces of the TB serve as a veritable superhighway for the spread of tumor, which varies as much in degree and extent as does the pneumatic pattern itself. The tympanic membrane (TM) offers some resistance to the medial spread of EAC pathology. The bone of the labyrinth is moderately resistant to tumor and serves as a temporary barrier. Along with the neurovascular structures, the foramen of Huschke, an incomplete closure of the tympanic ring, may also serve to permit tumor extent beyond the confines of the TB intracranially, into the parotid, into the IFTF, and vice versa. In addition to the major periauricular lymphatic drainage mentioned above, which is highly relevant in disease of the EAC, the ear is further served by upper cervical, deep jugular, postauricular, and posterior deep lymphatics. Whereas the inner ear has no known lymphatic drainage, the ME, mastoid, and ET drain into the deep jugular and retropharyngeal lymph nodes.[1] The significance of the lymphatics to TB tumors and their management is poorly understood.

TUMORS OF THE TEMPORAL BONE

A wide diversity of tumor types is encountered within the TB, each rarely; in fact, the occurrence of some tumors of the temporal bone is so isolated as to constitute case report material. An outline based on anatomic site serves to superficially classify these lesions:

I Tumors of the external auditory canal
   A. Benign
       1. Osteoma
       2. Exostosis
       3. Fibrous dysplasia
       4. Histiocytosis X
           (Langerhans' cell histiocytosis)
       5. Papilloma
       6. Nerve sheath neoplasm
       7. Paraganglioma
       8. Hemangioma
II. Tumors of the middle ear
   A. Benign
       1. Adenoma
       2. Meningioma
       3. Chordoma
       4. Paraganglioma
       5. Hemangiopericytoma
       6. Schwannoma
III. Tumors of the inner ear/petrous apex
   A. Benign
       1. Paraganglioma (glomus tumor)
       2. Lipoma
       3. Schwannoma
       4. Hemangiopericytoma
       5. Cholesterol granuloma

Next to the acoustic neuroma, the GT is the most common tumor encountered by today's neuro-otologists. Thankfully, TB carcinoma remains rare.

In general, benign TB lesions are slow-growing and insidious, producing minimal complaints until well advanced. The progression of these lesions can be so slow that neurologic symptoms undergo simultaneous compensation and therefore may be unnoticed by the patient. Inexorably and ultimately, these lesions produce cranial neuropathy and cause hearing loss, vestibular dysfunction, swallowing problems, dysphagia with glottic incompetence, facial nerve (FN) paresis, and ophthalmic disorders. The benign TB tumor is conceptually well represented by the GT, the diagnosis and management of which are applicable to rarer lesions.

Alternatively, patients presenting with otalgia, bloody or mucopurulent otorrhea, unresponsive external otitis, an EAC lesion/granulation tissue, or progressive cranial neuropathy, especially in the elderly with a long-term history of chronic otitis media, must be evaluated for malignancy and promptly biopsied. We deal with malignancy here generically only to differentiate it from its more benign counterpart.

Management of both benign and malignant disease is directed by disease type and extent. Complicated solutions are reserved only for complicated situations. Total tumor removal is paramount and, if possible, should be executed by protocols sufficiently flexible in scope to allow reasonable conservation of vital structures. When conservation is deemed impossible, strategies for defect reconstruction and cranial nerve rehabilitation must be planned preoperatively. A discussion of specific tumors follows the exposition of management concepts for benign lesions, as exemplified by the GT.

Glomus Tumors

Although GTs are generally benign and follow an indolent course, morbidity and mortality can occur by virtue of their location at the skull base adjacent to the posterior cranial fossa and the lower cranial nerves subserving coordination of deglutition and phonation.

Heretofore, the ability to diagnose these tumors far exceeded the ability to treat them. The evolution of treatment modalities has finally achieved parity with diagnostic technology. By consensus, the management of cranial-cervical GTs is surgical. The oncologically sound, primary objective is complete tumor resection for cure. Owing to the technical capacity of the day, issues of resectability have given way to issues of functional outcome, that is, the quality of postsurgical survival. The reconstruction of sizable defects, along with the rehabilitation of cranial nerve deficits, serves to minimize the most common ground on which surgery is most frequently criticized, the perceived risk of functional incapacity. Morbid consequences can be reliably predicted and outcomes controlled. Issues of intracranial extension (ICE) are well understood.

Nevertheless, the surgery versus radiation therapy (RT) debate continues to rage. The data to solve this dilemma do not exist. Radiation therapy proposes itself as a low-morbidity conservation management strategy that asks the patient to coexist with a biologically altered tumor. This chapter reviews the surgical standardization that conceptually dominates GT surgery. Intracranial extension, management, defect reconstruction, and cranial nerve rehabilitation are addressed. Radiation therapy is placed into perspective.

Glomus Tumor Classification

To direct surgical planning and provide standards for reporting surgical results, a GT classification is necessary.

Oldring and Fisch,[2] in 1979, recognized this need and proposed an A, B, C, and D tumor classification system. This system was upgraded in 1982[3] to include ICE as subclasses of Types C and D lesions.

The Glasscock-Jackson[4] system of GT classification retained the familiar and clinically utilitarian tympanic and jugulare subclasses, expanding subclasses by tumor extent. Intracranial extension is expressed as a superscript; for example, GJ-Type IV[2.0] refers to a Type IV lesion with 2.0 cm ICE (Table 36–1).

Glomus Tumor Biology

The nomenclature of GT is in some disarray. The term "glomus" is a misnomer.[5] The original thought that the tumor originated from true glomus complexes[6] has been discredited. It is now recognized that GTs arise from paraganglions, which are normally occurring structures usually found in close association with sympathetic ganglions along the aorta and its main branches. The chief cells of the paraganglions are of neural crest origin and are components of the diffuse neuroendocrine system (DNES). Glenner and Grimley[6] distinguished the adrenal paraganglion (the adrenal medulla) from extra-adrenal paraganglions. Paraganglion tumors (paragangliomas) also follow this classification. Recognizing the above, nonetheless the terms paraganglioma, GT, glomus tympanicum (GTy), and glomus jugulare (GJ) will be used interchangeably in this chapter.

The cranial-cervical (branchiomeric) paraganglions are distributed along the arterial vasculature and cranial nerves of the ontogenetic gill arches.[6] The branchiomeric paraganglions of prime interest to neuro-otologists are the jugulotympanic and intercarotid paraganglia. The intravagal paraganglion, as it is not intimately associated with arterial vasculature,[6] is not classified as a branchiomeric paraganglion.

Table 36–1 GLASSCOCK-JACKSON GLOMUS TUMOR CLASSIFICATION	
Type	**Physical Findings**
Glomus tympanicum	
Type I	Small mass limited to the promontory
Type II	Tumor completely filling middle ear space
Type III	Tumor filling middle ear and extending into mastoid process
Type IV	Tumor filling middle ear, extending into mastoid or through tympanic membrane to fill external auditory canal; may extend anterior to internal carotid artery
Glomus jugulare	
Type I	Small tumor involving jugular bulb, middle ear, and mastoid process
Type II	Tumor extending under internal auditory canal; may have intracranial extension
Type III	Tumor extending into petrous apex; may have intracranial extension
Type IV	Tumor extending beyond petrous apex into clivus or infratemporal fossa; may have intracranial extension

The jugulotympanic paraganglions are ovoid, lobulated structures measuring 0.1 mm to 1.5 mm in diameter.[7] Vascularized by the inferior tympanic branch of the ascending pharyngeal artery, they number on average three per side and are found in association with Jacobson's and Arnold's nerves. The number of paraganglions does not correlate with race or sex, and more than 50% are located in the region of the jugular fossa. They are innervated by the glossopharyngeal nerve, whereas those along Arnold's nerve are thought to be innervated by the vagus nerve. Intravagal paraganglions, as scattered cell groups, occupy the epineurium of the vagus nerve. The paraganglions are well vascularized and are composed of clusters (Zellballen) of chief cells supported by sustentacular cells and small blood vessels.[7]

The ultrastructural appearance of paragangliomas mimics that of their paraganglions of origin.[6] Their chief cells contain cytoplasmic granules that store catecholamines.[6] Two types of chief cells, light and dark, are identified ultrastructurally.

Biochemistry

The chief cells of the paraganglions are 1 of 40 distinct cell types of the DNES, the cells of which have the capacity to produce catecholamines and neuropeptides that may serve as neurotransmitters, neurohormones, hormones, and parahormones.[8,9]

The metabolism of tyrosine is key to the biochemistry of catecholamines.[5] Because paraganglions lack the enzyme phenylethanolamine-*N*-methyltransferase, usually norepinephrine accumulates[10]; however, a dopamine-secreting GT has been documented.[11] A GT secreting serotonin that provoked the carcinoid syndrome has been reported.[12] Neurohormones have been immunohistochemically documented in paraganglions and in paragangliomas, including neuron-specific enolase, substance P, cholecystokinin, bombesin, chromogranin, vasoactive intestinal polypeptide, somatostatin, calcitonin, S-100 protein, melanocyte-stimulating hormone, and gastrin.[5]

Clinical Correlates

The biochemical capacity of the GT is indeed rich. Its potential to produce neuroendocrine secretory products permits anticipation of a variable clinical symptomatology, and those tumors that secrete sufficient quantities are known as "functional" tumors or "secretors."

Every patient with a GT (except those with small GTy tumors) undergoes measurement of serum catecholamine levels and of urinary metabolites. Functioning paragangliomas occur in 1 to 3% of cases.[11] Norepinephrine levels elevated three to five times normal are generally required to produce the symptoms and signs of catecholamine secretion, such as headaches, excessive perspiration, palpitations, pallor, and nausea.[11] Rarely, the carcinoid syndrome may be encountered. The detection of elevated epinephrine levels mandates computed tomography (CT) of the adrenal glands or selective renal vein sampling to rule out pheochromocytoma.

Perioperative management is essential to safeguard against the mortal consequences of catecholamine overload on anesthesia induction or intraoperatively on tumor manipulation. Modern protocols for pharmacologic blockade employed for a pheochromocytoma are used. Alpha- and beta-blockade beginning 2 weeks preoperatively has been abandoned.

Paraneoplastic syndromes associated with other neurohormones (anemia, gastrointestinal symptoms, etc) must be sought and identified.

The presence of immunoreactive peptides can be used to diagnostic advantage. Scanning incorporating the somatostatin analogue I[123]-labeled Tyr3-octreotide (octreotide scanning) has been useful.[13] Histochemical markers may provide insight into the biologic aggressiveness of a tumor. Aggressive tumors have been proposed to have scarce sustentacular cell populations and produce fewer neuropeptides when compared to more benign lesions. Tendency toward malignant character has been implied by immunohistochemical analysis of relative ratios of chief cells to sustentacular cells and marker reactivity in the latter.[5]

The chief cells of GTs, as members of the DNES, are grouped with other cells of neual crest derivation and their associated neoplasms. Tumors known to occur in association with GTs include pheochromocytoma, thyroid neoplasms, and parathyroid adenoma. Glomus tumors have been noted in association with the multiple endocrine neoplasia syndromes.[5]

Glomus tumors are characteristically slow-growing and rarely metastasize. They spread from their sites of origin along tracts of least resistance, the most important of which are the air cell tracts of the TB. Vascular lumina, neurovascular foramina, the ET, and direct extension allow spread beyond the TB. Glomus tumors invade bone. Cochleovestibular destruction is caused by ischemic necrosis.[14,15] Spread along several fronts occurs simultaneously and is multidirectional. Intracranial extension into the posterior cranial fossa occurs directly through dura or along cranial nerve routes. The IAC is a frequent highway.

Cranial nerve paralysis occurs in 35% of jugulotympanic lesions and 57% of intravagal paragangliomas.[5] Cranial nerves VII through XII and the sympathetic trunk are most commonly involved.

Glomus tumors arise more often in Caucasians. Females are 4 to 6 times more commonly affected than males.[5] Tumors occur in infants and in the elderly, but usually occur in the fifth and sixth decades. A heredofamilial tendency has been outlined with an autosomal dominant mode of transmission. In familial tumors, the incidence of associated lesions is 25 to 50%.

A remarkable characteristic of GTs is their tendency toward multiplicity. In 10% of nonfamilial cases, another GT can be expected.[16] The additional tumor(s) may be ipsilateral or contralateral and involve any of the branchiomeric paraganglions.[17] The most common combination is a carotid body tumor with an ipsilateral GTy or GJ tumor.

Jugulotympanic paragangliomas rarely exhibit malignant degeneration, defined by finding paraganglioma tissue in locations other than those in which paraganglioma otherwise occur. Histologic evidence of malignancy is indeed rare. Lattes and Waltner[18] first reported a metastatic GT (to the liver) in 1948. The fraction of GTs that are malignant ranges from 1 to 12%, with the commonly cited figure at 4%.[19] The most common locations for metastatic deposits are the lymph nodes, skeleton, lung, liver, and occasionally spleen.[20] Glomus vagale tumors have a higher malignancy rate, estimated at 19%.[21] Symptomatology tends to be more severe and rapidly progressive in malignant GTs; they present at a more advanced state with a higher incidence of cranial nerve deficits. Treatment morbidity and mortality are higher than that for nonmalignant GTs. Nonetheless, prolonged survival is possible in the face of metastatic disease.[22]

The biology of the GT is indeed rich.[5] Its clinical evaluation involves not only delineation of tumor type and extent but also a comprehensive assessment of its unique biologic capacity.

Diagnosis

CLINICAL. Early diagnosis is key to conservation surgery, which ensures a high-grade postsurgical functional outcome.[23] The diagnostic process must be regarded as a treatment planning tool.

The clinical features of GT serve to alert the physician to a disorder of the ear, TB, and jugular fossa (Table 36–2). The patient with a GT usually complains of pulsatile tinnitus and/or hearing loss. Tumor growth into the mesotympanum manifests as a conductive hearing loss, whereas the extent of labyrinthine invasion determines the degree of the sensorineural component. Tympanic membrane erosion and bleeding are late symptoms. Cranial neuropathy suggests a more extensive process. Neurologic symptoms may, however, go unnoticed for a long time. Growth is slow, and neural degeneration occurs simultaneously with compensation. As cranial nerves are lost in aggregate, dysphagia, loss of airway protection, and shoulder, tongue, and voice weakness occur. "Idiopathic" cranial neuropathy, as it often reflects jugular or hypoglossal foramen disease, is an unacceptable diagnosis and mandates an aggressive search, with imaging studies, for a lateral skull base lesion. Facial paralysis is usually a late sign and an ominous omen for FN outcome. The aforementioned signs and symptoms of a "functioning" GT must be sought and differentiated from pheochromocytoma.

A mesotympanic vascular mass is characteristic but rarely may be absent. Superior mesotympanic masses can occur in GT but are rare and diagnostically confusing. Margins visible 360 degrees about the circumference of a mesotympanic mass permit the diagnosis of a tympanicum lesion (and its differential diagnoses). Without this physical finding, differentiation of a GTy tumor from a GJ tumor is insecure and impossible without imaging. When the margins of the mass are not clear, a GJ lesion should be expected until proven otherwise.

Myringotomy or tympanotomy for biopsy is mentioned in condemnation only. Such biopsy results in brisk bleeding that must be packed, risking damage to structures of the ear. Biopsy of an aberrant ICA cannot only be dramatic but also potentially catastrophic. Biopsy is rarely necessary in the face of good imaging. When indicated and unavoidable, a postauricular transmastoid approach, with all vital anatomy identified, is recommended.

The glomus vagale presents as an enlarging cervical or parapharyngeal mass characterized by a vague fullness high in the neck. Although inferior vagal paralysis is invariable and presents as aspiration or hoarseness, Horner's syndrome, other cranial neuropathies, and nasal and oropharyngeal signs can also emerge. Middle ear symptoms are rare.

The type and extent of tumor cannot be determined from physical examination alone.

LABORATORY. Treatment planning requires achievement of the following objectives[24]:

- Determination of the tumor size, type, and extent
- Evaluation of histochemical or multicentric associated lesions
- Identification and assessment of ICE
- Assessment of major vasculature involvement
- Assessment of intracranial collateral circulation

Most of these objectives are satisfied by defining a soft tissue mass and/or its associated bony destruction. A GTy tumor must be differentiated from a GJ tumor. Disease extent is then defined. The mainstay of this diagnostic phase is radiologic imaging.

The identification of air and/or bone between the tumor mass and jugular bulb characterizes the mesotympanic mass as a GTy tumor and is best achieved by CT of TB with bone windows in both the axial and coronal planes. Computed tomography also defines the tumor extent relative to the bony anatomy of the TB (Figures 36–1 to 36–3).

Tumor extent, ICE, and the relationship of the tumor to neural and vascular structures are best evaluated by magnetic resonance imaging (MRI). Magnetic resonance imaging of the head and neck of a known GJ tumor capably assesses multicentricity (Figures 36–4 and 36–5).

Bilateral carotid angiography is performed to evaluate ICA tumor involvement and is done preoperatively, at the time of tumor embolization. Angiography is particularly useful in determining tumor blood supply. This information is important in managing ICE, which can derive vascular supply from pial sources, the vertebral artery, the ICA, and AICA/PICA, in addition to usual

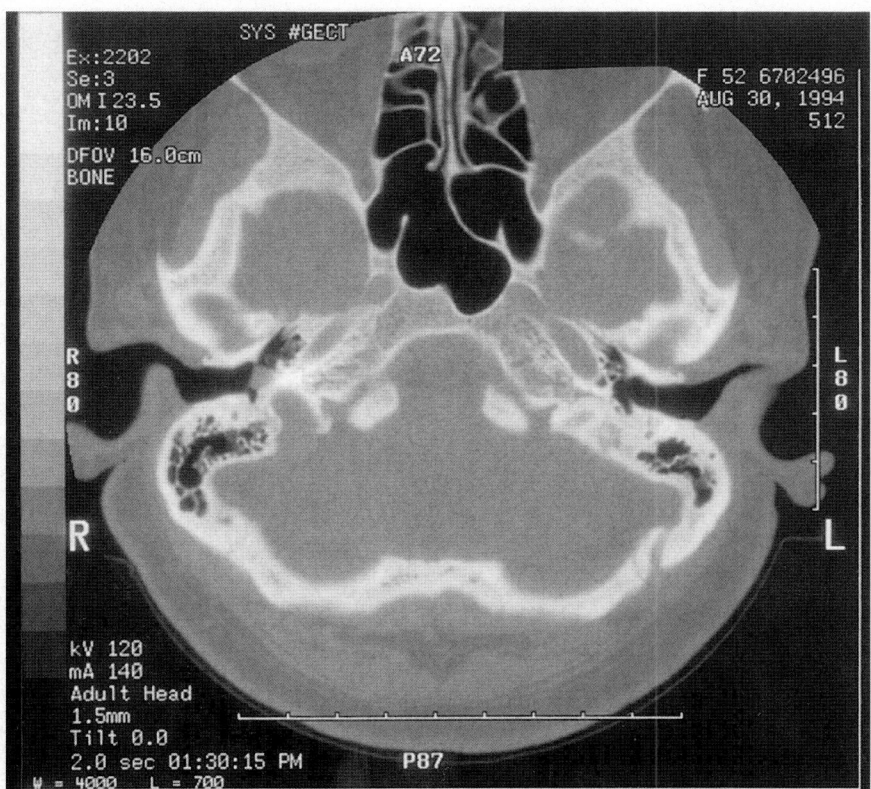

Figure 36–1 Axial computed tomographic scan shows right glomus tympanicum tumor and an uninvolved jugular bulb.

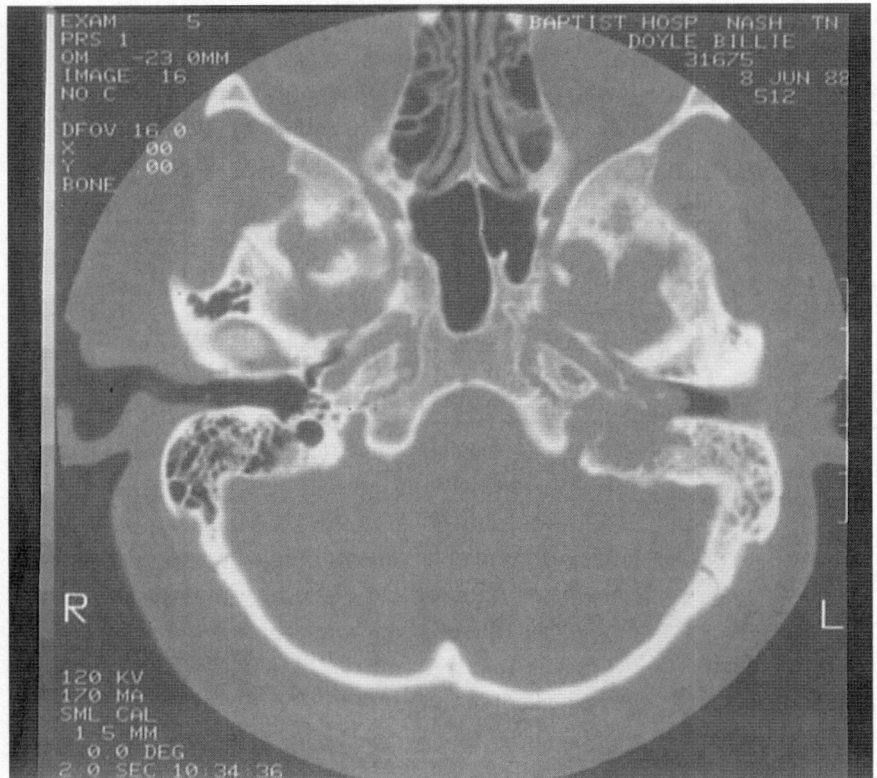

Figure 36–2 Computed tomographic scan shows tumor extent within the temporal bone.

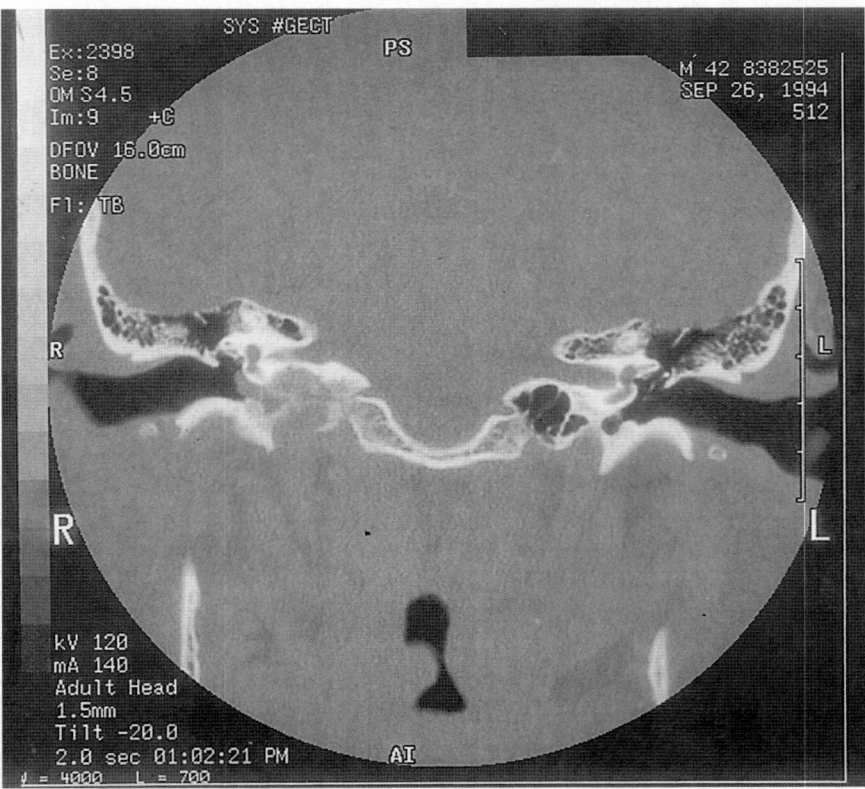

Figure 36–3 Axial computed tomographic scan shows right glomus jugulare tumor and extent relative to the petrous internal carotid artery.

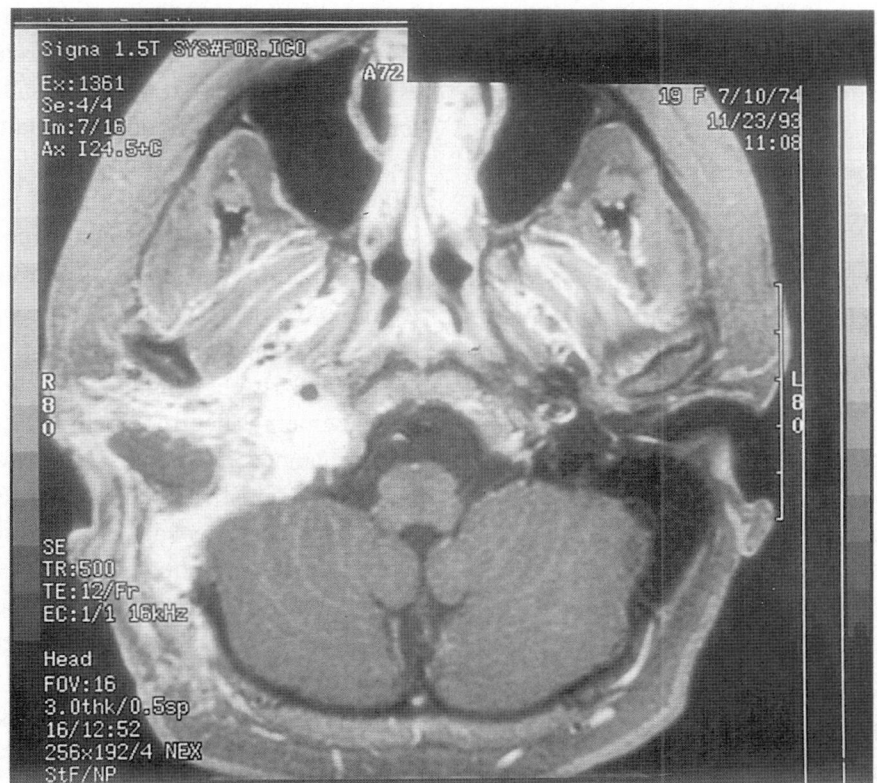

Figure 36–4 Magnetic resonance image shows typical appearance of a glomus jugulare tumor with flow voids of vessels within the tumor.

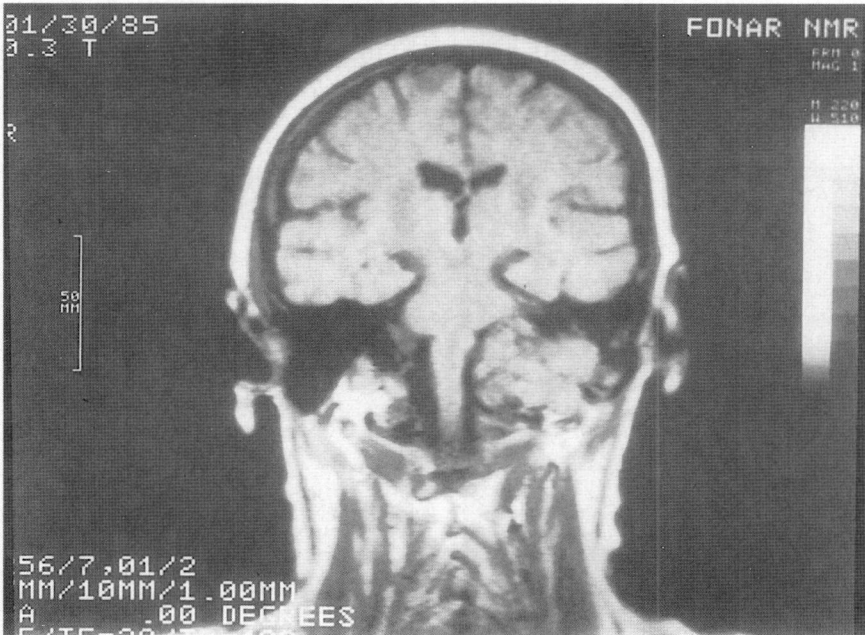

Figure 36–5 Magnetic resonance image shows intracranial extension.

external carotid artery (ECA) sources. The utility of embolization in limiting operative blood loss is documented.[24–27] The risks today are predictably low (Figures 36–6, A and B).

As ICA sacrifice is not done without revascularization, ICA sacrifice prediction testing is generally not done contemporarily.

The diagnostic laboratory evaluation of the GT patient is completed by catecholamine screening.

Treatment Planning

Treatment is palliative or definitive (curative). For the purpose of this chapter, RT is considered a palliative therapy. Definitive treatment is surgical.

No lesion is technically unresectable. Each treatment plan is based on data generated by the diagnostic evaluation yet must consider patient factors such as age, tumor type and natural history, and general medical health. The issue is whether in the natural course of the patient's remaining life, the tumor is likely to cause significant morbidity or mortality.

Palliation is reserved for the elderly, medically infirm, or those select, multicentric lesions in which definitive treatment is otherwise contraindicated. "Elderly" is best defined physiologically, yet approximates 65 to 70 years. A small GT in a 75 year old is unlikely to cause concern in his/her remaining years as GTs are slow-growing. In contrast, slow growth rate is not relevant to the typical 30-year-old woman in whom the GT is usually encountered. Surgery is offered to the latter and not recommended to the former. For the asymptomatic patient in whom palliation is elected, the GT is carefully observed with serial imaging. The symptomatic patient is irradiated.

In synchronous lesions, the most life-threatening lesion is operated on first. Neurologic outcome determines subsequent recommendations. Bilateral GJ tumors are particularly challenging. If one is operated on and the patient emerges neurologically intact, contralateral surgery is planned in 6 months. Extensive cranial nerve loss mitigates against such a plan because of the extraordinary risk of laryngeal denervation and pharyngeal deafferentation. Such an outcome represents a serious assault on quality of life attended by permanent tracheostomy, tracheal diversion, and/or artificial alimentary support. In such a case, the residual lesion is followed and palliated as indicated. Often no right answer exists.

Radiation Therapy

Resection of GJ tumors for cure has always represented a primary objective.[24] Owing to the technical capacity of the day, issues of resection or resectability have been minimized. Virtually any lesion is "resectable." The per-

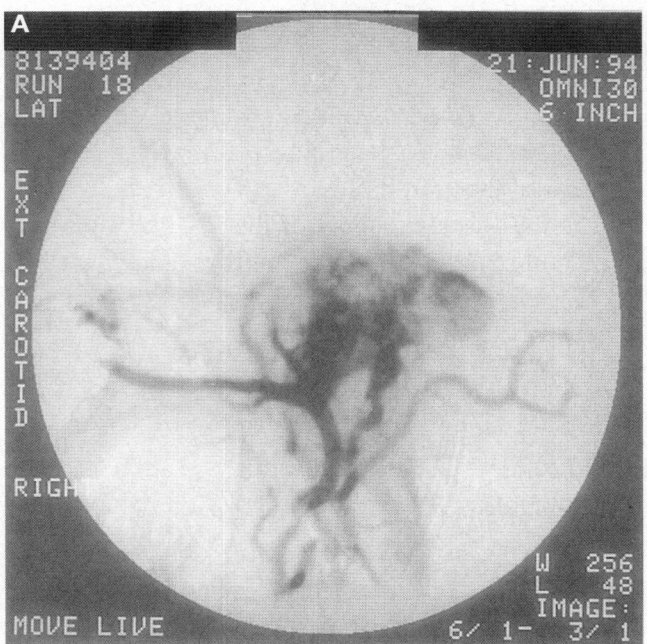
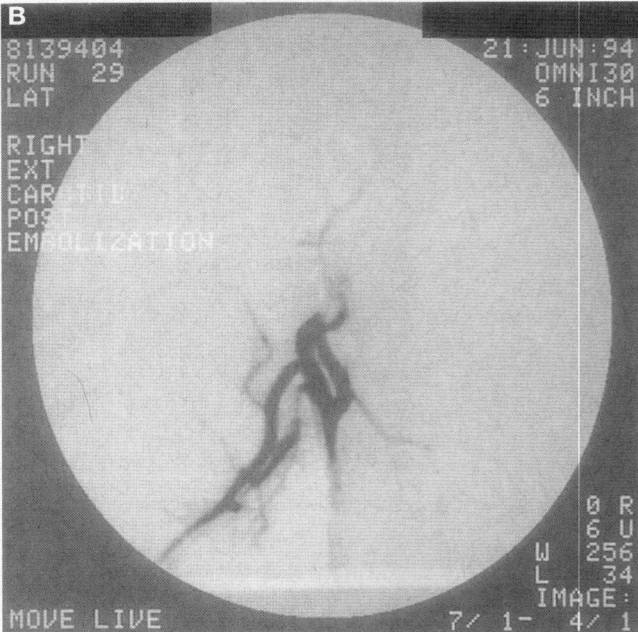

Figure 36–6 *A,* Angiogram blush before embolization. *B,* Successful embolization of this same tumor shown.

ceived risk of functional incapacity that attends lateral skull base surgery is the most common reason for which surgery is criticized. Today the success of conservation surgery and the operative rehabilitation of existing or iatrogenic phonopharyngeal deficits have gone far to mitigate such criticism.

As an alternative, RT proposes itself as a minimal, low-morbidity, low-cost conservation strategy. Recently, RT has received much attention.[28–30] Under the influence of managed care, it is expected that RT will continue to hold its prominent place in GT care.

As a result, a sharp controversy between surgeons and radiation therapists has emerged as to which modality is the best primary therapy for GT. The data to resolve this controversy do not exist. The RT position is summed by Cummings and colleagues,[31] who have noted "…the relief of symptoms and the failure of the tumor to grow during the remainder of the patient's lifetime is a practical measure of successful treatment." However, the assumption that irradiated tumor consists only of benign masses of inert cells is probably inaccurate.[32–34] Radiation therapy forces the patient to coexist with a biologically altered tumor. Because of the relative rarity of these tumors (which confounds statistical analysis), the protracted (15 to 20 years) natural history, and advancements in RT made over several decades, current data cannot support the contention of disease "control." The conceptual distinction between disease "control" and "cure" is more than semantic. In large tumors, no new cranial nerve deficits are generally created by GT tumor surgery, but in GJ tumor surgery, cranial nerve loss is a fact of life. Even though compensation and operative rehabilitation are effective, functional capacity is diminished. To the end of cure, the real risks of surgery are well defined, concurrent, and qualitatively documented.[35,36] Jackson and colleagues[35] reviewed the RT literature and compulsively sought the risks of RT with respect to hearing loss, central nervous system damage, osteoradionecrosis, and radiation-induced malignancy. They[35] concluded that the real risks of RT were ongoing, long term, and, as yet, undetermined.

The RT versus surgery debate continues to rage. In point of fact, RT as a minimally invasive protocol must continue to hold a prominent place in GT management. Glomus tumors are complicated treatment challenges. As data continue to be generated to properly quantify the risk/benefit ratio for each treatment modality, the patient's decision to tolerate coexistence with tumor or to seek freedom from it must be fully informed. Both options with available data need to be provided.

Surgical Treatment

BASIC PRINCIPLES. *ROUTES OF EXTENSION.* Glomus tumors originate from paraganglions that populate the ME and hypotympanum in the proximity of the jugular bulb. We have already discussed that from this regionally focused origin, routes of extension are along the lines of least resistance and are highly variable (Figure 36–7). An individualized surgical approach to each tumor and its ramifications within and beyond the TB must be represented by a coherent composition of surgical units as options (Figure 36–8). By definition, the strategy must be multidisciplinary and must accomplish the following:

- Exposure of all tumor margins
- Identification/control of vital regional anatomy
- Access to all margins of ICE

Following basic surgical principles,[24,36] the multidisciplinary approach maximizes the likelihood of complete tumor resection with the conservation of as much normal function as possible.

THE FACIAL NERVE IN LATERAL SKULL BASE SURGERY.

In lateral skull base surgery, the FN is an impediment to the fundamental principle of exposure. For the neuro-otologist, the FN is a structure to be dealt with rather than used. This general topic has been reviewed in detail in the surgical literature.[24,37,38]

It is the vascular supply of the FN that allows its successful relocation and manipulation and comprises extrinsic and intrinsic components. Facial nerve neural integrity monitoring (FNNIM) educates FN mobilization so as to promote the maintenance of vascular and neural integrity.

Facial nerve options in GT surgery are simple exposure, short or long mobilization, segmental resection, and selective division. The fundamental factors that determine which FN option is selected are tumor size and how much distal ICA control the tumor extent requires. Much attention has been given to protocols that involve simple FN exposure only, working between the lateral

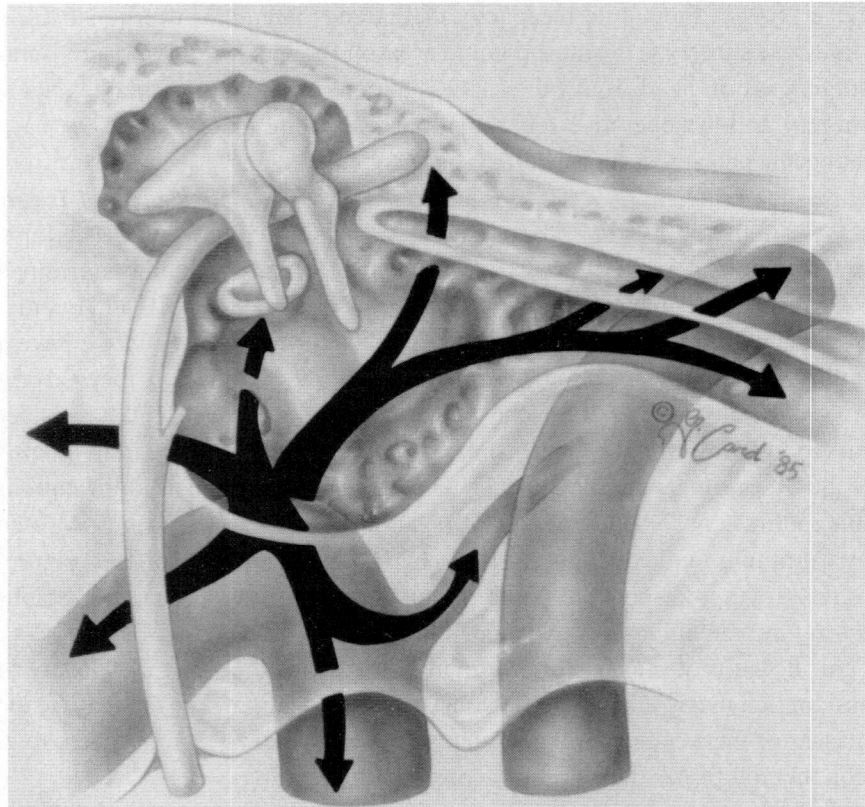

Figure 36–7 Glomus tumor extension route.

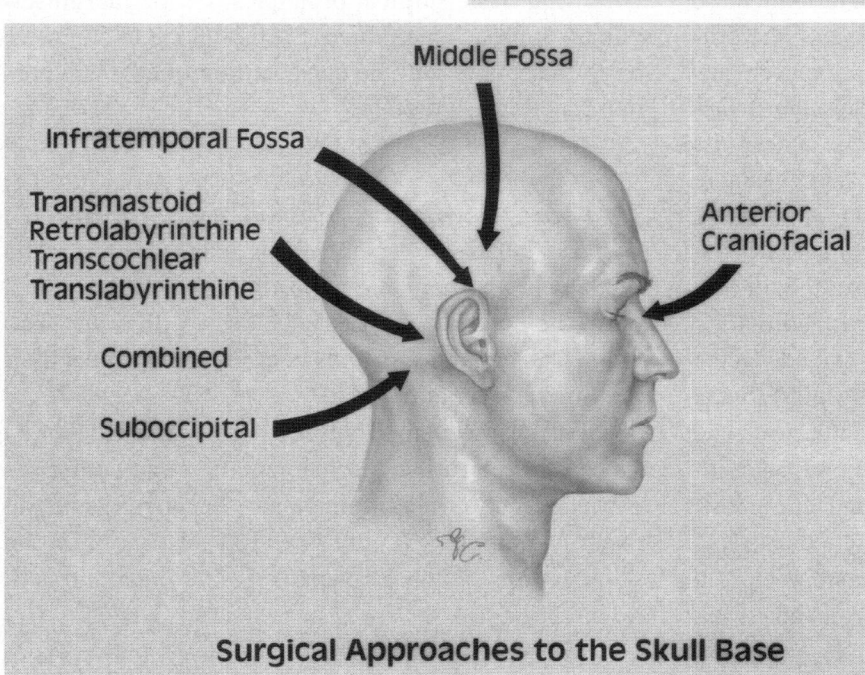

Middle Fossa

Infratemporal Fossa

Transmastoid
Retrolabyrinthine
Transcochlear
Translabyrinthine

Combined

Suboccipital

Anterior
Craniofacial

Surgical Approaches to the Skull Base

Figure 36–8 The surgical team must combine a variety of approach options.

process of C1 and FN. "Short" mobilization of the FN from the external genu laterally causes minimal morbidity, and nearly normal postoperative FN function is the rule. Long-term House-Brackmann (HB) recovery is excellent (Grades 1 to 2). For larger tumors, "long mobilization" is required from the geniculate ganglion (GG) distally. Long-term House-Brackmann outcome is also good. Selective division of the FN or its branches with

Table 36–2 PRESENTING SIGNS AND SYMPTOMS AMONG PATIENTS WITH GLOMUS TUMORS		
	Tumor Type	
Presenting Symptom	Glomus Jugulare (n = 106)	Glomus Vagale (n = 27)
Pulsatile tinnitus	84	8
Hearing loss	62	4
Otalgia	13	3
Aural fullness	32	3
Hoarseness	12	4
Dysphagia	8	5
Pharyngeal fullness	0	9
Vertigo	15	1
Facial weakness	15	1
Headache	5	0
Dysarthria	0	0
Aural bleeding	2	0

reanastomosis is rarely necessary today. Segmental resection is required when the FN is inextricable from the tumor, but this is rarely the case despite apparent involvement at the time of surgery. When FN function is normal prior to surgery, dissection of the FN from the GT should always be attempted. Facial nerve paralysis present preoperatively bodes poorly for FN salvation without resection and end-to-end anastomosis or interpositional grafting for reanimation.

INTERNAL CAROTID ARTERY. The ICA is fundamental to lateral skull base surgery as in every case the GT relates or attaches to it. The rate-limiting step in all lateral skull base surgery is the dissection of tumor from the ICA. The basic principles of vascular surgery—proximal and distal control—must be applied. "Control" means circumferential access to normal vessel. Access to the tympanic, petrous, and intracranial segments of the ICA must complement the generally easy access to the proximal vessel in the neck.

Guidelines for ICA sacrifice remain insecure, and prediction of outcome therefrom is less secure. When tumor inextricably involves the ICA, ICA continuity is restored by interpositional vein graft. Tumor behavior relative to the ICA cannot be preoperatively determined. If possible, when the need to sacrifice the ICA is determined preoperatively, and construction is not possible, extracranial bypass is performed.[39]

Internal carotid artery spasm is a dreadful intraoperative occurrence and occurs in response to longitudinal stretching of the vessel. When spasm occurs,

manipulation should cease immediately, pharmacologic measures should be taken (topical or ICA wall injection with papaverine), and the vessel should be observed.[40] In extreme cases, manual dilatation or segmental resection is required.

Internal carotid artery sacrifice by detachable, intravascular balloon, intra- or preoperatively, is still recommended by Fisch.[41] This extreme solution should be entertained only for extreme problems.

Surgical Technique
GLOMUS TYMPANICUM TUMORS. For a Class I tympanicum tumor (ie, a mesotympanic mass, the margins of which are visible 360 degrees, and with confirmatory imaging studies), complete resection can be accomplished by means of a transcanal tympanotomy. The mass is avulsed from the promontory, and bleeding is controlled by microbipolar coagulation or light packing.

For a Class II–IV GTy tumor, in which tumor margins cannot be visualized on otoscopy and in which radiologic differentiation from a GJ tumor has been accomplished, a transmastoid approach is elected. If imaging is found to have been unreliable and it is determined that the tumor is a GJ tumor, the procedure is aborted and definitive lateral skull base surgery is planned for another day.

The transmastoid resection is performed on an outpatient basis and comprises a complete mastoidectomy with extended facial recess exposure.[35,42] Hypotympanic exposure permits visual assessment of the GTy relative to the jugular bulb, ICA, and the structures of the TB (Figure 36–9). Once the GTy tumor is removed, necessary tympanoplastic reconstruction can be done. New technology employs the laser.[37]

GLOMUS JUGULARE TUMOR. The GJ tumor is removed by means of lateral skull base surgery and represents a multidisciplinary team effort.

Anesthetic goals in lateral skull base surgery include the following[24]:

- Maintenance of hemodynamic stability
- Prevention of increased intracranial pressure
- Maintenance of cerebral perfusion and oxygenation
- Maintenance of a still surgical field
- Facilitation of electrophysiologic monitoring

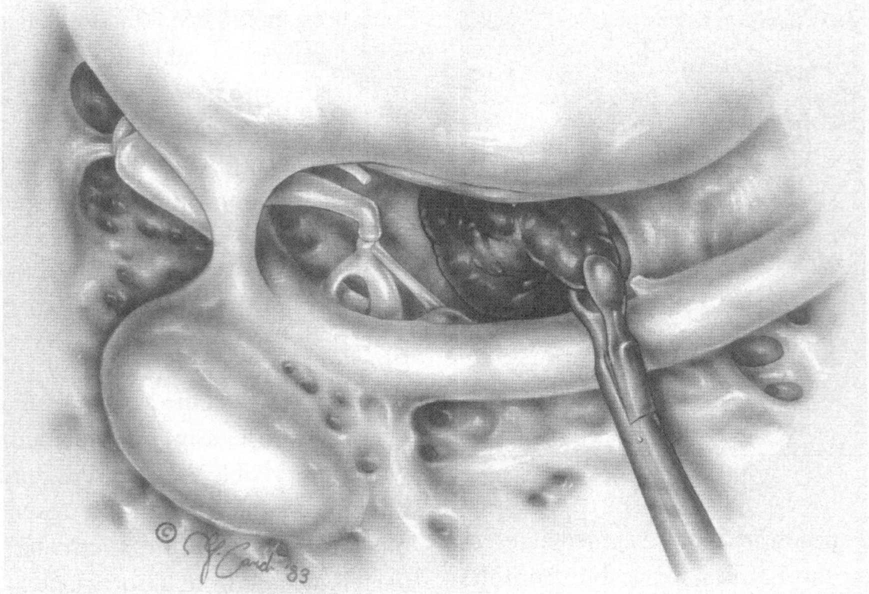

Figure 36–9 Facial recess and extensions provide wide exposure into the hypotympanum for tumor removal.

- Facilitation of surgical exposure and tumor removal
- Replacement of lost blood and prevention of transfusion-associated coagulopathies
- Provision of rapid emergence from anesthesia for the purpose of prompt establishment of a neurologic baseline
- Postoperative airway management

Invasive monitoring provides data regarding hemodynamic status, which is especially important during tumor manipulation and the fluctuant release of catecholamines. Blood replacement must keep pace with loss, and autologous blood is used whenever possible. Preoperative identification and treatment of "secretors" permit controlled induction and administration of anesthesia.

The surgical objectives are total tumor removal, with the preservation of structure and function to the greatest extent possible, that is, conservation surgery.

GLOMUS JUGULARE TUMOR CLASS I AND II (SMALL TO MEDIUM). The tumors are confined to the infra-labyrinthine chamber and involve the ICA only in its tympanic segment, and are amenable to a hearing conservation approach that conserves the EAC (provided that hearing is salvageable).[35]

The patient is in the supine position. An incision is outlined that permits access to the TB and neck and creates an anteriorly based flap (Figure 36–10). The vital neurovascular anatomy of the neck is isolated and controlled. Facial nerve extratemporal dissection is held to a minimum to protect vascular supply and neural integrity. The ICA is controlled and the internal jugular vein is ligated. Complete mastoidectomy, removal of the mastoid tip, inferior tympanic bone removal, and skeletonization of the inferior-anterior EAC allow access to the mesotympanum and complete dissection of the tympanic ICA to the ET for control (Figure 36–11). The FN undergoes "short" mobilization (Figure 36–12). Proximal control of the lateral venous sinus is achieved by intraluminal packing. With tumor dissected from the ICA, it is mobilized from the infralabyrinthine chamber. Within the jugular bulb, bleeding from the inferior petrosal sinus(es) is packed. Delicate dissection of the GJ tumor from the contents of the pars nervosa of the jugular foramen and the hypoglossal canal is rewarded by cranial nerve preservation in the smaller lesions.

GLOMUS JUGULARE TUMOR CLASS III AND IV (MEDIUM TO LARGE). When the GT extends out of the TB into the infratemporal fossa (IFTF) or when control of the petrous portion of the ICA is required, a modified IFTF approach, or its extension, is necessary. These approaches offer not only access to the deep recesses of the TB and IFTF but

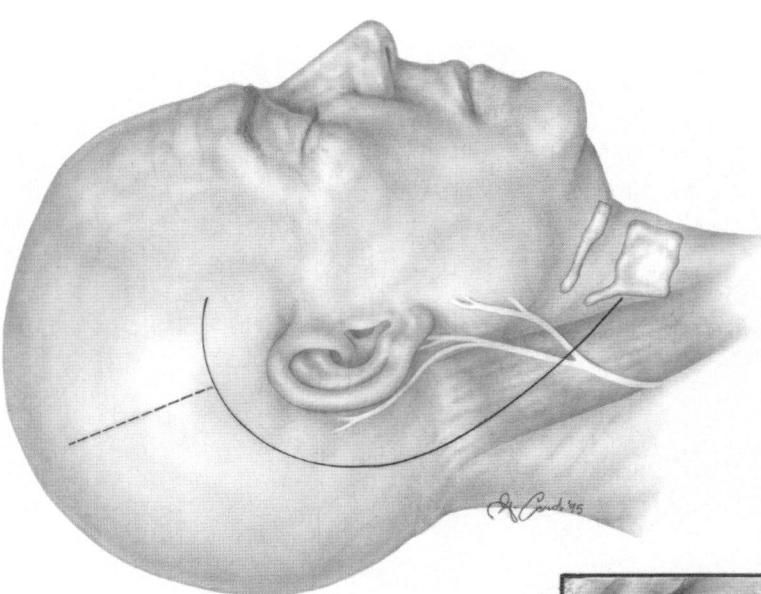

Figure 36–10   Incision minimizes superior flap necrosis and allows cephalic access for temporoparietal fascia.

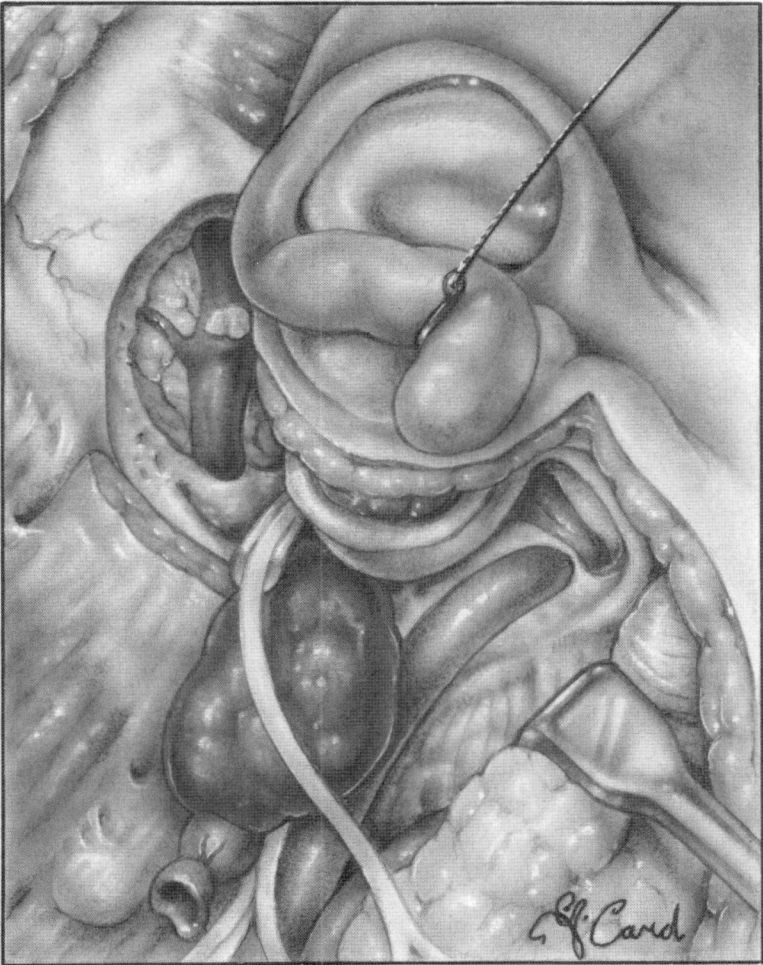

Figure 36–11   The infratympanic extended facial recess approach provides distal control of the internal carotid artery and allows hearing conservation.

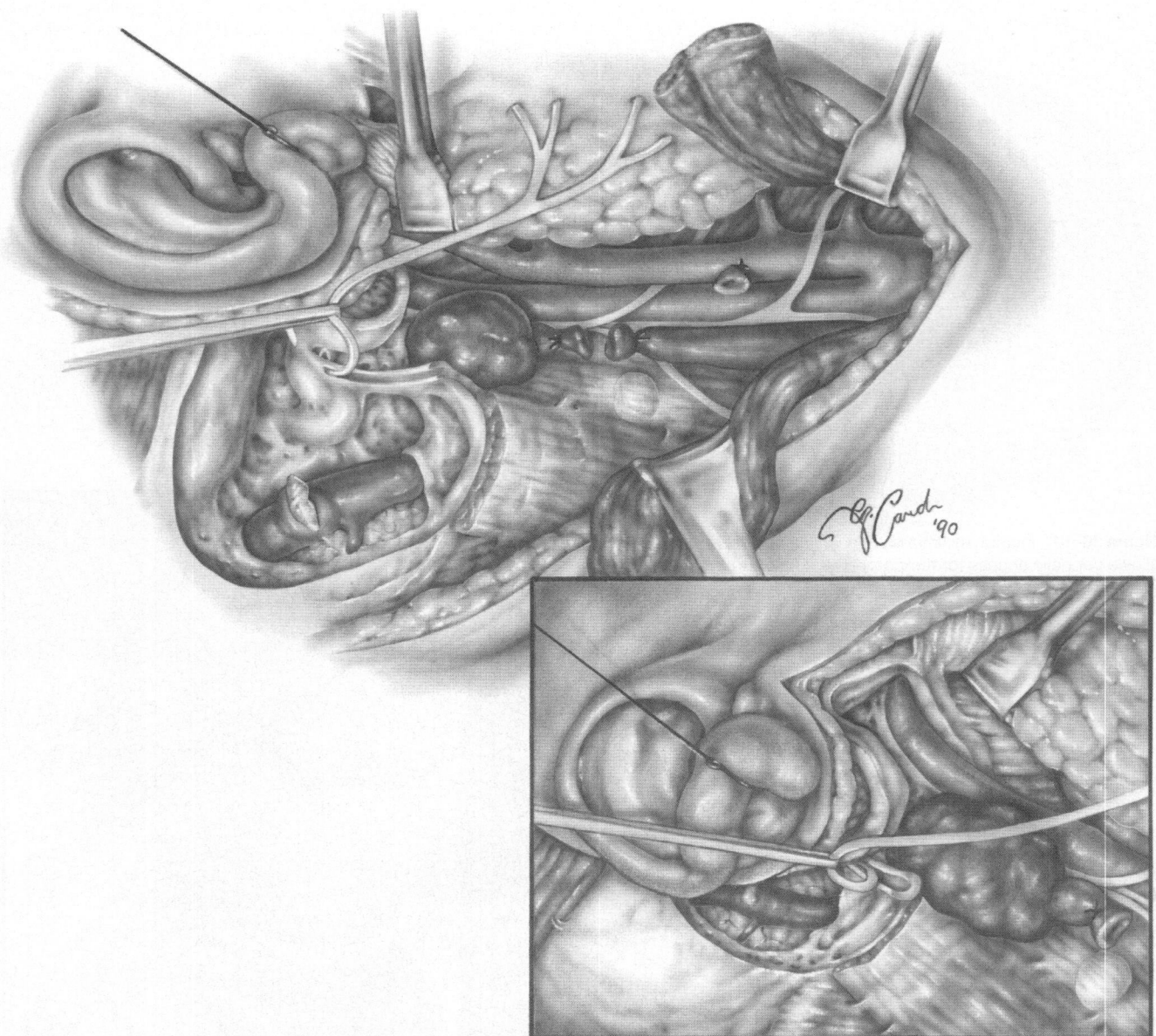

Figure 36–12 Tympanic bone removal, skeletonization of the external auditory canal, and facial nerve mobilization are basic.

also the clivus, the nasopharynx, cavernous sinus, and the posterior, middle, and anterior cranial fossae for removal of ICE. A complete conductive hearing loss is conceded.

The same incision is executed as for GJ tumor class I/II excision, but the EAC is transected and oversewn (Figure 36–13). The EAC, TM, and the contents of the ME lateral to the stapes are resected. Access to the petrous ICA and IFTF requires anterior and inferior dislocation of the mandible by dividing its anteromedial ligamentous attachments. The FN undergoes "long mobilization"

(Figure 36–14). More recent technique modifications leave the contents of the stylomastoid foramen and digastric attached to VII during translocation[43,44] (illustrations show the FN alone for illustrative clarity).

Retraction needs, to maintain exposure, are more formidable. The extirpation of tumor, with exposure achieved, proceeds as before.

When anterosuperior tumor extension or ICA dissection distally is extreme, this exposure is extended. By resecting the zygoma and TMJ unit and inferiorly reflecting the temporalis muscle with maximum anterior-

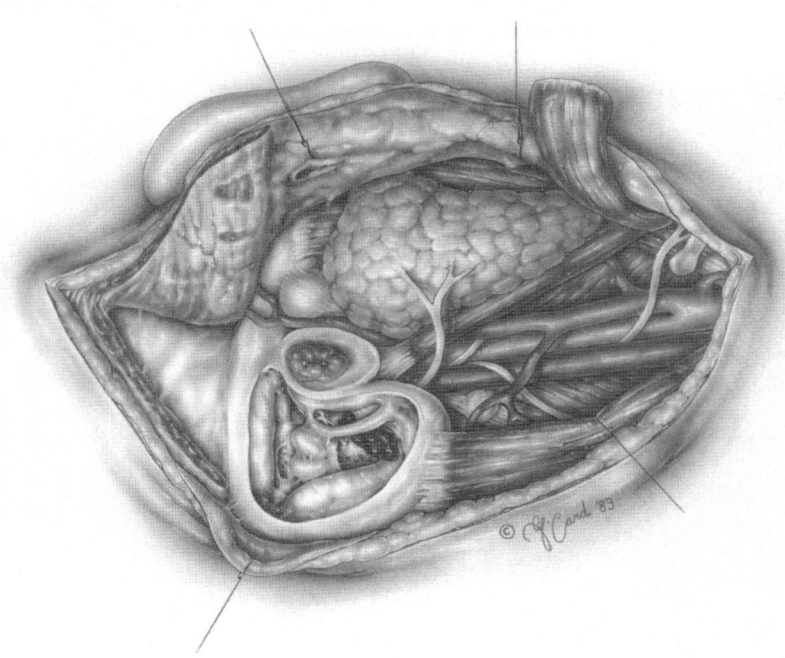

Figure 36–13   The external auditory canal is transected and oversewn in the infratemporal fossa approach.

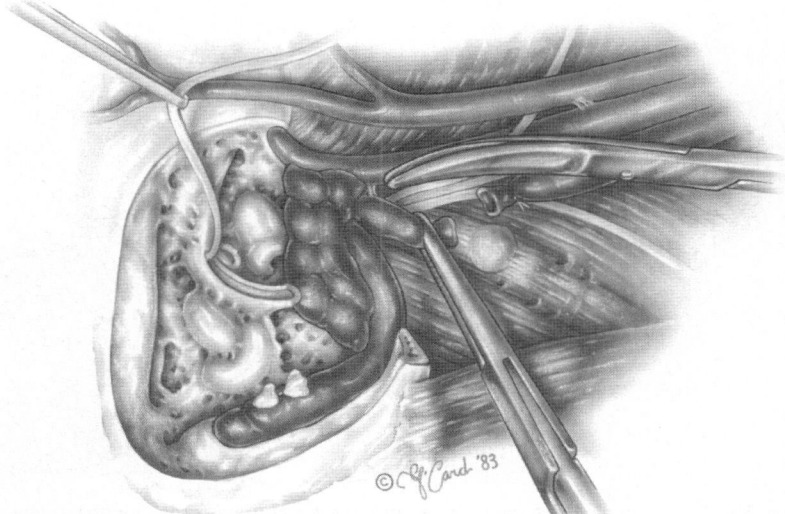

Figure 36–14   Facial nerve mobilization and mandibular dislocation provide proximal petrous internal carotid artery exposure.

inferior mandibular dislocation, the structures of the IFTF can be accessed (Figure 36–15). The ET is resected and the contents of the foramen spinosum managed on the way toward ICA dissection through the pterygoid region to its precavernous margin (Figure 36–16). Access to the middle cranial fossa, nasopharynx, foramen rotundum, clivus, posterior cranial fossa, and cavernous sinus is possible. Tumor resection proceeds as before.

Intracranial Extension

Intracranial extension is defined as the transdural spread of tumor through dura into the subarachnoid space. Intracranial extension was once regarded as a criterion for unresectability. The tumor and its ICE were often regarded as two separate lesions and managed as such. The modern trend is to correctly consider them a single unit with management in an unstaged procedure.

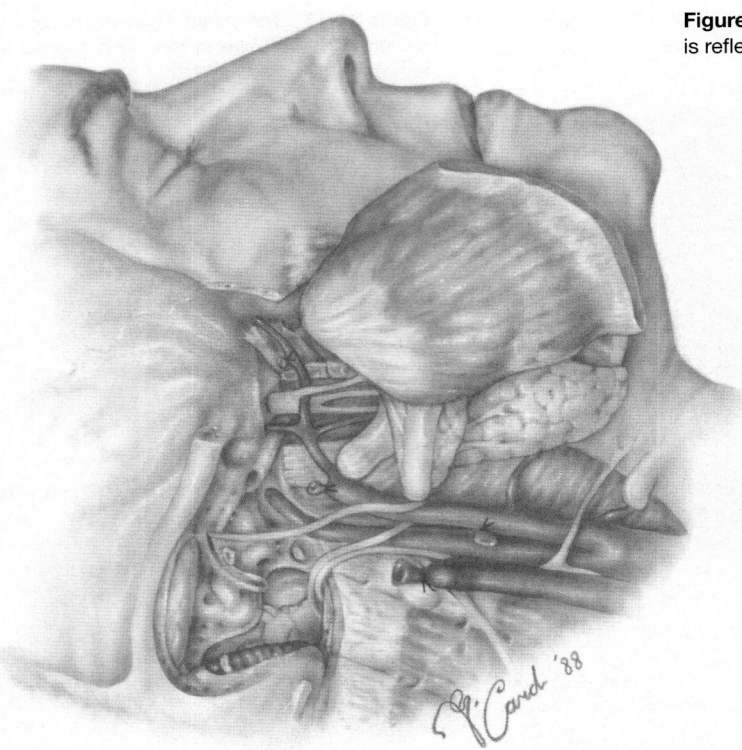

Figure 36–15   The mandible, temporal muscle, and zygoma unit is reflected to allow infratemporal fossa exposure.

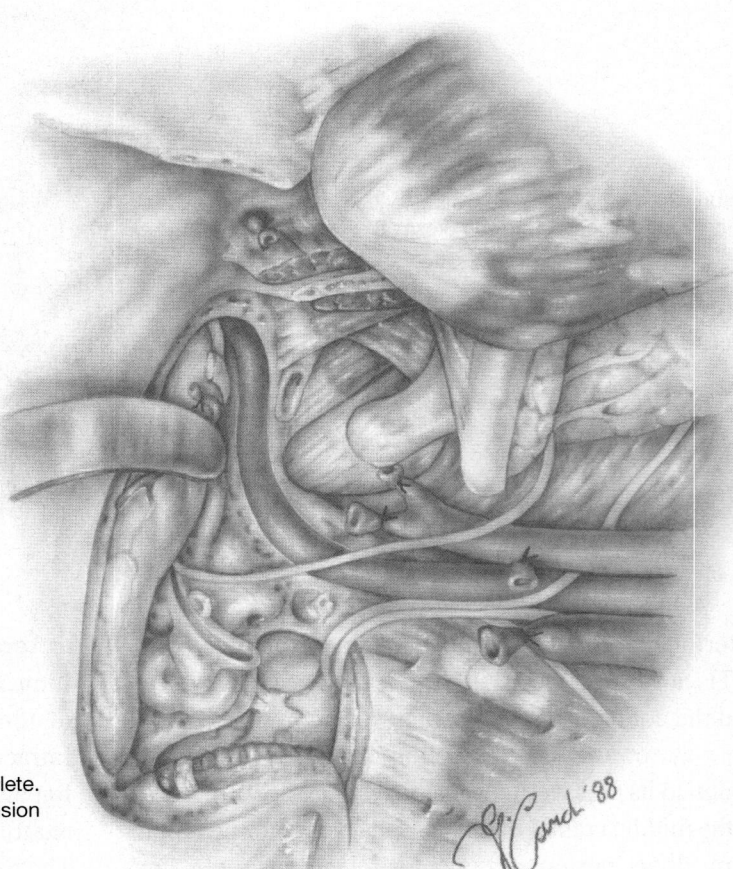

Figure 36–16   The internal carotid artery exposure is complete. Middle cranial fossa exposure is excellent. The maxillary division of cranial nerve V in the foramen rotundum is depicted.

The single-stage resection of ICE poses problems unique to lateral skull base surgery. Single-stage resection is complicated by problems of dural defect reconstruction and cerebrospinal fluid management far more complex than those posed, for example, by the resection of an acoustic neuroma. In neurotologic lateral skull base surgery, the following obstacles are unique[24]:

- Wider bony and soft tissue defects
- Local tissue usually rendered unavailable for reconstruction
- Cerebrospinal fluid (CSF) pressures enhanced by venous occlusion.
- Regional devitalization by RT, ICA exposure, and regional ischemia as a result of EAC ligation

Reconstruction schemes have as fundamentals the need for wide capacity ranging from simple to complex.

Intracranial extension usually occurs through the posterior fossa dura or along cranial nerve roots to the posterior cranial fossa (Figure 36–17) and is reliably detailed by MRI (see Figure 36–5). The management of a GJ tumor with ICE follows this sequence:

1. Tumor dissection from the ICA/IFTF
2. Tumor debulking from the TB down to the dura
3. Removal of the ICE
4. Defect reconstruction

Tumor removal from the posterior cranial fossa is usually not difficult through the exposure available once the lateral venous sinus (LVS) has been resected. Translabyrinthine and transcochlear adjunctive dissection expands the posterior cranial fossa exposure.

Resection of ICE limited to the area of the pars nervosa usually results in a small dural defect.

Defect Reconstruction

The size of the defect determines the complexity of the repair, which is modified by associated complicating factors such as the effects of RT.

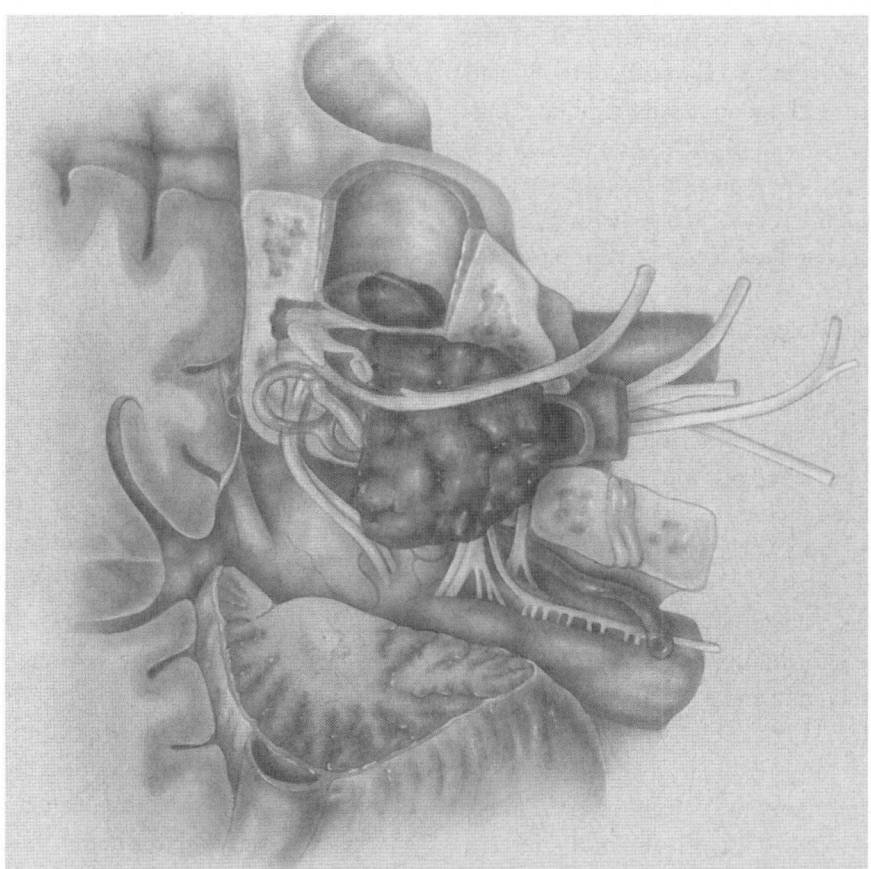

Figure 36–17 Transdural extension of tumor occurs into the posterior cranial fossa.

The following generalities apply[24]:

- Dural defect reconstruction by vascularized tissue
- Tissue bulk to reinforce the reconstruction and resist the CSF pressure head; also often vascularized
- CSF decompression by lumbar drain for 5 to 7 days
- Adherence to the basic principles of preservation and mobilization of local tissue to facilitate wound closure
- A prerequisite to successful resection of extensive tumors was the development of strategies to reconstruct the defects created and to prevent CSF leakage. In the face of significant tissue loss, the dura must be closed and ICA exposure addressed.

The successful reconstruction of these defects can be facilitated by the careful preservation and mobilization of tissues (Figure 36–18, A to C). The skin incision is outlined for access to the superficial temporalis fascia, the TB, and the neck. The neck skin flap is elevated deep to the platysma; elevation over the mastoid is superficial and subcutaneous to create a strong sternocleidomastoid (SCM) fascial flap, which is created by cutting along the temporal line up to or beyond the EAC if it is to be sacrificed. The SCM fascial flap is then mobilized posteriorly and inferiorly. This flap greatly facilitates closure through the reattachment of this tissue to the deep temporal fascia superiorly and parotid fascia anteriorly when the EAC has been transected. When the EAC is preserved, this flap is closed to the bony-cartilaginous junction of the EAC.

To preserve regional blood supply, the EAC is not divided.

Small dural defects are closed with vascularized superficial temporal fascia and a free abdominal fat graft.[24,35,37] This flap, described by Abul-Hassan and colleagues,[45] is vascularized by the EAC and requires careful dissection in the zygomatic region to maintain viable blood supply. Often referred to as a temporoparietal fascia flap, it is extensive. The superficial temporal fascia is left attached to the skin flap until it is determined it is needed. It is then detached and rotated into the defect to cover the dural defect (Figure 36–19). Even when the EAC is left intact and the ME open to CSF egress via the ET, this flap is ample enough to wrap around the intact EAC, facial recess, and antrum to allow for an aerated ME space. A lumbar drain remains indwelling for 5 to 7 days.

For medium-sized defects consequent to resection of more extensive lesions (more likely with malignancies of the temporal bone, ear, parotid, or meningioma, rather than the GT) more bulk is required,[46] such as that provided by a myocutaneous flap. In a young woman, the typical GT patient, a pectoralis donor site is unappealing; rather, the lower trapezius myocutaneous flap is preferred (Figure 36–20). Small defects in previously operated on or irradiated tissue may require this type of reconstruction. The flap is hearty and provides excellent coverage while maintaining trapezius function.

More massive defects require alternative flaps. The latissimus dorsi myocutaneous flap can be employed, but free-flap reconstruction is preferred. Of the multiple flaps available, the rectus abdominis muscle and its overlying tissue are preferred (Figure 36–21). Significant atrophy (40%) can be expected and is a drawback. The flap should be intentionally oversized to overcompensate for the atrophy. Overcompensation that persists can easily be corrected, more easily than additional bulk can be added. This flap has the added advantage of operative efficiency as harvesting can be begun by another team working in the abdomen as the final stages of lateral skull base surgery are completed.

It is emphasized that extreme solutions are applied only to extreme problems. The totipotential surgical capacity to customize resection and reconstruction ensures maximum possible functional outcome in these patients with dreadful lesions.

Rehabilitation of Cranial Nerve Loss

For small lesions, cranial nerve preservation can be achieved in over 90% of cases.[24,35–37] For preexisting cranial nerve deficits or for those created at surgery, a strategy must exist to ensure postsurgical outcomes that are of high quality. The lower cranial nerves function as a unit orchestrating phonopharyngeal function (Figure 36–22). Single nerve loss rarely causes a problem in airway protection, swallowing, or speech as most patients are able to compensate. Lateral skull base surgery exposes the patient to potential loss of cranial nerves IV through XII, as well as the sympathetic trunk. Acute loss of cranial nerves in aggregate is poorly tolerated but generally can be surgically rehabilitated. In the elderly, rehabilitation of swallowing may be impossible when combined cranial nerve loss occurs.

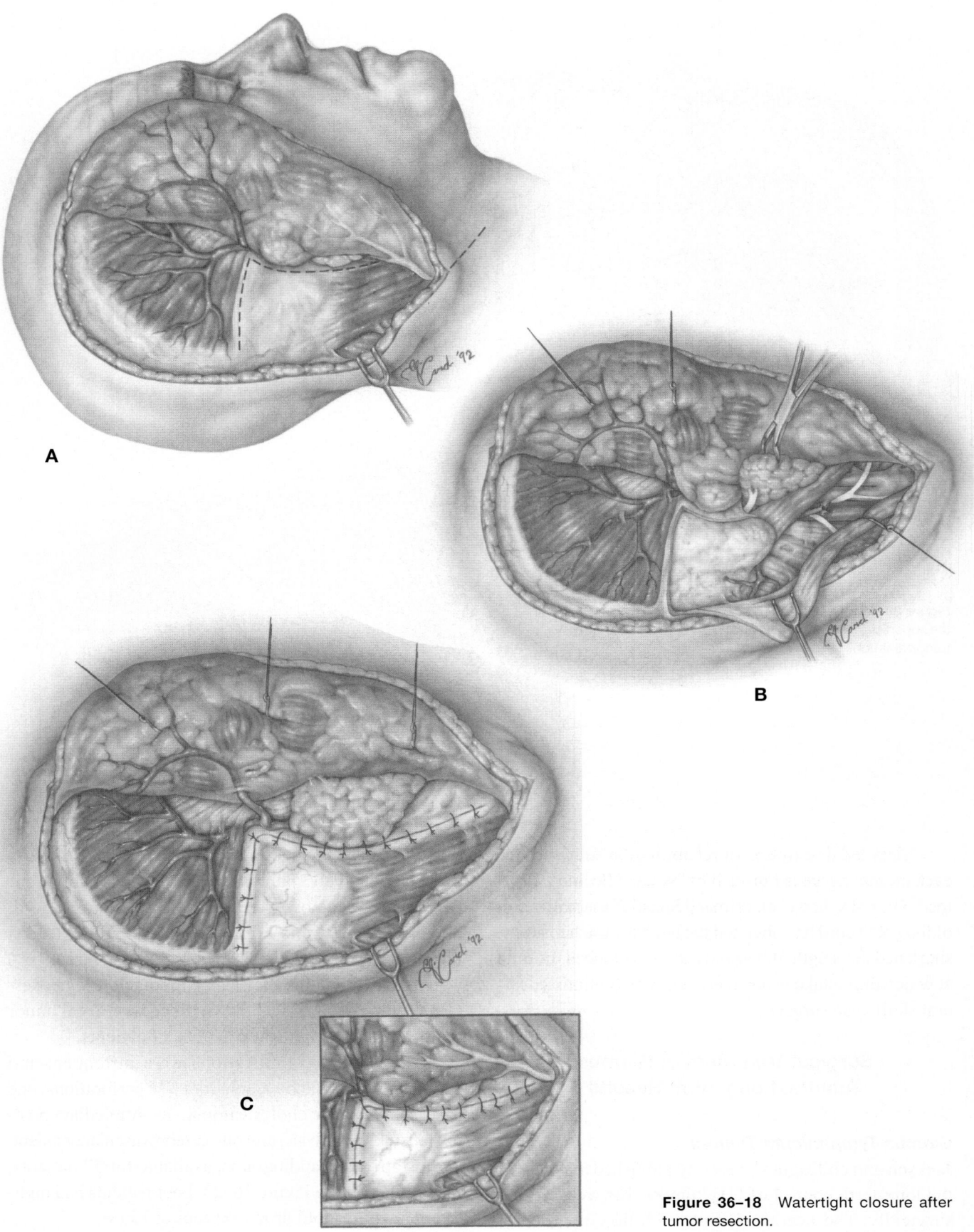

A

B

C

Figure 36–18 Watertight closure after tumor resection.

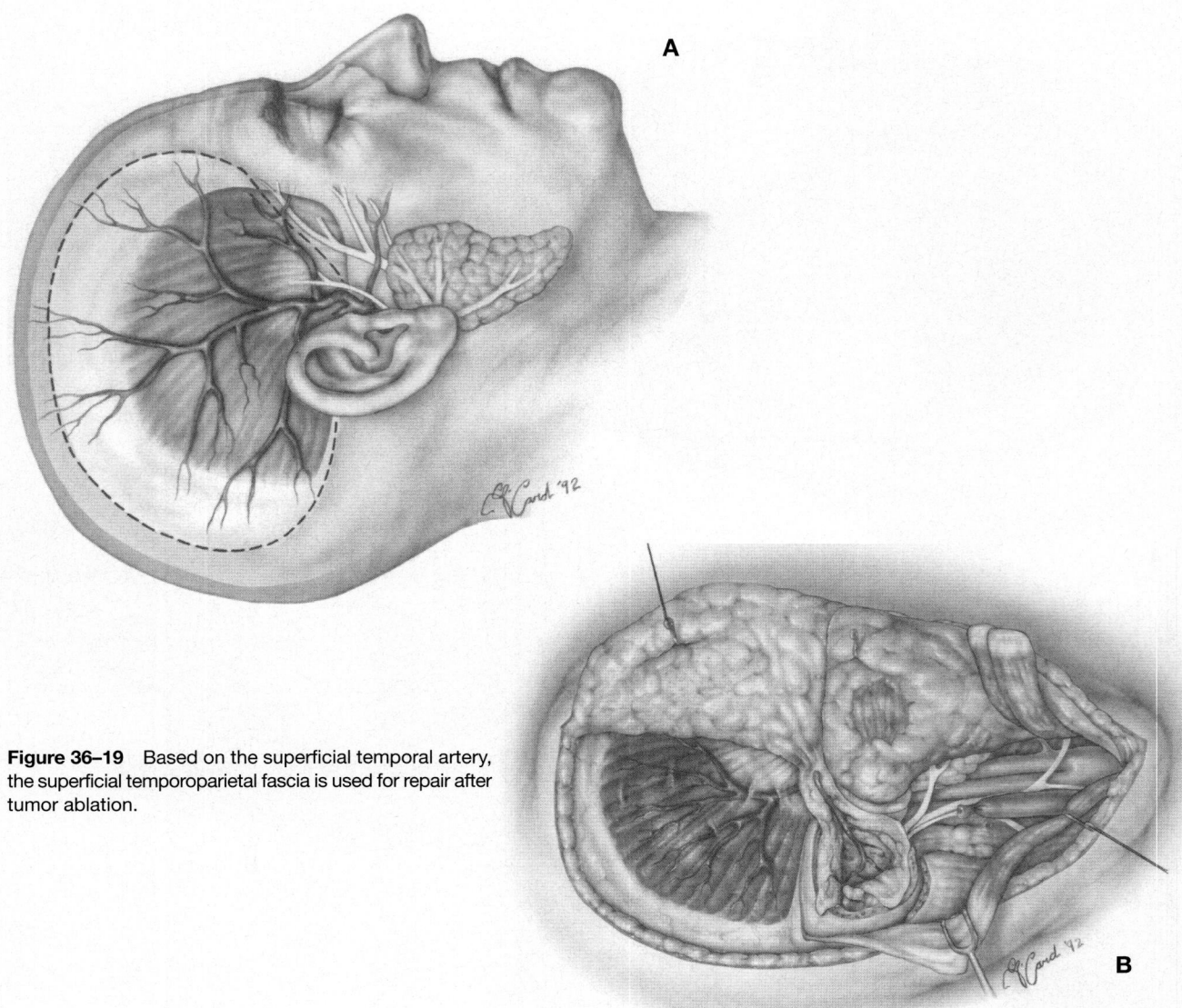

Figure 36–19 Based on the superficial temporal artery, the superficial temporoparietal fascia is used for repair after tumor ablation.

A detailed description of rehabilitation strategies for each cranial nerve is outlined by Netterville and Civantos.[47] Globally, however, primary Silastic® medialization of the vocal cord has obviated the need for tracheostomy, shortened the length of hospital stay, and reduced the time at which oral intake is resumed. It has revolutionized lateral skull base surgery.[47,48]

Surgical Treatment of Glomus Tumors: Long-Term Results

Glomus Tympanicum Tumors

Jackson and colleagues[49] recently published a review of the long-term control of GTy tumors that were treated surgically. The average length of follow-up was 55 months, and the average patient age was 53 years. Ninety-one percent of the patients were women. Thirty-four percent of the tumors were Stage I, 52% were Stage II, 3% were Stage III, and 11% were Stage IV. The extended facial recess approach was used in 73% of cases; 16% were removed via the transcanal approach. Eleven percent required a canal wall down procedure. Total tumor removal was accomplished in 95% of patients.

Postoperative complications were infrequent and included one wound infection, four TM perforations, one EAC stenosis, one cholesteatoma, one immediate postoperative FN paralysis, and one cerebrovascular accident.

Postoperative audiograms, available for 57 patients, are summarized in Figure 36–23. Four patients had high-frequency threshold drops exceeding 15 dB.

A

B

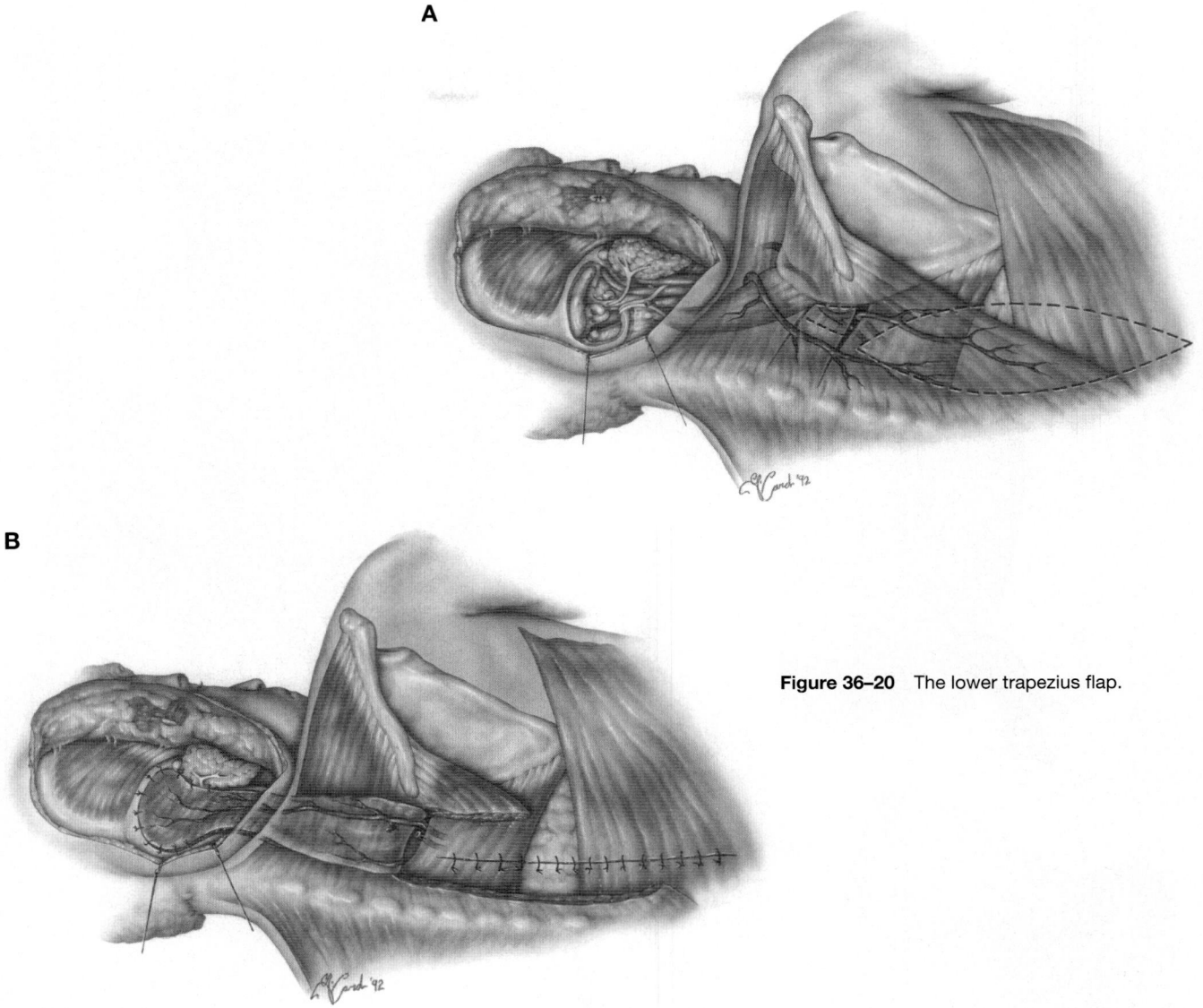

Figure 36–20 The lower trapezius flap.

There were two recurrences. Long-term tumor control was accomplished in 92.5% of patients.

In this series,[49] the GTy tumor was associated with other paragangliomas only once, in a patient with a history of familial paragangliomas. No patient exhibited symptoms of catecholamine, hormone, or parahormone secretion. Accordingly, we have modified our diagnostic protocol for GTy by eliminating routine biochemical analysis and urine sampling for catecholamines; biochemical survey is reserved for patients with GTy tumors with known multiple lesions and/or a family history of paragangliomas.

High-resolution CT of the TB, with and without contrast, is the definitive imaging study for GTy tumors. We employ MRI only when the diagnosis and/or the extent of the disease are in question. Extensive imaging evaluation is performed only in patients with GTy tumors with a known familial tendency and/or multiple lesions.

As one patient in this series developed a recurrence 14 years after surgery, long-term follow-up appears necessary. We follow our patients with GTy tumors yearly for 5 years and once every 5 years thereafter.

Skull Base Glomus Tumors

The long-term control of GTs managed by lateral skull base surgery has been recently reviewed.[50] This review contains current data regarding the incidence of major complications, surgical cranial nerve deficits, long-term

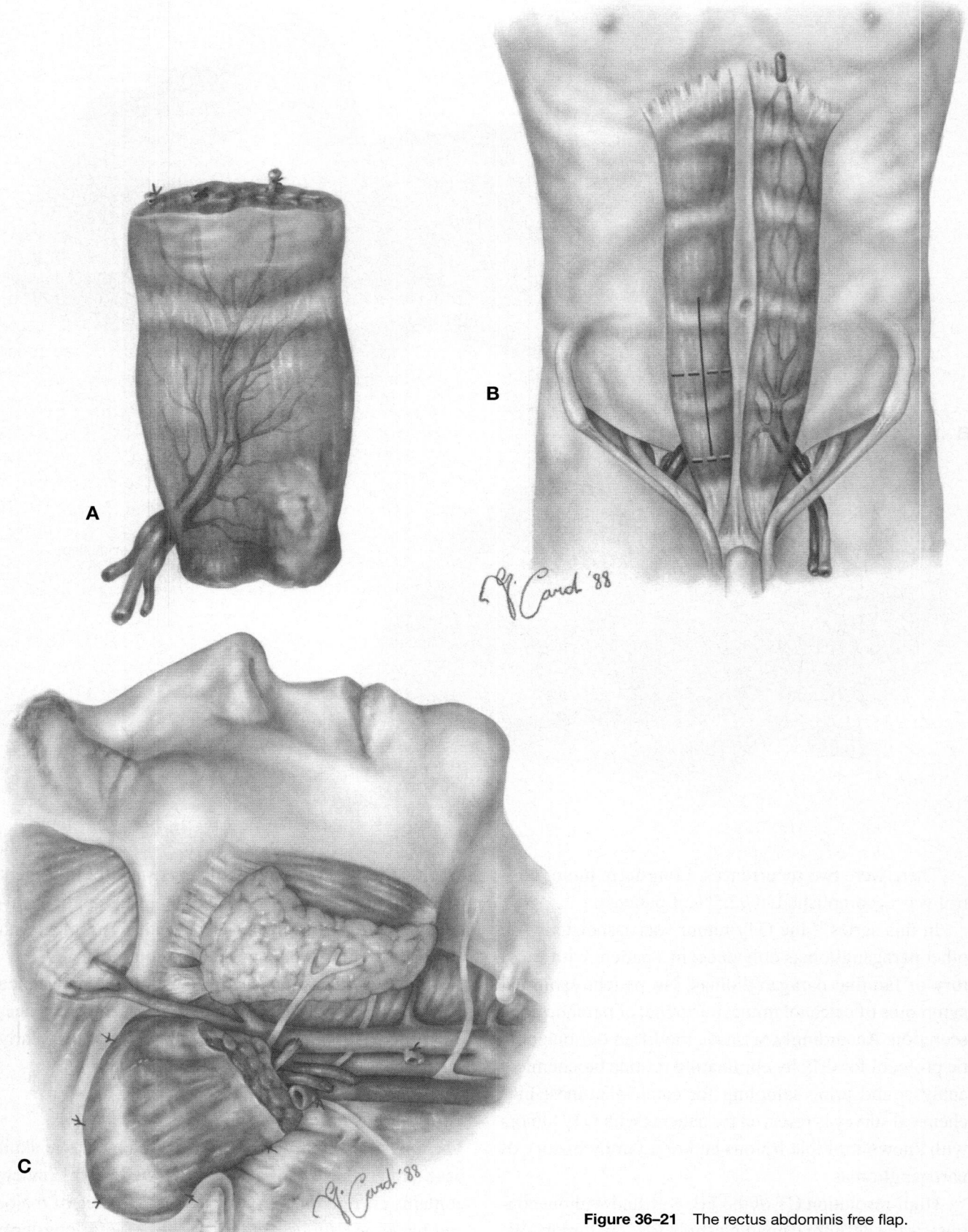

Figure 36–21 The rectus abdominis free flap.

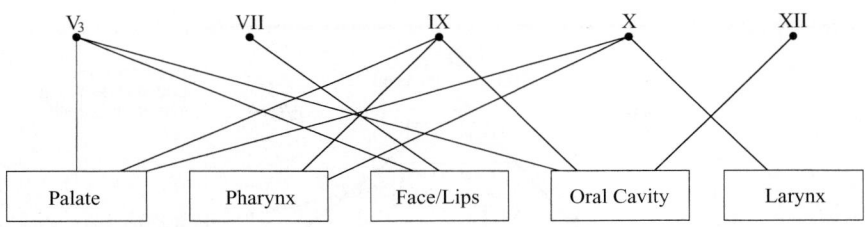

Figure 36–22   Interaction of lower cranial nerves in phonopharyngeal function.

surgical control rates, and recurrence risk of patients undergoing skull base resection for large paragangliomas using modern microsurgical techniques. Surgical control was defined as complete tumor removal with no evidence of recurrence over the follow-up period; coexistence with tumor was not considered control.

The review examined a total of 279 skull base procedures performed on 176 patients; 152 patients had GJ, 27 had GV (glomus vagale), and 3 had carotid body tumors that extended to the base of the skull. The average patient age was 41 years, and there was a 2.59 to 1 female-to-male ratio. The average length of follow-up was 54 months (range 1 month to 23.25 years).

Using the Glasscock-Jackson classification system, there were 27 (21.4%) Class I, 26 (20.6%) Class II, 44 (34.9%) Class III, and 29 (23%) Class IV tumors. Seventeen patients (9.7%) exhibited symptoms of catecholamine secretion, whereas 9% had multicentric tumors. The incidence of malignant GT in this series was 3.3%. (Regional or distant tumor developing in known glomus locations was regarded as a manifestation of multiple lesions, whereas tumor appearing in regional or distant nonglomus locations was viewed as a metastasis.)

Ten patients had previously undergone RT, whereas 77 patients had previously undergone surgery.

Surgical control was obtained in 164 of 182 patients (85%) (Table 36–3). Eighteen patients (9.9%) experienced subtotal resection, 4 of which were palliative procedures in elderly individuals. In accordance with preoperative patient preference, 14 procedures were planned as subtotal resections in order to maximize the preservation of cranial nerves or the ICA.

Nine cases (4.9%) developed recurrent tumor, defined as the reappearance of tumor in the resection field. Time to recurrence averaged 8.17 years; for this reason, postoperative surveillance is emphasized as appropriate throughout the postoperative life of the patient. Five of these patients ultimately underwent successful resection of the recurrent tumor, 1 was irradiated, 2 are under surveillance, and 1 was lost to follow-up.

The nerve most commonly affected was cranial nerve X. Preoperative cranial nerve dysfunction was associated with a significantly higher incidence of ICE. For the whole series, ICE was acknowledged in 36%. When a preoperative deficit in cranial nerves IX, X, XI, or XII existed, there was an ICE incidence of 68% 63%, 63%, and 56%, respectively. Intracranial extension resection was required, and accomplished in a single stage, in 36% of the cases.

The most common site of lower cranial nerve involvement was the pars nervosa of the jugular bulb, and this involvement was typically multiple. Involvement at the pars nervosa resulted in resection of cranial nerves IX through XII in 34.6% of the cases. Total tumor removal was possible without any cranial nerve resection in 31% of cases. In all cases of GV tumor resection, cranial nerve X was involved with tumor and was resected.

When ICE was present, 67% of cases had extensive pars nervosa tumor involvement resulting in resection of cranial nerves IX through XII. When there was a preoperative deficit of the lower cranial nerves, pars nervosa

Table 36–3 SURGICAL CONTROL		Number of Procedures	Percentage of Total
Subtotal resection		18	9.9
Palliation in elderly	4		
Carotid preservation	11		
Pars nervosa preservation	3		
Tumor recurrence		9	4.9
Complete resection		164	85.0
Total		182	

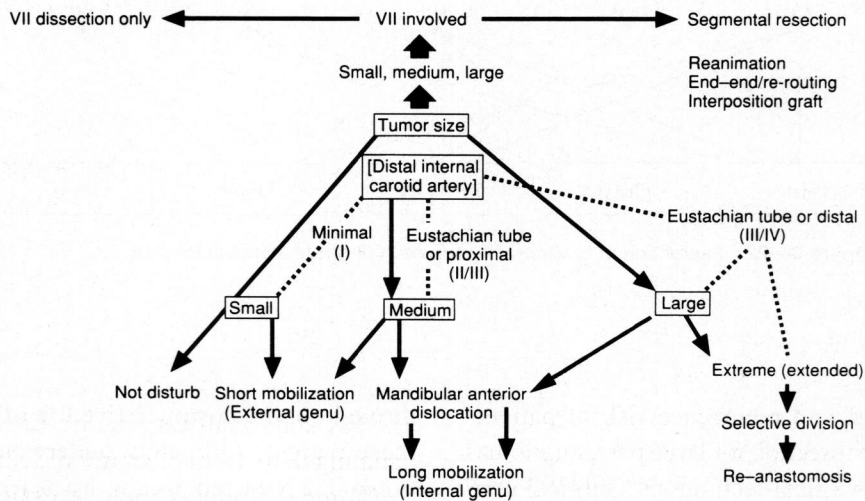

Figure 36–23. Postoperative hearing results.

tumor invasion and resection occurred in 61%. When preoperative exhibition of lower cranial nerve deficits and ICE were present, the pars nervosa was involved with tumor and resected in 87% of cases. When neither preoperative lower cranial nerve deficits nor ICE was present, only 11% had tumor involvement of the pars nervosa requiring resection. Pars nervosa tumor involvement and complete resection of cranial nerves IX through XII occurred in 100% of Class IV, 54% of Class III, 15% of Class II, and 0% of Class I tumors. Cranial nerve IX was taken alone in 19% of cases, not because of tumor involvement but in order to achieve distal control of the ICA.

Preoperative FN paralysis bodes poorly for its preservation as the FN could not be salvaged in any such case.

Complications included mortality (5 cases, or 2.7%), CSF leakage (3), tracheitis (1), wound infection (6), meningitis (4), ICA erosion and hemorrhage (1), CVA (4), hematoma (3), ileus (6), aspiration (19), pneumothorax (2), pneumonia (5), and TM perforation (4).

Because of their propensity for late recurrence and multicentricity, postoperative MRI surveillance should be conducted 1 year, 3 years, 5 years, and then every 5 years postoperatively for the life of the patient.

Selected Neoplasms

Endolymphatic Sac Tumors

In 1984, Hasserd and colleagues[51] reported the first endolymphatic sac tumor, which was discovered during endolymphatic sac surgery for presumed Meniere's disease; they described a highly vascular, lobular mass centered along the posterior portion of the TB. Both anatomic location and histopathology were highly suggestive of endolymphatic sac origin. Heffner,[52] based on microscopic (both light and electron) and immunochemical analysis of 20 similarly papillary-adenomatous tumors of the TB, proposed that the endolymphatic sac was indeed the site of tumor origin and that the tumor be designated as an "adenocarcinoma of the endolymphatic sac."

It is now generally thought that the endolymphatic sac, rather than the mucosa of the tympanomastoid compartment, is the source of low-grade, aggressive papillary tumors of the TB. These highly destructive tumors are centered between the sigmoid sinus and the internal auditory canal in the region of the vestibular aqueduct and frequently extend intracranially.[52] Macroscopically, the tumors are red, vascular, and polypoid. Microscopically, the tumors demonstrate a papillary-cystic architecture, with villus formation, a cuboidal or columnar lining epithelium, an underlying spindle or myoepithelial cell layer, and glandular lumens simulating a thyroid neoplasm.[52, 53]

Endolymphatic sac tumors must be differentiated from middle ear adenomas and adenocarcinomas (see Chapter 37), as well as carcinoid and choroid plexus tumors. Immunohistochemical analysis can help in the differential diagnosis. For example, Levin and colleagues[54] showed that, similar to normal endolymphatic sac tissue, endolymphatic sac tumors expressed cytokeratin, S-100 protein, neuron-specific enolase (NSE), and vimentin but not glial fibrillary acidic protein (GFAP). Mergerian and colleagues[55] found differential expression between choroid plexus papillomas and endolymphatic sac tumors for transthyretin, a known marker for choroid plexus epithelial tissue.

Endolymphatic sac tumors grow slowly and often are not diagnosed until extensive local destruction and intracranial extension have occurred; however, no tumor has been reported to have metastasized. Typical clinical manifestations include (sudden or progressive) sensorineural hearing loss and facial paralysis, with the diagnosis of the hearing loss preceding the diagnosis of endolymphatic sac tumor by an average of 10.6 years.[56] Endolymphatic sac tumors may mimic Meniere's disease, provoking hearing loss, tinnitus, and episodic vertigo.[56]

Gaffey and colleagues[57] documented a highly significant association of endolymphatic sac tumors with von Hippel-Lindau (VHL) disease (VHL is an autosomal dominant, hereditary phakomatosis consisting of retinal and cerebellar angiomatosis). Accordingly, the monitoring of the VHL patient should encompass a careful scrutiny of the endolymphatic sac region; early detection of an endolymphatic sac tumor may allow for tumor resection with hearing preservation.[58] Similarly, diagnosis of an endolymphatic sac tumor (if in conjunction with another major manifestation of VHL or VHL in at least one consanguinous relative) should prompt consideration of the diagnosis of VHL.[57]

On CT scanning, endolymphatic sac tumors appear as destructive lesions that are centered in the retrolabyrinthine portion of the TB and that contain areas of calcification.[59] Magnetic resonance imaging findings include areas of high signal intensity on T_1- and T_2-weighted images, as well as enhancement with gadolinium; tumors larger than 2 cm demonstrate flow voids.[58,59]

Complete surgical excision is the recommended management. Preoperative embolization of the tumor may expedite surgical excision.[60] Long-term follow-up is mandated as these tumors may recur as late as 10 years after resection.[56]

Choristoma

Choristomas consist of histologically normal rests of congenitally heterotopic tissue.[61] The most frequently reported choristoma of the ME[62] is made up of salivary gland tissue (approximately 26 cases), but a neural choristoma has also been reported.[61]

Choristomas typically present with a unilateral, conductive hearing loss and a tympanic mass; branchial cleft and FN abnormalities are also often present.[62] Differentiating them from other middle ear tumors is difficult.

Surgical findings include ossicular abnormalities and FN involvement, with the latter finding complicating excision of the choristoma.[62] Attempts at tympanoplasty and ossicular reconstruction have uniformly failed. Because the choristoma is not a true neoplasm and has no aggressive potential, conservative management (surveillance) is usually recommended.

Fibrous Dysplasia

Fibrous dysplasia consists of fibrous tissue, bony spicules that are undergoing resorption and formation, and islands of cartilage replacing bone marrow; it generally leaves the cortex intact.[63] There are monostotic and polyostotic forms, the latter exemplified by McCune-Albright syndrome (polyostotic fibrous dysplasia with precocious sexual development).

Radiographically, fibrous dysplasia has a "ground-glass" appearance. If it involves the TB, there may be progressive EAC occlusion,[64] as well as extension into the substance of the TB. Surgical excision may be indicated if there is progressive EAC obstruction, conductive hearing loss, recurrent infection, or EAC cholesteatoma.

Papilloma

Squamous papilloma is a benign neoplasm commonly occurring in the EAC. The lesion is typical of other papillomatous lesions and is usually exophytic and black or brown in color. It is believed to have a viral etiology. Excisional biopsy is often curative.

Schneiderian (inverting) papillomas, commonly encountered in the sinonasal tract, rarely involve the ME and mastoid.[65] Therapy for these papillomas of the

ME is surgical. Conservative surgery uniformly fails as these lesions have a very high propensity for recurrence. Attention should be directed to the eustachian tube as a primary highway from which extension from the sinonasal tract into the ME can occur. The danger of the inverting papilloma lies in its propensity for malignant degeneration and represents the primary impetus for early and aggressive surgical management.

Aberrant Internal Carotid Artery

Although not neoplasms, arterial anomalies of the TB figure conspicuously in the differential diagnosis of a ME mass. The incidence of one such anomaly, the aberrant (intratympanic) ICA has been reported[66] to be approximately 1%. Its clinical presentation has few distinguishing features, and on otoscopy it appears as a red, pulsatile, anterior mesotympanic mass. More than 50% of reported cases of aberrant ICA were diagnosed at the time of tympanostomy or biopsy, during which severe arterial bleeding resulted. High-resolution CT (axial and coronal) is the diagnostic imaging procedure of choice; magnetic resonance angiography can also demonstrate the aberrant ICA.

CONCLUSION

Paragangliomas are the most common lesions involving the ME and TB. The differential diagnosis of benign lesions of the TB, however, is broad. Myringotomy and biopsy, traditional solutions to this problem, should rarely be necessary given the wonderful imaging capacity afforded by high-resolution CT and MRI. The broad-based embryology of the TB contributes a potentially rich diversity in the variety of pathology exhibited within. We have the tools available to us to determine the type and the extent of the TB disease preoperatively. Only as the result of such detailed presurgical inquiry can treatment be individualized and postsurgical outcomes maximized.

REFERENCES

1. Anson BJ, Donaldson JA, editors. Surgical anatomy of the temporal bone. Philadelphia: WB Saunders; 1981.

2. Oldring D, Fisch U. Glomus tumors of the temporal bone: surgical therapy. Am J Otol 1979;1:7–18.

3. Fisch U. Carotid lesions at the skull base. In: Brackmann DE, editor. Neurological surgery of the ear and skull base. New York: Raven Press; 1982. p. 269–81.

4. Jackson CG, Glasscock ME, Harris PF. Glomus tumors: diagnosis, classification and management of large lesions. Arch Otolaryngol 1982;108:401–10.

5. Gulya AJ. The glomus tumor and its biology. Laryngoscope 1993;103 Suppl 60:7–15.

6. Glenner GG, Grimley PM. Tumors of the extra-adrenal paraganglion system (including chemoreceptors). In: Atlas of tumor pathology. 2nd series. Fascicle 9. Washington (DC): Armed Forces Institute of Pathology; 1974. p. 1–90.

7. Guild SR. The glomus jugulare, a nonchromaffin paraganglion, in man. Ann Otol Rhinol Laryngol 1953;62:1045–71.

8. Pearse AGE. The cytochemistry and ultrastructure of polypeptide hormone-producing cells of the APUD series and the embryologic, physiologic and pathologic implications of the concept. J Histochem Cytochem 1969;17:303–13.

9. Pearse AGE. The diffuse neuroendocrine system: historical review. Front Horm Res 1984;12:1–7.

10. Matsuguchi H, Tsuneyoshi M, Takeshita A, et al. Noradrenaline-secreting glomus jugulare tumor with cyclic change of blood pressure. Arch Intern Med 1975;135:1110–3.

11. Schwaber MK, Glasscock ME, Jackson CG, et al. Diagnosis and management of catecholamine secreting glomus tumors. Laryngoscope 1984;94:1008–15.

12. Farrior JB III, Hyams VJ, Benke RH, et al. Carcinoid apudoma arising in a glomus jugulare tumor: review of endocrine activity in glomus jugulare tumors. Laryngoscope 1980;90:111–9.

13. Myssiorek MD, Palestro CJ. [111]Indium pentreotide scan detection of familial paragangliomas. Laryngoscope 1998;108:228–31.

14. Myers EN, Newman J, Kaseff L, et al. Glomus jugulare tumor—a radiographic-histologic correlation. Laryngoscope 1971;81:1838–51.

15. Kinney SE. Glomus jugulare tumor surgery with intracranial extension. Otolaryngol Head Neck Surg 1980;88:531–5.

16. Spector GJ, Ciralski R, Maisel RH, et al. Multiple glomus tumors in the head and neck. Laryngoscope 1975;85:1066–75.

17. Ervin DM, Osguthorpe JD. Multicentric paragangliomas. Ann Otol Rhinol Laryngol 1984;93:96–7.

18. Lattes R, Waltner JG. Nonchromaffin paraganglioma of middle ear (carotid-body-like tumor, glomus-jugulare tumor). Cancer 1949;2:447–68.

19. Borsanyi SJ. Glomus jugulare tumors. Laryngoscope 1962;72:1336–45.

20. Davis JM, Davis KR, Hesselink JR, et al. Malignant glomus jugulare tumor: a case with two unusual radiographic features. J Comput Assist Tomogr 1980;4:415–7.

21. Druck NS, Spector GJ, Ciralsky RH, et al. Malignant glomus vagale: report of a case and review of the literature. Arch Otolaryngol 1976;102:634–6.

22. Irons GB, Weiland LH, Brown WL. Paragangliomas of the neck: clinical and pathologic analysis of 116 cases. Surg Clin North Am 1977;57:575–83.

23. Jackson CG, Cueva RA, Thedinger BA, Glasscock ME. Conservation surgery for glomus jugulare tumors: the value of early diagnosis. Laryngoscope 1990;100:1031–6.

24. Jackson CG, Marzo S, Ishiyama A, Lambert PR. Glomus and other benign tumors of the temporal bone. In: Canalis RF, Lambert PR, editors. The ear: comprehensive otology. New York: Lippincott Williams & Wilkins; 2001. p. 813–34.

25. Lasjaunais P, Berenstein A. Endovascular treatment of craniofacial lesions. In: Surgical neuroangiography. Vol. 2. Berlin: Springer-Verlag; 1987.

26. Schick PM, Hieshima GB, White RA, et al. Arterial catheter embolization followed by surgery for large chemodectoma. Surgery 1980;87:459–64.

27. Valavanis A. Preoperative embolization of the head and neck: indications, patient selection, goals, and precautions. AJNR Am J Neuroradiol 1986;7:943–52.

28. Cole JM, Beiler D. Long-term results of treatment for glomus jugulare and glomus vagale tumors with radiotherapy. Laryngoscope 1994;104:1461–5.

29. de Jong AL, Coker NJ, Jenkins HA, et al. Radiation therapy in the management of paragangliomas of the temporal bone. Am J Otol 1995;16:283–9.

30. Carrasco V, Rosenman J. Radiation therapy of glomus jugulare tumors. Laryngoscope 1993;103 Suppl 60:23–7.

31. Cummings BJ, Beale FA, Garrett PG, et al. The treatment of glomus tumors in the temporal bone by megavoltage radiation. Cancer 1984;52:2635–40.

32. Brackmann DE, House WF, Terry R, et al. Glomus jugulare tumors: effect of irradiation. Trans Am Acad Ophthalmol Otolaryngol 1972;76:1423–31.

33. Spector GJ, Compagno J, Perez CA, et al. Glomus jugulare tumors: effects of radiotherapy. Cancer 1975;35:1316–21.

34. Spector GJ, Maisel RH, Ogura JH. Glomus jugulare tumors. II. A clinicopathologic analysis of the effects of radiotherapy. Ann Otol Rhinol Laryngol 1974;83:26–32.

35. Jackson CG, Haynes DS, Walker PA, et al. Hearing conservation surgery for glomus jugulare tumors. Am J Otol 1996;17:425–37.

36. Myssiorek D, Jackson CG. Glomus tumors of the head and neck. Otolaryngol Clin North Am 2001. [In press]

37. Jackson CG. Surgical principles of neurotologic skull base surgery. Laryngoscope 1993;103 Suppl 60:29–44.

38. van Doersten PG, Jackson CG, Manolidis S, et al. Facial nerve outcome in lateral skull base surgery for benign lesions. Laryngoscope 1998;108:1480–4.

39. Awad IA, Spetzler RF. Extracranial-intracranial bypass surgery: a critical analysis in light of the International Cooperative Study. Neurosurgery 1986;19:655–64.

40. Smith PG, Killeen TE. Carotid artery vasospasm complicating extensive skull base surgery: cause, prevention, and management. Otolaryngol Head Neck Surg 1987;97:1–7.

41. Zane RS, Aeschbacher P, Moll C, et al. Carotid occlusion without reconstruction: a safe surgical option in selected patients. Am J Otol 1995;16:353–9.

42. Jackson CG. Infratympanic extended facial recess approach for anteriorly extensive middle ear disease: a conservation technique. Laryngoscope 1993;103:451–4.

43. Brackmann DE. The facial nerve in the infratemporal approach. Otolaryngol Head Neck Surg 1987;97:15–7.

44. Leonetti JP, Brackmann DE, Prass RL. Improved preservation of facial nerve function in the infratemporal approach to the skull base. Otolaryngol Head Neck Surg 1989;101:74–8.

45. Abul-Hassan HS, von Drasek Ascher G, Acland RD. Surgical anatomy and supply of the fascial layers of the temporal region. Plast Reconstr Surg 1986;77:17–28.

46. Netterville JL, Civantos F. Defect reconstruction following neurotologic skull base surgery. Laryngoscope 1993;103 Suppl 60:55–63.

47. Netterville JL, Civantos F. Rehabilitation of cranial nerve deficits after neurotologic skull base surgery. Laryngoscope 1993;103 Suppl 60:45–54.

48. Netterville JL, Jackson CG, Civantos F. Thyroplasty in the functional rehabilitation of neurotologic skull base surgery. Am J Otol 1993;14:460–4.

49. Forest JA III, Jackson CG, McGrew BM. Long-term control of surgically treated glomus tympanicum tumors. Otol Neurotol 2001;22:232–6.

50. Jackson CG, McGrew BM, Forest JA, et al. Lateral skull base surgery for glomus tumors: long-term control. Otol Neurotol 2001;22:377–82.

51. Hassard AD, Boudreau SF, Cron CC. Adenoma of the endolymphatic sac. J Otolaryngol 1984;13:213–6.

52. Heffner DK. Low-grade adenocarcinoma of probable endolymphatic sac origin. A clinicopathologic study of 20 cases. Cancer 1989;64:2292–302.

53. Batsakis JG, El-Naggar AK. Papillary neoplasms (Heffner's tumors) of the endolymphatic sac. Ann Otol Rhinol Laryngol 1993;102:648–51.

54. Levin RJ, Feghali JG, Morganstern N, et al. Aggressive papillary tumors of the temporal bone: an immunohistochemical analysis in tissue culture. Laryngoscope 1996;106:144–7.

55. Megerian CA, Pilch BZ, Bhan AK, et al. Differential expression of transthyretin in papillary tumors of the endolymphatic sac and choroid plexus. Laryngoscope 1997;107:216–21.

56. Megerian CA, McKenna MJ, Nuss RC, et al. Endolymphatic sac tumors: histopathologic confirmation, clinical characterization, and implication in von Hippel-Lindau disease. Laryngoscope 1995;105:801–8.

57. Gaffey MJ, Mills SE, Boyd JC. Aggressive papillary tumor of middle ear/temporal bone and adnexal papillary cystadenoma. Manifestations of von Hippel-Lindau disease. Am J Surg Pathol 1994;18:1254–60.

58. Manski TJ, Heffner DK, Glenn GM, et al. Endolymphatic sac tumors: a source of morbid hearing loss in von Hippel-Lindau disease. JAMA 1997;277:1461–6.

59. Mukherji SK, Albernaz VS, Lo WW, et al. Papillary endolymphatic sac tumors: CT, MR imaging, and angiographic findings in 20 patients. Radiology 1997;202:801–8.

60. Mukherji SK, Castillo M. Adenocarcinoma of the endolymphatic sac: imaging features and preoperative embolization. Neuroradiology 1996;38:179–80.

61. Gulya AJ, Glasscock ME III, Pensak ML. Neural choristoma of the middle ear. Otolaryngol Head Neck Surg 1987;97:52–6.

62. Buckmiller LM, Brodie HA, Doyle KJ, et al. Choristoma of the middle ear: a component of a new syndrome? Otol Neurotol 2001;22:363–8.

63. Schuknecht HF. Pathology of the ear. 2nd ed, Philadelphia: Lea & Febiger; 1993.

64. Nager GT, Kennedy D, Kopstein E. Fibrous dysplasia: a review of the disease and its manifestations in the temporal bone. Ann Otol Rhinol Laryngol 1982;91:1–52.

65. Wenig BM. Schneiderian-type mucosal papillomas of the middle ear and mastoid. Ann Otol Rhinol Laryngol 1996;105:226–33.

66. McElveen JT Jr, Lo WW, el Gabri TH, et al. Aberrant internal carotid artery: classic findings on computed tomography. Otolaryngol Head Neck Surg 1986;94:616–21.

37

Surgery for Malignant Lesions

MARK L. GUSTAFSON, MD
MYLES L. PENSAK, MD, FACS

Malignancies involving the temporal bone are rare but are associated with considerable morbidity and mortality, both owing to the disease processes themselves and the treatments patients undergo in hope of cure. The evolution of surgical treatments of these lesions coincides with the growing refinement and success of skull base surgery as a whole over the last half century. Temporal bone carcinoma was first reported histologically by Politzer in 1883.[1] Heyer described the first attempt at extirpation of a temporal bone malignancy in 1899.[2] For most of the early twentieth century, radical mastoidectomy followed by radiation was the standard treatment. It was not until the middle of the twentieth century that the idea of *en bloc* removal of all or a portion of the temporal bone was formalized. Campbell and colleagues raised the possibility of temporal bone resection,[3] but it was Parsons and Lewis who reported the first successful single-stage temporal bone resection in 1954.[4] Over the last 50 years, many authors have adapted and revised this concept.[5–13]

Despite the many advances, however, temporal bone malignancies still portend an ominous prognosis. Although surgical options are available for many of these lesions, often the physician and the patient must decide together not *what* can be done but what *should* be done. This chapter provides information for the physician treating patients with temporal bone malignancies but cannot provide answers to the many subjective concerns that come into play when deciding what treatment option, if any, is the right one for a particular patient.

ANATOMIC CONSIDERATIONS

The temporal bone is one of the most complex anatomic areas in the human body. It lies at the junction of the cranial cavity, skull base, and neck and contains the sensory organs of hearing and balance, cranial nerves VII (facial) and VIII (cochleovestibular), the internal carotid artery, and several dural sinuses draining ultimately into the jugular vein. Because of the large number of vital structures contained within or near the temporal bone, surgery in this area requires considerable training and experience. These structures are also at risk from the spread of tumors within this area. The detailed anatomy of the temporal bone and skull base is covered in Chapter 2. For assessment of malignancy in this area, the temporal bone can be imagined as four separate regions: the external auditory canal, middle ear space, mastoid cavity (or posterior petrous bone), and anterior petrous bone (or apex). Tumor spread (Figure 37–1) in each of these areas requires different surgical considerations and ultimately determines different outcomes.

The external auditory canal extends from the auricle to the tympanic membrane. The outer one-third of the canal is cartilaginous and the medial two-thirds is formed by the tympanic bone. The lateral one-third contains subcutaneous tissue with sebaceous and ceruminous glands as well as hair follicles. The skin of the medial two-thirds is extremely thin with no subcutaneous tissue. Anterior to the external canal are the parotid gland and infratemporal fossa, along with the temporomandibular joint more inferiorly. The incomplete closure of the tympanic bone anteriorly leaves the foramen of Huschke, which, along with defects in the cartilaginous canal (fissures of Santorini), allows tumor spread into these regions. Medially lie the tympanic membrane and tympanic cavity, which provide little resistance to invasion. The bony posterior wall and roof of the external canal provide some barrier to tumor spread but once breached lead to the mastoid cavity and facial canal posteriorly and the middle cranial fossa superiorly.

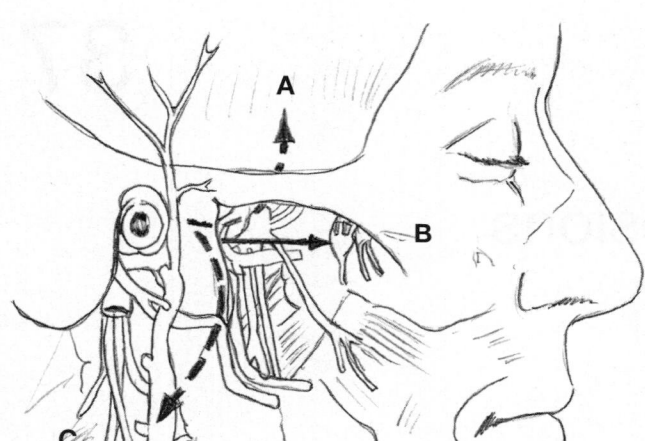

Figure 37–1 Tumors in the external auditory canal can spread easily through anatomic fissures in the anterior wall of the external auditory canal. Once beyond the confines of the canal, tumors can extend into the infratemporal fossa (A), the glenoid fossa or pterygomaxillary fissure (B), and the parotid gland (C). These anterior pathways are often sites of persistent or recurrent disease.

The middle ear contains the ossicles and the chorda tympani nerve. Its lateral extent is the tympanic membrane, and it is bordered inferiorly by the jugular bulb and internal carotid artery. Anteriorly lie the internal carotid in its vertical course through the anterior petrous bone and the eustachian tube leading to the nasopharynx. Superiorly is the middle fossa, posteriorly are the mastoid cavity and the vertical segment of the facial nerve, and medially are the inner ear and the horizontal segment of the facial nerve. The thick bone of the otic capsule provides some protection from direct tumor invasion, although cancer cells can still reach the inner ear through neurovascular channels.

Once a tumor enters the mastoid cavity, it can spread along the central mastoid tract and then into other pneumatized pathways, including the perilabyrinthine, retrofacial, subarcuate, perisinus, and epitympanic areas. The roof of the mastoid cavity is the tegmen of the middle fossa, which can be very thin and provides little resistance to the intracranial spread of tumor. The facial nerve usually runs in a bony canal, but

dehiscences in the canal can place the nerve at risk of tumor involvement.

The anterior portion of the petrous bone contains the internal carotid artery. Cranial nerves V (trigeminal) and VI (abduscent) run in close proximity to its medial ridge. The petrous apex can be pneumatized or may contain bone marrow, which can serve as a site for the hematogenous spread of metastatic disease from other areas.

The lymphatic drainage of the external auditory canal follows that of the auricle and includes the parotid, preauricular, and upper jugulodigastric nodes. The middle ear and mastoid can drain into lymphatics in the neck and to retropharyngeal nodes. The inner ear has no known lymphatic drainage.

EPIDEMIOLOGY/RISK FACTORS

Fortunately, malignancy of the temporal bone is rare. The reported incidence is 1 to 6 in 1,000,000.[13–15] The auricle is the site of origin of 60% of the cases of ear malignancy, with the external auditory canal giving rise to 28% and the middle ear or mastoid 12%.[13] The average reported age of patients presenting with temporal bone carcinoma ranges from 48 to 64 years, although it can occur in patients of all ages.[8,12,13,16–19] Sarcomas are more common in children, especially rhabdomyosarcoma (RMS), which is almost exclusively a pediatric disease.[20] Temporal bone cancer does not appear to have any gender predilection.[13]

Squamous cell carcinoma accounts for 60 to 80% of all temporal bone malignancies.[14] Basal cell carcinoma is a distant second followed by a variety of other tumors. Table 37–1 lists the frequencies of temporal bone malignancies compiled from several of the larger studies published over the last 40 years.[5–8,11,12,17,19,21–23] Differences in reported frequencies of each type of tumor likely arise from different referral patterns or patient populations (eg, children included or not).

The risk factors for temporal bone malignancy are not as well defined as they are for tumors arising on the auricle, owing to the inability to perform large risk assessment studies because of the rarity of the disease. It is frequently argued that chronic otitis media is a risk factor for temporal bone malignancy, especially squa-

Table 37–1 MALIGNANCIES OF THE TEMPORAL BONE	
Type	**Number (%)**
Epidermal	538 (82)
Squamous cell carcinoma	452 (69.2)
Basal cell carcinoma	74 (11)
Melanoma	12 (1.8)
Glandular	69 (10.6)
Adenocarcinoma*	28 (4.3)
Adenoid cystic carcinoma	25 (3.8)
Other†	16 (2.5)
Sarcomas	23 (3.5)
Rhabdomyosarcoma	9 (1.4)
Other‡	14 (2.1)
Other malignancies§	23 (3.5)
Total	653

Data compiled from Conley and Schuller,[5] Crabtree and colleagues,[6] Gacek and Goodman,[7] Lewis,[8] Kinney and Wood,[11] Pensak and colleagues,[12] Manolidis and colleagues,[17] Moody and colleagues,[19] Goodwin and Jesse,[21] Lesser,[22] and Pfreundner and colleagues.[23]
*Includes papillary cystadenocarcinoma.
†Includes mucoepidermoid and unspecified salivary malignancies.
‡Includes osteosarcoma, angiosarcoma, chondrosarcoma, and unspecified "sarcomas."
§Includes lymphoma, undifferentiated carcinoma, chordoma, malignant glioma, and metastatic renal cell carcinoma.

mous cell carcinoma.[11,24] Many patients with carcinoma of the external auditory canal or middle ear present with foul, purulent otorrhea. Differentiating between a chronically draining ear with associated inflammation and a malignancy can be difficult, especially given the rare occurrence of malignancy. Whitehead was the first to argue for a causal association in 1968.[25] Although a history of chronic otitis media is found in 40 to 60% of patients with temporal bone malignancy, it is less clear what role chronic infection may have in the development of malignancy. Carcinoma may arise, in a manner similar to Marjolin's ulcers, from epithelium damaged by chronic otorrhea or from bacterial toxins that can alter the normal mitotic activity of the epithelial cells. Some authors have found cholesteatoma associated with temporal bone malignancy, but a causal link has not been established.[15,21]

Unlike carcinoma of the auricle, carcinoma of the external canal and temporal bone does not appear to have a strong link to ultraviolet radiation, which, given the lack of exposure of the canal and middle ear to solar radiation, is not too surprising. There is an association between temporal bone malignancy and other forms of radiation, however. Radium dial workers in the 1940s and 1950s painted radium numerals on watch dials to make them visible in the dark, and as they did so, they would lick their brushes to keep a fine tip. A number of reported temporal bone malignancies have been connected with this practice.[26] In addition, external beam radiation can induce malignant transformation in cells, resulting in the appearance of cancer years later.[13,27] Human papillomavirus has been implicated in the development of carcinomas in other areas of the body and has been detected in temporal bone carcinoma.[28]

SQUAMOUS CELL CARCINOMA

Clinical Presentation/Diagnosis

The diagnosis of squamous cell carcinoma of the external auditory canal or temporal bone is often delayed owing to the nonspecific nature of presenting symptoms. The most commonly reported signs and symptoms are listed in Table 37–2.[12,17,19,29–33] The early symptoms of temporal bone carcinoma closely resemble those of chronic otitis externa or chronic suppurative otitis media, including purulent foul-smelling otorrhea, severe otalgia, bleeding, and pruritus. Patients with a chronic aural suppurative process that is unresponsive to antibiotic therapy should be evaluated closely for evidence of malignancy. Although the diagnosis is rare, early detection can have a considerable impact on outcome. Alterations in the character or volume of otorrhea in patients with chronic otitis media should be evaluated for malignancy, especially if the discharge becomes bloody or serosanguinous.

Other presenting symptoms of malignancy include hearing loss, headaches, tinnitus, vertigo, and aural fullness. There can be a secondary bacterial infection complicating the diagnosis. Cranial nerve palsy occurs late and is an ominous sign of tumor spread. The facial nerve can become involved either by invasion of tumor into the mastoid, invasion of the tympanic segment, or from extension into the parotid gland. Involvement of other cranial nerves can cause facial anesthesia, hoarseness, visual disturbances, and dysphagia. Spread into the glenoid fossa can result in trismus, and dural involvement can produce severe pain and headaches.

A full neurotologic examination should be performed of any patient suspected of having a temporal bone malignancy. Microscopic débridement and examination

Table 37–2 SIGNS AND SYMPTOMS OF TEMPORAL BONE MALIGNANCIES	
Sign/Symptom	Frequency at Presentation (%)
Aural discharge	80
Otalgia	80
Hearing loss	71
Facial palsy	32
Canal mass/lesion	26
Tinnitus	26
Periauricular swelling	22
Pruritus	20–39*
Headache	17–46†
Vertigo	15
Aural bleeding	3–28‡

The data of 710 patients summarized from multiple series of temporal bone malignancies are presented above (Pensak and colleagues,[12] Manolidis and colleagues,[17] Moody and colleagues,[19] Kuhel and colleagues,[29] Liu and colleagues,[30] Leonetti and colleagues,[31] Kenyon and colleagues,[32] Zhang and colleagues[33]).
Because some symptoms (pruritus, headache, and bleeding) were reported only in a few studies, the range of frequencies of those symptoms in the studies is provided rather than an overall frequency calculated using the entire group of patients.
*Data from Pensak and colleagues[12] and Liu and colleagues.[30]
†Data from Pensak and colleagues[12] and Leonetti and colleagues.[31]
‡Data from Pensak and colleagues,[12] Manolidis and colleagues,[17] and Liu and colleagues.[30]

of the external auditory canal are mandatory. Any suspicious canal wall masses, ulcerations, or polyps should be biopsied and sent for pathologic examination. Assessment for cranial nerve dysfunction, balance disturbance, trismus, and periauricular swelling can help clinically predict areas of tumor extension. Lymphadenopathy is uncommon with temporal bone malignancy,[12] but palpation of the neck, including the posterior regions, is important.

The use of imaging studies to assess tumor extent is critical. High-resolution computed tomographic (CT) scans show the bony anatomy of the temporal bone and demonstrate the extent of bony erosion. Computed tomographic scans of the neck may also reveal adenopathy that was clinically undetected. Magnetic resonance imaging complements CT scanning by providing a clearer image of soft tissue structures and the tumor itself; it is very helpful in evaluating dural involvement or frank invasion of brain parenchyma. In addition, it may show involvement of neural structures, the temporomandibular joint, or surrounding soft tissue planes. Arteriography is not routinely used unless there is a question of tumor invasion of the carotid artery or preoperative bal-

loon occlusion studies are required for planned surgical resection of the internal carotid artery.

Staging

There is no universally accepted temporal bone malignancy staging system. The majority of published series of temporal bone tumors do not use a staging system or do not provide enough detail in their materials and methods section to determine tumor stage. This lack of a uniform system makes comparison of data among studies difficult. The American Joint Committee on Cancer uses the same staging system as for cutaneous malignancies in other locations. Given the unique anatomy of the temporal bone, this staging system is inadequate and fails to provide valid prognostic information for tumors involving the temporal bone.

Several authors have proposed their own staging systems over the years. Goodwin and Jesse divided their patients into three groups.[21] Group I had disease confined to the cartilaginous ear canal, group II had involvement of the bony canal or mastoid cortex; and group III demonstrated invasion of the deep structures of the temporal bone (middle ear, facial nerve, tegmen, or mastoid air cells). A few years later, Stell and McCormick proposed a similar system based on the degree of invasion.[34] This system was modified by Clark and colleagues in 1991.[35] T1 tumors were limited to the site of origin with no evidence of bony destruction. T2 tumors demonstrated further invasion (facial palsy, bony destruction) but no extension beyond the temporal bone. T3 tumors were defined as those extending into the parotid, temporomandibular joint, or underlying skin and T4 tumors as those involving the dura, base of the skull, or brain.

More recently, Pensak and colleagues[12] and Arriaga and colleagues[36] have published more detailed staging systems. The Pittsburgh (Arriaga and colleagues) system (Table 37–3) is based on radiographic findings and has been correlated successfully with both clinical outcome and histopathologic examination of the involved temporal bones.[36,37] The University of Cincinnati (Pensak and colleagues) system (Table 37–4) incorporates radiographic and intraoperative findings and has been successfully used as a guide for determining the extent of temporal bone resection required. Ultimately, each of these systems emphasizes the detrimental effect of bony

Table 37–3 PITTSBURGH STAGING SYSTEM FOR EXTERNAL AUDITORY CANAL TUMORS[36]	
T1	Tumor limited to the external auditory canal without bony erosion or evidence of soft tissue extension
T2	Tumor with limited external auditory canal bony erosion (not full thickness) or radiographic finding consistent with limited (< 0.5 cm) soft tissue involvement
T3	Tumor eroding the osseous external auditory canal (full thickness) with limited (< 0.5 cm) soft tissue involvement or tumor involving the middle ear and/or mastoid or patients presenting with facial paralysis.
T4	Tumor eroding the cochlea, petrous apex, medial wall of the middle ear, carotid canal, jugular foramen, or dura or with extensive (> 0.5 cm) soft tissue involvement.
N status	Involvement of lymph nodes is a poor prognostic finding and automatically places the patient in an advanced stage (ie, stage III [T1N1] or stage IV [T2, T3, or T4, and N1])
M status	Distant metastasis indicates a poor prognosis and immediately places a patient in the stage IV category

invasion, middle ear involvement, and extratemporal spread on prognosis. Although a universally accepted system has not been agreed on, authors should at least provide a detailed description of patients in their series so that their data can be compared and effective therapies identified for these rare but dangerous tumors.

Surgical Treatment

The treatment of squamous cell carcinoma of the temporal bone comprises surgical excision possibly followed by radiation. The appropriate extent of the surgery is still very controversial, with some authors advocating total *en bloc* removal of the temporal bone[5,8–10,15,18,23,38] surrounding the tumor and others arguing for piecemeal removal of gross tumor with preservation of vital neurovascular structures followed by radiation therapy.[6,7,11,12,16,19,21,29,30,32,33] Historically, surgeons have used a radical mastoidectomy to treat temporal bone carcinomas. Parsons and Lewis[4] were the first to successfully

Table 37–4 UNIVERSITY OF CINCINNATI GRADING SYSTEM FOR TEMPORAL BONE TUMORS[12]	
Grade I	Tumor in a single site, 1 cm or less in size
Grade II	Tumor in a single site, greater than 1 cm in size
Grade III	Transannular tumor extension
Grade IV	Mastoid or petrous air cell invasion
Grade V	Periauricular or contiguous extension (extratemporal)
Grade VI	Neck adenopathy, distant anatomic site, or infratemporal fossa extension

demonstrate the use of more extensive resection of the temporal bone. Other authors expanded on their work, but the survival of patients with temporal bone carcinoma remained poor.[5] The primary reason for failure was local recurrence.

In an effort to improve local control, more extensive operations have been performed to obtain clear margins around the tumors. The *en bloc* resections advocated by Parsons and Lewis were limited by the intrapetrous carotid artery, and so the anterior portion of the petrous bone was left unresected. Graham and colleagues reported the first successful complete temporal bone and carotid artery resection in 1984.[9] Sataloff and colleagues[10] and Moffat and colleagues[18] have subsequently reported their own results with this procedure. The proponents of total temporal bone resection argue that the morbidity associated with advanced temporal bone tumors and the poor outcomes achieved previously with limited surgical resections make this procedure worthwhile. The surgery, however, results in significant postoperative morbidity, including multiple cranial nerve deficits and the risk of intracranial complications and stroke.

For early-stage tumors, especially those limited to the external auditory canal, *en bloc* resections can be achieved with minimal morbidity. Because of the morbidity of large *en bloc* resections for advanced neoplasms, however, many surgeons have advocated a piecemeal approach to these tumors. In 1987, Kinney and Wood described the difficulty in correctly identifying the true extent of temporal bone tumors.[11] They argued that many attempts at *en bloc* resections led to transection through a margin of tumor that had not been recognized preoperatively. Because of this finding, they proposed *en bloc* resection of the external auditory canal followed by piecemeal removal of tumor extending beyond this surgical margin. They argued that "the step by step procedures create less operative morbidity and mortality. The operation is sequential and allows for decision making and innovation. Often more bone is removed than in a classical temporal bone resection."[11]

The controversy over these differing philosophical surgical approaches to temporal bone tumors remains unresolved. Given the rarity of the disease and the variety of techniques employed, a conclusive study is unlikely to be published soon. A thorough understanding of the operations available to manage these tumors is needed, however, if one is to decide which approach to use. The classic operations include sleeve resection, lateral temporal bone resection, subtotal temporal bone resection, and total temporal bone resection. Pensak and colleagues,[12] based on the work by Kinney and Woods,[11] have advocated a modified lateral temporal bone resection for disease extending beyond the external auditory canal. Following is a detailed description of these operations along with our own personal views of when each should be employed.

Sleeve Resection

This operation should be used only for those rare tumors truly confined to the skin and soft tissue of the cartilaginous portion of the external auditory canal. An incision is first made medially to ensure that the bony cartilaginous junction is not involved. The lateral cut is made so that the resection encompasses the entire lesion. The involved skin and underlying cartilage are removed, resulting in a wide meatoplasty. The area can be lined with a split-thickness skin graft.

Lateral Temporal Bone Resection

For tumors that involve the bony and cartilaginous canal but have not violated the annulus and encroached on the tympanic cavity, a lateral temporal bone resection can be performed. The entire external canal is removed *en bloc* along with the tympanic membrane, malleus, and incus (Figure 37–2). First, the outer canal opening is outlined and an extended postauricular incision is made. The ear is reflected anteriorly and the resulting flap is extended to expose the parotid gland. The facial nerve is dissected from the stylomastoid foramen to the pes anserinus.

A cortical mastoidectomy with an extended facial recess approach is performed. The facial nerve should be skeletonized from its second genu to the stylomastoid foramen. The incudostapedial joint is disarticulated and the facial nerve is further exposed anteriorly along its horizontal segment. To remove the specimen *en bloc*, two surgical planes must be developed. The superior attachment of the osseous canal must be freed by opening the epitympanum and zygomatic root. The second plane is created in an anterior, inferior, and medial direction, transecting the tympanic bone medial to the tympanic annulus but lateral to the jugular bulb and facial nerve. This plane is continued anteriorly until the glenoid fossa is skeletonized. The specimen is now held by

the anterior tympanic bone, which can be fractured free with a medium osteotome. A radical cavity thus results. The specimen is left attached to the parotid gland and a superficial parotidectomy is performed. The eustachian tube can be plugged with muscle and the defect closed with split-thickness skin grafts.

Modified Lateral Temporal Bone Resection

If the tumor extends into the tympanic cavity or involves the mastoid air cells, further resection of involved areas can be performed. The facial nerve, if involved, should be sacrificed and biopsies taken to ascertain that the tumor is not tracking further along the nerve. A posterior petrosectomy can be performed to ensure removal of adequate bony margins. The cochlea and labyrinth are not sacrificed unless they are involved directly with the tumor. This piecemeal removal of additional bone allows more complete excision of tumors with transannular invasion or mastoid/petrous air cell invasion without the associated morbidity of a subtotal or total temporal bone excision.

The canal and postauricular incisions are made in a manner similar to the classic lateral temporal bone resection. A cortical mastoidectomy with extended facial recess approach is performed. The posterior petrosectomy consists of bone removal posteriorly back to the transverse-sigmoid sinus junction and the posterior fossa dura. Medially, the superior petrosal sinus at the middle fossa/posterior fossa dural interface is identified and exposed. The tegmen is removed below the temporal lobe. The perilabyrinthine and retrofacial air cells are opened down to the jugular bulb. The anterior dissection continues to the glenoid fossa in a manner similar to the classic lateral temporal bone resection and the lateral temporal bone specimen is removed in the usual manner. To close the more extensive defect created by the posterior petrosectomy, temporalis and sternocleidomastoid muscle flaps can be rotated in to obliterate the defect.

Subtotal Temporal Bone Resection

Traditionally, this procedure (Figure 37–3) is designed to remove the entire temporal bone lateral to the petrous carotid artery in an *en bloc* fashion. If necessary, portions of dura, sigmoid sinus, parotid gland, and mandible can be resected with the specimen. It has been used for tumors that extensively encroach on the tympanic cavity of the mastoid air cells.

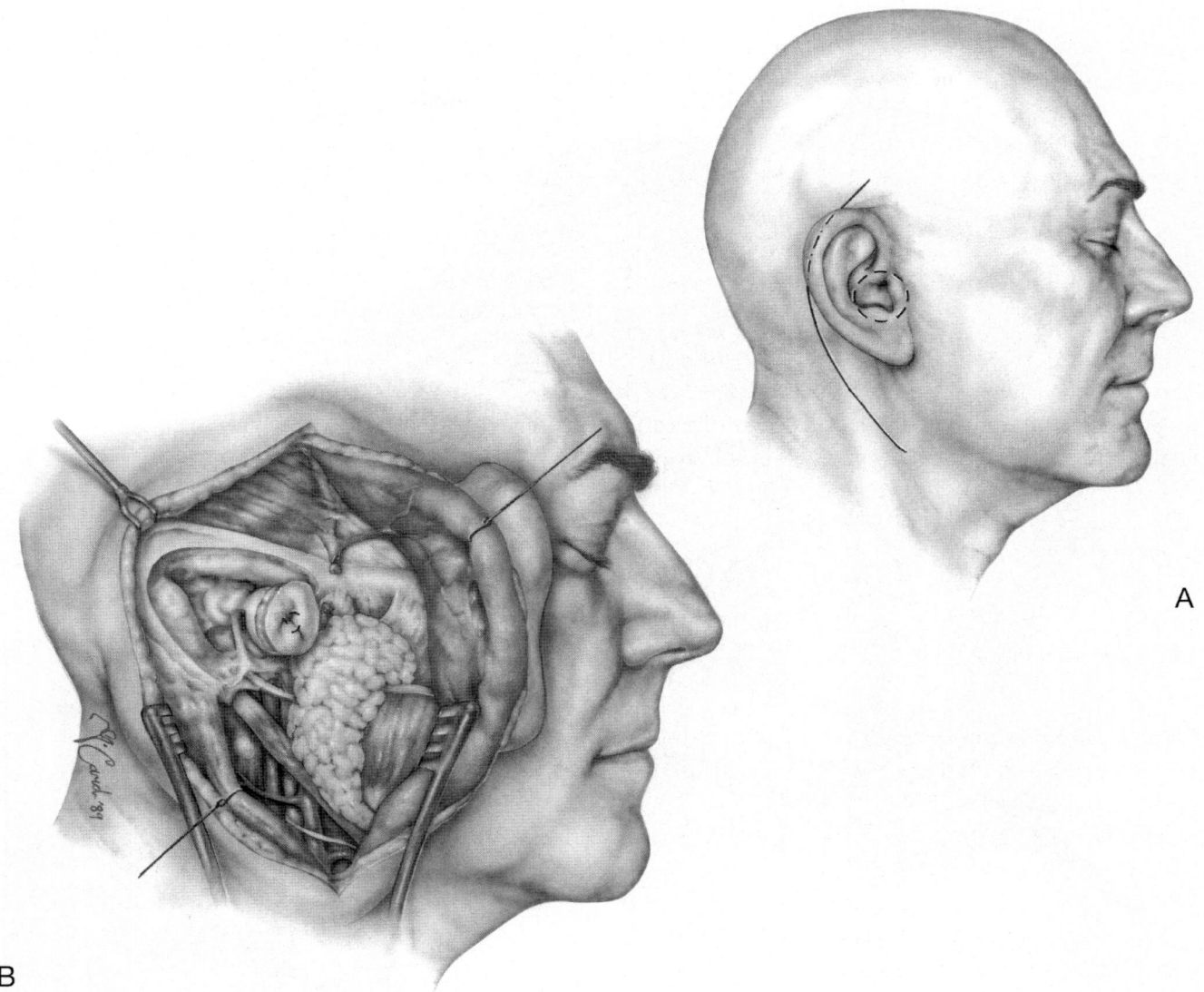

Figure 37–2 Lateral temporal bone resection. Canal and extended postauricular incisions are carried out (*A*). Anterior and posterior flaps are developed, showing the exposed parotid gland and facial nerve at the stylomastoid foramen. A mastoidectomy with extended facial recess approach is performed (*B*).

Continued on next page

The canal and postauricular incisions are made as described above. The inferior portion of the incision is extended into the neck and connected with a standard S-shaped vertical incision to allow adequate exposure for neck exploration. The great vessels and nerves of the neck are dissected out. The zygoma is transected, as is the ascending ramus of the mandible. The divided ramus and head of the mandible are removed and a subtotal parotidectomy is performed. The facial nerve is transected, but its distal stumps may be tagged for a subsequent hypoglossal-facial anastomosis. The sternocleidomastoid muscle and

the posterior belly of the digastric muscle are separated from the mastoid tip. The styloid process is transected. The external carotid artery is identified and divided.

A temporal craniotomy is performed to verify that there is no intracranial extension of the tumor. The temporal lobe is retracted medially to expose the petrous bone. A mastoidectomy is performed and the sigmoid sinus is skeletonized to the jugular bulb. Continuing anteriorly and superiorly, the internal carotid artery is exposed anterior to the jugular bulb and separated from the temporal bone. Looking from above, the internal

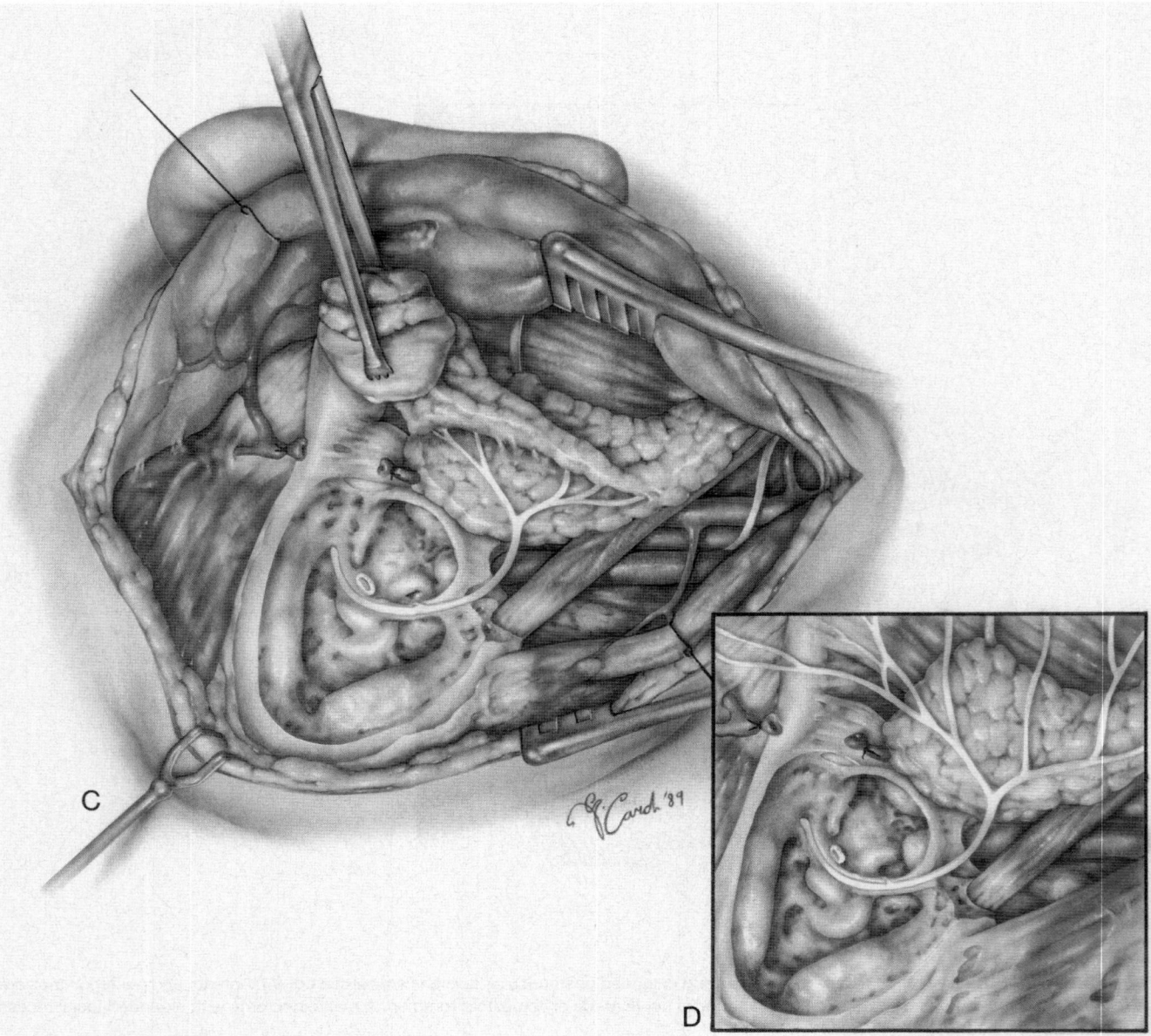

Figure 37–2 Continued. The external auditory canal and the tympanic membrane have been mobilized from the temporal bone. The specimen remains attached to the lateral lobe of the parotid gland. A lateral parotid lobectomy is completed (*C*). Appearance of a defect following removal of the specimen (*D*).

auditory canal is opened and the seventh and eighth cranial nerves are divided. The eustachian tube is divided anteriorly and the horizontal segment of the internal carotid artery is exposed. The only remaining attachment of the temporal bone is the anterior segment along the vertical face of the internal carotid artery. These osseous attachments can be fractured free with gentle rocking and careful use of osteotomes. The large defect can be filled either with regional muscle flaps or free vascularized grafts.

In lieu of an *en bloc* resection, we have used the modified lateral temporal bone resection with a posterior petrosectomy. Removal of the facial nerve, cochlea, and labyrinth is performed only when they are seen to be involved with tumor in the course of the operation. In this manner, vital organs can be preserved if possible.

Total Temporal Bone Resection

Graham and colleagues described their technique for total temporal bone resection with sacrifice of the carotid

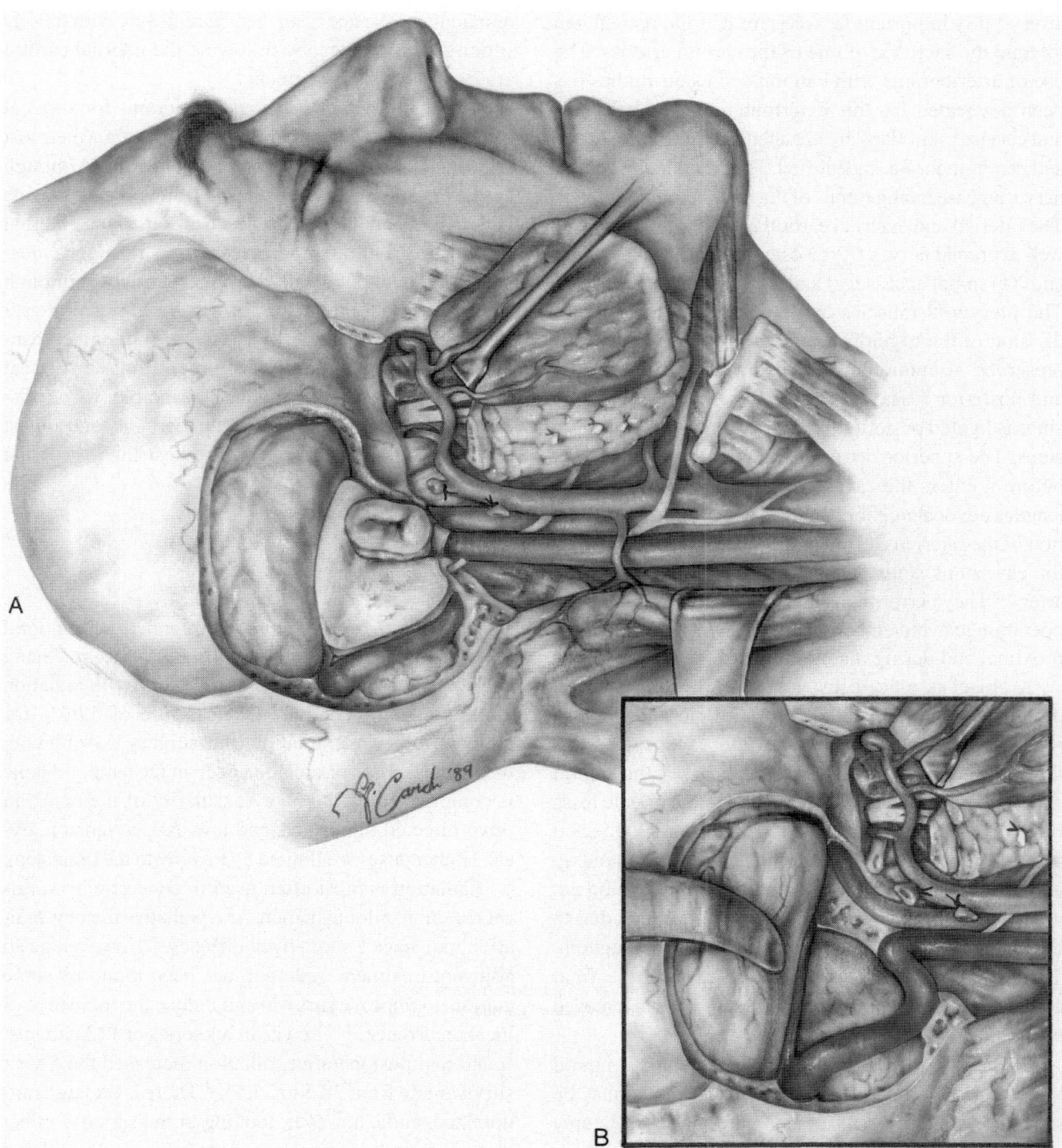

Figure 37–3 Subtotal temporal bone resection. The major neurovascular structures of the neck have been identified. The ascending ramus of the mandible is removed, and a subtotal parotidectomy has been performed. The common carotid artery is isolated, and the branches of the external carotid artery are sacrificed. The posterior and middle fossa dura are exposed (*A*). Appearance following removal of the specimen. The internal carotid artery has been exposed throughout its intratemporal course. The eustachian tube is obliterated and the cavity can be lined with split-thickness skin grafts (*B*).

artery.[9] It is important to ascertain that the patient can tolerate the sacrifice of one of the carotid arteries. The use of arteriograms with balloon occlusion studies has been advocated for this determination. The auricular and cervical skin flaps are elevated and the great vessels and nerves in the neck identified. The parotid gland, facial nerve, and ascending ramus of the mandible are resected. The internal and external carotid arteries are divided, as well as cranial nerves IX (glossopharyngeal), X (vagus), and XI (spinal accessory) and the internal jugular vein. The pterygoid muscles are divided. The mandibular division of the trigeminal nerve (V3) is identified and preserved. A craniotomy is performed, and the middle and posterior fossa dura are exposed. The transverse sinus is ligated posterior to its junction with the sigmoid sinus. The superior petrosal sinus is divided anteriorly before it enters the cavernous sinus. Sataloff and colleagues advocate ligation and division of the distal portion of the internal carotid artery intracranially between the cavernous sinus and the origin of the ophthalmic artery.[10] They perform this ligation prior to the rest of the operation to avoid emboli being thrown from the ligated proximal end during manipulation of the stump.

A chisel is placed just inside the foramen ovale, directed toward the ligated portion of the superior petrosal sinus. It passes lateral to the cavernous sinus through the carotid canal, the skull base, and lateral skull wall, freeing the anterior portion of the middle fossa floor. A posterior cut is made, lateral to medial, directed anteriorly and stopping posteromedial to the mastoid tip and posterior to the jugular foramen. A connecting cut is made from the posterior-lateral cut, going medial to the jugular foramen and lateral to the foramen magnum. The inferior petrosal sinus is divided with the final connecting portion of bone and the specimen is removed *en bloc*.

We have avoided performing total, *en bloc* temporal bone resection. If the entire petrous bone must be removed, we have performed an anterior petrosectomy along with the posterior petrosectomy procedure described above. A temporal craniotomy is done and the temporal lobe is retracted medially to expose V3, the middle meningeal artery at the foramen spinosum, the greater petrosal nerve, and the geniculate ganglion. The internal auditory canal is opened and Kawase's triangle is drilled out to the posterior fossa dura, after exposing the horizontal segment of the internal carotid artery. The

remainder of the apex can then be removed, with preservation of the cochlea, by following the internal carotid artery to its vertical segment.

Although there are a variety of options for surgical resection of temporal bone neoplasms, often the most important decision is not to operate at all. Although heroic efforts can be made, it is our feeling that patients with malignant invasion of the cavernous sinus, internal carotid artery, infratemporal fossa, or paraspinous musculature are not surgically curable. Similarly, although neck dissections can be performed for regional metastases, patients with distant metastases are not surgical candidates. Palliative radiation and more limited surgical procedures may be used to reduce the morbidity from disease, but large operations with high morbidity and almost no chance of cure are not in the best interest of the patient.

Radiation Treatment

The use of radiation for curative treatment of temporal bone malignancy has met with limited success. Zhang and colleagues reported a 5-year cure rate with radiation alone of 28.7% compared with a rate of 59.6% for patients receiving radiation and surgery.[33] Achieving tumoricidal doses of radiation deep in the temporal bone is complicated by the poor vascularity of the bone, an often infected tumor bed, and low oxygen tension levels. Higher doses are limited by toxicity to the brainstem.

Radiation is most often used in concert with surgical resection or for palliation. As a palliative therapy, radiation may have a short-lived efficacy.[39] However, as an adjuvant treatment, radiation has been found by some authors to improve survival and reduce the incidence of local recurrence.[11,16] Lewis, in his series of 132 patients, found that postoperative radiation increased the 5-year survival rate from 28.5 to 35.5%.[8] There is no large randomized study, however, looking at the specific effect that radiation has on survival or recurrence. Prasad and Janecka, in an extensive review of published series of temporal bone malignancies, concluded that radiation therapy offered no survival benefit for tumors confined to the external auditory canal and that the side effects may outweigh any advantage gained. For tumors involving the middle ear and mastoid, radiation improved survival over mastoidectomy alone, but no conclusions could be drawn when it was used as an adjuvant treatment with more extensive resections.[40]

When radiation is given, the protocol used must be individualized for the specific tumor. For carcinoma of the temporal bone, a wedged-pair photon radiation field is most often employed. The total dosage given is limited to 7,000 rads, with brain exposure held to 6,000 rads. Lesser and colleagues have found a trend toward better local control, with higher doses only for superficial squamous cell carcinomas. For larger tumors or those with deeper invasion, there does not appear to be a dose-response relationship.[22]

The side effects of radiation therapy are well recognized. They include desquamation, dryness, cartilage necrosis, eustachian tube dysfunction, hearing loss, vestibular dysfunction, and more serious complications such as osteoradionecrosis, facial nerve paralysis, and brain necrosis.[41] In addition, irradiation of the temporal bone has been associated with the development of aggressive temporal bone sarcomas many years later.[42]

Treatment of Metastases

Fortunately, the rate of regional and distant metastases from temporal bone malignancy is low. The reported rates for the presence of nodal disease at the time of presentation range from 9 to 18%.[3,16,18,22,23,33,36] When nodal disease is present, the upper jugulodigastric and parotid nodes are most commonly involved. Routine radical neck dissection has not been shown to improve survival. A superficial parotidectomy should be performed in every patient with more than superficial disease and neck dissection should be reserved for patients with known adenopathy.

Prognosis

The prognosis for patients with temporal bone malignancy has improved somewhat over the last few decades with improvements in imaging, surgical techniques, and radiation therapy.[38] Table 37–5 summarizes the overall results of several published series.[5,7,8,11,12,16,17,19,21,23,36,38] Given the heterogeneity of patients, tumor histology, and extent of disease and types of treatment, it is difficult to come to a firm conclusion. Overall survival rates

Table 37–5	TEMPORAL BONE MALIGNANCIES—SURVIVAL		
Source	No. of Patients	Survival (%)	Minimum Follow-up
Conley and Schuller[5]	61	61	2 yr
Gacek and Goodman[7]	31	61	2 yr
Lewis[8]	132	28	5 yr
Kinney and Wood[11]	30	69	6 mo (2.5 yr avg)
Pensak and colleagues[12]	39	51	5 yr
Austin and colleagues[16]	22	41	4 yr
Manolidis and colleagues[17]	81	58	3 yr
Moody and colleagues[19]	32	50	2 yr
Goodwin and Jesse[21]	136	46	5 yr
Pfreunder and colleagues[23]	27	61	2 yr
Arriaga and colleagues[36]	39	45	2 yr
Spector[38]	51	66	1.5 yr

Survival data reflect results regardless of staging, treatment modality, or pathology. Percentages are for overall survival, not disease-free or disease-specific survival.

range from 28 to 66%.[5,7,8,11,12,16,17,19,23,33,36,38] Given the age of most of the patients, many die of intercurrent disease. The disease-specific survival rates are therefore higher, ranging from 58 to 81.5%.[12,16,17]

These numbers, however, do not reflect the poor prognosis for patients with extensive disease. A patient with disease limited to the external auditory canal has a good chance of being cured. Most reported survival rates range from 80 to 100%. Once the disease extends into the middle ear and mastoid cavity, cure rates drop to 40 to 60% and plummet to 18 to 25% if the tumor extends beyond the temporal bone.[6,11,12,19,21,23,36,38]

Local recurrence is the most common reason for surgical failure.[40] Manolidis and colleagues found that 50% of T3 tumors (using the Pittsburgh staging system) and 86% of T4 tumors had positive margins following resection.[17] Malignancies can extend along nerves and vascular channels. The fissures of Santorini allow extension anteriorly into the parotid gland, infratemporal fossa, and glenoid fossa. Once the tumor has left the confines of the external auditory canal, it is very difficult to determine its full extent. Positive margins have been shown to reduce survival by nearly 50%.[17,23,36]

Proponents of *en bloc* excision argue that it allows for clearer surgical margins, thus improving survival. No randomized study has ever been done comparing piecemeal with *en bloc* excision, and, given the rarity of the disease, it is not feasible. Prasad and Janecka,[40] in their extensive review, concluded that there was no statistically significant difference seen between *en bloc* excisions and other procedures for tumors confined to the external canal. For lesions involving the middle ear and mastoid, there was a trend toward better cure rates for subtotal temporal bone resections versus lateral temporal bone dissections and radical mastoidectomy.[40] The limited number of patients, however, makes statistical analysis less reliable. Other authors have reported good results using piecemeal excisions for more extensive tumors.[11–13,19] Pensak and colleagues reported a disease-specific survival of 81.5% using a lateral temporal bone resection combined with anterior and posterior petrosectomies for more advanced disease.[12] At this time, no definitive statement can be made regarding which approach is best.

Several specific prognostic factors have been identified. The histology of the tumor affects survival. Malignancies other than squamous cell carcinoma are discussed later in this chapter. Dural involvement portends an ominous prognosis, with survival rates less than 10%.[19,40] Internal carotid artery, infratemporal fossa, and intracranial involvement likewise render the patient nearly incurable. Whereas nodal disease lowers survival to less than 30%,[36] radical neck dissection has not been shown to significantly affect outcome.[43] Other poor prognostic factors include pain, facial paralysis, and other cranial nerve deficits.[17]

OTHER EPITHELIAL MALIGNANCIES

Basal Cell Carcinoma

Basal cell carcinoma represents 11% of tumors of the external auditory canal and temporal bone (see Table 37–1). Temporal bone involvement most often occurs as tumors extend along the external canal from the auricle, particularly those originating in the preauricular and conchal areas. They rarely metastasize but can be very aggressive locally. They carry a better prognosis than squamous cell carcinoma, and even extensive tumors are usually amenable to surgical excision.[12]

Melanoma

Melanoma originating in the external auditory canal is rare. Unlike the external ear, which is exposed to a large amount of ultraviolet radiation, the ear canal is somewhat protected. When melanoma does involve the canal or temporal bone, it is often advanced and caries a poor prognosis. Treatment is surgical excision. The role of adjuvant radiation is still under investigation.

GLANDULAR MALIGNANCIES

Malignancies arising from the ceruminous glands of the external auditory canal are uncommon, representing approximately 10% of all temporal bone malignancies (see Table 37–1). There has been a great deal of confusion regarding the pathologic categorization of these tumors. Various names such as ceruminoma, apocrine carcinoma, papillary cystadenocarcinoma, and ceruminous adenocarcinoma can be seen in the literature. Recent publications have attempted to simplify this grouping, and two primary malignant glandular tumors are now identified: adenoid cystic carcinoma and ceruminous adenocarcinoma.[44,45] Other auditory canal glandular malignancies, such as mucoepidermoid carcinoma, are rare, found only in a few case reports.

Adenoid cystic carcinoma is the most common glandular malignancy found in the auditory canal.[45] It is characterized by slow but relentless growth and a predilection for perineural spread. Pathologically, the tumor consists of cords and islands of uniform darkly staining cells. There are several different cellular patterns seen including cribriform, tubular, and solid. The solid pattern carries the worst prognosis. Treatment of adenoid cystic carcinoma consists of surgical resection with wide margins. Tumor cells can spread proximally along nerves and therefore extend unnoticed beyond the surgical field. Postoperative radiation therapy is therefore recommended. Although short-term elimination of the tumor is often achieved, local recurrence is very common and often occurs 8 to 10 years after the initial surgery. This pattern of late local recurrence makes evaluation of many of the published studies difficult as standard 5-year outcomes are less meaningful for this particular tumor. Distant metastases do occur, predominantly to the lungs.[45] Patients, however, can live many years with active disease, and recurrences do not necessarily lead to a rapid demise.

Ceruminous adenocarcinoma has been divided by the Armed Forces Institute of Pathology into a low-grade form (papillary cystadenocarcinoma) and a high-grade undifferentiated type.[46] The low-grade variety is often slow growing, rarely metastasizes, and often can only be distinguished from a benign adenoma by pathologic evidence of invasion of surrounding tissue or bone. The tumor typically consists of double-layered cuboidal or columnar epithelial cells arranged in a glandular pattern. A variable amount of atypia and pleomorphism is present. The high-grade adenocarcinoma is characterized by undifferentiated cells that resemble metastatic disease from other sources. Wide surgical excision with postoperative radiation is the treatment of choice. These tumors tend to infiltrate along subcutaneous pathways, making margin analysis difficult. Chang and Cheung reviewed all published cases of auditory canal adenocarcinoma and found no long-term cures once the tumor had extended beyond the canal.[45]

SARCOMAS

Sarcomas are the most common temporal bone malignancy in the pediatric population. Although comprising a large percentage of pediatric temporal bone tumors, temporal bone sarcomas are rare and represent less than 5% of all temporal bone malignancies (see Table 37–1). Rhabdomyosarcoma is the most common variety, accounting for 30% of all sarcomas of the temporal bone.[13] Other types include fibrosarcoma, osteogenic sarcoma, Ewing's sarcoma, Kaposi's sarcoma, chondrosarcoma, and undifferentiated sarcomas.

Rhabdomyosarcoma

Rhabdomyosarcoma is the most common soft tissue sarcoma in children. The majority of tumors present before the child is 12 years old, and the average age at presentation is 4.4 years.[47] Forty percent of RMSs present in the head and neck. The majority of auricular RMSs arise from the middle ear.[20] The primary presenting symptoms are similar to those of chronic otitis media: purulent and bloody otorrhea, otalgia, canal polyp and granulation tissue, and hearing loss. Rhabdomyosarcoma originating in the petrous bone, however, may cause headaches and cranial nerve palsy without associated aural symptoms.

The natural history of RMS in the temporal bone is aggressive local destruction with a propensity for distant metastases. Up to 14% of patients with RMS in parameningeal sites present with distant metastases.[48] In the middle ear, the tumor quickly invades the fallopian canal, resulting in facial paresis or paralysis, and can then spread proximally to the internal auditory canal, other cranial nerves, and the meninges. It can also spread by destruction of the tegmen or along the eustachian tube.

Rhabdomyosarcoma arises from striated skeletal muscle cells. Four subtypes have been identified: embryonal, pleomorphic, alveolar, and botryoid. The embryonal variant accounts for nearly all of the head and neck RMS. The type of RMS significantly affects prognosis. Botryoid RMSs have the best survival rates, and embryonal RMSs are more favorable than alveolar RMSs, which have the worst prognosis.[47]

The Intergroup Rhabdomyosarcoma Study I (IRS-I) classification system is used to stage patients with RMS. The system is based on tumor resectability. There are four groups. Group I has completely resected localized disease. Group II has grossly resected disease with microscopically positive margins or regional disease. Group III has partially resected disease and Group IV has metastatic disease.

The treatment of RMS of the temporal bone historically consisted of aggressive surgical extirpation, which resulted in excessive morbidity and low cure rates. Until 1970, the cure rate for RMS of the head and neck was barely 20%.[48] Since 1970, three intergroup studies have been completed, and the approach to the treatment of these tumors has changed dramatically.[49–51] Currently, the standard treatment is surgical biopsy to confirm the diagnosis followed by chemotherapy and radiation therapy for cure. Using this approach, the 5-year survival rates for head and neck RMS have risen to 65%.[51]

Other Sarcomas

Sarcomas other than RMS are rare in the temporal bone. Prior radiation therapy may place a patient at risk for the development of these other sarcomas. Ewing's sarcoma responds best to radiation and chemotherapy, similar to RMS. Other sarcomas, including osteogenic sarcoma, fibrosarcoma, Kaposi's sarcoma, chondrosarcoma, and liposarcoma, should be treated with wide *en bloc* excision possibly followed by radiation. Their rarity makes survival and prognostic data unreliable.[47]

METASTATIC DISEASE TO THE TEMPORAL BONE

Metastases to the temporal bone are rare. The Armed Forces Institute of Pathology reported 31 cases of metastatic carcinoma in the temporal bone.[1] The most recent review of the literature found 141 reported cases.[52] Metastatic disease spreads primarily hematogenously to marrow-containing areas of the temporal bone. The most common cancers metastasizing to the temporal bone are the breast (25%), lung (11%), kidney (9%), stomach (6%), bronchus (6%), and prostate (6%).[53] The most usual presenting symptoms are hearing loss, facial paralysis, and vertigo.[53] The prognosis for patients with temporal bone metastasis is poor, and treatment consists mainly of palliative radiotherapy, if anything.

OTHER MALIGNANCIES

Other malignancies involving the temporal bone include those directly spreading from adjacent areas. Parotid, nasopharyngeal, auricular, and central nervous system tumors can invade the temporal bone, resulting in significant morbidity. Treatment is obviously dependent on tumor histology but often entails very aggressive surgical resection if the tumor is deemed resectable. Other rare tumors include extramedullary plasmacytoma, lymphoma, and hemangiopericytoma, all of which involve other areas of the head and neck much more frequently than the temporal bone.

Finally, mention should be made of Langerhans' cell histiocytosis (LCH), formerly called histiocytosis X. Although not truly a malignancy, LCH can present as a disseminated process with locally aggressive disease. Langerhans' cell histiocytosis typically affects children but can be seen in all age ranges. It consists of an abnormal proliferation and accumulation of Langerhans' cells, which are antigen-presenting cells located in the epidermis. Lesions grossly appear soft and granular with areas of necrosis and hemorrhage. Microscopically, there are clusters of Langerhans' cells, eosinophils, multinucleated giant cells, and other inflammatory cells. By electron microscopy, Birbeck granules, which are specific for LCH, can be identified in the Langerhans' cells. Classically, LCH has been divided into three progressively more aggressive groups, each with a different eponym: eosinophilic granuloma, Hand-Schüller-Christian disease, and Letterer-Siwe disease. Today descriptive terms are used to characterize these three groups (localized, multifocal, and disseminated disease). Approximately 25% of people with LCH develop aural symptoms.[54] Patients may present with granulation tissue in the middle ear or canal, otorrhea, and hearing loss owing to destruction of the ossicles. Associated symptoms include painful swelling of the calvarium, cervical adenopathy, and rash resembling chronic dermatitis. Other bony sites may be involved, and disseminated disease can be seen in other organs, especially in infants. Skull films may show characteristic hypolucent areas that can aid in the diagnosis. Biopsy of the lesions is critical, and any child, especially if younger than 3 years, with granulomatous or polypoid disease in the middle ear should undergo biopsy of the abnormal tissue to rule out LCH.

Biopsy and conservative curettage are often all that is needed to treat limited disease, and such tumors generally have an excellent prognosis. There is no reason to perform an extensive mastoidectomy or resection of the lesion.[55] For patients with multifocal or disseminated disease, adjuvant chemotherapy and radiation therapy play a vital role. Survival for patients with multifocal disease is 65 to 100%,[55] but infants with disseminated disease have a very poor prognosis. Mortality rates for these children range from 65 to 95%.[56]

SURGICAL RECONSTRUCTION

Surgical extirpation of a temporal bone malignancy can result in considerable skin and soft tissue defects of the lateral skull base. A variety of reconstructive options are available. The surgeon must decide which is best based on the defect, the need for observation of the surgical site, the use of postoperative radiation, and the viability of the blood supply to each flap.

Defects created by sleeve resection and mastoidectomy can be repaired with a canalplasty using split-thickness skin grafts. A large canal, similar to that following a canal wall down procedure, results. For lateral temporal bone resections, a similar strategy can be used. Split-thickness skin grafts can line the resulting cavity and allow for excellent monitoring of the surgical site for recurrence. In addition, a tympanoplasty can be performed over the remaining stapes to retain adequate postoperative hearing. Often it is difficult, however, to secure the skin graft over the irregular bony cavity. In addition, if the patient is to receive postoperative radiation therapy, the thin covering of skin may not provide much protection from the damaging effects of the radiation, which is especially true if dura was exposed during the procedure, as with a posterior petrosectomy. Obliterating the defect by rotating in a regional muscle flap, such as a temporalis flap, can provide both a protective layer and a viable base on which to secure a skin graft.

For larger defects that involve a substantial amount of soft tissue and skin, bulkier flaps are needed. The pectoralis major myocutaneous flap is typically used by otolaryngologists. It provides a substantial flap with a hardy blood supply. Its disadvantages include the resulting cosmetic defect on the chest and the inability of the flap to adequately reach the superior part of many lateral skull base defects. Another option is the trapezius flap, which can be rotated easily in to fill a lateral defect. Finally, free flaps, either the latissimus dorsi or rectus abdominis, can be harvested and used to fill the surgical bed. If the auricle was taken at the time of surgery, the patient can wear his/her hair long over the surgical site, or the prosthesis can be attached, both providing a fairly good cosmetic result.

CONCLUSIONS

Temporal bone malignancies are rare but potentially devastating tumors. Surgeons must be intimately familiar with the complex anatomy of the temporal bone and lateral skull base before attempting to treat these lesions surgically. Although great progress has been made in skull base surgery, heroic efforts at extirpation of an advanced temporal bone carcinoma often result in significant morbidity for the patient. More conservative surgical approaches, combined with adjuvant therapies, may allow preservation of vital organ and cranial nerve function. The ultimate solution, however, has yet to be realized. Physicians must consider social and emotional, as well as surgical, issues in order to work together with the patient to come to a solution that is best, both from a medical and a quality of life standpoint.

REFERENCES

1. Politzer A. Textbook of diseases of the ear. London: Balliere Tindall & Cox; 1883. p. 729–34.

2. Heyer H. Ueber einen Fall von Ohrencarcinoma, hehardelt mit Resection des Fesenbeines. Dtsch Z Chir 1899;50:552–3.

3. Campbell EH, Volk RM, Burkland CW. Total resection of the temporal bone for malignancy of the middle ear. Ann Surg 1951; 134:397–401.

4. Parsons H, Lewis JS. Subtotal temporal bone resection for cancer of the ear. Cancer 1954;7:995–1001.

5. Conley JJ, Schuller DE. Malignancies of the ear. Laryngoscope 1976;86:1147–63.

6. Crabtree JA, Britton BH, Pierce MK. Carcinoma of the external auditory canal. Laryngoscope 1976;86:405–15.

7. Gacek RR, Goodman M. Management of malignancy of the temporal bone. Laryngoscope 1977;87:622–34.

8. Lewis JS. Surgical management of tumors of the middle ear and mastoid. J Laryngol Otol 1983;97:299–311.

9. Graham MD, Sataloff RT, Kemink JL, et al. Total en bloc resection of the temporal bone and carotid artery for malignant tumors of the ear and temporal bone. Laryngoscope 1984;94: 528–33.

10. Sataloff RT, Myers DL, Lowry LD, et al. Total temporal bone resection for squamous cell carcinoma. Otolaryngol Head Neck Surg 1987;96:4–14.

11. Kinney SE, Wood BG. Malignancies of the external ear canal and temporal bone: surgical techniques and results. Laryngoscope 1987;97:158–64.

12. Pensak ML, Gleich LL, Gluckman JL, et al. Temporal bone carcinoma: contemporary perspectives in the skull base surgical era. Laryngoscope 1996;106:1234–7.

13. Kinney SE. Clinical evaluation and treatment of ear tumors. In: Thawley SE, Panje WR, Batsakis JG, et al, editors. Comprehensive management of head and neck tumors. Vol 1. Philadelphia: WB Saunders; 1999. p. 380–94.

14. Morton RP, Stell PM, Derrick PP. Epidemiology of cancer of the middle ear cleft. Cancer 1984;53:1612–7.

15. Arena S, Keen M. Carcinoma of the middle ear and temporal bone. Am J Otol 1988;9:351–6.

16. Austin JR, Stewart KL, Fawzi N. Squamous cell carcinoma of the external auditory canal: therapeutic prognosis based on a proposed staging system. Arch Otolaryngol Head Neck Surg 1994;120:1228–32.

17. Manolidis S, Pappas D Jr, Von Doersten P, et al. Temporal bone and lateral skull base malignancy: experience and results with 81 patients. Am J Otol 1998;Suppl 19:1–15.

18. Moffat DA, Grey P, Ballagh RH, et al. Extended temporal bone resection for squamous cell carcinoma. Otolaryngol Head Neck Surg 1997;116:617–23.

19. Moody SA, Hirsch BE, Myers EN. Squamous cell carcinoma of the external auditory canal: an evaluation of a staging system. Am J Otol 2000;21:582–8.

20. Wiatrak BJ, Pensak ML. Rhabdomyosarcoma of the ear and temporal bone. Laryngoscope 1989;99:1188–92.

21. Goodwin WJ, Jesse RH. Malignant neoplasms of the external auditory canal and temporal bone. Arch Otolaryngol 1980;106: 675–9.

22. Lesser RW, Spector GJ, Devineni VR. Malignant tumors of the middle ear and external auditory canal: a 20 year review. Otolaryngol Head Neck Surg 1987;96:43–7.

23. Pfreundner L, Schwager K, Willner J, et al. Carcinoma of the external auditory canal and middle ear. Int J Radiat Oncol Biol Phys 1999;44:777–88.

24. Moffat DA, Chiossone-Kerdel JA, Da Cruz M. Squamous cell carcinoma. In: Jackler RK, Driscoll CLW, editors. Tumors of the ear and temporal bone. Philadelphia: Lippincott, Williams & Wilkins; 2000, p. 67–83.

25. Whitehead AL. A case of primary epithelioma of the tympanum following chronic suppurative otitis media. Proc R Soc Med 1968;1:34–6.

26. Beal D, Lindsay J, Ward PH. Radiation induced carcinoma of the mastoid. Arch Otolaryngol 1965;81:9–16.

27. Lustig LR, Jackler RK, Lanser MJ. Radiation-induced tumors of the temporal bone. Am J Otol 1997;18:230–5.

28. Jin YT, Tsai ST, Li C, et al. Prevalence of human papilloma virus in middle ear carcinoma associated with chronic otitis media. Am J Pathol 1997;150:1327–33.

29. Kuhel WI, Hume CR, Slesnick SH. Cancer of the external auditory canal and temporal bone. Otolaryngol Clin North Am 1996;29:827–53.

30. Liu F, Keane TJ, Davidson J. Primary carcinoma involving the petrous temporal bone. Head Neck 1993;15:39–43.

31. Leonetti JP, Smith PG, Kletzker GR, et al. Invasion patterns of advanced temporal bone malignancies. Am J Otol 1996;17:438–42.

32. Kenyon GS, Marks PV, Scholtz CL, et al. Squamous cell carcinoma of the middle ear: a 25 year retrospective study. Ann Otol Rhinol Laryngol 1985;94:273–7.

33. Zhang B, Tu G, Xu G, et al. Squamous cell carcinoma of temporal bone: reported on 33 patients. Head Neck 1999;21:461–6.

34. Stell PM, McCormick MS. Carcinoma of the external auditory meatus and middle ear: prognostic factors and a suggested staging system. J Laryngol Otol 1985;99:847–50.

35. Clark LJ, Narula AQ, Morgan DA, et al. Squamous cell carcinoma of the temporal bone: a revised staging. J Laryngol Otol 1991;105:346–8.

36. Arriaga M, Curtin H, Takahashi H, et al. Staging proposal for external auditory meatus carcinoma based on preoperative clinical examination and computed tomography findings. Ann Otol Rhinol Laryngol 1990;99:714–21.

37. Arriaga M, Curtin HD, Takahashi H, et al. The role of preoperative CT scans in staging external auditory meatus carcinoma: radiologic-pathologic correlation study. Otolaryngol Head Neck Surg 1991;105:6–11.

38. Spector JG. Management of temporal bone carcinomas: a therapeutic analysis of two groups of patients and long-term followup. Otolaryngol Head Neck Surg 1991;104:58–66.

39. Harwood AR, Keane TJ. Malignant tumors of the temporal bone and external ear: medical and radiation therapy. In: Alberti PW, Reuben RJ, editors. Otologic medicine and surgery. Vol 2. London: Churchill Livingstone; 1988. p. 1389–408.

40. Prasad S, Janecka IP. Efficacy of surgical treatments for squamous cell carcinoma of the temporal bone: a literature review. Otolaryngol Head Neck Surg 1994;110:270–80.

41. Smouha EE, Karmody CS. Non-osteitic complications of therapeutic radiation to the temporal bone. Am J Otol 1995;16:83–7.

42. Lustig LR. Radiation induced tumors of the temporal bone. In: Jackler RK, Driscoll CLW, editors. Tumors of the ear and temporal bone. Philadelphia: Lippincott, Williams & Wilkins; 2000. p. 452–61.

43. Arriaga M, Hirsch BE, Kamerer DB, et al. Squamous cell carcinoma of the external auditory meatus (canal). Otolaryngol Head Neck Surg 1989;101:330–7.

44. Hicks GW. Tumors arising from the glandular structures of the external auditory canal. Laryngoscope 1983;93:326–40.

45. Chang CYJ, Cheung SW. Auditory canal: glandular tumors. In: Jackler RK, Driscoll CLW, editors. Tumors of the ear and temporal bone. Philadelphia: Lippincott, Williams & Wilkins; 2000. p. 84–102.

46. Hyams VJ, Batsakis JG. Pathology of tumors of the ear. In: Thawley SE, Panje WR, Batsakis JG, Lindberg RD, editors. Comprehensive management of head and neck tumors. Vol 1. Philadelphia: WB Saunders; 1999. p. 380–94.

47. Chandrasekhar SS. Temporal bone tumors in children: sarcomas. In: Jackler RK, Driscoll CLW, editors. Tumors of the ear and temporal bone. Philadelphia: Lippincott, Williams & Wilkins; 2000. p. 440–51.

48. Sutow WW, Sullivan MP, Reid HL. Three year relapse-free survival rates in childhood rhabdomyosarcoma of the head and neck: report from the Intergroup Rhabdomyosarcoma Study. Cancer 1982;49:2217–21.

49. Maurer HM, Beltangady M, Gehan EA, et al. The Intergroup Rhabdomyosarcoma Study–I: a final report. Cancer 1988;61:209–20.

50. Crist W, Garnsey L, Beltangady MS, et al. Prognosis in children with rhabdomyosarcoma: a report of the Intergroup Rhabdomyosarcoma Studies I and II. J Clin Oncol 1990;8:443–52.

51. Crist W, Gehan EA, Ragab AH, et al. The Third Intergroup Rhabdomyosarcoma Study. J Clin Oncol 1995;13:610–30.

52. Streitmann MJ, Sismanis A. Metastatic carcinoma of the temporal bone. Am J Otol 1996;17:780–3.

53. Brechtelsbauer PB, Telian SA. Metastatic and hematologic malignancy of the temporal bone. In: Jackler RK, Driscoll CWS, editors. Tumors of the ear and temporal bone. Philadelphia: Lippincott, Williams & Wilkins; 2000. p. 462–71.

54. McCaffrey TV, McDonald TJ. Histiocytosis X of the ear and temporal bone: review of 22 cases. Laryngoscope 1979;89:1735–42.

55. Angeli SI, Alcalde J, Hoffman HT, et al. Langerhans' cell histiocytosis of the head and neck in children. Ann Otol Rhinol Laryngol 1995;104:173–80.

56. Lahey ME. Histiocytosis X: an analysis of prognostic factors. J Pediatr 1975;87:184–9.

38

Partial Labyrinthectomy-Petrous Apicectomy Approach to the Skull Base

DAVID A. SCHESSEL, PHD, MD

LALIGAM N. SEKHAR, MD, FACS

The optimal surgical approach to any lesion incorporates the widest exposure of, and the shortest and most direct route to, the lesion such that retraction and ablation of vital structures are minimized. The resulting exposure should enable faster and more thorough treatment of the lesion with unchanged or preferably decreased morbidity.

The need for such an approach is perhaps no better exemplified than in the management of lesions in the most medial skull base. In the specific case of lesions in the area of the petrous apex, clivus, and Meckel's cave, the result has been a proliferation of approaches that incorporate portions of the retrosigmoid, transpetrosal, and middle fossa approaches.[1–9]

The partial labyrinthectomy-petrous apicectomy (PLPA) approach is a further modification of the standard transmastoid transpetrosal approach developed to access lesions in the petrous apex, mid- to upper clivus, Meckel's cave, and the extensions of posterior fossa lesions into the posterior cavernous sinus. This approach takes advantage of the recently demonstrated ability to reliably remove portions of the bony and membranous vestibular labyrinth while preserving hearing in the majority of patients.[8,10–12]

The types of lesion found to be optimally treated with the PLPA approach are exemplified by the tumors shown in Figure 38–1; note that these tumors extend into both the middle and posterior fossae and invade both Meckel's cave and the posterior cavernous sinus. A wide spectrum of pathologies is amenable to treatment via the PLPA approach including meningiomas, chordomas, trigeminal schwannomas, pituitary adenomas, and epidermoids. Large midvertebral-basilar artery aneurysms also have been accessed by the PLPA, which provides the space necessary for clip placement, bypass grafting, and trapping of the aneurysm. This chapter details and illustrates the surgical technique of the PLPA approach as it has been applied in over 100 cases. The utility of the approach is quantified using a morphometric analysis of three-dimensional computed tomographic (CT) scans, and the morbidity of the procedure, including issues relevant to risk to hearing, is reviewed. We believe that the PLPA approach offers advantages over the standard approaches used. The reliable capability to remove portions of the vestibular labyrinth and preserve hearing supports the use of the PLPA where hearing preservation is a consideration.

SURGICAL PROCEDURE

Surgeries incorporating the PLPA approach are typically performed with the patient in the supine position and the head rigidly fixed and turned 70 degrees away from the side of the lesion. Intraoperative electrophysiologic monitoring of the seventh nerve is mandatory.

Skin Incision

As the PLPA typically is carried out in association with other approaches, the skin incision may vary, depending

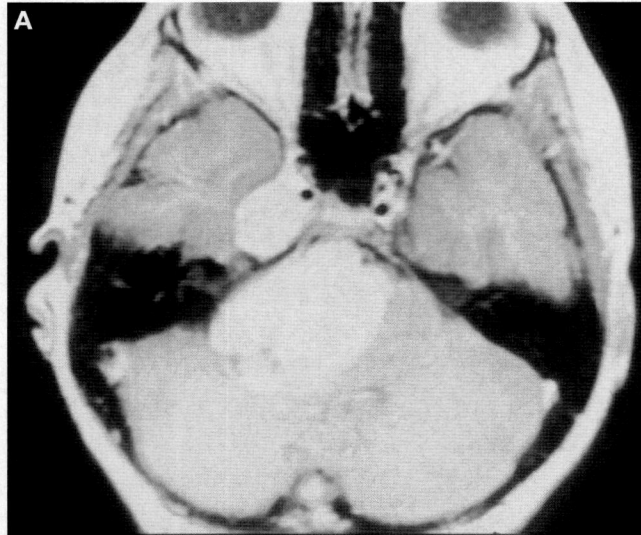

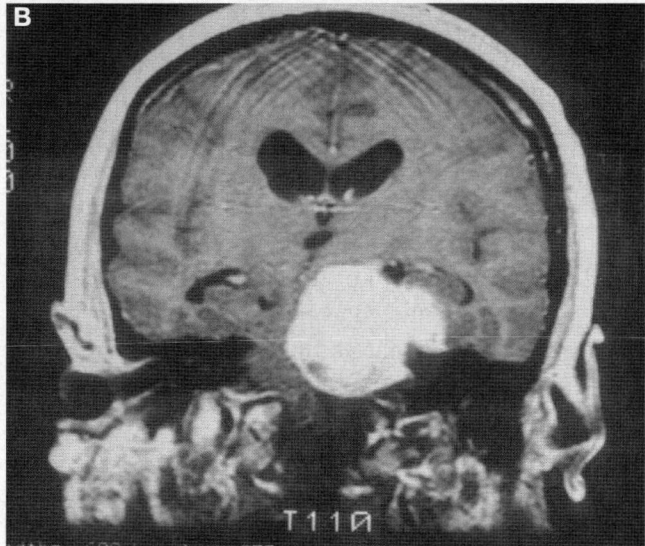

Figure 38–1 *A*, Gadolinium-enhanced, axial magnetic resonance image of a right trigeminal schwannoma in an 11-year-old boy. Note tumor extension into the middle and posterior fossa. *B*, Coronal magnetic resonance image of a right petroclival meningioma in a 58-year-old female.

on the degree of posterior fossa, middle fossa, and cavernous sinus exposure needed. In general, a curvilinear incision is used, which begins in the hairline above the ipsilateral eye and extends behind the ear about 4 cm posterior to the postauricular crease. The incision ends in the neck about 4 cm behind the mastoid tip (Figure 38–2). The sternocleidomastoid muscle is reflected inferiorly and the temporalis muscle is reflected anteriorly, taking care to preserve the frontal branch of the seventh nerve. The postauricular skin and mastoid periosteum are reflected anteriorly up to the suprameatal spine of Henle.

Elevation of external auditory canal skin medial to the spine is avoided as laceration of the thin canal skin typically results in postoperative cerebrospinal fluid (CSF) otorrhea.

Bone Removal

The first stage of the PLPA is an extended complete mastoidectomy (see Figure 38–2), exposing the temporal lobe from the zygomatic root back to the sinodural angle and, to a variable degree, the temporal lobe superior to the transverse sinus. This exposure permits linkage of the transpetrosal approach to a temporal craniotomy as needed. The sigmoid sinus is likewise decorticated, exposing a margin of retrosigmoid dura, enabling a retrosigmoid craniotomy, if desired, as well as retraction of the sinus to enhance the presigmoid exposure.

The configuration of the craniotomy is defined by the disposition of the lesion. It generally extends at least 2 cm beyond the limits of the tumor.

A standard transmastoid-transpetrosal approach is then completed (Figure 38–3), which involves removal of the tegmen medially to the plane of the bony superior semicircular canal (arcuate eminence) and removal of retrofacial and presigmoid bone to the plane of the posterior semicircular canal and jugular bulb. Retrolabyrinthine bone is removed to locate the endolymphatic sac and the endolymphatic duct entrance into the vestibule. The endolymphatic system is usually preserved. However, the endolymphatic duct can be transected if necessary, as is typically the case when the presigmoid surface area is reduced by an anteriorly displaced sigmoid sinus or a high-riding jugular bulb. Sectioning the endolymphatic duct substantially increases the presigmoid exposure with no additional morbidity. The vertical segment of the facial nerve is identified from its second genu to the stylomastoid foramen, leaving the nerve covered by a thin, protective shell of bone. Lastly, bone overlying the superior petrosal sinus is removed as far medially as possible, completing the transmastoid-transpetrosal approach.

The effect of the transmastoid approach with respect to visualization of the clivus is best demonstrated by a posterior view of the temporal bone (Figure 38–4). Note that the bone is removed medially to the level of the superior semicircular canal.

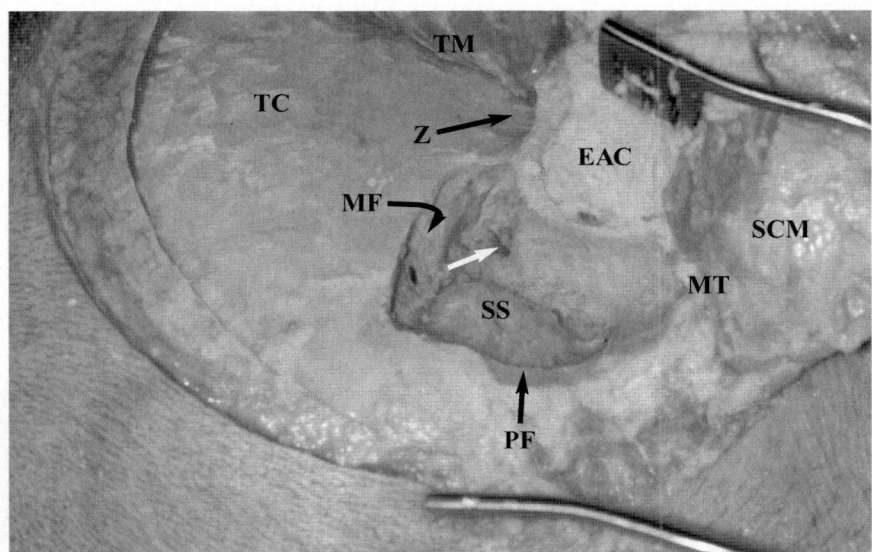

Figure 38–2 Cadaver study of partial labyrinthectomy-petrous apicectomy, right ear incision and simple mastoidectomy. The cadaver is in the surgical position; anterior is at the top of the figure. EAC = membranous external auditory canal reflected anteriorly; MF = middle fossa dura, tegmen removed; MT = mastoid tip; PF = rim of exposed posterior fossa dura; SS = sigmoid sinus; TC = temporal cranium; TM = anteriorly reflected temporalis muscle; Z = zygomatic root; *white arrow* = body of the incus in the aditus ad antrum.

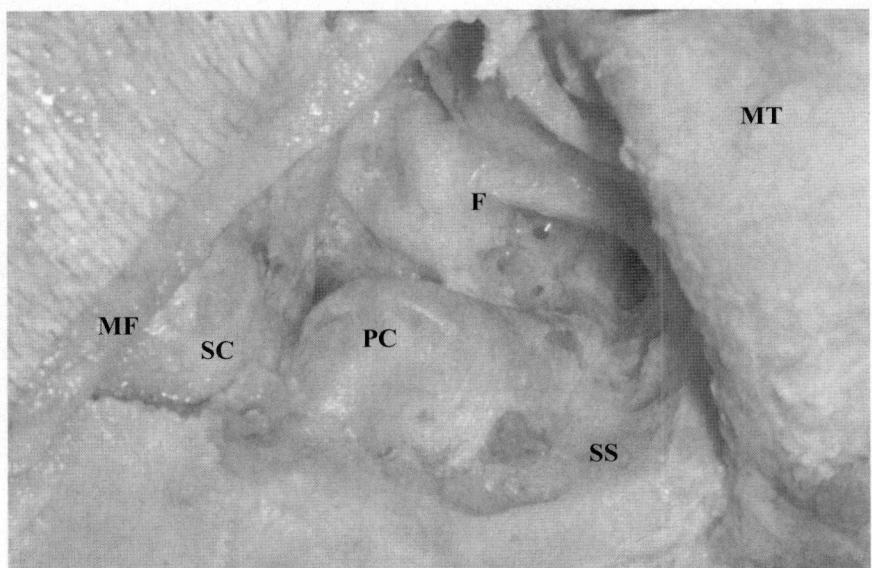

Figure 38–3 Standard transmastoid-transpetrosal approach. F = facial nerve; MF = middle fossa dura; MT = mastoid tip; PC = posterior semicircular canal; SC = superior semicircular canal; SS = sigmoid sinus.

Occlusion of the semicircular canals is then performed, as detailed by Hirsch and colleagues.[12] The bone encasing the superior and posterior semicircular canals is thinned until transparent (blue-lined). A small diamond bur is used to fenestrate the canals at four sites (Figure 38–5). Two fenestrations are in the bony canals adjacent to the posterior and superior canal ampullae. The other two fenestrations are made in the canals adjacent to the common

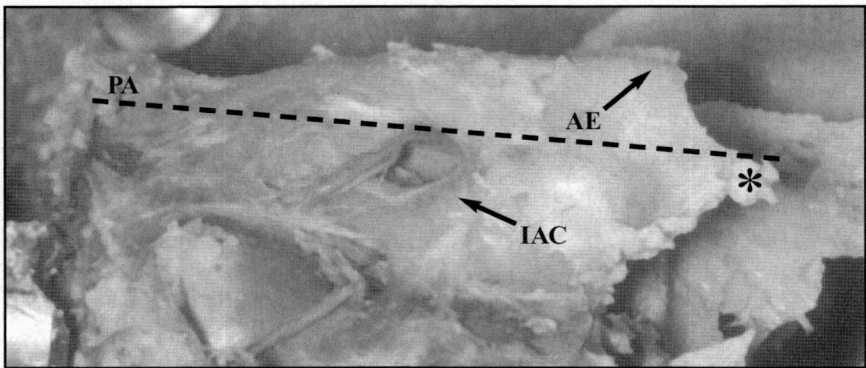

Figure 38–4   Posterior aspect of right temporal bone following the transmastoid-transpetrosal approach. Note that the dura has been removed from this specimen. The *dotted line* indicates the planned line of bone removal. AE = arcuate eminence (superior semicircular canal); IAC = internal auditory canal; PA = petrous apex; *asterisk* = vestibular aqueduct.

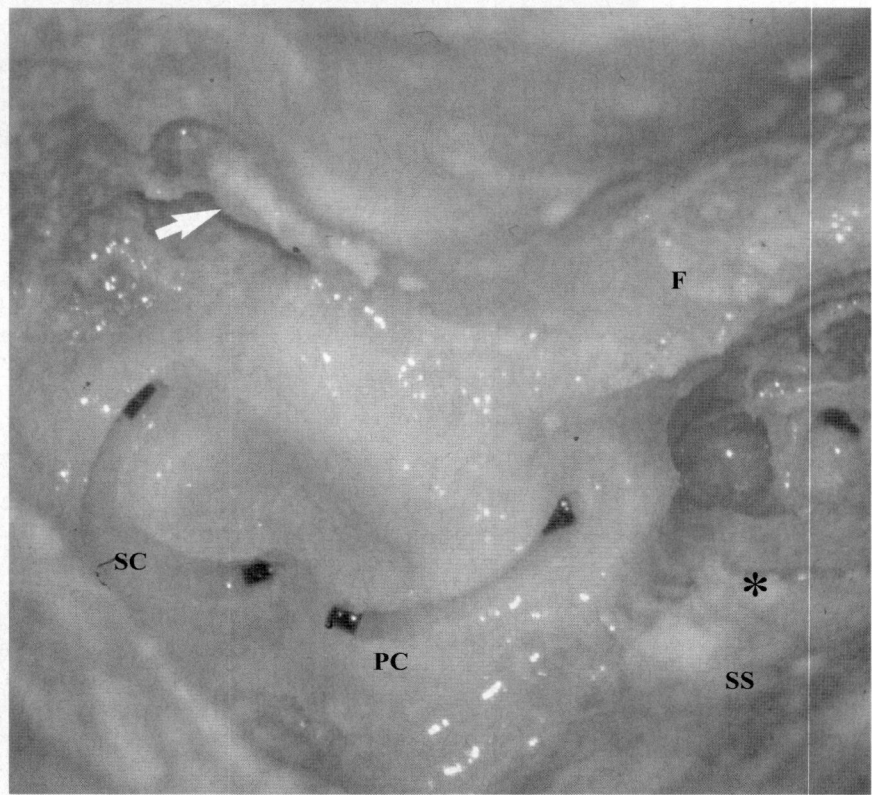

Figure 38–5   Sites of fenestration and occlusion of the semicircular canals. The fenestration sites are indicated by the *black dots* in the ampullated and common crus ends of the canals. F = facial nerve; PC = posterior semicircular canal; SC = superior semicircular canal; SS = sigmoid sinus; *asterisk* = endolymphatic duct; *arrow* = body of incus.

crus. As the canals are opened, they are occluded by packing the canal with bone wax using a gauze pledget.

In an effort not to disturb the membranous labyrinth before packing, care is taken not to drill through the canal or to apply suction directly to the exposed membranous labyrinth before it has been sealed. It is presumed that the packing procedure seals the membranous labyrinth, maintaining separation between the endolymphatic and perilymphatic spaces as well as the inner and middle

ears.[12] Once all four fenestrations have been occluded, the isolated bony and membranous semicircular canals can be drilled away. Note that the horizontal canal, vestibule, and three semicircular canal ampullae are not removed.

The petrous apicectomy is then performed, the goal of which is to remove the entire posterior-superior aspect of the temporal bone to the clivus. Initially, all bone superior to the line formed between the ampulla of the

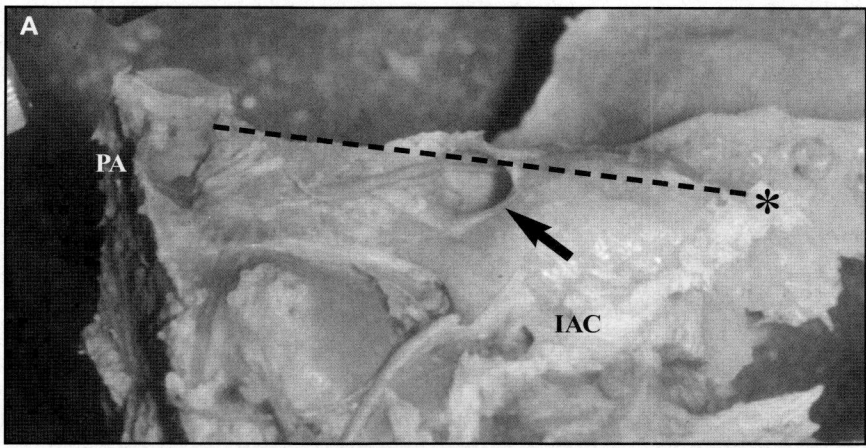

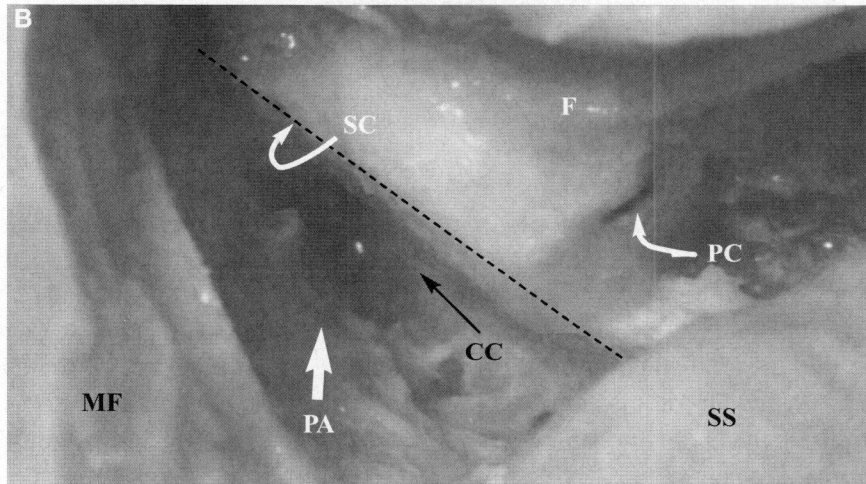

Figure 38–6 *A,* Temporal bone, posterior view. Note that all bone has been removed above the line between the endolymphatic duct (*asterisk*) and the superior semicircular canal ampulla. PA = petrous apex; IAC = internal auditory canal. *B,* Surgical view post-partial labyrinthectomy-petrous apicectomy. Note that all bone has been removed above the line formed by the superior semicircular canal ampulla (SC) and the endolymphatic duct (*asterisk*). The flat plane created is important for optimal exposure following dural incision (see text). CC = common crus; F = facial nerve; MF = middle fossa dura (tegmen removed); PC = posterior canal remnant (ampullated end); PA = petrous apex; *arrow* points to the apex in the depths of the dissection; SS = sigmoid sinus.

superior semicircular canal (SCC) and the entrance of the endolymphatic duct into the temporal bone is removed (Figure 38–6); this line defines the inferior limit of drilling. Note that the arch of the superior SCC and the superior portion of the posterior SCC are removed in this step.

Drilling further medially toward the petrous apex, the superior aspect of the internal auditory canal (IAC) is identified through the transparent bone. The seventh nerve, which runs in the superior aspect of the IAC, can be stimulated to verify IAC identification. The bone

overlying the IAC is blue-lined from the fundus to the porus (Figure 38–7).

Linking the line between the superior SCC ampulla and the endolymphatic duct with the IAC determines the plane used to guide the rest of the drilling medially through the petrous apex to the clivus. The establishment of this plane is important to guide the angle of further drilling as it is often done blindly, by feel. The effect of this final step is illustrated in Figure 38–8. Typically the dura is not violated during this stage of the procedure. Anecdotally, avoiding dural violation has been accom-

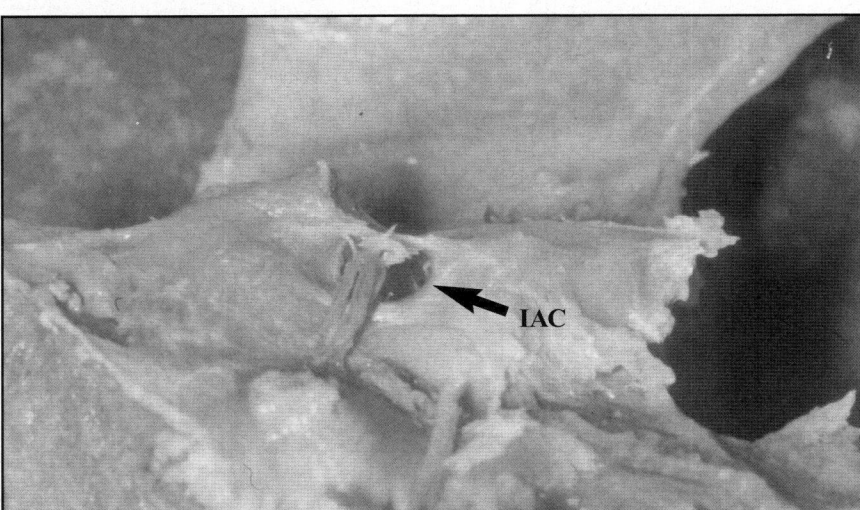

Figure 38–7 Posterior view of the temporal bone following bone removal to the internal auditory canal (IAC). Note the progressive removal of bone along the *dotted line* indicated in Figure 38–4.

plished by completing the labyrinthectomy, the exposure of the IAC, and the petrous apicectomy by hollowing out the temporal bone, leaving the overlying outer shell of the temporal bone in place. This shell serves to protect the dura and to provide excellent retraction medially, and its removal completes the procedure.

The posterior SCC inferior to the endolymphatic duct is removed to permit maximal, anterior reflection of the presigmoid dura (Figure 38–6). It is at this stage that the decision to transect the endolymphatic duct is made. Care is taken not to coagulate or occlude the remaining endolymphatic system.

The usual dural incision is carried through the presigmoid dura from the jugular bulb, along the medial edge of the sigmoid sinus, across the superior petrosal sinus, and anteriorly through middle fossa dura along the curvature of the temporal lobe. Once the tentorium is split, the dura is draped over the surface of the temporal bone. The exposure is thus maximized by creating a flat surface on the temporal bone during drilling.

Tumor removal proceeds in piecemeal fashion. Tumors are initially debulked, the normal structures at the margins of the lesion are identified, and the remaining tumor is dissected from this perimeter. Although total tumor excision is the goal, it is not always possible. Suffice it to say, the decision to leave part of the lesion behind is complicated and is based on both the individual patient and the structures involved. The details of tumor removal and aneurysm management can be found in a separate publication.[8]

Having dealt with the lesion, the dura is closed primarily or with a pericranial graft; however, a watertight closure is rarely accomplished. Therefore, the connection between the intracranial compartment and the eustachian tube must be blocked, which poses a particular problem in the PLPA approach. The middle ear/eustachian tube connection has to be broken, yet the middle ear must remain aerated to enable normal middle ear function for hearing. Temporary occlusion of the eustachian tube combined with blockage of the aditus ad antrum has proven the best means to accomplish this goal. The eustachian tube is occluded with Surgicel™ (oxidized regenerated cellulose, Johnson & Johnson, New Brunswick, New Jersey) inserted through the extended facial recess. Care must be taken not to perforate the tympanic membrane or dislocate the ossicles. The middle ear cannot be entirely filled with this packing material as swelling of the Surgicel can rupture the tympanic membrane. The aditus ad antrum is then packed with thin strips of Surgicel insinuated between the ossicles. Exposed temporal bone is coated with a very thin layer of bone wax and the mastoid is filled with fat. The conductive hearing loss produced by the packing typically resolves in 6 to 8 weeks.

OUTCOME AND CONSEQUENCES OF THE PARTIAL LABYRINTHECTOMY-PETROUS APICECTOMY APPROACH

Although the intent of this chapter is to describe the technical aspects of this approach, it is critical to understand what is gained by the addition of the PLPA, that is, when it becomes reasonable to include a procedure

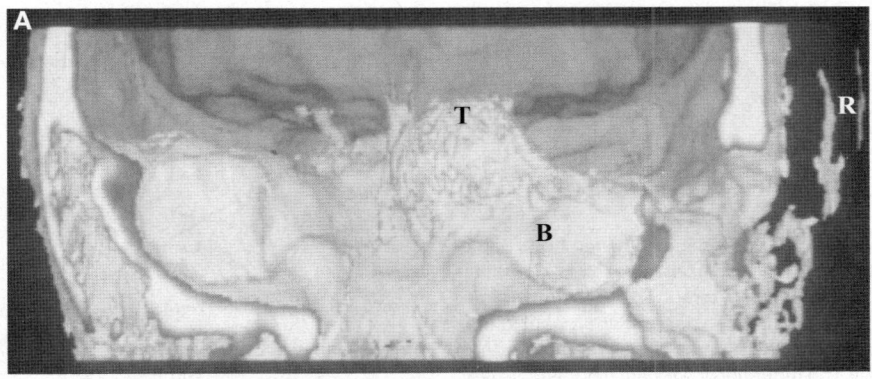

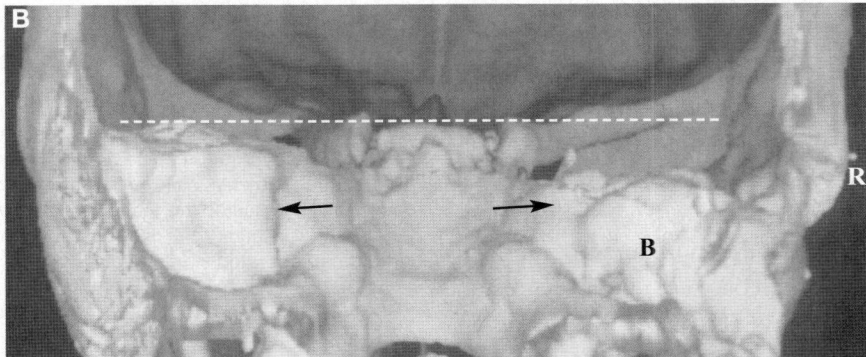

Figure 38–8 *A*, Three-dimensional reconstruction of skull base with right meningioma (same case as in Figure 38–1, B) following the partial labyrinthectomy-petrous apicectomy approach. The view is from the posterior fossa to the posterior aspect of the temporal bone. The occipital bone has been digitally subtracted. T = tumor (meningioma); B = left temporal bone. *B*, Tumor has been digitally subtracted demonstrating right partial labyrinthectomy-petrous apicectomy versus left (unoperated) bone. Note, as in the temporal bone dissections, that the bone of the petrous ridge has been removed down to the level of the internal auditory canal. *Arrows* indicate the position of the internal auditory canals.

that requires both added time and potentially adds morbidity to an already complex surgery. The ensuing discussion addresses the benefits of the PLPA approach through a morphometric analysis and its attendant morbidity, especially the risk of hearing loss. For a more complete discussion of patient outcomes, the reader is referred to Sekhar and colleagues.[8]

Surgical Outcome

The improved access gained by the PLPA, in comparison with nonpetrosal and the standard transmastoid-transpetrosal approaches, results from the reduction of vertical height of the temporal bone and the improved angle of approach, as illustrated by the case of a 58-year-old female with a large, right petroclival-cavernous meningioma (see Figure 38–1, B). The tumor was removed in two stages, with the approach temporally separated from tumor removal by 2 days. A three-dimensional recon-

struction of a contrast-enhanced CT scan of the patient following the PLPA but before tumor excision is shown in Figure 38–8, A. The tumor can be digitally subtracted from the image, allowing comparison of the bony anatomy of the right (unoperated) side with that of the post-PLPA side (Figure 38–8, B). Note the reduction in vertical height of the temporal bone of the operated side in comparison with that of the unoperated side. The vertical height reduction generally achieved is in the range of 1 cm, although the reduction can run the gamut from 5 to 10 mm.

More important is the change in the angle of approach afforded by the PLPA, which is quantified as follows: if the silhouettes of the surface of the operated and unoperated temporal bones are derived from the CT images (Figure 38–9), one can measure the angles necessary to contact points along the medial petrous apex, Meckel's cave, and the midline clivus. These points are representative of the locations of the lesions typically encountered.

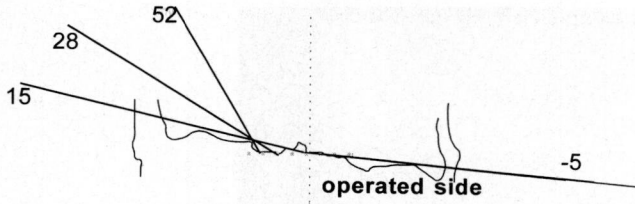

Figure 38–9 Silhouette taken from the surface of the temporal bone of Figure 38–8, B. Points have been added from the midline clivus laterally to encompass the typical location of tumor. The lines drawn indicate the angles necessary to contact these points if approaching the tumor from the lateral skull. Note the difference between the operated and unoperated sides. The reduction in vertical height achieved by the approach is indicated. In this case, it was about 1 cm.

As demonstrated on the left (unoperated) side, the minimum angle to get to the midline is 15 degrees above the horizontal. To approach tumor lateral to this, such as one in the petrous apex or Meckel's cave, temporal lobe retraction above this angle is required, as is illustrated by the larger angles to access the more lateral points in the unoperated side of the skull base (28 and 52 degrees). When a similar calculation is performed for the post-PLPA bone, it can be seen that similar points on the clivus and petrous apex are all approachable by the same angle, –5 degrees (see Figure 38–9). This angle is the same for all similarly drawn lines. In contrast to the variable reduction in vertical height gained with the PLPA, the angular improvement is always realized.

The reduction in the vertical height of the temporal bone and the increase of 20 to 57 degrees in the approach angle (the difference between operated and unoperated sides) following PLPA reflects the gain in working space achieved without additional brain retraction (see Figure 38–9).

The above calculation reflects what one would see when viewing the surgical field from a vantage strictly lateral to the head of the patient. As the surgeon uses a variety of angles about the head of the patient, the effect of the PLPA for the whole range of working angles was approximated by pitching the three-dimensional CT temporal bone image nose up and down. The same type, with the same or greater degree, of benefit was noted for over 40 degrees of rotation about the top of the head, encompassing those angles typically used. It is noteworthy that the real obstruction to surgical access is presented by the bone of the petrous ridge, which becomes more prominent as it extends medially to the clivus (Figure 38–10). As coronal images depict the petrous ridge, we have found them useful in preoperative planning.

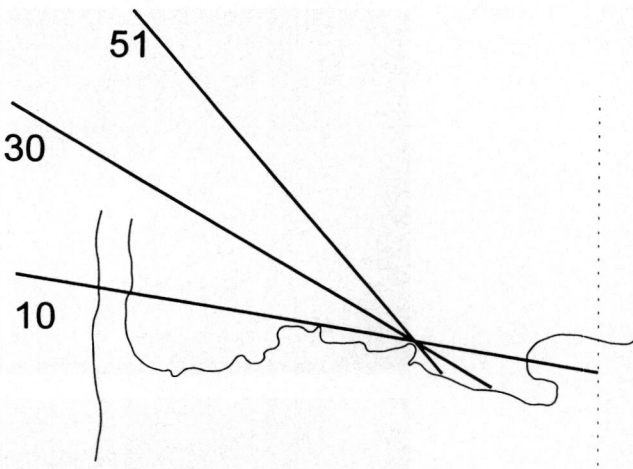

Figure 38–10 Surface projection of the right petrous bone following a standard transmastoid-transpetrosal approach (without partial labyrinthectomy-petrous apicectomy). The surface profile is derived from a three-dimensionally reconstructed computed tomographic scan. Angles indicated are those needed to contact points similar to those seen in Figure 38–9. Note that the approach angles are similar to the unoperated side of Figure 38–9.

Audiometric Outcome

Postoperative audiometric results are available for 84 of 100 patients operated by the PLPA approach (Table 38–1). Not all patients could be tested owing to geographic and practice logistical issues. The duration of follow-up ranges from 3 days to 50 months (mean 20 months).

Preoperative data were not always available; in these cases, the preoperative hearing was assumed to be perfect, with a pure-tone average of 0 dB and a speech discrimination of 100%. The pure-tone averages (mean of thresholds at 500 Hz, 1 kHz, and 2 kHz) and speech discrimination scores are presented. Because many of the patients were tested in the early postoperative period, bone conduction pure-tone thresholds are used to eliminate the effect owing to the temporary conductive hearing caused

Table 38–1 DEMOGRAPHICS		
N = 84		
Duration of follow-up (mean) 20 mo (3 d to 50 mo)		
Patients	Male 25	Female 59
Age (mean)	45.2 y (10 to 75 y)	
Pathology		
Meningioma		59
Vertebral basilar aneurysm/stenosis		7
Epidermoid		6
Chordoma		5
Trigeminal schwannoma		2
Chondrosarcoma		2
Craniopharyngioma		2
Trigeminal neuralgia (recurrent)		1

Table 38–2	HEARING OUTCOME (N = 84)	
	Preoperative	Postoperative
Pure-tone average		
Mean	12 dB	22 dB
Median	7 dB	19 dB
Speech discrimination		
Mean	89%	79%
Median	96%	92%
Retention of serviceable hearing (SD > 60%, PTA < 50 dB)	95% (76/80)	
Ipsilateral deafness		6% (5/84)

illustrated in Figure 38–11. Typically, there is a transient sensorineural hearing loss, with decreases in both the pure-tone threshold and speech discrimination early after surgery. A high-frequency hearing loss is usual, and the decrease in speech discrimination can be considerable. The hearing improves with time (several weeks), both with respect to speech discrimination and pure-tone thresholds; slow improvement has been observed. Some degree of high-frequency hearing loss is permanent.

by the middle ear packing. Air conduction stimuli were used in the measurement of speech discrimination. The preoperative and most recent postoperative audiometric results are summarized in Table 38–2. Note that 5 of 84 (6%) patients tested were completely deaf following surgery. Serviceable hearing was retained in 76 of 80 (95%) patients with serviceable hearing preoperatively; hearing improvement has been observed. Deafness as a result of surgery is noted immediately following surgery; gradual deterioration in hearing has not been observed.

A composite audiogram, including preoperative, early postoperative, and the most recent postoperative data, is

Vestibular System

Subjective reports of vertigo or associated vegetative symptoms are notably absent in the immediate postoperative period. Patients typically demonstrate bidirectional gaze nystagmus during the first postoperative day and may show typical (paralytic) vestibular nystagmus subsequently. This nystagmus is only first degree, is not associated with vegetative symptoms, and resolves within 2 weeks.

In long-term follow-up, it is difficult to separate the effects of the approach from the effects of treatment of the lesion, for example, oculomotor nerve and cerebellar/brainstem injury. Subjectively, patients are able

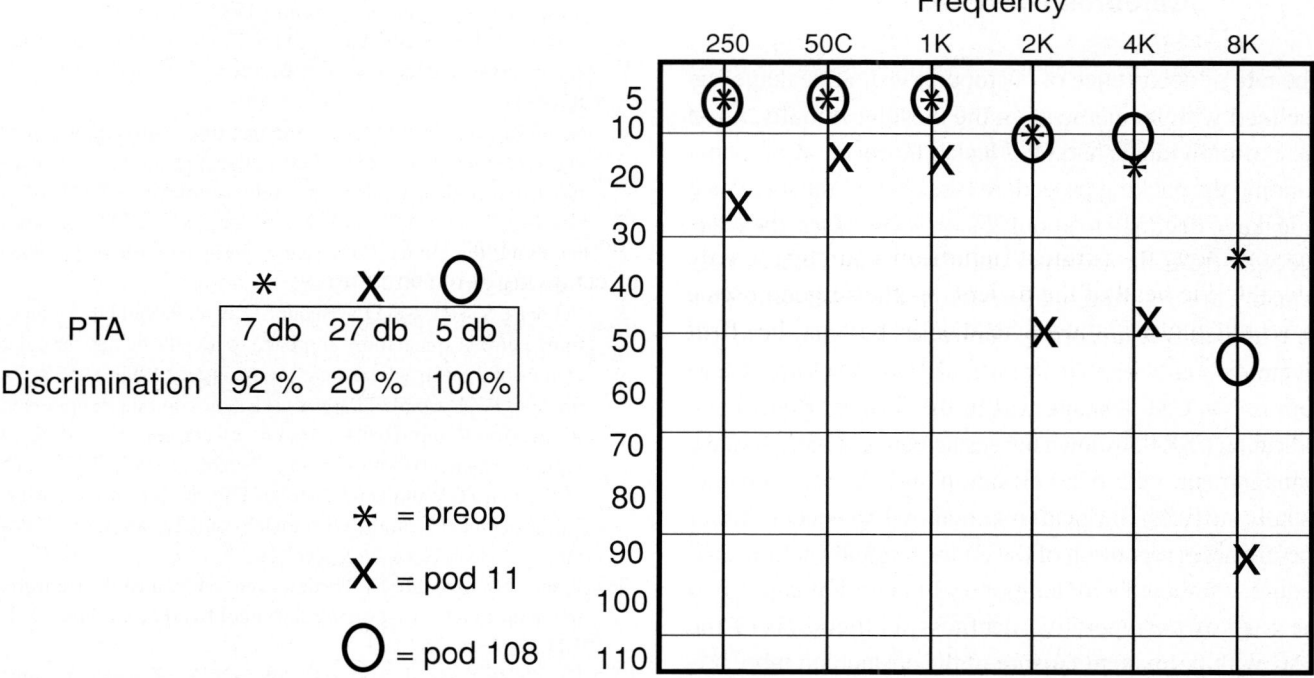

Figure 38–11 Composite audiogram of the patient illustrated in Figure 38–1, A, showing preoperative (preop) and 11 and 108 days postoperative (postop) results. PTA = pure-tone average.

to ambulate well, although some report persistent, episodic oscillopsia associated with rapid head movements. Two individuals developed benign paroxysmal positional vertigo (BPPV). In one of these patients, it was from the contralateral ear and resolved with canalolith repositioning maneuvers. In the second individual, the BPPV seemed to arise from the operated side; repositioning maneuvers, directed at both sides, were unsuccessful.

One individual developed delayed endolymphatic hydrops in the operated ear, which initially responded to diuretics. Eventually, however, intratympanic gentamicin was required to eliminate the vertigo. It is presumed that the hydrops reflected dysfunction of the endolymph absorption system.

Caloric testing (standard 30°C and 44°C irrigations) has been performed on three individuals; no vestibular response was recorded from the operated ear of any of these patients. Prolonged ice water stimulation evoked a typical, contralateral-beating horizontal nystagmus with a mean slow-phase eye velocity of 28 degrees/second. With 180-degree inversion of the patient (prone positioning), the direction of nystagmus reversed, lending credence to the conclusion that the responses originated from an at least partially intact horizontal SCC.

Cerebrospinal Fluid Leaks

The rate of occurrence of postoperative CSF leakage has declined with refinements in the closure. Initially, up to 23% of individuals had CSF leaks; however, after incorporating the packing procedure (see above), the incidence of leakage declined to about 2%. In some cases, the leakage was from the external auditory canal (EAC), presumably arising from a laceration in the EAC skin. This type of leak was uniformly controlled by 5 days of CSF diversion via a lumbar drain and EAC packing. More commonly, CSF leakage was in the form of rhinorrhea, indicating CSF flow down the eustachian tube; conservative management, with head elevation and lumbar drainage, usually suffices. Surgical treatment, when needed, either encompasses repetition of the entire surgical packing procedure, combined with temporary lumbar drainage, or, in the case of postoperative deafness, obliteration of the EAC with permanent closure of the eustachian tube. It is our impression that postoperative hydrocephalus predisposes the patient to the development of a CSF leak.

SUMMARY

The partial labyrinthine petrous apicectomy has been shown to provide improved access to lesions of the clivus, petrous apex, and cavernous sinus extensions of posterior fossa lesions. It has also been used to provide increased area for instrumentation of lesions in the posterior fossa, such as vertebral-basilar aneurysms. We believe that this increase in working room permits more controlled and thorough lesion management with reduced or unchanged brain retraction and acceptable morbidity to auditory and vestibular function. The ability to remove portions of the membranous labyrinth with no, or minimal, injury to hearing supports the use of the partial labyrinthectomy as a surgical adjunctive procedure.

REFERENCES

1. Al-Mefty O. Petrosal approach to clival tumors. In: Surgery of cranial base tumors. Sekhar LN, Janecka IP, editors. New York: Raven Press; 1993. p. 307–15.

2. Ammarati M, Ma J, Cheatham ML, et al. Drilling the posterior wall of the petrous pyramid: a microneurosurgical anatomical study. J Neurosurg 1993;78:452–5.

3. Bricolo AP, Turazzi S, Talacchi A, Cristofori L. Microsurgical removal of petroclival meningiomas: a report of 33 cases. Neurosurgery 1992;31:813–28.

4. Hakuba A, Nishimura S, Jang BJ. The combined retroauricular and periauricular transpetrosal-transtentorial approach the clivus meningiomas. Surg Neurol 1988;30:108–16.

5. Kawase T, Toya S, Shiobara R, Mine T. Transpetrosal approach for aneurysms of the lower basilar artery. J Neurosurg 1985;63: 857–61.

6. Samii M, Ammirati M. The combined supra-infratentorial presigmoid sinus avenue to the petro-clival region. Surgical technique and clinical applications. Acta Neurochir 1988;95:6–12.

7. Sekhar LN, Janetta PJ, Burkhart LE, Janosky JE. Meningiomas involving the clivus: a six-year experience with 41 patients. Neurosurgery 1990;27:764–81.

8. Sekhar LN, Schessel DA, Bucur SD, et al. Partial labyrinthectomy petrous apicectomy approach to neoplastic and vascular lesions of the petroclival area. Neurosurgery 1999;44:537–50.

9. Spetzler RF, Daspit CP, Pappas CTE. The combined supra- and infratentorial approach for lesions of the petrous and clival regions: experience with 46 cases. J Neurosurg 1992;76:588–99.

10. McElveen JT, Wilkins RH, Molter DW, et al. Hearing preservation using the modified translabyrinthine approach. Otolaryngol Head Neck Surg 1993;108:671–9.

11. Parnes LS, McClure JA. Posterior semicircular canal occlusion in the normal hearing ear. Otolaryngol Head Neck Surg 1991; 104:52–7.

12. Hirsch BE, Cass SP, Sekhar LN, Wright DC. Translabyrinthine approach to skull basetumors with hearing preservation. Am J Otol 1991;14:533–43.

APPENDIX

Surgical Anatomy of the Temporal Bone and Dissection Guide

DENNIS I. BOJRAB, MD

BEN J. BALOUGH, MD

FOREWORD

(Expanding on, the Material of G. E. Shambaugh Jr, MD)

It is easier to see today in the twenty-first century as we are on the shoulders of giants, with a much easier view of the terrain. The history of ear surgery is rich in dedication and resourcefulness. We owe much of our success to the many who have come before us, dedicated to ingenuity in research and development and teaching new generations of ear surgeons, allowing preceptorships and fellowships. All of the following otologists and many not mentioned encouraged and nurtured a collegial atmosphere of learning for all of us, many times through the relaxed atmosphere of a temporal bone laboratory. I would personally like to thank Dr. Michael E. Glasscock for my fellowship training and his encouragement to me in my endeavors. Dr. Howard House has too many achievements to cover in this format, but I would like to thank him for helping my career direction and for our many meetings during which he joyfully described to me the rich history of otologic surgery.

This Appendix is intended as an anatomic reference to the temporal bone and its structures, with a section on surgical dissection of the temporal bone. This resource is intended for the use of the otolaryngologist who wants a source that couples a basic guide to temporal bone anatomy, basic equipment knowledge of setting up a dissection bench (with microscope, drill, and suction irrigation), and a surgical dissection approach to the most common otologic procedures within the temporal bone.

The great pioneer otologist Bezold, in his *Textbook of Otology*, warned that "the danger to the patient of an incompetent operator, who does not know the many anatomical details crowded together in the narrow space of the temporal bone and their extreme variability, is much greater here than in any other region of the body." Only by cadaver dissections can the aspiring ear surgeon learn to safely traverse the perilous anatomy of the temporal bone so as to avoid injury to the many vital structures concealed in an area no larger than an olive.

Mastoid surgery was one of the most frequent surgeries in the 1930s for children with upper respiratory infections frequently developed acute otitis media followed by acute mastoiditis. Without antibiotics, mastoid surgery was required to combat disastrous complications such as meningitis, brain abscess, sinus thrombosis, and even death. The observation of Fleming, in 1928, of lysis of *Staphylococcus* colonies by *Penicillium* mold and the discovery by Domagk, in 1932, of the antistreptococcal effect of sulfanilamide progressively and dramatically reduced the mortality rate and indications for surgical intervention in acute ear infections. As the variety of antibiotics grew, ear surgery could evolve into a constructive rather than a destructive specialty.

In 1899, Körner suggested that in certain cases of chronic otitis, the tympanic membrane could be left in place during the radical operation, thus preserving useful hearing. In 1910, Bondy described the indication for and technique of a modification of the radical operation for cases of chronic otorrhea in which the pars flaccida perforation was accompanied by an intact pars tensa. Kessel, in 1879, performed stapes mobilization in an attempt to improve a conductive hearing loss. At the

1900 International Congress of Otology, leaders in the specialty united in condemning surgery for deafness as "not only useless, but dangerous to life." So complete was this rejection toward operations for improving hearing that earlier procedures such as stapes mobilization and stapedectomy for otosclerosis as well as operations for repair of tympanic membrane perforations and congenital aural atresia were discontinued. By 1919, Sir Charles Balance's book *Surgery of the Temporal Bone* failed to mention any sort of operation to improve hearing. In 1930, with *Diseases of the Ear*, Kerrison devoted less than a page to "Surgical Measures for the Relief of Deafness," concluding that "these operations mentioned for their place in otologic history are quite obsolete today."

With considerable courage in the face of this concerted opposition, Bárány, in 1911, Jenkins, in 1912, and Holmgren, in 1914, began to operate to try to improve hearing in otosclerosis. Nylén, in 1921, a young assistant in Holmgren's clinic, first employed a monocular operating microscope to assist in a radical mastoidectomy. Holmgren immediately recognized the advantage of magnification and began to use a binocular operating microscope for his operations on otosclerosis. Holmgren demonstrated that by careful aseptic technique, a semicircular canal could be opened safely and a temporary hearing improvement achieved.

In 1924, Sourdille observed Holmgren's operations and returned to France to devise his two- or three-stage operations called the tympanolabyrinthopexy. With this operation, Sourdille created a fistula in the horizontal semicircular canal and covered it with a skin flap from the meatus. For the first time, permanent hearing improvements in otosclerosis were achieved. In 1937, Sourdille's lecture to the New York Academy of Medicine prompted Lempert to apply the technique, using the endaural approach (rather than the postauricular) and a dental drill, for his one-stage approach to fenestrate the semicircular canal in otosclerosis. In 1938, G. Shambaugh Jr. became his first pupil and performed more than 5,000 fenestration operations (Lempert and Sourdille relied on the loupe for magnification). In 1940, Shambaugh Jr innovated the use of the operating microscope, continuous irrigation, enchondralization, and a diamond drill for construction of the fenestra; lasting hearing improvements were achieved in 80% of fenestrations. With Rosen's reintroduction of stapes mobilization surgery in 1953, the approach to otosclerosis surgery became the oval window area rather than the ampullated end of the horizontal canal. In 1956, Dr. John Shea introduced the stapedectomy procedure that is now used worldwide.

With this success, operations for congenital meatal atresia and then tympanoplasty to rebuild a sound-conducting system in the damaged ear began to rekindle. In 1950, Moritz used pedicled flaps to construct a closed middle ear cavity in cases of chronic otitis media, thus providing a sound shielding or protection for the round window preparatory to a later fenestration of the horizontal semicircular canal. In 1955, Dr. Fritz Zöllner and Dr. Horst Wullstein introduced their concept of myringoplasty and tympanoplasty, which was to allow restoration of hearing through reconstruction of ears with chronic disease or trauma. They reported the use of an oval strut of vinyl acrylic that acted as an acoustic transmitter between the mobile footplate and the tympanic membrane graft, but poor results with this material caused them to quickly abandon its use. They continued to enjoy great popularity in the United States for tympanoplasty and for connecting the incus to the oval window in stapedectomy. The use of ossicular repositioning by them and described by Hall and Rytzner became quite popular and are even to this day.

In 1958, Dr. William House applied the method of Clerc and Batisse of approaching the internal meatus and the geniculate ganglion from the middle cranial fossa. This led 3 years later to House's first operation to remove an acoustic neuroma by this approach. Soon House reported an impressive series of 47 acoustic neuroma operations without a fatality and with preservation of facial nerve function in the majority. Previous neurosurgical removals of similar tumors had carried a mortality rate of around 20% and permanent facial nerve paralysis in nearly all. House revived Portmann's operations for Meniere's disease and with Sheehy modified Jansen's operation for cholesteatoma without creating a radical cavity. House used the postaural approach to the temporal bone, whereas Lempert had taught that the endaural operation was best for nearly all ear surgery.

Temporal bone dissection has continued to play an important role in training the otolaryngologist to comprehend this complex anatomy. A foundation of normal anatomic dissection has become increasingly important in helping the surgeon coordinate the structural knowledge gained through dissection coupled with that of computed tomographic imaging to recognize and treat pathology. Anatomic knowledge provides the foundation for skillful and safe dissection of the temporal bone. The primary structure of interest in any dissection of the temporal bone is the facial nerve. Thus, locating and protecting this structure are essential aims in otologic surgery. The second key to achieving surgical proficiency is equipment knowledge. Understanding the mechanics and principles of the otologic drill and practice with that tool serves to facilitate dissection skills. Lastly, a road map that guides the surgeon through the dissections and provides a progressive course of more complex dissections built on familiar anatomy and procedures is the third step in mastering the temporal bone. Thus, this chapter will follow these guidelines and hopefully serve as a valuable bridge between the masters who came before and those who are just beginning their journey.

ANATOMY OF THE TEMPORAL BONE

External Anatomy

Lateral Surface

The lateral aspect of the temporal bone is the one most commonly encountered by the surgeon for operative procedures or during laboratory drilling. As such, special attention should be paid to the landmarks found here as they will be the ones identified during surgery after reflecting of the soft tissue. The tip of the mastoid process is easily palpated and is a landmark for the positioning of postauricular incisions. The zygomatic process is also readily identifiable. A prominent ridge known as the temporal line (linea temporalis) runs posteriorly and slightly superiorly from the root of the zygoma and defines the inferior border of the temporalis muscle. The temporal line also approximates the position of the floor of the middle cranial fossa. The squamous portion of the temporal bone (the squama) extends above the temporal line, whereas inferiorly and anteriorly is the tympanic ring and posteriorly the mastoid. Posterior and medial to the mastoid tip is a cleft for the posterior belly of the digastric muscle (digastric groove or mastoid incisure). The tympanomastoid fissure is anterior to the tip of the mastoid and can be traced medially to the stylomastoid foramen, which is the exit point of the facial nerve. Thus, caution must be exercised when dissecting

anterior to the mastoid tip during mastoid surgery, particularly in young children in whom the tip is not well developed. Anteriorly, the tympanic ring separates the external auditory canal from the glenoid fossa, which lies beneath the root of the zygoma. The tympanosquamous suture line is located in the anterosuperior part of the ring, and the tympanomastoid suture is located posterosuperiorly. The spine of Henle is a prominence of variable size that is found at the posterosuperior rim of the external auditory canal. Macewen's triangle (the fossa mastoidea), which laterally overlies the mastoid antrum, is delimited by the temporal line superiorly, a tangent to the posterior external auditory canal posteriorly, and the posterosuperior rim of the canal. Macewen's triangle is characterized by the presence of multiple small perforating vessels and hence is also known as the cribrose (cribriform) area (Figure A–1).

Superior Surface

The superior surface (tegmen) of the temporal bone is the floor of the middle cranial fossa, separating the tym-

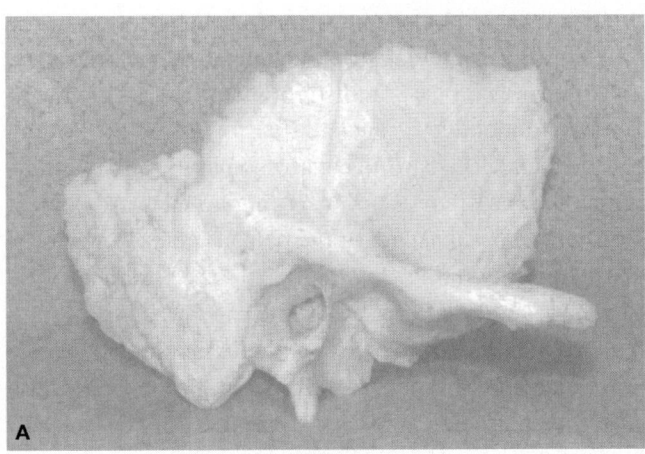

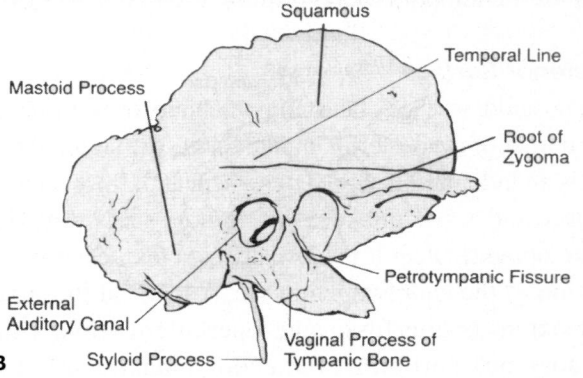

Figure A–1 Lateral surface anatomy: note the zygomatic process, tympanic annulus, temporal line, and mastoid tip.

panomastoid compartment from the temporal lobe. The tegmen can be divided into an anterior tegmen tympani (covering the tympanic cavity) and a posterior tegmen mastoideum (covering the mastoid air cells). The petrotympanic suture line forms the medial boundary of the tegmen. Further medially, the dense petrous bone (petrosa) runs an oblique course from lateral to medial. The petrous portion of the temporal bone is marked by depressions and eminences corresponding to the convolutions of the brain and the internal structures of the temporal bone. The arcuate eminence, present in about 85% of temporal bones, approximates the position of the superior semicircular canal (SSCC) and is a key landmark in middle cranial fossa surgery. The greater petrosal nerve (GPN) separates from the geniculate ganglion and emerges through the facial hiatus to run in a groove that is slightly medial to the petrotympanic suture and that parallels the petrous ridge. Lateral to and paralleling the greater petrosal nerve is the lesser petrosal nerve, which runs in the petrosquamous suture (superior tympanic canaliculus). The tensor tympani muscle is inferior to the lesser petrosal nerve.

The foramen lacerum, located at the junction of the base of the greater wing of the sphenoid, the petrous apex, and the basiocciput, is a false foramen that is filled with fibrous connective tissue and that forms the roof of the carotid canal. The carotid canal also parallels the petrous ridge. The gasserian (semilunar) ganglion lies in a depression at the lateral aspect of the petrous apex. Anteriorly, proceeding medially to laterally, are the foramen ovale (for the mandibular division of the trigeminal nerve) and the foramen spinosum (for the middle meningeal vessels and a recurrent branch of the mandibular nerve); these structures serve as surgical landmarks for the anterior limit of the temporal bone (Figure A–2).

Posterior Surface

The posterior surface of the temporal bone forms the anterior border of the posterior cranial fossa. The sigmoid sulcus is an indentation at the lateral aspect of the posterior surface and accommodates the sigmoid sinus. Anterior to the sigmoid sulcus is the foveate fossa for the intradural portion of the endolymphatic sac. A ledge at the superior extent of the fossa, the operculum, covers the intraosseous portion of the endolymphatic sac. The vestibular aqueduct runs anteriorly, superiorly, and medially from the operculum to end at the medial wall of the

vestibule. The superior petrosal sulcus, located at the interface of the posterior and middle cranial fossa plates of the temporal bone, carries the superior petrosal sinus from the sigmoid sinus to the cavernous sinus anteriorly.

The internal auditory canal penetrates the posterior surface of the petrous ridge, runs anteromedially to posterolaterally, and contains the cochlear, vestibular, and facial nerves, along with their blood supply. The canal extends approximately 1 cm from the porus medially to the fundus laterally. At the fundus, the canal is divided into an upper and a lower portion by the transverse crest (crista falciformis). The inferior compartment contains the cochlear nerve anteriorly and the inferior vestibular nerve inferiorly. A branch of the inferior vestibular nerve, the posterior ampullary nerve, which innervates the ampulla of the posterior semicircular canal, exits the internal auditory canal through the singular canal. A vertical crest of bone, Bill's bar, separates the superior

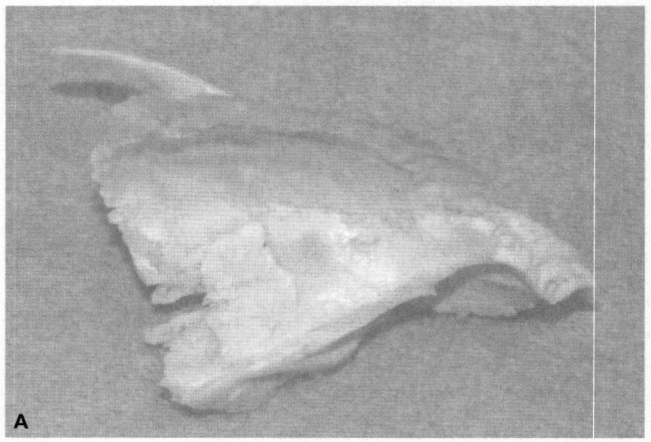

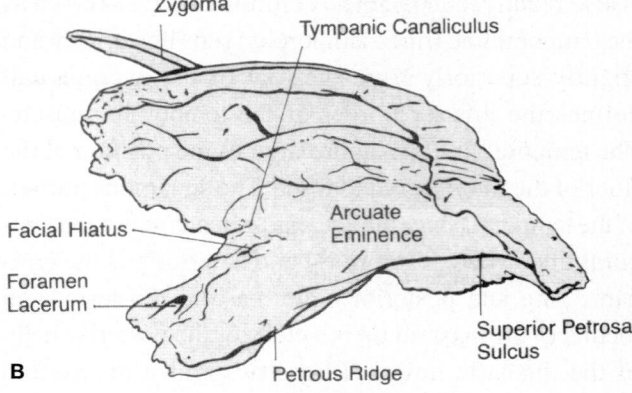

Figure A–2 Superior surface anatomy: important landmarks for the middle fossa surgeon are the temporosquamous suture line, facial hiatus (greater superficial petrosal nerve), tympanic canaliculus (lesser petrosal nerve), arcuate eminence (relative position of superior semicircular canal), and foramen lacerum (carotid artery).

portion of the canal into an anterior compartment, occupied by the facial nerve, and a posterior compartment containing the superior vestibular nerve (Figures A–3 and A–4).

Inferior Surface

The inferior surface of the temporal bone separates the upper neck from the skull base. Accordingly, many vital neurovascular structures traverse this surface. Anteriorly and medially, the external carotid foramen is the point at which the internal carotid artery enters the temporal bone. Posteriorly, a ridge of bone, the jugulocarotid crest, separates the carotid canal from the jugular foramen. Classically, the jugular foramen has been thought of as being divided into a posterolateral pars venosa,

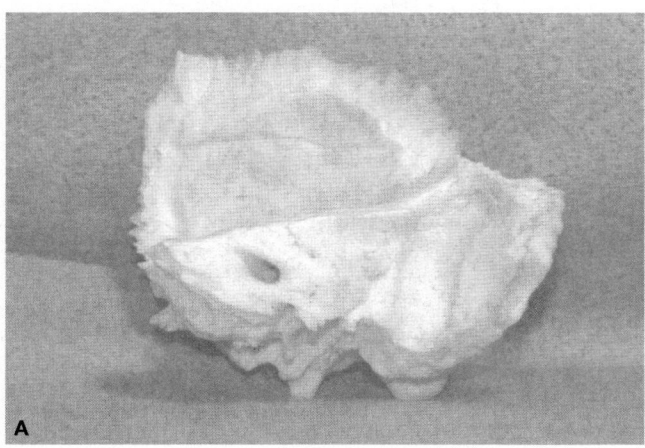

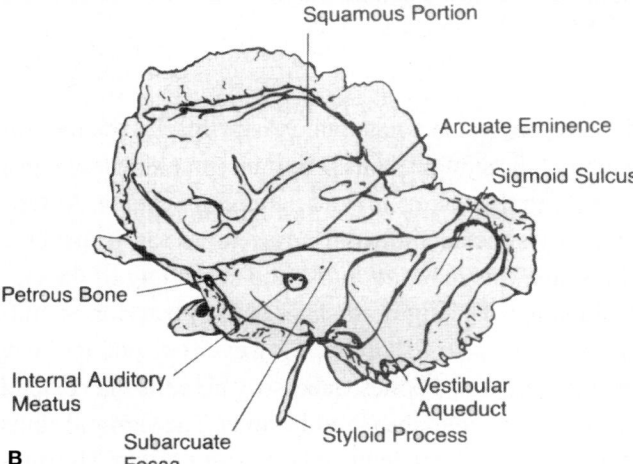

Squamous Portion

Arcuate Eminence

Sigmoid Sulcus

Petrous Bone

Internal Auditory
Meatus

Vestibular
Aqueduct

Subarcuate
Fossa

Styloid Process

B

Figure A–3 Posterior surface anatomy: the sigmoid sulcus forms a prominent depression on this surface. Anterior to the midportion of the sigmoid sinus is a lip of bone (operculum). Beneath the operculum is the opening for the vestibular aqueduct. Further anteriorly lies the internal auditory canal (IAC).

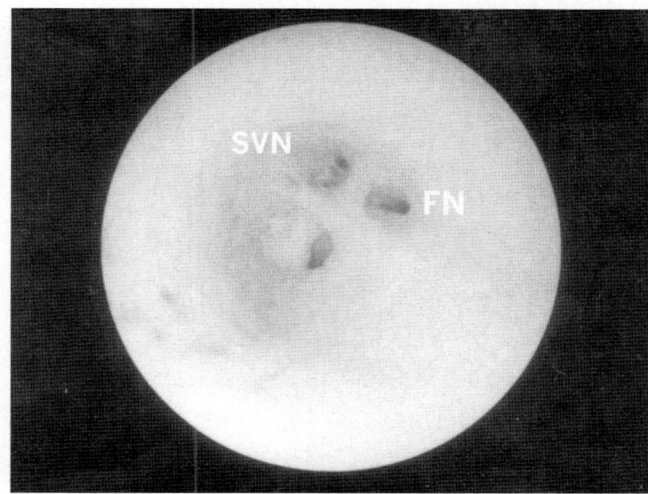

SVN

FN

Figure A–4 Endoscopic view of the left internal auditory canal (IAC). The transverse crest (crista falciformis) divides the lateral fundus of the IAC into superior and inferior compartments. The superior compartment is further divided by the vertical crest (Bill's bar), which separates the facial nerve anteriorly from the superior vestibular nerve posteriorly. The inferior compartment contains the cochlear nerve anteriorly and the inferior vestibular nerve posteriorly.

which is occupied by the jugular vein, and an anteromedial pars nervosa, which is traversed by the glossopharyngeal, vagus, and spinal accessory nerves. The hypoglossal nerve exits the occipital bone by the hypoglossal canal, medial to the pars nervosa of the jugular foramen. Lateral to the jugular foramen is the styloid process. Immediately posterior to the styloid process is the stylomastoid foramen, by which the facial nerve exits the temporal bone. Medial to the mastoid tip is the digastric groove for the posterior belly of the digastric muscle. The triangular opening of the cochlear aqueduct is located medial to the jugular foramen. The inferior tympanic canaliculus runs in the jugulocarotid crest and carries the inferior tympanic artery (a branch of the ascending pharyngeal artery) and the tympanic branch of the glossopharyngeal nerve (Jacobson's nerve) into the tympanic cavity (Figure A–5).

Anterior Surface

The petrous apex is the wedge of bone that separates the greater wing of the sphenoid from the occipital bone. The most prominent feature of this surface is the internal carotid foramen, through which the carotid artery exits the temporal bone. The impression for the trigeminal ganglion is located on the lateral surface of the petrous apex. The semicanal for the tensor tympani is lateral to the carotid canal; the bony portion of the eustachian

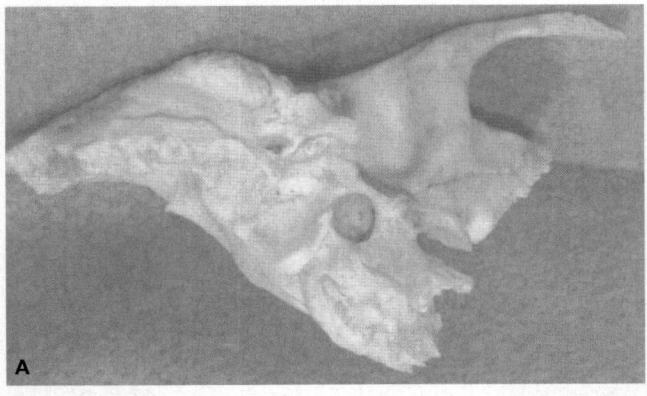

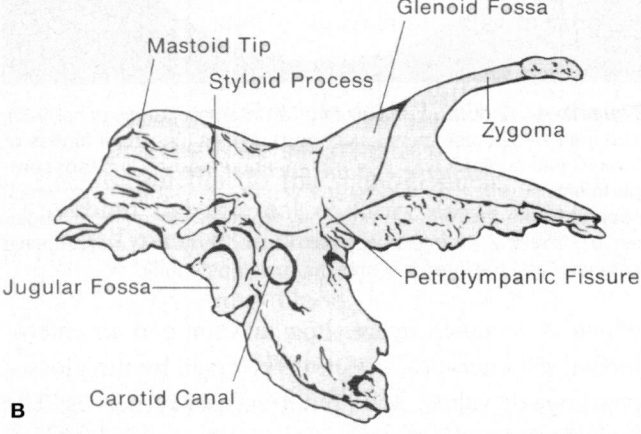

Figure A–5   Inferior surface anatomy: crucial relationships here for the skull base surgeon include the jugular fossa, stylomastoid foramen, and carotid canal.

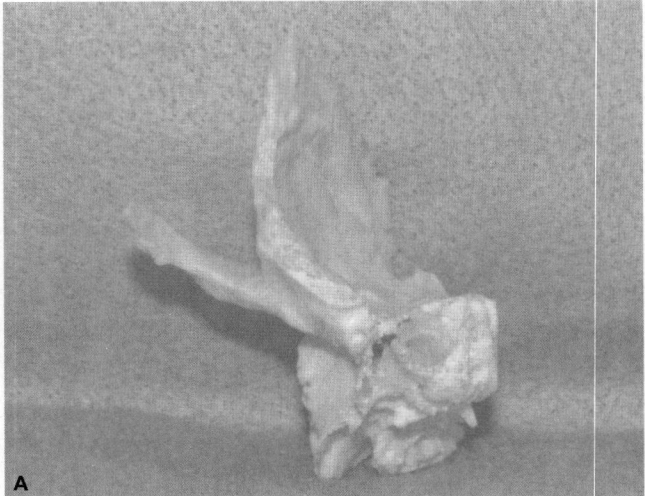

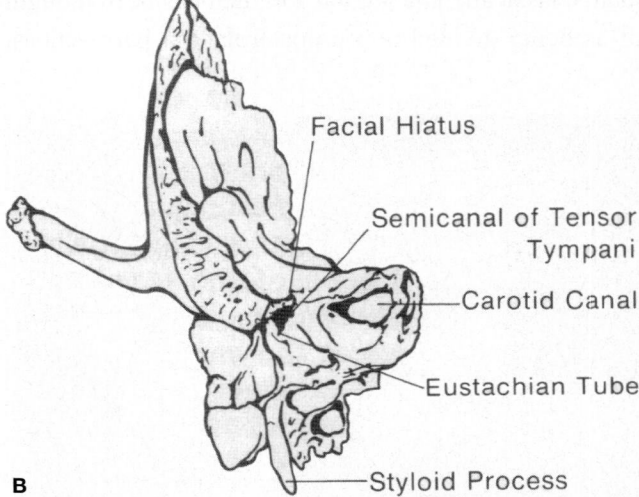

Figure A–6   Anterior surface anatomy: note the relationships of the facial hiatus, carotid artery, semicanal of the tensor tympani, and eustachian tube.

tube runs inferior and parallel to the tensor tympani muscle. The thin medial wall of the eustachian tube forms the lateral wall of the carotid canal and is frequently dehiscent. Thus, the carotid canal is vulnerable to injury in the course of surgical manipulations in the anterior tympanic cavity and in the medial wall of the eustachian tube (Figure A–6).

Vascular Anatomy

Several large dural venous sinuses are intimately associated with the temporal bone and comprise the principal venous drainage of the brain and cranial vault. The superior sagittal sinus and straight sinus merge at the internal occipital protuberance. The right and left transverse sinuses extend beyond this junction. The right transverse sinus is primarily the continuation of the superior sagittal sinus and thus is generally larger in diameter than the left transverse sinus, which is primarily the continuation of the straight sinus. The transverse sinuses lie just inferior to the tentorium and parallel its course. Anteriorly, the superior petrosal sinus joins the transverse sinus, and this junction marks the beginning of the sigmoid sinus. The sigmoid sinus is the posterior boundary of the mastoid cavity. However, in particularly well-pneumatized bones, accessory air cells may extend posteriorly beyond the sigmoid sinus. The sigmoid sinus is most superficial (lateral) at its superior origin. The middle fossa dura approximates the superior portion of the sigmoid sinus at the sinodural angle of Citelli. From the sinodural angle, the sigmoid sinus runs inferiorly and medially, with a variable relationship to the bony labyrinth. At its inferior extent, the sigmoid sinus rises to the jugular bulb. The jugular bulb exhibits considerable variability in its height, location, and relationship to the labyrinth, internal auditory canal (IAC), and tympanic cavity. The inferior petrosal sinus arises from the medial aspect of the jugular bulb and runs anteromedially to the cavernous sinus. The jugular vein exits the skull through the jugular foramen, accompanied by the vagus, glossopharyngeal, and spinal accessory nerves.

Emissary veins are drainage routes of the dural venous sinuses through the skull that communicate with the superficial veins of the scalp. A fairly constant emissary vein, the mastoid emissary vein, can be found at the junction of the temporal and occipital bones and usually communicates with the occipital or postauricular vein.

The internal carotid artery also travels through the temporal bone. Its entrance, the external carotid foramen, is medial to the styloid process and anterior to the jugular foramen. The internal carotid artery travels superiorly until it encounters the dense bone of the cochlea, at which point it makes a 90-degree bend to run anteriorly and medially. The carotid canal forms the medial wall of the eustachian tube; the internal carotid artery may be dehiscent and vulnerable to injury here. Rarely, the internal carotid artery may encroach on the tympanic cavity proper.

Cranial Nerves

The majority of the cranial nerves are in close anatomic relationship to the temporal bone. Knowledge of their location is not only important in surgical dissection but also serves the astute clinician as a diagnostic aid when cranial nerve deficits are encountered.

Fifth Cranial (Trigeminal) Nerve

The trigeminal (gasserian, semilunar) ganglion lies on the lateral aspect of the anterior petrous apex and indents its surface. This nerve supplies sensory and motor innervation to the face. The sensory root (portia major) pierces the lateral surface of the pons at the superior aspect of the cerebellopontine angle. The first two divisions of the trigeminal nerve, the ophthalmic and the maxillary, are sensory only. The motor branch (portia minor) lies medial to the sensory branch and joins the third division, the

mandibular, to supply the muscles of mastication; a small branch supplies the tensor tympani muscle within the middle ear.

Sixth Cranial (Abducens) Nerve

The abducens nerve innervates the ipsilateral lateral rectus muscle. It exits the brainstem from a groove between the superior medulla and inferior pons and then travels through Dorello's canal, which is formed by the petroclinoid (Gruber's) ligament and petrous apex. Inflammatory or neoplastic lesions in the petrous apex can present with lateral rectus palsy.

Seventh Cranial (Facial) Nerve

Preganglionic parasympathetic fibers destined for the pterygopalatine and submandibular ganglions and special sensory (taste) fibers comprise the nervus intermedius. This nerve joins the larger, motor root to form the facial nerve. In the cerebellopontine angle, the nervus intermedius lies between the facial and cochlear nerves. The facial nerve enters the temporal bone through the IAC, which it exits at the meatal foramen to travel anteriorly to the geniculate ganglion. This segment of the facial nerve, the labyrinthine segment, is the narrowest portion (0.61 to 0.68 mm) of the facial canal. At the geniculate ganglion, the GPN travels anteriorly, carrying parasympathetic fibers to the pterygopalatine ganglion. The main trunk of the facial nerve turns posteriorly, inferiorly, and laterally to continue in its tympanic (horizontal) segment. The nerve continues in this course until it turns inferiorly at the lateral semicircular canal (LSCC; the second genu), marking the terminus of the tympanic segment and the beginning of the mastoid segment. The facial nerve continues to travel inferiorly, posteriorly, and laterally until it exits the temporal bone at the stylomastoid foramen. For the majority of its course, the mastoid segment lies medial to the plane of the tympanic annulus; however, the nerve can cross the annular plane at any point as it travels inferiorly. Although the chorda tympani nerve usually separates from the mastoid segment of the facial nerve a few millimeters superior to the stylomastoid foramen, the exact location of this separation is quite variable. The chorda tympani nerve traverses the tympanic cavity to carry parasympathetic fibers to the submandibular ganglion and taste fibers to the anterior tongue. The motor component of the facial nerve supplies the stapedius, posterior digastric, and stylohyoid muscles, as well as the muscles of facial expression.

Eighth Cranial (Cochleovestibular) Nerve

The axons of the cochlear division of the eighth nerve arise from the bipolar cells of the spiral ganglion in the cochlea. From this ganglion, the fibers pass through the modiolus and the foramina of the tractus spiralis foraminosus and into the anterior-inferior portion of the fundus of the IAC, at which point they fuse to form the cochlear nerve. The vestibular portion of the eighth nerve divides into a superior and an inferior division in the IAC. The cell bodies for these nerves are in Scarpa's ganglion, also located in the canal. The superior vestibular nerve innervates the utricle, the SSCC and LSCC, and the superior saccule. The inferior vestibular nerve innervates the posterior semicircular canal and the inferior saccule.

Ninth Cranial (Glossopharyngeal) Nerve

The glossopharyngeal nerve exits the upper lateral medulla and passes through the jugular foramen, accompanied by the vagus and spinal accessory nerves. It carries preganglionic parasympathetic fibers to the otic ganglion and taste fibers from the posterior third of the tongue, general sensory afferents from the pharyngeal mucosa, and motor fibers to the stylopharyngeus muscle. After exiting the skull, the glossopharyngeal nerve descends between the internal jugular vein and the internal carotid artery and behind the styloid muscles before dividing into its several branches. One branch, the tympanic (Jacobson's nerve), is of particular interest to the otologist; this branch re-enters the temporal bone through the inferior tympanic canaliculus and emerges onto the promontory to merge with sympathetic fibers at the tympanic plexus, forming the lesser petrosal nerve. At the cochleariform process, the lesser petrosal nerve travels medial to the semicanal of the tensor tympani muscle to emerge on the floor of the middle cranial fossa.

Tenth Cranial (Vagus) Nerve

The vagus nerve is the longest of the cranial nerves. It arises as 8 to 10 rootlets from the medulla oblongata; these roots unite into the vagus nerve, which passes beneath the flocculus to the jugular foramen and exits the skull within a dural sheath shared with the spinal accessory nerve. Beyond its jugular and nodose ganglia, the vagus nerve travels through the neck and into the chest within the carotid sheath, between the internal jugular vein and common carotid artery. The vagus nerve carries sensory fibers from the hypopharynx and the larynx; its motor fibers supply the pharyngeal plexus and larynx. Additional sensory, motor, and parasympathetic fibers supply the alimentary tract to the splenic flexure of the colon.

Eleventh Cranial (Spinal Accessory) Nerve

Cranial and spinal rootlets combine to form the eleventh nerve. The spinal component extends to the level of C5 or C6. These rootlets ascend through the foramen magnum into the cranial cavity, cross the occipital bone, and exit through the jugular foramen. The spinal accessory nerve innervates the sternocleidomastoid and trapezius muscles.

Twelfth Cranial (Hypoglossal) Nerve

The twelfth nerve arises from the medulla and exits the brainstem as a series of rootlets located between the pyramid and olive. These rootlets fuse to form the hypoglossal nerve that exits the posterior cranial fossa through the hypoglossal canal of the occipital bone. The nerve then travels between the internal jugular vein and the internal carotid artery. Superior to the carotid bifurcation, the hypoglossal nerve passes lateral to both the internal and external carotid arteries and subsequently curves upward to innervate the intrinsic muscles of the tongue.

Tympanic Cavity

The tympanic cavity is divided into three portions: the attic (epitympanum), which lies above the tympanic annulus; the tympanic cavity proper (mesotympanum); and the hypotympanum, which is below the level of the tympanic annulus.

Superiorly, the middle ear cavity is separated from the brain by the tegmen tympani. Inferiorly, a thin bony covering separates the tympanic cavity from the jugular bulb. The tympanic membrane laterally delimits the tympanic cavity, and the inner ear is its medial boundary.

In adults, the tympanic membrane lies at a 45-degree angle to the long axis of the petrous pyramid. The ring of bone within which the tympanic annulus sits, the tympanic sulcus, is deficient superiorly at the notch of Rivinus. Two bands (the anterior and posterior malleal folds) extend from the notch and attach to the lateral process of the malleus. This notch and the malleal folds divide the tympanic membrane into two portions: superiorly, the pars flaccida (Shrapnell's membrane), and inferiorly, the main portion of the tympanic membrane, the pars tensa. The pars tensa averages 10 mm in diameter. The most medial portion of the eardrum, the umbo, lies at the tip of the handle (manubrium) of the malleus (Figure A–7).

Mesotympanum

The basal turn of the cochlea, in the form of its promontory, forms the majority of the medial wall of the mesotympanum. The tympanic plexus lies on the promontory. Superior to the promontory is the oval window (fenestra vestibuli), occupied by the footplate of the stapes. The round window (fenestra cochleae), sealed by the round window membrane (secondary tympanic membrane), is just inferior and leads to the scala tympani.

The tensor tympani tendon exits its semicanal at the cochleariform (spoon-shaped) process and inserts onto the malleus. Superior to the cochleariform process, the facial nerve makes a sharp bend (first genu) posteriorly and superiorly toward the IAC. The area superior to the cochleariform process approximates the position of the geniculate ganglion on the superior aspect of the temporal bone. From the cochleariform process, the facial nerve courses posteriorly and slightly inferiorly in the tympanic (horizontal) segment of its fallopian canal. The horizontal segment ends at the second genu of the facial nerve, which curves posterior and superior to the oval window and anteroinferior to the LSCC. The horizontal segment of the facial nerve and the cochleariform process medially define the superior extent of the mesotympanum.

The chorda tympani nerve enters the tympanic cavity through its posterior iter, which usually is located lateral to the pyramidal eminence and medial to the annulus, at the level of the round window and cochlear aqueduct; the facial recess lies between the facial and chorda tympani nerves. The chorda tympani nerve passes lateral to the long process of the incus and medial to the neck of the malleus before it exits the tympanic cavity through its anterior iter (the canal of Huguier) and the petrotympanic fissure.

Traveling along the posterior wall of the tympanic cavity, the first structure encountered below the posterior end of the tympanic facial nerve is the pyramidal eminence,

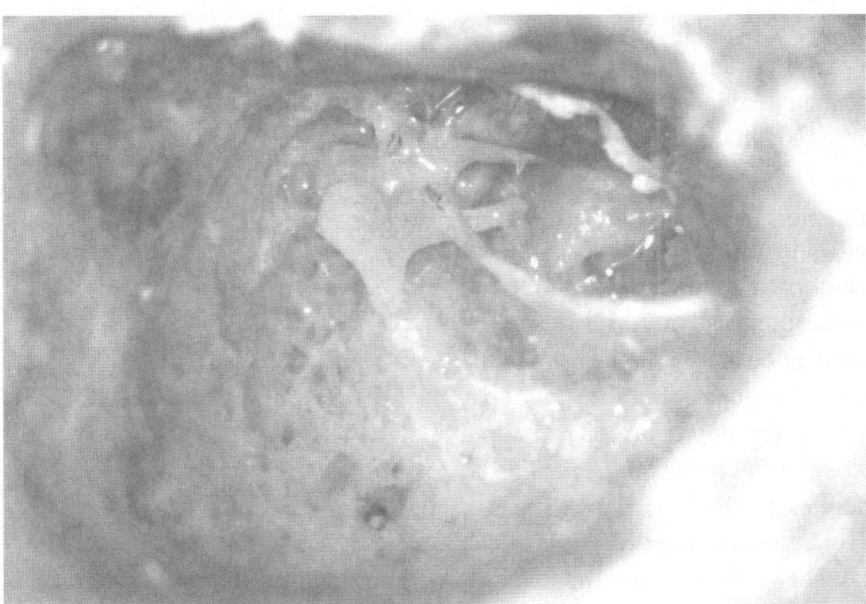

Figure A–7 Surgeon's view of the ossicles and middle ear with the external auditory canal removed. Note the positions of the umbo, chorda tympani, and the relationship between the lateral semicircular canal, incus, and horizontal facial canal.

traversed by the tendon of the stapedius muscle. The sinus tympani lies in the posterior mesotympanum, medial to the pyramidal eminence. The medial wall of the posterior mesotympanum is divided by two ridges, the ponticulus and the subiculum. The ponticulus runs from the oval window to the sinus tympani and defines its superior extent. The subiculum defines the inferior extent of the sinus tympani as it runs from the round window to the sinus.

Jacobson's nerve (the tympanic branch of the glossopharyngeal nerve) is a landmark on the promontory of the cochlea and "points" to the cochleariform process. As the facial nerve runs immediately superior to the cochleariform process, Jacobson's nerve can be used to locate the facial nerve.

The semicanal of the tensor tympani muscle is located in the anterior wall of the middle ear cleft and runs almost parallel to the eustachian tube. The tensor tympani muscle originates from the cartilaginous portion of the eustachian tube, passes along the cochleariform process, and inserts via its tendon, on the manubrium of the malleus. The eustachian tube connects the tympanic cavity with the nasopharynx, allowing passage of air between the two. In the adult, the upper one-third of the eustachian tube is bony, whereas the lower two-thirds is cartilaginous. In addition, the eustachian tube follows an inferiorly angled course to the nasopharynx. In infants and children, a greater proportion of the tube is cartilaginous; the tube is much smaller in diameter and follows a more horizontal course. These anatomic differences are thought to underlie the increased incidence of eustachian tube dysfunction in infants and children.

Epitympanum

The epitympanum (attic) leads to the aditus ad antrum and the mastoid antrum, the first area to be aerated in the process of pneumatization. The antrum leads to the remainder of the mastoid air cell system. The head of the malleus and the body of the incus are in the epitympanum. The fossa incudis in the posterior epitympanum houses the short process of the incus and serves as an important surgical landmark for the facial nerve. The cog, a bony projection from the tegmen superior to the cochleariform process, serves as an approximate landmark for the facial nerve. The cog also separates the anterior epitympanic space (the supratubal recess) from the remainder of the epitympanum.

Hypotympanum

The most variable region of the tympanic cavity is the hypotympanum. The depth of the tympanic cavity is largely determined by the height of the jugular bulb as the anterior jugular bulb forms the inferior and posterior borders of the hypotympanum. A more inferiorly placed jugular bulb creates a deeper hypotympanic space. Often the bone overlying the jugular bulb is thin or absent and the bulb can be visualized otoscopically as a purple, retrotympanic mass. Anteriorly, the carotid canal runs in the floor of the hypotympanum. The promontory delimits the hypotympanum superiorly. The infralabyrinthine cell tract runs inferior to the cochlea, between the jugular bulb and carotid artery, and can be used as a route to the petrous apex.

Auditory Ossicles

The ossicular chain consists of three bones connected by delicate articulations and ligaments. Passing from lateral to medial, the first ossicle encountered is the malleus, which has a head, neck, and three processes (anterior, lateral, and the manubrium). The head articulates with the body of the incus in the epitympanum. The tympanic membrane attaches to the malleal periosteum at the short process and at the umbo (the tip of the malleus). The incus consists of a body and two processes, short and long. On the anterior surface of the body of the incus, there is a facet that articulates with the head of the malleus by a synovial joint. The short process of the incus is tethered in the fossa incudis by the posterior incudal ligament. The long process, by means of its lenticular process, articulates with the stapes. The stapes comprises a footplate, anterior and posterior crura, a neck, and a head (capitulum). The stapedius tendon attaches to the neck. The footplate is secured in the oval window by the annular ligament (Figure A–8).

DISSECTION GUIDE

Temporal Bone Station Setup

The temporal bone dissection laboratory should provide a comfortable working space that is easy to set up and clean, which facilitates frequent use of the laboratory for dissection. Ideally, the equipment within the

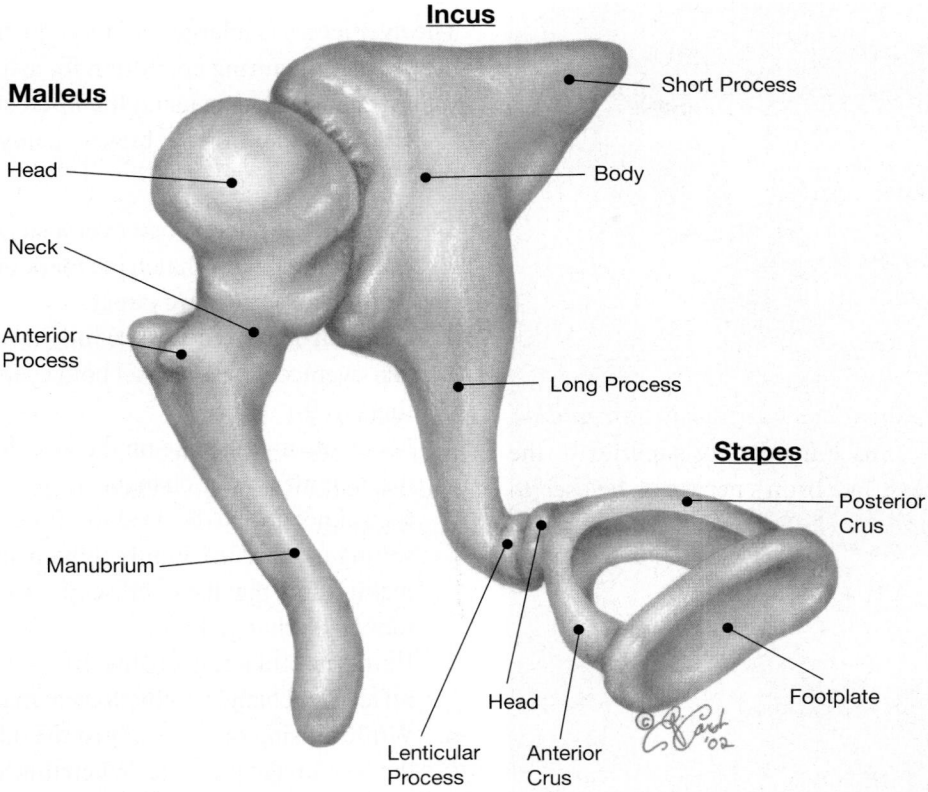

Figure A–8 Artist's depiction of the auditory ossicles under high magnification.

laboratory should closely resemble what is used in the operating room to simulate the operative experience realistically. The space itself should be well ventilated and lit and provide sinks for cleaning the equipment. Any flat working space can serve as a dissection station. Custom-built tables provide amenities such as integrated suction and water lines, electrical outlets, and drawers and cabinets for storage. A comfortable, adjustable chair enhances the ergonomics of the dissection station, which, as in the operating room, facilitates prolonged work without undue fatigue. Personal protective equipment such as gowns, masks, and gloves should be readily available. A temporal bone holder is essential to secure the bone during dissection. A holder that allows for movement in several planes, such as the House-Urban temporal bone holder, more closely simulates the surgical environment than a stationary holder and is thus preferred. Considerable additional instrumentation is essential and should be kept within the laboratory separate from that used in the operating room. Periosteal elevators, dissecting scissors, and scalpel handles and blades are useful in removing soft tissue prior to dissection. Middle ear

instruments, such as canal elevators, picks, alligators, cup forceps, and microscissors, are also required. Various sizes of plain and irrigating suction tips are essential to the dissection (Figures A–9 and A–10).

Operating Microscope

Carl Zeiss Inc (Oberkochen, Germany), working with Dr. Horst Wullstein, introduced the first operating microscope for otologic surgery in the late 1950s. Shortly afterward, Drs. Shambaugh and Kinney brought the first operating microscopes to the United States and, along with many other otologic surgeons, helped to popularize their use. Since the 1960s, operating microscopes have become an indispensable part of ear surgery. The microscope provides controlled magnification, stereoscopic vision, and coaxial illumination and protects the eyes during dissection. Modern amenities, such as video cameras and observer heads, expand the utility of the microscope for teaching and mainly were a result of the engineering genius of Jack Urban working with Drs. Howard and William House. Large, floor-mounted microscopes, such as those used in the operating room, are impractical for

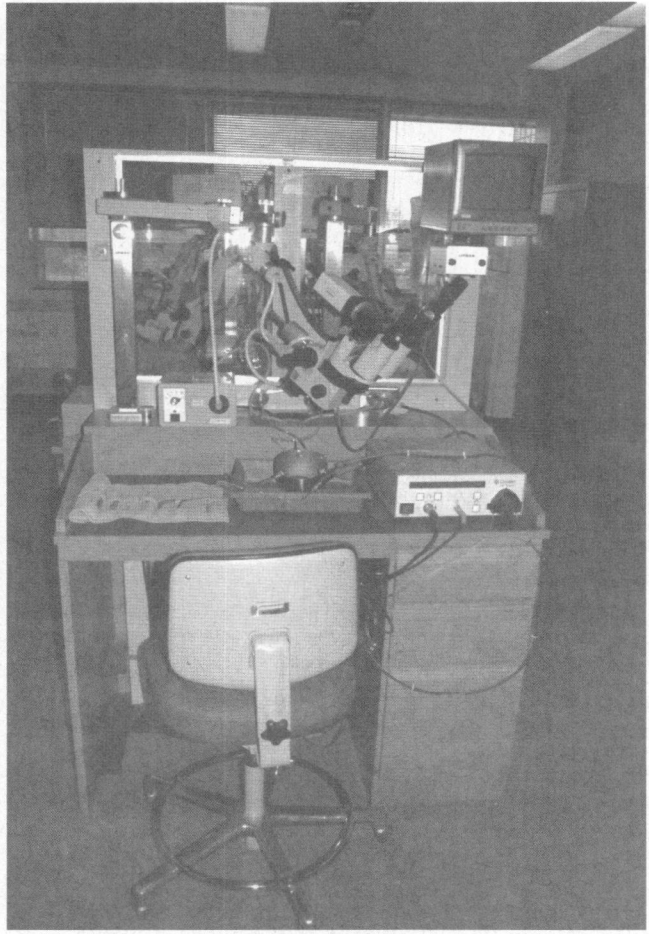

Figure A–9 Temporal bone dissection station at the Michigan Ear Institute depicting a microscope with an observer arm and a video monitor, an electric otologic drill system, a temporal bone holder, and a selection of instruments.

the laboratory. Many manufacturers provide microscopes that can be mounted to the workbench. The microscope selected should provide bright illumination, a variety of magnification settings, and adjustable binocular eyepieces. The eyepieces should offer adjustments for interpupillary distance and diopter setting. Optional items include exchangeable objective lenses with differing focal lengths or a variable focal length system and beam splitters to allow for the placement of teaching heads or cameras (Figure A–11).

The eyepieces contribute to the total magnification and compensate for operator visual acuity differences. It is very important that the eyepieces be correctly set and then locked, ensuring that the microscope is par focal. The major cause of eye fatigue, loss of convergence, and excessive refocusing is improper eyepiece settings.

The eyepiece has a large diopter adjustment range, but the operator requiring correction for astigmatism should wear eyeglasses when using the microscope.

Par focal vision is achieved using the following procedures*:

1. Position the microscope over a steady flat surface.
2. Make a small crosshatch (#) mark on white paper to be used as a focusing target.
3. Confirm that eyepieces are fully inserted into binocular eyepiece tubes and set both eyepiece diopter settings to 0.
4. Focus the microscope on the crosshatch target with the magnification changer at maximum. The fine focus knobs are to be used for this setting. When this setting is achieved, lightly tighten all tension knobs, making sure that the microscope is stable and has not moved or changed focus.
5. Being careful not to change focus, revolve the magnification changer to the lowest magnification.
6. While closing one eye, adjust the other eyepiece for the best image possible. When this has been accomplished for both eyes, tighten the diopter locks and make a note of the right and left eye settings for future use.
7. Adjust the eyepiece interpupillary distance for convergence.
8. To ensure that the microscope is par focal, revolve the magnification changer through each setting while viewing the target through the eyepieces.

Drill System and Burs

The drill is an important instrument for temporal bone dissection. Two equally important factors, the drill system and the drill bits, determine the ease and safety of bone removal. Modern, high-speed otologic drill systems allow for rapid, safe bone removal with relative ease. Both gas-driven and electric systems are used in the operating room, and each has its advantages and advocates. Ideally, a drill should be easy to handle, lightweight, and provide high speed and power, with little torque of the handpiece on initiation or cessation of drilling. Some surgeons prefer a drill bur to have a forward and a reverse mode.

---

*Courtesy of Larry K. Kleinberg from Urban Engineering.

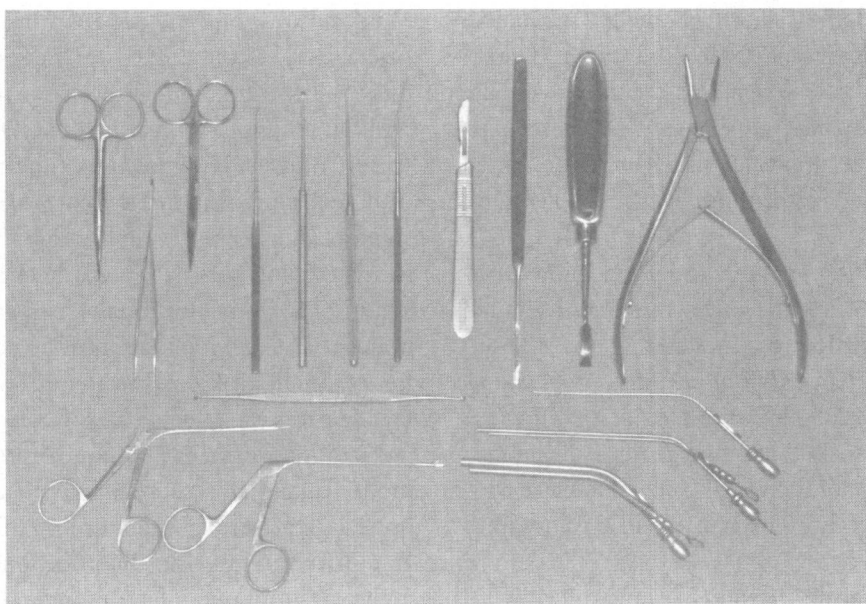

Figure A–10 In addition to the drill system, a variety of instruments are useful in the laboratory including plain and suction irrigators, forceps, scalpel handle, periosteal elevators, a selection of otologic picks, curette, and alligator scissors and forceps.

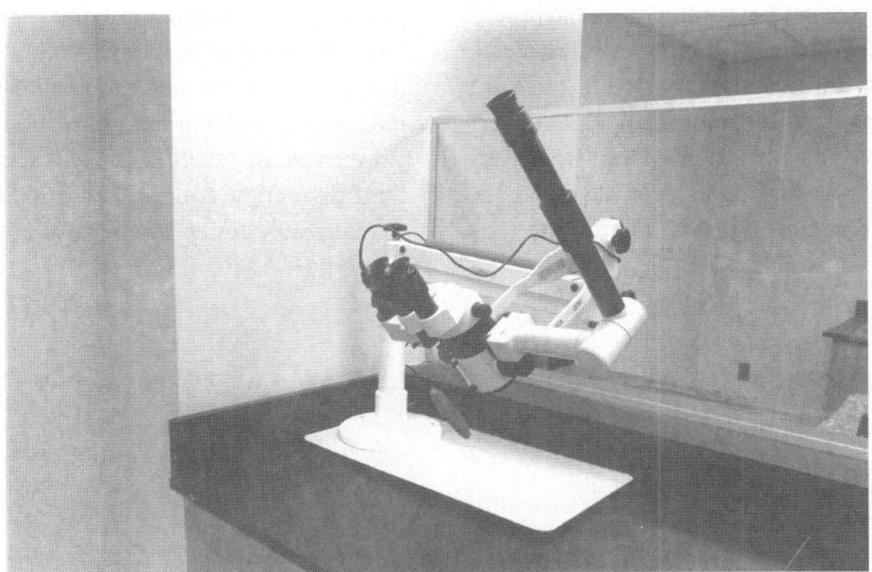

Figure A–11 Leica™ temporal bone dissection microscope with a monocular observer arm and a video camera.

Gas-driven drills traditionally have provided more power and speed, which helps in more rapid bone removal. The primary disadvantages of gas-driven systems are the need for dedicated high-pressure lines in the operating room (or compressed gas cylinders), the bulkiness of the delivery cord, and the noise level of the device. Electric drill systems allow for rapid setup, a thinner delivery cord, lower noise level, and ready power availability. The limiting factors of electric drills have been their lack of speed and torque, resulting in less efficient bone removal. Also, the handpieces tended to become hot during heavy use, further impeding dissection by requiring pauses, while the drill cooled. Recent advances in electric motor design have overcome these limitations. Electrically powered otologic drill systems are now available that provide speed and torque closely equaling that of gas-powered drills. Further innovations such as water-cooled drills enable prolonged use without overheating (Figure A–12).

The otologic drill is a versatile tool that enables millimeter-precise dissection of bone while leaving intact delicate underlying structures. Factors that can be modulated during drilling include bur size and type, speed, direction, and pressure. The specifics of using these variables are discussed below, but general guidelines are discussed here. A thorough familiarity with these variables must be gained through practice in the temporal bone laboratory.

A large bur contacts a greater surface area than a smaller bur. Thus, larger burs are generally more efficient in bone removal. Furthermore, the large surface area distributes the pressure of the bur tip, thus reducing the likelihood of the bur penetrating and damaging underlying structures. Hence, not only are larger burs more efficient, they are also "safer" and, accordingly, should be used whenever practical. The danger of larger burs relates to their limitation of visibility and the possibility of unintentionally contacting surfaces with the bur. As experience is gained, larger burs can be used more frequently.

Cutting, diamond stone, and "rough cut" diamond burs are currently available. Cutting burs provide the most rapid removal of bone but are more likely to injure soft tissue and fracture thin bone. Flute design is important; there is an optimal interflute space that allows a safe cut without clogging with bone dust. Diamond burs have a variety of uses. Their primary function is in the removal of bone approximating delicate structures, such as the sigmoid sinus, dura, or facial nerve. They can also be used to smooth and polish bony surfaces after dissection with a cutting bur. An additional use is to stop bleeding from bone surfaces, which can best be achieved with a gentle, pushing stroke and minimal or no irrigation. With practice, this can effectively stop bleeding from small temporal bone vessels. Diamond burs require relatively more irrigation than cutting burs. The irrigation cools the bone and bur, preventing burning of tissue; without sufficient irrigation, the diamond bur quickly becomes clogged with bone dust, dramatically reducing its usefulness. A third type of bit, the rough cut diamond, contains coarse particles of diamond stone. This bit can be used as an intermediate between the easy bone removal of a cutting bur and the relative safety of a diamond bur.

Drill speed is also an important variable. High speed equates to more efficient bone removal with less pressure, resulting in less operator fatigue. Higher speed also increases the likelihood that the drill will "run" and result in unintentional dissection and potential injury. Slower speeds result in improved control but less efficient dissection and greater drill pressure, potentially increasing operator fatigue. As a general rule, slower

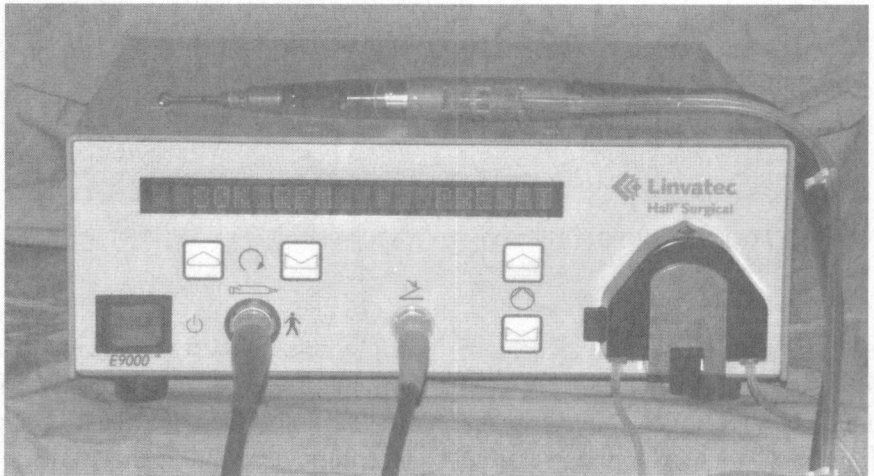

Figure A–12   Hall™ Linvatec otologic drill system and power supply. This electric drill provides a maximum speed of 80,000 rpm and has a unique water-cooling system.

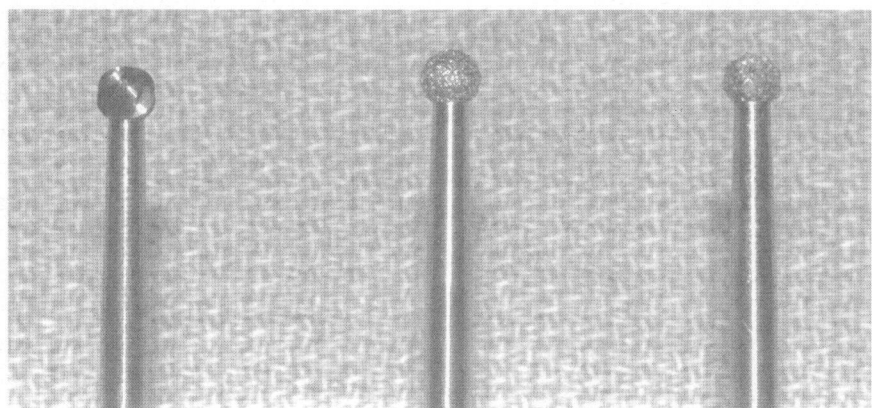

Figure A–13 Otologic burs, both cutting (*left*) and diamond (*middle*) styles, are available in a variety of sizes. The right bur is a rough-cut diamond; note the coarse texture.

speeds are best used for the final removal of bone over delicate structures and in confined spaces (Figure A–13).

DISSECTION MANUAL

Intact Canal Wall Mastoidectomy

The simple mastoidectomy is the basic approach to the temporal bone. As in soft tissue surgery, an intact canal wall mastoidectomy should provide adequate exposure to the deeper structures of interest, which are the antrum, the LSCC, and the incus. However, unlike soft tissue surgery, the structures of interest are located within dense bone that varies in thickness, shape, and pneumatization. Furthermore, other vital structures that occupy variable positions in the bone (eg, the sigmoid sinus and tegmen) can affect dissection and exposure. Therefore, the initial objective is to perform rapid, safe removal of bone to permit visualization of the antrum, LSCC, and incus.

Opening the Mastoid Antrum

After reflection of the soft tissues, the following landmarks are identified on the lateral surface of the bone: the root of the zygoma, the mastoid tip, and the external auditory canal (EAC). Using the largest cutting bur practical, a firm stroke is drawn posteriorly from the root of the zygoma paralleling the temporal line. By drawing the bur toward the surgeon, firm pressure can be applied in a controlled fashion. This cut roughly paral-

lels the middle fossa dura and defines the superior limit of the dissection. The next stroke is perpendicular to the first and tangential to the EAC. This cut defines the

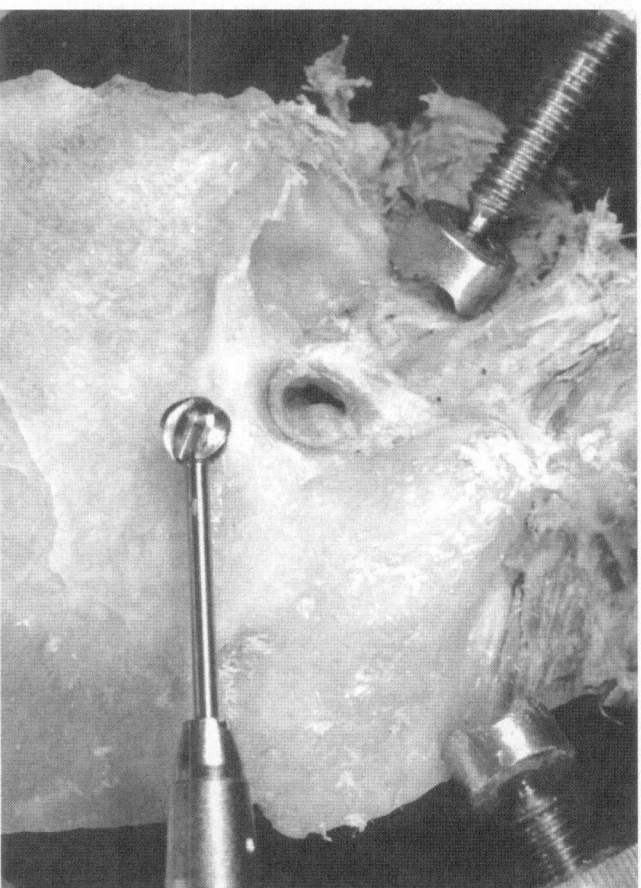

Figure A–14 Dried temporal bone specimen placed in the surgical position within the temporal bone holder.

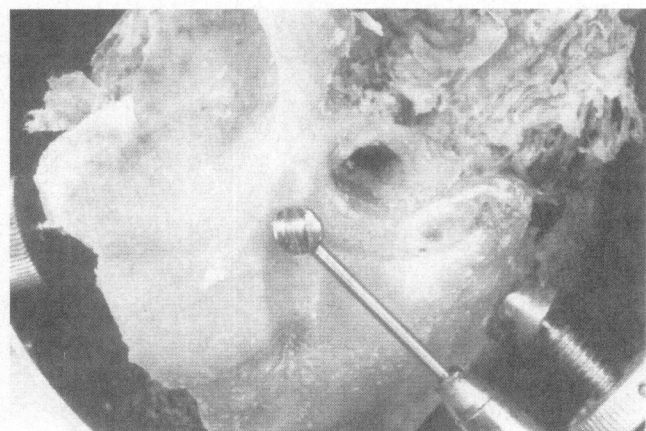

Figure A–15 Initial two cuts along the temporal line and tangential to the external auditory canal.

anterior limit of dissection. As the area of dissection is roughly triangular in shape, only the posterior boundary remains to be defined. The extent of the posterior boundary varies depending on the position of the sigmoid sinus (Figures A–14 and A–15).

As the dissection progresses, the surgeon identifies the tegmen mastoideum, the sinodural angle, and the area of the sigmoid sinus. Often adequate exposure can be obtained without skeletonizing the sigmoid sinus. The mastoid cortex is removed in a systematic, saucerizing (ie, eliminating bony overhangs) fashion. The surgeon may encounter a bony plate (Körner's petrosquamous septum) of variable prominence. The antrum is the next landmark of importance and displays considerable interindividual variability in size.

The antrum is our personal most valuable "safe" landmark as it opens to the important landmarks for otologic surgery: medially, the compact bone of the LSSC that allows exposure of the fossa incudis; the epitympanum anteriorly and superiorly; and the external genu of the facial nerve. The dense bone of the LSSC extends posteroinferiorly to the posterior semicircular canal.

To open the antrum, we use a small bur and, staying superior, dissect from medial to lateral to saucerize the antrum and visualize the LSCC and the body of the incus (Figure A–16).

Fossa Incudis, Facial Recess, and Facial Nerve

The next exposure to be mastered through dissection of the temporal bone is the facial recess approach. The boundaries of this triangularly shaped region are the

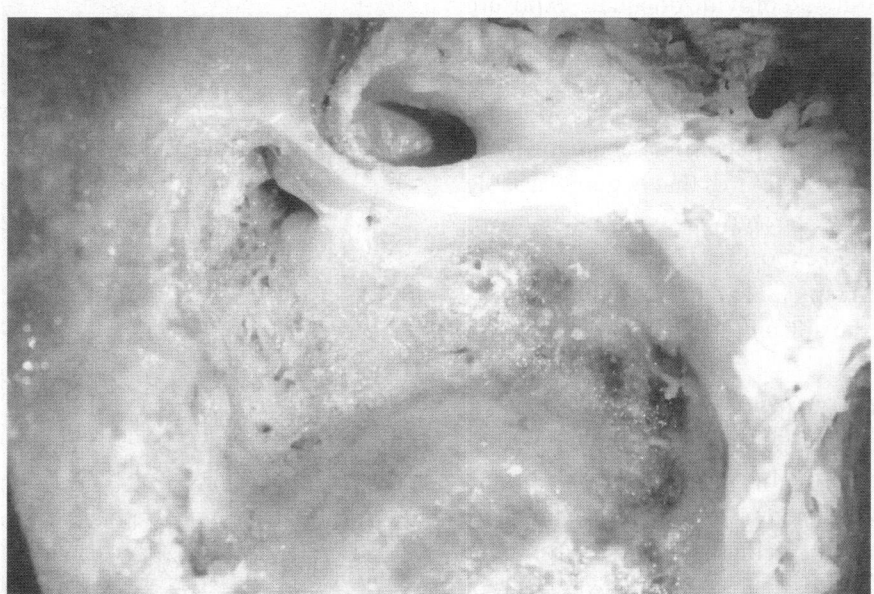

Figure A–16 Basic mastoidectomy completed. Initial cuts define the superior and anterior borders of the dissection. The posterior dissection is continued until the sigmoid sinus is identified. Further bone removal continues medially until the lateral semicircular canal and incus are identified.

facial nerve medially, the chorda tympani nerve laterally, and the fossa incudis superiorly. Opening the facial recess allows for positive and safe identification of the facial nerve as well as access to the tympanic cavity.

Dissection begins just inferior to the short process of the incus, in the plane of the incus, generally using a 3-mm diamond bur, and is carried inferiorly, paralleling the vertical segment of the facial nerve. Drilling is *never* perpendicular to the facial nerve (or, for that matter, any structure one wishes to preserve). With the high-intensity illumination and magnification afforded by the modern operating microscope, the surgeon can detect vital structures, such as the facial nerve, while a protective bony covering remains. Preferred surgical technique reveals anatomic structures and does not penetrate them. Since the tympanic segment of the facial nerve is medial to the incus, safe dissection is in the plane of the incus. Even in very sclerotic bones, a "herald" air cell is generally encountered just lateral to the second genu of the facial nerve. Once the facial and chorda tympani nerves are identified, smaller burs can be used to open the recess fully (Figures A–17 and A–18).

At the completion of the facial recess approach, the pyramidal process, stapedial tendon, stapes superstruc-

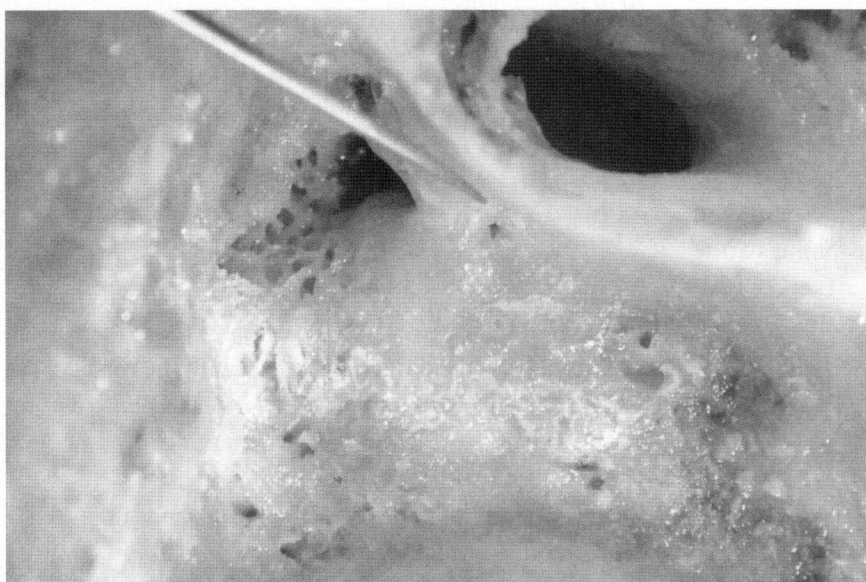

Figure A–17 Dissection inferior to the lateral semicircular canal and lateral to the incus develops the facial recess. Here the probe identifies the "herald" air cell that can be found even in very sclerotic bones.

Figure A–18 Facial recesses fully developed between the facial and chorda tympani nerves.

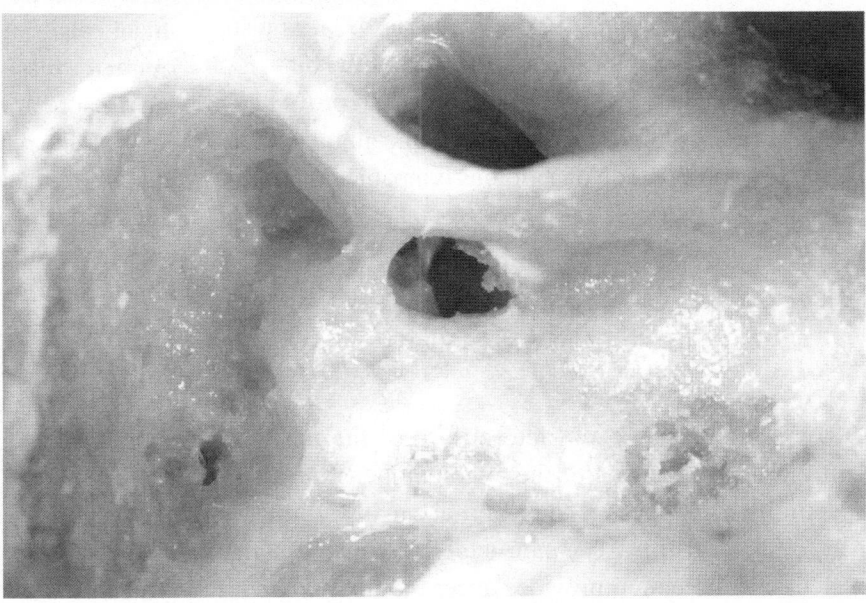

ture, long process of the incus, and oval and round windows can be visualized. This exposure provides access for dissection of cholesteatoma from the stapes and oval window, although the sinus tympani remains hidden. This approach also allows for accurate disarticulation of the incudostapedial joint and is used to provide access to the round window for cochlear implantation.

Caution: Care must be exercised when drilling close to the incus in the presence of an intact ossicular chain. Even slightly touching the incus with the bur can precipitate a substantial sensorineural hearing loss. The use of a small curette or pick to remove the last bit of bone can be quite useful in avoiding this complication.

Extended Facial Recess

Increased access to the hypotympanum can be obtained by extending the facial recess to the level of the tympanic annulus, which requires sacrifice of the chorda tympani nerve. The landmarks used in the dissection are the facial nerve, the chorda tympani nerve, the annulus, and the tympanic membrane. Inferiorly, the plane of the tympanic annulus tilts medially and the facial nerve courses laterally. Dissection begins at the point at which the chorda tympani nerve separates from the facial nerve. The chorda is transected at this site and the fallopian canal is followed inferiorly, carefully drilling with a small diamond bur. Occasionally, the facial nerve may pass lateral to the annulus before the inferior limit of the annulus is reached; by following the fallopian canal from a superior to inferior direction, facial nerve injury can be avoided. To avoid injury to the facial nerve, it is also important to use copious irrigation to cool the bur.

The extended facial recess approach can prove useful in accessing the hypotympanum and jugular bulb region (eg, for resection of a glomus tympanicum tumor) (Figure A–19).

Removal of the Incus and the Head of the Malleus

Dissection anteriorly and laterally from the mastoid antrum toward the root of the zygoma opens the attic. The limit of this space is the external canal wall inferiorly, and the tegmen tympani superiorly. Once completed, this dissection provides access to the body and short process of the incus, ossicular ligaments, and head of the malleus.

Removing the incus and head of the malleus affords access to the anterior epitympanic space and visualization of the entire tympanic segment of the facial nerve. This exposure also can provide access for decompression of the facial nerve lateral to the geniculate ganglion (Figure A–20).

Modified Radical (Canal Wall Down) Mastoidectomy

The modified radical mastoidectomy is used primarily to manage cholesteatoma, and the extent of the approach varies with the extent of disease encountered. Therefore, we describe a few specific approaches to be practiced in the temporal bone laboratory, recognizing that modification must be made for the individual patient. Furthermore, this approach can identify the extent of disease and simplify the surgical decision to continue with a more extensive procedure. Judicious dissection to provide adequate access to disease resection or exteriorization leaves a smaller cavity that better serves both the patient and surgeon. The dissection begins with the intact canal wall mastoidectomy already described. Identification of the antrum and LSSC gives a point of reference for the depth of the dissection.

Depending on the extent of disease, and if the ossicular chain is intact, a *Bondy mastoidectomy* (limited cavity) can be performed. In this procedure, a limited intact canal wall procedure is performed, staying superior in the dissection, identifying the antrum, and removing the superior and posterior canal wall until only a thin rim of bone remains over the ossicles. A medium-sized bur, drawn medially to laterally, facilitates bone removal. The final rim of bone is removed with a small curette to avoid traumatizing the intact ossicular chain. With experience, and in carefully selected patients, this procedure can be performed entirely from the canal side ("inside out"), thereby creating the smallest possible cavity. It is necessary to perform a meatoplasty to facilitate postoperative cleaning of the cavity (Figure A–21).

A modified radical mastoidectomy is used for more extensive disease and is designed to exteriorize all areas of the temporal bone. On occasion, the status of the tympanic cavity may allow for hearing preservation or

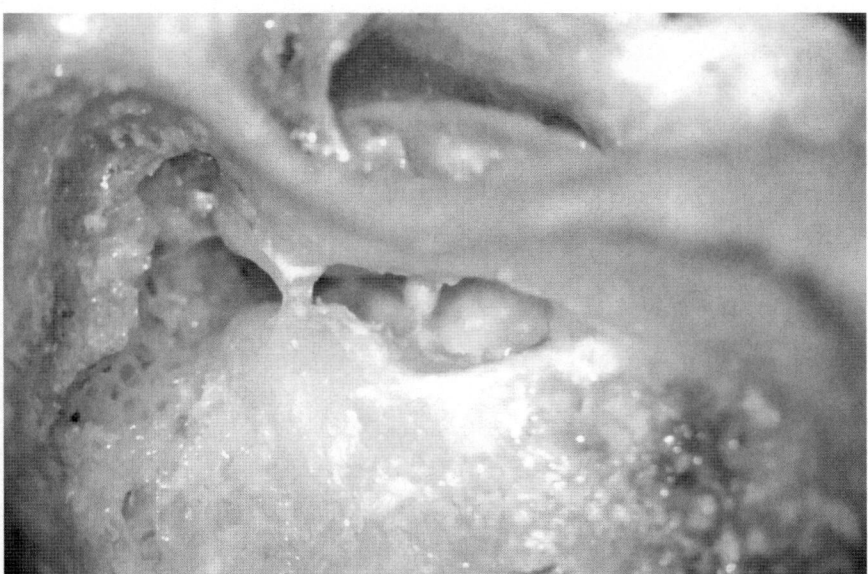

Figure A–19 Further expansion of the dissection into the extended facial recess approach. The chorda tympani nerve has been sacrificed. Note the delineation of the horizontal and vertical facial nerve and the improved access to the middle ear.

Figure A–20 High-power view of the epitympanum with the incus removed. Further removal of the malleus head will provide access to the anterior epitympanum, petrous apex, and complete horizontal facial nerve segment including the geniculate ganglion.

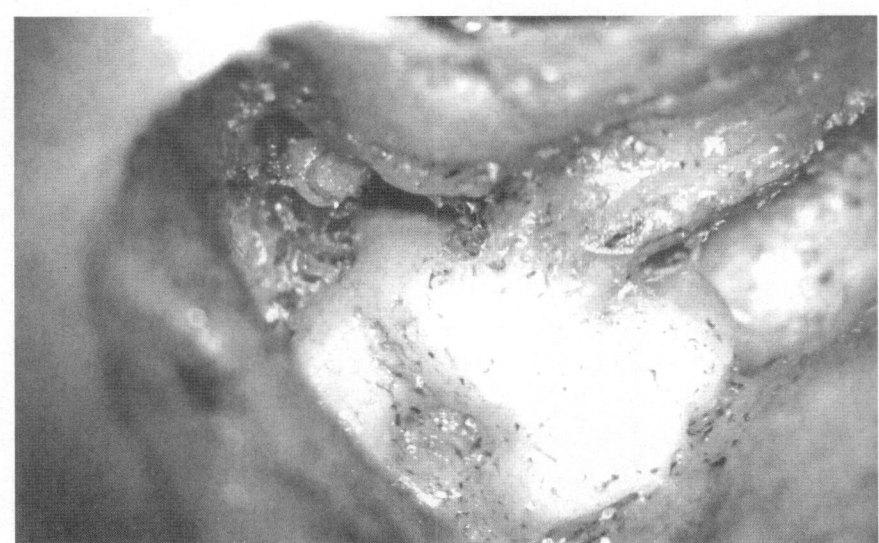

reconstruction, that is, tympanoplasty. An important landmark is the anterior buttress (the point at which the posterior bony canal wall meets the tegmen), which is totally removed to achieve a smooth continuum between the mastoid tegmen and the tegmen tympani. The posterior buttress, which marks the meeting of the posterior canal wall and the floor of the EAC lateral to the facial nerve, is also removed.

In the dissection laboratory, an intact canal wall mastoidectomy is performed. Removal of the incus reduces the potential for trauma to the ossicular chain, facilitating both the safety of the procedure and the speed with which it can be performed. The chorda tympani nerve is sacrificed, and the posterior canal wall is lowered to the fallopian canal (the "facial ridge"), improving exposure of the sinus tympani and the hypotympanum. At the completion of the procedure, the anterior epitympanic cavity is flush with the mesotympanum, and the floor of the mastoid cavity is flush with the floor of the bony EAC so that one large cavity is created. On occasion, the mastoid tip extends below the level of the bony canal, creating the potential for a "sink trap." To avoid the sink trap effect, the lateral (to the digastric ridge) mastoid tip

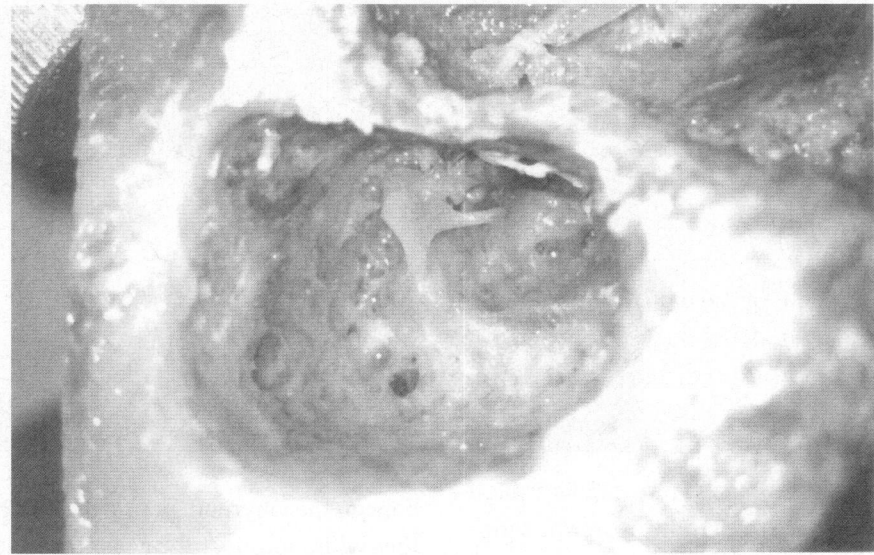

Figure A–21 Bondy modified mastoid cavity demonstrating removal of the external canal wall with preservation of the tympanic membrane and ossicular chain.

Figure A–22 Modified radical mastoid cavity. Compared to Figure A-21, the tympanic membrane has been removed and the canal wall lowered to the vertical facial nerve. Further saucerization of the cavity has also been performed, particularly anterosuperiorly and posteroinferiorly. The ossicular chain has been left intact for reference.

cells should be removed, resulting in a shallower mastoid cavity (Figure A–22).

A poorly performed modified radical mastoidectomy is characterized by incomplete removal of the posterior canal wall, superior canal wall, high facial ridge, and an inadequate meatoplasty.

Approach to the Endolymphatic Sac, Labyrinthectomy, and Translabyrinthine Exposure of the Internal Auditory Canal

This dissection begins with an extensively saucerized, intact canal wall mastoidectomy. Opening the facial

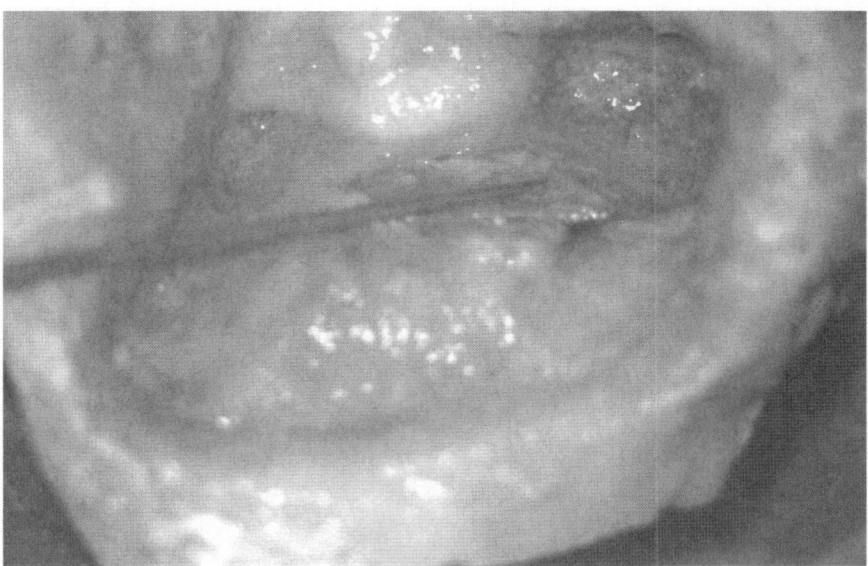

Figure A–23 The basic mastoidectomy is extended by removing the bone behind and over the sigmoid sinus in preparation for accessing the posterior fossa dura, endolymphatic sac, and labyrinth. The sigmoid sinus can now be compressed, allowing better access to these structures.

recess to identify the facial nerve facilitates dissection. The fallopian canal is traced from the LSCC to the digastric ridge. The sigmoid sinus is followed to the jugular bulb, medial to the fallopian canal. Air cells are removed and the semicircular canals are identified.

Access to the posterior fossa dura, endolymphatic sac, and labyrinth can be improved by decompressing the sigmoid sinus. Either complete or partial (leaving a bony island) removal of bone over the sinus works equally well. Having decompressed the sinus, the angle of approach to the semicircular canals is less acute, and broader strokes can be employed (Figure A–23).

Donaldson's line is an imaginary line drawn through the long axis of the LSCC, bisecting the posterior semicircular canal (PSCC). The endolymphatic sac is located inferior to this line and appears as a thickening of the posterior fossa dura. By opening the retrofacial air cells (medial to the facial nerve, inferior to the PSCC, and superior to the jugular bulb), the posterior fossa dura and the endolymphatic sac are exposed. Decompression (or drainage) of the endolymphatic sac is the only nondestructive surgical therapy for Meniere's disease (Figure A–24).

In addition to accessing the endolymphatic sac and jugular bulb, this posterior approach to the labyrinth can also be used for PSCC occlusion, used to treat BPPV.

Soft, judicious strokes with a small diamond bur, paralleling the canal, provide wide exposure of the canal.

A transmastoid labyrinthectomy is performed systematically and begins with an intact canal wall mastoidectomy and a limited facial recess dissection to establish the position of the facial nerve. If necessary, the sigmoid sinus is decompressed to provide better exposure. The semicircular canals are defined by removal of surrounding cancellous bone. Using a medium-sized bur and opening the LSSC, drilling from anterior to posterior, to expose the membranous canal begins the labyrinthectomy. An instructive exercise in the temporal bone laboratory consists of carefully removing the bone of the labyrinth, noting the color transition from yellow-white to bluish-gray as the bone is thinned. Familiarity with the varying appearance of the bone as it is thinned is useful in the operating room when trying to assess fistulization of the labyrinth in chronic otitis media. The open LSCC is followed to the PSCC, which is opened. The posterior canal is traced forward until the junction of the nonampullated ends of the posterior and superior canals is identified at the common crus (crus communis). The endolymphatic duct can be identified running from the endolymphatic sac to the common crus. A "cup" is formed, and drilling within this "cup" in a circular fashion is recommended to avoid bur slippage and consequent injury to the horizontal segment of

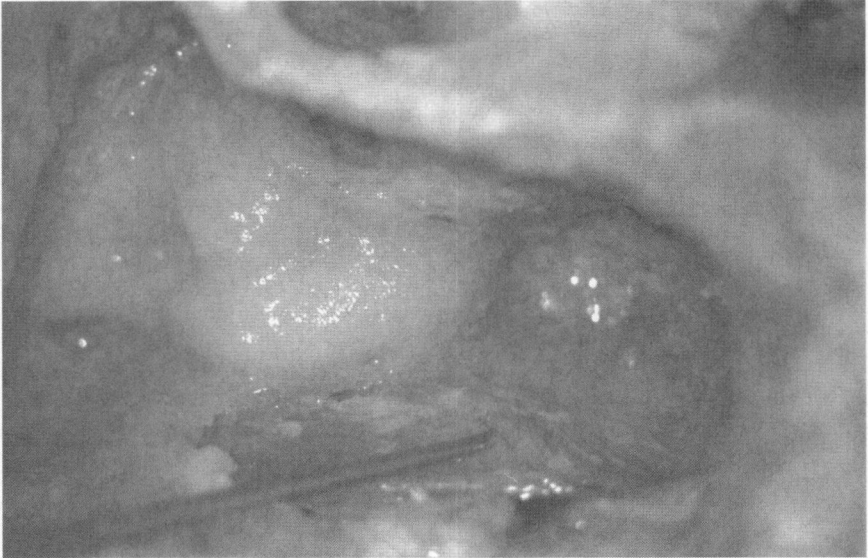

Figure A–24   Higher-power view of Figure A–23. The bone over the posterior fossa dura has now been removed. The probe is passed between the layers of dura into the superior limit of the endolymphatic sac. Anterior to the probe lies the endolymphatic duct as it travels to the crus communis.

the facial nerve. The superior canal is opened and followed anteriorly to its ampulla; the subarcuate artery is encountered as it courses within the arc of the superior canal. Lastly, the inferior portion of the PSCC is opened, taking care to avoid injuring the vertical segment of the facial nerve (Figures A–25 and A–26).

Each of the ampullae of the semicircular canals closely approximates a portion of the facial nerve. The labyrinthine portion of the facial nerve lies anterior to the ampulla of the superior canal. The ampulla of the lateral canal is just superior to the tympanic segment of the facial nerve. The posterior canal ampulla is just medial to the mastoid segment of the facial nerve.

Once all three canals are opened, drilling anteriorly from the ampulla of the posterior canal opens the vestibule. Within the vestibule, the elliptical recess (for the utricle) and the spherical recess (for the saccule) can be seen. The cribriform opening for the superior vestibular nerve (the macula cribrosa superior) is known as Mike's dot and serves as the landmark for the fundus of the IAC (Figures A–27 and A–28).

Once the labyrinthectomy has been completed, exposure of the IAC can begin and is done using a medium-sized bur. The superior boundary of the IAC lies inferior to the subarcuate artery. Thus, bone superior to this plane can be removed safely. The inferior border of the canal lies superior to the jugular bulb. With further medial and inferior dissection, the cochlear aqueduct is encountered. The cochlear aqueduct not only marks the inferior boundary of the IAC, it marks the medial extent of the canal as well. The bony plate of the posterior fossa is thinned until the porus of the IAC is defined. With the fundus and the porus thus defined, the bone of the IAC can then be thinned throughout its length. Finally, when eggshell thin, the remaining bone can be removed with a small hook, revealing the dural sheath and nerves within (Figure A–29).

From the translabyrinthine approach, the first nerves encountered within the IAC are the superior and inferior vestibular nerves, separated by a variable projection of bone, the transverse crest. Medial to the superior vestibular nerve, another small bony projection, the vertical crest (Bill's bar), can be palpated with a small hook; Bill's bar

Appendix: Surgical Anatomy of the Temporal Bone and Dissection Guide 791

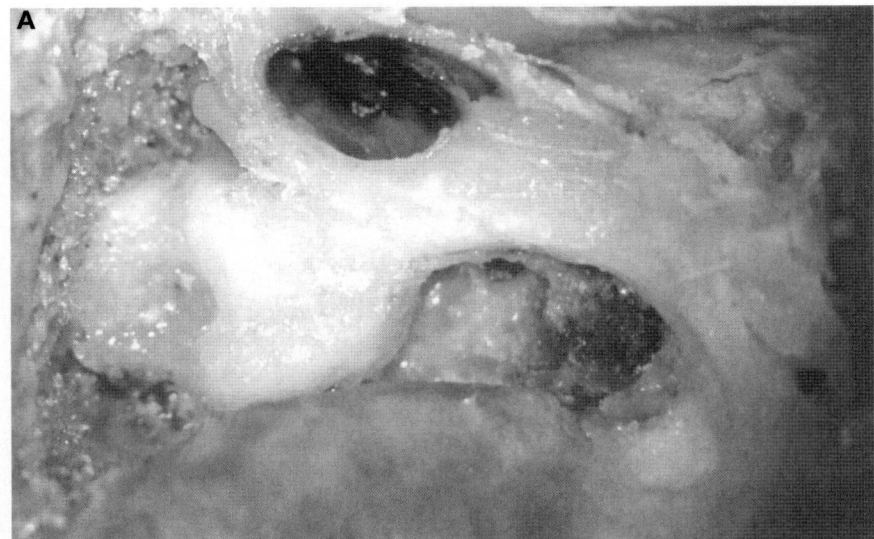

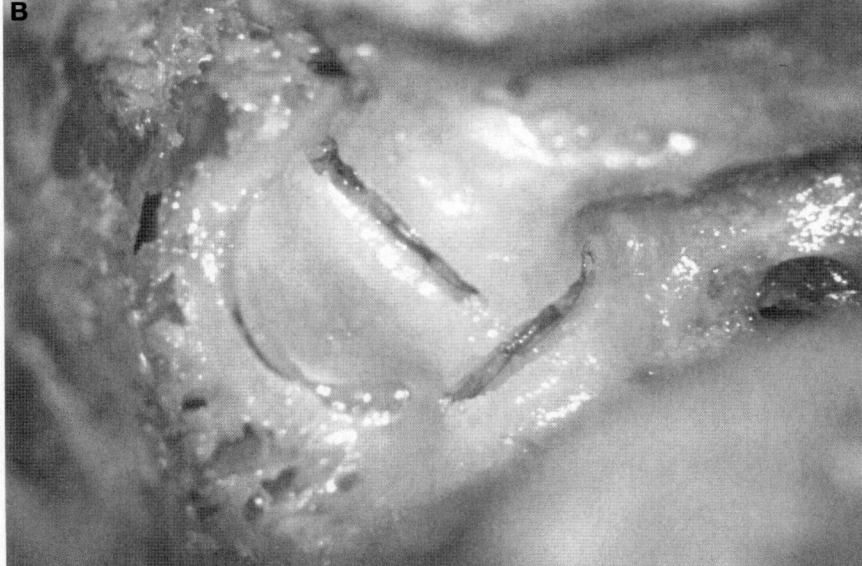

Figure A–25 Labyrinthectomy part one. *A,* The bone of the lateral, posterior, and superior canals is skeletonized. Note the position of the facial nerve in relation to the lateral and posterior canal. *B,* Canals opened within the same bone to demonstrate their orientation.

separates the superior vestibular nerve from the facial nerve. The facial nerve may, in fact, be difficult to visualize until the superior vestibular nerve has been avulsed and reflected posteriorly. The facial nerve is then visible, and the bone surrounding its labyrinthine segment can be removed until the geniculate ganglion is reached. The cochlear nerve is in the anterior/inferior compartment of the IAC and can be seen inferior to the facial nerve. Reflecting the inferior vestibular nerve posteri-

orly improves visualization of the cochlear nerve (Figure A–29).

Middle Fossa Approach to the Internal Auditory Canal

The temporal bone positioning used for a middle fossa dissection differs from the typical placement and warrants special mention. For middle fossa procedures, the

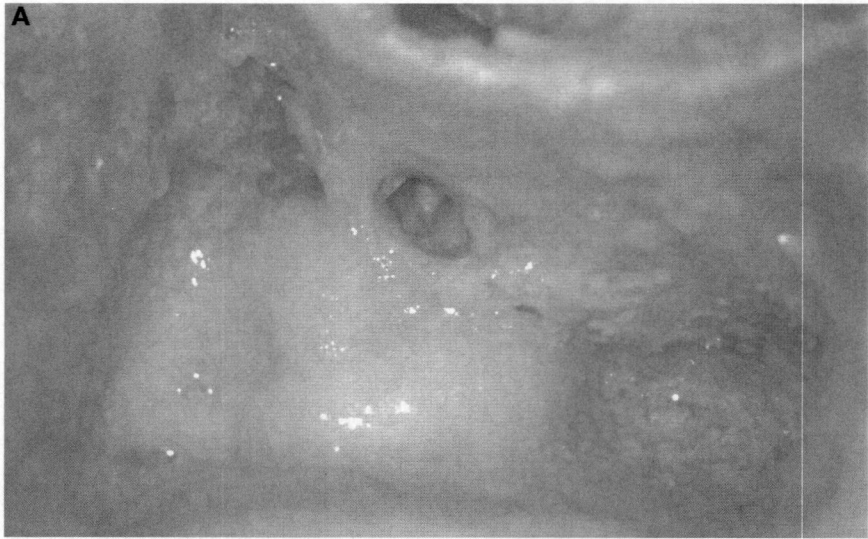

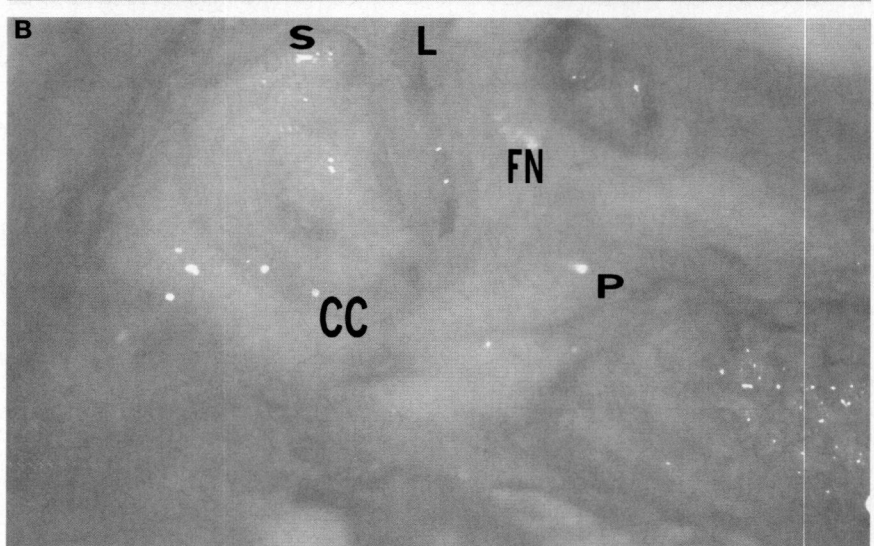

Figure A–26   Labyrinthectomy part two. *A,* Positions of bony canals. *B,* Canals have been traced and opened. CC = crus communis joining superior and posterior canals; FN = facial nerve; S, L, P = relative positions of ampullae's of superior, lateral, and posterior canals.

surgeon sits at the head of the patient looking toward the feet. In this position, the mastoid tip is pointing away from the surgeon. A 5-cm-square squamous craniectomy, centered on the zygomatic process and extending down to the linea temporalis (approximating the floor of the middle cranial fossa), is created. Dura is elevated in a posterior to anterior direction to avoid injuring an exposed geniculate ganglion and GPN (Figure A–30).

Middle fossa anatomic dissection, more so than transmastoid dissection, relies on the geometric relationships

of critical anatomic structures. Proceeding medially, the first structure encountered is the tympanosquamous suture line, medial to which is the facial hiatus for the GPN. The course of the GPN parallels the petrous ridge. The SSCC lies approximately 10 mm posterior and 5 mm medial to the GPN. At this point, the bone is thinned carefully until the superior SCC is blue-lined. The SSSC forms a right angle to the petrous ridge, and the IAC runs at approximately a 60-degree angle from the SSSC. The GPN is traced posteriorly until the geniculate ganglion

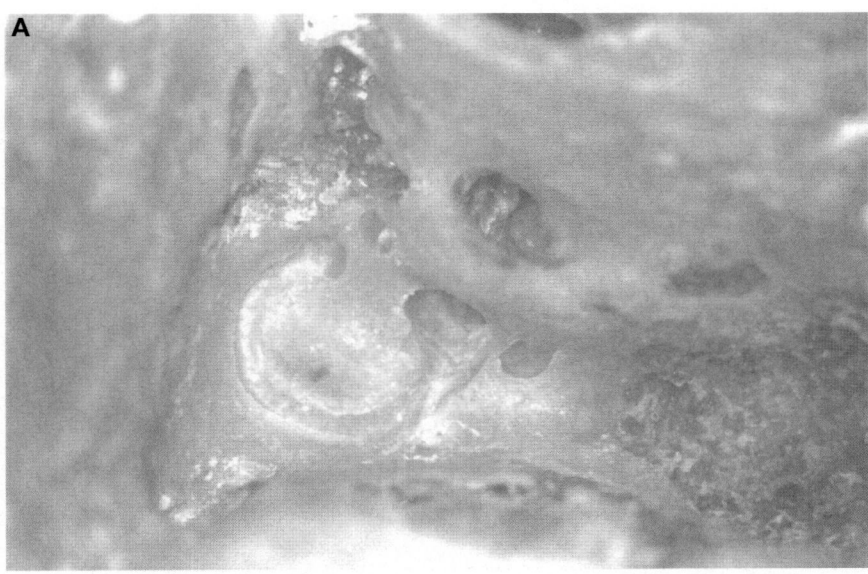

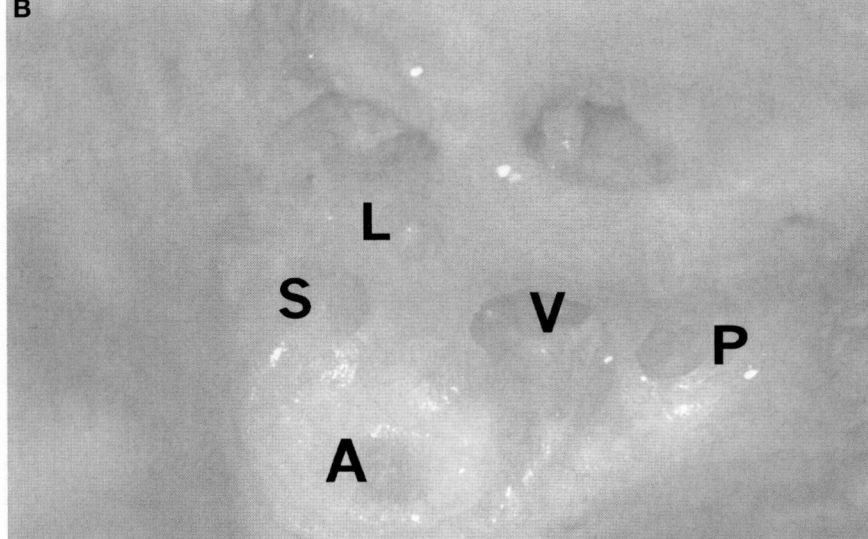

Figure A–27 Labyrinthectomy part three: the semicircular canals have been removed and the vestibule opened. This completes the labyrinthectomy. *A*, Low-power view. *B*, Higher-power view. A = subarcuate artery; S, L, and P = ampulla of superior, lateral, and posterior canals; V = vestibule.

Figure A–28 The superior and inferior limits of the internal auditory canal (IAC) have been defined. Inferiorly note the positions of the jugular bulb (JB) and cochlear aqueduct (A). Compare this view with Figure A-27, B, and note the position of the vestibule with respect to the lateral IAC.

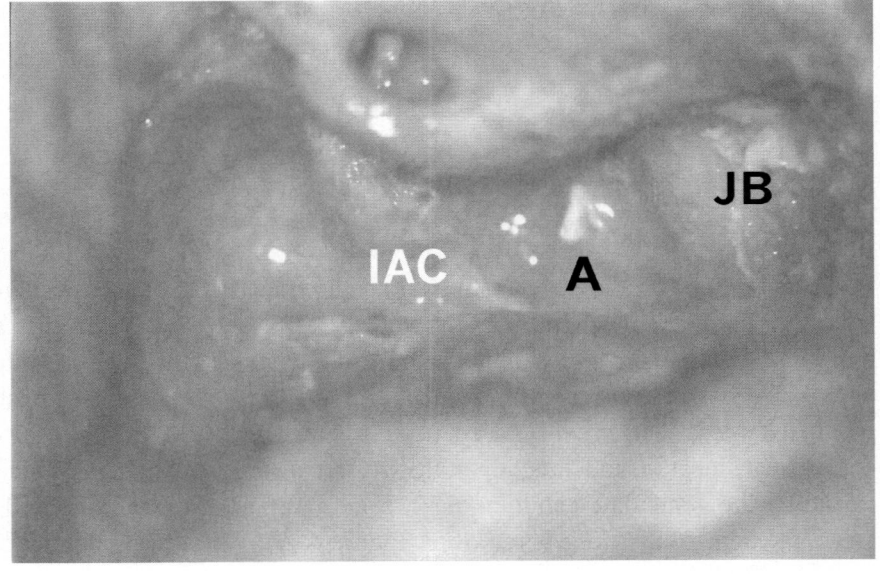

Figure A–29 The bone overlying the internal auditory canal (IAC) has been removed, exposing the neural structures contained within. The superior vestibular nerve has been removed to reveal the facial nerve (FN) beneath. The inferior vestibular nerve is also visible (IVN). TC = transverse crest.

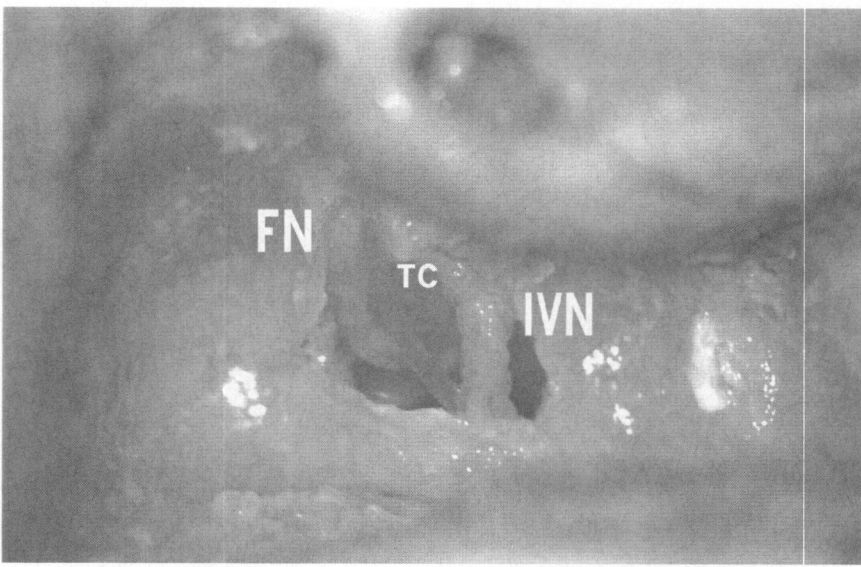

Figure A–30 Middle cranial fossa 1: the bone is placed in the surgical position and the window of squamous bone is removed. The shape of the bone flap has been altered to accommodate the specimen.

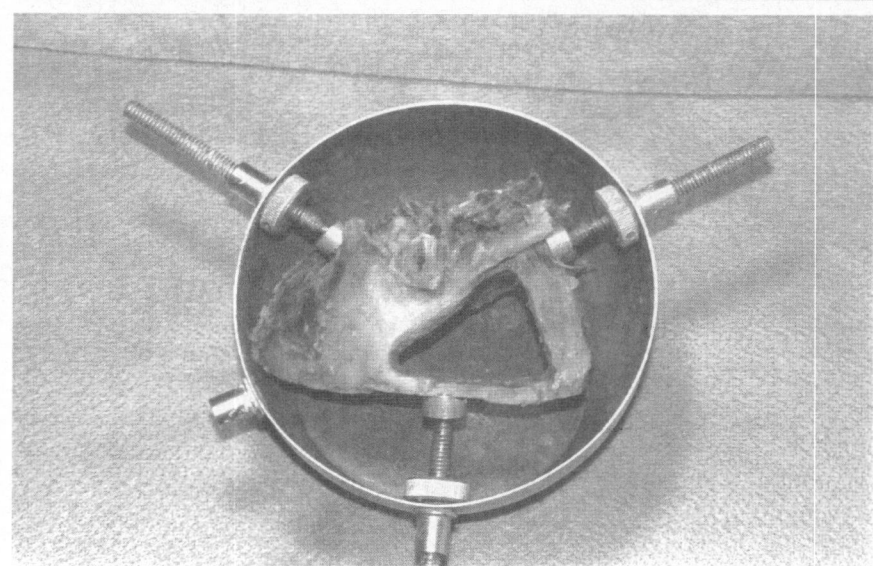

is encountered. Typically, only 4 mm separate the geniculate ganglion from the ampulla of the SSSC. Between these two structures lies the fundus of the IAC. Laterally, the IAC is relatively superficial but becomes deeper within the petrous ridge as it is traced medially. Once the approximate location and direction of the IAC are determined by the geniculate ganglion, SSSC, and petrous ridge, the bone of the ridge is removed (Figure A–31).

The safest area for dissection is medially as the critical structures are nearest to one another at the fundus. The basal turn of the cochlea lies just anterior and medial to the labyrinthine segment of the facial nerve. Medially, 180 degrees or more of the IAC can be exposed. When the bone overlying the IAC is sufficiently thinned, a small hook can be used to remove the final layer of bone and open the dural sheath. The

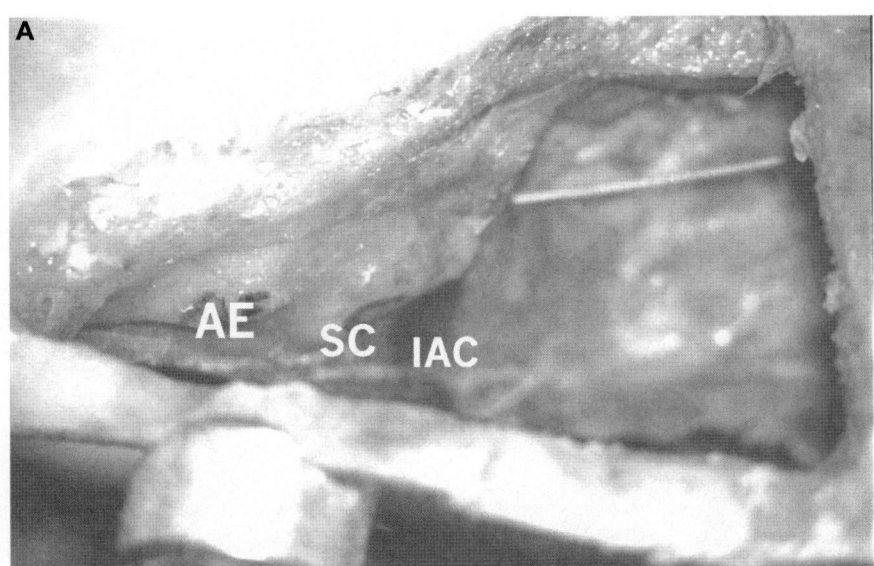

Figure A–31   Middle cranial fossa 2: the probe marks the facial hiatus for the greater superficial petrosal nerve. The relevant landmarks of the arcuate eminence (AE) and superior canal (SC) are labeled, and the relative position of the internal auditory canal (IAC) is noted. *A*, Surgical view and *B*, superior view.

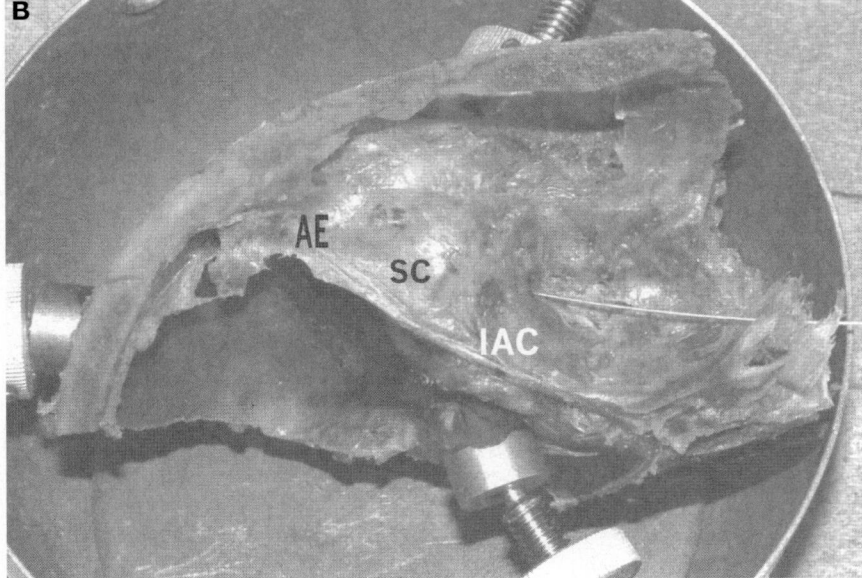

vertical crest (Bill's bar) can be identified at the fundus as it separates the facial and superior vestibular nerves. The facial nerve can be traced from the meatal foramen, through the geniculate ganglion, and to the tympanic segment. The fibers to the SSCC, LSCC, and the utricle can be seen passing through the macula cribrosa superior. The nervus intermedius (Wrisberg's nerve) can be seen traveling just inferior and posterior to the facial nerve. Inferior to these nerves is the transverse crest. The cochlear nerve and inferior vestibular nerve travel anteriorly and posteriorly, respectively, through this compartment. Finally, to complete the understanding of the anatomic relationships of this area, the SSCC and cochlea can be opened. Note that the cochlea is relatively closer to the IAC than is the SSCC. Thus, it is safer to begin delineating the IAC on its posterior surface (Figures A–32 and A–33).

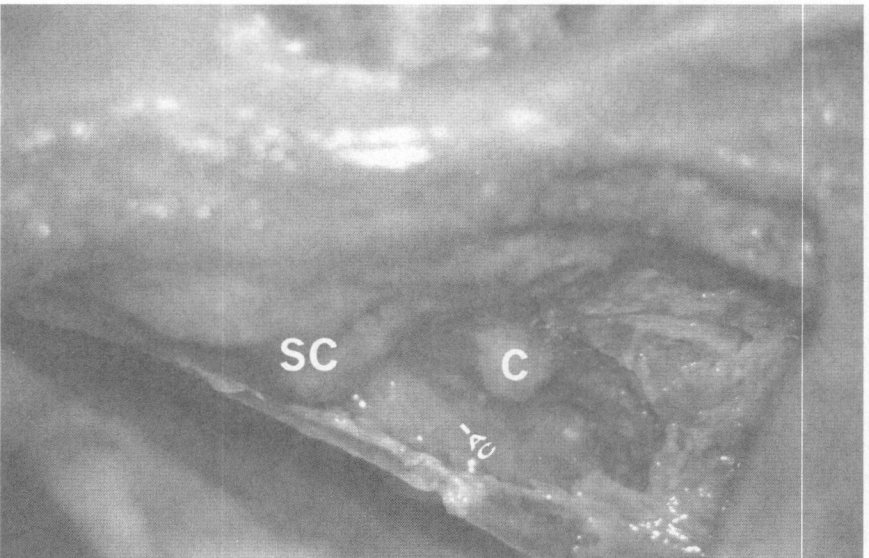

Figure A–32   Middle cranial fossa 3: the internal auditory canal (IAC) is developed. Note the depth medially and the relative superficial placement laterally. C = otic capsule containing cochlea; IAC = internal auditory canal; SC = superior canal.

Figure A–33   Middle cranial fossa 4: the internal auditory canal (IAC) is opened, as are the cochlea (C) and the ampulla of the superior canal (SC), for reference. Note the proximity of the meatal facial nerve (FN) to the basal turn of the cochlea and the wedge of bone, Bill's bar, separating the superior vestibular nerve from the facial nerve.

SELECTED READING

1.   Black B. Posterior geniculate artery: a surgeon's guide to the facial nerve. Am J Otol 1992;13:78–9.

2.   Donaldson JA, Duckert LG, Lambert PM, et al. Surgical anatomy of the temporal bone. 4th ed. New York: Raven Press; 1992.

3.   Gacek RR. Surgical landmark for the facial nerve in the epitympanum. Ann Otol Rhinol Laryngol 1980;89(3 Pt 1):249–50.

4.   Gulya AJ, Schuknecht HF. Anatomy of the temporal bone with surgical implications. 2nd ed. New York: Parthenon; 1995.

5.   Kartush JM, Kemink JL, Graham MD. The arcuate eminence. Topographic orientation in middle cranial fossa surgery. Ann Otol Rhinol Laryngol 1985;94(1 Pt 1):25–8.

6.   Litton WB, Krause CJ, Anson BA, et al. The relationship of the facial canal to the annular sulcus. Laryngoscope 1969;79:1584–604.

7.   Proctor B. Surgical anatomy of the ear and temporal bone. New York: Thieme Medical Publishers; 1989.

Index

THE LIBRARY
KENT & SUSSEX HOSPITAL
TUNBRIDGE WELLS
KENT TN4 8AT